Clinical
SURGERY

For W. B. Saunders:

Commissioning Editor: Ellen Green
Project Development Manager: Jim Killgore
Project Manager: Nancy Arnott
Designer: Sarah Russell
Index: J. R. Sampson

Clinical
SURGERY

Edited by

Michael M. Henry MB FRCS

Consultant Surgeon
Chelsea and Westminster Hospital and Royal Marsden Hospital
Honorary Consultant Surgeon
National Hospital for Neurology and Elizabeth Garrett Anderson Hospital
London

Jeremy N. Thompson MA MB MChir FRCS

Consultant Surgeon
Chelsea and Westminster Hospital and Royal Marsden Hospital
London

Illustrated by
Gillian Lee FMAA HonFIMI AMI RMIP and Louise Perks MIMI RMIP

 W.B. SAUNDERS

Edinburgh • London • New York • Philadelphia • St Louis • Sydney • Toronto 2001

W. B. SAUNDERS
An imprint of Elsevier Science Limited

First published 2001
Reprinted 2002

Standard edition ISBN 0 7020 1588 1
International edition ISBN 0 7020 2639 5
Reprinted 2002

British Library Cataloguing in Publication Data
A catalogue record for this book is available from the British Library

Library of Congress Cataloging in Publication Data
A catalog record for this book is available from the Library of Congress

Medical knowledge is constantly changing. As new information
becomes available, changes in treatment, procedures, equipment and
the use of drugs become necessary. The editors and contributors, and
the publishers have, as far as it is possible, taken care to ensure that
the information given in this text is accurate and up to date.
However, readers are strongly advised to confirm that the
information, especially with regard to drug usage, complies with the
latest legislation and standards of practice.

The
publisher's
policy is to use
**paper manufactured
from sustainable forests**

Printed in Spain

Contents

Contributors

Solomon Abramovich LRCP MRCS MSc FRCS
Consultant Ear Nose and Throat Surgeon
St Mary's Hospital
Central Middlesex Hospital
Honorary Clinical Senior Lecturer
Imperial College
London
Ear and nose

Shaun Appleton FRCS
Specialist Registrar in Surgery
Royal Marsden Hospital
London
The operation

Matthew Barry MS FRCS (Orth)
Consultant Orthopaedic Surgeon
The Royal London Hospital
London
Principles of orthopaedics

Rolfe Birch MA MB MChir FRCS
Orthopaedic Surgeon
Royal National Orthopaedic Hospital
Stanmore
Middlesex
Honorary Consultant appointment to:
National Hospital for Neurological Diseases;
Royal Postgraduate Medical School;
Hospital for Sick Children;
Reigmore Hospital;
Civilian Consultant to The Royal Navy
*Principles of management of fractures, joint injuries
and peripheral nerve injuries*

Jeremy Booth MB BS FRCS FFAEM
Clinical Director of Accident and Emergency
  Medicine and Surgery
Chelsea and Westminster Hospital
Honorary Consultant in Accident and Emergency
Royal Brompton and Harefield Hospitals NHS Trust
President (Accident and Emergency Section)
Royal Society of Medicine
Formerly Senior Examiner in Surgery to the University
  of London
London
Accident and emergency

Andrew W. Bradbury BSc MD FRCS (Ed)
Professor of Vascular Surgery and Honorary
  Consultant Vascular Surgeon
University of Birmingham
Birmingham Heartlands and Solihull NHS Trust
Birmingham
Arterial surgery

P. Declan Carey MB MCh FRCSI
Consultant Surgical Oncologist
Belfast City Hospital (Northern Ireland Cancer Centre)
  and Queen's University Belfast
Belfast
*Perioperative management and postoperative
complications*

Nicholas John William Cheshire MD FRCS
Consultant Surgeon
St Mary's Hospital
London
Surgical aspects of pancreatic disease

Richard Robert Harvey Coombs
MA DM MCh FRCS, MRCP, FRCS (Ed) ORTH
Consultant Orthopaedic Surgeon
Charing Cross Hospital
Imperial College School of Medicine
London
Principles of orthopaedics

David James Corless BSc MD FRCS (Gen)
Consultant General and Upper Gastrointestinal
  Surgeon
Leighton Hospital
Crewe
*Legal and ethical issues, and organisation of surgical
services*

A. Darzi MD FRCS FRCSI FACS
Professor of Surgery and Director of Academic
  Surgical Unit
Imperial College School of Medicine
St Mary's Hospital
London
The operation
*Perioperative management and postoperative
complications*

Clinical Surgery

R. J. Delicata MD FRCS (Ed)
Consultant Surgeon
Nevill Hall Hospital
Gwent Healthcare Trust
Abergavenny
Perioperative management and postoperative complications

Daryl Dob BSc, MB BS, FRCA
Consultant Anaesthetist
Magill Department of Anaesthesia
Chelsea & Westminster Hospital
London
Anaesthesia and pain control

David Paul Drake MA MB BChir FRCS FRCPCH
Consultant Paediatric Surgeon
Honorary Senior Lecturer
Great Ormond Street Hospital for Children NHS Trust
Institute of Child Health
London
Principles of paediatric surgery

Philip J. Drew
BSc, MD (Hons) MS FRCS (Ed, Eng & Glas) FRCS (Gen)
Senior Lecturer and Honorary Consultant
The University of Hull
Academic Surgical Unit
Castle Hill Hospital
Hull
Breast disease

Geoffrey Glazer MS FRCS FACS
Consultant Surgeon
St Mary's Hospital
London
Surgical aspects of pancreatic disease
Small bowel disease and intestinal obstruction

Pierre J. Guillou
BSc MD FRCS FRCPS (Glas) FMED Sci
Professor of Surgery
Dean of the School of Medicine
St James's University Hospital
Leeds
Principles of surgical oncology
Oesophagus, stomach and duodenum

Nagy Habib MB ChB FRCS ChM
Head of Liver Surgery
Imperial College School of Medicine
Hammersmith Hospital
London
Liver and biliary tree

Dimitri J. Hadjiminas
MPhil FRCS FRCS (Ed)
Consultant Breast and Endocrine Surgeon
St Mary's Hospital
London
Investigation of the surgical patient

Kevin M. Haire MB BS FRCA
Consultant Anaesthetist
Magill Department of Anaesthesia
Chelsea & Westminster Hospital
London
Anaesthesia and pain control

Raymond J. Hannon
MB BCh BAO MD FRCS (Ed)
Consultant Vascular Surgeon
Belfast City Hospital
Belfast
Arterial surgery

Michael M. Henry MB FRCS
Consultant Surgeon
Chelsea and Westminster Hospital and Royal Marsden Hospital
Honorary Consultant Surgeon
National Hospital for Neurology and Elizabeth Garrett Anderson Hospital
London
Co-editor
Surgery – what it is and what a surgeon does
Large bowel including appendix
Venous and lymphatic disorders

Michael Hershman
DHMSA MB MSc MS FRCS (Eng, Ed, Glas & Irel) FICS
Consultant Surgeon
Royal Liverpool University Hospital
Liverpool
Hernia

Arnold David Konrad Hill
MCh, FRCSI (Gen Surg)
Consultant General Surgeon and University Lecturer in Surgery
Department of Surgery
St Vincents University Hospital
Dublin
The operation

Andrew L. Hine MBBS MRCP FRCR
Consultant Radiologist
Department of Radiology
Central Middlesex Hospital
London
Investigation of the surgical patient

Rodney N. Juste MB ChB FRCA EDIC
Senior Registrar in Intensive Care Medicine
Royal North Shore Hospital
Sydney
The seriously ill and injured patient

Habib Kashi MB ChM FRCS (Ed)
Consultant Surgeon
Walgrave Hospital
Coventry
Organ transplantation

Vickie Lee FRCOphth
Specialist Registrar in Ophthalmology
Moorfields Eye Hospital
London
Ophthalmology in clinical surgery

Jonathan Nicholas Leonard BSc MD FRCP
Consultant Dermatologist
St Mary's Hospital
London
Surgical principles – skin disorders

John D. Lewis (deceased) MB BS FRCS (Eng)
Formerly Consultant Vascular Surgeon
Northwick Park Hospital
Harrow
Venous and lymphatic disorders

Martin D. Leyland BSc (hons) MBChB (hons) FRCOphth
Specialist Registrar in Ophthalmology
Moorfields Eye Hospital
London
Ophthalmology in clinical surgery

John Lynn MS FRCS
Endocrine Surgeon
Cromwell Hospital
London
Surgery of the endocrine glands

John McCall MBChB MD FRACS
Clinical Associate Professor
Hepatobiliary and Transplant Surgeon
Auckland Hospital
Auckland
Perioperative management and postoperative complications

Hamish A. Mclure MB ChB FRCA
Consultant Anaesthetist
Royal Marsden Hospital
London
Anaesthesia and pain control

Darren Vivian Mann MBBS FRCS MS
Fellow in Hepato-Pancreato-Biliary Surgery
Prince of Wales Hospital
Chinese University of Hong Kong
Hong Kong
Hernia

John R. T. Monson
MD FRCSI FRCS FACS FRCPS (Glas) (Hon)
Professor of Surgery and Head of Department
Academic Surgical Unit
University of Hull
Castle Hill Hospital
Hull
Perioperative management and postoperative complications
Oesophagus, stomach and duodenum
Breast disease

P. Paraskeva BSc (Hons) MBBS (Hons) FRCS
Lecturer in Surgery
Imperial College School of Medicine
St Mary's Hospital
London
The operation
Perioperative management and postoperative complications

Bryan Ronald Parry MD FRACS
Professor of Surgery
Consultant Colorectal Surgeon
University of Auckland
Auckland
Perioperative management and postoperative complications

Simon David William Payne
LLM FRCS (Ed) FRCS (Eng) FFAEM
Clinical Director of Emergency Medicine and Surgery
Ealing Hospital
London
Legal and ethical issues and organisation of surgical services

Graeme John Poston MB MS FRCS (Eng) FRCS (Ed)
Consultant Surgeon
Royal Liverpool University Hospital
Liverpool
Surgical aspects of pancreatic disease

Peter Richards FRCS FRCPCH
Consultant Paediatric Neurosurgeon
Radcliffe Infirmary
Oxford
Neurosurgery

Clinical Surgery

Peter John Saxby MBCLB FRCS (Plast) ChM
Consultant Plastic Surgeon
Royal Devon and Exeter Hospital
Exeter
Principles of plastic surgery

W. Edmund Schulenburg FRCS FRCOphth
Consultant Vitreo-Retinal Surgeon
Hammersmith Hospital
Western Eye Hospital
London
Ophthalmology in clinical surgery

David Scott-Combes MS FRCS
Consultant Endocrine Surgeon
King's College
London
Liver and biliary tree
Surgery of the endocrine glands

Philip John Shorvon
MB BS MRCP FRCR
Consultant Radiologist
Central Middlesex Hospital
North West London Hospitals NHS Trust
London
Investigation of the surgical patient

Dishan Singh
FRCS (Eng) FRCS (Orth)
Consultant Orthopaedic Surgeon
 and Honorary Senior Lecturer
Royal National Orthopaedic Hospital
Stanmore
Middlesex
Principles of management of fractures, joint injuries
 and peripheral nerve injuries

Shaw Somers
BSc (Hons) MD FRCS
Consultant Surgeon
Queen Alexandra Hospital
Portsmouth
Principles of surgical oncology

Neil Soni MD FRCA
Consultant Anaesthetist & Director of Intensive Care
Chelsea and Westminster Hospital
London
The seriously ill and injured patient

John Spencer
MS (London) FRCS (Eng)
Emeritus Reader in Surgery

Imperial College School of Medicine
Consultant Surgeon
Hammersmith Hospital
London
Acute abdominal conditions – surgical aspects

Allan David Spigelman MB BS MD FRACS FRCS
Professor of Surgical Science
School of Medical Practice
Faculty of Medicine and Health Sciences
The University of Newcastle
Newcastle
Australia
Acute abdominal conditions – surgical aspects

Nicholas D. Stafford MB ChB FRCS
Professor of Head & Neck Surgery/Otolaryngology
University of Hull
Hull
The neck and upper aerodigestive tract

Rex De Lisle Stanbridge MB BS FRCS FRCP
Consultant Cardiothoracic Surgeon
St Mary's Hospital
London
Chest and lungs
Cardiac surgery

Mr Nicholas J. Taffinder MA FRCS
Specialist Registrar in General Surgery
Academic Surgical Unit
Imperial College School of Medicine at
 St Mary's Hospital
London
Surgical infection

Jeremy N. Thompson MA MB MChir FRCS
Consultant Surgeon
Chelsea and Westminster Hospital and Royal Marsden
 Hospital
London
Co-editor
Surgery – what it is and what a surgeon does
Wound healing and management

James P. S. Thomson DM MS FRCS
Emeritus Consultant Surgeon, St Mark's Hospital
Emeritus Consultant in Surgery, Royal Navy
Honorary Civil Consultant in Surgery, Royal Air Force
Formerly Honorary Consultant Surgeon, St Mary's
Hospital and St Luke's Hospital for the Clergy
Anal and related disorders

Alison Waghorn MB ChB (Birm) FRCS FRCS (Ed) MD
Consultant Endocrine and Breast Surgeon
Royal Liverpool Hospital
Liverpool
Practical procedures

Christopher Margrave Ward BSc MA FRCS
Consultant Plastic Surgeon
Honorary Post at The Charing Cross Hospital
London
Principles of plastic surgery

Gordon Williams MS FRCS FRCS (Ed)
Consultant Urologist
Hammersmith Hospitals NHS Trust
London
Urology

Robin C. N. Williamson MA MD MChir FRCS
Professor of Surgery
Hammersmith Hospital
London
The spleen

Alastair C. J. Windsor MD FRCS FRCS (Ed)
Consultant Surgeon
St Mark's Hospital
Harrow
Anal and related disorders

John Winstanley BDS MD FDS FRCS
Consultant Surgeon
Royal Bolton Hospital
Bolton
Breast Disease

Acknowledgements

Clinical Surgery was originally conceived by MMH jointly with Professor Pierre Guillou (Leeds University) and Mr Michael Hershman (Royal Liverpool University Hospital), and we would like to acknowledge their important contribution to the early gestation of this book. For reasons of geography, it became impossible for them to play a major role in its production as the text developed.

We would also like to acknowledge the expert assistance and advice provided by Jim Killgore of Harcourt Health Sciences, without whose hard work and persistence this book would not have seen the light of day. We are also grateful for the support and encouragement of Ellen Green at Harcourt and her predecessors Margaret Macdonald and Seán Duggan. Elaine McNeela has provided expert assistance to both editors, and we are very grateful for her hard work. We would also like to acknowledge The Western Eye Hospital for kindly allowing publication of Figures 36.2 – 36.19.

Finally, we wish to thank the many authors who have contributed to this book and to acknowledge their patience during its production.

M. M. H.
J. N. T.

Preface

Clinical Surgery has been written to provide a comprehensive textbook of surgical disorders for both an undergraduate and a postgraduate readership. The book encompasses a wide range of surgical specialities within a single textbook, which sets it apart from other similar texts and makes it an attractive purchase from the student's point of view. Although the book is primarily aimed at medical students, the contributors have also made considerable efforts to provide updated information that will be of assistance to the young trainee embarking on a surgical career.

Clinical Surgery was originally conceived as a companion volume to Kumar and Clark's *Clinical Medicine*, and the text follows a similar style and format. Using this very successful medical textbook as our model, we have attempted to produce a book that is easy to read and readily understood. We hope the result will prove welcome and instructive to the next generation of medical students and surgical trainees.

The process of producing a major textbook takes a considerable amount of time and effort. We have tried to ensure that the text is fully up to date at the time of publication, but readers should always bear in mind that changes can occur quickly in any field, and textbooks can only provide a basis for further learning and clinical practice. We would welcome all comments and suggestions from readers.

Michael M. Henry
Jeremy N. Thompson

1

Surgery – what it is and what a surgeon does

The profession

Surgery is defined in the Oxford English Dictionary as:

The art or practice of treating injuries, deformities and other disorders by manual operation or instrumental appliances.

In modern jargon this is by the use of invasive procedures (although that phrase is a relative one, in that saying 'good morning' can, in some circumstances, be as invasive of peoples' psyche and privacy as taking a knife to them). The surgeon, therefore, is one who makes people better chiefly by the exercise of manual skills. In the development of medicine, surgeons have in consequence tended to be regarded as technical journey-people, in contrast to physicians who are seen as contemplative, analytical and devoted to the philosophical. To use modern terms again, the surgeon is labelled as more *action-orientated*, which, for those who regard surgery as a last resort, tends to be interpreted as 'operate first, ask questions later'. (Montaigne perhaps put it more felicitously when he wrote that 'the skill to embrace occasions in the nicke is the chiefest part of an absolute Captaine'.)

Although these polarities between the roles of physicians and surgeons are often expressed in the personalities of those who take to one or other of the major disciplines, the distinction is now becoming blurred. Invasive procedures are frequently done within medical subdisciplines which are only tangentially related to surgery. For example, a gastroenterological physician frequently carries out endoscopic procedures which are designed to deal, by manual operation, with disorders of, say, the biliary tract formerly regarded as needing a surgeon for their relief; an interventional radiologist will deal with a narrowed artery which was once bypassed using a surgical procedure. In addition to this, surgeons have skills in management that go beyond mere manipulative ones and, because of this, look after many patients who might possibly need an operation but in the event do not. Examples are those with head injury or acute abdominal pain.

A further stereotype of the surgical personality, derived, at least in part, from the need to take action in circumstances of uncertainty, has been the emergence of a dominant leader, ostensibly of a team, but more usually of the character expressed by the phrase: 'Follow me and when I say "charge", you charge too.' Anyone who dips into the biographical accounts of surgeons before the middle of this century, will find

1

many examples of men (although not women – see below) who fitted that template and who, even if they made notable contributions, were often dogmatic in their views and wrong as often as they were right. Again all this is changing – although some would say not as fast as it should be. The principal reasons are twofold: first, the increasing complexity of surgical procedures and their after-care makes a team essential, and although one individual may be dominant within this, leadership is by agreement rather than authority and is established by the needs of the patient rather than by the autocracy of an individual; and second, because society no longer favours the domineering personality. Most agree that the change to a more liberal view of leadership is right, but it has to be remembered that in surgical management, as in other affairs, there are occasions when someone has to take a decision when the facts are insufficient for certainty; this process is then best vested in an individual. Fortunately modern investigation, particularly imaging technology, has reduced the number of such occasions.

In law, as well as in society's perception, surgery is an *assault*, however deliberate and well-intentioned (see Ch. 2). The (usually) controlled violence of this has fostered a view that surgeons are unnaturally aggressive to the point of having well-nigh psychotic features in their make-up. To a minor extent this may well be the case, but to suggest that it goes beyond the bounds of normality is not supported by any evidence. There is no doubt that some of the characteristics described above are different in degree from those exhibited by, say, physicians or, for that matter, novelists but, particularly because of changes in society, the surgical personality is becoming more and more like that of any reasonably educated person in the modern world.

Because to a great, though not exclusive, degree, surgery has been and continues to be associated with manual skills, one-early 20th century surgical master (Berkeley Moynihan) remarked that it was necessary for the surgeon to have 'the eye of an eagle, the hand of a lady' and, he added (in that he saw himself as a leader whom all should follow), 'the courage of a lion'. In the development of surgery of new territories in Moynihan's time – the abdomen, the thorax and the head – this was probably true, but inbred dexterity and charismatic leadership have now largely given way to careful training and recognition by surgeons themselves of the limits of both their cognitive and their physical skills. It remains the case, however, that to carry out an operation successfully, either as a soloist or as part of an accomplished orchestral team, generates a sense of satisfaction, indeed elation. The surgeon may thereby attract considerable envy from colleagues who only rarely experience such a degree of personal achievement. The euphoria of success has to be balanced against the occasional depressing episode, when, because of unwitting surgical error or the bludgeonings

of chance, an operation may have disastrous consequences. In such circumstances there is not only the anguish of having harmed a patient but also the possibility of legal action (Ch. 2). In that surgeons remain, or are seen to remain despite the development of the team, first among equals, the accusing finger of the profession or of society may be pointed in their direction. News of surgical disasters travels fast and, in times past, did so mostly along the grapevine. Now, however, matters of technical and decision-making consequence are more formally regulated by audit which maintains a running peer-controlled check on the performance of individuals or teams. These matters are now being carried much further with the introduction, already the case in many Western countries, of periodic re-certification or revalidation of members of the surgical team and of penalties, such as restrictions on the type of operation that can be done, should performance not be regarded as up to standard. External inspection and quality control, and the development of national protocols and guidelines are currently proposed and will further limit an individual surgeon's freedom of activity. Despite these necessary controls, there is an in-built ethos of high quality of care amongst surgeons, so that technical competence is extremely high and disasters remain a rarity.

The surgical personality

For all the reasons discussed above, surgeons are on the whole moderately extroverted and optimistic people. Their culture has tended to attract the outgoing and the male personality and this pattern was until recently reinforced by the notable tendency amongst all medical people to cluster together according to their disciplines and interests. In the first half of the century a female surgeon was a rarity – perhaps reflecting the still somewhat frontier nature of the speciality where deeds of derring-do, akin to those of war, were undertaken. As a result of trends – both those in the profession of medicine as described above and those in society – this is no longer true, although the deficit in numbers of female surgeons will take many years to correct.

Surgery as an assault – psychological effects

The implied and legal view of surgery as an assault inevitably impinges on the relationship between the practitioner and the patient. The biological effects of a surgical procedure are increasingly well known and discussed in detail throughout this book (Chs 5–8), but there are important psychological and attitudinal matters that have been much less studied and frequently ignored by surgeons. Most patients are relatively ignorant about their body deep to their skin (one recent study showed, for example, that less than 10% of UK patients could accurately locate the gall bladder or define its function), so that a proposed attack on a structure or organ may inspire alarm or dismay out of proportion to what the surgeon knows to be appropriate. Irrespective of the organ or area which requires surgical attention, any physical invasion of the body creates fear and there is a lingering, although now rarely rationally justified, belief that surgery means a close brush with death. The surgeon must understand such misconceptions and balance them by a relationship of trust. This depends greatly on how the patient relates with the surgeon, which is in turn the outcome of the latter's ability to impart a feeling of confidence. Although it is true that some patients relish – and even require – ebullient surgical optimism, today most prefer to see in their surgeon and the team an attitude of self-assurance based on a sober assessment of the facts and experience of the procedure that is to be done.

In addition, surgeons must strive to recognise that certain operations have a particular psychological impact, although it is also important for them to understand that, such is the resilience of humankind, that adverse psychological effects are often relatively short-lived. Mastectomy for breast cancer is a good and obvious example of a severe injury to a woman's body image but one with which she usually comes to terms (Ch. 27). There are also more subtle threats such as removal of the womb (hysterectomy) or any organ removal that is associated, rightly or wrongly, with loss of capacity to handle life. The circumstances in which the operation is done are also of significance: to undertake an urgent total colectomy for toxic megacolon in a young woman and create a stoma (Ch. 24) may be life-saving but carries penalties in that she is unprepared for the psychosocial changes that are produced and the impact these may have on her sexual life.

One important maxim in informing the patient, over and above the standard processes of ensuring consent (Ch. 2), is that a surgical procedure should result in such benefit for the patient that the up-side outweighs any down-side. For example, in inflammatory bowel disease (Ch. 24), to have to put up with an ileostomy may be adequate recompense for years of endurance of 10–20 uncontrollable bowel motions a day. It can be difficult if not impossible to get messages of this kind across at the time of a surgical procedure, but the surgeon must have a feeling for the patient's long-term well-being, rather than the short-term matter of dealing with the presenting problem, and advise and act accordingly.

Training

Surprisingly, training in surgery differs between regions of the world. However, there are signs that these cultural differences are beginning to disappear. It is now uncommon for an individual to gain much practice in surgery during the period as an intern or house officer (immediately after graduation), although virtually all clinicians require at this time in their career development some manual dexterity in matters such as blood vessel cannulation. Such skills are needed to make a good job of looking after patients, and during this period graduates begin to learn whether or not they wish to have a career in manual-manipulative fields, of which surgery is an example.

In the UK, for those who feel surgery is their bent, training is currently a mix of craft apprenticeship to a number of individuals and formal learning assessed by examinations:

- *Craft apprenticeship* means acceptance onto a training programme approved by the professional bodies of the Royal Colleges of Surgeons (in England, the College of Surgeons of England; in Ireland the College of Surgeons in Ireland; in Scotland, the College of Surgeons of Edinburgh and the Royal College of Physicians and Surgeons of Glasgow; and in many other countries that derive their tradition from the UK, similar bodies). There follows over several years the gradual acquisition of skills and an increase in responsibility; during this period fixed duration appointments (usually 6 or 12 months) are

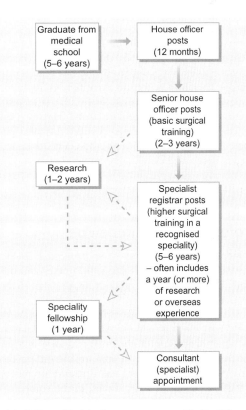

Fig 1.1 **Pattern of training in surgery proposed for the UK.**

held within institutions which are either part of or affiliated to the health service of the country in which training takes place. In the UK this pattern has now become standardised into 2 years of Basic Surgical Training and 5 or 6 years of Higher Surgical Training in a chosen speciality (Fig. 1.1).

- *Assessment* is by examinations in applied scientific knowledge and in clinical skills although these do not currently include manual dexterity. The first examination takes place after basic surgical training (leading to Membership of the Royal College of Surgeons in England or Associate Fellowship in the other colleges); the second examination is an exit test towards the end of Higher Surgical Training and success in this qualfies the trainee for full fellowship of a college as well as to become a consultant in the speciality chosen.

A further optional component of surgical (and also of most other specialist) training is to spend a period in *research*. All medicine has become increasingly based on applied science, or in the case of surgery, as one pioneer surgeon in the field put it, on surgical biology. It is argued that hands-on experience of scientific method and the production of new ideas at the scientific frontier make for a better and more perceptive clinician. How true this is in surgery is uncertain, but the prosecution of research by surgeons is regarded by most as essential to the progress of the discipline, however craft-based it may continue to be. For this to continue requires that some if not all surgeons gain formal training in science as applied to their discipline; most also find it exciting.

Given that the assessment hurdles are successfully surmounted, the surgical trainee who has been certified as properly trained is then in a position to apply for a permanent appointment within the health service or in a university that has a medical faculty and therefore health service responsibilities. The age at which this takes place is now often in excess of 35 years, especially if training in a highly specialised field is superimposed on basic training, although many think this is too long a period given the patterns that prevail in other professions.

Professional relationships

As mentioned above, there is an increasing development of *teams*, not only of surgeons, nurses and other health care workers but also of those who share a common interest in a group of disorders. Gastroenterology is one good example: both surgeons and physicians (*internists* in North America) investigate and look after patients with alimentary disease and both gain from joint activities. In spite of the difference in attitudes, to which reference has already been made, it is possible for the two disciplines, in the company of others, such as radiologists, to form a close and amicable working relationship. The same is true in the

care of cardiological and neurological patients. For such professional groupings to be effective, joint meetings must take place regularly at which the problems of patients and the results of investigations, such as imaging and pathological findings, are discussed and decisions reached on management. There is also often a place for seeing and managing patients together – for example, the surgeon may attend an endoscopy session run primarily by a gastroenterologist, or a neurologist may enter the operating room to view the problem that has been exposed. Patients requiring intensive care need close cooperation between surgeons and intensivists.

The same team approach is valid for the broader matters of patient care where the close incorporation of social workers, occupational and other therapists into the decision processes about a patient may simplify return to the community and work after a major operation.

Although the student of surgery increasingly sees the cross-disciplinary team at the centre of patient care, it still remains true that surgeons (and others) work and teach within small closely knit groups organised into a hierarchy of those who are fully trained and usually permanently appointed (*consultants* or *specialists* in the UK) and those at various levels of training (*house officers*, *senior house officers* and *registrars*). Such a group is often called a *firm* in England and has semi-autonomy in clinical decision-making, although increasingly it is subject to outside control by the surgeons in the institution as a whole (now often called a *directorate*).

FURTHER READING

Surgery in general

Douglas C (1975) *The Houseman's Tale*. Edinburgh: Canongate. (*A cynical but realistic novel on modern hospital practice based on the Royal Infirmary of Edinburgh.*)

Moore F (1995) *A Miracle and a Privilege*. Washington: National Academy Press (*Personal recollections of the growth of surgical biology.*)

Moynihan, Lord (1967) *Selected Writings*. London: Pitman Medical.

Starzl T (1992) *The Puzzle People – Memoirs of a Transplant Surgeon*. Pittsburgh: University of Pittsburgh Press.

Professional relationships and training

The Senate of Surgery of Great Britain and Ireland (1997) *The Surgeon's Duty of Care*.

General Medical Council (1995) *Duties of a Doctor*. London: General Medical Council.

Joint Committee on Higher Surgical Training (1988) *A Curriculum, Organisation and Syllabus for Higher Surgical Training in General Surgery and its Sub-specialities*.

2

Legal and ethical issues and organisation of surgical services

Legal and ethical issues for the surgeon

These issues are of increasing importance to surgical practice, for the following reasons:

- Advances in the techniques of investigation and management have created both new opportunities and new hazards for the patient.
- There is increased awareness among patients and relatives of the problems that may have to be surmounted to achieve a successful outcome and less tolerance of failure.
- Society has rejected the former paternalism of the profession of medicine.

All of these, plus (in the UK) the growing body of *case law* (accumulated legal experience which sets precedents) and *statute law* (rules generated by parliament) within which surgeons and others must work, have made the framework around the conduct of surgical procedures more complex and demanding. There are two areas in which the surgeon may encounter problems: negligence in treatment and consent for something to be done for the patient. They overlap, in that negligence may result from inadequate or inappropriate acts including the failure to obtain consent. In allegations of negligence, although not usually of consent, the surgeon may be jointly involved with the institution – usually a hospital.

Negligence

This a legal concept within the law of civil wrongs (*tort*) which has developed over the centuries to provide a system of compensation for loss when (and only when) it can be shown that this has occurred because of fault by others. When a professional skill is involved and negligence is alleged, the question that arises is: 'What level of skill and care does the law require?' The evolution of common law has, over the years, provided a number of guidelines of the standards of care expected so as to avoid or counter a charge of negligence.

The first and most general is:

A *fair*, *reasonable* and *competent* degree of skill is brought to the procedure

This does not seem to be contentious. However, to gauge the level of skill that was applied is often difficult although the operation of the 'firm' system (Ch. 1) should ensure that each member of the surgical team does only what is appropriate to his or her degree of training and experience. There is a duty of the less experienced to seek the advice of those with greater understanding. Those more knowledgeable (usually, but not always, more senior) must respond positively rather than opt out by delegation. Furthermore, there is a responsibility of all to keep abreast of advancing or changing surgical knowledge so that lessons learnt by others can be applied. The Hippocratian aphorism *ars longa, vita breva* (art is long, life is short) requires surgeons and others to keep up to date with the science and art of their speciality.

The second relates to circumstances in which there are alternative treatments for a given condition. Here the guideline is:

Failure to act in a way that a surgeon of ordinary skill would have done

This is sometimes expressed as the practice accepted as proper by a responsible body of medical people skilled in that particular area. This guideline could be turned round to say that if a surgeon has acted in a particular way then this is not negligent merely because there is a body of opinion who would take a contrary view. However, when an individual case comes under scrutiny it may be very difficult to establish what is 'accepted as proper', in that surgeons may differ both radically and dogmatically among themselves.

The third is the *causal chain*:

A direct causal link justified in terms of logic and medical knowledge must exist between the alleged negligent act and the damage or loss that has been sustained

For the patient undergoing surgical treatment, it can often be difficult or contentious precisely to define such a link, the more so when there has been complicated decision-making and difficult, often multiple, procedures. Here it is of great importance that record-keeping is comprehensive and that surgeons of all levels record their decisions at the time they are made. Another related factor that may make it difficult to claim negligence is the progress of the disease for which treatment was used.

Although there may be an established causal chain, if it contains too many conjectural links then *remoteness* may be invoked and, as a Master of the Rolls has said: 'It is wrong that the law should chase consequence upon consequence, possibility upon possibility, right down to a hypothetical line.'

Consent

It is a generally held tenet of law, and ethically unchallengeable, that an autonomous adult should have control in permitting what can be done to his or her body and mind. Thus anything that can be construed as invading these in any way without consent is unlawful and may attract proceedings for the crime of assault and battery (Ch. 2). However, although not exempt, a surgeon acting in good faith occupies a privileged position by virtue of the standing of the profession. A charge of assault requires the underlying attitude of hostile intent. This is rare in clinical practice but it is possible for mischievous and deluded patients to claim that an unauthorised or unnecessary contact has taken place during a medical examination or during recovery from an anaesthetic. The obvious tactic to guard against this possibility is the presence of an independent witness – in days gone by sometimes known as a *chaperone*.

In normal circumstances, consent to surgical procedures is a routine issue which is an integral part of the doctor– patient interaction as well as a formality for the case record. For trivial medical procedures, implied or verbal consent is adequate. 'Do you mind if I take a specimen of blood from your arm?' would nearly always prompt the patient to roll up a sleeve – a verbal request has produced implied consent.

However, the more complicated a procedure becomes, the greater is the risk of something going wrong. Important additions then need to be made to the process of consent and these apply to any surgical procedure that involves a general or regional anaes-thetic: written consent should be obtained on a standard form – both for operation and for anaesthesia.

The signature on such a form is merely evidence that the consent process has been completed. Legal action which alleges assault and battery may still ensue on the grounds that the consent was invalid. To some degree this possibility can be reduced if the form contains a statement that the patient has been *informed* of the nature and possible hazards of the procedure. However, this begs the question as to the meaning of 'informed'. It is a truism that fully informed consent is impossible, even if the patient is a colleague who knows as much about the operation as the surgeon, because emotional factors consequent upon being the patient may interfere with the perception of reality. This is more true of a lay person who may find it more difficult to understand technical terms in relation to, say, postoperative complications. In UK practice (although not in North America and increasingly Australasia), the requirement to fully inform patients about every possible complication of treatment is regarded as largely unnecessary.

What is necessary in English law is that sufficient information be given to patients to allow them to make

Information Box 2.1

Levels of risk and consent

Sideway v. Board of Governors of Bethlehem Royal Hospital (1985)

The patient underwent a cervical cord decompression because of spondylosis (see Ch. 33) but was not told before the procedure that there was a 1–2% risk of cord damage during the operation. She was made tetraplegic but lost her claim for negligence.

Reibl v. Hughes (1980)

Carotid endarterectomy (see Ch. 28) was done to prevent stroke but the patient was not told that there was a 4% mortality and a 10% chance of precipitating a stroke at operation.* Stroke and death ensued and the court ruled that he ought to have been informed of these specific risks to be able to form a balanced judgment about whether or not to undergo the procedure.

*These figures were correct at the time but would now be much lower.

a balanced judgment. A grave risk of adverse complications is judged by the standards of a reputable body of medical practice – a court of law uses *peer review* by experienced clinicians who form expert opinions after having appraised all the facts of the case. Some idea of the level of percentage risk that should or should not be disclosed can be gained from two recent leading examples that are much quoted (Information Box 2.1). It seems that the range is roughly from 2 to 10%.

Additional matters have emerged from the detailed judgments handed down in some leading cases and may be summarised as follows:

- The surgeon must weigh the balance of good and harm before treatment is recommended and is ethically required to provide information which is adequate to enable the patient to reach a balanced judgment.
- The patient is entitled to reject treatment and for that purpose must understand the possibility that harm may result.
- Information about the procedure may both (unduly) confuse and alarm.

Implicit in the above are that:

- The surgeon should take into account the nature and severity of the patient's condition in determining how much to disclose.
- Circumstances, e.g. urgency (see 'Consent in emergency care' below) and the effect of the condition to be treated on the patient's emotional state, must be taken into account.

- A judgment must be made on the patient's intellect and capacity to understand and deal with any information offered.

All the foregoing observations on consent are concerned with the legal issues. Surgeons, who tend to have a particular personality type, must also cultivate sensitive interpersonal skills to provide patients and their relatives with adequate information about management. Often this means giving a balanced (not wholly and falsely optimistic) view about the likely benefits as well as the possible side-effects and risks of a procedure. False hopes should not be implanted, but equally false fears – of pain, awareness during the operation or postoperative nausea – should be countered. The tentative pathway for the patient, e.g. the possibility of going to a high-dependency or intensive care unit (see above), should be outlined and the staff of such units are encouraged to introduce themselves to the patient before the procedure, as are others such as physiotherapists.

Age of consent
Above the age of 16, statute law (Family Law Reform Act 1969) empowers patients to provide valid consent for their own medical, surgical or dental treatment. For those younger than 16, tradition rather than law has vested consent in parents or guardians. However, in the 1980s, a Lord Justice said in a particular case:

provided the patient ... is capable of understanding what is proposed and expressing his or her own wishes, I see no good reason for holding that he or she lacks the mental capacity to express them effectively and to authorise the medical man...

In the light of this, the surgeon must make a clinical judgment in those under 16 as to whether:

- there is sufficient capacity in the patient to comprehend the implications of treatment
- it is sensible and proper for an agreement regarding treatment to be entered into directly with the patient, independent of the views of the parents.

Consent in emergency care
A clinical condition which requires urgent or immediate medical action does not obviate the need for consent although it can undeniably make gaining so-called informed consent more difficult, especially when the patient is confused, drunk or mentally ill. Such situations commonly occur in combination and late at night when junior medical personnel are first in line to deal with the matter.

Patients of sound mind
On the one hand, if a patient refuses treatment, however urgent, then unauthorised contact or invasion of the body is a *battery* and therefore a criminal offence.

On the other hand, inactivity in life-threatening circumstances breaches the surgeon's professional duty to provide necessary care and may lead to the possibility of an action in negligence. A further professional hazard is that the ethical duty of *beneficence* is also breached and disciplinary proceedings within the profession (in the UK by the General Medical Council) may result. This three-pronged horn – common in everyday practice – can usually be avoided by gentle persuasion with the assistance of more senior members of the surgical team. If alcohol or drugs is the cause of intransigence, management should be restricted to necessary life-saving measures until the effects of these substances have been dissipated.

Mental illness
In the presence of this, as shown by the patient's clinical state or past history, the provisions of the Mental Health Act (1983) may be invoked. However, in surgical circumstances, this is not of much value in that any treatment that may be forcibly applied relates only to the mental illness in question not to the needs of a surgical emergency.

Unconsciousness
The surgical team is entitled to assume that the patient consents to treatment for such procedures as are necessary to resuscitate and stabilise. They are however, not justified in assuming that they may proceed to immediate definitive treatment and should pause to endeavour to establish the wishes of the patient or gain guidance from next of kin.

Mental incapacity
A patient who is not mentally competent to reach a decision is usually helped by parents or others who can take responsibility for minor investigations or surgical procedures in which clear benefit is widely accepted, although such consent does not have validity in law. It is argued that it is impossible to know the true will of a patient with severe mental handicap and that treatment perceived as beneficial by others may not be so interpreted by the patient. The matter becomes complicated when a surgical procedure is proposed – such as female sterilisation – that has considerable or far-reaching effects and is virtually irreversible. In each and every case an application to the court should be made to obtain an *independent objective and judicial view* on the lawfulness of the procedure in the particular circumstance.

Jehovah's witnesses
Surgeons in particular face the occasion when a patient of sound mind who faces imminent death from haemorrhage refuses a blood transfusion because of religious conviction. This is a legal right but it is unlikely that any criminal proceedings would be brought against those who administer a blood transfusion to save life. However, that this is an area of difficulty is shown by a successful action by a Jehovah's Witness because of the mental trauma which followed a transfusion. Witnesses may also refuse blood transfusion for definitive procedures (such as cardiac surgery), but careful attention to detail can usually render replacement of lost blood unnecessary.

Decision in such circumstances should, if at all possible, be made by senior staff, in consultation with others and, on occasion, with the involvement of the legal profession. It is important to establish that the patient is of sound mind and, by inference, that the religious beliefs are genuinely held.

Undue influence

Children of Jehovah's Witnesses
If there is a threat to life, the surgeon is not entitled to assume that the parents' beliefs are shared by their offspring. There is a greater duty to act in the child's interests, protected by the view that the courts do not regard children as capable of forming profound religious beliefs.

Other forms of influence
When it can be shown that parental or other influence has caused the patient to withhold consent for life-saving treatment, the courts have taken the view that legal liability shall not attach to those who have acted in good faith.

Practical outcomes of legal issues

The foregoing pages may well have convinced the student that to practice medicine and particularly surgery in the 21st century is to walk unprotected through a legal minefield. To a degree this is true but there are some measures that can be taken to minimise the risks:

- Think, although not with apprehension, of the possible legal outcome of all clinical decisions.
- Avoid reaching clinical decisions that may have legal consequences without taking advice from those who have more experience and/or may have to take ultimate responsibility. It is always irritating to feel that you are clinically competent but nevertheless require protection, but this is a necessary condition for professional survival.
- Record carefully all decisions that may have legal implications, which means record *all* decisions.

- Make sure all other necessary paperwork is completed, especially forms of consent.
- Carry medical insurance (a necessary condition of employment in most medical cultures); in the UK this is through two agencies – the Medical Defence Union and the Medical Protection Society.

Death and bereavement

Death comes for us all in the end, but in a surgical context it may be sudden, unexpected and seem to be the direct outcome of the team's activities in attempting to cure. Sensitive and speedy handling of the physical and emotional turmoil, and awareness of cultural and social differences in those bereaved are essential.

Terminal care
All clinicians, including surgeons, are responsible in some way for the management of the last stages of life. The common aims are to allay suffering and maintain dignity, both of which require close and sympathetic contact with relatives. Although surgeons may feel the human and honourable need to strive against potential therapeutic defeat (see Ch. 1), it is not their task to wring the last drop of life out of all. For instance, in extreme old age, the correct management of an abdominal catastrophe may be pain relief rather than the hazards and discomforts of a major operation, although it should not be forgotten how well many octogenarians (and older) recover after taxing procedures. The difficult decisions needed require experience, consultation with others in the profession, the wishes of the patient, if these are available (including *living wills*), and those of relatives.

It is indubitably better to anticipate the special needs of the dying in consort with the general practitioner and sometimes a religious representative, especially if special care is going to be necessary.

Informing relatives
This task is often delegated to the most junior member of the team. Notwithstanding that we all need to learn, it means more to relatives if a more senior member of staff is involved. Nurses are often also helpful and questions posed should be answered honestly and directly provided the information is truly available.

Death certification
Junior staff are nearly always involved in the recording of death. The certificate is a legal document and also the basis of national population statistics. As such it should be completed accurately to avoid subsequent wrangles, anxieties and confusion for relatives and what may prove an unnecessary referral to a coroner

Information Box 2.2

Reasons for referral to the coroner or procurator fiscal

Physician

Did not treat the deceased in the final illness

Did not see the deceased in the last 14 days of life

Death in relation to surgical operation

During the procedure

Before recovery from anaesthesia

Within 24 hours

Circumstances

Suspected industrial cause of death

Patient in receipt of a war or industrial pension

Accidental death

Suspected or known
  violence
  neglect
  poisoning or administration of drugs

Medical mishap

Death in police custody

After abortion in mother and stillbirth of child

Within 24 hours of admission to hospital

Doubt and complaint

Doubt as to cause including sudden or unexplained death

Complaint by relatives

(in England, Wales and N. Ireland) or a procurator fiscal (in Scotland). Many other countries have similar procedures to observe. A cause of death should be recorded rather than the *mode* (e.g. ruptured aortic aneurysm rather than shock). Reasons for referral to a coroner or procurator are given in Information Box 2.2.

Postmortem examination
Opinions remain divided about the desirability of these examinations. Pathologists in particular point out that unexpected and instructive information is often forthcoming. Surgeons, in contrast, often feel that functional causes such as ARDS and multi-organ system failure are apparent during life and not well reflected by postmortem findings. If a death certificate cannot be issued, the death must be reported to the coroner or other official who will then decide. Otherwise it is better to have a team policy, although each instance must be considered on its merits and with sensitivity. In cases where a death certificate can be issued, the

consent of relatives must be requested if a postmortem examination is desired.

Organ donation

This is discussed in Chapter 13.

Organisation of surgical services

Some of the ways in which surgical work is organised have already been briefly introduced in the previous chapter, but if the student is to understand what is going on when entering the surgical environment during undergraduate training, some further information is necessary. This is particularly so at beginning of a new century in that marked changes and increases in the complexity of surgical organisation in the National Health Service (NHS) in the UK have recently taken place.

Autonomy

The view of the surgeon as leader of his 'firm' or 'team' outlined in Chapter 1 is still to some extent true. Formerly, such a core team included, in addition to surgeons, anaesthetists and a group of surgical nurses who worked in one place – a ward. However, this simple organisation has had to be radically modified in the last decade because of pressures of many kinds, including the following:

- Increasing complexity of care, which produces first the need to enlarge the team to include many other individuals or groups who are essential to optimum management, and second the need to concentrate skills and resources, such as equipment, where they are most applicable and will be fully used rather than lie idle.
- Allied to these, the development of new specialities and super-specialities (see below) with their own particular requirements.
- The development of health service management which seeks to make sure that money is wisely and efficiently spent but which, in consequence, reduces the autonomy of the individual clinical practitioner.

Funding of surgery

The United Kingdom currently spends less of its gross domestic product on health care in percentage terms than most European countries and the United States. Recent government administrations had tried to improve the efficiency of the funding and management of the Health Service by introducing competitive market principles at all levels of health delivery. Whilst some savings and improvements may have resulted, it

did not prove universally successful and has been largely disbanded. Fundamentally, it could not redress what became largely regarded as under funding compared to other developed countries. In the years to come it will be difficult to predict the level and mechanism of funding for the Health Service. Future labour governments may commit an increasing percentage of GDP to the Health Service with a parallel commitment to training more doctors whereas a Conservative government may emphasise a greater use of private health insurance.

Whatever the mechanism, the government allocates funding to each health authority and each NHS Trust has a budget set at the beginning of the year. The chief executive of each Trust has a legal obligation to balance the books of the Trust and not to overspend. Similarly, each Trust usually agrees, in the form of a contract, to provide emergency and elective surgical services to the patients of its local general practitioners who in turn are represented by their Primary Health Care Groups (PGCs).

Surgical community cover

In the NHS in the UK, the pattern is to have a *district general hospital* (DGH) (Table 2.1) which has a general surgical side staffed by two to three typical teams – gastroenterological, vascular and breast/endocrine – each (ideally) with three surgeons and often working in consort with physicians and others. Some modification of this is necessary for a *teaching hospital* which has an additional major role in undergraduate and post-graduate education; however, increasingly this distinction is becoming blurred as more teaching takes place outside major teaching hospitals.

This organisation of DGHs is supplemented either at the same site or elsewhere with more specialised surgical teams which may serve similar or larger (regional and supraregional) catchment areas: ortho-paedic, ear–nose– throat, urological, plastic and many others which are considered elsewhere in this book (and see also below in this chapter).

Surgical specialities and super-specialities

To bring the best care to patients requires the concen-tration of experience. If a condition is relatively rare,

Table 2.1
Organisation of surgical services

Level of care	Location
Primary	General practitioner clinic
Secondary	District general hospital – provides acute and elective medical and surgical services to the local population (200 000–500 000)
Tertiary	Subregional, regional or supraregional services usually in teaching hospitals – includes specialities such as cardiothoracic and neurosurgery

then it is logical to limit its management to centres where knowledge can be developed and skills refined (Table 2.1). Such a view tends to run counter to the growth of hospitals in the UK where there has always been the tendency to think that all services should be provided at the district level and that patients should not be asked to travel any distance to obtain care. In spite of this view, regionally organised specialities have developed over the years – in neurosurgery, burns, trauma and other fields – and in addition ad hoc units of excellence (sometimes also known as supraregional) have become established in many areas such as paediatric oncology, soft tissue tumours and the management of obesity. Some of these are well established and of wont draw in all the patients for which they can offer the best services, but others are not and attract only those whose surgeons recognise that a better quality of care can be offered at a site where there is a focus on a particular condition or technique (see also Ch. 10).

Multidisciplinary aspects of surgical care

As briefly touched on in Chapter 1, surgeons are always part of a team, the members of which vary with particular needs. Surgeons work most closely with anaesthetists, who increasingly manage aspects of post-operative care, such as pain relief (along with special-ised nurses – see Ch. 10), but also with physicians and other health professionals.

The patient's path to surgery (Fig. 2.1)

DEFINITIONS

An elective patient is an individual with a condition that may require surgical management but in whom the matter is not sufficiently acutely progressive to require immediate surgical action.

An emergency patient by contrast requires assess-ment at once, either because of the nature of the problem (e.g. acute injury or physiologically threaten-ing bleeding) or because of the possible rapid progression of the disorder that is thought to be present (e.g. an acute intra-abdominal condition).

Elective patients

Outpatient sessions

The majority of patients are seen in an outpatient department after referral by primary care physicians, consultant colleagues or from accident and emergency (A&E) departments using either letter, facsimile or telephone. Future developments in information tech-

nology are having an influence on the mechanics of this process: electronic mail (e-mail) is being increasingly used over conventional letters and details of investi-gations are being made available on networked computers.

The surgical specialist who sees such an elective patient is conventionally discouraged from a cross-speciality onward referral without the prior approval of the general practitioner unless an emergency is deemed to exist.

Surgeons usually prioritise elective referrals on the basis of the information provided into:

- *urgent* – see within a week
- *soon* – see within a month
- *routine* – see when the outpatient session has a vacant slot.

The ability to control a flow of patients is often limited and may result in long delays in initial assessment of patients who are judged to be in the routine category.

Open access sessions

In an attempt to give a more speedy service and where a particular focused need can be met, the patient may be managed by direct referral to a specific service. Examples are upper gastrointestinal endoscopy and flexible sigmoidoscopy, and some minor surgery although the latter is also increasingly dealt with by general practitioners. In addition to increased speed, the problem may often be dealt with in one visit rather than two.

One-stop sessions

A variant on open access is the one-stop session where again a focused need, such as the assessment of a breast lump, can be handled by a team which may include, in addition to the surgeon, experts in imaging, pathological examination, nursing and psychological care. Again the need for repeated visits is reduced and a quick answer to the patient's problem may reduce anxiety. However, this type of session is not suitable for the assessment of complex surgical problems which may need investigation by a wide variety of methods. When these appear necessary after the initial outpatient visit, the patient should always be given some idea of how long it will be before the investigations are complete and the results are available.

Elective surgery

If a decision is taken after an outpatient consultation that an operation is needed, the first question that is likely to be asked is 'when?'. Patients and conscientious purchasers and providers no longer accept the idea of a seemingly endless queue for simple procedures such as hernia repair, with the real possibility of being lost from the list. Ideally, it should be possible to book a patient for a given date, but the problems of resource and a fluctuating case load may make this difficult.

'Minor' procedures

The word 'minor' is somewhat ill-chosen because an operation is never minor for the patient. The removal of surface lesions ('lumps and bumps') is now often carried out by general practitioners who are trained in so-called minor surgery. Hospitals also usually organise sessions of such minor surgery, which can, provided there is careful case selection, fulfil a useful cost-effective role.

Day-care procedures

It is increasingly apparent that many problems can be dealt with without overnight admission to hospital and there is a long tradition, which began in paediatric surgery, of such day-care surgical procedures.

The use of day-care can be helpfully supplemented by *pre-management* clinics, which are also valuable even if eventually it is decided that hospital in-patient admission is required. Their purpose is to make sure that the appropriate anaesthetic and other preoperative assessments, including necessary documentation and investigations, have been carried out so that subsequent management can proceed smoothly and without delays.

The great majority of elective surgery which does not invade body cavities can be carried out in the day-case unit, including operations for groin hernia (Ch. 26) and varicose veins (Ch. 29), examinations under anaesthesia with or without biopsy, and excision of superficial lumps (Ch. 38). For some patients, however, concurrent medical problems or inadequate domestic circumstances may preclude day-case operation.

In-patient management

The two criteria are:

- *Major operations* associated with inevitable physiological disturbance which cannot be managed without recourse to medical care in an organised facility with access to intensive care (Ch. 10)
- *emergencies* which require preoperative assessment and stabilisation.

An additional third category includes those who cannot be satisfactorily looked after in the community because of lack of the appropriate social background for support during recovery. The consequence of an increase in day-case procedures is that operations on in-patients tend to concentrate on more major problems and that they may, in consequence, be more demanding on the surgical and nursing team. In addition, careful planning is needed for three purposes:

- to ensure that the patient comes to surgery with adequate attention to preoperative assessment and preparation

- to ensure that adequate back-up facilities are available for intensive care should this prove to be necessary
- to ensure that an operating list for a surgical team is of the appropriate size and can be completed within the time available and in the best order.

Planning is still requires skill and experience. Factors that need to be taken into consideration include the following:

- There should be sufficient advance planning to ensure an appropriate *case mix* in which the surgical team is challenged by different surgical needs so as to keep skills active.
- Planning should be sufficiently short-term so that new urgent patients can be accommodated.
- Especially complicated or major procedures should be scheduled for the start of a session so that not only is the team fresh but also, if complications are encountered in the immediate postoperative period, the senior surgeon and anaesthetist are still available in hospital.
- Patients with a fragile physiological status – such as diabetes – should be given a definite time so that their perioperative management can be adjusted.
- Children, if they do not have a session of their own, are better dealt with first so as to prevent prolonged and irritating starvation and also to allay their possible fears.

For complex surgery or that which requires a long period of recovery (such as adaptation to a stoma or the inevitable remobilisation after some forms of orthopaedic surgery), the pre- and postoperative activities of a team which includes nurses, physiotherapists and, in special circumstances, occupational and speech therapists are often essential. Elderly patients may need to adapt immediately to their home on discharge and anticipation and preoperative planning for the ultimate discharge time are means both of helping the patient and of cost control.

The operating suite (see also Ch. 6)

It has often been the case in the past that when the student takes a first step into an operating room suite, awe is inspired because everyone else seems to know what they are doing and to have an important and recognised role. These feelings can be overcome by a helpful attitude to the student, a major component of which is to be supportive and instructive.

The suite should ideally be geographically close to the accommodation where the patients are lodged and closely accessible to the A&E department (Ch. 3). Minor differences may be required between rooms used for particular types of procedure. Efficiency is improved by alloting specific rooms to surgical specialities such as:

- general/gastroenterological
- orthopaedics

- paediatrics
- super-specialities such as neurosurgery.

Surgeons and their teams also work better if they know each other and the group becomes expert in individual requirements.

Postoperative pathway for the patient

(Fig. 2.1)

After operations on in-patients, it is routine to take the patient into a *recovery unit* which is part of the operating suite. Here staff have the expertise to recognise early signs of problems in the recovery of consciousness, with the airway or from bleeding. Alternatively, a patient who is judged to need highly specialised postoperative care is transferred directly to one of the following:

- intensive care (ICU)
- high-dependency care (HDU).

Admission to such units is also often necessary as an early step in the management of a seriously ill or extensively injured patient even though no operation has been done (see also Ch. 10). Both for the post-operative individual and for those who suffer from critical illness or injury, the choice of unit depends on a judgement of the physiological state and the likelihood of complications.

ICU is generally used for those patients who need assisted ventilation (Ch. 10) and for whom control of ventilation, core temperature, and accurate fluid and electrolyte balance optimise recovery. Considerable nursing (1:1, nurse to patient) and medical expertise is required. Discharge from an ICU is determined by recovery of physiological normality, although the criteria for this are not clearly established. The surgeon should take an active role in decision-making but must defer to other specialists when discussing 'non-surgical' aspects of care (see also Ch. 10).

At one stage down from ICU is *high-dependency care*. Here are deployed intensive nursing skills (2:1, nurse to patient) without all the high-technology equipment of an ITU. The emphasis is on:

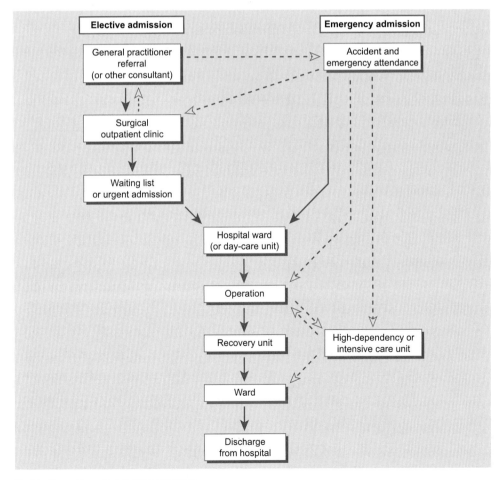

Fig 2.1 **The pathway to and from operation.**

- careful observation aided by a high ratio between staff and patients
- care suited to the continuing postoperative period – pain avoidance, special needs (e.g. paediatric patients).

Emergencies

The sources are:

- accident and emergency (A&E) departments
- general practitioner referrals
- inter-speciality referrals.

Patients attending an A&E department (Ch. 3) should be triaged and those who are considered to be possibly seriously ill should be managed initially in a resuscitation area. Facilities for intubation and control of the airway and for other forms of acute care are readily to hand and stabilisation is usually possible, although occasionally an emergency operation may be required in resuscitation (see Chs 3 and 17). If an emergency operation is necessary, direct transfer to an operating room is best, but preoperative imaging is often needed so that more accurate surgery can be undertaken. One of the pressing problems of modern A&E departments is to avoid delays in evaluation and transfer, which can result in mortality and morbidity.

Direct admission to an in-patient bed can often be avoided. Two commonly used alternatives exist:

- **Short stay/observation units** adjacent to the A&E and managed by the A&E staff (with a surgical representative) can effectively be used to screen for patients who may progress to require more intensive observation or investigation, especially by imaging (see Ch. 30); in addition, minor procedures which require general anaesthesia, such as manipulation of fractures or drainage of abscesses, may be dealt with in short stay units.
- **Admission units** are a different concept – all the acute patients for a defined period are taken into one adequately staffed ward which has the organisational advantage that doctors on duty know where to find all emergency admissions; confusion may arise when transfers take place subsequently, and at busy times congestion can be a problem.

The effective use of short stay and admission units is often hampered in the UK by the lack of available on-site senior surgical staff who are more able to make decisions about patient management.

Emergency and urgent procedures

Very few patients seen as an emergency need an operation within minutes. Penetrating wounds of the heart (Ch. 3) or the neck (Ch. 14) can be exceptions. Otherwise both traumatic and other emergencies are better handled as described in Chapters 3 and 10. Most surgical patients who require an operation do not need to be treated in the middle of the night. Formerly, pressure on operating time meant that many procedures were done in the small hours simply because no 'emergency' list was available the following day. This should no longer be the case and patients normally only undergo 'out of hours' operations when this is necessary on clinical grounds. The best organisation is to have an *emergency operating room* available throughout the day which has been shown to reduce out-of-hours operating and improve quality of outcome because of the increased availability of senior staff.

Trauma centres

These are considered in Chapter 10.

FURTHER READING

General

Joint Working Party of the British Medical Association, The Royal College of Physicians of London and The Royal College of Surgeons of England (1998) *Provision of Acute General Hospital Services – Consultation Document.*

Medicolegal aspects of surgery

Brazier M (1992) *Medicine, Patients and the Law.* Harmondsworth: Penguin.

Kennedy I, Grubb A (1994) *Medical Law.* London: Butterworths.

Skegg PDG (1988) *Law, Ethics and Medicine.* Oxford: Clarendon Press.

Mason JK, McCall-Smith RA (1994) *Law and Medical Ethics.* London: Butterworths.

3

Accident and emergency

The primary purpose of an accident and emergency (A&E) department is to diagnose and treat acute life-threatening injury and illness. Of necessity, such departments need always to be open – 24 hours a day – and adequately staffed. Inevitably, therefore, they also deal with large numbers of patients who do not, strictly, fall into the category of having a life-threatening illness.

Accident and emergency medicine is a rapidly expanding speciality in the UK and all A&E departments now have at least one consultant in charge with A&E accreditation. They should all have at least one senior house officer (more than a year qualified) per 5000 patients seen annually. A 6-month period in A&E medicine is often the first time a junior doctor has to make independent major clinical decisions. It follows, therefore, that training in A&E medicine is highly valuable regardless of the speciality that a graduate may ultimately enter.

One of London's medical schools has as its motto '*homo sum nihil a me aliem puto*' ('I am a man and all human calamities come home to me') – an appropriate description of the workload of an A&E department.

Because of its ready availability, all manner of patients pass through its doors: the lonely, the drug-addicted, society's misfits, and those who find conventional access to health care difficult. It is important that every medical student and junior doctor sees these patients because they have much to instruct us about the nature of humanity.

Surgical workload

Only about 1% of patients who attend an A&E department have suffered multiple trauma. A few more – although not many – come with surgical conditions which require urgent intervention: a leaking aneurysm of the abdominal aorta, a perforated abdominal viscus or a femoral artery blocked by an embolus. There is a much commoner third group of surgical patients: those who suffer from minor surgical conditions such as abscesses, paronychias and perianal haematomas.

Given this wide range of presentation, it is important for patients to be prioritised – a process known as 'triage' (from the French word meaning 'to sort'.)

Life-saving procedures in the A&E department

A number of surgical conditions demand immediate intervention if the patient's life is to be saved.

Airway

In all accident victims and in anyone who is unconscious, say after a head injury, care of the airway is paramount; for example, it is quite wrong to waste time dealing with a dislocated ankle if the patient is unable to breathe because of an obstructed glottis. Always deal with the airway first.

The common objects which obstruct the airway are the tongue, food and dentures. The most useful instrument to have to hand is a wide-bore (Yankers) sucker. The first action to be undertaken in dealing with an unconscious patient or an accident victim is to check that the upper airway – mouth to larynx – is patent, to suck out any food and to remove dentures if these are present.

Tongue

Because the tongue has its main muscular attachment to the posterior aspect of the body of the mandible, drawing the jaw forward automatically brings the tongue with it. Therefore, obstruction caused by the tongue falling back can be dealt with by either of two simple measures: chin lift or jaw thrust. An oropharyngeal airway (Guedel: Fig. 3.1) helps to keep the tongue forward. Alternatively, a nasopharyngeal tube can be inserted along the floor of the nose (Fig. 3.2). It is important to insert a safety pin at the nasal end to prevent the tube disappearing down the back of the patient's throat. Whenever it is feasible, the unconscious patient should be kept semi-prone (Fig. 3.3).

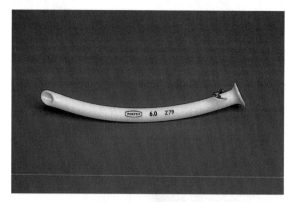

Fig 3.2 **Nasopharyngeal tube for airway maintenance.**

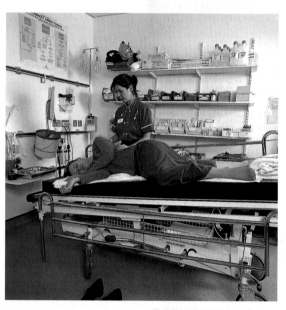

Fig 3.3 **The prone position for the unconscious patient.**

However, it is important to bear in mind that, in trauma cases, the cervical spine must be protected by means of a stiff-neck cervical collar, and the spine must be kept 'in line' until spinal trauma has been excluded.

If the foregoing measures do not work (as might be the case if there is severe maxillofacial trauma), *cricothyroidotomy* is the best way to restore an airway in an emergency. An incision is made directly over the cricothyroid membrane (Ch. 11) and an endotracheal tube is inserted into the upper trachea. Alternatively, the less experienced operator should pass a wide-bore intravenous trochar and cannula through the cricothyroid membrane and then remove the trochar. The stem of a Y-shaped connector is then attached to the cannula and one of the limbs of the Y is connected to an oxygen supply; insufflation of the lungs is achieved by intermittent obstruction of the remaining

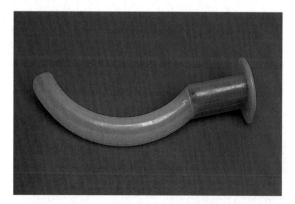

Fig 3.1 **Oropharyngeal airway** (Guedel).

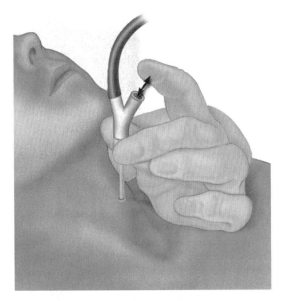

Fig 3.4 **Technique of jet insufflation.** Carefully palpate for the crico-thyroid membrane before insertion of the cannula.

vent (Fig. 3.4). This procedure, although crude, can buy very valuable time for more definitive management, usually by orotracheal intubation or tracheostomy (Ch. 14).

Breathing (ventilation)

Oxygenation of the tissues cannot be achieved even if the airway is patent if there is either absence of respiratory activity or impairment of cardiac output. There are four conditions commonly encountered in the A&E department:

- Tension pneumothorax
- Haemothorax
- Flail chest
- Acute cardiac temponade.

Tension pneumothorax

AETIOLOGY
There are two causes:
- closed trauma in which a fractured rib penetrates the lung
- rupture of an emphysematous bulla.

PATHOPHYSIOLOGY
More air passes out through a hole in the lung during inspiration than is returned on expiration and in the most acute examples there is one-way traffic only. With each inspiration the volume of intrapleural air increases, the intrapleural pressure rises and, in consequence, the lung collapses and the mediastinum is displaced towards the opposite side. The compressed lung causes a right-to-left shunt with cyanosis; the displaced mediastinum kinks the superior and, more importantly, the inferior vena cava, so reducing venous return and resulting in death from abolition of cardiac output.

CLINICAL FEATURES
History
There may be a story of closed injury or of previous emphysema and a conscious patient may complain of progressive dyspnoea.

Physical findings
There will be gasping attempts to breathe and, in the very final stages, cyanosis. There may be distended neck veins. Local physical signs on the affected side are:

- decreased chest wall movement
- a hyperresonant percussion note
- absent breath sounds.

In addition, although these are of late occurrence and difficult to detect, there will be:

- displacement of the trachea in the suprasternal notch away from the affected side
- movement of the apex beat – laterally in a right and medially in a left pneumothorax.

MANAGEMENT
A chest X-ray should not be done until urgent relief has been achieved by the insertion of a wide-bore needle through the second intercostal space in the midclavicular line (see Ch. 11). Formal chest drainage with an underwater seal can then be undertaken (Ch. 11) once deterioration of the patient has been averted.

Haemothorax

AETIOLOGY
The cause is usually trauma to the chest as the result of either penetration (knife or projectile) or blunt injury which is usually severe, such as a fall from a height or a crush by a vehicle.

PATHOPHYSIOLOGY
The usual cause of a haemothorax is rupture of one or more intercostal arteries. The intercostal vessels are segmental in nature and come directly off the thoracic aorta; hence haemorrhage is often brisk. Bleeding can also come from torn bronchial arteries or veins when the substance of the lung is itself lacerated.

Loss of blood can be severe and is combined with compression of the lung on the affected side to produce a right-to-left shunt.

CLINICAL FEATURES

Symptoms

In addition to a history of a physical injury, there may be chest pain and dyspnoea.

Physical findings

There will usually be general features of hypovolaemia and occasionally cyanosis. Local signs are:

- bruising of the chest wall
- evidence of fractured ribs including subcutaneous emphysema
- imprinting – a mark left on the skin by the object responsible for the injury, such as a tyre mark or other evidence of cause
- an entry wound, perhaps with, in a projectile injury, a complementary exit wound
- dull percussion note on the affected side
- absent or reduced breath sounds also on the affected side.

INVESTIGATION

Provided there is not urgency to restore ventilation, a chest X-ray often shows shadowing on the affected side with a fluid interface with the lung. If there is also a pneumothorax, an erect film reveals a horizontal fluid level.

MANAGEMENT

Treatment is different from that of a tension pneumothorax; a needle is inadequate for drainage. A wide-bore chest drain must be inserted and positioned so that it lies in the dependent part of the chest cavity.

Drainage and re-expansion of the lung are frequently followed by cessation of the bleeding. However, if the rate of blood loss is greater than 200 mL/h or there is marked hypotension uncorrected by rapid infusion of blood and plasma expanders, urgent thoracotomy is indicated.

Flail Chest

AETIOLOGY

Trauma is the only cause and, once again, may be open or closed – usually the latter.

PATHOPHYSIOLOGY

The injury is always serious and very frequently associated with an underlying contusion of the lung. The chest wall injury is a fracture of one rib (but usually more) at both the anterior and posterior ends. Thus a segment of chest wall moves independently in a *paradoxical* manner – inwards on inspiration and outwards on expiration. The size of the involved segment determines the degree of reduction in respiratory efficiency, which is made worse by any lung contusion which causes a right-to-left shunt.

CLINICAL FEATURES

Symptoms

The symptoms are these of hypoxia and respiratory distress.

Physical findings

The physical findings are:

- dyspnoea
- paradoxical respiration in the involved segment of chest wall.

DIAGNOSIS

Early recognition can be surprisingly difficult, particularly when breathing is shallow, but is important in that the whole thrust of management is to avoid tissue hypoxia. The majority of those with a flail chest that is causing respiratory insufficiency require positive pressure ventilation which can be established in the A&E department by intubation of the trachea and either hand or mechanical ventilation. The procedure must be continued until the flail segment has stabilised which may take several weeks. Surgical fixation of the chest wall is only occasionally indicated.

....

Circulation

Acute cardiac tamponade

AETIOLOGY AND PATHOPHYSIOLOGY

Blood accumulates within the pericardial sac and compresses the heart so that cardiac output is decreased. The source is a leak from the heart either because of a penetrating injury, such as a knife wound, or from blunt trauma. The outcome is a low cardiac output which will eventually cause death; venous return is reduced so that there are features of right heart failure.

CLINICAL FEATURES

History

Penetrating or blunt trauma is usually obvious. The victim becomes progressively ill from low cardiac output, with confusion and eventually unconsciousness.

Physical findings

Apart from an external injury in penetrating trauma, physical findings are few. Dilated neck veins are universal and loss of a palpable apex beat may be suggestive, but this may be difficult to evaluate.

MANAGEMENT

Unless there is prompt relief, continuing hypoxia and death result. Tamponade caused by a stab wound requires immediate thoracotomy, if necessary at the place where injury occurred or in the A&E department.

The thorax is entered via the left fifth rib space, the bulging pericardial sac is incised longitudinally avoiding the phrenic nerve, the blood is evacuated, and a finger is placed over the myocardial wound to arrest further bleeding while preparations are made to close the wound with simple sutures. This dramatic management results in survival of at least a quarter of victims. For those untrained in thoracotomy time may be bought by performing needle pericardiocentesis.

Imaging in the trauma patient

Any imaging must be related to the clinical state of the patient and, in particular, a competent clinical individual should accompany the patient during the procedure.

There are three standard radiological views which, in trauma, should be taken namely:

- cross-table view of the cervical spine
- chest X-ray
- anteroposterior pelvis.

Cervical spine

Firstly, and most importantly, a cross-table cervical spine X-ray which shows all seven cervical vertebrae and the cervicothoracic junction is mandatory to avoid the possibility of a missed diagnosis of a cervical spine injury. Unrecognised, this may lead on to damage to

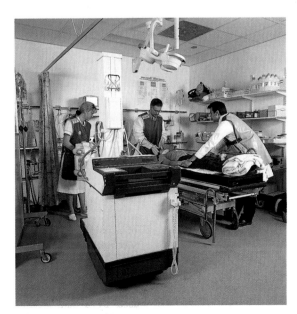

Fig 3.5 **Method of obtaining a cross-table X-ray of the cervical spine.**

the spinal cord. Such views are facilitated if the patient's shoulders are pulled down (Fig. 3.5). If the cervical spine cannot be completely imaged, then a *swimmer's view* can be obtained, where one arm is extended over the patient's head, the X-ray tube is brought into the axilla, and a plate is placed on the opposite side and then exposed. There are four lines on a lateral cervical spine X-ray:

- prevertebral
- the anterior aspect of the vertebral bodies
- the posterior aspect of the vertebral bodies
- the spinous processes.

All of these must be smooth curves. A feature which is commonly missed in interpreting these X-rays is a haematoma deep to the prevertebral fascia which clearly shows as a soft tissue swelling. Odontoid peg fractures are also commonly missed and it is important to check that the distance between the posterior aspect of the body of the first cervical vertebra and the anterior aspect of the odontoid peg is no greater than 3 mm.

Chest X-ray

An upright (Ch. 4) chest X-ray should be obtained in any patient who has sustained trauma to the trunk – chest or abdomen. There are numerous possible abnormalities, but commonly missed diagnoses include:

- pneumothorax (see above) where it is important to check that lung markings go right out to the periphery of the lung field
- ruptured diaphragm
- traumatic aortic dissection (Ch. 28) which often reveals itself as a widened mediastinum.

Pelvis

A *diastasis* (abnormal widening) at the symphysis pubis may indicate damage to the urethra (Ch. 32), which can be confirmed by urethrography. This is easily performed in the resuscitation room by inserting a urinary balloon catheter (Ch. 11) and securing it in the meatal fossa by gently inflating the balloon and instilling contrast medium under gentle pressure.

Concurrent with or subsequent to the information derived from these basic imaging techniques, other methods may be indicated (Fig. 3.6).

Computed tomography (CT)

This technique has transformed radiological practice, particularly in neurotrauma (Ch. 30). Spiral CT makes imaging more rapid than was previously the case.

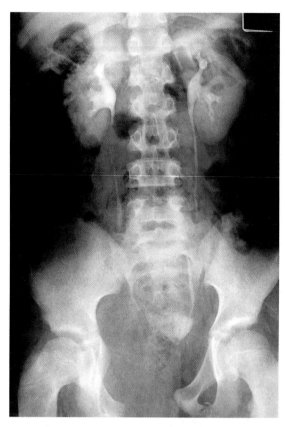

Fig 3.6 **Abnormal widening of the pubic symphysis with an associated rupture of the urethra and high-riding bladder.**

Urgent surgical conditions which cause hypovolaemic shock

The commonest causes of *non-traumatic* massive blood loss are:

- ruptured abdominal aortic aneurysm (Ch. 28)
- ectopic pregnancy
- gastrointestinal haemorrhage (usually from the upper GI tract) (Ch. 22).

In civilian A&E practice in the UK, the common *traumatic* causes are:

- Ruptured spleen.
- Rupture of other intra-abdominal viscera such as the liver and tearing of the mesenteric vessels.
- Long bone fractures – a single femoral shaft fracture leads to the loss of 1.5 L of blood which is 30% of the total blood volume.
- Pelvic fractures – several litres of blood may be lost and the patient may rapidly die from hypovolaemia.

Hence, if a pelvic fracture is suspected clinically, very urgent resuscitation is required and the haemorrhage can often be abated by applying an external fixator to the pelvis in the resuscitation room.

Ectopic pregnancy

This condition should be considered in any woman who presents to the A&E department with acute abdominal pain and who may, even as a remote possibility, be pregnant. A denial of recent sexual intercourse is not a guarantee that the patient is not pregnant.

CLINICAL FEATURES

History

There is frequently (90%) a short history of lower abdominal pain followed by more generalised and constant pain which may also be felt in the shoulder if blood tracks up the paracolic gutters to the under-surface of the diaphragm. Dysuria is also common. Vaginal bleeding is absent in 25%.

Physical findings

General features of bleeding are often apparent – pallor, circulatory collapse and air hunger may be present together with abdominal tenderness and rigidity, initially most marked in the lower abdomen. Cervical excitation also causes pain.

MANAGEMENT

In any patient in which an ectopic pregnancy is likely, two large intravenous cannulae should be inserted even if the circulation is apparently stable; in such circumstances it may be possible to confirm the diagnosis by obtaining a positive pregnancy test. A patient with signs of hypovolaemia should go immediately to the operating room for surgery, preferably by a gynaecologist who may be able to save the affected fallopian tube.

Common surgical conditions seen in the A&E department

Soft tissue abscesses

These represent a very considerable component of the surgical work of an A&E department. An abscess is defined simply as a collection of pus and the pain of an abscess is caused by the build-up of pressure in the inflamed soft tissues. It is true to say that the smaller the abscess, the greater the pain and, because an abscess may appear small, this is not a reason to underestimate the distress caused.

An abscess in the finger (e.g. a pulp space abscess) is much more painful than, say, an abscess on the scrotum, because in the former there are strong fibres which connect the pulp of the fingertip to the periosteum of the distal phalanx and also pressure rises in a confined space. Thus there is little opportunity for the abscess to expand and the tension in the affected area is high.

DIAGNOSIS

This is usually straightforward. The symptoms are of inflammation, the signs of which are heat, redness, tenderness, swelling and loss of function of the affected part. In addition there is often fluctuation .

MANAGEMENT

Once an abscess has been diagnosed, the correct treatment is incision and drainage rather than recourse to antibiotics, although these may be administered to deal with the possibility of spread when a surgical procedure is undertaken, or any associated cellulitis.

Before incision is performed, an appropriate method of anaesthesia needs to be established. For pulp space abscess and those beside the fingernail (paronychia), ring block regional anaesthesia is suitable. A solution of 1% lignocaine is introduced on either side of the base of the digit to anaesthetise the digital nerve. It takes 5 or 10 minutes for the anaesthetic to take effect; then an incision is made over the chosen point where the abscess is at its most prominent. In all abscesses, it is a cardinal error to make the incision too small.

There are some abscesses which are better dealt with under general anaesthesia, e.g. the breast, the axilla and the ischiorectal fossa.

There is now a school of thought that maintains that after drainage and the use of appropriate antibiotics, the drainage site can be closed primarily. There is certainly a case for this but caution should be observed unless drainage and excision of dead tissue are indubitably complete.

Traumatic haematoma

There are two small haematomas (which cause severe pain) that can easily be dealt with in an A&E department:

Subungual haematoma
This usually occurs when the extremities of either a finger or a toe have been damaged: blood oozes out beneath the affected nail and, because there is initially little room for expansion, the pain soon becomes severe

and requires urgent release. The old fashioned method of *trephine*, in which the red hot end of a paper clip is pushed down on the nail in order to bore a hole and allow the escape of blood, is very effective but ring block anaesthesia should be used.

Perianal haematoma
See Chapter 25.

Minor wounds

Relatively simple lacerations to the skin and underlying tissues are common in the A&E department, but a wound should never be regarded as *minor*. It is imperative that the basic principles of wound management are observed (Ch. 8). Chemoprophylaxis is required for all animal (including human) bites.

Tetanus prophylaxis

In dealing with a laceration in the A&E department, consideration should always be given to whether or not the patient is immune to the effects of *Clostridium tetani* (Ch. 9). Tetanus is rare in developed countries but is a major cause of mortality in developing communities. The very low rates of tetanus in the UK are attributable to an effective immunisation programme and good standards of hygiene. However, previous and often repeated immunisations, as took place during the 1940s, have produced a population which is now ageing and in whom resistance to *C. tetani* may be on the decline.

Table 3.1
Immunisation against tetanus

Wound	Immunisation	Action
Clean wound	Last of three-dose course or reinforcing dose within last 10 years	None
Tetanus-prone wound	Last of three-dose course or reinforcing dose within last 10 years	None – although a dose adsorbed vaccine may be given in high risk, e.g. contamination with stable manure
	Last of three-dose course or high reinforcing dose more than 10 years previously	Reinforcing dose of adsorbed vaccine with reinforcing dose of anti-tetanus immunoglobulin
	Not immunised or immunisation status not certain	Full three-dose course of adsorbed vaccine given at monthly intervals, plus anti-tetanus immunoglobulin

In a patient who has never been actively immunised and who has a contaminated wound, possibly with a source of *C. tetani* (soil-contaminated wounds or those associated with severe tissue damage), *passive* immunisation with human anti-tetanus immuno-globulin (HATI) 250 IU by intramuscular injection is essential. Table 3.1 gives guidelines for specific anti-tetanus treatment.

Antibiotic prophylaxis

There are some wounds which, by definition, will be heavily contaminated by bacteria, e.g. agricultural injuries, and human and animal bites. These should not be primarily sutured (see below) but should be thoroughly washed out with normal saline, left open and prophylactic antibiotics (Ch. 9) prescribed.

INITIAL EXAMINATION

Examination must include that part of the body distal to the wound to ensure that nerves, blood vessels and tendons have not been damaged. For example, in a laceration to the hand caused by a broken glass, all the fingers must be carefully examined to ensure that nerve and tendon function is intact. It is inadequate merely to ask the patient to make a fist – each finger must be examined and flexor digitorum profundus and flexor digitorum superficialis tendons must have their integrity established.

The possibility that there might be a foreign body should always be considered.

MANAGEMENT

The principles of excision and suture are outlined in Chapter 8. Lacerations over the pretibial (shin) area should not be sutured because the skin is already quite tight and additional tension easily results in ischaemia of the wound edges. The correct management is for the wound edges to be approximated only, often by means of sterile adhesive plastic strips (Steristrips; see also Ch. 6) and a light dressing applied. These wounds usually heal well, although they can take many months to do so.

Head injury

Definitive management is considered in Chapter 30. Initial decision-making and management in the A&E department are vital to subsequent success.

Every year, 3 per 100 000 of the population are admitted to hospital with head injuries; they make up approximately 20% of acute surgical admissions. The majority are admitted under the care of general surgeons and therefore it behoves those in training to have a thorough working knowledge of their initial management and to be able to detect warning signs of deterioration. They must be fully conversant with the

in-house arrangements for the procedures to be under-taken with such patients and must also know the lines of referral to their local neurosurgical unit.

HISTORY AND PROGRESS

For every victim of a head injury, the following clinical matters must be recorded, if necessary with the help of witnesses and family:

- time of injury
- time seen by the examining doctor
- mechanism of injury
- evidence of loss of consciousness
- period of amnesia both before (retrograde) and after sustaining the injury and whether the patient now has a continuous memory of events
- any visual disturbance
- vomiting
- headache
- fits
- an alcohol and drug history; (if possible).

CLINICAL FEATURES

Physical findings

Urgent findings are:

- presence of blood behind the eardrum (haemotympanum)
- cerebrospinal fluid coming from the nose or ears, often blood-stained (rhinorrhoea and otorrhoea)
- pupillary signs, including inequality between the two sides and dilatation, particularly if it is unresponsive to light.

The first two findings are an indication of a fracture of the base of the skull.

The pupillary signs are possible indications of compression of the ocular motor (third cranial) nerve against the edge of the tentorial hiatus from critically raised intracranial pressure perhaps because of an expanding supratentoreal extradural haematoma.

Level of consciousness

This is recorded against the Glasgow Coma Scale (GCS) scoring system (see Ch. 30). The initial and subsequent estimates must be, together with the time, recorded in the notes both as individual scores and as a total.

Indications of a severe head injury are given in Information Box 3.1

URGENT MANAGEMENT

Any patient known or suspected to have a head injury is dealt with according to the protocols laid down by the advanced trauma life support (ATLS) system. As in every other circumstance of injury, the airway is of overriding importance – however severe the injury to the head, the airway always comes first in an attempt to ensure survival.

Indications of a severe head injury

- A GCS of 12 or less
- Evidence of a fractured skull in combination with confusion, focal neurological signs, fits or a depression in the level of consciousness
- Coma continuing after correction of other possible causes, such as hypoxia and profound hypotension from blood loss
- Apparent or suspected open injury of the vault or base of the skull
- Depressed fracture
- Deterioration – includes those who have a GCS of 15 on admission which then drops to 14; it is better to act on such a small change than to wait until the patient is comatose
- Pupillary signs (see text)

Any of the foregoing requires the urgent presence of an anaesthetist and the neurosurgical team must be contacted.

As is also emphasised above, arterial hypotension in the presence of a head injury should not be presumed to be caused by damage to the head. Although scalp lacerations can bleed profusely, intracranial bleeding of itself does not produce hypotensive shock; the systemic response to raised intracranial pressure caused by an expanding intracranial haematoma is usually brady-cardia with later hypertension. Therefore, other causes for hypotension should sought.

For further discussion on management of head injuries, see Chapter 30.

Some aphorisms in A&E medicine

- *Always introduce yourself to the patient*
In the AED, patients are nearly always frightened and in pain. When there is time and a pressing state of emergency does not exist, an early rapport is established by introducing yourself to the patient. The patient will forgive most things related, for example, to delay if you are perceived as being a kind and caring doctor. By contrast, forgiveness is uncommon for one who is seen to be offhand. Being kind does not require any special training and is therapy needed by every patient you meet.

- *Do not be distracted by the spectacular*
Spectacular injuries are not uncommonly seen in a busy A&E department. It is easy to become distracted by a patient with bilateral fractured femurs with the bone ends clearly visible, but concentration on the local injury may divert attention from a need to attend to the airway or to make sure that there is a channel for fluid replacement. The injury that is spectacular is not necessarily the one that should be attended to first.

- *Clinical notes are a medicolegal document, and legible, timed and signed records should be taken in every instance*
This good professional practice is easy to forget in the hurly-burly of an A&E department. However, these records are a legal document (see Ch. 2) and may later have to be made available to the patient or legal advisors, not necessarily because legal action is being taken but perhaps because an insurance claim is pending (sometimes years after the accident) which can only be dealt with properly if clear notes were taken initially. Further, if, at a later date, malpractice (Ch. 2) is alleged, comprehensive and legible clinical notes are a necessary part of the defence; by contrast, absence of a record or its incomplete nature makes defence difficult.

- *The diagnosis of a fracture is clinical, not radiological*
A normal X-ray should not lead to a false sense of security that a fracture is absent. A classical example of this is after a fall onto the outstretched hand (Ch. 34) when there is a fracture of the head of the radius or of the scaphoid. Similarly, an elderly lady who has fallen on her hip and is complaining of local pain could have a fracture that is impacted and permits walking (Ch. 34), even if the initial X-ray looks normal – *never make a diagnosis of a bruised hip*; admission to hospital is the best course.

- *Never diagnose drunkenness*
It is unsatisfactory and sometimes very dangerous for both the patient and the medical attendant to make a diagnosis of alcohol intoxication in the A&E department. Other conditions such as head injury and hypoglycaemia must be excluded. If the patient has sustained a head injury, then it is prudent to assume that confusion is caused by the head injury and is not the result of alcohol. The correct course of action is to admit the patient to hospital, and make regular neurological observations until the situation has declared itself. If the patient's neurological condition deteriorates, then urgent CT scanning is indicated with appropriate airway management.

- *Never diagnose hysteria*
It has been known for a patient, usually a young woman, to be labelled 'hysterical' after a minor chest injury: she is then given a paper bag to breathe into and put into a cubicle, only to be found dead some time later from a tension pneumothorax. *A diagnosis of psychological problems in A&E should only be made after physical causes have been properly excluded.*

If the patient's neurological condition deteriorates, then urgent CT scanning is indicated with appropriate airway management.

● *Assume the presence of pregnancy in any woman capable of being pregnant*
Any woman of child-bearing age who complains of abdominal pain must have a diagnosis of ectopic pregnancy seriously considered (see above). Denial of sexual intercourse is no guarantee.

● *The likelihood of morbidity of a wound is in inverse proportion to its size*
The smaller the wound, the more likely it is that complications will be discounted or overlooked. A compound fracture of the tibia and the fibula after a motorcycle crash is not easily missed, but a tiny cut on the finger sustained while washing the dishes may be followed by failure to detect a divided digital nerve. Serious and permanent morbidity may then result. The term minor injury should never be used. All injuries have a potential for morbidity and should be dealt with in this light.

● *If there is abdominal pain, examine the chest*
Myocardial infarction not infrequently presents with epigastric pain, and pleural involvement in lower lobe pneumonia can also cause referred pain to the abdomen.

4

Investigation of the surgical patient

Decision-making in the surgical patient is not often based on clinical findings alone. More frequently, investigations are undertaken to support or refute a clinical suspicion. Any investigation increases the cost of health care and often carries a risk both to the patient and to health care workers (e.g. exposure to X-rays). In consequence, investigations should only be undertaken if they are thought to contribute significantly to patient management (see also Ch. 7). It has now become customary to grade investigations by their degree of invasiveness (Ch. 1). There is not an agreed scale to define this, but the amount of compromise of the body surface and the likelihood of complications (both morbidity and mortality) are a rough guide; for example, a venepuncture is regarded as less invasive than an arterial puncture.

Objectives

There are three objectives to carrying out investigations:

- To establish a diagnosis which includes the determination of the extent of the pathological process and the planning for its surgical correction.
- To assess system physiological impairment (e.g. pulmonary or cardiac) and therefore the possible risk which is present if surgical treatment is needed.
- To screen for disorders that are common but without symptoms; however, this is only worthwhile if their presence results in a change in management (e.g. previously undiagnosed hypertension, diabetes mellitus or coronary artery disease in those who require operations for vascular disorders).

There is an additional meaning of the word 'screen'. It can be, and often is, a synonyn for a group of tests designed to detect a specific abnormality such as in clotting (see below). When the word is used in this sense, the surgical student should understand the difference.

Efficacy

A given investigation (just as with any clinical or laboratory observation) has a given *degree of association* with an underlying disease or disorder. This degree is a measure of the probability that, in a run of patients with disease X, the investigation will be positive in a given fraction of those who actually have X. For example, in patients with perforated peptic ulcer (Ch. 18), an upright chest X-ray reveals gas under the diaphragm in 60 out of a 100 consecutive patients – a probability of 0.6. Observations of this kind can be incorporated into mathematical formulae using Bayes' theorem (see 'Further reading') to calculate the likelihood that a given set of observations which include clinical findings and investigations implies the presence of a particular disease/disorder.

Sensitivity, specificity, positive and negative predictive values

Sensitivity describes the ability of the clinical test to identify patients with a particular abnormality, even though it may also select patients who do not actually have the condition. It is calculated as:

$$\frac{\text{true positives}}{\text{true positives} + \text{false negatives}}$$

Specificity describes the ability of the test to identify the healthy individuals who do not have that particular abnormality, even though it may miss some patients who have the condition. It is calculated as:

$$\frac{\text{true negatives}}{\text{true negatives} + \text{false positives}}$$

Positive predictive value describes the probability of an individual who tested positive actually having the abnormality and is calculated as:

$$\frac{\text{true positives}}{\text{true positives} + \text{false positives}}$$

Negative predictive value describes the probability of an individual who tested negative actually not having the abnormality and is calculated as:

$$\frac{\text{true negatives}}{(\text{true negatives} + \text{false negatives})}$$

False negatives are those patients who truly have the condition but were not detected by the clinical test, and false positives are those who, on subsequent analysis, turn out not to have the condition under study but had a positive test.

The ideal investigation is one whose sensitivity and specificity approach unity. In practice, however, there is a trade-off between the two ratios – the greater the sensitivity, the less the specificity and vice versa. This matter is particularly important in screening for early disease.

Haematological investigations

Full blood count

The diagnostic use of full blood count in surgical patients is less common than in assessment and screening, e.g. to ensure that the patient has a haemoglobin level sufficient for oxygen carriage during anaesthesia (see Ch. 6) and a platelet count which ensures adequate haemostasis. Nevertheless, the full blood count is the commonest haematological investigation ordered in surgical patients (Table 4.1).

In diagnosis, the mean corpuscular volume (MCV) helps to identify the cause of anaemia, because chronic occult bleeding produces a low MCV (microcytic anaemia) whereas acute haemorrhage is associated with a normal value but a low haemoglobin. A high MCV may be encountered in chronic alcoholism and vitamin B_{12} or folate deficiency (past total gastrectomy without vitamin B_{12} replacement, Crohn's disease [Ch. 23] of the terminal ileum or previous resection of this part of the gut). High haemoglobin and red blood cell counts are commonly the result of severe dehydration and compensation for chronic respiratory failure. Occasionally they direct attention to the possibility of polycythaemia rubra vera.

White cell count

A raised white cell count with neutrophilia may be indicative of the presence of bacterial infection or necrotic tissue (Ch. 9). A severe septic response, however, may be associated with an abnormally low count. Eosinophilia may be a manifestation of parasitic infestation or allergic reaction and a high lymphocyte count can indicate the possibility of viral infection. Low white cell counts follow cytotoxic chemotherapy. Patients with AIDS may have low numbers of lymphocytes.

Table 4.1
Full blood count

Component	Normal value
Haemoglobin	
Male	12.5–16.5 g/dL
Female	11.5–15.5 g/dL
Haematocrit	
Male	0.42–0.53
Female	0.39–0.45
Red blood cell count	
Male	4.4–6.5×10^{12}/L
Female	3.9–5.6×10^{12}/L
White blood cell count	4–11×10^{9}/L
Platelet count	150–400×10^{9}/L
Mean corpuscular volume (MCV)	80–98 fL
Mean corpuscular haemoglobin (MCH)	27–32 pg

Platelets

Thrombocytopenia may be the result of a drug reaction (e.g. heparin), hypersplenism, an autoimmune process (idiopathic thrombocytopenic purpura), leukaemias or excessive consumption (disseminated intravascular coagulation). Thrombocytosis is seen in chronic sepsis and after splenectomy (Ch. 20) or haemorrhage.

Coagulation

In certain surgical patients, disorders of the clotting mechanism are more common. A coagulation screen should be obtained in:

- obstructive jaundice in which absence of vitamin K absorption leads to lack of prothrombin synthesis (Ch. 19)
- those on anticoagulants for the management of other disorders
- patients who have undergone significant haemorrhage, e.g. during operation or after trauma
- patients who appear, during operation, to have coagulation defects, i.e. those with unexpectedly heavy bleeding.

Coagulopathies are not common but can occur in the course of other serious illness which may require surgical management.

Disseminated intravascular coagulation (DIC)

This condition is usually part of another severe illness or widespread malignancy and is characterised by activation, within the intravascular compartment, of both the coagulation and the fibrinolytic cascades. Clotting factors are consumed at a higher rate than they are replaced. The results are:

- depletion of clotting factors and coagulopathy characterised by high prothrombin time and a low platelet count and fibrinogen levels
- increased circulating products of fibrin degradation (FDPs).

The cause of the syndrome is probably the activation of the vascular endothelium in capillary beds, which assumes a *pro-coagulant* state and initiates the coagulation cascade. Many bacterial products such as endotoxin and cytokines (e.g. tumour necrosis factor, interleukin-1) are capable of inducing a pro-coagulant state in endothelial cells, but it is not known which combination of mediators operates in the clinical syndrome.

Biochemical tests

Table 4.2 lists the most commonly used biochemical tests.

Blood levels

Previously well patients who are not taking medication can undergo minor surgery without any biochemical studies other than routine urinalysis for the presence of glucose (see below). Levels in the blood are, however, important screening tests for many surgical patients: those with a cardiovascular disorder, on diuretic treatment or with known diabetes mellitus, should always have their blood levels of sodium and potassium determined before an anaesthetic. Potassium changes (usually hypokalaemia) make patients vulnerable to cardiac arrhythmias; correction is necessary and usually easy. Elevated serum urea concentration is common with dehydration or renal insufficiency, whereas serum creatinine concentration is a more reliable marker of renal disease and is usually not affected by moderate dehydration. Elevation usually signifies the loss of 50% of renal function. Creatinine clearance is an accurate measure of glomerular filtration rate and should be done in those who are to undergo major vascular reconstructions (e.g. aortic aneurysm repair), when it may reveal asymptomatic renal insufficiency.

Postoperative abnormalities in serum electrolyte concentrations are very common, chiefly because, in many surgical circumstances, the gastrointestinal tract cannot be used for the administration of maintenance fluids and electrolytes. In addition, postoperative requirements may be difficult to calculate when losses

Table 4.2
Commonly used biochemical tests and enzymes

	Normal value	Enzymes	Normal value
Sodium	135–146 mmol/L	Total protein	62–80 g/L
Potassium	3.5–5.5 mmol/L	Albumin	35–50 g/L
Urea	2.6–6.7 mmol/L	Bilirubin	<17 mmol/L
Creatinine	60–120 mmol/L	Alkaline phosphatase	25–120 U/L
Calcium	2.2–2.6 mmol/L	Aspartate aminotransferase	10–40 U/L
Glucose	3.9–5.6 mmol/L	Alanine aminotransferase	5–30 U/L
Urate	0.18–0.42 mmol/L	Lactate dehydrogenase	40–195 U/L
		Creatinine phosphokinase	24–195 U/L

are complicated – fistulae, nasogastric suction and fluid sequestration into either the intestine or large inflamed areas. Although sepsis and inappropriate ADH secretion can cause a low serum sodium concentration (hyponatraemia), the commonest cause of this is water overload. If the patient is dependent on parenteral fluid therapy, the levels of electrolyte and urea in the blood should be measured at least every second day and preferably daily.

Changes in serum potassium concentration are particularly likely in patients with an unusually high urine output (low potassium – hypokalaemia) or pathologically low output (raised potassium – hyperkalaemia). Prompt correction of the underlying cause is mandatory. Renal blood flow may be reduced during and after prolonged hypotension caused by uncorrected loss of blood volume or in patients with systemic sepsis. Postoperative elevations of urea and/or creatinine concentration are often the consequence of this. Serial measurements of urea concentration may provide an early warning of the development of renal failure.

Other blood levels, such as calcium and enzyme concentrations, are dealt with under the heading of the disorders or disturbances which cause their change.

Urinalysis

Testing of the urine has been greatly simplified by the use of dip stick and other prepackaged tests. Relevant finding in surgical patients are:

- *glucose* as an indicator of diabetes and the need for further preoperative investigation
- *nitrates* – particularly in acute undiagnosed abdominal pain: a positive test should lead to microscopy for the presence of leucocytes and bacteria indicative of a urinary tract infection
- *blood* (haematuria) suggests disease of the urinary tract, but the test is likely to give a false positive result in a woman who is menstruating
- *bilirubin* – see Ch. 19
- *human beta-chorionic gonadotrophin* – pregnancy.

Twenty-four hour collections of urine are sometimes diagnostically valuable.

Microbiological investigation

Routine preoperative testing is indicated in the following circumstances:

- multiple antibiotic screening for carriage of resistant bacteria (e.g. MRSA – see Ch. 10)

- urinary infection in patients undergoing urological operations
- hepatitis virus infection (B and C) in patients from high-risk areas.

Tumour markers

See Chapter 12.

Imaging

Surgery is a discipline based largely on anatomy and the function of anatomically discrete organs. In consequence it is highly dependent on techniques which can give insight into the position and activity of organs and systems. Until the 1970s, this was achieved largely by the use of X-rays. However, although most hospitals still have organisations which are usually known as X-ray or radiology departments, many other techniques of imaging are now practised both in these departments and elsewhere. For this reason, 'departments of imaging' would now be the more appropriate phrase.

Imaging now has a central role in the management of patients and image guidance is widely used for both diagnosis and treatment. Therapeutic procedures carried out utilising an imaging technique are called interventional although they are no more – and are usually less – invasive than surgical techniques.

In addition, some methods and their physical basis (ultrasound, radioisotope imaging and functional MRI) overlap with studies of organ function.

Requests for imaging

Because there are so many different ways of performing all types of imaging and also many specific contraindications and complications, it is essential that adequate clinical information is given when requests are made. This ensures not only that the test is carried out in the optimal way to answer the question posed, but also that any action is avoided that may be, at best, inappropriate and, at worst, dangerous. It is also important that whoever makes the request is aware of what is involved, the contraindications and the possible hazards. If the surgical team is in any doubt, then a discussion with the imaging department is mandatory.

Finally, to make intelligent decisions on requests, it is also essential that the team has a general understanding of the physical basis of the various forms of imaging – their capabilities and limitations.

There are currently many different types of imaging, some of which interact with each other:

- radiological – plain X-rays (including tomography), contrast studies and computed tomography

- ultrasound (US)
- magnetic resonance imaging (MRI)
- isotope scanning.

All have a place in surgical diagnosis and they are discussed separately below.

··

Radiological imaging

PHYSICAL BASIS

X-rays and gamma rays (γ-rays) are part of the spectrum of *electromagnetic radiation* (Fig. 4.1); both have short wavelengths and are therefore of high frequency. All electromagnetic waves travel through space at approximately 3^{10} metres per second and are identified either as fluctuations of electrical and magnetic fields (waves) or as the effect of discrete photons (particles) on sensitive receptors. Their short wavelength and high frequency are associated with a large *photon energy*. To produce X-rays, electrons which have been accelerated to a high velocity by a potential difference (known as the peak kilovoltage, kV_p) across a vacuum tube strike a suitable target such as tungsten or molybdenum. On impact, the electrons lose energy which, for the most part, is dissipated as heat. However, a small proportion is converted into X-rays and the target can be arranged so that these pass through tissues. The higher the kilovoltage, the greater is the penetration but the smaller the differential absorption by tissues, and hence the *inherent contrast* produced in the receptor device on the far side of the structure towards which the X-rays are directed.

Interaction of X-rays with matter

In the energy range of diagnostic (as distinct from therapeutic) X-rays, three interactions occur:

Coherent scattering

In this interaction the incident photon undergoes a change of direction without a change in wavelength. Only a small proportion of the radiation interacts in this way.

Photoelectric effect

The photon is completely absorbed by an atom with ejection of an electron and ionisation; the so-called characteristic radiation of a fixed and typical wavelength is released. This occurs more commonly with low-energy X-rays.

Compton scattering

A photon strikes an outer shell electron of an atom, ejects it and leaves an ionised atom; the incident photon is deflected but retains some of its energy. Compton scattering accounts for most of the scattered radiation encountered in diagnostic radiology.

SAFETY

The photoelectric and Compton effects cause ionisation which leads to breaking of chemical bonds with, importantly, damage to DNA. Large amounts of X-rays produce so-called *non-stochastic* (which roughly means non-random) or *deterministic* (consequent on a known biological effect of given frequency) effects: cell death, bone marrow suppression, cataract formation and hair loss. However, all of these occur at levels in excess of those used in diagnostic radiology. Stochastic (chance)

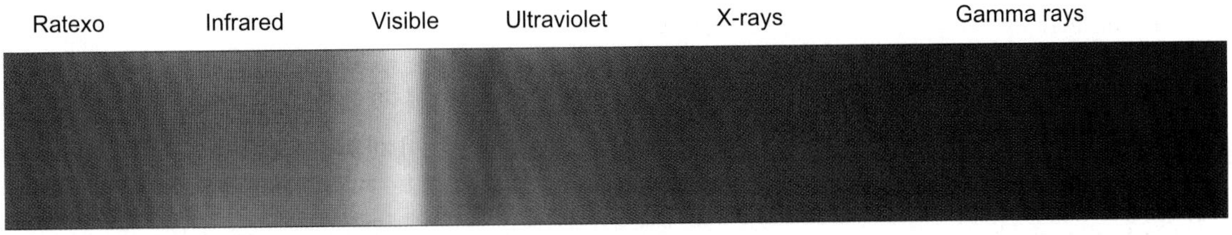

Fig 4.1 **The position of X-rays and gamma rays on the electromagnetic spectrum.**

Table 4.3
Typical risks from X-ray examinations (per million). (From Plaut 1993)

Irradiation examination	Hereditary effect		Effect on fetus	
	Paternal	**Maternal**	**Childhood cancer**	**Mental retardation**
Lumbar spine	0.2	16	200	1560
Abdomen	2	11	170	1300
Pelvis	24	6.3	100	740
IVU	23	19	220	1610
Barium meal	0.8	9.4	220	1620
Barium enema	5.4	26	960	7200

effects, however, can also occur and include the induction of malignancy (including that of the bone marrow) and genetic mutations in germ cells (Table 4.3). Some tissues are more radiosensitive than others, in particular the ovaries, testes, thyroid and bone marrow. There is often a long (up to 30 years) latent period before these effects come to light. In consequence, any X-ray examination is not without risk, however small that may be. The higher the dose the greater the risk, although this has to be placed in context with life's other hazards (Information Box 4.1). In any proposed X-ray examination there is a duty to weigh up the risk of irradiation against the benefit that may ensue. There is no such thing as a routine X-ray or one performed out of interest only. It is also important to be particularly cautious before performing X-ray examinations in:

- infants and children
- pregnant women
- those who have been much exposed in the past.

Proposed examinations in all such patients must be discussed with radiologists. In addition, X-rays which expose specially sensitive structures, such as the gonads, thyroid and bone marrow, should be kept to a minimum.

Information Box 4.1

Effective dose equivalent of X-ray examinations and the comparative risk. (From Plaut 1993)

Examination	Effective dose equivalent (millisieverts*)
Chest X-ray	0.02
Abdomen X-ray	1.0
Barium meal	3.8
Barium enema	7.7
CT chest	9.0
CT abdomen/pelvis	9.5
CT lumbar spine	6.0

Relative contribution to deaths in the UK

Smoking 10 cigarettes/day	1 in 200
Influenza (all ages)	1 in 5000
Road traffic accidents	1 in 8000
Radiation dose equivalent of 10 millisieverts	1 in 10 000
Accident at work	1 in 43 500
Being hit by lightning	1 in 10 mil

*The sievert is the SI unit of dose equivalent, which is a compound measurement derived from absorbed dose, the type of radiation and other modifying factors; it has replaced (or is replacing) other measures such as the rem and the roentgen.

DETECTION

The original method of detection was by the effect the beam of X-rays emerging from the patient had on a photographic plate – the less absorption there is by body tissues, the greater the electrochemical conversion on the plate and the darker the image. This method is still widely used in plain film radiology.

Image amplification using image intensifiers, colloquially known as screening, has been available for many years. Initially this was by a fluorescent screen in a darkened room during face-to-face encounters between radiologists and their patients. However, more complex methods are now routine which subject the raw output after tissue passage to recognition by photon detectors and amplification by photoelectronic techniques. These can include digital methods that allow storage in a form which is available for subsequent manipulation by computer (see also 'Digital subtraction' below). Real-time images can be stored, replayed from film or video-disk and be modified (post-processed) to aid in interpretation by highlighting areas of interest and increasing their contrast.

Plain X-ray films

These are images taken without any modification by the clinician or radiologist. Because the beam is differentially absorbed as it passes through the body, a two-dimensional impression of a three-dimensional structure is created on the output device. The X-rays alone can form a spatial image but this requires a higher radiation dose than the commonly used practice of having a fluorescent plate in contact with an X-ray film, which amplifies the effect of the X-rays and reduces the overall dose.

Tomography

This is an X-ray technique that allows imaging of a defined section of the body. There are two types:

- *analogue* – using plain films
- *digital* – using computation as in computed tomography (CT) (also known as computed axial tomography or CAT).

Plain film tomography

In this technique, images are produced using an X-ray source and film combination that move with each other, so that only a single plane (slice) of interest is unaffected by the movement and all other planes are blurred out. It is now not commonly used except as part of intravenous urography.

Computed tomography

This technique uses a rotating X-ray beam to acquire tomographic slices, the information being detected by multiple receptors. By mathematical processing of the output (rendered possible by the high speed of the digital computer) an *attenuation value* is assigned to each small volume (voxel) of tissue that the beam has traversed. By combining these, a digital picture of the slice of the body at which the beam is directed is assembled and this can be further converted into grey scale values to be displayed on a screen or printed onto a film. By altering the centering point and the range of units ascribed to each grey scale point, images which demonstrate soft tissue, bone or air-containing structures to the best advantage can be produced (Figs 4.2 a–c). The most recent scanners use *slip ring* techniques to allow the continuous transfer of data while the X-ray beam is rotated and therefore a spiral pattern of data acquisition as the patient is moved slowly through the scanning aperture. Images can be obtained in a short space of time over quite large sections of the body – e.g. the whole chest while the patient stops breathing for less than 30 seconds. Because of the design principles outlined above and also the practical constraints of positioning the patient, most CT scans are performed in the axial plane (Fig. 4.5) – hence the original name, computed axial tomography (CAT). However, limited variation in the scanning plane can

be achieved so that direct coronal scans of some anatomical sites are possible, e.g. the paranasal sinuses. Two-dimensional reformatting of axially acquired data into any plane (Fig. 4.3a) and three-dimensional reconstruction (Fig. 4.3b) are also possible, although this has, up to now, resulted in some loss of quality of the image. However, in that spiral CT produces volume rather than axial data, loss of quality has now become less of an issue. Reconstruction is of particular use to the surgeon who wishes to judge the relationship of structures to each other.

Radiological cross-sectional studies of this kind have revolutionised imaging and are now supplemented by similar techniques using ultrasound and magnetic resonance imaging (MRI) both of which are considered later in this chapter.

Contrast studies

It is a common practice to enhance contrast in an X-ray, including CT, usually by the use of radio-dense substances which outline organs or areas of interest: in the biliary, vascular and urinary tracts, iodine-containing compounds are used, and in the gastrointestinal tract

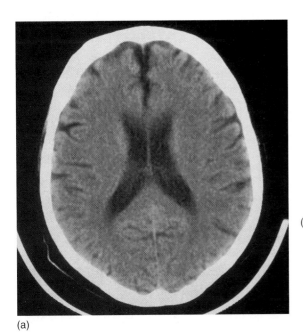

(a)

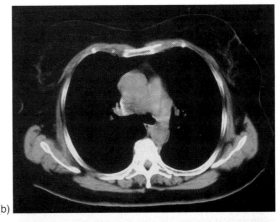

(b)

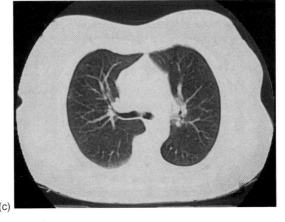

(c)

Fig 4.2 **(a) Axial image of brain at the level of the third ventricle.** The CSF, ventricles and sulci are of low density (black) and the cerebral substance – cortex and medulla – are of intermediate density (grey). The bone is high density (white). **(b) Axial CT image of the chest with the grey scale set to show soft tissues of the mediastinum and chest wall.** The lungs are not shown due to the position and width of the grey scale. **(c) The same CT image (as b) with the grey scale set to show the lungs.** Note that the mediastinum and chest wall are poorly seen with the grey scale setting.

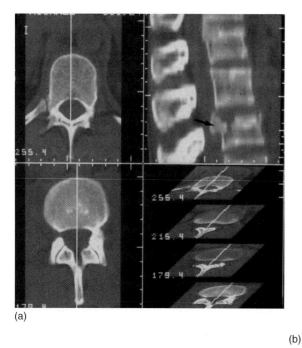

(a)

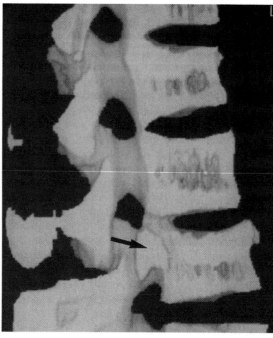

(b)

Fig 4.3 **Example of two-and three-dimensional reconstruction. (a) Sagittal reformatted image. (b) Three-dimensional reformatted image showing a large fragment of bone displaced posteriorly (arrow) into the canal.**

both iodine-containing compounds and barium sulphate. These materials are known collectively as contrast media or agents, although this is sometimes shortened to 'contrast' (used as a noun). The term dye is often applied but it is incorrect and should be avoided. Although contrast media are usually substances containing atoms of high atomic number that strongly absorb X-irradiation (positive media), fat-containing and gas-containing (negative media) contrasts are occasionally employed, and in the gastrointestinal tract double contrast with barium sulphate and gas is commonly utilised. Many examples of the use of contrast media are found in other chapters of this book, such as the gastroenterological and urinary tracts (Chs 18 and 25); the cardiovascular system (Chs 18 and 28) and the neurological system (Ch. 30).

As indicated above, plain films are relatively insensitive in distinguishing minor changes in radio density (as opposed to photon detectors used in computed tomography and in digital subtraction). Enhancement can be achieved by:

- Opacifying the organ or tissue by adding an agent to the blood which perfuses it, e.g. the brain in computed axial tomography.
- Specifically outlining blood vessels so as to demonstrate these either directly on a record such as a film or after removal of the tissue background by digital subtraction (see below); both a normal vascular supply and unusual circulations such as that to a tumour (neovascularisation) can be

demonstrated. The technique is also used in the direct study of blood vessels (angiography – see Ch. 28).

- Administration of a contrast agent that is selectively concentrated by the organ as part of its function, e.g. uptake and concentration of contrast medium by the kidney for urography (see Ch. 32).

When the uptake and distribution of intravascular contrast agents is studied sequentially by ordinary X-ray exposures or CT, the investigation is often called

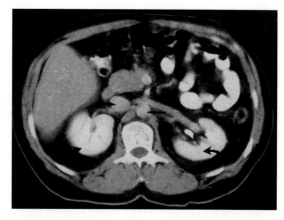

Fig 4.4 **Axial CT slice of the upper abdomen during the injection of intravenous contrast medium.** Oral contrast medium opacifies the bowel. The blood vessels (arrowed) and kidneys (curved arrows) are also opacified, making them of high density (white).

'dynamic' and can give useful information on patterns of blood flow in normal and diseased tissues (Fig. 4.4).

Intravascular contrast media

The objective is to deliver large amounts of substances containing atoms of high atomic number into the vascular system. The molecules must be:

- water-soluble
- ultimately excreted from the body
- associated with a low incidence of adverse effects.

To date, only iodine atoms packaged in various organic molecules have proved satisfactory. There are three broad groups of intravascular contrast agents:

- conventional
- ionic low osmolar
- non-ionic low osmolar.

These are discussed further in Table 4.4.

Reactions. In general, intravenous administration of contrast media is more liable to be associated with severe reactions than is intra-arterial injection. Severe life-threatening anaphylactic reactions to intravascular agents are idiosyncratic and occur in about 0.1% of intravenous administrations of conventional agents and 0.001% of low osmolar non-ionic agents. The risk is greater in allergic individuals, particularly those with asthma, and such patients should have 24 hours of steroid prophylaxis before a contrast study. Other relative contraindications are given in Table 4.5. If a patient with one of these conditions is thought to require investigation, the matter should be discussed with the imaging department.

Other uses

Intravascular agents can also be used for investigations outside the vascular system.

Table 4.5
Relative contraindications to intravascular contrast media

Condition	Problem
Sickle cell disease	Sludging and thrombosis
Phaeocromocytoma	Paroxysmal hypertension
Myeloma	Renal tubular blockage
Asthma	Induction of bronchospasm
Renal failure	Exacerbation
History of idiosyncratic reaction	Further reaction

Intravenous injection
This is used for:

- contrast enhancement during CT scanning
- urography (IVU, see Ch. 32)
- venography (see Ch. 29).

The contrast is administered as either a fast bolus or a slow infusion, or as a combination of the two. A bolus creates an almost immediate high peak concentration which is often suitable for high uptake and concentration in an organ such as the kidney. For some dynamic studies, however, a high concentration must be maintained in the bloodstream. Because most contrast agents move relatively freely into the interstitial space and are also excreted by the kidney, following a bolus injection an additional infusion may be needed.

Arterial injection
This is now almost always done by the Seldinger technique (Ch. 11). It is widely used for:

- *Direct imaging* of the arterial tree (Ch. 28) and the heart (Ch. 12) to provide fine and precise details of vascular anatomy, both normal and abnormal, and to outline organs and abnormalities such as tumours.
- *Interventional procedures*
  - after a lesion has been identified it may be possible to treat it by the intra-arterial route

Table 4.4
Types of intravascular contrast agents

Class	Nature	Examples	Problems
Conventional (up to 8 × concentration of plasma)	Salts of triiodinated benzoate anion	Sodium and meglomine iothalomate or metrisoate	Nausea and vomiting Endothelial and red cell damage Vasodilatation
Ionic low osmolar	Mono- and dimer compounds that can package the same amount of iodine at half the osmolarity	Sodium and meglumine ioxaglate	Much reduced osmolar effects. Have an overall incidence of 0.05% of urticaria and mild hypertension (compared with 0.1% with conventional agents)
Non-ionic low osmolar	Replacement of carboxyl group by a non-ionising radical	Iopamidol Iohexol Iopromide	Bronchospasm, urticaria and mild hypotension – 0.02% compared with 1% with conventional agents Life-threatening reactions – 0.001% compared with 0.1% with conventional agents

Table 4.6
Relative contraindications to arteriography

Condition	Risk
Pregnancy	Radiation dose
Bleeding disorders	Bleeding from arterial puncture site
	Peri-arterial haematoma
Disorders involving vascular fragility (systemic sclerosis)	Arterial injury
	False aneurysm
Severe degenerative arterial disease	Arterial injury
	False aneurysm
	Thrombosis
	Distal embolus
Previous reactions to contrast media	Recurrence

- dilatation of coronary and peripheral arteries (angioplasty Chs 12 and 28)
- stenting of stenoses in peripheral vessels (Ch. 28)
- embolisation of bleeding lesions in the gastrointestinal tract (Ch. 18) and arteriovenous malformations.

There are no absolute contraindications to arteriography but special precautions are needed in some patients (Table 4.6).

Intraluminal contrast agents for the bowel

Barium sulphate

Barium sulphate is relatively inert and is insoluble in water, characteristics that have made it the contrast medium of choice for bowel examination for more than 50 years. There are two types of study: *single contrast* (Fig. 4.5) and *double contrast* (Fig. 4.6). Both include examples of the four different images that can result, but the proportions differ. These images are double contrast (in which air is the other contrast medium), full column, compression and mucosal relief images.

In single contrast studies, full column, mucosal relief and compression views are utilised, with few double contrast images; double contrast studies consist mostly of double contrast images with some full column and mucosal relief images. The barium required for double contrast studies is generally of much higher density than that for single contrast films. In double contrast, a fine layer of radiographic density is required, whereas in single contrast the X-ray beam attempts to penetrate the barium column in order that protrusions of the wall into the lumen (*filling defects*) can be seen as dark (greater radio penetrance) areas within the barium image; conversely, ulcers and diverticulae contain barium and appear as white (reduced radio penetrance) foci.

Double contrast techniques have the potential to identify smaller abnormalities than single contrast

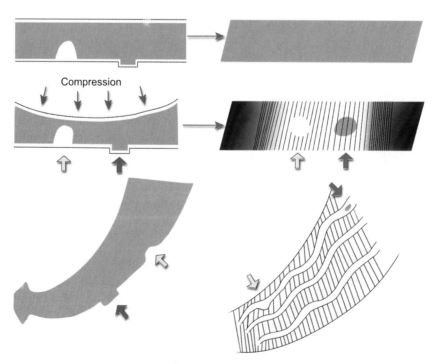

Compression

Fig 4.5 **Single contrast barium images.**

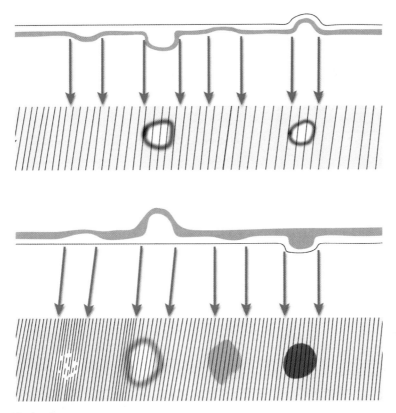

Fig 4.6 **Double contrast barium images.**

studies but with the disadvantage of being more difficult to interpret (Fig. 4.7). The accessibility of the gastrointestinal tract to endoscopic study has led, inspite of the lack of good comparative data to indicate that the slightly safer barium studies are diagnostically significantly inferior, to an inexorable increase in the use of endoscopy (see below). Endoscopy has the advantage that diagnostic biopsy is possible and

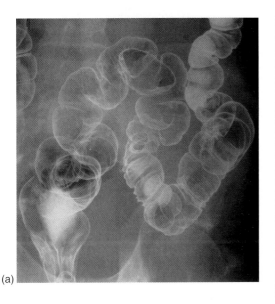

(a)

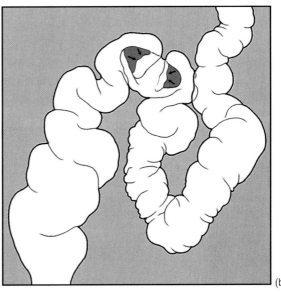

(b)

Fig 4.7 **This double contrast study shows a carcinoma of the sigmoid colon with a saddle outline.** It is recognised only by the presence of abnormal line or edge densities, emphasising that the double contrast technique is the most sensitive but also the hardest to interpret.

Table 4.7
Comparison between barium contrast studies and endoscopy in the gastrointestinal

Factor	Barium contrast	Endoscopy
Safety	Higher	Lower
Overall diagnostic accuracy	Slightly lower	Slightly higher
Detection of superficial mucosal lesions	Lower	Higher
Detection and management of bleeding lesions	Lower	Higher
Biopsy	Not possible	Usually possible
Ionising radiation	Inevitable	Present only if X-ray examination is used as an adjunct
Hard copy	Automatic	Only if still photography or tape recording is used; video-endoscopies easily produce a permanent record
Subtle strictures	Better	May be missed
Overall topography and surgical mapping	Better	Poorer
Study of distal duodenum and small bowel	Prime method	Not possible as routine

therapeutic action, such as relief of oesophageal obstruction, can follow on direct observation. Comparisons between radiological and endoscopic techniques in the gastrointestinal tract are given in Table 4.7. An important, but underused, advantage of barium studies over endoscopy is that they can also assess motility in addition to structure. A radiological study can also better demonstrate some subtle strictures (Fig. 4.8).

Other agents

The excellent handling characteristics, safety and low cost of barium sulphate suspensions make them nearly always the contrast media of choice. However, barium preparations are contraindicated where there is a risk of contamination of serous surfaces, in particular when an intraperitoneal perforation is suspected or impending. Barium in the peritoneal cavity causes a high mortality from peritonitis and survival may be followed by extensive fibrosis. Barium sulphate is also regarded by many surgeons as not the best medium if an emergency or an early operation is contemplated, in that it remains for some time in the bowel and may become inspissated. The other contraindication to the administration of barium by mouth is when there is a risk of respiratory aspiration.

Water-soluble contrast media can be used when barium is inappropriate. They are the same as urographic contrast agents and, if spilled into the peritoneum, are absorbed and excreted by the kidneys. The commonest is a mixture of sodium and meglumine diatrizoate (Gastrografin), although it is hyperosmolar and, if aspirated, causes pulmonary oedema. When this risk is present, the more expensive but safer low osmolarity agents are used. Only basic single contrast studies can be performed with water-soluble agents and, for the most part, their use is limited to the demonstration of perforation, fistula and obstruction.

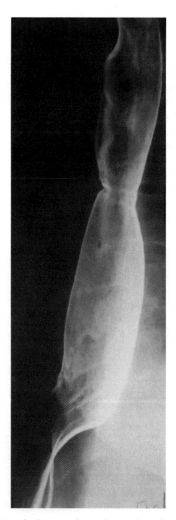

Fig 4.8 **Stricture in the oesophagus in a patient who presented with difficulty in swallowing.** Endoscopy had failed to reveal any narrowing.

Digital subtraction

The data that constitute an X-ray image may be either analogue or digital. Manipulation and comparison are much easier with the latter because arithmetic addition or subtraction within each small zone that has been assigned a numerical value based on digital code (a *pixel*) becomes possible. In consequence, an original analogue image must first be converted into pixels, although a digitally acquired image is already in that form. Once the image is digital, a preliminary plain film can be subtracted from a subsequent contrast study of the same region so that the background is removed and the contrast is enhanced. The technique is widely used in vascular studies.

Radiological interpretation

PRECAUTIONS AND PRELIMINARIES IN INTERPRETATION

Many of these guidelines apply to all images, but some are specific to plain X-rays:

- Always look at the label that gives the patient's name and the date; it is very easy for films to find their way into the wrong packet.
- Always check the marker that indicates side – right or left.
- Make an assessment of the adequacy of the film: does it include the entire part being examined; is it sufficiently penetrated; is it correctly positioned?
- Make a conscious effort to decide in what position the film was taken. Appearances may be altered dramatically by whether:
  - patient was supine or erect

- the part was weight-bearing or not
- exposure was made in inspiration or expiration
- the X-ray beam was horizontal or vertical – this is important because the demonstration of air–fluid or fat–fluid interfaces depends primarily on the orientation of the beam and not on the position of the patient (Figs 4.9 and 4.10).
- When fractures and dislocations are examined radiologically or when they are suspected, two films are needed, preferably taken at right angles to each other to allow a mental reconstruction of a three-dimensional assessment (Fig. 4.11). Some fractures are only visible on one of the two views.
- With a contrast enhanced study, always remember that an opacity may have been present before the agent was administered and review any plain films, which normally are taken initially (Fig. 4.12).

PRINCIPLES

As already indicated, X-rays are interpreted by a biological or artificially created difference in contrast. This reflects the difference in penetration of the beam after its encounter with tissues and therefore its ability to reach the detection device. There are biological contrasts – the difference in penetration of an air-filled organ such as the lung – which can be interpreted on plain films. However, from the point of view of differentiating many structures of comparable radiographic density (contrast resolution), plain films are not so adept. For practical purposes, four radiographic densities are distinguishable on plain films:

- *gas* – dark
- *fat* – relatively dark

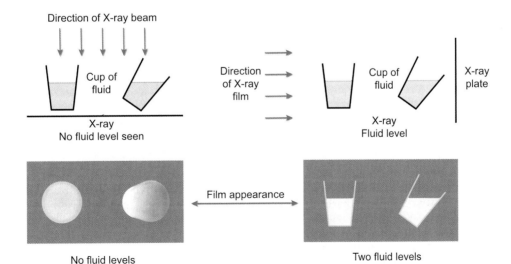

Fig 4.9 **For fluid levels to be shown on a film, it is the direction of the X-ray beam (which must be horizontal), rather than the position of the patient, that is important.**

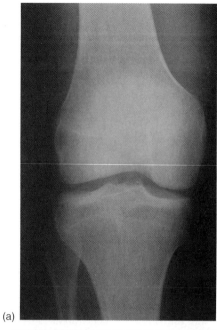
(a)

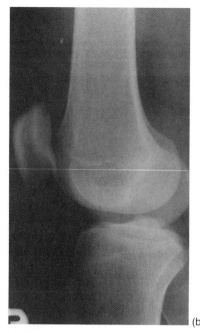
(b)

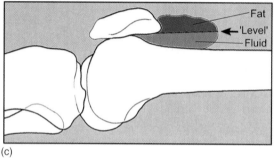
(c)

Fig 4.10 **(a) This AP view of a knee, taken after trauma, was considered normal. (b & c) A horizontal beam film was taken later and a clear fat-fluid level was seen in the suprapatellar pouch of the joint.** This indicated that there is a fracture, with blood and liquid bone marrow fat escaping into the joint space. A tibial plateau fracture was later confirmed.

- *other soft tissue and body liquids* – relatively light
- *calcium/bone* – light.

They can only be distinguished by contrasting one with another, e.g. an interface between gas and fat or liquid.

A basic radiographic maxim is the *silhouette sign*. Paraphrased, this states that if structures of similar radiographic density are contiguous with each other, then a radiographic boundary between them is not seen. At first sight, this seems obvious, yet it is difficult to explain in situations such as that illustrated in Figure 4.13. The rule was initially formulated for the interpretation of chest X-rays, to explain, for instance, why a consolidated middle lobe (soft tissue density) can be inferred from loss of definition of the right heart border (also soft tissue density). However, it can also be used to explain signs such as the loss of the psoas border in acute pancreatitis because the fatty tissue adjacent to the psoas, which is normally responsible for delineation of the border of that muscle, becomes oedematous and necrotic with a density closer to soft tissue than to fat. Applying the silhouette sign, the two adjacent tissues are now of the same radiographic density and can no longer be distinguished. The application of this sign will also avoid radiographic misinterpretation such as believing you can diagnose a cyst within liver parenchyma without contour deformity or calcification.

Ultrasound

PHYSICAL BASIS

To create an ultrasound image, wave energy at a frequency above 20 kHz (the level of audibility to the human ear), but usually in excess of 3 MHz, is directed at tissues, liquids and gases from a transducer – often a small probe. Some reflection takes place which varies with the nature of the tissue and can be detected by a separate sensor at the ultrasound source. Because the velocity of sound in soft tissue is a constant, the time delay for an echo to return to the detector is an indication of the depth at which reflection takes place. After electronic processing these echoes can be displayed on a screen.

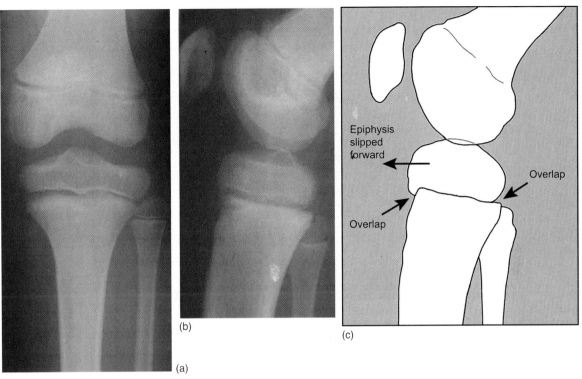

(b)

(c)

(a)

Fig 4.11 **X-rays give only a two-dimensional representation of a three-dimensional object.** In many circumstances, particularly skeletal trauma, it is essential to obtain two views, ideally in orthogonal (right angle) planes. There is an injury to the epiphysis of the upper tibia: the AP view **(a)** appears to be normal but the lateral projection **(b & c)** shows a forward slip of the epiphysis.

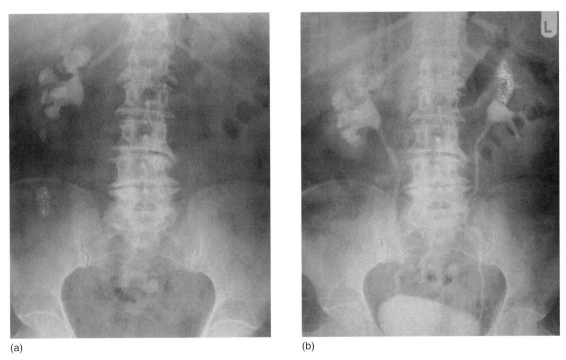

(a)   (b)

Fig 4.12 **It is important in many clinical circumstances to obtain a plain film (a) before contrast (b) is administered.** In this patient undergoing an IVU, the large staghorn calculus is almost obscured by the medium that is being excreted by the kidney.

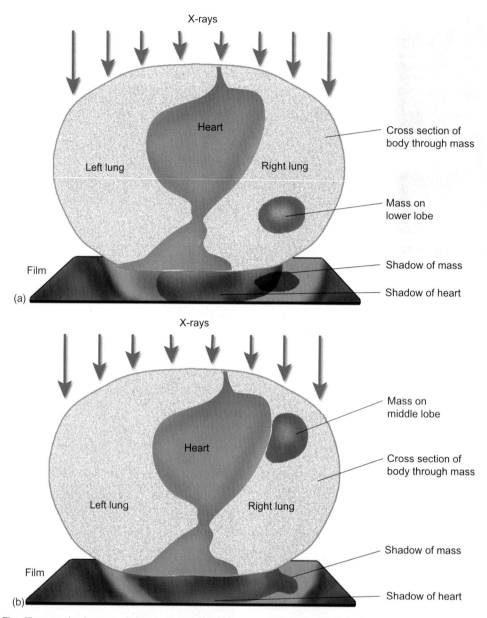

Fig 4.13 **The silhouette sign is not as obvious as it sounds. (a) The mass in the right lung is in the lower lobe and a border is seen between the heart and the mass on the film. (b) The same size mass is in the middle lobe abutting the heart and a border is not seen between the mass and the heart.** In both instances, however, the X-ray beam has passed through the same mass of tissue.

The *resolution* of the image is directly related to the frequency of transmission – the higher the frequency, the better the resolution. However, *penetration* into tissues is inversely related to the frequency, which means that for reasonably deep penetration, as is needed in, say, the abdomen, a low frequency of between 3 and 5 MHz has to be used with some consequential limits on resolution. However, for small parts such as the thyroid, scrotum, eye and breast, it is possible to use higher frequencies (7–15 MHz) in that the probe can be placed very near to the area of

interest. The development of *endoluminal* probes has also permitted higher-frequency scanning and hence better resolution of organs within the body: transvaginal for ovaries and uterus; transrectal for prostate and rectum; and transoesophageal for heart and oesophageal wall and transgastric for stomach wall, pancreas and biliary tree.

Doppler effect

The movement of red blood cells towards or away from a transducer can be detected by the well-known

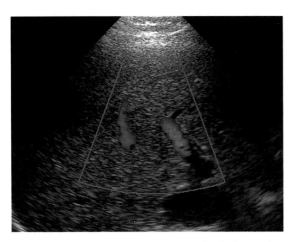

Fig 4.14 **Duplex Doppler of the liver showing flow in the portal and hepatic veins.**

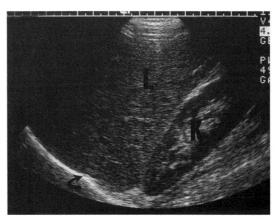

Fig 4.15 **Example of a real-time Doppler image.** A sagittal image of the right upper abdomen showing the right hemidiaphragm (curved arrow), liver (L) and right kidney (K).

frequency shift of returned echoes. The amount of shift is related to both the velocity and the angle of incidence of the ultrasound beam to the direction of flow. With *duplex Doppler* equipment, the imaging and Doppler analysing capability are combined into one probe so that it is possible simultaneously to image a blood vessel and to measure the flow within it. The disadvantage is that it is only possible to assess flow in a small segment of a single vessel. Colour images are produced by detailed analysis of the frequency shifts over the whole area under study and such images allow flow in all blood vessels within the field of view to be displayed. Blood is shown as varying shades of blue and red, depending upon the direction of flow with respect to the transducer and also the velocity (Fig. 4.14). The method has become of considerable importance in the investigation of the vascular system (see Chs 28 and 29).

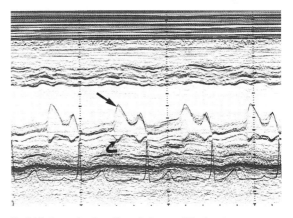

Fig 4.16 **Example of an M-mode image of the heart (echocardiogram) showing normal movement of the anterior (arrow) and posterior (curved arrow) cusps of the mitral valve.** The ECG recording is shown at the bottom of the tracing.

DETECTION AND DISPLAY

The most usual method of display is *brightness (B) mode* in which the intensity of the spot on the screen is related to the amplitude of the echoes. By fast mechanical or electronic sweeping of the transmitted sound waves through a sector or rectangle, a real-time ultrasound image can be built up. Its anatomical plane is determined by the angle at which the probe is placed to the skin surface. The thickness of the imaged slice depends on the width of the ultrasound beam, which in practice is a few millimetres (Fig. 4.15). *Motion (M) mode* display is used to assess movement but without an accompanying real-time image. Echocardiography, for example, produces traces in which motion of the heart valves and other intracardiac structures is displayed as a varying position of the reflected echo from the moving structure (e.g. the cusp of heart valve) with respect to the baseline (Fig. 4.16).

With advances in the technical performance of probes and in processing of the signals, the quality of ultrasound images has improved substantially over the past 30 years. Three principles are important:

- The sound waves must be transmitted into the tissues by good contact between the transducer and the skin, which is achieved by using a contact jelly.
- Gas and areas of calcification (e.g. bone) do not transmit sound waves; in consequence, the position and angle of the probe have to be constantly adjusted to avoid both (e.g. the bowel in abdominal examination) and to obtain the best image of a particular anatomical region and any disorder within it.
- The examination is taking place in real time, and therefore there is constant change in the image.

Endoluminal probes can also be used to overcome some of the obstacles to external ultrasound imaging.

The information obtained from an ultrasound examination and its interpretation are related to multiple real-time images. Static or snap images are taken during the course of any real-time session but the ultrasound operator eventually gives a report based on all the information that has been accumulated during the examination. Real-time ultrasound is thus very operator-dependent in both the acquisition and interpretation of data.

SAFETY

There is currently no evidence that ultrasound waves have any deleterious biological effects. However, an open mind must be kept because methods of detection of cell damage are still quite crude. Nevertheless the perceived safety of ultrasound over X-rays, the lack of ionising radiation and the low cost make it the investigation of first choice in many circumstances, such as suspected biliary disease (Ch. 19), neonatal brain problems and gynaecology.

Magnetic resonance imaging

The production of an image by magnetic resonance imaging (MRI) involves more complex physics than the production of radiological plain images, CT or ultrasound scans. Therefore only a brief description is given here, but further information can be obtained from texts listed in the 'Further reading' section.

PRINCIPLES

MRI is based on the fact that nuclei spin and that those with uneven numbers of protons (particularly hydrogen which is the most abundant nucleus in biological tissues) behave like small magnets with a north and south pole. They align themselves along the main magnetic field to which they are exposed but can be sent 'off balance' by a radiofrequency pulse; they then subsequently resonate and realign. As this takes place, a radiofrequency pulse is emitted which can be detected by receiver coils. These can be exactly located in relation to the slice of tissue targeted. One great advantage of MRI is that any anatomical plane can be chosen for acquisition and consequently the most diagnostically helpful orientation is employed for different clinical circumstances – sagittal and axial images of the spine; sagittal and coronal images of the pituitary; similar views for the knee; and oblique coronal and axial views for the shoulder (Fig. 4.17).

DETECTION AND DISPLAY

The signal produced from the targeted tissue depends on a number of variables, including the density of protons within the sample volume, and the way in which resonance stops when the radiofrequency pulse is switched off (relaxation). These determine two main phenomena which are used in clinical practice:

- *T1 (longitudinal) relaxation time*, which is the result of the resonating nuclei transferring energy to larger non-resonating macromolecules in the environment

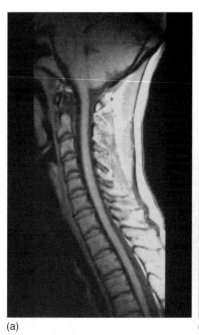

(a)

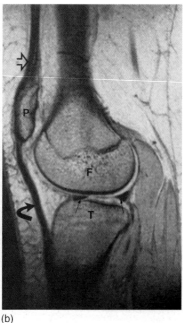

(b)

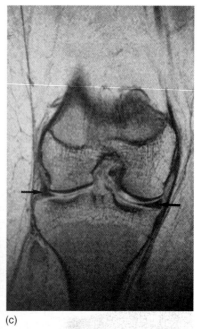

(c)

Fig 4.17 **Examples of different planes achievable with MRI. (a) A sagittal T1 weighted image of the cervical spine. (b) Sagittal image of a knee showing the black triangular-shaped anterior and posterior portions of the medial meniscus (arrows) lying between the medial femoral condyle (F) and the medial tibial plateau (T).** The patella (P), patellar tendon (curved arrow) and quadriceps tendon (open arrow) are seen anteriorly. **(c) Coronal image of a knee showing the menisci as black triangles (arrows).**

- *T2 (transverse) relaxation time*, which is the interaction of energy transfer (dephasing) of the resonant nuclei with other adjacent nuclei.

Both of these occur simultaneously but, by varying the scanning criteria (so-called pulse sequences), it is possible to produce MR images with different tissue contrast – T1 and T2 *weighted* images. Furthermore, because different tissues have variable macromolecular contents, they can be differentiated on one imaging sequence or another; the intrinsic contrast resolution of MRI is thus very high. The way that a tissue behaves with different sequences also gives some idea of its water content. Another useful variant in MRI is to use sequences which cause fat saturation or fat suppression in which the signal from fat-containing tissues is suppressed, thus highlighting signals from adjacent non-fatty tissues. The general appearances of tissues on MRI are given in Table 4.8 and representative examples of T1 and T2 weighting are shown in Figures 4.18 (a) and (b).

An MRI system comprises:

- a main magnet of extremely high and uniform magnetic field (0.2–2 Tesla, which is 4000 to 40 000 greater than the Earth's magnetic field)
- gradient coils which can superimpose minor magnetic gradients on the main magnetic field in a defined manner along the x, y and z axes; these are turned on and off rapidly during imaging to produce spatial localisation
- radiofrequency transmitting and receiving coils which send, with great precision, radiofrequency pulses into slices of the patient and detect the resultant signal;

Table 4.8
Appearances of tissues and their contents on MRI

Tissue or content	T1 weighted image	T2 weighted image
Air	Black	Black
Liquid (CSF, urine, bile)	Dark grey to black	White
Bone cortex Fibrous tissue Tendon	Black	Black
Fat Fatty bone marrow	White	White
Cellular bone Marrow	Dark grey	White
Neoplasms	Dark grey to grey	White
Haematomas	Variable (met-haemoglobin white)	Variable
Muscle	Grey	Grey
Brain		
White matter	Light grey	Dark grey
Grey matter	Dark grey	Light grey

these coils can be either large body or small surface for increased resolution of small areas of tissue
- computational facilities to process the raw data and provide storage, image display and manipulation
- methods for display of 'hard copy.'

SAFETY
MRI has no known deleterious biological effects (contraindications, see Information Box 4.2)..

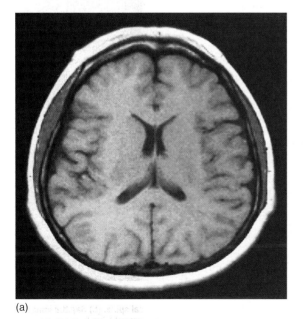

(a)

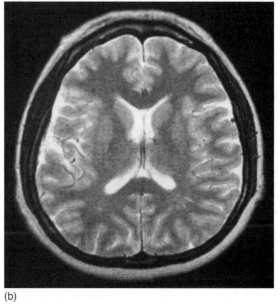

(b)

Fig 4.18 **(a) A T1 weighted axial image of the brain at the level of the lateral ventricle showing CSF in the ventricles and cerebral sulci as low signal intensity (black). (b) On the corresponding T2 weighted image, the CSF is high signal intensity (white).**

ADVANTAGES AND DISADVANTAGES

MRI has the *advantage* that it:

- is without ionising radiation
- can image in any plane
- provides very good images of soft tissues – better than CT.

MRI also provides images of blood vessels and is capable of producing angiograms without intravascular injections (Fig. 4.19). Their quality is improving with technological advance and they are beginning to replace some conventional techniques.

The main *disadvantage* of MRI is that it is relatively slow and expensive compared with other techniques. Each sequence has until recently taken between 2 and 15 minutes to perform depending on:

- magnet strength
- pulse sequence
- image quality required.

With these times of scanning, movement of the patient, respiration and cardiac motion are all problems. Faster scanning is being developed and has already allowed some MR images to be obtained in seconds rather than minutes. Interventional MRI techniques are also under development and, when combined with fast scanning, are beginning to allow the possibility of surgical procedures under real-time MRI control.

Comparison with other methods of cross-sectional imaging

The availability of CT, ultrasound and MRI for the creation of cross-sectional images makes the choice of method for individual circumstances quite difficult

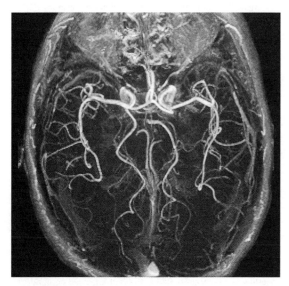

Fig 4.19 **MR angiogram of intracranial blood vessels.**

Information box 4.2 gives a comparison of the features of the three methods.

Radioisotope imaging

PRINCIPLES

Radioisotope imaging studies provide information more about function rather than structure. Radioisotopes are isotopes which emit radioactivity, and most of the radioisotopes in medical usage emit γ-radiation, identical to X-rays, but a few emit particulate radiation in addition (α- or β- radiation). Radioisotopes in common usage include Tc^{99m} (technetium), I^{123}, I^{131}(iodine), In^{111}(indium), Ga^{67}(galium) and Th^{201}(thalium). Radioisotopes may be administered to the patient as ions (e.g. pertechnetate (Tc^{99m}) scan for Meckel's diverticulum), but may also be incorporated onto more complex molecules (radiopharmaceuticals). These substances mimic a metabolic or biochemical pathway and localise in the target organs of interest, and their sites of distribution may be visualised using a special detector called a gamma camera. Although the radioisotopes produce radiation in all directions, spatial localisation is achieved by collimators permitting only radiation in one direction to interact with a large sodium iodide crystal (scintillation) detector in the camera. The radiation impact produces photons in the crystal which are then amplified by photomultiplier tubes. Tomographic techniques can be used to improve spatial resolution, but in general such resolution is inferior to cross-sectional imaging techniques.

With SPECT (single photon emission computed tomography), images are acquired in a similar manner to planar studies except that the camera head or heads rotate around the patient collecting data over 180 or 360 degrees, and the data is analysed using similar computing techniques (backprojection) to those used in CT. The SPECT studies take longer to acquire than conventional planar studies, but this disadvantage is often countered by administering a greater dose of the radiopharmaceutical.

PET (position emission tomography) is a newer and more expensive technique. Some radiographic substances emit positrons which combine with an electron to convert their energy into two back-to-back photons. If these photons are detected in opposite detectors at the same time (coincidence), their position of origin in a line connecting the detectors can be assumed. Computer techniques are used to reconstruct a large number of these 'coincidences' into a cross-sectional image. Positron emitters are produced by cyclotrons and incorporated into biologically relevant and stable compounds, and physiological metabolism can be evaluated. PET is proving useful in imaging of physiological brain metabolism, tumour detection and functional cardiac imaging.

ℹ Information Box 4.2

Comparison of cross-sectional imaging techniques

	Computerised tomography	Ultrasound	Magnetic resonance imaging
Uses ionising radiation	Yes	No	No
Speed	0.5–20 s	Real time	2–15 min
Imaging plane	Axial but coronal in some circumstances	Variable at time of scan	Multiplanar
Portable	No	Yes	No
Capital cost (£)	200 000–600 000	20 000–150 000	500 000–2 000 000
Operator dependency	Low	High	Low
Image degradation	Metal implants	Bone and gas and patient movement	Metal implants
Images			
Bone	Yes – cortex	No	Yes – medulla
Lungs	Yes	No	No
Solid organs	Yes	Yes	Yes
Gall bladder calculi	Only if radio-dense	Yes	No
Head and spine including neonate	Yes	No – except neonatal and intraoperatively	Yes – best method
Liquid collections	Yes	Yes	Yes
Blood vessels	Yes but needs contrast medium	Yes with Doppler	Yes and does not always require contrast medium
Fetus with safety	No	Yes – ideal for routine scanning	No – research only at present time
Guided biopsy and drainage	Yes	Yes	Feasible and likely to increase
Contraindications	Same as for all X-rays	None known	Heart pacemakers; clips on intracranial aneurysms; metal in eye

SAFETY

The risks of radioisotope imaging are those of ionising radiation. The dose depends on the type of examination and the activity of isotope used, but in general many of the examinations have doses in the mid or high range compared to other radiological examinations. The incidence of allergic reactions to injected radioisotopes is exceedingly small.

ADVANTAGES AND DISADVANTAGES

Although spatial resolution is poor, radiopharmaceuticals can be tailored to be handled in different ways by various organs, and the amount of radioactivity passing through different systems can be quantified. Transport, distribution, metabolism and clearance can all be measured. The functional information supplied is unique and examples include:

- the demonstration of osteoblastic activity for the detection of skeletal metastases before radiographic changes

- distinguishing a dilated non-obstructed renal collecting system from an obstructed one
- localising foci of infection or segments of active inflammatory bowel disease with labelled leucocytes
- localising active gastrointestinal bleeding when angiography is negative.

Endoscopy

Endoscopy ranks as one of the most important technical advances in medicine of the last few decades. Not only has it added a new precision to gastrointestinal and pancreaticobiliary diagnosis, particularly when used in conjunction with cytology or biopsy, but it has also been one of the earliest tools, along with interventional radiological techniques, in the advances of minimally invasive therapy.

There are two types of endoscope: rigid and flexible. Rigid instruments are usually more basic in design. Typical examples of rigid instruments are the proctoscope (for the anal canal; Ch. 25) and the sigmoidoscope (for the rectum up to the rectosigmoid junction; Ch. 24). Rigid bronchoscopes (Ch. 16) and oesophagoscopes (Chs 14 and 18) are now only infrequently used. The rigid cystoscope is still useful for diagnostic purposes, but most urological units rely on flexible cystoscopy for inspection of the bladder and reserve the rigid instrument for operative intervention (Ch. 32). Laparoscopy (inspection of the peritoneal cavity; Ch. 5) and arthroscopy (Ch. 33) are performed with a rigid instruments partly because it is easier to work with a rigid instrument in a cavity which has been distended by gas (carbon dioxide) as is done in both instances.

The modern flexible endoscope is a complex but robust precision instrument varying in diameter from 7 mm (bronchoscope, arthroscope) to 15 mm (colonoscope). It has the following features:

- Light source – in the handle with a fibreoptic bundle for the transmission of light to the area under investigation.
- Viewing system – originally a second bundle arranged coherently to transmit an image to a lens system; more recently, a silicon-based photosensor made up of a grid of photosensitive elements. Photons impacting on this are converted into a digital video signal which can then be viewed on a screen; the endoscopist no longer needs to peer down an eyepiece. The video image can easily be stored for use in teaching and can be enhanced by electronic processing.
- Control and manipulative elements which are still mechanical and allow the tip to be deflected and instruments such as snares, stents, biopsy forceps, balloons and baskets to be passed along a working channel.

Flexible endoscopes are used in the following investigations:

- upper GI endoscopy (Ch. 18)
- retrograde biliary and pancreatic endoscopy (ERCP) (Chs 19 and 21)
- sigmoidoscopy and colonoscopy (Ch. 24).

Because endoscopy can be physically and emotionally unpleasant for the patient, most procedures are performed under sedation (which may vary from a small dose of a benzodiazepine to heavy sedation with a combination of a narcotic with a benzodiazepine) and, where necessary, local anaesthesia. The use of sedation means that patients need help to return home and need to take a day off work. Sedation itself does carry some risks: continuous monitoring of arterial oxygen saturation with pulse oximetry is now used routinely because, particularly in the elderly, there is a high incidence of hypoxia and cardiac dysrhythmias. Because of these concerns there is increasing use of thinner and less traumatic endoscopes without sedation in upper gastrointestinal endoscopy.

COMPLICATIONS

Diagnostic endoscopy is generally a safe procedure provided the endoscopist and his team are well trained.

Cross-infection

As with any procedure in which patients with potential pathogens are investigated, there is a risk of these being carried by instruments from one individual to another. Endoscopes are not the easiest of tools to clean but there are satisfactory regimens and the hazard is currently low.

Transmission of viral disease appears to be virtually non-existent.

Bacteraemia

Any instrumentation of a tract that normally contains organisms may cause transient bacteraemia, but the rate is low and the clinical manifestations are usually absent or minimal. The number of organisms in the blood is increased during procedures that require much tissue manipulation, such as dilatation of a stricture in a contaminated hollow tube. Particularly at risk and for whom antibiotic prophylaxis must be seriously considered are those with:

- prosthetic heart valves
- other prostheses, although the exact hazard is not fully established
- previous rheumatic fever with damage to heart valves
- immunosuppression.

There is a further theoretical risk of cross-infection because of a contaminated instrument, but careful cleaning eliminates this hazard.

Perforation of hollow viscera

This is commonest following dilatation of strictures and during a difficult colonoscopy. The latter is particularly dangerous because symptoms of perforation are often delayed so that a high morbidity and mortality may result.

Other hazards

Other hazards of gastrointestinal endoscopy include:

- aspiration of upper GI contents into the lungs
- haemorrhage from mucosal injury.

Therapeutic endoscopy

There is now a wide range of therapeutic procedures that can be carried out under endoscopic (and sometimes additional fluoroscopic or ultrasound) control. These are considered throughout this text and include a variety of methods to control haemorrhage (Chs 18 and 20), dilatation (and stenting) of strictures in the gastro-intestinal tract and its tributaries (Chs 18, 19 and 21). Removal of foreign bodies is greatly facilitated (Chs 14 and 25) and percutaneous gastrostomy has made sup-plementary enteral feeding (Ch. 7) much more accept-able. Polypectomy for colonic lesions (Ch. 24) and injection therapy for oesophageal varices (Ch. 20) have changed management.

In addition to these specialised endoscopic tech-niques, endoscopes (usually rigid) form the basis of minimal access surgery which is considered in Chapter 5.

Tissue sampling

Cells for examination under the microscope may be obtained in four ways:

- *Body fluids*, e.g. sputum (Ch. 16), urine (Ch. 32), effusions in the pleural and peritoneal spaces.
- *Brushings or smears*, e.g. cervical smear.
- *Fine needle aspiration* (FNA).
- *Tissue biopsy*, which can be either an open removal of a sample or of the whole identifiable lesion, or a core biopsy using a large-bore specially designed needle. This yields a core of tissue that can reveal not only the type of cells within a lesion but their position in relation to other elements such as the basement membrane and vessels.

Brushing (or scraping) and fine needle aspiration (FNA)

Brushing is suitable for the skin and endoscopically accessible parts of the gastrointestinal tract. FNA is applicable to organs near the surface (such as the breast) but, under image control, can be applied to many deeper organs (see Box 4.1). Both techniques yield cells only from the organ being sampled and do not establish how these cells are related to tissue architecture.

Both may show cells that are obviously abnormal with unusual nucleocytoplasmic ratios, increased mitotic activity and structural changes in the nuclei and nucleoli. Also, the presence of obviously malignant epithelial cells in an aspiration sample from a tissue which does not normally have epithelial elements (e.g. pleural cavity or lymph node) is as effective in confirming the presence of carcinoma as is a biopsy.

FNA has some disadvantages:

- Positive results are the only ones that can be evaluated with confidence; false negatives due to sampling errors are possible but can be reduced if

---

Box 4.1

Fine needle aspiration 5

- A 22G needle is attached to a syringe inserted into the target issue (usually a lump) and aspiration is achieved by withdrawing the barrel of the syringe
- If the lesion is a cyst, liquid flows and the structure is emptied, if necessary by changing the syringe until no more can be aspirated
- If solid tissue is encountered, negative pressure allows a number of cells and tissue fluid to be aspirated into the needle, which can then be expelled onto microscopy slides and analysed cytologically.

---

the area of interest can be precisely targeted, e.g. under ultrasound control.

- In a solid organ, such as the breast, it is not possible to distinguish in situ from invasive cancer.
- In the thyroid (Ch. 31) it is not possible to distinguish between follicular adenoma and carcinoma.

Biopsy

There are two forms:

- *Closed biopsy* – this is an extension of FNA in which a wide-bore needle is used with the aim of removing a core of tissue which is suitable for histopathological examination (Fig. 4.20). Advances in imaging guidance have made this technique more widely applicable to organs such as the prostate and the pancreas.
- *Open biopsy* – a lesion is targeted and a formal incision is used to expose it and obtain a segment of tissue.

If the target of open biopsy is a lymph node, it is better to excise this intact rather than to cut into it so as to avoid spillage of possible malignant cells which can cause a local recurrence. An intact node is also helpful to the pathologist because its architecture can be assessed (see Ch. 29).

In contrast to FNA, a biopsy may reveal that abnormal cells are transgressing natural boundaries such as the basement membrane of a mucosal surface or are invading blood vessels or lymphatics.

Biopsy may be contraindicated when it possibly transgresses the field of resection of a malignant growth.

Frozen section biopsy

Occasionally histological diagnosis is required urgently while the patient is under an anaesthetic, because confirmation of malignancy may change the type of

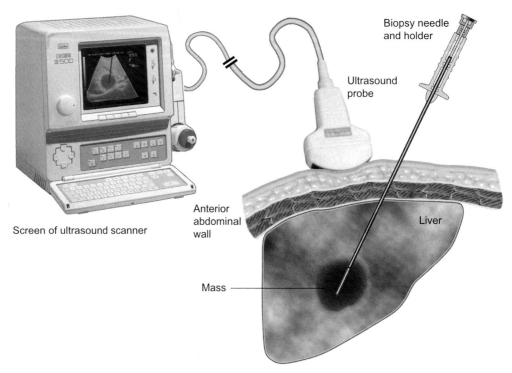

Fig 4.20 **Closed needle biopsy.**

operation that the patient should undergo. In such circumstances, the usual tissue fixation techniques are too slow. Instead the biopsy is frozen in liquid nitrogen which makes slicing and staining for microscopy possible within minutes.

Decisions based on frozen sections should be made only in broad categories such as malignant or benign; pathologists should not be asked to make fine distinctions on frozen sections.

Function tests

To measure the functional capacity of organ systems, with or without visualisation of anatomical structure, can provide a more accurate assessment of the risks of an operation. Assessment of cardiovascular, respiratory, renal and, in some circumstances, liver function are evaluations that can be useful.

Cardiovascular risk

Electrocardiogram and stress electrocardiogram

An electrocardiogram (ECG) should be obtained routinely for all elective surgery in those over 40 years of age. Younger patients require ECG if they are symptomatic or in a high-risk group for coronary artery disease. However, the sensitivity of an ECG in demonstrating asymptomatic coronary artery disease is not high. Major vascular operations (e.g. aortic aneurysm repair) often impose a specific physiological strain on the cardiovascular system; in consequence the presence of asymptomatic coronary disease may be of significance. If present, correction prior to the vascular procedure should be undertaken.

In a stress ECG, clinical evaluation and serial readings are made while the patient walks on a treadmill at increasing speeds and may reveal subclinical myocardial ischaemia – angina induced by, a fall in blood pressure, changes in the ST segment and ventricular ectopic beats.

Similar stress can be induced by administration of inotropic agents such as dobutamine.

201-Thallium (or ^{99m}Tc-sestamibi) perfusion scintigraphy

The procedure is a relatively non-invasive method which identifies areas of myocardial hypoperfusion which may include infarcts. Other areas, apparently normal at rest, may not show increased uptake on exercise and are therefore supplied by coronary arteries with narrowing that are unable to allow the increased flow that is physiologically demanded by exercise. Such abnormalities should be investigated by more detailed studies of left ventricular function (see labelled red cell ventriculography below) and by coronary angiography; when a major procedure is under consideration, a preliminary angioplasty or coronary bypass operation may be necessary.

Technetium-labelled red cell ventriculography (MUGA)

If there are significant areas of abnormal isotope uptake on a perfusion scan, then ^{99m}Tc-labelled red cell ventriculography is indicated and provides information about left ventricular function, including ejection fraction and the presence of aortic regurgitation during diastole.

Echocardiography

This non-invasive investigation can also provide some assessment of the function of the left ventricle but it is not as accurate as radionucleide ventriculography.

Regional blood flow

See Chapter 28.

Lung function

Upper abdominal and thoracic operations produce the greatest impairment of respiratory function, but all procedures associated with general anaesthesia and pain cause some abnormality of respiratory function (Ch. 6). The risk of postoperative respiratory complications increases in:

- smokers
- obesity
- the elderly
- those with pre-existing respiratory disease – chronic bronchitis and emphysema, asthma and mucoviscoidosis.

In some circumstances, pre-existing respiratory dysfunction may require special measures or even contraindicate operation.

Function is assessed by the measurement of:

- arterial blood gas concentrations
- peak expiratory flow rate
- occasionally, the lung volumes.

Criteria for prediction of postoperative risk of respiratory complications include:

- forced vital capacity (FVC) less than 70% of that predicted
- forced expiratory volume in the first second (FEV$_1$) less than 70% of that predicted
- FEV$_1$/FVC less than 65% of that predicted
- arterial blood CO_2 tension (P_aCO_2) greater than 45 mmHg

- in upper abdominal procedures, a vital capacity of less than 1l.

Gastric and intestinal function

See Chapters 18 and 23.

Pancreatic function

See Chapter 21.

Endocrine function

See Chapter 31.

Screening for surgical disease

Screening for malignant disease

See Chapters 12, 18, 24 and 27.

Other surgical disorders

The general principles of screening outlined in Chapter 12 for malignant disease are applicable to all screening programmes. Current endeavours under consideration or subject to pilot studies include:

- abdominal aortic aneurysm by ultrasound (Ch. 28)
- prostate cancer by prostatic-specific antigen (Ch. 32).

FURTHER READING

Armstrong SJ (1990) *Lecture Notes on the Physics of Radiology*. Bristol: Clinical Press.

Bretland PM (1978) *Essentials of Radiology*. London: Butterworths.

Cardoza JD, Herfkins RJ (1994) *MRI Survival Guide*. New York: Raven Press.

Grainger RG, Allison DJ (1993) *Diagnostic Radiology*, 2nd edn. Edinburgh: Churchill Livingstone.

Plaut S (1993) *Radiation Protection in the X-ray Department*. Oxford: Butterworth Heinemann.

Westbrook C, Cout C (1990) *Practical Gastrointestinal Endoscopy*, 3rd edn. Oxford: Blackwell Scientific Publications.

5

The operation

For those entering the operating department for the first time it can be a daunting experience (Ch. 2). It is an unfamiliar environment, there are specific regimented procedures that must be followed, a multitude of new terms, and unfamiliar techniques and equipment that have to be understood. In this chapter some of these matters will be demystified through discussion of the following: the working of the operating department including its design and the way patients pass through it; the techniques used in operations in general; and the current role of the recently introduced *minimal access surgery*.

Surgical terms

A list of commonly used suffixes in surgery is provided in Information box 5.1.

Design of the operating department

Principles

Although the physical features of operating depart-ments often differ, they are all designed around some widely accepted principles which are the outcome of the experience of surgeons and the impact of the biomedical sciences. In the UK, they have been promulgated by the Department of Health.

The individual principles upon which the design of each operating department is based are as follows:

- *Scope of service* – this depends on which surgical services are to be catered for.
- *Workload* – this is largely the outcome of the scope of service, an estimate of which determines the number of operating rooms (known in the UK as theatres).
- *Needs of special services* – for example, the implantation of orthopaedic devices requires systems for ultraclean and smooth air flow; ophthalmic and plastic surgeons use operating microscopes and lasers; and the cardiac surgical team may need a pump room in which cardiopulmonary bypass equipment can be prepared.

51

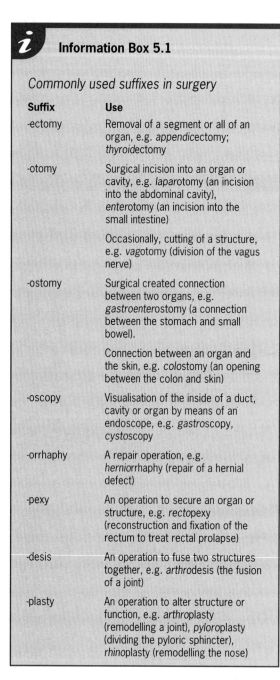

Information Box 5.1

Commonly used suffixes in surgery

Suffix	Use
-ectomy	Removal of a segment or all of an organ, e.g. *appendic*ectomy; *thyroid*ectomy
-otomy	Surgical incision into an organ or cavity, e.g. *laparo*tomy (an incision into the abdominal cavity), *entero*tomy (an incision into the small intestine) Occasionally, cutting of a structure, e.g. *vago*tomy (division of the vagus nerve)
-ostomy	Surgical created connection between two organs, e.g. *gastroentero*stomy (a connection between the stomach and small bowel). Connection between an organ and the skin, e.g. *colo*stomy (an opening between the colon and skin)
-oscopy	Visualisation of the inside of a duct, cavity or organ by means of an endoscope, e.g. *gastro*scopy, *cysto*scopy
-orrhaphy	A repair operation, e.g. *hernio*rrhaphy (repair of a hernial defect)
-pexy	An operation to secure an organ or structure, e.g. *recto*pexy (reconstruction and fixation of the rectum to treat rectal prolapse)
-desis	An operation to fuse two structures together, e.g. *arthro*desis (the fusion of a joint)
-plasty	An operation to alter structure or function, e.g. *arthro*plasty (remodelling a joint), *pyloro*plasty (dividing the pyloric sphincter), *rhino*plasty (remodelling the nose)

- *Accessibility* – there needs to be a speedy access to the intensive therapy unit, the accident and emergency department, the imaging department, local X-ray and the places where patients are accommodated both before and after an operation.

Supplies

Repeatedly used and disposable equipment (instruments, drapes and other special items) come either from an adjacent dedicated theatre sterile supply unit (TSSU) or the central sterile supply department (CSSD) which supplies the whole hospital.

The operating complex must also provide for:

- teaching
- catering and rest facilities for staff
- changing facilities.

Management

There is usually a theatre manager with overall charge of the smooth day-to-day running and optimal use of the available operating rooms. Each speciality will have routine elective (i.e. designated) lists, but in the past, and to a considerable extent still today in the UK, emergencies have had to be inserted into this routine flow. However, operating rooms and personnel are being increasingly set aside exclusively for emergency work (Ch. 3).

The manager is also responsible for the staffing of each list by appropriately trained staff (Box 5.1). With the current expansion of a market-led health service (Ch. 2) the role of the theatre manager has expanded to include involvement in the costing and budgeting of theatre services and equipment.

Patient flow

In well designed departments, patients enter at a central reception area (Fig. 5.1). There they are handed over by the team responsible for preoperative care (Ch. 6) to the theatre staff and a check is made to ensure the patient is properly ready:

Box 5.1

Theatre personnel

Theatre manager – usually a senior nurse in overall charge of normal day-to-day running of the department

ODA (operating department assistant) – trained in all aspects of operating theatre technique, ODAs typically assist the anaesthetist, especially during induction of anaesthesia and positioning of the patient

Scrub nurse – a nurse trained in theatre techniques who prepares the instruments and assists the surgeon during the operation

Runner – a nurse or health care assistant who prepares the theatre for each operation and fetches equipment required during the procedure

Porters – they transport patients to and from theatre and often assist in their transfer and positioning in the operating theatre

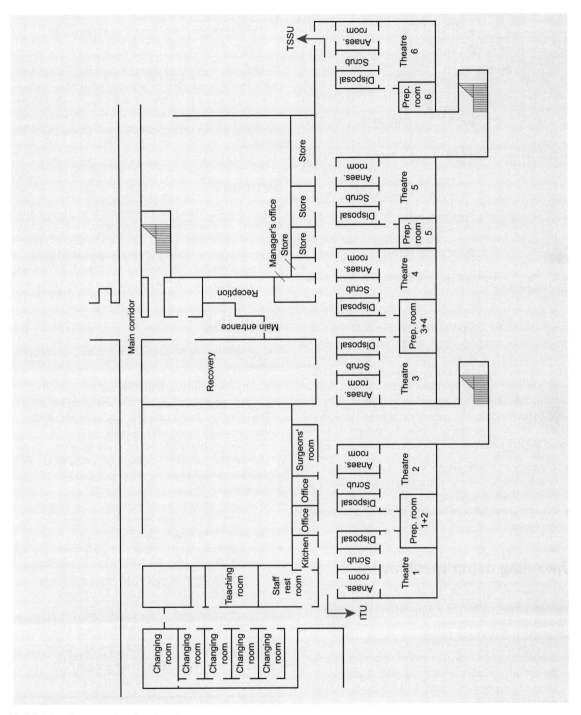

Fig 5.1 **Plan of an operating department.**

- completed and correct identity bracelet
- consent form (Ch. 2) completed
- time of last food and drink
- impediments to safety, such as false teeth, make up, nail polish and jewellery, all removed.

From this point the patient may be transferred to a theatre trolley and then taken to the anaesthetic room. Before or after anaesthesia has been induced (Ch. 6), transfer is made to the operating table, but anaesthesia is usually induced in the anaesthetic room. Once the patient has been prepared for operation, he or she is

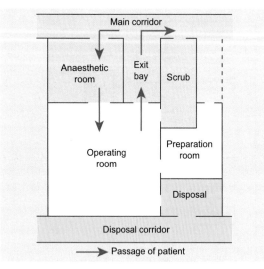

Fig 5.2 **Plan of an individual operating theatre with clean, sterile and disposal zones.**

transferred to the operating theatre (Fig. 5.2). Once the procedure is complete, exit to the recovery area is usually through a different path from that of entry. This one-way flow of traffic through the operating room prevents congestion, allows a continuous flow of patients and allows the anaesthetist to deal with the next patient while the previous patient is leaving theatre. From the recovery room, the patient is transferred back to wherever it is thought appropriate, e.g.

- in-patient accommodation after major operations, which may be either to a routine bed or to intensive or high-dependency care
- a holding area before returning home after day-case operations.

Operating department layout

An important aspect of theatre design is to keep bacterial contamination to a minimum – the concept of *asepsis*. Operating areas (Figs 5.1 and 5.2) can therefore be divided into zones, as follows:

- *Transfer zone* – includes the reception area where the patient arrives, the recovery and staff changing areas and the points of entry to the department from the rest of the hospital.
- *Clean zone* – a transition area between the transfer and sterile zones which includes the corridor to each operating room, the anaesthetic room, the scrubbing up and gowning areas and the rest areas for theatre staff. It must also incorporate storage areas for theatre and pre-sterilised equipment.
- *Sterile zone* – the operating room and sterile preparation room where the equipment for individual operations is assembled.

- *Disposal zone* – the least clean area where the detritus, such as swabs, dirty instruments and human waste, are dealt with.

Although there is no strong bacteriological evidence that adhering to zones, or isolating each zone, reduces infection rates, it is a concept that should nevertheless be observed. Unnecessary movement between zones, especially the operating and disposal zones, should be avoided.

Structure

The operating complex is designed so that a high standard of cleanliness can be maintained. Junctures between walls, ceilings and floors are curved to prevent the collection of dust. All equipment should be movable so that the theatre can be cleared for cleaning and all surfaces should be smooth and easily washable.

Ventilation

The ventilation system of the operating department permits:

- Control of temperature and humidity – typical figures are 20–22°C and 60% relative humidity; lower temperatures carry the risk of hypothermia for an anaesthetised patient in whom vasoconstriction is abolished, and higher ones make the work of the operating team uncomfortable (see also the special needs of neonates – Ch. 35).
- Air filtration to remove microorganisms.
- Movement of air from clean to less clean areas within the department by creating overpressure in the most clean zones.
- Rapid and non-turbulent air change in the operating room: 20–30 changes per hour is usual and dilutes the concentration of microorganisms inevitably released from patients and staff. In circumstances where infection of a wound is disastrous, e.g. orthopaedic prosthesis insertion (Ch. 9), special systems are used which direct a stream of clean air over the operating zone (laminar flow enclosures) at a rate of change of 500–600 changes per hour.

Infection control

Antisepsis places a barrier which destroys organisms between the wound and the external environment and was the original method introduced by Lister when it was first realised in the second half of the 19th century that infection was the outcome of bacterial contamination and growth. In surgical operative practice it has been entirely replaced by asepsis, the objective of which is to have as few organisms as possible in the immediate vicinity of the operating field. This is achieved partly by ventilation control (as described above) but principally by ensuring that everything that comes into contact with the field is first rendered sterile by the complete destruction of all microorganisms including bacterial spores. A number of methods of infection control are available (Box 5.2). There are three major factors of importance in the operating field:

- sterilisation of instruments and equipment
- skin preparation and draping of the patient
- preparation and clothing of the operating team.

Sterilisation

There are two types of sterilisation: heat and cold (Box 5.3). The process applies to instruments and equipment for use in a procedure where the skin is breached but not necessarily to gastrointestinal endoscopy (Ch. 18). Skin cannot be sterilised (see below).

Heat sterilisation

Steam under pressure
An increase in ambient pressure raises the boiling point of water. The higher the temperature, the greater the lethal effect on microorganisms and so sterilisation is dependent on the temperature attained and the length of time that this is maintained. This process is carried out in an *autoclave*. The instruments or drapes to be sterilised are usually pre-packed in a container which is permeable to the steam but which will not subsequently let in organisms. Air is sucked out to create a vacuum and the instruments are then exposed to moist heat under pressure. Typical cycles are:

- $134°C$ and 30 lb/in^2 (20×10^3 N/m^2) for 3 min
- $121°C$ and 15 lb/in^2 (10×10^3 N/m^2) for 15 min.

Large autoclaves are usually located in the CSSD, to supply the needs of the whole hospital, or in the TSSU, usually situated next to the operating department. Smaller autoclaves may be found in the preparation room of each operating department for dealing with dropped instruments or those required for consecutive operations.

Dry heat
In this type of sterilisation a higher temperature for a longer period is required, e.g. $160°C$ for 2 hours. It is thereforesnient as an autoclave but is suitable for sterilising airtight containers and fine instruments that are susceptible to corrosion.

Low-temperature steam/formaldehyde
A combination of dry saturated steam and formaldehyde sterilises at a lower temperature ($73°C$) and is therefore suitable for heat-sensitive materials and equipment. It is important to remove all traces of formaldehyde at the end of the process.

Cold sterilisation

Irradiation
Gamma rays at high intensity are lethal to cells, including those of microorganisms. The method is not feasible in a hospital setting but is used by industry for the sterilisation of mass-produced disposable items such as syringes, catheters and sutures.

Ethylene oxide
This is a highly penetrative gas that, under controlled conditions, has good sterilising properties, killing most bacteria, spores and viruses. It is ideal for heat-sensitive, delicate items such as electrical equipment or endoscopes but is largely an industrial process for sterilising single-use plastic items.

Glutaraldehyde
Alkaline glutaraldehyde (Cidex) is a liquid chemical

disinfectant used to clean lensed instruments such as flexible endoscopes or cystoscopes, which have many heat-sensitive components. It is, however, a highly toxic, irritant and allergenic substance and its use should be carefully controlled by trained staff.

Preparation of the patient's skin

Up to half of all wound infections are caused by bacteria resident on the skin. Their quantity can be reduced by having the patient shower on the morning of the operation with an antiseptic substance such as chlorhexidine. At the start of the operation a wide area of skin around the incision site is cleaned with a povidone-iodine or chlorhexidine solution. Either of these combined with ethyl alcohol gives better disinfection but organisms still persist in hair follicles and sweat glands. Pools of residual alcohol must be avoided because they can be ignited by a spark from an electrocoagulation instrument and cause a burn.

Shaving

Hairs get in the way during closure of the skin wound. Patients have traditionally been shaved for operations but when a razor is used it can cause minor nicks and scratches so bringing bacteria to the surface and increasing the incidence of wound infections. If the skin has to be shaved, then ideally clippers should be used as close to the start of the operation as possible.

Isolation of the operation field

The area to be operated on is isolated using heat-sterilised surgical drapes. These are usually cotton sheets, although cotton can quickly become wet and lose its protective ability. Newer impermeable materials and disposable drapes have been introduced but they are more expensive. Self-adhesive plastic drapes are often used for irregular or extensive operation sites but there is no evidence that they reduce wound contamination or infection rates.

Drapes also serve to identify the aseptic operating zone in which the surgeon, assistants and scrub nurse work; any equipment, instruments or staff that come into contact with the drapes must also be sterile.

Preparation of the operating team

Scrubbing up

Scrubbing up is the term given to the hand and arm cleaning process undertaken at the start of an operation. It was formerly a ritualised process of alternate scrubbing and rinsing of the fingers, hands and arms with a brush for a defined period of time. This is now known not to be necessary and that brisk scrubbing of the skin with a brush can cause microtrauma to the epidermis and increase the bacterial count at the skin surface. An initial scrub of the fingernails at the start of an operating list is all that is required and should take about 3–5 minutes.

All jewellery is removed. The fingers, hands and forearms are cleaned thoroughly using a medicated detergent such as chlorhexidine gluconate (Hibiscrub) or povidone-iodine (Betadine). Chlorhexidine is rapidly effective and has a prolonged action but is ineffective against bacterial spores. Povidone-iodine kills all organisms including spores but does not have a prolonged effect and has a higher incidence of allergic reactions. After washing, the hands are dried thoroughly with a sterile towel; this further decreases the bacterial count and makes donning of gowns and gloves much easier.

Gowns and gloves

Both of these are donned with a closed technique (i.e. the skin does not touch anything on the outside surface) so that the chance of contamination of a surface which is in contact with the patient's tissues is reduced.

Conventional sterile cotton gowns can soon become wet and pervious to bacteria. They also allow contamination of the surgical team by the patient's body fluids. One partial solution is to wear a disposable plastic apron beneath the gown. Newer materials such as Gortex or close-woven polyester have been developed to overcome the problem of permeability but have two drawbacks: they are expensive and their impermeability may cause discomfort. However, some form of impervious gown is essential when operating on high-risk patients (hepatitis B and C; HIV – see also below) to prevent transmission of the infective agent in the patient's body fluids to the surgical team.

Gloves were formerly lightly coated or the hands dusted with talc so as to make them easy to put on. However, talc is irritant and a particularly difficult form of adhesive small bowel obstruction (Ch. 23) may follow contamination of the peritoneal cavity. Starch was then substituted but it is now clear that there are individuals who are starch-sensitive who also form abdominal adhesions. Most surgeons therefore now use starch-free gloves.

Infected and other high-risk patients

Patients themselves can be a source of infection and pose particular problems when their tissues are exposed. The simplest instances are when infected patients, e.g. those having drainage of an abscess or those with infected open wounds, contaminate the operating room, which can lead to contamination of subsequent patients. It was previously common practice to put those regarded as being able to disseminate infection at the end of elective operating lists. However, if the theatre is adequately cleaned between each procedure, then this practice is not essential.

Specialities, such as orthopaedics or transplant surgery, which require ultraclean conditions should have dedicated theatres that are not used by others.

Dressings or bandages from infected patients and disposable equipment used in their operation should be carefully disposed of in plastic sacks. These should only be filled to three-quarters of their capacity (in case overfilling results in rupture) before being sealed and disposed of by incineration.

The term 'high-risk' has now become applicable to other specific groups positive for:

- HIV
- hepatitis B
- hepatitis C.

These agents are of most concern to the surgical team because of the risk of transmission through the chance that the patient's blood may enter the body of a member of the team during an operation by a surface injury such as a needle stick or a minor nick with a knife. The same applies to a lesser extent to other body fluids. Other transmissible agents may appear in the future.

The usual measures to prevent *cross-infection* within the operating suite include:

- use of impervious gowns and drapes so that the operating table or surgical team do not come into contact with the patient's blood or body fluids
- a plastic apron under the operating gown if heavy contamination is anticipated
- latex operating gloves, although these provide little or no protection from injuries by sharp instruments such as knives or needles
- operating room discipline, e.g. passing needles or scalpels between the scrub nurse and surgeon in a transit dish to prevent injury from hand-to-hand passage
- careful disposal of all contaminated material at the end of the procedure into plastic sealable bags for incineration.

At present, routine testing of patients for HIV or hepatitis B antibodies is not performed in the UK (except in private institutions). The ethical and moral issues which relate to testing preoperative patients continue but currently the only way to identify high-risk patients is by the patient's own admission of infection, a history of high-risk behaviour or the detection of significant physical signs, such as multiple injection marks from intravenous drug abuse.

The safest policy to adopt would be to consider all patients to be high-risk, but this adds to costs and may slow down the work of the operating team. However, the majority of surgeons do take extra precautions when they are known or likely to be needed and modify their techniques to decrease the likelihood of injury by knives and needles.

Extra precautions when operating on high-risk patients include:

- *Double gloving.* Wearing two pairs of gloves reduces the likelihood of glove perforation; it is usual to wear the inner glove a half-size larger than the individual's normal size.
- *Eye protection.* Goggles or visors are essential to prevent splash contamination of the conjunctiva. They are most important when power tools are being used because these can create a fine aerosol mixture of body fluids with a theoretical risk of viral transmission.
- *Surgeon.* The most experienced surgeon available should do the operation.
- *Staples.* Stapling devices (Ch. 8) should be employed for anastomoses and skin closure to reduce the risk of needle pricks.
- *Needles.* Hand-held needles should be avoided because the incidence of glove perforation is so high as to be unacceptable. Needles have been designed with blunted ends that will penetrate fascia but should not pierce gloves and are particularly useful during mass closure (Ch. 8) of laparotomy wounds when the incidence of needle injury and glove perforation is greatest.

Prevention of cross-infection and the infection of health care workers by viral diseases depends on the efficacy of the barrier between patients and the surgical team; this consists of both the mechanical barrier (as outlined above by the use of impervious materials) and that resulting from good surgical practice. At present there is no satisfactory prophylaxis against either HIV or hepatitis C. Hepatitis B can be protected against by immunisation and this should be mandatory for all health care workers.

Positioning of the patient

Once anaesthetised, patients lose the protective reflexes generally taken for granted in daily life. It is the responsibility of the operating room staff and, in particular, the surgeon and anaesthetist to make sure that no harm comes to the patient as a result. The surgeon is also responsible for positioning the patient so that good exposure may be achieved during the operation.

The operating table

In most rooms this is free-standing and may be moved out during cleaning. Some rooms have a fixed base built into the floor with removable top sections which can be changed according to the operation being done. The table must be heavy and stable enough to support the patient but also highly adjustable. The top of the table is divided into sections each of which can be adjusted independently. The central section should be radiolucent, which is especially important in urological and general surgery when perioperative abdominal X-rays or the image intensifier are used. Operating tables have a soft sorbo-rubber padding on top so that pressure is widely distributed to avoid pressure points which could lead to skin breakdown. The common positions and their terminology are listed in Table 5.1

Precautions

Rigorous care must be taken to avoid:

- unintentional contact of the patient with metal – if monopolar diathermy (Ch. 8) is being used and the patient is in contact with metal, such as a part of the operating table or a support, the current will pass to earth through the exposed skin and metal and a burn (usually full-thickness) at the point of contact will result

- possible points of pressure – padding should be placed around areas at risk of pressure such as the elbows or heels; in the supine position a rubber pad is placed under the ankle joints to relieve pressure on the skin of the heels and to avoid compression of the deep veins of the calf muscles.

Avoiding nerve and joint injuries are two other matters which depend on careful positioning.

Nerve injuries occur as a result of traction or pressure. It must be remembered that muscle paralysis may impose forces different from those in the un-anaesthetised state. The nerves particularly at risk include:

- *brachial plexus* – abduction of the arm to greater than 90∞ can stretch the plexus
- *ulnar nerve* – from compression by a table support or other hard surface as the nerve passes behind the medial epicondyle at the elbow
- *radial nerve* – risk of compression where it winds around the shaft of the humerus
- *common peroneal nerve* – may be damaged by lithotomy supports where the nerve winds around the neck of the fibula.

Joint injuries. These are avoided by maintaining natural joint positions and not forcing the limbs to conform to what seems best for the surgical team; for example, hip joints can be damaged when putting a patient in the lithotomy position unless care is taken to lift both legs smoothly and together. Particular care should be taken in transferring patients with known back or joint problems or those at particular risk such as patients with rheumatoid arthritis or those who have had a joint replaced.

Temperature control

The unconscious patient has lost the ability to regulate body temperature because of vasomotor paralysis and also possibly inhibition of central mechanisms. Hypothermia will follow if the ambient temperature falls below 21°C for more than an hour or two. Measures to prevent this include:

- minimising the time the patient is left uncovered
- limiting the exposure of large areas of tissue to the atmosphere, particularly the contents of the abdomen or chest
- placing a heating mattress between the patient and the operating table consisting of multiple long tubes which are electrically heated or filled with circulating warm water

Table 5.1
Common positions for operations

Position	Use
Supine	Suitable for many operations
Tendelenburg Supine, but the patient is tilted 30–40° head-down	Operations of pelvic organs: small intestine moves out of the way with gravity
Reverse Trendelenburg As Trendelenberg but the tilt is head-up	Operations on upper abdominal organs
Lithotomy Supine with hips and knees fully flexed and the feet in stirrups or straps	Access to the anal and perianal regions and the external genitalia, vagina and uterine cervix, urethra and bladder (endoscopic)
Lateral Position of extension on the right or left side with the uppermost arm raised above and in front of the head. The centre of the table may be angled (broken) to improve access	Operations on the kidney and in the chest
Lloyd–Davies As Trendelenburg but with the legs abducted and the hips and knees slightly flexed and the legs in rests	Combined procedures which involve the abdomen and perineum (usually on the distal large bowel)
Bowie Prone with flexion at the hips	Access to the perianal area

- placing space blankets or warm air heated blankets over the patient and beneath the drapes, leaving only the area being operated on exposed
- humidification of inspired anaesthetic gases
- use of warming devices for the administration of blood or other fluids.

Access and common incisions

In order to do an operation well, the correct incision must be made. The most important aspect is that it allows adequate access to the operating field. Other important considerations are:

- sound healing
- minimum pain during the course of healing
- minimum complications
- satisfactory cosmetic result.

The ability to extend an incision to allow greater access is also necessary when unexpected problems or findings are encountered. In the abdomen, the classic example is when the appendix is exposed for appendicitis but a carcinoma of the caecum is found and a right hemicolectomy is needed. Some operations are approached through a standard incision (thyroidectomy, Ch. 31) while others may be done through a variety of approaches (see 'Abdominal incisions' below). For example, an open cholecystectomy (Ch. 19) may be performed via a right upper paramedian or midline incision, a transverse upper right incision or an oblique subcostal incision, depending to a certain extent on the surgeon's preference.

Skin incisions

Although exposure is the most important principle in surgical access, cosmesis is also desirable because the skin incision is the patient's only visible reminder of the operation. The cleavage lines or lines of Langer show the 'grain' of the skin and represent the parallel sheets of collagen and elastic tissue fibres in the dermis. They run transversely or obliquely on the trunk and neck and longitudinally on the limbs (Fig. 5.3). Incisions made along the lines will heal with fine scars and minimal contraction, whereas those made across them retract maximally to leave ugly scars.

Joint crease lines are areas where the skin is more firmly attached to the underlying fascia and are more marked on the flexor aspects of the joint. As with skin cleavage lines, they should not be crossed perpendicularly because tethering of the skin may result in impaired joint function.

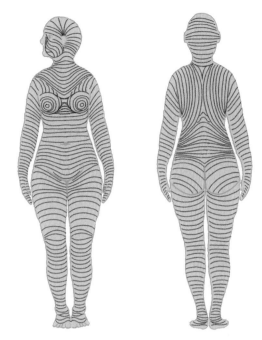

Fig 5.3 **Skin cleavage lines (Langer's).**

Abdominal incisions

The abdominal incision chosen depends on the diagnosis or the organ involved and may be vertical, horizontal or oblique (Fig. 5.4).

Vertical incisions

Upper midline
This incision allows access to the stomach, duodenum,

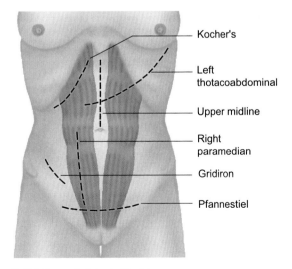

- Kocher's
- Left thotacoabdominal
- Upper midline
- Right paramedian
- Gridiron
- Pfannestiel

Fig 5.4 **Types of abdominal incision.**

liver, gall bladder, pancreas and spleen. It divides the skin, subcutaneous fat, linea alba, preperitoneal fat and peritoneum; it is relatively bloodless and is also quick to make and close.

Lower midline
This allows access to the pelvic organs. As with the upper midline incision, it can be extended for greater exposure.

Full midline
This incision is used when greater exposure of the abdominal contents are required; e.g. for an abdominal aortic aneurysm

Paramedian incision
A paramedian incision is made 2 cm either side of the midline depending on which organ or portion of the bowel is to be operated on. The skin and anterior rectus sheath are incised; the rectus muscle is retracted laterally and the posterior rectus sheath and peritoneum are then divided in the same line as the skin. It takes longer to open and close than a midline incision but is said to have a lower incidence of wound problems as the rectus abdominis muscle acts like a shutter to prevent hernia formation.

Horizontal incisions

Transverse abdominal incision
This type of incision heals well with fine scars and less pain. It allows good access to the abdominal contents; They are either *muscle-splitting* or *muscle-cutting* the former taking longer to open and close. Transverse abdominal incisions are often used in neonates or infants.

Pfannenstiel incision
This is a transverse incision 1 cm above the pubic symphysis. It is widely used by gynaecologists because it gives good access to the pelvic organs.

Oblique incisions

Right subcostal (Kocher's)
This type of incision begins below the xiphisternum and runs laterally 2 cm below and parallel to the costal margin, dividing all layers in the line of the incision. It gives access to the gall bladder.

Gridiron
This is the classical approach to the appendix, centred on McBurney's point, which is two-thirds of the way along a line from the umbilicus to the anterior superior iliac spine. The incision passes obliquely downwards from lateral to medial and splits the aponeurotic and muscle layers in the line of their fibres.

Closure of abdominal incisions

Midline incisions may be closed with a mass closure, which employs a strong, slowly absorbable (or non-absorbable) suture in a continuous over-and-over stitch, taking bites of all layers of the incision deep to the skin 1cm from the wound edge and 1 cm apart. To reduce the incidence of wound dehiscence or postoperative hernia after mass closure, the ratio of suture material used should be four times the length of the wound.

The closure of abdominal incisions is discussed in more detail in Chapter 8.

Haemostasis in surgery

See Chapter 8.

Drains

Drains are inserted either to evacuate established collections of pus, blood or fluid or to drain potential collections that may follow operation because of continued oozing of blood or inflammatory exudate. They range from a simple gauze wick to low-pressure suction applied to tubes.

The use of drains is contentious. Advocates maintain that:

- drainage of fluid collections removes a potential source of infection
- drains guard against further fluid collection
- drainage content may alert the surgeon to the presence of an anastomotic leak or to the possibility of secondary haemorrhage)
- when removed, a track is left for any residual collection to discharge.

Opponents argue that:

- the presence of a drain increases the chances of infection by acting as a route for bacterial entry
- damage can be caused by mechanical pressure and through the use of suction
- healing is delayed and, in certain circumstances, complications (such as leakage from an intestinal anastomosis) are more common
- In the peritoneal or pleural cavities, the majority of drains are sealed off within 6 hours and are therefore ineffective.

There are many different types of drain, which may be either *active* or *passive* (Fig. 5.5). In active drainage, suction forces provided by vacuumed containers (disposable, e.g. Redivac, or reusable) are used to draw

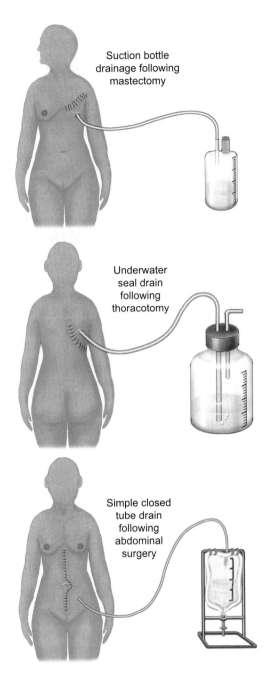

Suction bottle drainage following mastectomy

Underwater seal drain following thoracotomy

Simple closed tube drain following abdominal surgery

Fig 5.5 **Different types of drain.**

Drains may also be *open* or *closed*. Open passive drains lead directly into dressing or stoma appliances (Ch. 24). They may be tubes or sheets – often corrugated – of rubber or plastic. Closed tube systems drain directly into a container with or without suction and avoid spillage and soiling of dressings and minimise the hazards if the drainage material is contaminated.

For many years tube drains were made from soft red rubber, but because this substance is irritant (bioreactive) it has largely been superseded by newer material such as polyvinylchloride, Silastic or polyurethane. All have the advantages that they are relatively inert and are transparent so the colour of the drainage fluid can be seen. However, a degree of reactivity can sometimes be advantageous because the fibrosis leaves a track when the drain is removed down which residual drainage can occur. T-tubes to drain the common bile duct after exploration (Ch. 19) are often still made of rubber for this reason.

Drains are discussed further in Chapter 7.

Minimal access surgery

The term minimal access surgery partially overlaps with several others, including:

- endoscopic surgery
- minimally invasive surgery
- laparoscopic surgery.

Lay people refer to it as *keyhole surgery*. The student should realise that these words and phrases are often used interchangeably but that individual surgeons and surgical teams may have their own preferred definition.

Types of procedure
Laparoscopy

Laparoscopy, i.e. minimal access to the abdomen for diagnosis and later for therapy, was invented in 1910 by a Russian gynaecologist (Isaac Ott). The peritoneal cavity is distended with a gas (usually carbon dioxide) and instruments, including a telescope, introduced through trocars via small puncture wounds known as *ports*. It took some decades for surgeons (as distinct from gynaecologists) to adopt the technique for diagnosis, but it has been used by a few for the past 20 years.

out any collection. Passive drains function by differential pressures between the body and the exterior and are dependent on gravity or capillary action to drain fluid. Because these differential pressures are sometimes reversed, with intraperitoneal or intrapleural pressures lower than atmospheric pressure, fluid movements along the drain can be reversed, thereby increasing the risks of the introduction of bacteria from the outside.

Therapeutic application in areas other than gynaecology began in 1987 when a French surgeon (Philippe Mouret) performed the first laparoscopic cholecystectomy. Soon after, and with the advent of high-definition televideoscopy, a revolution began in abdominal and also in thoracic surgery (thoracoscopy) which is still in progress. The advantages of laparoscopic access for cholecystectomy (Ch. 19) are now well recognised. Its place in both diagnosis and management of the abdomen is discussed elsewhere in this book.

DIAGNOSIS

Advances in the quality of view that can be achieved with the laparoscope now allow surgeons to perform an abdominal exploration that approximates very closely to that achieved through a large laparotomy incision. Applications include:

- assessment of liver disease
- unknown causes of ascites
- the acute abdomen, including acute appendicitis
- detailed diagnosis and staging of intra-abdominal malignancy
- diagnosis and staging of lymphoma
- preoperative assessment of both blunt and penetrating trauma

MANAGEMENT

Laparoscopy is used in the management of the following:

- cholecystectomy
- oesophageal reflux
- gastro-esophageal malignancy
- colon malignancy
- pancreatic malignancy
- splenectomy
- retroperitoneal procedures, e.g. adrenalectomy.

In all but the first of these, the exact place of laparoscopy is still under close scrutiny. Also under development are flexible laparoscopes and ultrasound probes that can be introduced into, and manipulated within, the abdomen. These devices should add significantly to thorough evaluation not only of the peritoneal cavity but also of the retroperitoneum.

Thoracoscopy

See Chapter 16.

Urological minimal access surgery

See Chapter 32.

Advantages and disadvantages of minimally invasive surgery

Advantages

- The large painful wound of open access is avoided.
- The instruments used for dissection are small and fine and so the tissue trauma of surgical dissection is further reduced.
- The operation is carried out inside the closed confines of the body cavity which avoids cooling, drying, excessive handling and extensive retraction of internal organs.
- The overall disturbance to the patient, including pain and discomfort, is reduced.
- Recovery to full activity is accelerated.
- There is considerable reduction in all complications related to the wound; dehiscence and incisional hernia disappear (although too large an incision to create a port may result in a later port site hernia).
- There is reduced contact with the patient's blood and a consequent reduction in the risk of transmission of viral diseases (Ch. 9).
- There is a reduction in postoperative complications associated with recumbency and pain; e.g. chest problems (Ch. 16), deep vein thrombosis Ch. 29).
- There is a possible reduction in postoperative peritoneal adhesions.

Disadvantages

These fall into categories of general, organisational physiological and pathological constraints.

General and organisational constraints

- *Time*. Procedures performed laparoscopically are generally slower, especially when setting-up time is included. This has important effects on scheduling and costs.
- *Skills*. Special technical expertise is necessary and it is only recently that training centres have been set up.

Physiological and pathological constraints.

- A large pneumoperitoneum may compress the diaphragm and lung bases and cause postoperative hypoxia.
- Previous adhesions may make a pneumoperitoneum impossible.
- There is a risk of gas embolism, although this is very small.
- Tactile feedback to the operating team is lost; this is important in some aspects of the evaluation of local disorder,
- Precise control of bleeding is undoubtedly more difficult to achieve through an endoscope because the bleeding point often retracts within surrounding

tissues. Bleeding during minimally invasive surgery can considerably obscure the field of vision.

- Organ extraction: in some instances use is made of natural pathways, such as the mediastinum for the oesophagus or through the rectum for the colon. Other organs, such as the gall bladder or appendix are small enough to be removed through a port site after they have been put in a bag to stop the consequences of rupture and possible contamination. Yet others (spleen) can sometimes be broken up (*morcellised*), but for some circumstances the matter remains unresolved.

Conversion from laparoscopy to open exposure

Minimally invasive surgery is only as safe as the skill and judgement of the surgeon. Conversion from a laparoscopic to open procedure does not constitute a failure. Part of the success of minimally invasive surgery rests on the ability of the surgeon to determine that the patient's interest are best served by converting a laparoscopic procedure to the same operation performed with open access.

6

Anaesthesia and pain control

The speciality of anaesthesia has expanded to take in many areas of hospital practice which now include not only the operating rooms (Ch. 5) but also the intensive care unit (Ch. 10), chronic pain clinics and the midwifery labour ward. However, this chapter concentrates on the management of patients who undergo surgical procedures.

The administration of a safe anaesthetic is the central purpose of the speciality, but equally important are careful preparation and appropriate post-operative care. This chapter includes information to help undergraduates not only during their anaesthetic attachments but also in their general understanding of the care of the surgical patient. Detailed descriptions of practical procedures are not given, in that these are best learned during a clinical attachment. Throughout, drugs are referred to which may be initially unfamiliar and these are described in some detail (see 'Drugs used in anaesthesia' below).

History and principles of anaethesia

The introduction of anaesthetics in the 19th century was a major advance in the practice of surgery. Before it took place, the range and extent of procedures possible were limited. The first anaesthetic reported was given on the 16th October 1846 by W.T.G. Morton of Boston in the United States. The patient was anaesthetised by inhaling ether. The practice spread rapidly and in the UK the first anaesthetic was given later that same year to a patient undergoing dental extractions. Chloroform and nitrous oxide were soon added to the range of anaesthetics available and initially simple techniques were used. Since then there has been a steady evolution of the speciality; some of the more notable landmarks are shown in Information Box 6.1.

What is anaesthesia?

It is difficult to give an all-encompassing definition for the term. The phrase *reversible unconsciousness* has been popular but obviously does not include regional anaesthesia. A brief description of the purpose of anaesthesia is the best way to describe the scope of the subject.

Information Box 6.1

Key points in the history of anaesthesia

1846	W.T.G. Morton, a Boston dentist, demonstrated the use of ether
1853	John Snow, a London physician, gave chloroform analgesia to Queen Victoria at the birth of Prince Leopold
1884	Koller, Viennese ophthalmologist, demonstrated local anaesthetic properties of cocaine
1898	Angus Bier, first use of spinal analgesia
1917	Edmund Boyle, Guy's Hospital, described an early anaesthetic machine
1934	J.S. Lundy, US anaesthetist, popularised thiopentone
1935	Introduction of the intravenous drip
1949	Introduction of muscle relaxants
1956	First use of halothane clinically at the Manchester Royal Infirmary
1972	Royal College of Anaesthetists formed

Purpose

The purpose of anaesthesia is to allow patients to undergo surgical or investigative procedures in a safe and pain-free way. With general anaesthesia, the patient is unconscious and should not be aware of what is happening. This state, when associated with techniques to reduce the perception of painful stimuli, is now called *balanced* anaesthesia. The term recognises the fact that a number of different techniques and agents (drugs) can be used in combination to produce the desired state. Many procedures include the use of muscle relaxants, either to allow intubation of the trachea for protection from obstruction of the airway and to permit safe administration of inhaled gases or to aid surgical access (e.g. laparotomy). Paralysis is therefore often a feature of an anaesthetised patient but is not essential.

In the use of local or regional anaesthesia, it cannot be said that the patient is generally unaware. Rather there is a selective state of lack of recognition of what is being done in the area of the procedure. In this, as in all forms of anaesthesia, there is always a balance between ensuring a pain-free subject and the potential undesirable effects of high concentrations of anaesthetic agents.

How do anaesthetics work?

Despite the highly scientific and technical growth of the

speciality over the past 150 years, it is still not possible to give a definitive description of how general anaesthetics work in the way that, for example, an endocrinologist can often describe the chemical pathways which account for the action of, say, insulin. However, there are a number of factors that allow some reasonable assumptions about the possible action of anaesthetic agents:

- The potency of anaesthetic agents is closely related to their lipid solubility – this points to the cell membrane as the likely site of action.
- Anaesthetic agents probably interfere with the propagation of nerve impulses through central nerves by an effect on the neuronal cell membrane at synaptic junctions.

Many of the assumptions made about the actions of general anaesthetics come from observing their effects on patients. The difficulty of defining exactly how anaesthetics work has made the measurement of the level of anaesthesia in individual patients difficult. Much research is currently looking at this area.

The actions of local anaesthetics are more readily explicable, as will be described later in this chapter.

Preoperative preparation

A crucial factor in the administration of safe anaesthesia is the correct preparation of the patient. The aim is always to have the optimum condition for an operation. For simple day-case procedures, preparation is relatively straightforward. However, in more complex circumstances, admission may be necessary several days in advance to organise investigations and optimise underlying medical conditions. The anaesthetist visits the patient during this period to make an assessment of likely problems; this is now usually known as pre-assessment.

Pre-assessment

The elective patient is evaluated by a review of the history, physical examination and available investigations in the context of fitness for both anaesthesia and the operative procedure. If required, further investigations may then be ordered and specific therapy initiated to optimise the patient's condition before the procedure. This period also provides an opportunity to discuss the anaesthetic and to explore postoperative issues such as the need for analgesia, intravenous infusion and high-dependency care (Ch. 10). Most importantly, the preoperative visit gives patients an opportunity to voice any fears about the anaesthetic, and to receive informed reassurance from the person responsible (the anaesthetist) for their care during and often after the operation.

The assessment often begins with questions to assess the patient's understanding of the proposed procedure. Most individuals can understand the diagnosis and relate this to the site of the lesion; this is adequate for most minor and routine surgery. However, in unusual or major cases, the anaesthetist must always be in contact with the surgical team to discuss the intended procedure, how it might have to be extended and the requirement for blood products or more intensive postoperative care. It is not unusual for the simple closed reduction of a bone fracture, intended to finish in a few minutes, to progress to open fixation and nailing over several hours with considerable blood loss and the need for postoperative high-dependency care. Similarly, to know the site of the lesion and route of surgical access is important because operations on various sites – from lung and larynx to bladder and feet – require very different airway and anaesthetic management. For example, to maintain the airway in an anaesthetised patient by a mask over the face is not possible if the surgeon requires to work inside the mouth.

Assessment of medical fitness

With the nature of the procedure clarified, the patient's present medical status may then be evaluated. Details of the past medical history should be recorded and existing disease documented with respect to duration, severity, medication, complications and hospital admissions.

Consideration may then be given to the requirement for further investigation and treatment. Within each of the physiological systems there are many conditions which influence anaesthetic management. Lack of cardiorespiratory reserve is a great concern because surgical procedures elicit a stress response with neuroendocrine changes which lead to alterations in metabolic function and, in major surgery, elevations in cardiac demands and oxygen requirements. Lack of cardiorespiratory reserve may mean that these demands cannot be met without decompensation in spite of the most effective balanced anaesthesia and most minor surgery. Therefore, for those with significant disease, the anaesthetist may require further investigations, specific treatment (even coronary artery bypass grafting before a major procedure on another system such as the gastrointestinal tract), more invasive peroperative monitoring and intensive or high-dependency postoperative care.

Assessment of the adequacy of cardiac and respiratory function is of overriding importance in that both are disturbed by anaesthesia and surgery and both may determine postoperative complications. Impair-

ment is assessed clinically by evaluation of exercise tolerance to activities of daily living, such as walking, climbing stairs and carrying shopping. Known cardiovascular disease – congestive cardiac failure, angina, previous myocardial infarction (particularly within the last 6 months), arrhythmias, hypertension and valvular lesions (particularly aortic stenosis) – need not lead to cancellation, but it is helpful if the anaesthetist is given ample warning in advance so as to formulate an appropriate plan. Hypertension is defined as a systolic pressure greater than 160 mmHg and/or a diastolic pressure of greater than 90 mmHg. Hypertension so defined occurs in approximately 10% of the adult population and constitutes a serious perioperative risk to the patient of stroke or renal dysfunction. Hypertension is therefore a contraindication to elective surgery and patients found to be hypertensive should be referred for a cardiological opinion which, if unfavourable, should lead to the search for alternatives to operation.

Respiratory competence is assessed initially by clinical means – exercise tolerance and the occurrence of breathlessness under physical stress – and, for even minor surgery, it is essential that obstructive airways disease, asthma and infection should have been investigated and measures taken to reduce adverse factors. There is a higher incidence of perioperative and postoperative complications (e.g. hypoxic episodes, pneumonia) in patients with respiratory disease. The incidence increases significantly if the disorder is not controlled.

Pathological disturbances within other physiological systems may also be pertinent. A history of gastrooesophageal reflux warns of patients who may have a hiatus hernia and who are therefore at much higher risk of aspiration. Such individuals can benefit from acid suppression prophylaxis (e.g. ranitidine) and from early tracheal intubation to protect the lower airway. A history of epilepsy may alter anaesthetic medication in that some anaesthetic drugs lower the seizure threshold. Evidence of peripheral nerve damage or neuropathy may dissuade the anaesthetist from employing regional techniques of nerve blockade. Patients with diabetes require varying degrees of management, dependent on the severity of the condition and the magnitude of the procedure; management ranges from simple monitoring of blood glucose by the BM stick procedure to precise metabolic control with frequent blood glucose determinations, intravenous infusions of dextrose, insulin and potassium which may begin some hours preoperatively.

Cerebrovascular disease is common. Stroke is responsible for death in 9 and 15% of the general population of adult men and women, respectively. A history of previous stroke, particularly in the presence of hypertension, means that particular attention should be paid to the state of the peripheral circulation and the patient should undergo examination of the carotid pulse (palpation and auscultation) at the least before operation. If there have been recent transient disturbances of cerebral function, these patients should be referred for duplex Doppler examination with a view to possible carotid angiography.

Other system disease, such as renal failure, liver disease, haematological or musculoskeletal abnormalities, must also be defined because all may influence anaesthetic technique.

Existing medical treatment

An accurate medication and allergy history is vital. Diuretics may cause electrolyte imbalance which can lead to cardiac arrhythmias or dehydration, which on induction of anaesthesia may lead to hypotension. Beta-blockers may prevent cardiovascular compensation for hypotension caused by either bleeding or loss of sympathetic vasomotor control during both regional and general anaesthesia. Anti-arrhythmics (e.g. digoxin, amiodarone) may potentiate the bradycardic effects of anaesthetic drugs such as propofol, fentanyl or vecuronium (these agents are discussed later).

Bronchodilators and other sympathomimetics may increase the incidence and severity of tachyarrhythmias. If a course of systemic steroids has been taken within the last year, consideration needs to be given to steroid supplementation as prophylaxis against an adrenal crisis (Ch. 31). Those on monoamine oxidase inhibitors may experience severe cardiovascular and neurological disturbances if sympathomimetics (e.g. adrenalin) or opioid analgesics such as pethidine are used.

Those on the oral contraceptive pill may require measures to reduce the risks of developing deep vein thrombosis and pulmonary emboli (Ch. 16). In circumstances in which the patient is likely to be ambulatory soon after the operation (the majority of modern procedures), the risks of an unwanted pregnancy usually outweigh the chances of thrombotic complications; however, operations for malignant disease are an exception. Oral anticoagulants may need to be adjusted to a reduced dose, changed to intravenous heparin or stopped altogether. Drugs such as anti-hypertensive, anti-arrhythmic bronchodilator agents should be maintained at their usual schedule up to the induction of anaesthesia, and so may need to be included in the premedication.

Details of past anaesthetics should be sought from both the patient and the notes. A history of difficult intubation, allergy, malignant hyperthermia (a serious allergic reaction to certain anaesthetic agents) and postoperative nausea and vomiting are of great interest and influence the plan for subsequent anaesthesia. For those previously not exposed to an anaesthetic, a review of family experiences of anaesthesia complications may reveal congenital conditions of note, e.g. malignant hyperthermia, suxamethonium apnoea (see below) and sickle cell disease.

Questions should be directed towards cigarette and alcohol consumption, a social history which may yield very useful information about unrevealed problems, as well as indicators of the response to an anaesthetic. Premenopausal women should be asked if they could be pregnant, to avoid exposing the fetus to potentially teratogenic anaesthetic drugs. However, the indication for surgery is usually a greater risk to the fetus than the anaesthetic itself.

A check that an appropriate period of fasting will have elapsed before induction of anaesthesia should be mandatory. A period of 6 hours following solid food and 4 hours following clear liquids is standard in most hospitals.

Airway examination

Examination of the airway is mandatory for the anaesthetist, particularly if the use of an endotracheal tube is contemplated – patients have died after induction of anaesthesia where there was, because of lack of previous knowledge, inability to ventilate the patient or site an endotracheal tube. Conditions that lead to difficulties with intubation are shown in Table 6.1.

The airway examination should include:

- mouth opening (two finger breadths or less is likely to lead to problems)

Table 6.1
Conditions which predispose to difficult endotracheal intubation

Congenital	Anatomical	Acquired
Pierre–Robin sequence	Reduced mouth opening	Airway instability: trauma, rheumatoid arthritis
Treacher–Collins syndrome	Reduced neck movement	Trismus, fibrosis: causing reduced movement of temperomandibular joint
Achondroplasia	Small mandible	Reduced neck movement: arthritis, hard collar
Marfan's syndrome	Prominent teeth	Swelling: tumour, abscess, haematoma
Noonan's syndrome	Obesity	Airway obstructed: bleeding, vomitus
Cystic hygroma		Scarring: burns, radiation

- jaw protrusion – can the lower incisors be placed in front of the upper?
- neck flexion and extension
- the presence of prominent or loose teeth
- a view of the posterior pharyngeal structures – this has been shown to be a valuable indicator of the ease of laryngoscopy.

Very occasionally additional investigations of the airway are needed, such as lateral X-rays of the neck, flow-volume pulmonary function tests or awake fibre-optic examination. The known difficult intubation seldom causes severe problems, but the unexpected one may quickly become a medical emergency. Therefore patients who are known to be at risk of a difficult intubation should be referred to senior anaesthetists at pre-assessment.

Investigations

Further investigations may be required, the common indications for which are listed in Table 6.2. The list is not exhaustive and many other examinations may be necessary. In addition, few of the indications are absolute and, if an investigation has recently been performed, then it is not, unless circumstances have changed, of value to repeat it.

Table 6.2
Indications for preoperative investigations

Investigation	Indication
Full blood count	History of bleeding, major surgery, cardiorespiratory disease, premenopausal women, Asians
Electrolytes	History of vomiting, diarrhoea, renal disease, cardiac disease, diabetes, diuretics, ACE inhibitors, anti-arrhythmics, steroids, hypoglycaemics
Glucose	History of diabetes, abscesses, steroids
Liver function tests	History of liver disease, alcoholism, bleeding, pyrexia of unknown origin
Clotting studies	History of liver disease, bleeding
Sickle cell test	Afro-Caribbeans if sickle cell status unknown.
Electrocardiogram	History of hypertension, cardiorespiratory disease, age > 55 years
Chest X-ray	History of cardiorespiratory disease, heavy smoker, potential metastases, recent immigrants from area where TB is endemic
Pulmonary function tests	Respiratory disease, thoracic surgery
Arterial blood gases	Respiratory disease, thoracic surgery
Cervical spine X-ray	Rheumatoid arthritis, trauma

Box 6.1

Preoperative grading system of the American Society of Anesthesiologists

ASA I	Healthy patient
ASA II	Mild systemic disease, no functional disability
ASA III	Moderate systemic disease, functional disability
ASA IV	Severe systemic disease, constantly life-threatening
ASA V	Moribund patient, unlikely to survive 24 hours with or without an operation

Preoperative grading

Following this assessment, the anaesthetist will be able to grade the patient. A commonly used system is that described by the American Society of Anesthesiologists (ASA) in which patients are allocated to one of five categories (Box 6.1 – addition of an E denotes an emergency procedure, usually of higher risk). The scoring system allows easier communication between anaesthetists and is also a useful research tool. However, it gives only limited prognostic information about the chances of an individual surviving an operation. Significant factors, including the type of procedure, a history of difficult intubation and of obesity, are not included in the classification.

Immediate preoperative preparation

Although reflexes which protect the lungs are lost only under general anaesthesia, the requirements for preparation for general, local and regional anaesthesia are the same. An adequate history and examination must have been taken, fasting protocols adhered to, drugs and fluids for resuscitation and also a defibrillator must be readily available, and suction, oxygen and airway equipment must be to hand. Except for the simplest of procedures, it is sound to ensure that there is someone available other than the anaesthetist to monitor the patient, including pulse, blood pressure and oxygenation.

Medication

In the early days of anaesthesia, premedication before the patient left the ward, room or other place of

Table 6.3
Commonly used premedications

Indication	Class of drug used	Example
Sedation	Benzodiazepines	Temazepam, diazepam, lorazepam
	Opioids	Morphine, papaveretum, pethidine
	Butyrophenones	Droperidol
Acid aspiration prophylaxis	H₂ antagonists	Ranitidine, cimetidine
	Prokinetics	Metoclopramide
	Antacid	Sodium citrate
Reflex activity prophylaxis	Bronchodilators	Salbutamol
	Bradycardia prophylaxis	Atropine
Anti-sialogues	Anticholinergics	Hyoscine, glycopyrronium, atropine
Anti-emetics	Phenothiazines	Trimeprazine, promethazine
	Butyrophenones	Droperidol
	Antihistamines	Cyclizine
Analgesics	Opioids	Morphine, papaveretum, pethidine
	NSAIDs	Diclofenac
Amnestic	Benzodiazepines	Lorazepam
	Anticholinergic	Hyoscine

accommodation was essential to reduce anxiety and dry airway secretions before induction with ether. Now, sedation and an anti-sialogue premedication are no longer an absolute necessity. Premedication is usually only prescribed to individuals for specific reasons, although a small dose of a benzodiazepine is frequently given. Common premedications are shown in Table 6.3, and for each patient details of dose, route of administration and the time must be given. Timing is particularly difficult because staff are often busy, premedication is frequently given a low priority and times to completion of preceding operations are highly variable. Poor adherence to timing can lead to a short-acting premedication (such as some inhaled bronchodilators) wearing off before the patient reaches anaesthesia. Anti-sialogue premedication reduces the profound salivation which may occur with instrumentation of the airway (e.g. during awake fibreoptic intubation) and its omission can lead to difficulties.

The route varies from oral to dermal, intramuscular, nasal, rectal or sublingual, although oral tends to be favoured because it avoids a further injection and the medication can be found at most drug stations. If the oral route is inappropriate, e.g. in intestinal obstruction, then an intramuscular or intravenous injection must be used. In addition to pain from such injections, there are other disadvantages with some methods of premedication:

- unexpected excessive sedation in those who have been inadequately assessed
- dry mouth with anti-sialogues
- nausea and dysphoria with opioids
- prolonged postoperative sedation.

The practice of general anaesthesia

There are a number of ways to anaesthetise a patient and the technique used depends on a number of factors, some of which have already been considered. The most important are:

- clinical condition and general health
- the type and extent of the procedure
- protection of the airway.

The last of these is integral to safe anaesthesia and should be an essential part of undergraduate practical training.

Management of the airway

After the induction of general anaesthesia, the patient's ability to maintain the airway is lost. There are many contributory factors but the relaxation of the muscles of the tongue is central and can lead to physical obstruction of the airway which may be partial or complete. To avoid both, anaesthetists rely on careful positioning of the patient and special equipment.

Patient position

The patient is usually supine, with the head resting on one pillow and the shoulders flat on the theatre trolley or bed – the head is thus extended on the neck and the jaw is elevated (Fig. 6.1). This position lifts the base of the tongue away from the posterior wall of the pharynx and is sometimes called *sniffing the air*.

Equipment

Anaesthetic mask

All masks must fit snugly against the face to produce an airtight seal to ensure the precise delivery of gases. As with all apparatus it is important to select the right size: the average adult male requires a size 5 mask, adult females size 4 (Fig. 6.2).

Oral and nasal airways

These are the simplest aids to airway management. Oral airways (e.g. Guedel) come in different sizes and

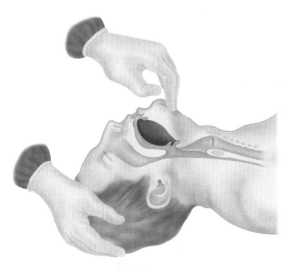

Fig 6.1 **Supporting the airway.**

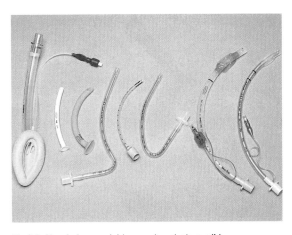

Fig 6.3 **Nasal airways. (a)** laryngeal mask airway; **(b)** nasopharyngeal airway; **(c)** different types of endotracheal tubes (with and without cuffs).

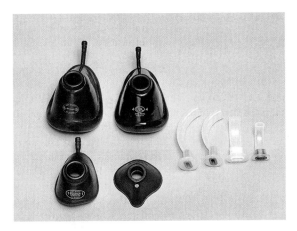

Fig 6.2 **Anaesthetic masks and oral airways.**

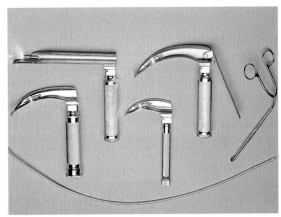

Fig 6.4 **Different laryngoscopes and aids to intubation.**

help to keep the tongue away from the posterior pharyngeal wall (Fig. 6.2). Nasal airways are useful if it is impossible or inappropriate to use an oral airway (Fig. 6.3)

Laryngeal mask airway (LMA)

The LMA is a more complicated oral airway than the Guedel. Because of its design it can be directly attached to an anaesthetic circuit (Fig. 6.3). However, it is still an airway and although it has an inflatable cuff, its position above the vocal cords does not provide protection against aspiration into the trachea.

Laryngoscopes

These are instruments used to facilitate tracheal intubation and many types have been designed (Fig. 6.4) to suit many different situations (examples are paediatric and fibreoptic instruments for children and for difficult intubations).

Tracheal intubation

A specially designed tube is passed across the vocal cords into the trachea and guarantees a clear upper airway free from the risk of aspiration, particularly if, as is usually the case for adults, the tube has an inflatable cuff (Figs. 6.3 and 6.5). Intubation is an essential skill for those involved in airway management and students should gain hands-on experience during clinical attachments. This includes familiarity with equipment for intubation and the safeguards used to check that the tube is correctly placed in the trachea.

Induction, maintenance and recovery from anaesthesia

Induction

Induction usually takes place in an anaesthetic room adjacent to the operating room. Patients will have been

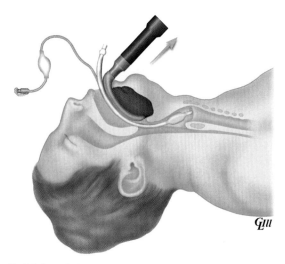

Fig 6.5 **Use of a laryngoscope to insert an endotracheal tube.**

checked to ensure they are properly prepared for surgery. The anaesthetist normally has an assistant who may be another specialist or a nurse. On arriving in the anaesthetic room, monitoring equipment is attached and, in most instances, an in-dwelling intravenous catheter is inserted at this stage. Usually an intravenous agent such as thiopentone is used to induce anaesthesia, although occasionally induction is by breathing anaesthetic gases (inhalational induction). While the patient is breathing 100% oxygen, the intravenous agent is injected slowly. Once the patient has lost consciousness, the anaesthetist places an anaesthetic mask on the face and changes the gases to deliver an anaesthetic mixture which usually includes oxygen, nitrous oxide and a volatile agent such as isoflurane. During this period, the concentration of anaesthetic gases in the patient's tissues increases as the concentration of the intravenous agent decreases – induction gives way to maintenance. At this stage any additional ancillary procedures are done, such as

---

Box 6.2

Indications for endotracheal intubation

Provides clear airway

Protects against aspiration

Allows positive pressure ventilation

Protects airway if operative site is near

Patient in awkward position, e.g. prone

Airway maintenance by mask difficult

Box 6.3

Indications for the use of muscle relaxants

Facilitate intubation

Facilitate ventilation

Allows surgical access e.g. laparotomy

Allows control of CO_2 levels

---

intubation (the indications for which are in Box 6.2) or the insertion of additional intravascular lines for cardiovascular monitoring. During this time, attachment to an anaesthetic machine is usually necessary and, if paralysis has been induced (indications in Box 6.3), a ventilator is necessary.

Maintenance

The patient is either transferred into the operating room with the anaesthetic machine or reconnected to one in the room. The maintenance of anaesthesia requires constant vigilance (Fig. 6.6). It is essential to

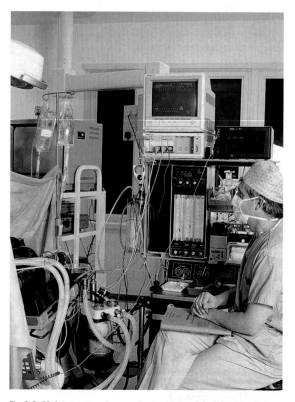

Fig 6.6 **Maintenance of anaesthesia.** Note the extensive monitoring and vigilant anaesthetist.

Box 6.4

Signs indicating inadequate depth of anaesthesia

Dilated pupils

Tears

Sweating

Tachycardia and hypertension

Patient movement

Increased respiratory rate

Box 6.5

Common complications of anaesthesia

Hypoxia

Hypercapnia

Hypotension

Arrhythmias

Pulmonary embolism

Allergic reactions

Hypothermia

Awareness

Minor trauma, e.g. sore throat

Headache

Malignant hyperpyrexia

Nausea and vomiting

ensure that anaesthesia is deep enough (Box 6.4) to avoid the risk of awareness. The patient is monitored so that any complications of the surgery or anaesthesia not obvious clinically can be detected early and treated. During this period the anaesthetist tries to keep the patient's general condition in balance, which includes fluid management, replacement of blood loss, cardiorespiratory support and maintenance of body temperature. During the procedure other drugs are administered to supplement anaesthesia. In most instances an analgesic (e.g. morphine) and an anti-emetic (e.g. cyclizine) are given.

Recovery

As the operation comes to an end, the anaesthetist steadily reduces the concentration of anaesthetic gases and, once the last active painful stimulus is withdrawn, the anaesthetic agents are turned off and replaced with 100% oxygen. At this point it may also be necessary to give a drug to reverse residual muscle paralysis; this injection does not have any effect on the concentration of anaesthetic gases in the body and therefore does not influence wakening. Gradual awakening occurs as the concentration of gases is reduced by expiration. If possible the recovery position is adopted until full control of the airway has been achieved. As this occurs, adjuncts such as an endotracheal tube are removed and a more simple oxygen mask applied. Transfer to a recovery area then takes place for further care.

Complications of anaesthesia

Emergency surgery and that undertaken at the extremes of age are more dangerous than that done as a routine on healthy subjects. Box 6.5 lists some of the more common complications. Here two potentially fatal matters are considered.

The difficult airway

In certain instances the airway may be difficult to maintain and therefore the delivery of adequate oxygen becomes a problem which can be life threatening. Prediction may be possible, and if a problem is anticipated, senior members of staff should be involved even though all anaesthetists are trained to cope with an airway problem, both one that is expected and one that comes out of the blue. There are a number of techniques and instruments to help deal with these matters.

Aspiration of stomach contents

With the onset of anaesthesia, the reflexes that protect the airways – especially cough and gag – are lost. Therefore it is possible for stomach contents to reflux up the oesophagus and enter the lungs. The repercussions can be serious: either acute asphyxiation or aspiration 'pneumonia' (a progressive bronchopneumonic inflammation). Therefore elective patients are fasted to ensure that the stomach is empty. In an emergency where the stomach may be full, either because of a previous meal or because of the presenting condition (e.g. intestinal obstruction), an endotracheal tube is passed to avoid reflux and inhalation. However, there is a short period of time after the patient has become unconscious and before the endotracheal tube is sited when the lungs are still potentially at risk. A procedure known as *cricoid pressure* is used during this period. Pressure sufficient to occlude the upper oesophagus is exerted anteroposteriorly on the cricoid ring just below the larynx. Those in attendance on the induction of anaesthesia in such circumstances require training and the technique is not without hazards.

Local and regional anaesthesia

While most patients and many doctors will assume that anaesthesia automatically implies a state of unconsciousness, such loss of awareness is not always necessary or even desirable. Many procedures can be performed safely and comfortably under local or regional anaesthesia; under regional anaesthesia with sedation; or with a combination of regional and general anaesthesia. Regional anaesthesia is the term used to describe local anaesthetic blockade of a group of nerves or nerve roots (e.g. the brachial plexus) to produce anaesthesia of a specific area. There is often no clear-cut advantage of one technique over another: Table 6.4 shows some of the factors that influence the decision.

How does a local anaesthetic (LA) work?

Local anaesthetics block the generation and propogation of nerve impulses at several sites – the spinal cord, spinal nerve roots or peripheral nerves – by inhibiting sodium channels in nerve fibres which are essential for the propogation of nerve impulses. In general, they are *membrane stabilisers.*

Local anaesthetic toxity

As with any group of drugs, overdosage of local anaesthetics leads to toxic side-effects. Box 6.6 shows the maximum dosage allowed of some commonly used agents. Local anaesthetics are presented for use as percentage strengths, which can easily be converted into milligrams (mg) if it is remembered that a 1% solution contains 10 mg of drug per millilitre (mL). Hence 10 mL of 2% lignocaine contains 200 mg.

Table 6.4
Factors affecting the choice of regional anaesthesia

Advantages	Disadvantages
Avoid complication of GATs	Toxic effects of local anaesthetics
Contributes to post-operative analgaesia	Patient unhappy to be awake
Less nausea and vomiting postoperatively	Inadequate anaesthesia
Patient satisfaction (e.g. caesarian section)	Possible nerve damage
Reduces incidence of DVTs	Can be slow onset

Box 6.6

Maximum safe doses of local anaesthetics
Lignocaine 4 mg/kg
Bupivicane 2 mg/kg
Prilocaine 5 mg/kg
NB: 1% solution of drugs = 10 mg/mL

During a toxic episode, inhibitory cell membranes are first blocked which leads to unopposed excitatory activity manifest as seizures. Other excitable cell membranes are also inhibited, most notably those of the conducting system of the heart, which results in arrhythmias such as ventricular tachycardia or fibrillation. Eventually coma and cardiovascular collapse ensue.

Routes of administration

Topical
EMLA (eutectic mixture of local anaesthetic) or Ametop cream may be used to provide skin analgesia before venepuncture, although the effect is best on the relatively soft skin of children. The conjunctivae, and the mucosa of the nose, throat and urethra can also be anaesthetised topically.

Subcutaneous infiltration
This is used, for example, before venepuncture and in the suturing of wounds. When local agents are infiltrated circumferentially around an extremity (the toe or finger) a *ring block* is produced which can have implications for the circulation.

Bier's block
Also known as intravenous regional anaesthesia, this has been classically used for reduction of Colles' fractures (Ch. 34) and is the exception to the rule that local anaesthetic should never be injected directly into the circulation. Systemic toxicity is prevented by the use only of prilocaine (the least toxic LA) and by separating the intravenous local anaesthetic in the limb from the general circulation by a tourniquet until the agent is bound in the tissues – about 20 minutes. Deaths have resulted as a consequence of tourniquet failure.

Nerve block
Individual nerves can be anaesthetised if local anaesthetic can be introduced close enough to the nerve; in theory, any nerve can be blocked, but in practice some nerves are difficult to reach even for those who are

skilled and enthusiastic. In that most nerves pass close to arteries, these vessels can be used as markers to position the injection. A peripheral nerve stimulator can also be used if the nerve carries motor fibres: a small electrical current is produced which elicits muscle twitching if the needle to be used for the block is close to the nerve. Blocks can be one-off single injections or flexible catheters can be inserted to allow repeated injections ('top-ups') or continuous infusions. In this way, the block can be continued for as long as the catheter remains in situ.

Epidural and spinal anaesthesia

In relation to nerve action, the introduction of local anaesthetic into the epidural or subarachnoid (spinal) spaces is similar to regional blockade, although the timescale and intensity differ. Both techniques involve the insertion of a needle into the midline between the spinous processes of adjacent vertebrae (Fig. 6.7). This form of anaesthesia is especially useful for surgery below the waist; blocks can be made as high as the mid-thoracic region, but associated abdominal and

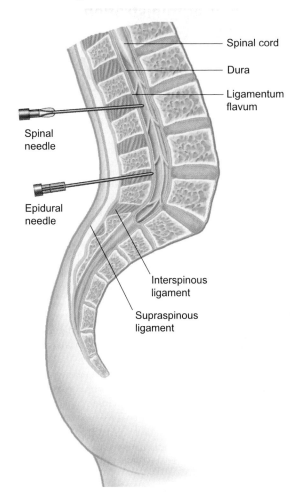

Fig 6.7 **The anatomy of spinal and epidural anaesthesia.**

intercostal muscle weakness can interfere with the ability to breathe or cough.

The epidural space is the more superficial of the two and is classically identified by the loss of resistance to injection of air or saline. Because an epidural injection does not puncture the dura, and therefore is well clear of the spinal cord, it can be done at any level in the vertebral column. In addition, wider bore needles can be used, which allow the passage of a catheter into the epidural space and either 'top-ups' or continuous infusions. The local anaesthetic introduced into the epidural space has to diffuse through the epidural fat towards the nerve roots as they emerge from the dura; as a result, the block can take up to 20 minutes to become effective and may miss some nerve roots, leaving unblocked segments. It is generally less dense than a spinal anaesthetic. Larger doses of anaesthetic agent are also needed than for a spinal because the anaesthetic is injected further from its eventual site of action.

With spinal anaesthesia, the dura is deliberately punctured to enter the subarachnoid space. The resulting persistent hole can lead to leak of CSF and be a cause of debilitating 'spinal' headache. To minimise this complication, very fine needles are used and catheters must not be inserted. Spinal anaesthetics are therefore 'single shot' and usually last up to 2 hours. The spinal cord ends at the level of the body of L1: at or above this level, the cord is tethered and is at risk of being skewered by a needle; below this, there is the freely floating cauda equina and a needle tends to push the nerves away.

In consequence, spinal anaesthetics are administered below the level of L1. The anaesthetic introduced is close to the nerves and very small volumes can produce satisfactory blocks with very rapid onset. The agent introduced into the subarachnoid space can be 'floated' in the CSF towards the desired level of block above the level of insertion by appropriate positioning of the patient.

Epidural and spinal anaesthesia carry the same hazards as all other nerve blocks but local complications in the central nervous system can be catastrophic, as follows:

- Infection in the vertebral column can result in meningitis or cord compression secondary to abscess formation.
- Haematoma can also lead to cord compression.
- Epidural cannulae can shift over time or be misplaced from the beginning so that inadvertent epidural venous cannulation can lead to rapid onset of local anaesthetic toxicity and an unrecognised spinal tap can lead to an epidural dose being injected spinally, with dangerously high levels of block.
- Epidural and spinal anaesthetics block not only motor and sensory nerves but also vasomotor

control; vasodilation and and a fall in the blood pressure may result.

Such anaesthetic blockade should never be performed without the same preparation and monitoring as for a general anaesthetic.

Monitoring and charting

All patients undergoing anaesthesia or sedative techniques should have their vital signs monitored. The range of monitoring information available to anaesthetists is vast, from fairly simple parameters such as temperature to complex data such as integrated electro-encephalograms. In this section we will concentrate on what are now accepted as standard monitoring requirements. We can usefully divide monitoring into devices that monitor the patient and those that monitor the anaesthetic machine and its function. However, in all cases the best monitor is the constant presence and vigilance of the anaesthetist (Fig. 6.6). The anaesthetist should view the information he or she receives from the monitors in the context of the individual patient and the procedure the patient is undergoing.

Monitoring the patient
Clinical observations

The anaesthetist can obtain useful information by direct observation and examination. A warm, well perfused, pink patient who is passing good volumes of urine is unlikely to be hypovolaemic. Likewise, observations of the pupils will guard against awareness (see Box 6.5). It is important for the anaesthetist to be aware of what is going on surgically. Measuring blood loss and predicting further losses will enable a more controlled replacement by transfusion if required.

Equipment

Standard monitoring is aimed at the cardiorespiratory systems (Box 6.7). The continuous recording of the ECG is mandatory and gives information on the heart rate and rhythm. Measurement of blood pressure is usually automated. The machines use the same principle as a manual blood pressure cuff used at the bedside. The automated mechanism and detecting devices allow the pressure to be measured at regular intervals (e.g. every 2 minutes). The pulse oximeter (Fig. 6.8) gives the anaesthetist a continuous measurement of oxygenation. The device measures the percentage of haemoglobin which is in oxygenated form, and isolates that measurement to arterial blood. These three devices give a lot of

Box 6.7
Standard monitoring
ECG
Non-invasive blood pressure
Pulse oximetry
End-tidal carbon dioxide levels
Temperature
Degree of muscle relaxation
Inspired oxygen concentration

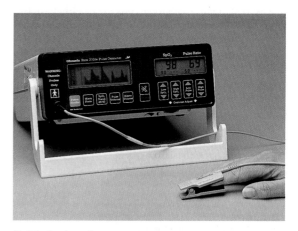

Fig 6.8 **A pulse oximeter.**

information about the patient's well-being. They are safe, easy to use and accurate. However, their interpretation requires some knowledge of physiology. For example, the oxygen saturation is related to the partial pressure (the important parameter) of oxygen in the blood by the relationship shown in the oxyhaemoglobin dissociation curve (Fig. 6.9). It can be seen from this diagram that, when the saturation falls below 90–91%, there is then a rapid decline in the partial pressure of oxygen. Before use these devices are programmed with what are considered normal limits for the patient. If the measurements fall outside these limits an alarm will sound.

Standard monitoring also includes measurement of the concentrations of gases exhaled from the lungs (i.e. alveolar gas, which has a higher than ambient level of carbon dioxide). A *capnograph* enables measurement of the level of CO_2 in expired alveolar gases. In turn, this indicates if ventilation is adequate and also, importantly, whether controlled or spontaneous ventilation is happening at all.

In addition to the standard monitoring outlined above, anaesthetists have a number of other tools at

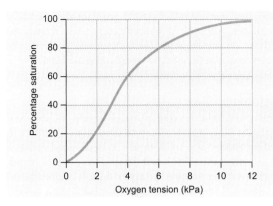

Fig 6.9 **Oxyhaemoglobin dissociation curve.**

their disposal. The degree of muscle paralysis can easily be assessed. In complex cases, the function of the cardiovascular system can be followed invasively with intra-arterial catheters, central venous lines and cardiac output devices. These also allow frequent blood sampling for measurement of haematological and biochemical variables.

However, one measurement which is not easy to make is the depth of anaesthesia. Current research into the effects of anaesthesia on the electroencephalogram (EEG) may produce a device that will be clinically useful for this purpose.

Throughout the procedure the anaesthetist charts the information received from the monitors; this allows observation of developing trends and also acts as a permanent record of events.

Monitoring the anaesthetic machine

Once again the anaesthetist's vigilance is most important. The function of the machine will have been checked before the procedure is embarked upon and regular observation throughout should detect problems. Within the machine there are devices to detect changes in pressure and flow throughout the system. Importantly, incorporated with the capnogram described above are devices which measure the concentration of gases that enter the patient. In particular, it is vital to know that a safe concentration of oxygen is delivered. The device also measures the concentrations of anaesthetic agents which leave the patient's lungs, so enabling approximate adjustment of the depth of anaesthesia.

The anaesthetic machine (Fig. 6.10)

The anaesthetic machine at first glance appears to be a baffling collection of cylinders, gauges, valves and monitors. However, it is really the modern descendant

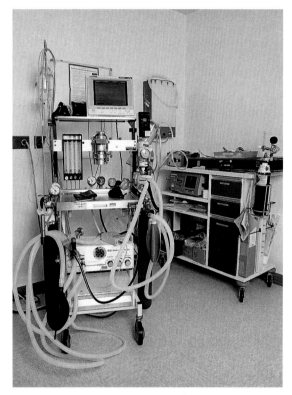

Fig 6.10 **Anaesthetic machine (left) and a difficult airway trolley (right).**

of the very simple systems used to deliver anaesthetics in the 19th century. At that time agents such as ether were dripped onto simple masks held over the patient's face, allowing the inhalation of the vapour produced. The modern machine is designed to deliver highly accurate concentrations of vapours and gases to maintain appropriate levels of anaesthesia while at the same time avoiding rebreathing of expired CO_2.

Flow meters
Anaesthetic gases are delivered to anaesthetic machines from pipelines connected to a central source or from cylinders at high pressures. The pressure is reduced by a series of valves and the flow meters then accurately deliver the gases at atmospheric pressure at the flow rates required.

Vaporisers
The liquid but volatile anaesthetic agents (e.g. halothane, isoflurane) are kept on the anaesthetic machine in vapourisers which allow delivery of accurate concentrations into breathing systems.

Breathing systems
The anaesthetic machine produces a mixture of gases and vapours. To deliver these to the patient without dilution by air, a breathing system (circuit) is used.

There are a number of systems available that have different characteristics and are designed for different circumstances (e.g. paediatric anaesthesia). The details of these systems are outside the scope of this chapter. Two of the most commonly used are the Magill and Bain circuits.

Ventilators
A ventilator is a device that takes over the work of breathing from the patient. Most use a phase of positive pressure to blow gases into the lungs. There are many different types with different characteristics. All ventilators are able to deliver a set volume of gases to the lungs at a set rate and usually have safeguards to prevent too high a pressure being delivered.

Drugs used in anaesthesia

Intravenous induction agents
Ideally the agent used should have a rapid onset of effect, with rapid production of unconsciousness. It should have few side-effects on the cardiovascular and respiratory systems and be quickly metabolised to aid speedy recovery.

Thiopentone
Introduced into clinical practice in 1932, this drug is a sulphur analogue of pentabarbitone (a barbituate). It produces unconsciousness in less than one brain–arm circulation time (about 30 seconds). It is then redistributed to the fat and muscle compartments so its effects wear off relatively quickly. Unfortunately it needs to be used very carefully because too large a dose can cause a severe fall in blood pressure, especially in those who have other factors which can contribute, e.g. hypovolaemia and impaired vasomotor tone. In common with all anaesthetic induction agents, it causes marked respiratory depression. Although painless on intravenous injection, extravasation into the tissues or accidental intra-arterial injection can cause pain and distal ischaemia.

Propofol
This simple molecule (2,6-di-isopropylphenol) has become extremely popular. It has a fast onset of action and is metabolised very rapidly by the liver and other organs. This means that the agent has very few hangover effects and results in a very bright, clear-headed recovery – it is ideal for day-care surgery. Its rapid metabolism also allows use as a continuous infusion, either for a short anaesthetic or as sedation on the intensive care unit. In common with thiopentone it

can cause marked falls in blood pressure and markedly depresses respiration. Unfortunately it is sometimes painful on intravenous injection, and to prevent this, many anaesthetists add a small dose of local anaesthetic (lignocaine) to the solution.

Ketamine
This phencyclidine derivative is somewhat different from the other agents. It can be used as a sedative or to induce anaesthesia. Interestingly, systolic blood pressure is usually raised by ketamine and respiration is not depressed except by very large doses. It is also a good analgesic. Unfortunately it is associated with a high incidence of postoperative hallucinations. It may be used as the sole anaesthetic agent in those with shock and thus has a role in military surgery.

Inhalational maintenance agents

Once anaesthesia has been induced, it must be maintained, usually by inhalational agents. These are mainly ether derivatives (methyl-ethyl ethers) and hydrocarbons (halothane). They are mostly liquids at room temperature and are administered through special vaporisers on the anaesthetic machine, which are calibrated to allow specified concentrations of the vapour to be added to the oxygen and other gases in use for ventilation.

Halothane
This is a halogenated ethane which is pleasant to smell and results in concentrations that reach the required levels in the brain within a few breaths. Like all the volatile agents it depresses respiration and, if given in too high a concentration, can also decrease cardiac output and cause falls in blood pressure. It may sensitise the heart to endogenous or administered catecholamines and so cause arrythmias.

Sevoflurane, desflurane, isoflurane and enflurane
These modern ether derivatives are all useful agents because they have a rapid onset and offset of action. Sevoflurane is pleasant to inhale and is often used to induce anaesthesia by the inhalational route in children who are intolerant of needles. Desflurane is less pleasant but, because it has a very rapid offset of action, is quite frequently used in day-case surgery, where rapid recovery is desirable. Isoflurane is an older agent in common use which has a relatively quick offset of action and has less cardiovascular side-effects than halothane. Enflurane is very similar to isoflurane.

Nitrous oxide
The gas is supplied in blue cylinders which can be connected to the anaesthetic machine. It is an analgesic

gas (colloquially known as laughing gas). Special meters on the anaesthetic machine allow it to be mixed in known proportions with oxygen. Because of its analgesic properties it is widely used in childbirth.

Neuromuscular blocking agents

Muscle relaxant drugs are often used as part of a balanced anaesthetic to allow intubation of the trachea and controlled respiration by intermittent positive pressure ventilation. This is usually necessary for prolonged or major surgery, particularly in the abdomen or thorax. It is also necessary in some emergency situations.

Muscle relaxants may also be used to facilitate assisted ventilation for long periods of time in the intensive care unit.

There are two main types of agent:

Depolarising. These first stimulate contraction by their action at the neuromuscular junction and then produce paralysis. The only clinically important depolarising muscle relaxant is suxamethonium chloride.

Non-depolarising. By contrast, these do not cause any muscle activity before relaxation. These are competitive blockers (see below) at the acetylcholine receptors on the neuromuscular junction. Drugs such as atracurium, vecuronium and pancuronium are examples.

The effects of these drugs can be reversed by the administration of acetyl cholinesterase inhibitors such as neostigmine which increase the concentration of acetyl choline in the neuromuscular junction by preventing its breakdown. The increased concentrations of acetyl choline then compete with neuromuscular blocking drugs (hence the term competitive blockers) for receptors at the neuromuscular junction and muscle power returns.

Suxamethonium

Suxamethonium is a depolarising neuromuscular blocking agent which provides very rapid muscle relaxation (within 30 seconds). It is therefore very useful in emergency work where rapid control of the airway is essential to avoid aspiration of stomach contents. Its effects usually wear off in 2–3 minutes. It is metabolised by plasma cholinesterase (also known as pseudocholinesterase). It does have side-effects as follows:

- postoperative muscle pain
- bradycardia
- release (e.g. in the severely burned) of potassium from muscle cells into the bloodstream which may cause cardiac arrest
- suxamethonium apnoea – approximately 1 in 3000 of the population have an inherited defect in

cholinesterase which causes the muscle paralysing effects to be prolonged, and anaesthesia and respiratory support must be maintained until the effects wear off

- acute anaphylactic shock (rare)
- malignant hyperpyrexia – a condition in which temperature control fails and death may follow.

Vecuronium, atracurium and pancuronium

These are longer-acting, competitive muscle relaxants. They take longer than suxamethonium to relax the muscles (approximately 2–3 minutes) but their effects last longer (sometimes between half an hour and 1 hour). Vecuronium is a useful muscle relaxant with very few side-effects. It is metabolised in the liver and excreted via the kidneys.

Atracurium is also commonly used but can, as a side-effect, release histamine; however, it has the advantage that it is degraded spontaneously in the bloodstream by a process called Hoffman degradation, which is dependent on the temperature and the pH of the plasma and is independent of liver and renal function. It can therefore be used in patients with renal or hepatic failure.

Pancuronium is a much longer-acting muscle relaxant often used during prolonged procedures.

Analgesics

Opioid analgesics

Most balanced anaesthetic techniques use opioids for analgesia. Opioid analgesics mimic endogenous opioid compounds which act at opioid receptors. There are three types of receptor:

- μ (mu)
- δ (delta)
- κ (kappa).

The mu-receptor agonists are most commonly used. Drugs such as morphine and diamorphine have medium-term effects which last 2–4 hours. Shorter-acting opioid derivatives, such as fentanyl and alfentanil, are used intraoperatively for shorter procedures. Opioids can be administered by a number of different routes (see the section on postoperative analgesia).

Morphine

Morphine has potent analgesic and euphoric effects. It also depresses respiration by decreasing the respiratory response to increased levels of carbon dioxide in the blood, and respiration may stop altogether. Among a host of other effects, morphine also causes nausea and vomiting and should be given with an anti-emetic. The effects of morphine and other mu-agonist opioids may be antagonised by naloxone (Narcan). Morphine is metabolised in the liver to active metabolites which are excreted via the kidneys.

Diamorphine

This drug is the di-acetyl ester of morphine and has very similar effects. It is more potent than morphine because of its greater lipid solubility and is therefore given in lower doses. It is said to have less emetic effects and to cause more euphoria than morphine.

Fentanyl

This is a synthetic opioid which is commonly used intraoperatively. It crosses the blood–brain barrier rapidly and its effects wear off within a relatively short time (~ 30 minutes). It is a potent respiratory depressant. In common with the other opioids it also causes nausea and vomiting.

Alfentanil

This short-acting opioid has an even faster onset of action than fentanyl. It is also a very potent respiratory depressant.

Simple analgesics

Although simple analgesics such as paracetamol and aspirin are of limited value on their own after major surgery, they are a useful adjunct to analgesic regimens and may reduce the dose of opioid drugs required.

Paracetamol

The combination of this with codeine formulations is extremely useful in the management of day surgical operations and also if given on a regular basis for more extensive procedures (e.g. Co-dydramol contains 500 mg of paracetamol and 10 mg of codeine).

NSAIDs

This group of drugs is playing an increasing role in the management of postoperative pain. They are effective analgesics and, as part of a balanced approach to pain control, reduce markedly the requirements for opioids. They can now be delivered by all routes (oral, rectal, intramuscularly, intravenously and topically). Caution must be applied when using these drugs as they have well recognised, serious side-effects in the vulnerable patient (e.g. gastric ulceration with bleeding [Ch. 22] and renal failure). The most popular drugs in current use are diclofenac sodium and ketorolac trometamol.

Miscellaneous drugs

Many other drugs are used as part of a balanced technique.

Benzodiazepines

These drugs are used for premedication (e.g. temazepam) and for short-acting intravenous sedation during procedures carried out under regional anaesthesia (e.g. midazolam).

Anti-emetics

Different classes of anti-emetics are used to prevent and treat postoperative nausea and vomiting. Metaclopromide and domperidone act at dopamine receptors in the midbrain. *Anticholinergic agents* (hyoscine) affect the so called vomiting centre, also in the midbrain. *Antihistamines* (e.g. cyclizine) are effective but can cause sedation. A relatively new group of drugs is the *5HT$_3$ antagonists* (e.g. ondansetron).

Postoperative care

Recovery from anaesthesia

Immediate recovery occurs at first in the operating room and then continues as the patient is transferred into the recovery unit which should be a dedicated one, designed, staffed and equipped to deal with all aspects of recovery. Patients are managed in separate bays, each equipped with oxygen, suction and monitoring equipment and adequately staffed by specially trained personnel skilled in management of the unconscious patient, particularly in airway management. As recovery proceeds, vital signs are monitored and the management of fluid balance and oxygenation continues. A check is kept on the operative site to detect any immediate problems such as bleeding. Pain control is also assessed and treatment instituted in consultation with anaesthetic staff. Before a patient is considered fit to leave the recovery room and return to the ward, a number of criteria must be met (Box 6.8). Those who have undergone major procedures or who have

---

Box 6.8

Criteria for discharge from the recovery unit

Awake and cooperative

Cardiovascular stable

Well oxygenated

Pain controlled

Surgical site uncomplicated

Postoperative fluids and drugs charted

complex medical problems may need transfer to a high-dependency unit (HDU) or an intensive care unit (ITU).

Special features of recovery from day surgery

In the UK there has been a considerable increase in day surgery in recent years (Ch. 5). In some hospitals, 60% of routine surgery is done in day care units. It is crucial to the success of this type of service that recovery is sufficiently rapid to allow a safe return home. It is essential that suitable patients are chosen and that the procedures they are to undergo are relatively brief and unlikely to result in significant postoperative pain. The criteria used to discharge patients home after day surgery are similar to those used to discharge in-patients back to hospital wards. However, it is essential that patients and their carers are informed about what to expect when they are at home. In particular, they should be given clear instructions on the analgesia that has been prescribed. With careful patient selection and preoperative education, even fairly complex operations (e.g. laparoscopic hernia repair) can be carried out successfully without in-patient hospital admission.

COMPLICATIONS DURING THE RECOVERY PERIOD

Hypoxia

There are a number of causes:

- Respiratory depression caused by anaesthetic agents and analgesics
- Unconsciousness with airway obstruction
- Ventilation/perfusion mismatch – poorly controlled pain with inadequate expansion particularly of the lung bases, and unresolved pulmonary collapse; most resolve in a relatively short time and can be treated easily with supplementary oxygen.

The requirement for oxygen after operation varies with the the type of operation and the patient's pre-existing condition. However, all patients should receive postoperative oxygen even after minor surgery and the decision to discontinue oxygen should be taken with care and in the light of objective evidence of adequate oxygenation.

Postoperative nausea and vomiting (PONV)

Both of these are common and distressing and are the result of a combination of many factors. Anaesthetic agents and analgesics are often implicated. It is recognised that certain procedures have a very high incidence of PONV (e.g. middle ear operations and gynaecological procedures). A past history of PONV is a common feature. Management is with the agents discussed above.

Postoperative pain

One widely used definition of pain is an unpleasant experience caused by a noxious substance, tissue damage or anticipated tissue·damage: this produces a reaction consisting of withdrawal response, metabolic response, hormonal response and conscious aversion. To discuss treatment it is necessary to look briefly at how pain is produced. Tissue damage (e.g. surgical operation, trauma) causes the release of chemicals – so-called pain mediators (e.g. histamine, bradykinins) – at the site of injury. These stimulate nerve fibres which transmit the sensation of pain via the spinal cord to higher centres where the pain is experienced. Therefore it seems logical that there are several points along this pathway where it might be possible to interrupt and alter the pain message. Anti-inflammatory agents inhibit the release of pain mediators at the site of injury. Local anaesthetic agents can block peripheral and central nerves to prevent the impulses reaching the brain. Opioids (e.g. morphine) act centrally to alter the perception of pain.

Why should pain be treated?

This seems to be a rather simple question. However, the effects of pain on the postoperative patient are diffuse. There is of course the unpleasant experience for the patient and the psychological upset this causes. However, poorly controlled pain can lead to a number of other unhelpful sequelae. Patients who have undergone abdominal or thoracic surgery find breathing and coughing difficult and painful. The consequent inadequate ventilation can lead to hypoxia in the immediate postoperative period and chest infections subsequently (Ch. 16). Chest infections can seriously complicate the recovery period. There is something of a vicious circle here because the prophylaxis and treatment of chest infection involve vigorous physiotherapy, which further exacerbates the problems of pain control. Postoperative pain can lead to hypertension and tachycardia which may stress a vulnerable myocardium. Poor pain control can lead to a slow recovery and delayed mobilisation with increase in the risk of other complications such as deep vein thrombosis (Ch. 29).

How should pain be treated?

A number of techniques and drugs are used. The drugs have been described earlier. Important underlying principles before prescription are as follows:

- Each patient should be treated as an individual and likely needs assessed preoperatively.
- The patient should be involved in and understand the decisions taken.
- Patient confidence in the plan for pain control is vital.
- An important part of pre-assessment is to evaluate which analgesics are safe and whether any technique (e.g. an epidural) is contraindicated.

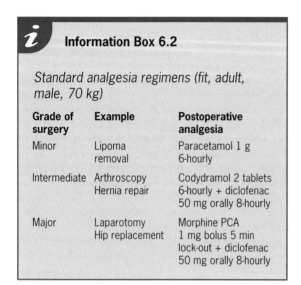

Information Box 6.2

Standard analgesia regimens (fit, adult, male, 70 kg)

Grade of surgery	Example	Postoperative analgesia
Minor	Lipoma removal	Paracetamol 1 g 6-hourly
Intermediate	Arthroscopy Hernia repair	Codydramol 2 tablets 6-hourly + diclofenac 50 mg orally 8-hourly
Major	Laparotomy Hip replacement	Morphine PCA 1 mg bolus 5 min lock-out + diclofenac 50 mg orally 8-hourly

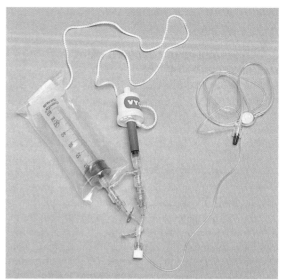

Fig 6.11 **A device for patient-controlled analgesia.**

There are two other important matters. First, postoperative pain is much easier to manage if the patient wakes up with pain already minimised; management should therefore begin during or even before surgery, so-called preemptive analgesia. Secondly, there are a number of different groups of drugs that are analgesic in action; good analgesia can best be achieved by a combination of these, which in turn enables smaller doses of each type to be used, so lessening the risks of side-effects (balanced analgesia).

A fairly simple guide to postoperative pain management is given in Information Box 6.2. It is obvious that the major operations are those where the problems are most difficult.

MANAGEMENT OF PAIN AFTER MAJOR OPERATIONS

A combination of drugs usually produces the best results. This may include the use of local anaesthetic agents either at the site of surgery or as part of a regional nerve block (e.g. epidural) with NSAIDs and opioids. The administration of opioids has changed in recent years and a closer examination of the place of morphine is a useful example.

For many years, morphine given intramuscularly at regular intervals was the mainstay of control, but recently the method has been the subject of criticism. Nevertheless, if morphine is given at regular intervals and at a correct dosage, good analgesia can be achieved. The method is also cheap and safe; however, on a busy surgical ward it can be difficult to make sure that administration is sufficiently frequent and adjusted to individual needs. Therefore other techniques have been developed. Morphine by bolus intravenous injection is a good way of rapidly controlling acute postoperative pain but its use further into the postoperative period is limited by safety factors and the intermittent nature of the analgesia achieved. Morphine

by intravenous infusion allows a steady concentration to build up in the blood. Although this smoothes out some of the breakthrough pain experienced with intramuscular injections, it is difficult to select the correct infusion rate and altering the infusion rate takes a significant time to achieve results. This has led to the widespread introduction of patient-controlled devices (patient-controlled analgesia, PCA).

PCA

The morphine is housed in the reservoir of a pump system and connected to an intravenous cannula; the patient controls the delivery of the drug by pressing a button which causes the device to deliver a predetermined dose (Fig. 6.11). There follows a period (*lock-out time*) when a further press is ineffective, which protects against overadministration. Use of such a device allows the patient to determine analgesic dose according to perceived pain. The device also gives the patient confidence that analgesia is readily available when necessary.

Opioids can also be administered as part of an epidural regimen, usually in combination with a local anaesthetic. However, it is important to note that more involved pain management techniques such as this need more intensive nursing and are probably unsuitable for most general surgical wards. The adverse effects of opioids are discussed above. Box 6.9 lists some suggested doses.

MANAGEMENT OF CHRONIC PAIN

There is a large group of patients who have continuous pain. The types, sites and causes of this pain are many and varied and most specialities have some patients

Box 6.9

*Standard opioid doses
(fit, 70 kg, male)*

Morphine (i.m.)	10 mg 2-hourly PRN
Morphine (PCA)	1 mg bolus 5 min lock-out
Diamorphine (i.m.)	5 mg 2-hourly
Pethidine (i.m.)	75 mg 2-hourly

who experience chronic pain. Anaesthetists have now developed a major interest in this group. The practical skills and the knowledge of analgesics required for standard anaesthetic practice are readily transposed into the management of chronic pain. Most large hospitals now have a chronic pain clinic headed by an anaesthetist. However, it is important to note that the initial management of any patient with chronic pain is to endeavour to achieve a diagnosis and then to treat the underlying cause. A chronic pain specialist uses the skills of a number of other practitioners to treat patients, e.g. psychologists, physiotherapists and acupuncturists.

In most cases, the management of chronic pain involves a multifaceted approach. In chronic back pain (a common condition), an epidural injection may be followed by a course of physiotherapy. At the same time, various analgesics may be prescribed and amitriptyline used for depression. Antidepressants, at the dosages used in chronic pain, seem to have several effects. They have a direct and indirect analgesic effect, the mode of action being unclear. They also help the patient to sleep and the direct antidepressant effect is helpful.

FURTHER READING

Aitkenhead AR, Smith G (1996) *Textbook of Anaesthesia*, 3rd edn. Edinburgh: Churchill Livingstone.

Atkinson RS, Rushman GB, Lee JA (1987) *A Synopsis of Anaesthesia* 10th edn. Bristol: Wright.

Heining, MPD, Bogod DG, Aitkenhead AR (1996) *Essential Anaesthesia for Medical Students*. London: Arnold

7

Perioperative management and postoperative complications

This chapter deals with the maintenance of patients before, during and after an operation and the complications which may ensue. For this purpose, an understanding of the physiological responses to injury (which are common to surgery, trauma and sepsis) is an essential foundation because the changes that occur influence management. The 20th century, particularly after 1930, has been noteworthy for the widespread application of new scientific knowledge and technology to improve perioperative care. Among the areas involved are anaesthesia (Ch. 6), ventilatory support (Chs 6 and 10), blood transfusion, renal dialysis, cardiopulmonary bypass (Ch. 17), antibiotics (Ch. 9) and parenteral nutrition (Ch. 10). Advances in all these and other areas have permitted major surgical procedures to become commonplace with minimal morbidity and mortality.

The growing therapeutic complexity of surgical care has led, as recounted in Chapter 1, to increased specialisation among doctors and the necessity for teamwork. However, the surgeon retains the primary responsibility for perioperative care.

Most complications that follow soon after operations are directly related to the operative procedure. Many can be avoided by good surgical technique. Careful perioperative care, however, can also decrease the incidence of complications and enhance the patient's chance of recovery.

Physiological basis for surgical care

The biological response to injury can be thought of as a wake-up call to optimise performance and integrate the action of body systems (homeostasis) in the face of a potential threat to survival. Priorities are to ensure:

- oxygen delivery (Chs 6 and 10)
- tissue perfusion (Chs 6 and 10)
- acid–base equilibrium (Ch. 6)
- water and electrolyte conservation, balance and replacement
- availability of energy.

The injury response is initially short (hours) but leads on to secondary longer-acting (days to weeks) events, notably restrictions on the excretion of sodium and water, increased metabolic rate and protein catabolism. These distinctive consecutive periods were originally described by Cuthbertson in the 1920s and 1930s, who dubbed them the *ebb* and *flow* phases of metabolism, respectively. They were originally thought to be mediated mainly by the counter-regulatory hormones (catecholamines, cortisol and glucagon); however, it is now clear that the pro-inflammatory cytokines (tumour necrosis factor-alpha [TNF-a], interleukin-1 [IL-1] and interleukin-6 [IL-6]) have more fundamental, although as yet poorly understood, additional regulatory roles. Evidence is also accumulating that, at the tissue level, arachidonic acid metabolites, oxygen-free radicals, nitric oxide and the amino acid glutamine have important controlling effects.

Water and electrolyte metabolism

In a 70 kg male, body composition is approximately:

- fat (15 kg)
- protein (12 kg)
- water (42 kg)
- glycogen and minerals (1 kg).

Total body water (TBW) is divided into two main compartments (Fig. 7.1):

- water around cells (extracellular fluid, ECF) – 19 L
- water in the cytoplasm (intracellular fluid, ICF) – 23 L.

The ECF (Fig. 7.2) is further subdivided into:

- interstitial – 15 L
- intravascular (plasma) – 3 L

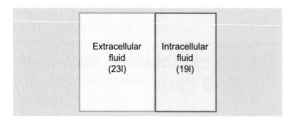

Fig 7.1 **Total body water.**

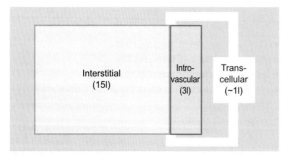

Fig 7.2 **Extracellular water.**

- third space (transcellular – gastrointestinal and renal) – small (~1 L) at any one moment but with a large rate of turnover: approximately 12 L/day for the GI tract and 170 L/day for glomerular filtration; an abnormal third space may develop if the normal transcapillary exchange is interfered with by, say, inflammation so that exudation exceeds reabsorption.

Extracellular fluid contains sodium (Na) at 124 mmol/L and potassium (K) at 4 mmol/L. ICF has concentrations of Na and K opposite to that of ECF: Na at 10 mmol/L and K at 150 mmol/L maintained by the energy-dependent Na/K pump in the cell membrane. With the exception of 1 L of non-exchangeable water enfolded in the quaternary structure of protein molecules, all water molecules in the various compartments and most non-ionised small molecules (e.g. urea) are freely diffusable. The result is that osmolality (overall osmotic concentration in mmol/kg) is maintained uniform throughout the body except at special sites such as the transcellular water in the kidney.

The 24-hour intake and output of water in health is shown in Table 7.1. Sodium intake varies widely with diet, but in the developed world is between 50 and 100 mmol/day. Excretion, mainly via the kidneys, is regulated by the distal renal tubule which is the effector organ of the *renin–angiotensin–mineralocorticoid* endocrine axis. If input of Na falls, so does renal output and, in consequence, the volume of the ECF and tissue perfusion are maintained. If extrarenal losses – vomit, diarrhoea, increased sweating – occur, compensation is not possible (except by replacement by therapy) and the ECF shrinks. Requirements for K are of similar magnitude, approximately 40–80 mmol/day. Excretion is via the kidney and, in contrast to Na, persists even when intake is reduced.

During the perioperative period in major procedures, intravenous (i.v.) fluids are often required for

Table 7.1
Twenty-four hour intake and output of water and electrolyte in health

Substance	Intake	Excretion and route
Water	2000–2500 mL (further 500 mL of water of oxidation which must be taken into consideration if renal excretion is limited)	Kidney (1500 mL) and insensible loss, (respiratory and sweating, 1000 mL)
Sodium	100 mmol	Kidney (although sweat may also contain substantial quantities at up to 120 mmol/L)
Potassium	Up to 100 mmol	Kidney; restricted input is not followed by fall in excretion

a variable period until oral intake can be re-established. As part of the response to injury, the secretion rate of cortisol, aldosterone and antidiuretic hormone (ADH) is increased with the effects in the first 24–48 pos-operative (or post-injury) hours of:

- reduction in renal excretion of Na and consequently of water so that osmolality remains constant
- increase in renal excretion of K, some of which is the result of the amount of tissue damage and breakdown of cells
- decreased renal water excretion with a urine of low volume and high concentration, unresponsive to the normal effect of any increase in water intake.

After this time, and depending on the degree of surgical trauma and the presence or otherwise of sepsis, Na (and water passively) retention may continue, with increased K excretion.

MANAGEMENT
Water and electrolyte therapy (indexed to a 70 kg adult male) are divided into maintenance needs, restoration of pre-existing deficits and replacement of ongoing losses.

Provision of maintenance requirements
- Water – 100 mL/hour, adjusted upwards for fever and/or high ambient temperature
- Sodium – 75 mmol/day but can be further reduced over the first 2 days
- Potassium – 60 mmol/day.

Replacement of pre-existing deficits
Loss of extracellular fluid is combined loss of sodium and water (commonly called dehydration in clinical practice although that word literally means loss of water alone) and is replaced with fluids which have a sodium content close to that in the extracellular space, e.g. normal saline or Hartmann's (Ringer lactate) solution.

Loss from the stomach has special features. Although hydrogen ions are lost, renal compensation takes place with reabsorption increased by the kidney and excretion of potassium and bicarbonate also raised. In con-sequence, hypochloraemic alkalosis and hypokalaemia may develop and slightly more complicated therapy is required.

Pure water loss occurs only when either access to water is impossible (trapped patients after injury) or there is a high obstruction to the gastrointestinal tract (usually oesophageal). Replacement is enteral if the obstruction can be bypassed or by isotonic (6%) dextrose solution given intravenously.

Replacement of ongoing losses
The commonest of these are:

- gastrointestinal – nasogastric aspirate or vomit, fistula and diarrhoea
- loss into an abnormal third space (see above) usually the result of inflammation, e.g. the retroperitoneal effusion that occurs in pancreatitis (Ch. 21)

Assessment is by careful recording of fluid balance, supplemented where possible by daily weighing. Measured upper gastrointestinal losses are replaced with isotonic sodium-containing solutions – normal saline or Ringer lactate – supplemented by potassium.

In losses from gastrointestinal fistulas or diarrhoea, increased amounts of potassium are usually required in that the more distal in the intestine the source, the higher the potassium content.

Third space losses (which are not directly assessable) are replaced with Ringer lactate; the volume administered is determined by observation of those clinical features which indicate a normal ECF volume (adequate filling of the veins and normal central venous pressure; satisfactory perfusion, including renal perfusion and normal urinary output).

Favourable or unfavourable responses to a fluid challenge may also be helpful.

Energy requirements

Assessment of energy requirements in surgical patients must be undertaken with the factors indicated in Box 7.1 in mind. Body energy stores contain approximately 2000 kcal of glucose as glycogen (liver and muscle) and 125 000 kcal of free fatty acids (FFAs) and glycerol hydrolysable from fat.

Tissues, which are largely obligate users of glucose (red blood cells, renal medulla, brain and healing wounds), adapt gradually over some days of starvation to the use of ketones derived from FFAs. Once glycogen stores are exhausted (approximately 24–36 hours), a minimum of 500 kcal/day of glucose is generated by gluconeogenesis from amino acids (plasma protein, muscle and visceral sources). The term 'body protein reserves' is inaccurate; any but the most trivial loss of

---

Box 7.1

Factors affecting energy requirements in the postoperative period

Body weight (at fat-free mass)
Degree of surgical trauma
Sepsis
Nutritional status

protein leads to impairment of function, e.g. muscle weakness and immune deficiency. The theoretical benefit of providing glucose in standard intravenous regimens, which reduces protein breakdown during starvation to a minimum, cannot be relied on in practice adequately to prevent or reverse gluconeogenesis from amino acids because of the altered metabolic milieu of the injured surgical patient.

Energy expenditure

In health, total energy expenditure (TEE) is approximately 40 kcal/kg body weight per day. Resting energy expenditure (REE) is the baseline level of the body's metabolic machinery, i.e. basal metabolic rate (BME) plus the thermic effect of ingested food (dietary induced thermogenesis, DIT) – approximately 25 kcal/kg body weight per day. The difference between TEE and REE (15 kcal/kg body weight per day) is the net energy cost of exercise (activity energy expenditure, AEE).

Elevations of REE between 10 and 30%, often loosely referred to as hypermetabolism or hypercatabolism, are seen in the surgical patient and depend on the degree of surgical trauma and the presence of underlying sepsis. In surgery of low or intermediate severity, this increased REE is compensated for by a fall in AEE (the main cause is that ambulation is reduced perioperatively) and thus the energy requirement is unchanged, at 40 kcal/kg body weight per day. In the more critically ill, considerable expansion of total body water (up to as much as 10 L) can be present; the energy requirement should then ideally be related to the metabolic body size, for which fat-free mass (FFM) is a good substitute, to give a figure of approximately 50 kcal/kg FFM per day. However, accurate methods of body composition analysis are not widely available and body weight remains the usual index. Caution to avoid inadvertent overprescription of nutritional support is therefore required particularly in the obese and/or oedematous.

MANAGEMENT OF ENERGY PROVISION

In most nutritional enteral or parenteral regimens, glucose and fat are usually delivered in roughly equal proportions, although for short-term supplementation (2 weeks), glucose as the sole energy source is acceptable. However, in major injury and sepsis, FFAs appear to be the preferred fuel source and for this reason some fat should be provided. After 3–4 weeks, glucose-only regimens result in the clinical effects of essential FFA deficiency (a rash is the first sign) and subclinical effects are best avoided by the early provision of fat. Energy replacement may be enteral, provided that the gut is functioning, or parenteral, i.e intravenous nutrition. Enteral nutrition has the advantage that the function of the cells of the gut is preserved, which may be of significance in the preservation of their metabolic role and also possibly in the prevention of mucosal atrophy and translocation of bacteria.

Respiratory function in relation to operation

The set of often connected circumstances that threaten respiratory function in surgical patients includes:

- Preoperative respiratory disease.
- Anaesthesia which may, because of a combination of positive pressure ventilation (PPV) and the agents used, result in ventilation–perfusion (V/Q) mismatch and a fall in the arterial oxygen saturation (see also Ch. 6).
- Correction of lowered P_ACO_2 by an increased fraction of inspired oxygen. This reduces the biologically passive nitrogen skeleton of the inspired gas mixture and leads to a patchy collapse of the bronchiolar–alveolar complex; further V/Q defects follow and a vicious cycle is established.
- Hypoventilation and a reduced cough impulse after surgery because of inadequate pain control, supine posture in bed, and the after-effects of anaesthesia and analgesia. Poor expansion of the lungs results, with the formation of mucus plugs to occlude bronchioles leading to further collapse.

Pre-existing respiratory disorders are common because of cigarette smoking and the advanced age of many surgical patients. Restrictive and obstructive (reversible or otherwise) patterns are identifiable in patients with chronic emphysema, bronchitis and asthma. Otherwise healthy patients who have existing, or who are convalescent from, upper respiratory tract infections (URTIs) often have protracted periods of unusual bronchial hyperreactivity which puts them at increased risk of respiratory complications – these are avoidable if elective surgery is deferred. Preoperative treatment with incentive spirometry and chest physiotherapy appears to be of some value to improve overall pulmonary status in preparation for operation. Underlying pulmonary infections such as bronchitis or pneumonia should always be treated and operation delayed if possible because the ciliary paralysis that occurs with anaesthesia may cause severe postoperative pneumonia.

Routine preventative respiratory therapy is frequently used postoperatively to prevent pulmonary complications. Early mobilisation after operation is believed to improve the patient's overall respiratory status.

In high-risk patients, routine postoperative prophylactic chest physiotherapy has been shown to decrease the frequency of pulmonary infection significantly.

In seriously ill patients on respiratory support in the intensive care unit and who are on intravenous nutrition (IVN), high-energy infusions which utilise glucose as the sole energy source may lead to difficulty in disconnection from the ventilator; the cause is the high output of carbon dioxide when energy supply is from glucose (respiratory quotient 1) as compared with fat (respiratory quotient in the region of 0.75). The acidosis produced results in hyperventilation.

Features of preoperative assessment

Preoperative work-up

What is now commonly called a work-up allows:

- screening (Ch. 4) to identify unexpected conditions or medications which may add to the risk and complexity of perioperative management
- evaluation of existing co-morbid conditions and their potential impact on risk
- assessment of these co-morbidities in planning the most appropriate operative procedure and care
- optimising pre-existing conditions to reduce the risk of operation
- initiation of standard perioperative regimens (e.g. preventative antibiotics [Ch. 9] and prophylaxis of deep vein thrombosis).

A routine history of the present complaint(s) and the illness for which surgery is planned must be recorded together with a past history of other conditions and enquiry in relation to other body systems. During physical examination it is important both to confirm that the indications for surgery have not changed and to undertake a comprehensive examination particularly of the cardiovascular and respiratory systems. Investigations are considered in Chapter 4.

Assessment of risk

General and specific risk factors for operation are shown in Box 7.2 (see also Ch. 6.)

Patient preparation for theatre

(see also Ch. 6)

Psychological preparation

To undergo an operation is a major life event. In addition to the procedure itself, the underlying disease may be a cause of considerable stress, especially in patients with malignancy, those needing to undergo life-threatening procedures such as coronary artery bypass (Ch. 17) and transplantation (Ch. 13), and those in whom the diagnosis is uncertain. These situations evoke a natural response of fear and anxiety with which even a well adjusted individual with good support may find it difficult to cope. Surgeons,

---

Box 7.2

Risk factors for operation

General factors
Extremes of age
Poor nutritional status
Cardiovascular disease
Diabetes mellitus
Chronic respiratory disease
Systemic infection
Dehydration or other metabolic abnormalities
Renal impairment
Hepatic disease
Obesity
Malignant disease

Specific factors
Previous operation at the same site – increased operative difficulty and complication rate
Local infection – wound or deep infection
Bladder outflow obstruction – urinary retention
Chronic airways disease – pneumonia
Thrombotic tendency – deep vein thrombosis/ pulmonary embolism
Haemorrhagic disorder or anticoagulant therapy – wound haematoma or postoperative haemorrhage
Previous radiotherapy – poor wound or anastomotic healing/dehiscence
Steroid treatment or cytotoxic chemotherapy – infection, impaired wound healing
Peptic ulcer disease or NSAID treatment – gastrointestinal haemorrhage

---

naturally enough, have a tendency to focus on the technical surgical problem but must also be able to recognise and respond appropriately to psychological distress. Excessive fear and anxiety are often the result of inadequate communication. The importance of clear and honest interchange of views and a willingness to spend time discussing the issues of greatest concern to the patient cannot be over emphasised. Sometimes specialised input will also be required, e.g. from support nurses or psychologists, and is best sought at an early stage. Such assistance is usually accepted if presented in a non-threatening way.

Specific traps for the surgeon include a well recognised, although rare, syndrome in which surgical conditions are mimicked for the purpose of procuring an operation (Munchausen's syndrome). Somatisation – the exaggeration or invention of physical symptoms – is more common and an operation should not be lightly recommended if symptoms are atypical. However, it is imperative to remember that people with psychological and mental disorders are not immune from physical illness and are entitled to the same consideration as others who present with similar clinical features.

Skin preparation

This is discussed in detail in Chapter 5.

Diet and bowel preparation

Any patient who is to have a general anaesthetic should not have anything by mouth for 6 hours beforehand so as to minimise the risk of vomiting and aspiration. Obviously this is not always either possible (emergencies) or effective (bowel obstruction, gastric stasis) and in these cases anaesthetists take specific measures to protect the airway, especially during induction (Ch. 6). For most operations, other specific dietary constraints are not necessary preoperatively. Elective operations on the large bowel are usually preceded by bowel preparation to reduce the risk of septic complications which may follow faecal contamination of the operative field. Recently, several randomised studies have called into question the need to do this for elective large bowel resection when systemic antibiotic prophylaxis is used; nevertheless most surgeons employ bowel preparation routinely, at least for left-sided resections. Methods of bowel preparation are divided into two broad categories:

- mechanical – getting rid of faecal mass
- chemoprophylactic – reduction in the bacterial concentration in the faecal residue.

Mechanical preparation combine a low-residue diet with either purgatives, isotonic lavage solution (e.g. polyethylene glycol) or osmotically active agents. The disadvantages of mechanical preparations include poor patient tolerance and fluid and electrolyte disturbances. Those who receive mechanical bowel preparation and who have cardiovascular or renal impairment are also given maintenance intravenous fluids with potassium supplementation overnight before operation to prevent dehydration and hypokalaemia.

Chemoprophylactic. The evidence regarding the need to supplement systemic antibiotic prophylaxis with oral antibiotics for elective large bowel surgery is conflicting. Many surgeons, particularly in North America, continue to use both. Oral regimens commonly include neomycin in combination with either metronidazole or erythromycin.

Informed consent

This is discussed in detail in Chapter 2.

The postoperative period

POSTOPERATIVE ORDERS

Good communication between the team in the operating room and those responsible for postoperative care is essential. Verbal communication alone is not adequate and a handwritten note of the procedure should be made immediately and leave the operating room with the patient accompanied by the anaesthetic chart and notes (Information Box 7.1). The procedures to be followed must be stated precisely, in uniform terms and with clear legibility. The team (including the anaesthetist) states the specifics of postoperative management to nurses and other members of the health care team via the postoperative orders. The pre-operative work-up should already be available in the notes (whether these are held in hard copy or on a

---

i

Information Box 7.1

Sample postoperative orders

Date	Signatory	Notes
13/5/98	Hardy	*Operation:*
		Surgeon: Mr Laurel
		Assistant: Dr Hardy
		Findings:
		Tumour upper rectum
		No evidence of metastatic disease or other abnormalities. Bowel preparation adequate
		Procedure:
		Anterior resection; stapled colerectal anastomosis; leak test OK, not defunctioned. Pre-sacral drain. Blood loss = 600 mL. Patient stable throughout
		Postoperative orders:
		i.v. fluids as charted
		NG tube free drainage
		Ice to suck
		Routine observations & hourly urine output measurement. Maintain output at greater than 30 mL/h
		Epidural analgesia – see anaesthetic chart for protocol
		Chest physiotherapy as ordered s.c. heparin to continue
		Early mobilisation in conultation with house staff
		i.v. ranitidine as prescribed

NB. No rectally administered medications and no NSAIDs.

14/5/98		Check FBC, urea & electrolytes, creatinine

computer) the preoperative work-up to which has been added the operative procedure performed and postoperative orders.

Postoperative observations

CLINICAL SIGNS

A variety of physical signs are important to recognise in the postoperative period (Table 7.2). Other physical signs may be present after specific operative procedures, e.g. changes in pulse characteristics after vascular procedures or neurological changes after neurosurgical procedures. The postoperative instructions must be sufficiently clear so that the nursing staff can notice and report the development of such specific features.

Monitoring

This is the term commonly used for routine observations undertaken on the assumption that deviations from normal values, particularly if they are progressive, indicate that something may be amiss. What is measured is guided by a thorough understanding of the preoperative status and medical history, the diagnosis that led to the operation, what procedure was done and the circumstances. The variables chosen (often called 'vital signs') are mostly in the cardiovascular and respiratory systems (Table 7.3).

If the patient is sent to the intensive care unit (ICU) this usually implies that there are grounds for believing that the postoperative course may be complicated and that additional monitoring is required. Table 7.4 shows the additional vital signs frequently used.

Table 7.2
Specific signs that may be important in the early postoperative period

Sign	Possible meanings
Respiratory distress Tachypnoea Cyanosis	Hypoxia
CNS depression	Oversedation Carbon dioxide retention
Agitation	Blood loss Hypoxia Pain
Disorientation	Inappropriate sedation Hypoxia
Severe inappropriate pain	Local complication at site of operation – bleeding, leakage of secretions, ischaemia
Wound Bleeding Soft tissue haematoma	Uncontrolled blood vessel Clotting disorder
Irregular pulse	Unrecognised cardiac disorder Hypoxia
Skin pallor, empty veins hypotension, tachycardia	Hypovolaemia

Table 7.3
Routine postoperative monitoring of clinical signs

Measurement	Possible significance
Temperature	
Low	Excessive heat loss during surgery Reduced metabolic rate possibly from poor peripheral perfusion
High	Core but not peripheral – peripheral vasoconstriction possibly from blood loss Core and peripheral – 1–2∞ normal in first 24 hours but thereafter may mean sepsis
Pulse rate, blood pressure	Changes beyond minor variations imply possible circulatory instability
Central venous pressure	Usually a sensitive guide to venous return to the heart
Respiratory rate Increased	Possible carbon dioxide retention or hypoxia
Decreased	Oversedation
Urine output (hourly)	Indirect measure of renal perfusion and therefore of organ blood flow
Fluid intake/output	Necessary to ensure that neither over – or under infusion takes place

Table 7.4
Additional vital signs often measured in the ICU

Sign	Possible significance
Direct measurement of arterial pressure (indwelling catheter usually in radial artery)	Earlier detection of changes in blood pressure
Continuous monitoring of CVP	Assessment of venous return
Pulmonary artery pressure (indwelling pulmonary catheter)	Detection of left heart strain (myocardial failure or artery over-infusion) Determination of cardiac output by dilution techniques
Pulmonary artery wedge pressure pressure (Swan–Ganz catheter)	As for pulmonary artery
Pulse oximetry	Arterial oxygen saturation
Continuous ECG	Detection of arrythmias

LABORATORY INVESTIGATIONS

A variety of laboratory tests may be routinely obtained postoperatively to assess the patient's course and detect changes that may require management to be altered (Table 7.5). However, these should not be a substitute for careful physical examination.

In interpreting laboratory findings after major surgical procedures, the following are important:

● A surgical procedure always tends to make diabetics more hyperglycaemic although this does not

Table 7.5
Laboratory investigations in routine postoperative management

Investigation	Purpose	Frequency
Blood glucose concentration in diabetics	Control of insulin administration	4–6 hourly
Haemoglobin concentration	After blood loss in excess of 500 mL	Once after lapse of 24–36 hours and also after transfusion
White cell count	If there is suspicion of sepsis	Daily if initial value raised
Platelet count	Unexplained bleeding	Daily if thrombocytopenia identified
Serum sodium, potassium and urea concentrations	When parenteral fluids are required, e.g. after some gastrointestinal operations	Daily
Arterial P_{O_2}, P_{CO_2} and pH	In borderline respiratory insufficiency	Daily or more frequently if respiratory failure is imminent or identified

necessarily mean that either insulin or an increase in the dose usually being administered is required.

- Haemodilution after haemorrhage takes up to 24 hours. A continued fall in haemoglobin after this time means that there is further bleeding (see 'Postoperative haemorrhage' below).
- The white blood cell count normally increases slightly after operation for 2–3 days; persistent elevation only becomes significant after this time.
- Mild thrombocytopenia normally accompanies major injury, massive transfusion and major operative procedures (e.g. cardiac bypass).
- In healthy individuals with normal renal function there is a slight fall in serum sodium concentration for the first 2–5 days after a major operation, which may be exaggerated or prolonged if there is overinfusion of water. In patients with chronic renal or hepatic disease or an illness that causes electrolyte derangement, concentration changes are difficult to predict and frequent measurements are indicated so that life-threatening hypo- and hyperkalaemia can be rapidly corrected.

Intravenous (parenteral) fluids

The major (normal) changes in water and electrolyte metabolism which influence management are:

- secretion of antidiuretic hormone (ADH) in response to pain and other stimuli so that the normal response to water administration is suppressed and urine of high concentration and low volume is inevitable; the duration of such obligatory oliguria is 24–36 hours
- reduction in renal sodium excretion, for 36–48 hours
- increase in potassium excretion which may be greater if there is a considerable amount of tissue damage.

For two reasons nearly all patients return from the operating room with an intravenous infusion in place:

- replacement has been considered necessary because of losses (insensible water, blood) sustained during the procedure
- a route is required for the administration of drugs or other pharmaceuticals such as antibiotics.

Continued parenteral therapy is required only until normal enteral absorption is restored. In general this is no more than 24–36 hours and often less. Normal postoperative circumstances in which a more prolonged period of intravenous therapy may be required are:

- gastrointestinal procedures where recovery of absorption of fluid may be delayed
- unconsciousness.

In an adequately hydrated patient who has undergone a procedure with minimal blood loss and for whom the postoperative recovery period is expected to

---

ⓘ Information Box 7.2

Standard daily postoperative maintenance fluids

Nature	Amount (L)	Time period (h)
Dextrose 5% + 30 mmol/L potassium	1	8
Sodium chloride 0.9% (normal saline)	1	8
Dextrose 5% + 30 mmol/L potassium	1	8

	Totals
Water	3 L
Sodium	140 mmol
Potassium	90 mmol

Table 7.6
Effects of postoperative pain

Effect	Outcome
Decreased respiratory excursion	Hypoventilation Pulmonary collapse/consolidation
Gastrointestinal atony	Ileus, nausea and vomiting
Bladder atony	Urinary retention
Catecholamine release	Vasoconstriction; increased blood viscosity, clotting activity and platelet aggregation; raised cardiac work

be short, maintenance fluids are sufficient (Information Box 7.2).

Pain and its relief (see also Ch. 6)

Surgical intervention almost always causes pain. Because it can have serious physiological and psychological consequences (Table 7.6), prevention is best, but if that cannot be completely achieved, rapid and adequate relief is essential. The intensity of postoperative pain that is perceived by the patient is influenced by:

- cultural and family background, upbringing, personality, constitution, past experiences and motivation
- amount of information provided preoperatively – the more the better is a good guide
- psychological factors which are often situation-specific, such as emotional arousal and fear; a calm reassuring attitude from the team is of great value and is helped by close interpersonal relations with the patient
- preoperative and postoperative support provided by the whole team, which includes nurses and physiotherapists.

MANAGEMENT

Management has increasingly become a specialised province of either the anaesthetist or a pain management team (Ch. 6).

Prevention

A caring, sympathetic and informative approach by the team does much to reduce the patient's perception of pain, as does assurance that any pain felt will be relieved at once. Physical methods for preventing pain include:

- gentle surgical technique with minimal tissue damage
- adequate immobilisation of areas that have been operated on when this is possible – limbs in particular and after orthopaedic procedures
- blockade of nerve impulses which may be achieved at a number of sites on the afferent pathway.

Therapy

All agents are better given on a regular basis rather than withheld until relief is asked for.

Non-steroidal anti-inflammatory agents and drugs such as aspirin and paracetamol are often sufficient for mild postoperative pain provided the patient can swallow.

Narcotic (opioid) analgesics have long been the main agents used to counteract postoperative pain and morphine sulphate remains the drug most widely used. Immediately after operation they are given by the parenteral route either intramuscularly or intravenously. It is now common for a continuous infusion to be used so that saturation of opioid receptors in the brain is achieved. Such an infusion may be supplemented by patient-controlled analgesia in which the patient can trigger the administration of a small bolus of drug by a syringe driver which is programmed so as to avoid excessive self-administration. This technique has obvious advantages in terms of satisfaction and in reducing the load on the nursing staff. More complicated regimens are considered in Chapter 6.

Tubes and drains

The nature of tubes and drains placed at operation varies with the operation performed and the individual surgeon (Table 7.7). A more detailed consideration is given in Chapter 5.

Table 7.7
Tubes and drains after surgical procedures

Purpose	Nature	Indications
Gastrointestinal decompression	Medium-bore nasogastric tube; gastrostomy	Controversial – see text: operations on the GI tract; need for enteral nutrition
Removal of blood and serous fluids	Open drainage by soft rubber or plastic wicks Closed drainage by tubes, preferably with suction	Extensive dissections Large dead space
Drainage of pus found at operation	Wicks or (preferably) tubes	Persistent infected cavity
Channel for exit if leakage occurs	Usually small- to medium-bore tubes often with suction	Suture lines in the GI tract (often routinely used but little evidence to support this)

Decompression of the gastrointestinal tract

The rationale is that, in abdominal procedures, a period of gastrointestinal paralysis follows:

- abdominal incisions and handling of abdominal organs
- retroperitoneal dissection.

As a result, gastrointestinal secretions accumulate in the stomach and proximal small bowel and may cause vomiting and aspiration into the respiratory tree.

However, in spite of a good deal of study, the exact circumstances when this occurs have not been accurately established and there is little clinical evidence to support the routine use of either nasogastric intubation or gastrostomy. Nasogastric tubes in particular are uncomfortable for the patient and may contribute to respiratory complications by making coughing more difficult. Surgical teams now usually adopt a highly selective policy. Nasogastric decompression is appropriate in any patient in whom nausea, vomiting or gastric distention cannot be otherwise controlled.

Urethral drainage

A balloon urethral catheter (Foley) is commonly used after major procedures and serves two main purposes:

- alleviates discomfort and prevents urinary retention
- allows measurement of hourly urine output.

When hourly or frequent assessment of urine volume is no longer required and the patient is thought able to void spontaneously, the catheter is removed. Voiding is affected by postoperative pain, drugs (opiates, anticholinergics), regional anaesthesia (caudal, spinal, epidural blockade) and any pre-existing prostatism (Ch. 32). Males need to be comfortable enough to stand out of bed. Once the catheter is removed, documentation of adequate voiding is required. Even if voiding is successful, it is important not to allow the bladder to become overdistended, because this delays recovery of detrusor tone and may even necessitate the discharge of the patient with a catheter in situ and subsequent return for a retrial of voiding.

Parenteral and enteral feeding

This type of feeding is discussed in detail in Chapter 10.

Postoperative complications

All operations have a risk of complications, both general and local. Some can occur after any operation, irrespective of its site, while others are the consequence of a particular surgical procedure.

Classification may be into early and late, by pathophysiological nature or by relation to specific site or nature (infection, circulation or respiration); a mix of all these is used here. House officers (interns) play an essential part in the recognition and management of impending or actual complications, as do nursing staff. In consequence, students, all of whom will become preregistration house officers, must understand what may happen in the immediate aftermath of a surgical procedure.

Prophylaxis

Pre-emptive action is an essential feature of perioperative care. Ideally it should be:

- cost-effective
- without additional risk to or discomfort for the patient.

Prophylaxis has become the leading indication in surgical patients for the prescription of antibiotics (Ch. 8). Although their judicious use can reduce overall costs and prevent morbidity, inappropriate use is expensive and leads to the emergence of multiresistant strains of bacteria. Use must therefore be based on sound principles and evidence derived from properly conducted clinical trials.

Wound infection

Surgical wounds are categorised into four classes:

- clean
- clean-contaminated
- contaminated
- dirty.

A clean wound is achieved by aseptic technique (Ch. 5) and is not exposed to any additional contamination during the procedure (e.g. inguinal hernia repair, thyroidectomy). A clean-contaminated wound is produced either where a violation of aseptic technique occurs or where there is exposure during the procedure to known or potentially infected material (e.g. appendicectomy for uncomplicated appendicitis, elective bowel resection). A contaminated wound is exposed to more major contamination (e.g. after entry into the unprepared gastrointestinal tract or into an infected urinary or respiratory tract). A dirty wound is one which is contaminated by established sepsis (e.g. laparotomy in peritonitis, thoracotomy in empyema).

In general, the rate of infection is lowest for clean and highest for dirty wounds; however, other patient factors (e.g. immunosuppression, shock) and surgical factors (e.g. duration of the operation, wound haematoma) also have an influence.

SURGICAL PREVENTATIVE MEASURES

Wound management
Occasionally in contaminated wounds or if there is a delay in instituting management, the risk of wound sepsis is high and it is more effective initially to leave the wound open and then undertake delayed primary or secondary closure (Ch. 8).

Skin preparation
Any surgical wound, including abdominal wounds, can become infected with skin organisms such as *Staphylococcus aureus* (pus-forming) or *Streptococcus pyogenes* (wound cellulitis). Measures to reduce the risk are considered in Chapter 5.

Antibiotics
For clean and clean contaminated wounds, antibiotic prophylaxis – by saturating the tissues with the agent before (in the case of an operation) or as soon as possible after the wound has been sustained (injury) – has been shown to reduce the incidence of wound infection by about two-thirds. The important issues to consider are:

- choice of agent
- route of administration
- timing
- duration of prophylaxis.

The choice of agent must reflect the likely spectrum of contaminating organisms. For operations which involve the upper gastrointestinal tract, this is predominantly facultative aerobic Gram-negative bacilli such as *Escherichia coli*. Examples of antibiotics which provide prophylaxis against Gram-negative organisms include second- and third-generation cephalosporins, aminoglycosides and clavulinic acid/amoxicillin. In the lower gastrointestinal tract, additional cover for anaerobes (mainly *Bacteroides*) is required. Selected second- and third-generation cephalosporins have some activity against anaerobes but metronidazole is usually given in addition. Clavulinic acid/amoxicillin provides good prevention against anaerobes but the aminoglycosides do not. Gram-negative bacilli often contaminate the obstructed urinary tract and the spectrum of normal vaginal flora is similar to that found in the lower gut.

The route of administration depends on the drug and the patient. A non-functioning gut or a poorly absorbed drug contraindicates oral administration. Rectal administration is cheap and effective for some antibiotics (e.g. metronidazole). However, the intravenous route is most commonly used. Timing is important as the aim is to achieve adequate tissue levels at the time of contamination. Rectal or orally administered antibiotics may be given with the premedication (about 1 hour preoperatively), whereas intravenous antibiotics are usually given on induction of anaesthesia.

In the past, prophylactic antibiotics were often continued for up to 72 hours postoperatively. However, more recent trials have shown that a single dose with a drug whose half-life is long enough to maintain effective levels for 6–8 hours is just as effective. In prolonged procedures a second dose should be administered after 6 hours.

Prosthesis infection

A wide variety of biomechanical devices are implanted surgically. These include:

- artificial heart valves (Ch. 17)
- vascular grafts (Ch. 28)
- joint replacements (Ch. 33)
- vascular access devices (e.g. for administration of drugs or renal dialysis)
- cardiac pacemakers.

Prosthesis infection can be life-threatening (e.g. an infected prosthetic heart valve) and is a disaster for the patient which at least necessitates removal of the infected device. Therefore, whenever possible, prosthetic devices are inserted via surgical incisions made under ideal conditions (Ch. 5). Many surgeons, particularly for orthopaedic implantations (Ch. 33), routinely use antibiotics even though the procedure is clean. The most common contaminating organisms are derived from the skin or, more exceptionally, from the operating room environment. Infection subsequent to implantation may also occur from transient bacteraemia. Organisms which have become implanted in a prosthesis may remain silent for months or years before giving rise to symptoms.

PROPHYLAXIS
Antibiotic prophylaxis against prosthesis infection is combined with meticulous care to protect the operating field (Ch. 5). The agent should cover staphylococcal species, including *Staph. epidermidis*. The principles which govern timing, route and duration of therapy are similar to those for prophylaxis of wound infection. A patient with a prosthesis already in place should be given antibiotics if any procedure which might cause transient bacteraemia (e.g. a dental extraction) is necessary.

Taking all of these factors into account, there are a number of different antibiotic prophylactic regimens suitable for any given procedure. The final choice is usually dictated by local hospital policy taking into account:

- cost
- known local antibiotic sensitivities
- need to reserve important therapeutic agents for use in therapy and avoid the ever-present risk of the emergence of resistant strains.

Most hospitals have an Infection Control Committee which monitors local trends and conditions and provides guidelines (Ch. 9).

Respiratory complications

PATHOPHYSIOLOGY

Pulmonary complications are common after general surgery and other operative procedures. In addition to any exacerbation of infection already present, the primary event is pulmonary collapse. In one study, dependent atelectasis (3–4% of lung volume) developed in 100% of patients 5–10 minutes after administration of anaesthesia; 1 hour later, collapse was present in 90%; and at 24 hours, it was still a feature in 50%. Up to 40% of the obese show evidence of basal pulmonary collapse on initial postoperative X-ray. Once an unrelieved segment of collapse is present, secondary infection is almost inevitable and pneumonia ensues. Factors which contribute to postoperative pulmonary collapse are shown in Box 7.3.

Those with pre-existing chronic lung disease and who smoke are particularly likely to progress to respiratory infection because they commonly harbour organisms in the lower respiratory tract, including *Pneumococcus* and *Haemophilus* species. If collapse persists, pneumonia in non-ventilated bronchoalveolar units is likely to follow.

PROPHYLAXIS

Prophylaxis is aimed at interrupting the sequence of events culminating in postoperative respiratory infection at several levels:

- At-risk patients are identified preoperatively (Ch. 6) and, for elective procedures, every effort is made to improve respiratory function; physiotherapy, bronchodilators and specific antimicrobial therapy based on sputum cultures may all have a role.

Box 7.3

Factors which contribute to postoperative pulmonary complications

Wound pain, particularly in the upper abdomen and chest

Limitation of respiratory excursion

Ciliary paralysis

Drying of bronchial secretions

Oversedation

Obesity

- Antibiotic prophylaxis with an agent which covers most common pathogens in the gut, e.g. second- and third-generation cephalosporins, usually also provides adequate perioperative respiratory protection; established respiratory infection requires specific therapy (Ch. 9).
- Adequate pain relief is essential in the postoperative period (Ch. 6) and is combined with early mobilisation, chest physiotherapy and regular incentive spirometry.

MANAGEMENT

Chest physiotherapy and appropriate antibiotic treatment are used for established pulmonary collapse and infection. Oxygen supplementation and other forms of respiratory support may also be necessary (see Chs 6 and 10).

Deep vein thrombosis

This is discussed in detail in Chapter 29.

Complications associated with indwelling vascular catheters

Central venous catheters (single or multiluminal) and arterial catheters may be associated with perforation of the vascular system, thrombus formation and infection. In one study, complications related to initial catheter placement occurred in 5.7%, sepsis in 6.5% and mechanical difficulties (commonly major venous thrombosis or nursing mishaps) in 9%. Careful technique and monitoring and the use of heparin-coated catheters can help keep the incidence low.

Complications of placement are haemorrhage and, for central venous catheters, pneumothorax (Ch. 11).

MANAGEMENT

Central venous thrombophlebitis and/or sepsis usually require immediate removal and parenteral antibiotic therapy; absolute indications are:

- continued fever without other cause
- repeated positive blood cultures despite antibiotic therapy.

An effective method of assessing catheter contamination in patients with central lines in place is routine catheter exchange and culture.

Urinary complications

Although a urinary catheter has advantages, its placement can lead to a number of complications, the most common of which is urinary tract infection. The distal urethra is normally colonised with bacteria and even a single catheterisation results in urinary tract infection in 1% of ambulatory patients. Infection develops within 3–4 days of catheterisation in 95% of those managed with indwelling catheters attached to open drainage systems. In general surgery patients, the overall infection rate after operation is 10% and a quarter of these occur secondary to urinary tract infections; for example, 50% of orthopaedic infections and 75% of urological and medical infections are related to a urinary tract cause.

Escherichia coli is by far the most common pathogen, although other Enterobacteriaceae are also frequent. Staphylococci, streptococci and enterococci also cause urinary tract infection.

MANAGEMENT
The catheter should be removed as soon as it is no longer necessary. Appropriate antibiotic therapy and the maintenance of a high-volume urine output usually suffice unless urinary tract obstruction is present (see Ch. 32).

Upper gastrointestinal bleeding

Before the routine administration of antacids, life-threatening upper gastrointestinal bleeding was a common problem in those with major stress, particularly head injury, burns or multiple trauma. Standard prophylaxis is now 30–60 mL of antacids by nasogastric tube every 1–2 hours to maintain gastric pH above 4. With adequate prophylaxis, the incidence of massive upper gastrointestinal bleeding is almost zero.

Diabetes mellitus

The diabetic patient presents a number of management problems in the postoperative period. Precise control of blood glucose levels is necessary to avoid hypoglycaemia or hyperglycaemia with associated complications such as diabetic ketoacidosis and dehydration secondary to glycosuria.

Uncontrolled diabetes has a significant negative impact on wound healing. For patients whose disease is managed by diet alone, additional measures are usually unnecessary. In the postoperative period, careful monitoring, including finger-prick glucose measurements every 4–6 hours, is appropriate with a sliding scale of regular insulin administered as needed. In those who are receiving oral hypoglycaemic agents, the medication is discontinued on the day before operation and insulin used as necessary to control hyperglycaemia. In those who normally require insulin, an intravenous dextrose infusion and one-half of the total daily dose of insulin as regular insulin is given on the morning of the operation.

Glucose is administered throughout the operation, as guided by repeated measurement of glucose levels. In those who require major procedures and extensive fluid administration, blood glucose is measured frequently during operation and insulin given intravenously as necessary. Postoperatively, glucose levels in some patients are well controlled by administration of insulin on a sliding scale based on finger-prick monitoring of blood glucose.

Acute parotitis

Although now rare, this complication can occur in serious illness if mouth hygiene is deficient and dehydration develops. The gland swells rapidly with signs of local infection and early pus formation.

Initial management is by intravenous antibiotics. If there is no response, pus is likely and the gland should be incised using Hilton's method. Attention to mouth hygiene and a dental consultation are also required.

Pressure sores

Although not restricted to the postoperative period, age, obesity and immobility after operation do contribute to what should be regarded as a preventable condition.

Psuedomembranous enterocolitis

This complication may follow prolonged (and often inappropriate) use of systemic antibiotics. The cause is colonisation of the large bowel with *Clostridium difficile* and the acute, sometimes fulminant, infection that follows.

The clinical features are diarrhoea usually 3–4 days after operation which may be associated with abdominal distension, hypotension and shock. Blood and mucus, sometimes with a cast of the distal large bowel, may be passed per rectum. Diagnosis is confirmed by identification of *Clostridium difficile* exotoxin in the stool. Initial management is non-operative and with intravenous fluid replacement and metronidazole and vancomycin. The development of *toxic dilatation* may necessitate emergency colectomy.

Intraperitoneal abscess

The two common anatomical sites for this type of abscess are pelvic and subphrenic. Both are usually the consequence of leakage from the gastrointestinal tract or from operations for intestinal perforation and peritonitis, e.g. perforated peptic ulcer (Ch. 18), perforated appendicitis (Ch. 24) and perforated diverticulitis (Ch. 24). The organisms involved are of

Table 7.8
Specific findings in intraperitoneal abscess

Features	Pelvic	Subphrenic	Elsewhere

Symptoms	Urgency of defection
	Mucous diarrhoea
	Sometimes blood in stool
	  if abscess ruptures into rectum
		RUQ pain (but often absent)
		Respiratory complications
		Hiccough
			Vague
			Subacute intestinal
			  obstruction

Findings	Abdominal – nothing or slight
	  lower distension from coils
	  of bowel above the abscess
	PR – tender (referred to
	  anterior abdominal wall)
	  boggy mass also felt PV in
	  female
		Upper abdominal tenderness
		Diminished diaphragmatic
		  movement on affected side
		  (usually right)
		Collapse/consolidation of lung,
		  and pleural effusion
			Nil or those of intestinal
			  obstruction

Supplementary investigations	Straight X-ray for intestinal
	  obstruction
	Ultrasound/CT scanning
		Straight X-ray for lung signs
		  and presence of gas under
		  the diaphragm
		Ultrasound/CT scanning
			Straight X-ray for
			  intestinal obtruction
			Ultrasound/CT scanning
			Labelled leucocyte scan

Special points	Postoperative diarrhoea must
	  be investigated
		Pus somewhere, pus nowhere
		  else = pus under the
		  diaphragm
			Re-exploration must be
			  considered if there is
			  poor recovery and features
			  of sepsis after an
			  abdominal procedure

enteric origin: *Bacteroides* (anaerobic) and usually *E. coli* (aerobic).

The clinical features common to either site are malaise and persistent or recrudescent fever from after the fourth postoperative day. The specific findings are in Table 7.8.

MANAGEMENT

In the early stages, systemic antibiotics are given. However, evidence of obvious failure of the infection to resolve requires drainage either by percutaneous means or at open operation. Pelvic abscesses can usually be drained into the rectum.

Wound dehiscence

Wounds fail to heal and may then burst open because of:

- sepsis
- failure of adequate progression of healing
- distractive forces, especially in the abdomen.
- poor surgical technique.

There are three types of wound dehiscence:

- *Superficial and revealed* – occurs at about 2 weeks when the skin sutures are removed and the skin and subcutaneous layers separate; the cause is most often a wound haematoma or cellulitis
- *Deep and concealed* – occurs at any time in the postoperative period and gradually, with separation of all layers of the abdominal wall with the exception of the skin. If not recognised while the

patient is in hospital and given that the skin unites, an incisional hernia always develops at a later date. The cause is usually a combination of faulty technique and impaired healing, usually with emphasis on the first.

- *Complete and revealed* – occurs on about the 10th day gradually or suddenly with the protrusion of a knuckle or loop of bowel or a portion of the omentum through a wound which is completely separated in the whole or part of its length (burst abdomen).

Burst abdomen was once a relatively common event in general surgery. The incidence is now very low as a result of mass closure of the abdominal wall using an appropriate suture material (slowly absorbed or non-absorbable, strong) and good technique (large, closely spaced bites of tissue). Rarely, abdominal disruption may be the consequence of a paroxysmal rise in intra-abdominal pressure (coughing) or the rapid accumulation of ascites (cirrhosis).

A complete dehiscence is usually heralded by sero-sanguineous or blood-stained discharge from the wound. In some instances, a concealed disruption may become obvious when superficial sutures are removed and bowel or omentum protrudes through the wound.

MANAGEMENT

This depends on the type of dehiscence (see Table 7.9)

Enterocutaneous fistula

This is characterised by a communication between the gastrointestinal tract and the skin surface. The most

Table 7.9
Management of abdominal wound dehiscence

Type	Management
Superficial and revealed	Lay skin and subcutaneous tissues open; treat infection. Once wound is granulating either allow this to proceed to healing by secondary intention or carry out secondary suture
Deep and concealed	Usually only recognised late in convalescence; provided the skin remains intact, repair is deferred until recovery is complete unless there is a high risk of a strangulation through the incisional hernia
Complete and revealed	Urgent re-suture of all layers by mass closure

common aetiological factors are listed in Box 7.4. The clinical features are usually systemic sepsis followed by the development of inflammation on the abdominal wall or in the abdominal wound. Initially, pus may be discharged, but this is rapidly followed by intestinal content, the quantity of which varies according to the level of the fistula.

Clinically fistulae are usually classified as of either high or low output. The former occurs predominantly in the upper gastrointestinal tract from stomach to terminal ileum, where output may be a litre or more a day and is further increased if distal obstruction is present. The latter is characteristic of large bowel fistulae or those which are not associated with complete division of the bowel or distal obstruction.

The local effects of fistulae are variable, but if the effluent contains digestive enzymes (stomach to terminal ileum), rapid digestion and secondary septic infection of the abdominal wall take place. The general effects are:

- water and electrolyte loss
- malnutrition from failure of absorption and the increased catabolism of the septic state.

Box 7.4

Aetiological factors in enterocutaneous fistula

Wound pain, particularly in the upper abdomen and Anastomotic dehiscence (see Ch. 000)

Intestinal obstruction (distal to anastomosis)

Chronic inflammatory disease (e.g., Crohns, Tuberculosis)

Previous irradiation

Intestinal ischaemia

MANAGEMENT
The management of fistulae is often complex, although many close spontaneously unless there is distal obstruction, mucocutaneous union or a persistent infective focus. Until closure takes place, nutritional and electrolyte support is necessary as is protection of the skin from digestion. If any of the factors which prevent closure are present, operation is required once the fluid and electrolyte losses, malnutrition and sepsis have been corrected.

Postoperative circulatory failure

Correct diagnosis of circulatory failure (rapid low-volume pulse, hypotension) in the postoperative period is essential because management can be life-saving and has to be instituted as a matter of considerable urgency. The possible aetiological factors which need to be considered are listed in Box 7.5.

Haemorrhage
Major postoperative bleeding can be recognised by:

- evidence of overt bleeding including heavily bloodstained fluid from a drain
- cold and wet (clammy) peripheries
- distension after abdominal procedures.

Usually the diagnosis is self-evident but occasionally it may not be apparent that major bleeding has occurred, particularly if the patient is obese or if the drain malfunctions because of obstruction by clot. In such circumstances the diagnosis may need to be confirmed by urgent, repeated haemoglobin estimation and by ultrasound examination.

Management
The loss is stopped by control of the source of bleeding or by correction of coagulopathy. Either at the same time or immediately subsequently, transfusion, guided in rate and quantity by the circulatory indices, corrects the deficit. Re-operation may be required to control a bleeding point.

Box 7.5

Causes of postoperative circulatory collapse

Haemorrhage

Severe sepsis including septicaemia

Myocardial infarction

Pulmonary embolism

Hypersensitivity reaction

Severe sepsis and septicaemia

Septic circulatory failure is associated with:

- surgical procedures carried out in the presence of sepsis
- technical failure (anastomotic dehiscence) with intraperitoneal or intrathoracic leakage of gastrointestinal contents
- general spread from a focus, particularly if there is a reduced ability of the body to resist the multiplication of the organisms (impaired immunity, leucopenia)
- bloodstream contamination from a device, most commonly a central venous cannula.

A direct effect of circulating cytokines and other inflammatory mediators is to cause arteriolar dilatation so that, in contrast to other forms of circulatory failure, the peripheries may be warm. In addition there is loss of circulating blood volume as a result of capillary leak. If the infection is overwhelming the blood pressure is profoundly reduced and the circulation resembles that of profound hypovolaemia.

Usually the clinical features are:

- high pyrexia
- hypotension
- tachycardia
- a warm periphery.

Investigation

Venous blood is sent for culture, but even if this proves negative the diagnosis of severe sepsis may still be correct and treatment should be begun with a best guess antibiotic combination. A search is made for a focus, e.g. a central catheter or an undrained abscess.

Management

Resuscitation is with intravenous fluids and intravenous antibiosis. Re-exploration may be indicated to deal with a septic focus or a technical failure.

Myocardial infarction and pulmonary embolism

This is not the appropriate place for a detailed description of these important central causes of shock. In those at risk, baseline measurements of ECG may help comparisons and so the diagnosis. Prolonged preoperative immobilisation may suggest that the likely cause of postoperative collapse is a pulmonary embolism (Ch. 29).

Hypersensitivity reaction

This may develop as an immune response to a blood infusion or to drug administration, e.g. intravenous antibiotic. There is usually pyrexia and the circulatory collapse may also be accompanied by respiratory distress and urticaria. Treatment includes discontinuing the drug/infusion, intravenous corticosteroids and circulatory support.

8

Wound healing and management

Any breach in the surface of the body (which includes the gastrointestinal tract) or any tissue disruption deep to the skin produced by the application of *energy* is a wound – *open* in the first instance, *closed* in the second (see also Ch. 34 for the application of the same classification to fractures of bones). Most often the energy is physical, but a burn (Ch. 10) is as much a wound as is an incision made with a knife and follows the same course towards the restoration of normality – generally known as healing. The similarity of the response of the body to different modes of injury makes the student's and the surgeon's task of understanding and controlling the process that much easier.

Primary wound healing

Healing is a natural and spontaneous phenomenon which occurs irrespective of (and sometimes despite) the surgeon. Although the basic events have been observed for many years, the factors which initiate and control the process remain incompletely understood. The pattern of wound healing may be affected by endocrine or pharmacological manipulation of the wound's environment.

Some wounds heal completely without surgical intervention. These include not only small lesions but also some larger tissue craters produced, for example, by drainage of an abscess or excision of a pilonidal sinus. Even if, as is often the case, such wounds are too heavily contaminated with bacteria for immediate surgical closure, they often contract surprisingly quickly. However, a further important influence on the behaviour of open wounds is the manner in which they are locally treated.

Phases of healing

The overall healing process is illustrated in Figure 8.1. A number of different terms are used by experts on the subject but healing can be divided into three generally agreed phases:

- *Inflammatory* (preparative) – in this phase the early cellular reactions to injury take place. As the name implies these are the responses which prepare the site of injury for repair and are similar to the

101

Wound healing and management

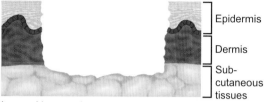

Epidermis

Dermis

Sub-
cutaneous
tissues

Large skin wound

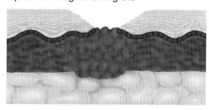

Wound fills with granulation tissue.
Epidermis begins to migrate

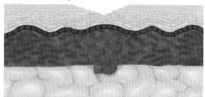

Wound contraction takes place.
Epidermal migration almost covers defect

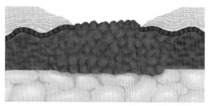

Wound now healed with mature scar covered
by epidermis which has migrated across from
skin margins

Fig 8.1 **Phases of wound healing.**

responses of tissues to acute inflammation from any
cause.
- *Reparative* – the redevelopment of structural integrity.
  This does not usually mean the regeneration of
  functioning cells; rather it is by the laying down of
  collagen, and in epithelium by migration of living
  cells, to close a defect.
- *Consolidative* – once the tissue is knitted together by
  collagen, this substance undergoes changes which
  include reorientation and contraction to ultimately
  form a mature and relatively inactive scar.

These phases are not wholly separate but merge
seamlessly one into the other.

Inflammatory

Tissue and cell injuries lead to a cascade of events:

- bleeding followed by clotting and then clot lysis

- inflammatory cytokine release with cell swelling,
  increased capillary permeability, intercellular oedema
  and migration of leukocytes into the damaged area
- phagocytosis by macrophages of dead cells and
  other debris.

The duration is about 3 days. Any factor which
interferes with the progress of the cascade may interrupt
or delay healing.

Reparative

The following take place from about day 3 onwards:

- New capillary loops form in the damaged area to
  provide a blood supply for subsequent events.
- New cells appear – *fibroblasts* – capable of producing
  strands of collagen; their origin is uncertain but may
  be either from the pericapillary cuff or from
  wandering macrophages.
- Extracellular collagen is deposited – at first
  provisional and apparently untidy but gradually
  becoming orientated along any lines of stress
  applied to the wound.
- The mass of capillaries, fibroblasts and collagen
  (known collectively as *granulation tissue* because of
  its visual appearance in an open wound) starts to
  contract, probably through the effects of specialised
  myofibroblasts.

The combination of alignment of collagen fibrils,
their cross-linkage and their subsequent contraction is
vital to the restoration of tensile strength. In addition,
in an open surface wound, epithelium at the margins
migrates across the surface of granulation tissue to
cover the naked area. As with the preparative phase,
anything that interferes with or delays the steps
described slows the whole process down. A distinction
is drawn between this active process of contraction of
the whole wound mass and the later shrinkage of
mature collagen which may lead to distortion of a
healed area – known by the general term *contracture*.

Consolidative

As collagen deposition is completed, the vascularity of
the wound gradually decreases and any surface scar
becomes paler. Although collagen turnover never ceases
completely, the wound becomes relatively quiescent.
The amount of collagen that is finally formed – the
ultimate scar – is dependent upon the initial volume of
granulation tissue. In an open wound with an epithelial
gap, this may be large and, although the size is reduced
by contraction, scarring may be considerable or made
worse by the slow pace at which the wound is covered
by inward migration of epithelium. By contrast, too
vigorous epithelial cellular activity is also not in the
interests of a good cosmetic result. In some, the normal
equilibrium between collagen synthesis and degradation
is disturbed: instead of maturation with subsidence

of cellular activity over a period of about 12 months, collagen may continue to be produced and results in a red, lumpy, hypertrophic appearance. If there is extension into the surrounding tissues this is a true *keloid*.

Recovery of tensile strength

In some circumstances – such as the fascial layers of the abdominal wall after a surgical incision and at the site of tendon repair – the ultimate tensile strength (i.e. resistance to disruptive stresses) is of importance to tissue stability. During the preparative phase in any wound, the opposed edges are merely adherent as a consequence of fibrin, and the intrinsic tensile strength is effectively zero. As collagen accumulates during the reparative phase, strength increases rapidly but it is many months before a plateau is reached at about 80% of the original tissues (Fig. 8.2). Until this time, the wound requires extrinsic support from the method used to bring it together – usually sutures (see below). By contrast, in a wound in a viscus, e.g. the liver or intestine, where significant disruptive forces are not usually present, the scar formed rapidly exceeds the strength of the tissue.

Clinical factors

The account given above is of the biology of wound healing. In surgical practice, wounds vary in four ways:

- causation
- contamination
- time interval between wounding and initial treatment
- biological factors in the individual.

Causation
The amount of damage within a wound is directly proportional to the force applied. An incised wound made by the deliberately applied scalpel of the surgeon

causes very little surrounding damage; modern surgical technique is based on delicate incision and dissection to minimise tissue injury and so to permit smooth and rapid healing. At the other end of the scale are those wounds caused by large transfers of energy: shock waves are generated, tearing tissues or distracting them from their blood supply. Cells are destroyed and the tissue disrupted by bleeding. Such features are typical of wounds made by the weapons of war such as high-velocity missiles.

Contamination
Once the skin or other epithelial surface, for example the mucosa of the gastrointestinal tract, is breached, a way is opened for the entry of bacteria. The circumstances in which the wound is sustained clearly influences what organisms enter on their own or are carried in on foreign bodies. Injuries sustained in the garden or in agriculture (including war wounds where the battle has taken place over cultivated land) are at high risk of contamination by the spores of *Clostridium* which can produce tetanus and gas gangrene (see Ch. 9). In hospital, surgical wounds may be inoculated not only with organisms that originate from the patient's or other skin areas explored (e.g. the gastrointestinal tract) but also from cross-infection in the environment. The most important current cause is infection with a difficult organism – methicillin-resistant *Staphylococcus aureus* (MRSA) – which can lead to failure of prostheses and other wound complications although these are not usually fatal. Other contaminating bacteria in hospital are streptococci and *Bacteroides* (Ch. 9).

Time
Healing begins the moment a wound is sustained. However, in a contaminated wound, particularly if there is dead or damaged tissue, the division and growth in numbers of organisms that may be present also take place from the outset. In most wounds, the first 4–6 hours is a period when organisms are present but not in sufficient numbers to influence the healing cascade greatly, and if they can be eliminated or their environment made unattractive during this time then healing proceeds normally. From 6 to 18 hours, the balance tends progressively to tip in favour of the proliferating organisms, which by this time are themselves influencing the inflammatory process, so that by now the wound must usually be regarded as infected.

Biological factors
Both local and systemic factors affect wound healing.

Local (Box 8.1)
Bacterial infection as a consequence of contamination leads to further tissue damage and prolongs the inflammatory phase; abscess formation separates the wound edges and may be associated with dehiscence. If the

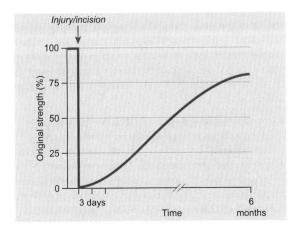

Fig 8.2 **Recovery of tensile strength in a fascial layer.**

local blood supply is inadequate there will be relative hypoxia which slows the rate of cell division; well vascularised wounds on the face and neck heal quickly whereas those on the lower limb are slow and may be prone to breakdown. Ischaemia may also result from excessive tension applied for closure, from peripheral vascular disease (particularly in the lower limbs) and from an increase in tissue tension either secondary to infection or as a result of a compartment syndrome. A foreign body within a wound can both separate healing tissues and, if it is contaminated, act as a focus for persistent infection and inflammation. Tissues infiltrated by malignant disease do not heal, e.g. a squamous carcinoma in a varicose ulcer or a pathological fracture of bone.

Systemic (Box 8.2)

Malnutrition slows the healing process, and specific deficiences such as vitamin C (necessary for collagen synthesis and cross-linkage), zinc (an enzyme cofactor) and vitamin A delay the healing course. Old age probably slows down the reparative response to injury, although this is not a contraindication to a necessary operation. Diabetes mellitus carries an increased risk of wound infection as well as being often associated with microvascular disease which reduces tissue perfusion and oxygenation. Jaundice is associated with delayed angiogenesis and reduced collagen synthesis. Renal failure suppresses cell division, neoepithelialisation

and the formation of connective tissue. Treatment with corticosteroids or cytotoxic agents inhibits the inflammatory response and collagen synthesis. Radiotherapy interferes with cell division but its effect is also to cause chronic damage to small blood vessels so that previously irradiated tissues are relatively ischaemic. Other general causes of reduced tissue perfusion and oxygenation are cardiac failure, chronic respiratory disease and severe anaemia. Haemorrhagic diatheses may lead to wound haematoma, delayed apposition of tissues and possible infection.

Pathways of wound management

The objective of management is to ensure uninterrupted progress to healing with the minimum amount of scar. How this is achieved is dictated by the clinical factors described above. Wounds can be divided into four classes:

- *Incised* – of recent origin and without significant contamination.
- *Lacerated* – of recent origin with tissue damage and/or contamination.
- *Late* – either incised or lacerated; strictly with a time interval of greater than 6 hours between injury and treatment but this may be extended up to 18 hours in some circumstances such as well vascularised, lightly contaminated wounds in the face and scalp.
- *Infected* – wounds seen beyond 18–24 hours must be regarded as, and are often seen to be, infected, i.e. they are the site of an inflammatory response to the organisms that are resident rather than the normal cascade of wound healing.

Incised wounds

Typical examples of these are surgical incisions and accidental wounds from sharp agents such as knives and glass. After arrest of bleeding (haemostasis) they can be closed. This is known to surgeons as *primary closure*. However, all but the most superficial wounds must also be gently explored. There are two reasons for this:

- *unsuspected foreign body* – apart from the possibility of later complications there may be medicolegal consequences
- *unsuspected penetration* with damage to deeper structures which requires either immediate or later treatment, e.g. nerves, blood vessels and viscera – a wound should be regarded as having penetrated a vital structure until this has been proven not to be the case.

Lacerated wounds

All dead and damaged tissue, visible contamination and foreign bodies must be removed by a combination of mechanical lavage and surgical excision using the knife or scissors. British surgeons used to call this 'excision' because sharp dissection is used to remove devitalised tissue and adherent foreign bodies. However, today it is more usually known as *debridement*. It may be difficult to be certain of viability especially if the tissues are bruised and swollen as a result of injury; skin may be sheared off deep fascia in degloving injuries and so lose its blood supply; fat which initially appears normal may undergo late necrosis. Judgement may also be difficult if there has been much interstitial bleeding and swelling. In such circumstances the wound is best left open and reinspected at intervals before closure (delayed primary closure). However, if a thorough debridement can be achieved, the wound is now similar in biological nature to an incised one, and after exploration and arrest of bleeding it can be closed. This whole process is known as *excision (debridement) and primary closure*.

Late wounds

In the grey area of time between 6 and 18 hours, debridement and closure may be possible, particularly if antibiotic therapy is used (Ch. 9). However, it is now likely that organisms that are dividing cannot be wholly eliminated so that the circumstances for their further proliferation should be made as unfavourable as possible. Bacteria welcome warmth, moisture and darkness – conditions that are found in a closed wound. If, after debridement and haemostasis, the wound is left open, the first two (and on occasion also the third – see Ch. 10) are less available. Provided infection does not become apparent within 3 days it is then biologically and practically reasonable to close the wound. This is known as *debridement and delayed primary closure* and is almost always used for war wounds and increasingly for complicated circumstances in peacetime. A wound managed in this way pursues the same path to healing as one closed primarily, because it enters the reparative phase at the same time as a primarily closed wound – therefore nothing is lost.

Later than 18–24 hours, a wound is almost always infected. All that should be done is to open it widely, remove foreign bodies and detached tissue and treat the infection with systemic antibiotics. Because of the time involved, the wound now contains granulation tissue; the two granulating surfaces can then either be coapted or covered in some other way (e.g. grafting). This is known as *secondary closure*. In some circumstances, the amount of contraction of the wound during the management of infection makes formal closure unnecessary; perianal wounds such as those following incision of a perianal or ischiorectal abscess (Ch. 25) are a good example.

Infection

PREVENTION AND MANAGEMENT

Bacteria can be assumed to be present in all accidental wounds and in those sustained at a surgical operation when an area that is colonised by organisms is involved (e.g. the colon).

Good wound care is the first essential for the prevention of infection. In accidental injury, debridement and delayed primary closure are the two most important procedures. Incisions made by surgeons do not need debridement, but if there is contamination at operation (as may occur in an operation on the gastrointestinal tract), delayed closure of the superficial layers is sometimes used. Many wounds can be assumed to be contaminated the moment they are sustained, e.g. when the abdomen is opened to deal with an intraperitoneal infection or when a limb is wounded in an accident. In the early part of the preparative phase when bacterial proliferation is just beginning, it may be possible to eliminate these organisms by establishing a high concentration of antibiotic in the tissues by parenteral administration. This prophylactic use of antibiotics over a short period of time is now common in many circumstances

An established local bacterial infection, other than the special circumstances of *Clostridium* (Ch. 9), is dealt with as described above.

Arrest of bleeding (haemostasis)

A dry wound – i.e. one with minimal oozing – is an essential prerequisite for successful closure to achieve the best result with minimal formation of fibrous tissue. Failure to achieve adequate control of bleeding:

- keeps the wound edges apart and thus requires a larger gap to be bridged, which leads to a greater deposition of fibrous tissue
- may result in a haematoma – an accumulation of clot which is lysed and may require release before the wound edges can be opposed
- may lead to infection – a haematoma is an ideal place in which bacteria can multiply.

The three main techniques used to stop bleeding are:

- compression
- ligation
- thermal coagulation.

Compression

Packing a bleeding cavity or applying pressure to a bleeding area are both particularly useful if there is widespread oozing. Five minutes of compression allows

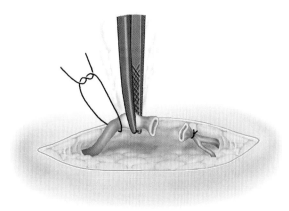

Fig 8.3 **Ligation of a bleeding vessel.**

normal haemostasis to take place by contraction of the mouths of small vessels, platelet aggregation and clotting. However, these processes must be normal for the effective arrest of bleeding.

Ligation

The mouth of the divided vessel which is bleeding is picked up with special forceps (haemostats, see Fig. 8.3) and tied off with a ligature; either absorbable or non-absorbable materials may be used. Absorbable sutures have a clear advantage in that, once the vessel has been occluded and has thrombosed behind the point of ligature, the suture ultimately disappears so that foreign body reaction is minimal. However, the rate of disappearance may be too fast, particularly in the presence of sepsis and, in consequence, *secondary haemorrhage* may occur, particularly if there is infection which accelerates lysis of the suture material and interrupts the normal healing process. For this reason, large vessels are more often ligated with non-absorbables which may be braided for easy handling.

Blood vessels and other small tubes (e.g. the cystic duct) may also be closed with stainless steel clips carried on a special forceps (Fig. 8.4). Larger vessels may be transected using vascular stapling instruments.

Thermal coagulation

Boiling oil and the hot iron have both been used since ancient times, although the amount of tissue damage they produced induced a famous surgeon of the 16th century (Ambrose Pare) to abandon them in favour of more bland wound care which was equally successful.

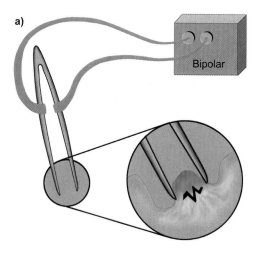

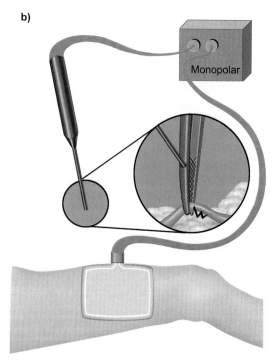

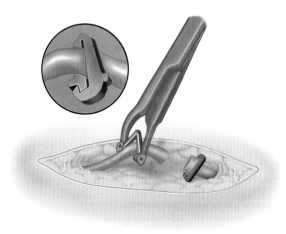

Fig 8.4 **Application of a clip to a bleeding vessel.**

Fig 8.5 **(a) Unipolar diathermy. (b) Bipolar diathermy.**

The modern, and much more refined, equivalent is high-frequency electric current – *diathermy* in Europe and *cautery* in North America. The pathway of current is either from the point of application through the body of the patient to a large area contact plate and thence to earth (*unipolar*, Fig. 8.5a); or between two points of the instrument (*bipolar*, Fig. 8.5b).

Small blood vessels can be precisely dealt with using either technique and the method is also used for cutting soft tissues with minimal bleeding when a continuous waveform is produced and an arc is generated between the electrode and the tissue. Vaporisation of the water in the cells occurs with disruption of tissue continuity (so-called cutting diathermy).

Other haemostatics

Many attempts have been made to mimic the body's own method of achieving haemostasis through the conversion of prothrombin to thrombin. The disadvantage is that, in nature, this takes place within a blood vessel whereas applications of coagulant mixtures act only at the surface. However, development continues for specialised applications.

Wound closure

The methods of wound closure are as follows:

- suture with needle and the appropriate material (traditional method)
- techniques that mimic suturing, e.g. tapes and staples
- plastic procedures – mainly to close defects that cannot be dealt with by the above two methods.

Needles and sutures

This classical method of bringing tissues together is based on the long established techniques of the seamstress and tailor.

Needles

Straight needles are very similar to those used in ordinary sewing and are intended to be held in the hand. The two main differences from the housewife's needle are as follows:

- The thread is *swaged* inside the hollow blunt end (Fig. 8.6) instead of being passed through an eye.
- For closure of the skin and other tough collagen-containing tissues, the point has a triangular cutting edge behind it (Fig. 8.6).

Curved needles in modern surgical practice are designed for use with a needle holder (Figs 8.6 and 8.7) and can either have a cutting edge or be round-bodied. Curved cutting needles may be large and are employed

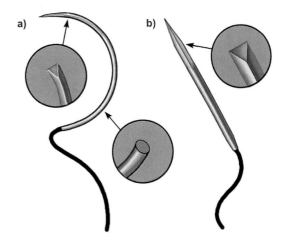

Fig 8.6 **(a) The swaged attachment of the suture material to an eyeless needle. (b) Profile of a straight needle with a cutting edge.**

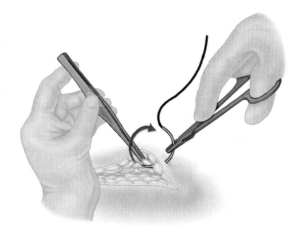

Fig 8.7 **Principle of the use of curved needles with a needle holder.**

for closing wounds where they may have to penetrate tough fascial layers. Round-bodied needles push the tissues aside and are often smaller and designed for precise work on viscera (such as the intestine), nerves and blood vessels. Microsurgical sutures, e.g. for vascular and ophthalmic surgery, are of this type.

Sutures

These are used both for the arrest of bleeding by ligation and for closure. They may be either absorbable or non-absorbable.

Absorbable materials are broken down by proteolysis (catgut) or by hydrolysis (the newer synthetic absorbable polymers or monomers such as polyglycolic acid). Absorbables have the obvious theoretical advantage that they do not persist as a foreign body and therefore, if a wound becomes infected, organisms cannot use the suture as a permanent hiding place. For many years, catgut (treated sheep intestinal submucosa

– effectively denatured collagen) was the only absorbable material and it is still widely used because it is cheap, supported by surgical tradition and has handling characteristics that many surgeons find attractive. However, its rate of dissolution is such that it is unsuitable for wounds that are subject to any form of distraction because it does not last long enough for intrinsic tensile strength to recover. Furthermore, in an infected wound catgut may disappear too quickly, which may result in secondary haemorrhage.

The synthetic absorbables can have their rate of dissolution adjusted so that they can be used in such circumstances, although some surgeons do prefer non-absorbables because of the reassurance they provide about the maintenance of tensile strength until wound healing has progressed to an adequate intrinsic tensile strength.

Non-absorbable materials are not subject to attack by proteolysis or hydrolysis and therefore retain their tensile strength for long periods – virtually permanently. However, they do promote a variable foreign body inflammatory reaction, which is greatest in natural materials such as linen or silk and least with synthetic materials such as polyamide (Nylon) and polypropylene (Prolene). Natural materials are available only in braided form which, although it makes them easy to handle, also provides a potential nidus in which organisms can lurk. Infection which occurs in a wound with buried natural non-absorbables does not resolve until these are removed and the same is also largely true for synthetic materials. However, synthetic non-absorbables are usually monofilaments, which means that they slide easily through the tissues and do not form such effective hiding places for organisms.

Suture gauge

The original definition of suture diameter was based on 'gauge 1' which was, at the time, the finest available with the numbers increasing for thicker threads. The development of finer sutures led to the introduction of gauge 0, 00 and so on down to 10/0, used in microsurgery. The modern metric gauge is 10 times the diameter of a suture material in milimetres: thus metric 3 corresponds to the old 000 or 3/0 and is 0.3 mm in diameter.

Other methods of closure

Although needle and suture closure has stood the test of time, surgeons are constantly looking for other methods either for novelty or to improve the quality of the end result.

Staples

Adaptations of the familiar office stapler have been developed which semi-automatically introduce a row

or a circle of stainless steel staples. They have found application in:

- *Skin* – where they reduce the time taken for closure
- *Intestine* – where joining two cut ends of gut (anastomosis) in anatomically difficult circumstances is easier and quicker
- *Lung* – resections can be done using a stapler which delivers a staggered row of staples so that the line is airtight.

Stapling is a growth industry in that surgeons are not only fascinated by the possibility of new technology but are also keen to adopt methods which will remove the tedium of painstaking hand-sewing. Stapling techniques can also assist in minimal access surgery (see Ch. 5).

Tapes

These are applicable only to skin closure. They are useful in minor wounds and also where the cosmetic outcome is critical (e.g. the face) because the skin puncture marks of sutures are avoided. Once the wound has healed they can be peeled away rather than having to be removed.

Adhesives

Tissue glues, particularly enbucrilate preparations (Histoacryl), are sometimes used for the closure of minor skin wounds. They avoid suture marks and are particularly useful in children because injection of local anaesthetic can be avoided. Their mechanism is polymerisation on contact with tissue moisture to form a firm adhesive bond. A thin layer is used to avoid burns from the exothermic reaction. Their disadvantage is that incorrectly opposed tissues cannot be realigned.

Techniques of closure

The choice should be the simplest and safest; more complex and therefore more hazardous procedures are chosen only when the simpler methods do not meet reconstructive (and occasionally aesthetic) requirements.

Great attention to detail is required to ensure the most acceptable scar is achieved: haemostasis must be meticulous, tension must be absent and suture material should be of narrow diameter unless high extrinsic strength is required.

Simple closure

The wound should first be converted to an ellipse whose long axis lies parallel to the skin creases – failure to do so may result in unsightly *dog ears*. The wound is closed so that the edges are precisely matched and slightly everted (Fig. 8.8). Fine-toothed forceps and skin hooks are used to minimise crushing damage by instruments to the skin edges. Tension is avoided by

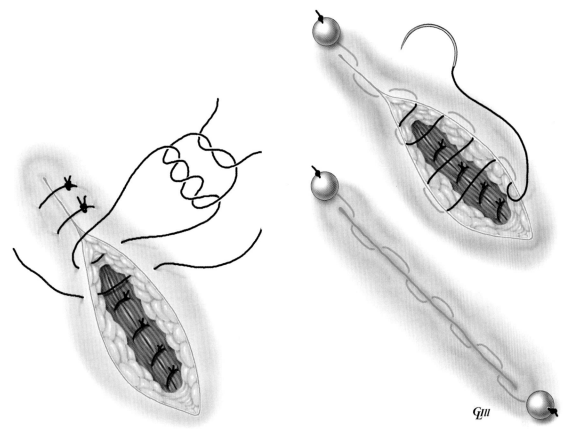

Fig 8.8 **The technique for closure of superficial wounds. (a) Simple suture. (b) Subcuticular suture.**

making sure that the tissues approximate easily; the support of buried subcutaneous sutures and the distribution of stress with adhesive tapes can both contribute to this. Given attention to these matters, the quality of the final scar is determined by the wound healing characteristics of the individual.

Closure of the abdominal wall

After a laparotomy (Ch. 5), the incision is under tension. A different closure technique is required to resist the tendency for the wound to pull apart. Heavy sutures are inserted through all layers deep to the skin so that the disruptive forces are distributed over a large suture–tissue interface (Fig. 8.9).

Dressings

Surface wounds that are open or that have been closed are commonly covered. Apart from avoiding what may be a disturbing sight for the patient and others, the main purposes of dressings are:

- protection from further contamination
- absorption of discharge from a raw surface

- application of substances which may help eliminate infection and dead or damaged tissue and thus accelerate healing.

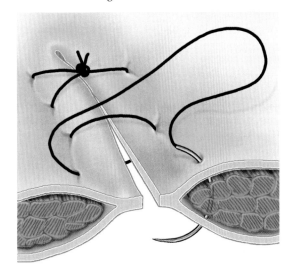

Fig 8.9 **Suturing of the abdominal wall with a continuous non-absorbable suture.** Unlike most suturing, which aims to be fine and delicate, an abdominal wall suture line is subject to distraction and the bites are deliberately made large so that the forces are distributed over a large suture–tissue interface.

Protection and absorption

In a sutured wound, protection from further contamination after 48 hours is not usually required and hence many surgeons expose suture lines after this time; patients are often less enthusiastic, feeling (wrongly) that their wound is then at an unnecessary risk.

A wound which has not been closed for one or more of the reasons discussed above requires a barrier between it and the outside. Common ones are:

- plain cotton gauze with an outer layer of absorbant material – cotton wool is still the mostly widely used
- alginate mesh – an absorbant which is biocompatible and most suitable as a dressing for the donor site from which a split-skin graft has been taken
- gauze soaked in or impregnated with a bactericidal – an example is dressing of a burn with silver compounds.

Plain gauze has the disadvantage that it adheres to the wound so that, if it is removed without anaesthesia, pain occurs in addition to surface injury. Both can be avoided if the dressing is moistened and removed only under general anaesthesia. Non-adherent dressings (e.g. gauze impregnated with petroleum jelly) are easily changed but they have little absorptive capacity and are unsuitable if discharge is profuse. In that circumstance, special polymer absorptive substances in bead form (Debrisan and Iodosorb) have a place when there is a cavity but are expensive. An alternative is an occlusive dressing which contains a water-absorbing compound (Sorbsan or Granuflex).

Therapeutic dressings

It has always been a goal of surgical management to find substances which hasten healing, but down the centuries this has been more of a search for the surgical equivalent of the philosopher's stone than a rational objective. Apart from the barrier function of certain materials in special circumstances (e.g. silver compounds in burns), dressings which contain ingredients thought to be active in removing dead tissue or promoting the formation of granulation tissue have not so far been shown to add anything to simple and rigorous surgical and nursing care.

FURTHER READING

Ellis B (ed.) (1995) *Emergency Surgery*, 12th edn. Oxford: Butterworth-Heinemann.

Surgical infection

'Every operation in surgery is an experiment in bacteriology'.

Berkely Moynihan (1920)

This chapter is in two parts. The first is an introduction to infection in general. The second is about specific infections that are common or important in surgical practice; it is not an exhaustive account and the comparable chapter in the companion volume (see 'Further reading') has a more complete coverage of infectious diseases.

Surgical infections include both those which are established and present to surgeons and those that result from surgical interventions (often called iatrogenic).

Infection in general

Importance of infection

History

As recently as 100 years ago, surgeons had few methods for the elimination of contamination from potential causes of infections. There were no antibiotics to combat established infections and no supportive treatments that are now available for patients with severe sepsis (Ch. 10). Infected wounds were treated by radical operations, in the knowledge that amputation was often essential to save life.

Antisepsis and asepsis

A series of 34 amputations performed during the Franco-Prussian war of 1870 had a reported 100% mortality from infection. Louis Pasteur hypothesised that organisms caused infection by being carried through the air. Joseph Lister (1827–1912) discovered that meticulous technique and a spray of carbolic acid into and around the wounds of compound leg fractures reduced the incidence of infection and could make amputation avoidable. This use of the technique of *antisepsis* (destruction of infective organisms by physicochemical means) was followed by the development of *asepsis* (the absence of infective organisms) in surgical procedures. Amongst others, William Halsted (1852–1922) promoted handwashing, the use of surgical gloves and the donning of clean clothes before an operation, as did Lord Moynihan (1865–1936). The discovery by Paul Ehrlich (1854–1915) of chemical agents which could kill organisms changed for ever the treatment of infection. In 1929, Sir Alexander Fleming (1881–1955) discovered that a mould (penicillium) inhibited bacterial growth, published on its therapeutic effect in 1940 and won the Nobel prize in 1945.

Technical improvements have now led to almost absolute sterility in the operating theatre and the deployment of many powerful natural and synthetic antibiotics.

Incidence

The incidence of postoperative infection has fallen because of advances in sterilisation techniques, antibiotic prophylaxis and surgical awareness. The risk is related to the type of surgery performed and the physiological status of patient. In general surgery, operations have been classified into four risk groups (Table 9.1).

Morbidity and mortality

Postoperative infections are responsible for high morbidity, significant mortality and a prolonged stay in hospital. Many deaths after operation are the result of uncontrolled or unrecognised sepsis. Prevention relies to a large extent on attention to detail in the perioperative care of the patient (Ch. 7).

Cost

An estimate of a 5% postoperative infection rate, with each incident resulting in an average increase of 7 days in hospital, leads to a cost of approximately £183 million a year in the UK. Thus any method of reducing postoperative infection rates has the potential of being cost-effective.

Biology of infection

Infection is defined as the proliferation of organisms in tissues and their invasion of various bodily pathways such as the blood. Colonisation of parts of the body – e.g. the gastrointestinal tract and upper respiratory passages – is normal and usually without harm; in some instances it is important for health. So-called *commensal* organisms may have a role in production of essential metabolites. There is also frequent exposure of the body to contamination by other potentially invasive organisms but infection remains comparatively rare. Its development requires interaction between the organism, local factors and host defences (Fig. 9.1).

Organisms

Load

Experimental studies have shown that a certain concentration or quantity of organisms is required

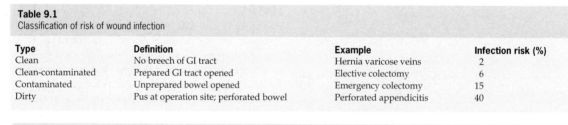

Table 9.1
Classification of risk of wound infection

Type	Definition	Example	Infection risk (%)
Clean	No breech of GI tract	Hernia varicose veins	2
Clean-contaminated	Prepared GI tract opened	Elective colectomy	6
Contaminated	Unprepared bowel opened	Emergency colectomy	15
Dirty	Pus at operation site; perforated bowel	Perforated appendicitis	40

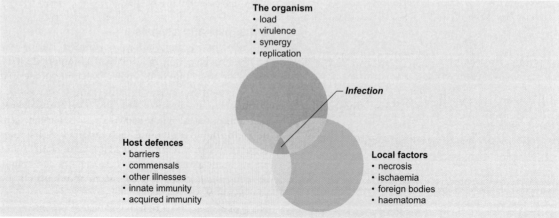

The organism
• load
• virulence
• synergy
• replication

— *Infection*

Host defences
• barriers
• commensals
• other illnesses
• innate immunity
• acquired immunity

Local factors
• necrosis
• ischaemia
• foreign bodies
• haematoma

Fig 9.1 **Interaction between the factors that produce infection.**

before infection results. For example, more than 100 000 *Staphylococcus aureus* organisms are needed in a wound for an abscess to develop. Any wound is inevitably contaminated from the surrounding environment. The application of agents to a wound that selectively kill the organisms (antiseptics), decrease the load and reduce the chance of the development of an infection: this is the basis of simple first aid in traumatic wounds.

Pathogenesis and virulence

Organisms capable of causing infection (pathogens) have varying virulence or power to proliferate and spread within the body. The factors responsible include:

- *Direct growth*, which damages surrounding structures by pressure and/or ischaemic effects, e.g. hydatid disease of the liver.
- *Production of bacterial toxins* which cause a variety of effects – e.g. bacterial spread (streptokinase), cell damage (haemolysins), interference with metabolism (cholera toxin), stimulation of nerve impulses (tetanus toxin), activation of cytokine cascades (Gram-negative endotoxin).
- *Synergy and interaction* – e.g. combined promotion of infection by beta-haemolytic streptococci and anaerobic bacteria to produce rapid spread in cutaneous gangrene (necrotising fasciitis) where hyaluronidase from the streptococci cleave the fascial planes and allow the infection to spread rapidly.
- *Replication* – doubling rates of organisms can vary from less than 1 hour for most bacteria and viruses, to many days (tuberculosis) and even to years for some of the slow virus (prion) infections. Before antibiotics, a pneumococcal infection was a race between bacterial multiplication and host immune response. The patient died if the response did not keep up with bacterial replication.

Local host factors

The local environment has an impact on the chance of contamination resulting in an infection. Factors include:

- *Tissue death* – dead tissue can easily become infected, often with anaerobic organisms; in the absence of a blood supply, the host response is non-operative and removal of necrotic tissue is essential in both the prevention and treatment of such infection.
- *Reduction in oxygen supply (ischaemia)* reduces the effectiveness of phagocytes and also aids the growth of anaerobic bacteria. Improvement in local tissue oxygen concentrations (e.g. the treatment of gas gangrene with hyperbaric oxygen and the management of infection in the lower limb by bypass grafting) can halt invasion.

- *Diabetes mellitus* is particularly associated with skin and soft tissue infections – the mechanism is multifactorial: local hyperglycaemia, microvascular disease and peripheral neuropathy.
- *Haematoma* provides an ideal environment for bacterial growth – absence of blood supply and nutrition for the organisms. Prevention is by careful haemostasis during operations and appropriate use of drains.

Host defences

Mechanical, physical and chemical barriers

Invasion is discouraged wherever a natural interface occurs between the tissues and surrounding environment.

- Skin is a mechanical barrier against organisms and also secretes acidic sebum which can kill many pathogens.
- Cilia in the respiratory tract keep contaminated secretions in constant movement towards the exterior and so discourage local proliferation.
- The acidic pH in the stomach destroys many organisms so that the proximal small bowel is largely sterile.
- Peristaltic movement discourages local organismal growth.
- A competent ileocaecal valve prevents reflux from the large to small bowel.
- Secretions such as tears and urine have a flushing action.
- Normal endogenous (commensal) flora on the skin and the gastrointestinal tract provide a physical barrier by preventing the adherence of foreign organisms and some also secrete mucus to produce a chemical barrier.

Concomitant illnesses

The general state of the patient can affect resistance to infection. The exact mechanisms are poorly understood but the disorders thought to influence the incidence and course of infection through effects on host defences are given in Box 9.1.

Box 9.1

Factors predisposing to infection

Malnutrition
Malignancy.
Jaundice
Age
Obesity
Diabetes

Table 9.2
Complement proteins and their action

Active molecule	Action
C3a	Chemoattractant for neutrophils
	Liberates histamine
C3b	Enhances phagocytosis
C5a	Opsonisation
C8	Causes cells to leak
C9	Lyses antigens
C5–9	Chemoattractant for neutrophils

Table 9.3
Cytokines and their actions in relation to infection

Factor	Source	Actions
IL-1	Macrophages	Pro-inflammatory
IL-4	T cells	T- and B-cell proliferation
		Macrophage activation
IL-6	T cells	B-cell differentiation
Il-9	T cells	Mast cell growth
IL-10	T and B cells	Cytokine inhibition
	Macrophages	
IFN-a	Multiple	Antiviral
IFN-g	T and NK cells	Antiviral
		Macrophage activation
		MHC induction
TNF-a	Monocytes	Cytotoxicity
		Cachexia, fever
TNF-b	T cells	Inhibits T- and NK-cell
	Macrophages	activation
G-CSF	Macrophages	Granulocyte growth

Natural immunity

Phagocytic cells: the macrophage and the neutrophil

Organisms that overcome the mechanical barriers of the skin or the respiratory and GI tracts are first attacked by these cells which ingest and then kill them using either oxygen-dependent methods (free radicals and superoxide molecules) or oxygen-independent mechanisms.

The complement system

A cascade of active proteins attract phagocytic cells, increase vascular permeability and directly lyse pathogens (Table 9.2). Activation is either by the classical (antibody-mediated) or alternative (endotoxin-mediated) pathways. Defects in this system can lead to infection from normally non-pathogenic commensals.

Acquired immunity

There are two types of acquired immunity: antibody-mediated and cell-mediated.

Antibody-mediated

Not all organisms can be overcome by natural immunity. Those that evade the first lines of defence encounter lymphocytes. B lymphocytes secrete antibodies which are classically divided into five classes: IgM, IgG, IgA, IgD and IgE. Stimulation of antibody production is most often T-cell-dependent but some polysaccharides can stimulate B-cells directly. Antibodies protect the host by simply binding to the foreign antigen or act with complement proteins to opsonise, lyse and kill invading organisms. The classical pathway for complement activation involves Clqrs binding to IgG or IgM, which leads to the activation of C3 and consequent amplification of protein production; this in turn causes an increase in vascular permeability, attracts neutrophils and lyses foreign cells.

Cell-mediated

Two different processes are involved:

- CD8 T lymphocytes kill cells which contain replicating invaders, usually viruses
- CD4 T lymphocytes help macrophages to kill phagocytosed organisms.

Cytokines

Cytokines are small peptides, released by white blood cells, which act like hormones for the immune system. They allow communication between the different cell populations and control the response to infection (Table 9.3).

Immune deficiency syndromes

Defects in the innate or adaptive immune systems illustrate the importance of both in protection from infection:

Innate
- Primary
  - complement disorders
  - phagocytic cell deficiencies: chronic granulomatous disease, Chediak–Higashi syndrome
- Secondary
  - burns
  - trauma (including surgical procedures)
  - presence of foreign bodies
  - therapeutic corticosteroids.

Adaptive
- Primary
  - B-cell deficiencies: Bruton type agammaglobulinaemia
  - T-cell deficiencies: DiGeorge syndrome
  - combined: severe combined immune deficiency (SCID).
- Secondary
  - humoral: immunosuppressive drugs
  - cell-mediated: AIDS
  - generalised: malnutrition, neoplasia.

Postsplenectomy

The spleen is part of the reticuloendothelial system and has three functions which oppose infection:

- specific immunity – T and B lymphocyte production
- phagocytosis of foreign antigens by macrophages
- opsonin production – two proteins (tuftsin and properidin).

Removal of the spleen leads to an increased risk of overwhelming infection by encapsulated organisms such as pneumococci (overwhelming postsplenectomy infection [OPSI]). If the spleen is to be removed electively, vaccination against pneumococci, meningococci and *Haemophilus influenzae B* should be done at least 2 weeks before operation. After operation, all patients need to be on lifetime prophylactic penicillin or amoxycillin (which is active against *H. influenzae*).

Infection control and prevention

Measures are required to protect the patient, other patients and health care personnel from infections which may be encountered during surgical management. Risks arise both from the environment and from the patient's own endogenous flora.

Disinfectants
Disinfectants are substances that can kill most pathogenic organisms but not bacterial spores or slow viruses. Their main use is for cleaning instruments (e.g. endoscopes) and surfaces which cannot be sterilised by other means. Examples in common use include:

- aldehydes, e.g. glutaraldehyde (Cidex)
- ethyl alcohol – 60–90%
- chlorine-releasing agents, e.g. sodium hypochlorite (bleach)
- clear phenolics, e.g. Clearsol

Antiseptics
These are disinfectants that can be used on living tissue. Common examples include:

- aqueous or alcoholic 0.5% chlorhexidine
- aqueous or alcoholic 10% providone-iodine.

Sterilisation
This process involves the complete destruction of all organisms, including spores and slow viruses. A number of methods are available and the choice depends on the resistance of the material to be sterilised and the quantity involved, (for methods and details, see Ch. 5).

Protection for the patient

The risk of infection of the surgical site (wound, anastomosis, peritoneal and other cavities) may be reduced in a number of ways. Four factors associated with increased risk of infection are:

- operation of more than 2 hours' duration
- abdominal procedures
- contamination, either endogenous or exogenous
- more than three diagnoses for the patient.

When one or more of these is present, additional preventive measures should be considered. Prominent among these is the use of prophylactic antibiotics, although these are no substitute for sound surgical aseptic techniques. An assessment of the risk is made, based on the patient's medical state and the type of surgery to be done. Of the above four factors; if only one is positive, there is an increased risk of less than 3%, and if all four are positive, there is an increased risk of 30%.

Theatre design and sterilisation of instrument and prostheses

This is discussed in detail in Chapter 5.

Aseptic surgical technique

Handwashing (Ch. 5) reduces the number but does not eliminate all organisms found on the hands. Gloves (also Ch. 5) are put on with minimal contact between their external surface and the hand. Likewise, surgical gowns are put on in such a way that the outside surface is never touched. Hair cover and masks are traditionally worn although their role in preventing infection has been questioned.

Preparation of the skin and bowel
Skin
Antiseptics are used for the preparation of the skin before operation. Adherent plastic film placed onto the patient's exposed skin may further reduce the chance of contamination from skin organisms.

Gastrointestinal tract
This is discussed in Chapters 18–25.

Antibiotic prophylaxis
Identification of patients at risk
Patients who are at high risk of infection or in whom the risk may be low but infection would have serious consequences should be given prophylactic antibiotics. There are operative and patient-related factors to consider.

Operative
- High risk of an infection – contaminated or dirty surgery (e.g., colectomy, trauma surgery)
- Placement of foreign materials, e.g. heart valve, arterial graft, joint replacement.

Patient
- Immunosuppression
- High-risk patients, e.g. previous foreign body implants, heart valve disease, peripheral vascular disease.

Choice of antibiotic

This is determined by the likely infecting organisms. Most units have agreed protocols tailored to suit the type of operations carried out and the local prevalence of particular organisms. The chosen antibiotic must be:

- effective for the likely organisms
- economical
- unlikely to promote resistance.

Cephalosporins are widely used for orthopaedic and general surgery, often in combination with metronidazole. Penicillins and aminoglycosides are also popular choices (Table 9.4).

Dose and timing

The highest tissue concentration of antibiotic is required at the moment of tissue contamination. For most procedures, parenteral administration at the time of induction of anaesthesia produces high local concentrations at the moment of incision and provides a satisfactory tissue level for the duration of the procedure. Two further doses at appropriate subsequent intervals completes 24 hours of prophylaxis which is sufficient. Some argue that one dose is enough. Certain patients may require a longer course, such as those in intensive care units (Ch. 10), those with heart valve replacements or those with peripheral vascular disease undergoing arterial operations.

Route of administration

Intravenous
Adequate serum concentrations are guaranteed but the method is the most expensive.

Oral
The oral route is not widely accepted as effective except for prophylaxis in high-risk patients undergoing minor procedures, e.g. dental work on patients with prosthetic heart valves in whom an infection has serious consequence.

Rectal
Metronidazole suppositories are still popular with gastrointestinal surgeons and have the advantage of low cost. However, absorption kinetics are variable.

Topical
This route is used for specific circumstances:

- gentamicin-impregnated cement for orthopaedic prostheses
- beads which contain gentamicin implanted locally at sites of persistent sepsis
- tetracycline lavage of the peritoneal cavity.

Long-term prophylaxis

Certain groups of patients are at continuing risk of infection and long-term prophylaxis may be appropriate to prevent overwhelming infections (see 'postsplenectomy'. The hazard of the development of resistance can be overcome by rotation of those agents which are effective.

Protection for others
Other patients

Continuous accurate monitoring of infections in the hospital environment as a whole can give important early warning of potential epidemic infections and so allow early measures to be taken such as temporary cessation of operations, isolation of patients and change in antibiotic regimens.

The routine and specially indicated measures used in the operating room are discussed in Chapter 5. On the ward those who are highly infectious to others are isolated in side bays. Clear instructions for staff and visitors about barrier nursing and the use of gloves, aprons and masks must be given.

After inspecting a wound (or indeed touching a patient or his/her belongings), all health care staff should wash their hands before doing anything else.

Table 9.4
Examples of antibiotic prophylaxis

Operation	Infection site	Likely organisms	Prophylactic antibiotics
Colectomy	Wound	E. coli Anaerobes Bacteroides	Cefuroxime Metronidazole
Hip replacement	Prosthesis	Staph. aureus	Cefuroxime
Bladder instrumentation	Urinary tract	E. coli Klebsiella	Gentamicin
ERCP	Biliatry tract	E. coli	Piperacillin
Vascular graft	Graft	Staph. aureus Staph. albus	Cefuroxime

Patients who are admitted for elective joint surgery (Ch. 33) should not be placed next to someone with an infected wound.

In outpatient clinics, standard hygienic measures are common sense: paper covers to the examination couches; washing, disinfecting or sterilising examination instruments such as endoscopes; and, on microbiological if not economic grounds, the use of disposables.

Health care personnel

The spread of HIV has drawn attention to the protection of health care personnel, although hepatitis B has killed far more health care workers over the years. There have been very few instances of HIV seroconversion following occupational injury. Almost all have been from hollow (syringe) needle injuries often with deep penetration.

Surgical technique
This is discussed in Chapter 5.

Vaccination
All staff at risk (which implies all medical and paramedical personnel) should be vaccinated against hepatitis B, and have had a recent serological test to show adequate antibody levels is desirable. While the vaccine for hepatitis B is very effective, other transmissible diseases such as hepatitis C and HIV do not yet have vaccines available.

Monitoring and reporting events
In order to monitor the incidence of occupationally acquired infection, injuries caused by sharps – knives and needles – must be reported and a serum sample obtained at the time with another planned at 3 months. The use of AZT prophylaxis against HIV after injury from a high-risk patient remains controversial. Health care workers can contract many of the diseases associated with work in the same way as the general population; to prove a work-related cause, Evidence of seroconversion following a reported injury is essential.

Diagnosis and management of infection

Prompt identification of the source of infection and initiation of correct treatment are crucial to avoid the morbidity and mortality associated with delay. Blind treatment with broad-spectrum antibiotics before the causative organism is identified should, if possible, be avoided although severe infections demand prompt

antibiotic treatment on a best guess basis while efforts are made to define the cause.

CLINICAL FEATURES OF INFECTIONS IN GENERAL
History
The timing of a postoperative infection gives clues as to its cause. Wound infections do not usually become clinically manifest in the first 48 hours and chest infections are a more likely cause in the early period after operation. A gastrointestinal anastomosis that leaks often presents with continuing low-grade fever after 4 or 5 days. Deep-seated prosthetic infection may be delayed for weeks or months.

Direct questions for cough, dysuria or abdominal pain may focus further enquiry and investigation.

Established infections not necessarily associated with surgical events prompt the search for a history of recent travel, administration of antibiotics and determination of occupation. Evidence of immunosuppression or reasons for breakdown in the normal barriers to infection (e.g. intravenous drug abuse, diabetes) should be identified.

Physical findings
General
An assessment, with measurement of pulse, blood pressure and temperature, gives an indication of severity. Signs of systemic disturbance increase the urgency of treatment and may change the management plan. Resuscitation and consideration of transfer to an intensive care unit are necessary in severe instances, particularly if septic shock is present (see Ch. 10). In the elderly or those on corticosteroids, usual clinical features may be masked until circulatory failure develops.

Specific
Full rigorous examination is essential in a surgical patient with a pyrexia of unknown origin (PUO). Non-infective causes of PUO (deep vein thrombosis, haematoma, malignancy) should at this time be kept in mind. Likely causes include:

- chest infection
- the surgical site (wounds, anastomoses) or areas adjacent to it (e.g. subphrenic spaces, pelvis)
- urinary tract infection, often secondary to catheterisation
- infection of intravenous lines.

INVESTIGATION OF INFECTION
Blood sampling
Full blood count. A raised white blood cell count suggests the presence of infection and occasionally is the first sign of a deep abscess. Severe infections can suppress the bone marrow and cause leucopenia, anaemia and thrombocytopenia.

Blood culture. It is essential to take blood for both aerobic and anaerobic culture (and occasionally other samples such as CSF) before antibiotics are started because interpretation of results afterwards may become difficult.

Serological examination to detect antibodies can identify specific infections in their recovery phase but is seldom useful for therapy (viral infections, hydatid disease).

Microbiological analysis

All possible samples should be sent for microbiological analysis, e.g.:

- swabs from contaminated or infected wounds
- drainage fluid
- urine
- stool
- tissue biopsies, particularly in chronic infections such as suspected tuberculosis (see also amoebic disease of the bowel).

Methods of analysis include:

- **Direct microscopy.** Instant analysis can be performed but the information may be limited.
- **Gram-staining of fluids** can guide urgent treatment before a formal culture and sensitivity report is available.
- **Culture and sensitivity** currently takes 24–48 hours. Ideally the organism responsible for the infection should be grown and identified and the sensitivity of that organism to a range of antibiotics tested. In severe infections, the time delay may not be acceptable and treatment must be started according to likely sensitivities.

New microbiological techniques

Enzyme-linked immunosorbent assay (ELISA) is used to detect antibodies to a particular organism and is the current technique to identify HIV and other viruses.

Blotting for DNA and the polymerase chain reaction for microbial DNA are not at the moment in routine clinical use but may become techniques for the future.

Imaging

Localisation of the source of infection is often a challenge and details of the techniques available are given in Chapter 4. Because of its precision and simplicity, ultrasound has become the first line of imaging in many circumstances, but other techniques such as CT scanning may be needed in individual circumstances. Radionuclide imaging with labelled leucocytes has the particular advantage that it is a direct determinant of the presence of infection (or inflammation).

MANAGEMENT OF INFECTION

General measures

Resuscitation. See Chapter 10.

Symptomatic. Measures include analgesia for pain, anti-emetics, paracetamol and cooling fans for high fever.

Specific measures

Antibiotics. The decision as to which antibiotics to start and when to start them is not always easy. It may be beneficial to withhold antibiotics until the cause becomes apparent if the patient is not systemically unwell. Some fevers do not require antibiotics (e.g. postoperative pyrexia caused by DVT) and certain infections respond poorly to antibiotic therapy (e.g. an abscess). Antibiotics are covered in more detail at the end of this chapter.

Drainage. A local collection of pus contains organisms that are inaccessible to systemic antibiotics. In addition, it acts as a toxic focus and may also exert pressure effects on surrounding structures. The collection should be removed, usually by external drainage. This can be achieved by:

- *Simple needle aspiration.* For abscesses that can be reached with a needle, aspiration and antibiotic therapy may be all that is required. The technique is particularly useful for areas where a scar is undesirable, such as on the face or breast. The disadvantage is that adequate drainage is often hard to achieve and the small puncture site is quick to close over, so allowing a collection to reform.
- *Guided drainage.* Under image control with radiological or ultrasound techniques a tube drain can be inserted and left until the cavity has collapsed.
- *Surgical drainage.* This is the most certain method; not only can all loculi (subcavities with varying communication with the main one) be reached, but also dead tissue (slough) can be removed. The cavity is then dressed regularly and left open to heal by secondary intention (see also 'Gas gangrene').

Systemic effects and syndromes

Bacteraemia

The word 'bacteraemia' means simply bacteria in the blood. Blood is normally sterile but any minor trauma to a colonised area (even brushing teeth) can lead to transient contamination. This does not usually cause systemic colonisation but in patients with a diseased heart valve or a valve prosthesis, bacterial endocarditis can result.

Septicaemia

In cases of septicaemia, bacteria are not just present in the blood but are using it as a culture medium and multiplying. The clinical manifestations are the response of the body to the event: fever, tachycardia, hypotension, oliguria, respiratory failure (ARDS) and multiple organ failure. Blood cultures are often positive but the absence of a detectable organism does not preclude the diagnosis, because the clinical effects can be produced by the products of bacterial metabolism and their interaction with defence mechanisms such as cytokines (endotoxaemia). Other causes of a negative blood culture include:

- low concentrations at the time of sampling – after the initial spike of fever
- prior administration of systemic antibiotics which prevent organisms in the blood sample from growing in culture.

Endotoxaemia

In some instances of severe sepsis, often with shock, organisms are not found but circulating Gram-negative endotoxins can be demonstrated. Translocation of Gram-negative material from the gut and sub-sequent cytokine activation (notably tumour necrosis factor, TNF) have been proposed as the cause of this apparently sterile septic state.

CLINICAL FEATURES

Symptoms
Confusion and worsening general features of malaise during the course of a surgical illness are warning signs. There may be symptoms related to a focus from which the bloodstream has become involved.

Physical findings
Fever, hypotension and oliguria are common findings. Focal sepsis may be evident, e.g. inflammation around the entry point of a central venous line. See also systemic inflammatory response syndrome (SIRS).

INVESTIGATION
Repeated blood culture is vital but may not always be positive even if there is generalised sepsis. Raised white cell count is usual unless there is some systemic suppression of white cell production (immuno-compromise by drugs or underlying illness).

MANAGEMENT
Best guess antibiotic therapy should be started immedi-

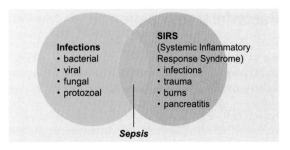

Fig 9.2 **Relationship between infection and systemic inflammatory response syndrome (SIRS).**

ately after local and blood samples have been taken. Costly newer agents are often used (e.g. piperacillin or imipenem, because of its current broad-spectrum efficacy). Restoration of the circulation is considered below. Any focus discovered should be eliminated as soon as possible, usually by drainage.

Systemic inflammatory response syndrome (SIRS)

NOMENCLATURE
The systemic inflammatory response syndrome (SIRS) is the name given to a physiological state of septic collapse. It is often caused by an infection, but not always (Fig. 9.2). It therefore embraces the terms 'sepsis', 'septic shock' and 'toxic shock'.

PATHOPHYSIOLOGY
The central mechanism appears to be activation of macrophages and release of tumour necrosis factor (TNF). Oxygen supply to the tissues is reduced and the situation is aggravated by cell injury which leads to deficient uptake of oxygen. The result is general tissue hypoxia and a build-up of lactic acid. Cytokine activation also occurs; TNF can produce this clinical pattern experimentally. The clinical picture is characterised by fever, hypotension, respiratory failure, oliguria and multiple organ failure, with hepatic and bone marrow suppression occurring as late events.

Generalised fungal infections

Causes are as follows:

- a severely compromised immune system as in leukaemia, lymphoma or HIV infection
- extensive burns where immunocompromise may also be a factor
- prolonged administration of multiple antibiotics.

The commonest infection is with *Candida*.

Bacterial translocation

Some clinicians believe that ischaemic damage to the gut in the critically ill allows translocation of bacteria and toxins to maintain the appearances of sepsis; indeed the GI tract has been called the undrained abscess of the abdomen. Once bacteria have crossed the bowel wall, they may translocate to the respiratory system which becomes colonised with enteric organisms whose toxins can more easily escape into the systemic circulation.

PREVENTION

Selective decontamination

To reduce the endogenous bacterial load, selective decontamination of the digestive tract with topical, oral and intravenous antibiotics has been used. However, the technique has not lessened mortality and, in consequence, has not been widely adopted.

Immunomodulation

Artificial enhancement of immunity to endotoxins, and thus prevention of the systemic response, is an attractive idea that has yet to make a clinical impact. Immunoglobulins raised against the cell walls of Gram-negative organisms (anti-endotoxin antibodies) have been protective in animal studies but have not improved mortality in humans.

Important infections in surgical patients

Infections which particularly concern the surgeon and surgical patients can arise as a result of surgical interventions or present as established infections that require surgical management. The infections considered here are particularly common or important to surgical practice. Bacteria, fungi, viruses and protozoa all cause infection that can present to the surgeon.

Use of antibiotics

When to use antibiotics and which ones to choose is not always clear (Information Boxes 9.1 and 9.2). Blind (rather than best guess) treatment is often needed for sick patients, but may obscure the bacteriological diagnosis.

The selection of an antibiotic rests on:

- severity of the infection
- likely organisms and their sensitivities
- patient factors – allergies, pregnancy, renal function
- hospital policy.

More expensive antibiotics have a broader spectrum of activity but encourage bacterial resistance and are kept in reserve for severe infections or as second-line treatment.

Once the antibiotic has been decided upon, samples such as blood cultures must be taken before treatment is begun. Other factors to take into account are:

- dose
- route of administration (i.v., oral, rectal),
- duration (up to 5 days' treatment is usually sufficient for common bacterial infections)
- potential side-effects.

Acquired infections

Some infections arise as a consequence of an intervention or because of hospital admission. Common causes include:

- *The operative site* – the wound, any anastomosis, the cavity in which the operation was done (e.g. abdomen, pleura or within the central nervous system).
- *In relation to a prosthesis* – joint, cardiac, other vascular or more recently the mesh used to repair a hernia.
- *Respiratory or gastrointestinal tract* from translocation.
- *Urinary tract* from procedures such as urinary catheterisation.
- Infection from *intravenous lines.*
- *Cross-infection* at any site, particularly methicillin-resistant *Staphlylococcus aureus* (MRSA).

CLINICAL FEATURES

Most wound infections can be identified by simple inspection for erythema and palpation which should be done whenever there is postoperative pyrexia.

A deeper infection may present insiduously, again with pyrexia, a rise in the white blood count or organ dysfunction such as prolonged postoperative ileus. Some deep infections are hard to detect and require special imaging techniques (Ch. 4) or exploratory laparotomy.

MANAGEMENT

Prevention

The following represent the ideal situation:

- Meticulous technique to inflict minimal damage to tissues and to avoid a haematoma.

Information Box 9.1

Common antibiotics and their uses

Antibiotic	Common uses	Notes
Penicillin	All cocci: *Strepto- Staph- Pneumo-*	85% of staphylococci are resistant because of beta-lactamase production Allergies are common: effects range from a simple rash to fatal anaphylaxis
Flucloxacillin	Active against staphylococci: should be included in treatment of cutaneous infections	
Methicillin	Similar antibiotic to flucloxacillin	Used to test bacterial sensitivity to flucloxacillin
Co-amoxiclav (Augmentin)	Broad spectrum: soft tissue, infections, pneumonia, UTI and for antibiotic prophylaxis	Combination of amoxycillin and clavulinic acid: latter acts to prevent action of beta-lactamases
Amoxycillin	Active against both Gram-negative and -positive organisms: urinary tract and respiratory infections	An amino group added to the basic penicillin molecule gives increased antimicrobial activity
Piperacillin	Prophylaxis for biliary procedures such as ERCP	Later generation penicillin that has activity against *Pseudomonas*
Tazocin	Reserved for severe infections in combination with gentamicin (for Gram-negative resistant organisms)	
Ticarcillin + clavulinic acid (Timentin)	Same uses as Tazocin	
Cefuroxime	Broad spectrum: prophylaxis for bowel and biliary operations; treatment of GI conditions – cholecystitis, appendix mass, diverticulitis	Second-generation cephalosporin: in common use in GI surgery often in combination with metronidazole; 10% of those allergic to penecillin are similarly affected by cephalosporins
Cefotaxime or ceftazidime	Second-line treatment for sepsis insensitive cefuroxime	Third-generation cephalosoporin: some improvement in activity against Gram-negative organisms but slightly poorer against staphlyococci
Imipenem	Broad spectrum – reserved for use in ITU	A carbapenem – thienamycin beta-lactam best combined with cilastin – an enzyme inhibitor of its metabolism by the kidney
Tetracycline	Pelvic inflammatory disease; other sexually transmitted diseases	Bacteriostatic rather than bactericidal; however, active against *Chlamydia*
Gentamicin	Severe sepsis (in combination with penicillin or metronidazole) Prophylaxis during urinary tract instrumentation	Aminoglycoside active against Gram-negative organisms and *Pseudomonas*; inactive against anaerobes and streptococci Potentially nephrotoxic and serum levels must be regularly checked
Erythromycin	Soft tissue and chest infections	Active against staphylococci and *H. influenzae* Useful in those allergic to penicillin
Clarithromycin	Similar to erythromycin	Used for *Helicobacter pylori* infections of the upper GI tract
Vancomycin	Gram-positive infections resistant to penicillins and cephalosporins (MRSA and pseudomembranous colitis)	

- Prophylactic antibiotics as already discussed.
- Avoidance of complications such as anastomotic breakdown.

Treatment

Antibiotics treat cellulitis surrounding a wound but cannot penetrate into an abscess. There is no substitute for drainage in presence of pus.

Drainage. An infection of the wound can simply be laid open, the infection allowed to run its course and the wound left to heal by secondary intention (Ch. 8). More complex collections require drainage radiologically or surgically.

Continued spread. The common form of this is peritonitis. If the infection has not localised, the only effective treatment is to re-explore and remove products of infection by lavage and control the cause of the infection. This is likely to be a leakage from an anastomotic suture line which requires repair or exteriorisation.

Prostheses. Infection is a disaster. Although high-dose systemic antibiotics may work, the most effective treatment is to remove the prosthesis and not replace it until the infection has been controlled. Some prostheses cannot be removed without being immediately replaced (e.g. heart valves and peripheral vascular grafts with critical ischaemia beyond) and special measures may be necessary.

Respiratory tract

DEFINITION

Infection of the respiratory tract includes a range of conditions: bronchitis, pneumonia, lung abscess and empyema. An element of alveolar underexpansion after operation is common (Ch. 6), can cause mild pyrexia.

ORGANISMS

The commonest organisms are *Pneumococcus* and *Haemophilus influenzae*. Gram-negative organisms can also be found in postoperative chest infections (see also 'Translocation').

CLINICAL FEATURES

Symptoms
- Fever
- Cough
- Breathlessness
- Confusion from hypoxia.

Physical findings
- Cyanosis
- Green sputum
- Consolidation on chest examination.

INVESTIGATION
- Chest X-ray
- Culture of sputum or bronchial washings
- Arterial blood gas tensions.

MANAGEMENT

Prophylaxis
- Do not undertake elective surgical procedure in the presence of uncontrolled respiratory infection.
- In the postoperative period, provide adequate postoperative analgesia, physiotherapy and early mobilisation.

Treatment
- Initial administration of oxygen with the aim of restoring normal blood gas tensions.
- Antibiotic administration; most hospitals have a policy on the treatment of chest infections – a combination of penicillin and erythromycin is a common first-line treatment which can be altered on the outcome of sputum culture.
- Drainage of focal collections such as purulent pleural effusion or an empyema.

Urinary tract (see also Ch. 32)

DEFINITION
Bacterial contamination of the urine is common and the clinical picture needs to be taken into account. Urinary tract infection (UTI) encompasses a range of clinical conditions which include cystitis, pyelonephritis and perinephric abscess.

ORGANISMS
Escherichia coli is the most common organism. Other Gram-negative bacteria include *Klebsiella, Streptococcus faecalis, Pseudomonas* and *Proteus mirabilis*. Coagulase-negative staphylococci are an occasional cause.

DIAGNOSIS
The urine of those with an indwelling catheter frequently contains organisms but not white cells. Unless the patient is systemically unwell this does not require treatment. The urine will not become sterile until the catheter is removed.

CLINICAL FEATURES

Symptoms
Smelly urine, dysuria and, if a catheter is not in place, increased frequency and nocturia are all symptoms of a UTI.

Physical findings
In cystitis these are unusual. If proximal spread is taking place, tenderness in the renal angles may be found and is accompanied by fever. Established urinary tract infection can mimic an acute abdomen and be confused with appendicitis (Ch. 24).

INVESTIGATION
Midstream or catheter drainage specimens must be taken before any treatment is started, but the results of cultures do not have to be awaited before best guess antibiotic therapy is begun.

MANAGEMENT
Common first-line antibiotics are trimethoprim, gentamicin, ciprofloxacin or co-amoxiclav until antibiotic sensitivities are known.

Pseudomembranous colitis

This condition has appeared in the last two decades and seems to be on the increase in surgical patients who have a prolonged stay in hospital.

AETIOLOGY AND ORGANISMS
Disturbance of the normal colonic bacterial flora because of use of antibiotics leads to colonisation with *Clostridium difficile*, an anaerobic spore-forming organism which produces an enterotoxin. Certain patients are at risk:

- prolonged admission (more than 4 weeks)
- elderly
- malignant disease
- broad-spectrum antibiotic treatment.

CLINICAL FEATURES

Symptoms
The patient develops profuse mucous diarrhoea after continued or repeated courses of antibiotics.

Physical findings
Fever and non-specific features of toxicity are common findings. The abdomen may be distended and slightly tender. Sigmoidoscopy reveals diffuse inflammation with contact bleeding and, in severe instances, the typical yellow plaques of membrane.

INVESTIGATION
Culture of *C. difficile* is difficult (hence the name) and, although useful for research, it is not of practical value for diagnosis. A water-soluble contrast enema may give a characteristic picture of ulceration and mucosal plaques.

   The diagnosis is made by the detection of the toxin in the stool.

MANAGEMENT
Prompt recognition and treatment are necessary to avoid significant mortality and morbidity associated with toxic dilatation of the colon (see 'Ulcerative colitis', Ch. 24) and progressive systemic toxicity.

   Stopping the antibiotics may be all that is needed in mild attacks. Oral metronidazole or vancomycin are the antibiotic treatments of choice. Colectomy may be needed for:

- failure to respond to medical treatment
- toxic dilatation
- perforation.

Methicillin-resistant *Staphylococcus aureus* (MRSA)

Methicillin is an antibiotic now only used to test bacterial sensitivity to flucloxacillin in the laboratory. Infection or colonisation with MRSA poses problems in management. Patients become colonised while in hospital, possibly by staff acting as carriers. The organism itself is no more virulent than its flucloxacillin-sensitive counterpart but the increase in MRSA since 1990 has had considerable financial implications for the control and treatment of colonisation.

MRSA is particularly prevalent amongst elderly long-stay hospital in-patients, and is now endemic in UK hospitals.

CLINICAL FEATURES

A patient may be colonised but have no signs of infection. Manifestations are those of low-grade staphylococcal infection, with wounds and prostheses being particularly affected.

INVESTIGATION

Swabs for culture from the wound, throat, nose, perineum, axilla and groin of the patient should be taken.

MANAGEMENT

Most hospitals have a policy to deal with occurrences of MRSA which consists of:

- isolation
- barrier nursing including skin antiseptics
- topical mupirocin – an antibiotic agent related to vancomycin (Information box 9.2) for local use only
- regular samples from the patient to ascertain if eradication has been achieved
- intravenous vancomycin or teicoplanin (an analogous agent) to treat serious infections.

Eradication of MRSA is possible by these methods but lack of compliance with the treatment or ineffective barrier nursing methods leads to failure in over 50%. Colonisation of the throat is particularly difficult to eradicate. The problem is an important issue in orthopaedic, vascular surgical and cardiothoracic patients. Standard antibiotics used for prophylaxis do not deal with MRSA.

Pyrexia of unknown origin (PUO)

The cause of fever in the postoperative recovery period is not always apparent. Fever can be caused by exogenous factors such as Gram-negative endotoxin or by endogenous factors such as some cytokines (Table 9.3). Nevertheless a hidden infection is the cause in 50% of cases and should be looked for vigorously:

---

i Information Box 9.2

Examples of typical antibiotic choices for particular clinical infections

Infection	First choice	Alternatives
Chest infection	Penicillin + erythromycin	Co-amoxiclav (Augmentin)
Wound infection (cellulitis)	Penicillin + flucloxacillin	Co-amoxiclav
Wound infection (abscess)	Drain collection	Flucloxacillin
Intra-abdominal infection (endogenous organisms likely)	Cefuroxime + metronidazole	Cefotaxime Gentamicin
Cholecystitis – cholangitis	Cefuroxime + metronidazole	Piperacillin Tazocin
Urinary tract infection	Trimethoprim	Gentamicin Co-amoxiclav
Pelvic inflammatory disease	Tetracyclines + cefuroxime + metronidazole	
Severe sepsis	Gentamicin + metronidazole + penicillin	Imipenem Ticarcillin
MRSA	Vancomycin	Teicoplanin
Pseudo-membraneous colitis	Metronidazole	Vancomycin
Gas gangrene	Penicillin+ metronidazole	Metronidazole

- intravenous lines
- abscess
- cholecystitis/pancreatitis in those convalescent from other disorders, particularly severe trauma
- pneumonia
- viral infections, e.g. cytomegalovirus.

Other less common causes of PUO include:

- unresected tumour
- factitious (Munchausen's syndrome)
- collagen diseases (SLE, rheumatoid arthritis).

Established infections in the surgical patient

Cellulitis

This presents as a diffuse reddening, usually of connective tissue, without pus formation (although cellulitis is present around an abscess). It can affect any part of the body but is commonly encountered as a primary event in the cutaneous or subcutaneous planes of the legs or face. Two special types, both uncommon, are worthy of mention:

- *Erysipelas* – intradermal infection with streptococci. The organism produces streptokinase and spreads rapidly. The facial skin is often involved, and before penicillin the condition was potentially fatal.
- *Ludwig's angina* – submandibular cellulitis, secondary to dental infection.

    Secondary cellulitis from intravenous lines or infected sutures is common.

ORGANISMS
Causative organisms are streptococci, staphylococci and occasionally Gram-negative rods.

CLINICAL FEATURES

Symptoms
Pain and fever are common, often with tenderness in the regional lymph nodes.

Physical findings
These include a hot, tender, erythematous but non-fluctuant swelling with ill-defined margins and tender enlarged lymph nodes. There may be red lines leading proximally as a consequence of lymphangitis.

INVESTIGATION
It is rarely possible to obtain tissue or fluid specimen for culture.

MANAGEMENT
Treatment with appropriate antibiotics – penicillin for streptococci, flucloxacillin for staphylococci – should be started. Hospital admission for intravenous administration of antibiotics and pain control may be necessary.

Established abscesses

DEFINITION
An abscess is a collection of liquefied leucocytes, dead tissue (slough) and organisms.

ORGANISMS
The commonest pathogen is *Staphylococcus aureus*. Depending on the site of the infection, other organisms are also common, such as gut bacteria (e.g. *E. coli* and enterococci in perianal and intra-abdominal collections). Tuberculous abscesses are a special case.

CLINICAL FEATURES

Symptoms
Abscesses close to the surface of the body cause pain from tension within the cavity. Deep-seated collections cause illness, fever and local pressure symptoms which depend on the site involved.

Clinical findings
A tense, painful, red, hot and occasionally fluctuant swelling in a patient with a fever is almost infallibly diagnostic. If there is any doubt as to whether pus is present (cellulitis can often mimic an abscess), needle aspiration of pus confirms the diagnosis and can sometimes be definitive treatment (e.g. breast abscess).

INVESTIGATION
Ultrasound and CT are useful to delineate deep-seated collections. A raised leuckocyte count is usually present.

MANAGEMENT
Treatment is governed by the site and size of the abscess:

- Needle aspiration – used for abscesses on the face or breast to avoid unsightly scars
- Guided drainage – an interventional radiologist can insert drains under ultrasound or CT guidance
- Incision and drainage allows the abscess cavity to heal from the base (secondary intention).

    Antibiotics are relatively ineffective in an established abscess but can partially control the surrounding cellulitis.

Gangrene

DEFINITION

Gangrene is the presence of dead tissue nearly always colonised by bacteria. Two types are described:

- non-infected or *dry* (often colonised by bacteria)
- infected (organisms are proliferating) or *wet*.

Infected gangrene can be subdivided into clostridial and non-clostridial.

Clostridial gangrene (gas gangrene)

ORGANISMS

Although other clostridia species can be involved, the predominant one is *Clostridium perfringens* (formerly called *Cl. welchii*) often in association with other anaerobes. The anaerobic Gram-positive clostridia are found in the gastrointestinal tract of herbivores and omnivores and produce spores which survive in soil and faeces. In consequence, gas gangrene is likely to occur in contaminated wounds and was once common in wars fought over cultivated land. Modern surgical techniques and antibiotics have made it now almost unknown where proper facilities are available for the management of wounds.

The organisms multiply in dead muscle so that for the most part removal of this is an effective method of prophylaxis and also management.

CLINICAL FEATURES

Symptoms

In 50% of instances in civilian life, there is no history of trauma. The clostridia come from the GI tract of the patient affected. Severe pain and systemic illness lead rapidly on to the features of septic shock and death if untreated.

Physical findings

Findings include a characteristic musty odour blackening of the overlying skin and watery brown discharge from a wound or sinus. Digital palpation may suggest, from the sensation of *crackling*, the presence of gas (surgical emphysema) in the subcutaneous tissues. Prompt diagnosis is essential to avoid the high mortality associated with the condition.

INVESTIGATION

X-ray or ultrasound can demonstrate the presence of gas in the tissues. Gram-staining of wound discharge or tissue removed at operation shows the characteristic large Gram-positive rods and these can be grown in anaerobic culture.

MANAGEMENT (see also Box 9.2)

Treatment is begun before the bacteriological diagnosis.

Box 9.2

Prophylaxis of gangrene and tetanus

The text deals with the management of established gas gangrene and tetanus. However, real advances have come from the recognition that good practice can prevent nearly all infections. For *gas gangrene* and *non-clostridial gangrene*, early adequate excision of dead and damaged tissue, avoidance of primary suture and systemic prophylactic antibiotics have made the conditions vanishingly rare. For *tetanus*, immunisation programmes are in place. All children are immunised and adults are recommended to receive boosters every 10 years (ideally for the rest of their life). Emergency departments systematically enquire about the vaccination status of patients who present with wounds and give HTIG (250 units) if immune status is considered currently inadequate (see Ch. 3). Wounds are cleaned with antiseptics and antibiotic prophylaxis is given if contamination is judged severe. Subsequent active immunisation is recommended. Groups at high risk (armed forces, agricultural workers) are carefully supervised to ensure that active immunisation is up to date.

- Resuscitation.
- High-dose penicillin usually with metronidazole.
- Urgent surgical debridement of all necrotic tissue back to bleeding and viable structures; urgent amputation may be needed.
- Oxygen therapy in hyperbaric chambers has been used to raise local oxygen tension and so kill the clostridia.

Non-clostridial gangrene

A number of different names have been used to describe this condition. The two main groups are:

- *Synergistic bacterial gangrene (Meleney's gangrene)* (a mixed infection with a microaerophilic *Streptococcus* and *Staphylococcus aureus*) – spreads relatively slowly and affects chiefly the skin.
- *Necrotising fasciitis (Fournier's gangrene)* (streptococci and anaerobes) – spreads quickly and causes necrosis of fat and fascia with overlying secondary necrosis of skin.

ORGANISMS

Streptococcus releases toxins such as streptokinase and hyaluronidase which aid the spread of infection through the tissue planes.

CLINICAL FEATURES

Symptoms

In Meleney's gangrene, there is failure to control an

episode of surface infection by conventional means. In Fournier's, there is very rapid development of severe toxaemia.

Physical findings
Black discoloration and break down of the skin without the crepitus of gas-gangrene. Fournier's often affects the perineum (where it may have started as a small perianal collection).

MANAGEMENT
- Wide surgical debridement
- Penicillin and metronidazole.

There is no role for hyperbaric oxygen in either of these conditions.

Tetanus

Tetanus is a state of muscle spasm caused by an exotoxin (tetanospasmin) produced by the anaerobe *Clostridium tetani*. As with gas gangrene, wounds contaminated with soil or faeces are the main predetermining cause and the disease is therefore more likely to be a complication of war wounds or agricultural work. Neonatal tetanus is caused by contamination of the umbilicus with organisms at division of the cord and is found only in developing countries where ritualistic dressing practices persist.

ORGANISMS
Clostridium tetani survives as a spore in soil and multiplies in the absence of oxygen.

CLINICAL FEATURES
The condition has an incubation period between an injury and the development of symptoms which varies from days to 3 months. A better prognosis is associated with a longer incubation period.

Symptoms
A sense of apprehension followed by jaw stiffness may be the first symptom, progressing to facial spasms (*risus sardonicus*) and back-arching convulsions with impaired ventilation. Autonomic dysfunction can present as arrythmias and labile blood pressure.

Physical findings
Between episodes, findings may be normal. During an attack, muscle tone is increased and muscle spasm may be local or general. An obvious neglected injury may be present but may have healed. There is a high risk of cardiorespiratory arrest with brain damage or death.

INVESTIGATION
Drumstick spores can be found in wound tissue. However, treatment should be undertaken on the clinical diagnosis alone.

MANAGEMENT (see also Box 9.2)
The disease only occurs after the migration of toxin along nerves to the central nervous system and its (irreversible) fixation to motor neurons. Nevertheless it is customary to give human tetanus immunoglobulin (HTIG) intravenously in doses of 5000–10 000 units. Any neglected wound is treated and systemic penicillin administered. The spasms should be controlled by medical means: sedation with diazepam in mild coses, full respiratory paralysis and ventilatory support in severe cases.

Candida infection

Candida is an omnipresent fungus which can cause an opportunistic infection in patients who are ill for other reasons or who are taking antibiotics. A generalised fungal infection is life-threatening (overall mortality 30%).

PATHOLOGICAL FEATURES
The commonest sites are:

- oral and oesophageal – the elderly, the young, patients with AIDS or those on chemotherapy
- perianal – a cause of pruritis
- vaginal – the contraceptive pill, in pregnancy and in diabetes
- endocardium – endocarditis in intravenous drug abusers
- generalised – immunosuppression (post-transplant, blood disorders such as leukaemia), multi-organ failure.

CLINICAL FEATURES
Symptoms
Symptoms are usually those of the accompanying disease or disorder.

Physical findings
Findings include clinical appearance of white plaques or white discharge. In generalised Candida infection, features of toxaemia and lack of response to conventional antibiotic treatment may be seen.

INVESTIGATION
- Microscopic evaluation of swabs or scrapings
- Blood culture.

MANAGEMENT
Local infection
Topical nystatin cream, mouthwash or pessaries suffice, accompanied by a general review for any underlying disorder and consideration of changes in therapy.

Generalised infection

This is normally treated with intravenous agents, such as amphotericin, and correction of pre-disposing disease or treatments.

Tuberculosis

ORGANISMS

Tuberculosis is mainly caused by *Mycobacterium tuberculosis*, a Gram-positive non-sporing bacillus.

PATHOLOGICAL FEATURES

The disease can affect the lung, skin, lymph nodes, bones, joints, genitourinary system, gut and the CNS. Two pathological types are recognised:

- *proliferative* – affects solid organs (lungs, kidney)
- *exudative* – affects serous cavities (pleural, peritoneal and pericardial cavities).

In both forms there is a slowly progressive inflammatory process which produces *granulomas*. In the proliferative form these tend to aggregate into an inflammatory mass. This leads to tissue breakdown, sterile caseation and a cold abscess which contains pus which may become secondarily infected if exposed on the surface of the body. In the exudative type, the granulomas cause inflammatory reaction on the affected surface with effusion into the involved cavity – peritoneal, pleural or subarachnoid. Haematogenous spread from a primary focus of either the proliferative or exudative type may set up metastatic foci or lead to generalised blood stream invasion (*miliary disease*).

The disease is not on the decline as many would have hoped with the advent of chemotherapy in the years after World War II. Undernutrition, poor and overcrowded housing and the spread of HIV infections have kept the incidence high in both developing and developed communities and this has been helped by undertreatment and the emergence of strains resistant to antibiotics.

About 90% of affected patients have lung involvement, but the common forms of surgical presentation are:

- cold abscesses in lymph nodes anywhere in the body but most frequently in the neck with a 'collar-stud' abscess
- scrotal sinuses from testicular disease
- acute or chronic tuberculous peritonitis (often regarded as miliary because it has arisen from haematogenous spread)
- renal disease.

CLINICAL FEATURES

These are the consequence of the site of infection and are considered elsewhere.

INVESTIGATION

Histological examination of tissue obtained from an infected site may show classical granulomas and caseation. Staining by the Ziehl–Neilson technique may identify acid-fast bacilli (AFB). The tuberculin skin reaction is positive with infection or with previous vaccination with TB antigens and is generally unhelpful in making a diagnosis in an individual.

MANAGEMENT

Prophylaxis

This is generally beyond the scope of this text, although in the developed world, reduction in drug abuse and HIV infection are relevant.

Therapy

A current medical protocol is 6 months' therapy with a combination of:

- isoniazid
- rifampicin
- ethambutol.

Surgical management is outlined for individual organs and systems throughout this book.

Human immunodeficiency virus

Surgical presentation is the result of complications and is partially dependent upon the stage of infection. The risk of cross-infection to the health care team, although real, is very small provided certain precautions are taken (Ch. 5).

Early infection (Centre for Disease Control [CDC] groups I and II) with the virus does not present with the disease itself but with problems linked to the lifestyle of those at risk:

- anal diseases – warts, perianal abscess and carcinoma, herpetic ulceration (Ch. 25)
- complications of injection of drugs – abscesses in relation to sites of injection, septic venous thrombosis and false arterial aneurysm.

Late infection (CDC III and IV)

- Achieving and maintaining i.v. access for systemic antimicrobial therapy (Ch. 11)
- Enteral access for nutritional support – percutaneous endoscopic gastrostomy (PEG – Ch. 4)
- Various abdominal procedures – splenectomy for thrombocytopenia, bowel resection for obstruction from deposits of Kaposi sarcoma or for bleeding from infections (cryptosporidium, tuberculosis)
- Lymph node biopsy for the diagnosis of associated disorders – tuberculosis, lymphoma and persistent generalised lymphadenopathy (PGA)

● Operations for other complications – cerebral abscess (Ch. 30); endocarditis (Ch. 17).

Hydatid disease

The disease is endemic in the Mediterranean, South America, South Africa and Australasia. It is still seen occasionally in the UK wherever humans, dogs and sheep co-exist or in immigrants from endemic areas. The dog is the definitive host of the parasitic worm *Echinococcus granulosus* while sheep are the inter-mediate host. Close contact between an infected dog and humans allows humans to act as the intermediate host. Ingested ova hatch in the upper gut, enter the portal system and pass to the liver where they settle to form cysts.

PATHOLOGICAL FEATURES
Cysts in the liver and secondarily in other sites such as the peritoneum and the lung contain clear fluid; although many have become sterile over the years, they may contain active brood capsules which are the starting point for new scolices. The outer layer of the cyst is made up of compressed fibrous tissue. Cysts occasionally become secondarily infected by pyogenic organisms.

CLINICAL FEATURES
Symptoms
The patient may present with symptoms of a mass or of epigastric discomfort. Occasionally there is rupture into the peritoneum or biliary tree, the first of which causes an abdominal emergency and the second an attack of obstructive jaundice. Anaphylaxis may complicate either event.

Physical findings
Unless one of the above complications develops, physical findings are usually absent. The liver and/or an abdominal mass may be palpable.

INVESTIGATION
A plain abdominal X-ray occasionally shows calcification in the wall of a cyst but ultrasound is more accurate in delineation. Eosinophilia is common but non-specific. Serological tests for the antibodies to hydatid are available but they have high false-positive and false-negative rates. Immunoelectrophoresis has a place in following medical treatment. CT gives detail on the site and size and is often used before a surgical procedure. The septae of the cysts can be clearly seen.

MANAGEMENT
Prophylaxis
● *Control of dogs* – Limiting the number of strays, repeated worming and denying access to offal have succeeded in almost completely abolishing the condition in New Zealand.
● *Chemotherapy* – Albendazole is effective and may cause immunoelectrophoresis to return to normal, but it is a hepatotoxic compound that has to be used with caution.
● *Percutaneous aspiration* and instillation of alcohol to kill the brood capsules
● *Conservative surgery* – cystectomy, marsupialisation again using alcohol to avoid spread
● *Radical surgery* – partial hepatectomy.

FURTHER READING

Pollock AV (1992) *Postoperative Complications in Surgery*. Oxford: Blackwell Scientific Publications.

Taylor EW (1992) *Infection in Surgical Practice*. Oxford: Oxford University Press.

10

The seriously ill and injured patient

Some features of organisation for care of the surgical patient have been given in Chapter 2. There is, in the late 1990s, an increasing tendency to direct patients deemed to be critically ill or injured to special units either initially or after rapid assessment in the A&E department (see Chs 2 and 3). Postoperative patients may also required planned or unexpected admission to critical care.

Among patients for whom critical care may be required are those with:

- Burns – usually to a regional or supraregional unit which specialises in both the early (shock phase) care and later skin cover, plastic and reconstructive procedures (see Ch. 37)
- Neurosurgical problems (especially head and spinal injury)
- Transplantation – particularly in relation to liver and heart where urgent action may be necessary to save life (Ch. 13)
- Neonates and older children with critical illness or injury
- General, vascular and other surgical problems with acute physiological disturbance and those with multiple injuries.

Critical care units

A number of sites for the care of critically ill patients are available (Box 10.1).

Burns units

These units comprise facilities for the management of the whole range of burn injuries, from minor burns requiring little or no resuscitation and no plastic surgery to those needing major resuscitation and extensive surgery. This specialist unit requires good critical care management associated with appropriate specialist burns treatment from plastic surgeons. As the results from well-run units are very good, there is no place for the management of occasional cases in non-specialist units.

> ### Box 10.1
>
> *Sites for the care of the critically ill*
>
> **Intensive care/therapy unit (ICU/ITU)**
>
> An area where patients are treated for actual, impending or potential organ failure who require a high degree of organ support, including mechanical ventilation.
>
> *Work style* – 1:1 nursing; medical cover immediately available
>
> **High-dependency unit (HDM)**
>
> An area where patients at high risk are continuously and invasively monitored. Mechanical ventilation is not normally required.
>
> *Work style* – 1:2/3 nursing; medical cover immediately available
>
> **Ward**
>
> Intermittent clinical monitoring.
> Variable nurse: patient ratio.

High-dependency units (HDUs), intensive care units (ICUs) and the future

With the increasing use of day-case surgery and out-patient management of patients who would previously have been admitted, it is inevitable that in-patients as a group will become an increasingly dependent and generally sicker population. As a result of this change, the level of nursing dependency will increase as will the dependence on manpower-saving monitoring. Continuous monitoring on wards will become standard and so part of the differentiation between the HDU and the ward which currently exists will disappear. A gradation of illness will still exist but the emphasis of applying appropriate care will relate to the availability of nursing and medical input rather than to the prescence of monitoring. Interventions will remain in designated areas such as ICU and HDU.

ICU and HDU admission criteria

This is a highly controversial area. Patients should receive a level of monitoring, nursing and medical care appropriate to the severity of their illness. However, the ability to sustain life in intensive care cannot be the only consideration; other important factors must be addressed:

- reversibility of the illness
- patients' and relatives' wishes
- quantity and quality of resources.

In light of the fact that 15–25% of patients admitted to general ICUs die – and in certain subgroups the mortality is much greater – it is important to pursue attainable and relevant goals. One approach is to apply intensive care medicine on the basis that the outcome realistically sought is to return patients to a state similar to that prior to their acute illness. This requires an assessment of the probability of achieving a successful outcome, not in isolation, but against the difficulties and discomfort likely to be imposed on the patient and the potential benefits to be accrued by the patient. Many individuals are unwilling to submit themselves or their family members to prolonged hospitalisation in the ICU, with its inherent discomfort, if the physician cannot state that there is a reasonable chance of survival. The physician must learn to predict when survival is possible and when death is inevitable. Despite attempts to approach this problem systematically, this remains a difficult endeavour.

The use of resources is a contentious issue. If a patient has advanced malignancy with limited life expectancy and a severe acute illness, it may mean that the acute illness can be treated but that it will take as long or longer than the life expectancy of the patient to return that person to a semblance of health. Age is not an issue but is part of the assessment of potential benefit. Each case needs to be sensibly appraised on its own merits. It is inevitable that intensive care will always be a limited resource and therefore it should be used efficiently and not abused.

Patient management

The nature of critical illness means that patients have complex, life-threatening conditions and the level of medical input should be appropriate to these problems. A multidisciplinary approach is required but this has to be focused or it is counterproductive. The only way of achieving this is to have a team primarily involved in management who take consultancy advice from the various specialities involved. This implies that the primary team are trained and effective in the care of the critically ill patient, and in many countries intensive or critical care medicine is a recognised speciality.

Scoring systems

How sick is sick? Can we determine the likely outcome from the appearance of the patient on admission? Patients from a wide range of specialities develop critical illness and need intensive care. In such a heterogeneous group of patients it has always been difficult to compare clinical management and audit outcome, either between patients or between intensive care units. An essential prerequisite is a common language and measurement system by which one can gauge illness severity. A sickness severity score can also be used to predict outcome and to compare actual outcome with predicted outcome.

Any scoring system has to allow for particular diagnoses which influence outcome, the physiological derangement at the time of admission, the health background of the patient prior to admission and, in more sophisticated systems, the way that the illness progresses once treatment has been initiated. On recovery, the quality of survival may need to be measured.

The APACHE II (Acute Physiological and Chronic Health Evaluation) scoring system is one of the most commonly used systems in intensive care (Table 10.1). The acute physiology score is derived from the worst values of 12 basic physiological indices in the first 24 hours, to which is added a chronic health evaluation. By evaluating outcome in large populations, the admission diagnosis can be given a prognostic value, which in combination with the Apache II score can give an indication of the likelihood of death, the 'risk of death'. The predicted risk of death in a cohort of patients can then be compared with the actual death rate for that cohort and a standardised mortality ratio (SMR) can be derived. This provides a means of assessing the therapeutic efficacy of an intensive care unit.

It is important to appreciate that the efficacy of a scoring system is heavily dependent on the individual who enters the data.

The number of scoring systems available is large and steadily increasing. In trauma a commonly used system is called TRISS, derived from the Revised Trauma Score (RTS) and the Injury Severity Score (ISS). The RTS is the score at the point of injury, scoring 1–4 for the Glasgow Coma Score, 1–4 for the systolic blood pressure and 1–4 for respiratory rate, giving a maximum score of 12 for a normal individual; a score of less than 4 indicates very severe injury. In the ISS, each injury sustained by a trauma patient is allocated a value from a large 'catalogue' of over 1000 injuries. The scores run from 1 to 6, where 1 is minimal and 6 is not compatible with life. The highest scores from all three body regions are taken, squared and added together, giving a maximum score of 75. A single score of 6 automatically leads to a maximal score of 75. The two scores are combined to produce TRISS which can then be used to predict and audit outcome. Other scoring methods are being developed to measure the quality of life (QOL). This latter method is in its infancy but may be useful in determining the efficacy of health care as assessed by the condition of the patient after critical illness.

During admission to the ICU there are methods such as the Therapeutic Intervention Scoring System (TISS), which can be used to quantify the amount of intervention needed by a patient. This system lists all the interventions, drugs, procedures and monitoring used for that patient and produces a score. This score can be costed and the amount of financial and other resources consumed by a particular patient derived. Many of these methods can be used as an audit system of the cost-effectiveness of health care. They are not, at present, used to determine suitability for ITU admission.

History and examination of the critically ill

As with every other area of medicine, the clinical history is extremely important but frequently overlooked while focusing on the specific episode (Box 10.2). The acute events leading to illness are important: why did the patient present for surgery; was it an elective or emergency procedure; if the patient presented with an acute abdomen, how long had the problem been there? In trauma, the mechanism of injury is very important: how fast was the car going; did it stop gradually or did it hit a wall and stop immediately? In shooting incidents, other questions are relevant: what was the type of gun, the muzzle velocity and distance of point of impact; how far did the patient fall? All these factors give indications as to the mechanism of injury, which may suggest the extent of damage.

Postoperatively the nature, extent and duration of surgery are important. Was there contamination of the peritoneum? Was the surgery definitive? Was the bleeding stopped? Are there surgical packs in situ?

It is essential to have a clear idea of the mechanism and the full nature of the injury. The background of the patient is important; previous medical history, chronic illness and age may all impact on management and outcome.

In the examination of the critically ill patient it is important in the first instance to follow the ABC of resuscitation and assess the adequacy of respiratory and cardiovascular function. A quick glance will allow you to assess the patient's colour and identify obvious hypoxia and sweating, and whether the patient is pale, distressed, agitated or exhausted. The quick glance should tell you if the patient looks ill.

The airway and respiratory system must be evaluated for evidence of hypoxia, difficulty with breathing or abnormal patterns of breathing (Table 10.2). When the immediate problems have been corrected, examine the whole patient.

The history alerts one to the potential problems but the examination should allow the clinician to decide if the patient is sick, how sick and where the problem lies. In the critically ill, the initial history and examination are part of the introduction to the patient, but management of that patient requires frequent re-evaluation of symptoms and signs throughout the course of the

The seriously ill and injured patient

Table 10.1
Acute physiological and chronic health evaluating (APACHE II) scoring system

Physiological variable	High abnormal range				0	Low abnormal range			
	+4	+3	+2	+1	0	+1	+2	+3	+4
Temperature – rectal (°C)	≥41°	39°–40.9°		38.5°–38.9°	36°–38.4°	34°–35.9°	32°–33.9°	30°–31.9°	≤29.9°
Mean arterial pressure – mmHg	≥160	130–159	110–129		70–109		50–69		≤49
Heart rate (ventricular response)	≥180	140–179	110–139		70–109		55–69	40–54	≤39
Respiratory rate (non-ventilated or ventilated)	≥50	35–49		25–34	12–24	10–11	6–9		≤5
Oxygenation: A–aDO$_2$ or P_aO_2 (mmHg) a. F_iO_2 ≥0.5 record A–aDO$_2$	≥500	350–499	200–349		<200				
b. F_iO_2 ≥0.5 record only P_aO_2					P_{O_2} > 70	P_{O_2} 61–70		P_{O_2} 55–60	P_{O_2} <55
Arterial pH	≥7.7	7.6–7.69		7.5–7.59	7.33–7.49		7.25–7.32	7.15–7.24	<7.15
Serum sodium (mmol/L)	≥180	160–179	155–159	150–154	130–149		120–129	111–119	≤110
Serum potassium (mmol/L)	≥7	6–6.9		5.5–5.9	3.5–5.4	3–3.4	2.5–2.9		<2.5
Serum creatinine (mg/100 mL) (double point score for acute renal failure)	≥3.5	2–3.4	1.5–1.9		0.6–1.4		<0.6		
Hematocrit (%)	≥60		50–59.9	46–49.9	30–45.9		20–29.9		<20
White blood count (total/mm^3) (× 1000)	≥40		20–39.9	15–19.9	3–14.9		1–2.9		<1

Glasgow coma score (GCS): score = 15 minus actual GCS

A Total acute physiology Score (APS): sum of the 12 individual variable points

Serum HCO$_3$ (venous-mmol/L) (not preferred, use if no ABGs)	≥52	41–51.9		32–40.9	22–31.9		18–21.9	15–17.9	<15

B Age points Assign points to age as follows:

Age (years)	Points
≤44	0
45–54	2
55–64	3
65–74	5
≥75	6

Table 10.1 – *continued*
Acute physiological and chronic health evaluating (APACHE II) scoring system

C Chronic health points
If the patient has a history of severe organ system insufficiency or is immunocompromised, assign points as follows:
a. for non-operative or emergency postoperative patients – 5 points
b. for elective postoperative patients – 2 points

DEFINITIONS
Organ insufficiency or immunocompromised state must have been evident prior to this hospital admission and must conform to the following criteria:
Liver: biopsy-proven cirrhosis and documented portal hypertension: episodes of past upper GI bleeding attributed to portal hypertension: or prior episodes of hepatic failure encephalopathy/coma.
Cardiovascular: New York Heart Association Class IV.
Respiratory: chronic restrictive, obstructive or vascular disease resulting in severe exercise restriction, i.e. unable to climb stairs or perform household duties: or documented chronic hypoxia, hypercapnia, secondary polycythaemia, severe pulmonary hypertension (>40 mmHg) or respirator dependency.
Renal: receiving chronic dialysis.
Immunocompromised: the patient has received therapy that suppresses resistance to infection, e.g. immunosuppression, chemotherapy, radiation, long-term or recent high-dose steroids, or has a disease that is sufficiently advanced to suppress resistance to infection, e.g. leukaemia, lymphoma, AIDS.

APACHE II SCORE
Sum of *A* + *B* + *C*
A, APS points _____
B, Age points _____
C, Chronic health points _____
Total APACHE II _____

Box 10.2

Clinical history

Acute

When – time to presentation at hospital
Where – place of injury/illness
How – mechanism
Drugs/medications taken
Episodes of hypoxia or hypotension
Other events

Chronic

Age
Immunosuppression
Malignancy
Drug therapy – cytotoxics, steroids
Normal health status and mobility

Table 10.2
Signs of respiratory failure

	Signs
Pattern of breathing	Rapid shallow gasping
	Very slow, large-volume, sigh-like
Colour	Cyanosis, peripheral or central
Skin	Sweating, cool periphery
	Sweating, warm periphery
	(CO_2 retention)
Accessory muscles	Neck muscles, shoulders, abdominal
Saturation	Low
Arterial blood gases	$P_aO_2 < 7.5$ kPa, $P_aCO_2 > 6.4$ kPa
	Respiratory acidosis, CO_2 retention
	Metabolic acidosis or mixed with
	hypoxaemia

---

illness. From frequent reassessment the clinician is rapidly able to interpret trends, which facilitates greater sensitivity to any changes occurring in what is always a dynamic situation.

The cardiovascular system

The sympathetic system is very effective, especially in younger patients, at compensating for impaired cardiovascular function. Look for signs not only of decompensation, i.e. tachycardia, hypotension and poor peripheral perfusion, but also that the sympathetic system is working well. The normotensive, tachycardic, peripherally shut-down young patient is potentially misleading.

The important cardiovascular signs are:

- perfusion and capillary filling; warm or cold; peripheral cyanosis
- pulse rate, volume, rhythm
- jugular venous pressure (JVP) – up or down
- blood pressure
- urine output.

Assessment of the pulse is always useful. The rate and nature of the pulse and their presence both centrally and peripherally can be used, in conjunction with the state of peripheral perfusion, to assess intravascular volume. Tachycardia, a low volume or thready pulse with cold hands and feet may indicate hypovolaemia. Hypotension, if present, always signifies cardiovascular derangement, i.e. hypovolaemia, pump failure or acute vasodilatation. However, a normal blood pressure can be misleading, especially in young patients, and may mask underlying hypovolaemia.

Look at the jugular venous pressure. If it is absent, it is a useful sign of potential hypovolaemia. If it is high with engorged veins, it provides information either on cardiac function and failure or on excessive fluid administration.

Feel the apex beat. In hyperdynamic septic patients with high cardiac output, there may be a bounding left ventricle which is easily palpable. Heart sounds may indicate rate and rhythm and there may be a high-output systolic flow murmur. It may be possible to detect the murmur of tricuspid incompetence in a dilated heart. This would be associated with a large V wave on the JVP.

The central nervous system

Assessment of a patient's level of consciousness is an essential part of the initial examination. An unconscious patient is at risk for many reasons, but in particular there is a risk of aspiration and airway obstruction. Confusion, agitation or loss of consciousness may be indicators of poor cerebral perfusion or cerebral injury, both of which are important considerations in the injured patient. The critically ill patient with severe sepsis may present with a 'toxic' confusional state.

The conscious level can be evaluated using the Glasgow Coma Scale and it is a reasonable way of appraising the critically ill (Table 10.3). Examine the peripheral nervous system. Motor and sensory function is particularly important after trauma.

Table 10.3
Glasgow Coma Scale

Signs	Evaluation	Score
Eye opening	Spontaneous	4
	To speech	3
	To pain	2
	None	1
Best verbal response	Oriented	5
	Confused	4
	Inappropriate	3
	Incomprehensible	2
	None	1
Best motor response	Obeys commands	6
	Localises pain	5
	Withdrawal to pain	4
	Flexion to pain	3
	Extension to pain	2
	None	1

Abdominal examination

In the unconscious patient, abdominal examination may be misleading and classical signs are not dependable. In the conscious patient, look at the shape and size of the abdomen and whether it is normal for that individual. Assess for guarding, rebound and localised pain. Are there any masses? Check the liver and spleen. Always examine the inguinal area. Look for lymph nodes and check for occult hernias. Bowel sounds are a difficult sign to interpret in the critically ill but a change in the bowel sounds may be important, so a baseline assessment is essential.

Examine the patient's back. It is often forgotten and there may be important signs, such as bruising or septic lesions.

The urological system

It is important to ascertain whether the patient is passing urine – if so what does it contain? The volume of urine is important. Following trauma, blood is an indicator of potential problems. Muddy urine may indicate the presence of myoglobin.

The patient should be looked at from head to toe: look at the skin, look for rashes and assess their colour.

Diagnosis

There are two aspects to diagnosis: the first relates to identification of all the physiological disturbances which need urgent correction if life is to be sustained; and the second to identification of the underlying problem that resulted in the patient becoming critically ill.

As with any medical diagnosis, history and examination should provide the general diagnosis. Defining the specific problem is important. The methods available are the same as those available to other specialities and should be used. However, some investigations such as CT scanning, require the patient to be moved which, in the critically ill, may be hazardous. Nevertheless, it may provide the information required to plan definitive treatment and so should not be ruled out. There is always a balance to be struck between the usefulness of the information that might be gained by an investigation and the cost, in terms of morbidity, of acquiring that information.

Aetiology of critical illness

Any patient from any speciality can become critically ill, although it is more likely in some specialities than in

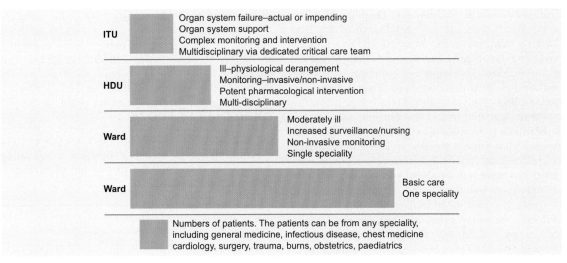

Fig 10.1 **Aetiology of critical illness**

others. As the severity of illness increases, so do the levels of monitoring and intervention required. As a very general statement, the physiological derangement tends to follow common pathways, irrespective of the original speciality. Obviously there will be aspects of the original problem which will have an influence on the development and pattern of critical illness (Fig. 10.1).

Shock

Shock is a descriptive term based on the symptoms and signs which are secondary to one or more of a wide range of problems. Traditionally, each 'type' of shock was described by the symptoms and signs seen in that particular situation. It is more fruitful to look at the final common pathway and work back to the myriad causes. The final pathway is failure to adequately supply the peripheral tissues and cells with oxygen. At the cellular level it is the situation where cells are breaking down more ATP for energy than they are making because the oxygen supply is inadequate to maintain oxidative metabolism at an adequate rate.

When groups of cells become threatened with a reduction in oxygen supply, the body reacts vigorously to prevent this from happening. The manifestations of shock are partly those of the specific mechanism causing shock, partly the consequences of tissue hypoxia and partly those of the physiological protective mechanisms instituted to maintain oxygenation. These physiological mechanisms are the signs of sympathetic activity.

Shock should be considered in terms of:

- causes of shock
- consequences of shock
- physiological responses
- treatment.

MECHANISMS

Anything that impairs the passage of oxygen delivery from the outside environment through to the oxidative metabolic system in the mitochondrion can result in shock. This can be at any stage in the process, for example from breathing hypoxic air (e.g. at altitude) or through airway obstruction or ventilatory failure from causes such as muscle paralysis. Impairment of oxygen delivery sometimes occurs between the lungs and the tissues: there may be difficulty in the transfer of oxygen from the alveoli to the capillaries, as with oedema, or failure to transfer the oxygen-carrying blood from the capillaries to the rest of the body. Exsanguination or hypovolaemia from any cause may reduce circulating volume. Cardiac failure may reduce the blood and therefore effective oxygen supply to the tissues. At the tissue level, oedema in the interstitium may impede oxygen transfer from the capillaries to the cells, and at the mitochondrial level toxins such as cyanide may impede oxygen uptake by the cytochrome system. In short, any mechanism preventing a significant population of cells from receiving and using oxygen will result in a state of shock.

CONSEQUENCES

The consequences of shock start at the cellular level. Cells need energy (ATP) and use up their supplies very rapidly, producing hydrogen ions as a by-product:

$$ATP = ADP + P + H^+$$

H^+ ions are taken up during oxidative metabolism at a rapid rate but only very slowly in anaerobic metabolism. If anaerobic metabolism increases, the rate of production of hydrogen ions from the cell using ATP far exceeds the ability of anaerobic metabolism either to use hydrogen ions or to produce ATP. There is a build-up of H^+ which coincides with a build-up of the base (lactate) from anaerobic metabolism. An acidosis develops intracellularly and this moves out of the cell and is buffered. Eventually the buffering is used up and a systemic acidosis develops. This is known as lactic acidosis.

Other signs may reflect the primary cause. If the myocardium is deprived of oxygen, cardiac failure will ensue. Hypotension is the sign of losing intravascular volume or pump failure. If hypovolaemia occurs from blood loss there will be signs of tissue hypoxia and poor perfusion associated with a fall in blood pressure. In sepsis, profound vasodilatation may result in a hot periphery, bounding pulses and hypotension. Usually these signs will be influenced heavily by the compensatory mechanisms that swing into action to protect the tissue oxygen supply.

RESPONSES

The responses to cellular hypoxia are aimed at improving oxygen supply. The changes occurring from the mechanism of injury combined with the responses geared to increasing oxygen supply are the signs of shock. Air hunger and tachypnoea are attempts to increase gas exchange and oxygen availability. They also serve to excrete CO_2 and compensate for an advancing metabolic acidosis from cell hypoxia.

The cardiovascular system is stimulated to try to deliver more oxygen by delivering more blood to the tissues. This is achieved by increasing the heart rate and improving contractility, thereby increasing the cardiac output. All of this is mediated by the sympathetic system. Blood is diverted to perfuse vital organs. The periphery is non-vital and therefore it becomes cold. The pulses tend to be rapid and of low volume in most situations, the exception being septic shock where vasodilatation is part of the underlying problem and the patient may have a large-volume, low-pressure pulse. With massive sympathetic compensation this may later become low in volume and low in pressure. Sweating is part of the sympathetic response, so the patient becomes cold and clammy. Renal perfusion is reduced and urine output ceases.

The patient in shock is very agitated. Failure to supply oxygen to the brain adds a picture of confusion and eventually loss of consciousness. This is superimposed on the agitation and irritation caused by the sympathetic system.

TREATMENT

Treatment is aimed at restoring oxygen delivery to the cell as rapidly as possible and this is the primary intention. The cause of the shock should be determined and treated while ensuring the pathway between oxygen outside the body and the cell is unimpeded at all levels. The basic principles are to increase ambient,

oxygen, ensure a clear airway, facilitate adequate ventilation, guarantee an adequate circulating blood volume and improve cardiac performance – essentially the ABC of resuscitation: airway, breathing and circulation.

Examples of shock

Three patients with shock of different aetiologies are described below to illustrate how the precipitating mechanisms may be different but the physiological pathways come together.

Myocardial infarction – cardiogenic shock

A 50-year-old man collapses at work complaining of severe chest pain and increasing shortness of breath. On arrival he is grey, cold and clammy with beads of perspiration on his forehead and he is extremely anxious. He has peripheral cyanosis. His pulse is 120/min, regular but very weak and thready in nature. His JVP is markedly elevated. His blood pressure is low at 80/50 mmHg.

He has a myocardial infarct with reduced left ventricular function and his heart is failing to pump. Tissues are not getting enough oxygen. His sympathetic system is trying to compensate by increasing oxygen delivery. He is breathing faster to try to acquire more oxygen. His heart is failing and blood is backing up in his lungs and he is getting pulmonary oedema which worsens his oxygen transport further. His poor ventricular function is inadequate and so he is developing a tachycardia to compensate. He is shutting down peripherally to divert blood to the central organs.

Management will involve treating both the shock and the condition: increasing oxygen, aiding breathing and improving cardiac output. Oxygen should be given, by mask and a diuretic administered to try to reduce the fluid building up in his lungs. Perhaps also administer streptokinase to reverse the infarct. A dilator may help, so that the heart is pumping against less resistance. An inotrope may be needed to boost left ventricular function if the BP is too low, but it has the negative effect of increasing the work on the heart which may make the infarct worse.

Trauma – hypovolaemic shock

A 24-year-old man rides his motorbike into a bus. He sustains injuries to his pelvis, fractures his femur and tears his femoral artery. When the ambulance arrives he is lying in a pool of blood – conscious, in pain and very pale. He is sweating profusely. He is cool peripherally and feels clammy. He is breathing fast and he is agitated. His pulse is 150/min and his BP is 70/50 mmHg. JVP is not detectable and his conjunctivae are white.

He has lost his circulating blood volume and cannot deliver oxygen. He compensates by pushing it all round faster courtesy of his sympathetic system and a fit young heart. Agitation is a function of sympathetic outflow and to some degree hypoxia. He has diverted all his remaining blood to vital areas. Other areas will be getting hypoxic rapidly. His ability to compensate falls as his blood volume reduces.

The paramedics give him oxygen, and stop the bleeding. They insert large drips into him and pour in fluid to give him a circulating volume. You only need a few red cells to carry oxygen but they have to be carried by fluid. With adequate fluid he will get a circulating volume and will be able to deliver oxygen to the tissues. Extra blood will help.

Meningococcal septicaemia – septic shock

A 24-year-old girl on a working holiday in the UK and living in a crowded flat in Earls Court develops a flu-like illness. She has temperature and sore throat. Her flatmates go to work and she rings them there later to say she is feeling worse. When they get home she is lying on a sofa, very drowsy and confused. She feels hot all over. They notice a nasty purplish rash on her feet. The ambulance takes her to hospital and she is unrousable on arrival. Her breathing is rapid and laboured and she is hot and sweaty. She has photophobia and obvious neck stiffness. Her pulse is 150/min and her BP is 80/60 mmHg. Her neck veins are not visible.

She has septic shock. 'Toxins' are causing profound vasodilation and they are probably affecting her cardiac contractility. At cell level, although oxygen is available, her cells either cannot get it or cannot use it as effectively as they would like. Her white cells are activated and are using oxygen to produce oxygen radicals to combat infection. This all leads to increased oxygen requirements. Despite her heart working as fast as it can and a huge amount of blood being pushed around the circulation, her tissues are feeling oxygen-deprived and need more. Her sympathetic system is struggling. It can push her heart but her toxaemia prevents her blood vessels from constricting to divert the blood to vital organs. With all the vasodilation, her blood volume is inadequate to fill the space and her blood pressure falls.

Antibiotics will treat the meningococcus. Treatment is by support of her circulation and provision of oxygen to try to help her organs through a period of relative hypoxia. As inotropes will not work well at vasoconstriction, the only alternative is to try to fill the circulation with enough fluid to enable it to work in its dilated state and deliver oxygen. Inotropes may be necessary to push the toxic heart. The block of oxygen utilisation will improve as the septicaemia comes under control.

SIRS, sepsis and septicaemia

Following a wide range of insults, patients can develop a pattern of illness that has been defined as the systemic inflammatory response syndrome (SIRS) (see also Ch. 9). These patients demonstrate very similar problems to those with septicaemia and for many years they were described as septic. However, while occasionally a causative organism was found, most of the time no organisms were found. This inflammatory response was probably sterile.

SIRS does not require an infective cause. Some of the features of SIRS include having more than one of the following:

- body temperature > 38°C or < 36°C
- heart rate >90 beat/min
- tachypnoea >20 or a P_aCO_2 < 4.3 kPa
- white cell count of either >120 000 or < 4000 with more than 10% of these being due to immature neutrophils.

Sepsis as a subset of SIRS can be defined in the same way but with the presence of infection.

Septicaemia is a term that has outgrown its usefulness. Bacteraemia is the presence of bacteria in the blood and sepsis is the systemic inflammatory response to infection.

It has been suggested that SIRS is caused by an inflammatory cascade. A trigger factor – which can be a bacterial agent, another microbiological agent or an insult such as trauma, toxins, damaged cells or damaged tissue – can result in the activation of active mediators from macrophages and other cells, including cytokines, prostaglandins and various peptides. These in turn lead to stimulation and release of other factors and mediators from other cells – a cascade.

The haemodynamic response in sepsis is vasodilation, which is frequently described as a reduction in systemic vascular resistance associated with a fall in blood pressure, often with an increase in heart rate but not necessarily with any change in filling pressure. Changes in membrane permeability and a tendency to form oedema in various organs, especially the lungs, are examples of occasional features of the syndrome.

In practical terms, the vasodilation and membrane permeability seen in sepsis mean that patients not only have a far bigger intravascular space than usual, but are also losing fluid from that space into the interstitium. They have inadequate fluid in the intravascular compartment. The nature of sepsis means that the vasodilatation does not respond to their sympathetic system as it should, so they become hypotensive. These changes influence their haemodynamic management. With all the sympathetic activity, raised cardiac output and cardiac work, and increased white cell activity, the oxygen requirements of these patients rise. All of these features can exist with SIRS.

Having defined the term SIRS; it is important to appreciate that it is just a name and does not obviate the necessity of determining, if possible, the cause. The problem of acronyms in ICU is a serious one. It is easy to try to treat the acronym rather than the patient. Too often a diagnosis of, for example, ARDS seems to imply that a set pattern of treatment is now appropriate and the underlying cause is no longer important. Nothing could be further from the truth. These acronyms should be an aid to description not an end-point in diagnosis and management.

One of the reasons for defining these syndromes cautiously is that they often lead on to the development of other non-specific syndromes (which carry acronyms).

SIRS is a systemic insult and potentially leads to problems throughout the body. Each and every organ system can be affected and damaged, each to a greater or lesser degree. As all organs are exposed to the generalised insult and some are overtly injured, this is grouped under the descriptive term of multiple organ system failure (MOSF). This is now called MODS (multiple organ dysfunction syndrome) because it implies that the alteration in function in each organ is not absolute at any particular point in time but describes some degree of malfunction or dysfunction which may be changing with time. Organ system dysfunction can be primary, as in an immediate response to a specific localised insult, e.g. contusion of the lung causing lung dysfunction. Alternatively, lung injury may occur as a consequence of repeated insults to all organs, including the lungs. In the first situation the injury is localised and, unless it triggers SIRS, will only affect the lung, while in the second situation all organs are affected to varying degrees and the acute lung injury is the manifestation of the generalised injury to that organ. Each organ will respond to a particular insult in an individual manner, with some organs being more susceptible than others. An example of this is hypotension and the kidney: a period of sustained hypotension will affect any perfused organ, but the kidney responds physiologically with a visible change in function. It may also be more sensitive. The effects of renal failure are easily seen, while liver or lung dysfunction may be less visible but still present.

As a non-specific insult results in a describable series of events, therapeutic strategies have been developed which aim to intervene in those patterns of events. If an initial insult liberates a cascade phenomenon, it gives us a rationale for treatment. The insult itself, whether infection, trauma, toxin or something else, should be contained and controlled and the impact of the insult minimised. For example, when treating hypovolaemia from haemorrhage, stopping the bleeding removes the insult and prompt volume replacement minimises secondary effects. These simple measures may inhibit initiation of any cascade while sustained hypovolaemia may trigger the cascade.

If the cascade has started, there may be ways of impeding its development, i.e. mopping up the trigger factors. Endotoxins have been implicated and there is considerable interest in the use of various antibodies for mopping up endotoxins, but to date the results are unconvincing.

An alternative approach is to block mediators within the cascade. Attempts have been made to use antibodies to block either the cytokines themselves, e.g. anti-TNF antibodies, or the cytokine receptors or to inhibit their production with the use of agents such as pentoxifylline. Prostaglandins have been implicated in the sepsis syndrome and agents which inhibit them, such as ibuprofen, have been tried.

At capillary level, local production of nitric oxide is involved in capillary reactivity. This is often abnormal in sepsis. In the pulmonary vasculature, vasoconstriction can be reversed using exogenous nitric oxide which may be helpful in oxygenating the patient. Paradoxically, there may be too much nitric oxide peripherally and agents which block its production are being investigated.

Free radical production is another area of current interest. White cell activation increases in SIRS. Oxygen radicals are produced and may account for some of the increased oxygen utilised in SIRS. Free radical scavengers and antioxidants have been tried, but while there is a lot of evidence that free radicals are involved in some aspects of organ system damage, there is little or no data showing the efficacy of free radical scavengers.

An important part of the management of the critically ill with or without SIRS is preventing the primary problem from recurring and preventing or reducing secondary insults. These insults include nosocomial infection, haemodynamic instability and hypoxaemia. Management also involves minimising catabolism and trying to provide nutritional support.

Monitoring (see also Ch. 6)

It is important to consider what monitoring is for and what it is not for. Assessment and monitoring are in the first instance a 'hands-on' phenomenon. Equipment facilitates and supports clinical monitoring. From field to hospital, into the resuscitation room, to wards, operating theatre or ITU, the personnel looking after the patient are responsible for continual reassessment and monitoring of physiological parameters and should act on these assessments.

Monitoring systems provide several additional benefits (see Box 10.3). However, they are always an adjunct and a help to the clinicians, not a replacement; they do not substitute for clinical acumen. This is in contrast to the alternative view that patient management requires total body monitoring and total body pan-scanning to provide maximum information and

---

Box 10.3

Advantages of monitoring systems

Confirm and support clinical monitoring; enhance accuracy and frequency
Detect changes early
Guide and follow clinical interventions
Free up clinicians from repetitive, time-consuming tasks

early warning of problems. This latter approach presumes that any kind of monitoring provides information and that all information is intrinsically beneficial. But remember: a small amount of relevant information is infinitely preferable to any amount of irrelevant information.

Monitoring is an adjunct to management, not vice versa, and a careful balance has to be struck when deciding which monitors to use, based on a cost–benefit analysis. One then has to decide what constitutes minimal requirements and build from that starting point. The question should be 'what do I need?' not 'what would I like?'. Monitoring should always assist and never hinder.

There are many monitoring facilities which can help considerably and, given the fundamental provisos discussed above, they can make management very much more effective.

Monitoring by organ system

The central nervous system

Clinical appraisal is most important. Scoring is usually by the Glasgow Coma Scale, which gives a reasonable indication of level of consciousness irrespective of cause. Localising or lateralising signs may indicate the need for a CT scan providing the patient has been assessed and is stable in other respects. This is particularly pertinent in neurotrauma (see Ch. 3). CT scans provide anatomical information but do not indicate function. MRI scanning has a limited place in the critically ill but may be of assistance in the specific diagnosis of certain types of lesion. Intracranial pressure (ICP) monitoring may be useful in situations where there is intracranial damage and swelling or oedema is anticipated, e.g. following a closed head injury. Monitoring the ICP identifies and characterises the problem and may facilitate interventions designed to reduce the pressure. High pressure may impede the blood supply to the brain. If the ICP is known then the cerebral perfusion pressure (CCP) can be calculated (mean blood pressure – ICP). Currently a CPP of greater than 60 mmHg is thought best to ensure adequate perfusion.

Electroencephalograph, (EEG) may be helpful in determining if there is evidence of fitting or to assess the level of electrical activity. Cerebral function monitors, which allow continual assessment of electrical activity, are used in some situations to monitor the level of cerebral electrical activity.

Evoked potential monitoring involves providing a stimulus and measuring the response to determine whether the central nervous connections are intact and the speed of response. These are specialised measurements and require careful expert interpretation.

The respiratory system

Clinical monitoring is of paramount importance. The pattern and rate of breathing, whether ancillary muscles have been recruited, the patient's colour and general condition all provide information as to the adequacy of respiratory function. Clinical awareness of 'tiredness', when a patient is struggling to breathe but seems too 'tired' to breathe effectively, is an important sign both off and on a ventilator. These clinical signs are of greater value than blood gases, which will usually help confirm a clinical impression.

Pulse oximetry (See Ch. 6) measures, by light absorption methods, the saturation of haemoglobin in arterial blood. It is non-invasive and easy and rapid to apply. It indicates oxygenation and pulse rate. Indirectly it indicates perfusion as a trace, which is an indication of blood flow. However, as most oximeters compensate for the signal and amplify low output, the trace is not a direct measurement. Therefore the presence of a trace indicates perfusion but the compensatory mechanisms prevent extrapolation of the trace into qualitative values. There are several situations where the trace may be misleading. It is a late indicator of hypoxia so desaturation means that hypoxia is present. Peripheral perfusion may influence accuracy. The presence of carboxyhaemoglobin in significant amounts will give an artificially high value at about 85% even if the oxyhaemoglobin is much lower. It is also unreliable in a very anaemic patient. The values from the oximeter must be checked by evaluating against clinical assessment. Genuine changes and artefacts are common but it is still a very useful monitoring tool. In current practice it is extremely useful in ventilated patients and reduces dependence on blood gas analysis.

Airway pressure monitoring will show the peak pressures in the upper airway and give an indication of the pressures to which the lungs are exposed. High pressures (greater than 40 cmH$_2$O) are associated with barotrauma manifested as alveoli breakdown and pneumothoraces. This technique will also indicate and monitor residual pressure in the lungs when using positive end expiratory pressure (PEEP) or continuous positive airways pressure (CPAP) modes of respiratory support. All patients on ventilators should have their airway pressures monitored routinely.

End-tidal carbon dioxide is easily measured on a breath by breath basis. The presence of carbon dioxide helps to confirm both tube placement and ventilation. It is also an indirect indicator of cardiac output, as the carbon dioxide delivered to the lungs falls with falling cardiac output.

The chest X-ray is also a monitor of the respiratory system, not just for acute events, e.g. pneumothorax or aspiration, but more importantly for following trends such as the development or resolution of pneumonia or oedema.

Arterial blood gases are a standard measurement in the critically ill patient. The partial pressures of oxygen and carbon dioxide are measured, as is the acid–base status. The carbon dioxide pressure indicates efficacy of ventilation. Oxygenation is indicated by the arterial oxygen partial pressure. The pH and the base deficit indicate the acid–base status and the likely cause of an acidosis, whether metabolic (low bicarbonate value) or respiratory (high carbon dioxide value). These measurements are invaluable in assessing a patient's condition. These measurements can also be used in combination with others, such as cardiac output, to measure oxygen delivery to the tissues.

The cardiovascular system

A simple cardiograph gives heart rate and rhythm which is a valuable continuous clinical sign. The trace itself may give warning of ischaemia by monitoring the ST segment.

Manual blood pressure monitoring is labour-intensive, very intermittent and often unreliable. Automatic non-invasive systems are relatively cheap, easy to apply and an excellent example of how monitoring can be done more frequently and accurately and free up personnel at the same time. The monitors do not treat but their presence gives clinicians more time. They are temperamental in the very unstable situation but useful once there is an element of control. They enable regular and reliable monitoring on an almost continual basis.

Invasive arterial monitoring is extremely helpful where there is instability. It is immediate and continuous. The trace can provide useful information as well as the absolute values. Fluctuations in amplitude with respiration show the reliance of cardiac output on venous return which is accentuated in hypovolaemia.

Central venous pressure (CVP) monitoring can be helpful. A catheter placed in a central vein will give a pressure indicative of the pressure in the venous system returning blood to the heart, as does estimating the jugular venous pressure: low may indicate hypovolaemia while high may indicate overfilling. However, clinical judgement based on the signs of pulse rate (high), blood pressure (low) and peripheral perfusion (poor) tell you when a patient is 'empty' and confirmation with CVP is not necessary. The value may be helpful with control of fluid administration. With rapid refilling it helps to prevent pushing the filling pressures too high and this is its main use.

It is very important to remember that the CVP measures pressure not volume and does not indicate volume status of the patient. A young exsanguinated patient can compensate with vasoconstriction. A normal CVP can be achieved easily while that patient is tightly vasoconstricted, but if vasodilation occurs, as with analgesia, the fluid deficit is rapidly and sometimes disastrously exposed. It is the assessment of CVP in association with other signs such as peripheral perfusion which gives some indication of intravascular volume status.

Monitoring of the left side of the heart gives an indication of left ventricular function, which may be significantly different from that indicated by the right side pressures in some circumstances. A pulmonary artery catheter can be introduced for this purpose, usually through a central vein, through the heart and into the pulmonary artery. If flow into the vessel containing the catheter is obstructed by inflating a balloon in that vessel, the pressure measured distal to the ballon reflects the pressure of the left atrium.

Oxygen delivery and consumption can also be measured. Oxygen delivery is the volume of blood (cardiac output) multiplied by the amount of oxygen it contains (determined by knowing the haemoglobin, the saturation and the binding coefficient of haemoglobin). Cardiac output can be measured with a pulmonary artery catheter, the arterial blood gases will give the saturation and the haemoglobin can be measured. The binding coefficient is a known constant. It is then easy to calculate the quantity of oxygen delivered by the heart per minute, i.e. the oxygen delivery. After passing around the body, the blood comes back to the lungs, depleted of oxygen. This can be measured by sampling a mixed venous sample from the pulmonary artery through the catheter. The difference between that delivered and that returned is the oxygen consumption.

The gastrointestinal system

Gastrointestinal functional assessment starts with the physical examination of the abdomen. Conscious level is important, as in the unconscious, unresponsive or intubated patient, the flat, soft abdomen can be misleading. Passing a nasogastric tube can be informative in terms of stomach contents, the presence of gastric emptying with low volume residue and also gastric pH. Some sources recommend using gastric tonometry, which measures intraluminal pH, to indicate gut perfusion. Intraluminal acidosis indicates poor mucosal perfusion, the implication being that increasing blood supply to that area may be of benefit. The value of gastric tonometry is controversial.

The urological system

Renal function is easily monitored with a urinary catheter. The presence of albumin glucose or blood in the urine can be ascertained. Urine volume is a useful indicator of general renal function. Tests such as short-term creatinine clearance measurements can give more accurate assessment of function, as can monitoring plasma urea and creatinine.

In impaired renal function the urea and creatinine both rise. In a dehydrated patient the urea may be reabsorbed while creatinine is not, leading to a greater rise in urea than in creatinine. Other causes of this are increased urea absorption from other sites, the most common example being gastrointestinal bleeding.

Other monitoring

Temperature

Temperature is always measured in the critically ill. Core temperature is more useful than peripheral temperature. The differential between core and periphery is an indirect measure of general perfusion and can be a useful tool.

Pregnancy

Pregnant patients are rarely discussed and yet they present a particularly difficult problem: there are two patients involved, mother and fetus. Both should be monitored as early as possible as this may influence decisions regarding delivery. Monitoring can be clinical in the first instance, preferably with obstetric medical involvement, but use of continuous fetal heart monitoring assists during the various phases of resuscitation. It does not take priority over the ABC of resuscitation. Monitors will not save patients, but may prevent them from dying.

Therapeutics

In the ICU every therapeutic intervention is performed to achieve benefit. Each and every intervention will have both positive and negative attributes. It is essential that each is evaluated in terms of potential benefits against potential harm prior to use. To do this, both positive and negative attributes need to be understood. The other fundamental principle is that it is better to prevent than to treat.

There are two parallel approaches necessary in the critically ill: resuscitation and diagnosis. It is essential to resuscitate the patient and correct life-threatening physiological disturbances. It is also vital to make a diagnosis so that the cause can be treated. All too often the diagnosis is ignored while the patient is salvaged, or alternatively the patient lost while the diagnosis is made. Both are essential in the management of the critically ill.

The goals of treatment are to:

* correct physiological disturbance and support normal physiology
* treat the underlying cause
* prevent secondary problems.

The respiratory system

Adequate oxygenation is fundamental. It is important to ensure that the patient is ventilating adequately and that the inspired oxygen is adequate to ensure oxygenation.

Ventilatory failure

Ventilatory failure is brought about by the inability of the chest wall to generate a negative pressure and therefore to ventilate adequately (Box 10.4). Management involves reversing the cause. An example of this is apnoea secondary to opiate overdose depressing ventilation. Naloxone reverses the opiate-induced respiratory depression allowing the patient to breathe. Another example is apnoea due to airway obstruction: clearing the airway allows spontaneous ventilation.

Alternatively the patient may be ventilated. Mechanical ventilation is extremely effective for ventilatory failure, whether mechanical or neurological.

Respiratory failure (see Box 10.5)

This is lung failure or the inability to take oxygen up from the lung and to excrete carbon dioxide from the lung due to problems within it. This occurs either because there is mismatch between ventilation (V) and perfusion (Q) or because there is an effective barrier between the gas space and the blood which inhibits gas exchange. In the case of a mismatch there may be parts of the lung which are well ventilated but have no blood supply; a pulmonary embolus would do this. Alternatively there may be a good blood supply but no ventilation; severe pneumonia or atelectasis will cause this.

A barrier may be formed by fluid, pulmonary oedema or inflammatory or cellular infiltrates. There is

---

Box 10.4

Causes of ventilatory failure

CNS failure and loss of respiratory drive – CVA, sedative drugs, head injury, spinal cord injury, infections (e.g. meningoencephalitis), sleep apnoea

Peripheral nerves – phrenic nerve damage, neuromuscular blockade, myasthenia, Guillain–Barré

Muscular problems – dystrophies, electrolyte disturbances (hypokalaemia, hypophosphataemia), disrupted diaphragm, disuse atrophy

Chest wall – fractured ribs, thoracic surgery, kyphoscoliosis, obesity

Airway – bronchospasm, obstruction, pulmonary fibrosis, air trapping

---

Box 10.5

Causes of respiratory failure

Hypercapnic (ventilatory) failure
Central nervous system
Peripheral nervous system
Chest wall/musculoskeletal
Upper airways
Lower airways
Hypoxaemic 'lung' failure
Alveolar hypoventilation
V/Q abnormality
Diffusion defects
Right-to-left shunt

---

a condition termed, adult respiratory distress syndrome (ARDS), or more recently acute lung injury (also known as non-cardiogenic pulmonary oedema), which is essentially hypoxaemia in the presence of low cardiac filling pressures; it is associated with diffuse alveolar infiltrates apparent on chest X-ray. In fact, the original definition was radiological. Any insult involving the lung (either local to the lung or general) may result in acute lung injury (ARDS, see Box 10.6).

The main problems with ARDS lie in determining the underlying diagnosis in order to treat the problem and dealing with oxygenation. The pathophysiology is a combination of V/Q mismatch, some shunting and a barrier effect. Therapeutic measures include:

- methods to reverse the pathology by recruiting alveoli, thereby increasing the surface area of gas exchange
- methods to alter local perfusion by vasodilatation

Box 10.6

Causes of acute lung injury (ARDS)

Local insult

Smoke inhalation
Airway burns
Aspiration of gastric acid
Near-drowning

Parenchymal insults

Confusion
Infection (bacterial and viral)

Systemic insults

Septicaemia and SIRS
Shock of any cause
Pancreatitis
Amniotic fluid embolus

- methods to improve the blood supply to ventilated alveoli, such as inhaled nitric oxide
- more simple methods such as increasing the inspired oxygen concentration.

Where gas exchange is poor, ventilatory failure is likely to become superimposed on respiratory failure and ventilation may help to alleviate the ventilatory component. Unfortunately it may aggravate part of the respiratory component as the balance of V/Q abnormality is unpredictably altered by positive pressure ventilation.

Lung failure is almost always a combination of different pathophysiological factors and is far more difficult to treat than ventilatory failure.

Methods of ventilation

Spontaneous breathing is the physiological norm. The chest generates a negative pressure and entrains air. The negative pressure assists venous return to the heart. Ventilation and perfusion of areas within the lung are controlled by intrinsic mechanisms.

Mechanical ventilation is not physiological. It creates positive pressure in the chest, forcing air into areas that are most compliant (easily distendable). A number of modes of respiratory support and ventilation are used, as summarised in Table 10.4. However, it should be noted that there are negative aspects of positive pressure ventilation:

- impairs venous return and depresses cardiac output
- induces endocrine changes, e.g. raised ADH
- worsens V/Q abnormality and gas exchange
- produces barotrauma
- creates a need for increased sedation or relaxants
- creates a potential for infection.

In very severe cases, it may be possible to manage oxygenation by putting the patient on extracorporeal membrane oxygenation (ECMO), but this is largely experimental at the present time.

The cardiovascular system

Support of the cardiovascular system is a fundamental part of management of the critically ill patient. This is the system that delivers oxygen from the lungs to the tissues and ultimately to the cells. Failure of this system, either locally or globally, leads to tissue hypoxia. The areas which may be influenced are the heart and the vascular system.

The heart may fail for a number of reasons, including the failure to maintain adequate performance, either through impaired contractility or through an inefficient rate, whether high or low. Another mechanism of heart

Table 10.4
Modes of respiratory support and ventilation features

Spontaneous

Continuous positive airway pressure (CPAP)	Positive pressure overcomes resistance to inspiration, opens and keeps open alveoli which may otherwise collapse. Reduces work of breathing, recruits alveoli and improves oxygenation

Ventilation

Continuous positive pressure ventilation (CMV)	Machine provides all ventilation
Intermittent mandatory ventilation (IMV)	Machine provides set number of breaths and the patient breathes between
SIMV	Patient can trigger machine breaths as well as breathe between mandatory breaths
Assists spontaneous breathing (ASB)	Patient triggers machine which applies a preset pressure to assist the patient's breathing
Inverse ratio ventilation (IRV)	The inspiration : expiration (I : E) ratio is usually 1:2 but this reverses the ratio to 2:1. A longer inspiratory time allows longer for pressure to expand the lung and recruit alveoli. Helps oxygenation. Higher mean pressure in the airway
Positive end expiratory pressure (PEEP)	Applied with most ventilation modes. Maintains positive pressure in the airway and helps prevent collapse of alveoli. Better oxygenation, worse venous return.

Table 10.5
Cardiac inotropes: their effects on the heart and peripheral vasculature

Drug	Contractility	Rate	Vaso-constriction	Vaso-dilatation
Adrenaline (high dose)	+++++	+++	++++	
		+		
Adrenaline (low dose)	+++	++		++
Noradrenaline	+++	+	+++++	
Dopamine (high dose)	+++	+++	++++	
Dopamine (low dose)	+	+		+
Dobutamine	+++	++		+++
Dopexamine	+++	++		+++
Milrinone	++	++		++++

failure is where, despite performing well, the heart fails to meet the excessive requirements imposed upon it. The intravascular volume is a fundamental part of cardiac performance and any cause of hypovolaemia will reduce cardiovascular performance.

Vascular changes influence the work that the heart has to perform. Vasoconstriction will tend to increase the work of the heart. Profound vasodilatation will reduce the work against resistance but may necessitate a larger cardiac output to sustain blood pressure.

The cardiovascular system obeys the rule $V = IR$, where V is pressure, I is flow or cardiac output and R is the resistance of the system. Each can be influenced by disease and each can be therapeutically manipulated. The key question is the volume status of the patient. This needs to be optimal. Assessment of volume is performed by evaluating perfusion (e.g. a warm periphery) and filling pressure (the JVP). This can be measured directly, as the CVP. The CVP does not indicate volume, only pressure, and an assessment of perfusion must be made.

If a patient is hypovolaemic, this should be corrected. The optimal filling pressure for the heart should be found. An easy test is to administer fluid to the patient until filling appears to be adequate. Then give small incremental boluses of fluid (200 mL in an adult) to see if the blood pressure improves. At the point where there is no improvement in blood pressure, the filling is probably optimal.

Cardiac performance can be improved by influencing contractility and, sometimes, rate. Various inotropes have effects on cardiac performance and on the vasculature (Table 10.5). The vasculature can be influenced by the vasoconstrictors listed in Table 10.5, but it is also possible to use a direct alpha-agonist such as phenylephrine or metaraminol as a potent vaso-constrictor. Vasodilators currently used include glyceryl trinitrate (GTN), sodium nitroprusside and prostacyclin.

Over the last few years there has been considerable emphasis on measuring oxygen delivery and attempting to increase delivery if thought inadequate. The difficulty is that, when grossly inadequate, it is obvious, but it has proved very difficult to define when a small enhancement of oxygen delivery might be of benefit. One of the problems is that there is a cost for increasing oxygen delivery by virtue of the other effects of the drugs used.

Methods of improving oxygen delivery

There are various methods of increasing the oxygen supply. At the lungs the inspired oxygen concentration can be increased. In the lungs, V/Q may be influenced by CPAP, ventilation pattern (Table 10.4) or by agents such as nitric oxide. In the blood, oxygen carriage can be increased by changing haemoglobin concentration and guaranteeing intravascular volume. The delivery of oxygen can be enhanced by increasing cardiac output. This is achieved by volume loading or inotropes, or both. In the periphery, delivery may be influenced by venodilators such as GTN or prostacyclins.

An alternative approach to improving the ratio of supply to requirements is to reduce requirements by reducing consumption. The work of breathing is reduced by using a ventilator. Good temperature control, either by reducing hyperthermia or by generating hypothermia, will also cut the oxygen requirement.

The kidneys and renal failure

While the critically ill may develop renal failure for any of the reasons seen in the normal population, some causes are far more commonly seen. The mechanism is frequently prerenal due to effective hypovolaemia and hypoperfusion of the kidneys. Common causes include dehydration from poor fluid intake and inadequate replacement, and loss of fluid from any cause e.g. diabetes mellitus and insipidus, bleeding, burns, diarrhoea and vomiting. Renal causes, including diseases such as glomerulonephritis, are relatively uncommon although nephrotoxicity from drugs is frequently a component of renal failure in critically ill patients. Postrenal causes should always be excluded, usually by ultrasound.

As with many situations in the critically ill, there may be multiple causes. A kidney damaged by prerenal failure is more susceptible to nephrotoxicity, and potent and potentially dangerous drugs are more likely to be used in the critically ill. Due to alterations in drug kinetics, the use of these drugs is also far less predictable in this setting.

The principles of managing renal dysfunction are simple. Try to identify the cause of the problem while ensuring that there is no prerenal element by maintaining a well perfused patient with adequate blood pressure. An adequate blood pressure is one that is preferably close to the patient's normal value. This may require aggressive fluid management and sometimes inotropes. As perfusion is also important, it may be necessary to add a vasodilator to improve this.

There are also some other time-honoured methods of encouraging urine output. Diuretics should only be used if the patient is normovolaemic as they can aggravate hypovolaemia. Osmotic diuretics are sometimes used especially if there is jaundice when patients are particularly susceptible to renal injury. Frusemide is also often used and acts by affecting the Na/K pump in the loop of Henle, encouraging a diuresis. It is currently thought that, at low dose, frusemide also reduces the oxygen requirement of the tubules and protects them from hypoxia. These methods are frequently advocated and regularly used, but remain of unproven benefit.

In the critically ill, renal failure is usually associated with generalised injury, and if the kidneys are failing there is usually damage to other organs although it may be less easily detected. When renal failure is secondary to severe injury it carries a poor prognosis and the mortality in the critically ill with renal failure is high, claimed to be between 50 and 70% in most series and unchanged by recent advances. If the renal failure is genuinely an isolated phenomenon, associated with, for example, a nephrotoxic drug, it usually has a good prognosis.

Renal replacement

The principles of renal replacement are simple. The object is to remove toxic materials such as urea, creatinine and potassium from the blood. This can be done in two ways. The first of these is to remove or filter all the fluid containing the toxic waste and replace it with clean replacement fluid. This is filtration and the removal of fluid parallels the glomerular filtration rate (GFR). A GFR of 20 mL/min needs $20 \times 60 = 1200$ mL/h or 28.8 L/day of replacement fluid.

The second method involves the use of the osmotic gradient (*dialysis*). If the plasma with toxic waste is exposed to similar fluid with no toxins across a semipermeable membrane, the toxins will pass down a concentration gradient into the clean solution. If a countercurrent is used, there is rapid transit of both urea and creatinine and this is similar to the mechanism in the tubule. No replacement fluid needs to be given and there is no contact between body fluid, plasma and the dialysis fluid except across the semipermeable membrane. Creatinine clearances of 25–30 mL/min are easily achieved.

The blood flow through the filters can be driven either by blood pressure using an arteriovenous shunt or by venovenous pump. The latter is more dependable, independent of blood pressure and has minimal haemodynamic consequences. Standard dialysis with high flows can be used for much more rapid clearances but is more likely to result in haemodynamic instability.

The central nervous system

The central nervous system is very susceptible to injury and, in particular, to hypoxia. Once damage has occurred, reversal of damage is difficult or impossible. The main thrust of intensive care management of brain injury is to limit the damage that is taking place, prevent further damage and then attempt to reverse injury or at least provide an environment where recovery is more likely.

Fitting

There are two potential problems: hypoxia both from poor ventilation and from localised hypoxia around the area of the epileptiform activity in the brain, and injury from fitting itself. Treatment involves protection of the airway, ensuring adequate oxygenation and control of the fits. The latter is achieved with anticonvulsants, but while they may control the fits, they may also depress ventilation.

Table 10.6
Factors affecting intracranial pressure (ICP)

ICP	Intervention
↑ ICP	↑ Blood pressure
	↑ Fluids
	↑ P_aCO_2
	Head-down posture
↓ ICP	↓ Blood pressure
	↓ P_aCO_2
	Head up posture
	Barbiturates ?
Ideal ICP	Prevent hypoxia and hypercarbia
	Normocarbia or mild hypocapnia
	Maintain cerebral perfusion pressure (CCP)
	Avoid acute changes in blood pressure

Table 10.7
Factors involved in the gut which can become a source of problems in the critically ill

H_2 antagonists	Reduced pH	Increased colonisation
Nil by mouth	Reduced gastric emptying	Increased colonisation Cholestasis?
	Altered upper GI dynamics	Changed flora
	Reduced substrates in gut	Reduced biosynthesis
Antibiotics	Changed flora	Pathogenic organisms increased
		Reduced biosynthesis
Stasis	Overgrowth	Translocation?
	Villous atrophy	Toxaemia
	Immunological incompetence	Infection
Poor perfusion in gut and liver	Barrier incompetence (morphological and immunological)	Barrier incompetence Toxaemia and translocation

Cerebral injury and cerebral oedema

The brain is in an enclosed space. Most kinds of injury result in localised oedema and, if this is extensive, the brain will swell and then be constrained by the skull. Pressure in the brain will rise and blood flow will fall (Table 10.6). Tissue hypoxia will result, accentuating the injury. The approach to treatment is to prevent a rise in intracranial pressure (ICP) but to try to ensure that the cerebral perfusion pressure (i.e. systolic blood pressure – ICP) remains adequate to perfuse the brain.

Several mechanisms are likely to cause a rise in ICP (Table 10.6). Acute rises in blood pressure must be prevented. Hypercapnia also causes a rise in ICP. Excess fluid administration may increase oedema formation, as may a head-down posture. These should be avoided but the cerebral perfusion pressure must be maintained, so hypotension must be avoided. Hypocapnia can result in cerebral vasoconstriction and reduced cerebral flow, so that should also be avoided.

Mechanisms for reducing intracranial pressure include diuretics such as mannitol. This will reduce pressure acutely and is useful in a crisis, as is hypocapnia, but sustained use of either will cause problems. In severe situation, using agents to reduce cerebral oxygen requirement to help protect the cells has been advocated and drugs such as barbiturates have been used. The penalties associated with prolonged iatrogenic coma almost certainly outweigh the perceived benefit.

The key to cerebral treatment is cerebral protection.

The gastrointestinal system

Intestinal function consists of the absorption of nutrients, and the colon may also be involved in biosynthesis of short-chain fatty acids and branch-chain amino acids. The bowel is full of organisms and, in the critically ill, has been described as 'the sewer within'. The organisms are usually commensals with which the host lives comfortably under normal circumstances. Table 10.7 lists a number of factors which affect intestinal function in the critically ill.

The gut often becomes quiescent in the critically ill and the milieu of the contents changes in terms of the substrates present. Antibiotics decimate gut flora and allow overgrowth of any organisms which are unimpaired by them. The flora changes completely to one which may be potentially hazardous to the host. An example of this is the high incidence of *Enterobacter faecalis* seen in ICUs since cephalosporins became routine for surgical prophylaxis, as this organism is resistant to cephalosporins.

Furthermore, in critically ill patients, gastric stress ulceration is a potentially lethal complication which is occasionally seen and, to prevent this, H_2 antagonists are used to reduce acid secretion. This increases intragastric pH and allows bacterial overgrowth of the upper GI tract, colonised from organisms which usually cannot thrive in the upper intestine. This may in turn, by spilling over into the respiratory tract, increase the incidence of nosocomial ('hospital-acquired') pneumonia. The stagnant gut also tends to undergo epithelial atrophy. The morphological and immunological barrier which exists in the gut wall may become impaired and translocation of toxins and even bacteria may increase across the gut wall. These effects are accentuated by poor gut and liver perfusion in critically ill patients. Toxaemia and sepsis may then arise from the gut.

Various strategies are used to reduce these potential problems. H_2 antagonists are avoided by using mucosa-protecting agents such as sucralfate to prevent stress ulceration without altering pH. Early feeding prevents gut atrophy, reduces translocation and helps to sustain immunocompetence of the gut wall. Antibiotics should be avoided when possible to preserve commensal bacteria. Enteral feeding and the use of carbohydrates, live yoghurt and other agents which may encourage friendly flora to colonise the gut are strategies that may be used in the future – so-called probiotic therapy.

Early feeding

After major surgery the small bowel often starts peristalsis very rapidly – within a couple of days as can be demonstrated with ultrasound. Unfortunately gastric emptying is frequently delayed and so feeding via nasogastric tube may be futile. Some drugs, including dopamine, impair gastric emptying without influencing small bowel motility. Tubes may be placed in the jejunum from the nose via the stomach (nasojejunal) or a feeding jejunostomy catheter may be placed at operation. The benefits of early enteral feeding are better colonisation, less small bowel atrophy, better immunological function and less translocation.

Any approach to nutrition must take into account the pathophysiology of the patient at the time. There are three main categories of patient:

- the starved patient
- the hypercatabolic injured patient
- the starved hypercatabolic patient.

The starved patient has a specific response to starvation with a general slowing of metabolic rate, an adaptation to fat utilisation and an endocrine profile concomitant with this. Such patients are tuned to being able to survive by conservation of resources. Their energy expenditure is relatively stable and therefore predictable. These patients will adapt readily and rapidly to nutritional support and will utilise it efficiently. They will utilise both fats and glucose but are very well adapted to fat utilisation. In this regard, total parenteral nutrition (TPN) reverses starvation catabolism in skeletal muscle.

The injured patient has an increased metabolic rate and a hormonal profile which enhances metabolic activity. While there is an adaptation of normal tissues towards fat utilisation, there is also an increased glucose requirement by the injured tissues. The endocrine profile is described as a stress response. The energy utilisation is extremely variable and unpredictable; indeed the calculated energy utilisation by indirect calorimetry can vary by 30% on consecutive days.

Under these conditions an overall change in metabolic status occurs. There is an increase in resting oxygen consumption, with a respiratory quotient (RQ) of 0.8–0.85, reflecting a mixed fuel source. Energy is derived from available glucose, proteins and some fats. There is an increase in all these substrates, but as fat utilisation increases there is a relative decrease in the ratio of calories derived from glucose and from amino acids.

Nutritional support

There are two principles underlying nutritional support:

- everyone needs food
- the easiest, most normal route is best.

Nutrition is important not only because a small but significant proportion of patients are malnourished but also because the stress of major surgery or illness rapidly depletes nutritional resources. It is well known that operating on severely malnourished patients carries a high morbidity, and the fact that malnutrition is associated with poor outcome has led to the sensible assumption that nutritional support and correction are probably beneficial. Preoperative correction of malnutrition is probably relevant in less than 5% of patients admitted for major surgery, but it is important to note that it takes some time, probably about 10 days or longer, to make any impact on nutritional status.

In the critically ill, support of the catabolic patient during the acute phase of the illness may be crucial to survival. Malnutrition reduces the resistance to infection and slows down most healing processes. There is also an associated reduction in oxidation of pyruvate and an increase in release of alanine and lactate with oxidation of C_2 fragments from fat and amino acids. Carbohydrate metabolism is characterised by increased glycogenolysis, not suppressible with exogenous insulin or glucose, and an increase in glucose flow and utilisation by peripheral tissues, especially those that are injured. Insulin is increased but so is the glucagon: insulin ratio. The peripheral lactate by-product is recycled through the liver. Fat metabolism is increased with an increase in lipolysis and decreased lipogenesis. There is increased mobilisation of long- and medium-chain fatty acids with a reduction in clearance of fatty acids. The increase in protein catabolism has already been mentioned with the resultant massive mobilisation of amino acids. There is increased use of branch-chain acids, in particular glutamine, which is produced to transport available amino acids to sites of utilisation both as amino acids and as a calorie source to produce ATP via the Krebs cycle. Glutamine can be easily used as a primary substrate by many organs including the gut.

Nutritional assessment can be done at the bedside and should be part of the physical examination. Look for signs of weight loss. More sophisticated methods use arm muscle circumference, arm circumference and triceps skinfold thickness. This last measurement can indicate loss of muscle bulk but is better as a trend measurement than as an isolated reading as it takes 3–4 weeks to show nutritional change. Measurements of serum albumin, total non-binding capacity (TIBC), transferrin, thyroxine-binding pre-albumin and retinol-binding protein can all be used to assess nutritional status.

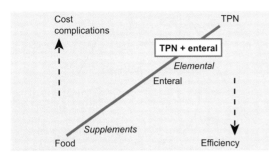

Fig 10.2 **Nutritional methods and their relationship to cost, complications and deficiency.**

Administration

The route of nutrition is important. Enteral feeding is cheaper, safer and more efficient than parenteral feeding (Fig. 10.2). There should be a gradation from normal food at one end of the spectrum through to total parenteral nutrition (TPN) at the other. Efforts should be made to keep nutrition as simple as possible: simple is safe.

Enteral feeding

Enteral feeding keeps the gut functional, helps to maintain normal gut flora and may reduce the incidence of sepsis. The gut can assimilate and use nutrition from the gut lumen and this may play a part in keeping the intestinal mucosa healthy. Current practice is to encourage early and aggressive enteral feeding. A number of different enteral feeds are available and they may be delivered into the stomach or proximal jejunum.

Parenteral feeding (TPN)

Intravenous supplementation should seek to provide the optimal combination of water, calories, protein, vitamins and trace metals for an adequate diet. This is in the context of the underlying problem and the ability of the patient to cope with not only the fluid load but also the nutritional load.

The two main components are calories and protein – the former as glucose or fat, and the latter as amino acids. In starvation, large calorie loads can be used, e.g. 55 kcal/kg per day with a kcal:N ratio of 200:1. In catabolic septic or injured patients, a calorie input of 30 kcal/kg per day and a kcal:N ratio of 100:1 (0.3 g/kg per day) are more appropriate.

Energy requirements are a controversial issue. After elective surgery, peak metabolism increases by 10–13% and returns rapidly to normal. After burns it may increase by 50%, largely determined by the temperature gradient between the patient and the ambient environment as the calories are largely used to sustain body temperature. A calorie requirement of 34 kcal/kg per day is not unreasonable.

Glucose is a good calorie source, but after a maximum of about 5 mg/kg per minute there is a tendency for glucose to become lipid through lipogenesis with a high output of CO_2 in the process. Glucose yields about 4 kcal/g. Lipid is easily administered and effectively used. Fat-soluble vitamins as well as essential phospholipids can be given with the lipid. The emulsion has chylomicron size globules which are cleared from the circulation.

Protein is given in the form of amino acids at a rate of about 0.3 g N_2/kg per day. The range of available amino acids should include branch-chain amino acids, in particular glutamine.

Vitamins and trace elements should be supplemented in the critically ill. Folate deficiency is relatively common as is thiamine deficiency. Selenium is also recognised as being commonly deficient and may play a significant role in prostaglandin pathways and in leucocyte function, via glutathione reductase. Zinc, iron, copper, manganese, cobalt, iodine, chromium and molybdenum are also important.

Complications of TPN

The complications of TPN are all the complications of venous access, including pneumothorax, arterial puncture and, most importantly, infection. TPN is associated with sepsis and line infection is a common problem with a significant morbidity. Disciplined asepsis when dealing with TPN lines and rigorous surveillance are both essential. Other problems include cholestasis, which is also seen in the critically ill patient without TPN.

Coagulation

There are many causes of coagulopathy in critically ill patients. Postoperatively the commonest cause after a large haemorrhage and massive blood transfusion is exhaustion of clotting factors, often including platelets. This coagulopathy will respond to replacement therapy.

Abnormal coagulopathies include disseminated intravascular coagulopathy (DIC). In patients with major sepsis complicating the surgery, DIC may develop. Other causes include devitalised tissue or gross disruption of tissues. Brain contains cerebral thromboplastins and massive disruption of cerebral tissue may result in release of thromboplastin and cause DIC; this is seen as deteriorating clotting studies with falling platelets and raised fibrin degradation products (FDPs). Clinically there may be bleeding from puncture sites, and blood samples taken fail to clot. Treatment is twofold: firstly, correction of the precipitating cause; and secondly, support, with replenishment of the clotting system.

Infection

While relatively few patients present with infection as a primary diagnosis, infection is a major problem in ICU

Box 10.7

Patient surveillance

Clinical – clinical behaviour, temperature, white cell count, CRP

Blood cultures – through central lines, peripheral sites

Wound culture – wound sites

Sputum – regular sputum culture

Skin – skin swabs for methicillin-resistant *Staphylococcus aureus* (MRSA)

Nares – nasal swabs

Urine – midstream urine

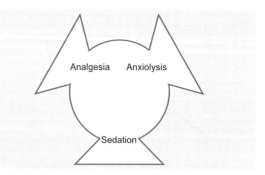

Fig 10.3 **Overlapping objectives in an intensive care unit.**

because it is a very common secondary complication in ill patients. Whatever the primary cause of their illness, whether trauma, major surgery or infection, the severe stress imposed tends to threaten their immunocompetence. These patients undergo multiple procedures and have many breaches of their integument, such as wounds, intravenous lines and endotracheal tubes, all of which can serve as conduits for infection.

Because of the serious nature of infection in the ICU and the heavy use of powerful antibiotics, the unit tends to harbour pathogenic and often resistant organisms. The high intensity of nursing and medical attention predisposes to cross-infection. Handwashing is not only simple and sensible but is the only easily applied method of preventing cross-infection that has been shown to work.

General microbial surveillance is important so that the prevalent organisms in the ICU and in individual patients are known by both the microbiologist and the intensive care staff (Box 10.7). When a patient becomes infected it is better to be able to treat an identified organism than to be forced to use broad-spectrum therapy that may miss the relevant organism. It is also difficult to grow organisms from patients on antibiotics, and so avoiding antibiotics and using intensive surveillance constitute a logical approach to treatment.

The traditional approach in ICU of the widespread use of broad-spectrum antibiotics both prophylactically and to treat probable and possible infection may be partly responsible for the increasing emergence of super-resistant organisms. Cautious, controlled organism-specific use of antibiotics is more efficacious and less likely to lead to resistance.

Analgesia and sedation

Patients in the ICU are frequently in pain, e.g. due to surgery or acute problems such as peritonitis, and they may suffer lesser discomfort from flatulence or constipation. Perceived oxygen lack or problems in the lung such as pulmonary oedema create anxiety and discomfort. Physical interventions such as intubation and positive pressure ventilation are at best uncomfortable. There are three aspects of management that overlap, all of which need to be considered (Fig. 10.3):

- analgesia for pain
- anxiolytics for anxiety
- sedation for awareness.

The relative quantities of each are determined by the specific requirements of each patient at the particular point in his or her ICU management.

Sedation is a loosely used term to describe keeping a patient comfortable in ICU. In some circumstances it may be appropriate for this to mean unconsciousness, in others immobility, while at other times it may mean wide awake but not in discomfort and able to move, breathe and in particular to coordinate with the ventilator. There are several scoring systems available to attempt to quantify the level of sedation of a patient. While none is perfect, it is important to have some means of describing a level of sedation to aim for.

Pharmacological considerations

The level of pharmacological control and the length of time it is required determine the choice of agent (see Information Box 10.1). Frequently a combination of agents works well because it enables smaller doses of individual drugs with differing pharmacodynamic profiles to be used.

Sedation

If rapid reversible sedation is required then propofol is preferred. For longer periods the benzodiazepine, midazolam, may be more cost-effective, although it takes longer to wear off, especially in the presence of liver dysfunction.

Information Box 10.1

Features of sedative, analgesic and anxiolytic agents

Sedatives agents	Advantages	Disadvantages
Propofol	Rapid onset Rapid offset	Expensive Haemodynamic disturbance
Midazolam	Rapid onset Accumulates Slow offset	Accumulates and can be a negative inotrope
Barbiturates	Rapid onset Long half-life Reduces metabolic rate	Accumulates Long time to wear off Haemodynamic effects
Analgesics		
Opiates		
Diamorphine	Good analgesia Long action	Accumulates
Fentanyl	Good analgesia Long action	Chest wall rigidity Accumulates
Pethidine	Good analgesia Long action	Accumulates, especially with renal dysfunction Neurological effects
Alfentanil	Good analgesic Short action	Expensive Accumulates if used by infusion
Ketamine	Good effect Long action	Hallucinations Agitation
Non-steroids	Anti-inflammatory Helpful adjunct No respiratory depression	Renal failure
Anxiolytics		
Benzodiazepines	Good effect Drowsiness	Tolerance develops rapidly
Haloperidol	Effective Long half-life	

Barbiturates are unpopular but have their uses. They provide good sedation and, at high dose, may reduce the metabolic rate. They are cardiodepressive and they have a long half-life.

Analgesia

Opiates are powerful analgesics. They all work rapidly but cause respiratory depression. Diamorphine may have additional euphoric effects. For short-term requirements, alfentanil is effective and wears off rapidly. Most analgesic requirements are longer term in ICU and so diamorphine, morphine and pethidine are effective and cheap.

In renal failure, the metabolites of the opiates, especially pethidine, accumulate and cause neurological excitation. In some patients, ketamine, which is less cardiovascularly depressive, and in fact may increase the blood pressure, may be of benefit. However, it can cause hallucinations and dysphoria.

Relaxants

There are occasions when immobility is important. In critically ill patients who are difficult to ventilate or when delicate practical procedures are being performed, it may be safer to paralyse the patient with muscle relaxants. For rapid control of the airway, the depolarising muscle relaxant suxamethonium is useful and produces a rapid onset of full paralysis. For longer term relaxation, a non-depolarising agent such as atracurium of vecuronium can be used. As these agents are short-acting, a continuous infusion can be used. Atracurium is broken down by Hofmann degradation and is not dependent on renal or liver function for its metabolism, so it does not accumulate; however, it can release histamine, causing bronchospasm which may be a problem. Vecuronium is haemodynamically neutral, very unlikely to release histamine, but it is renal- and liver-dependent and can accumulate.

Pancuronium has sympathomimetic properties (increases heart rate) and this can be useful in cardiovascularly compromised patients. It is relatively long-acting but can be used by giving intermittent boluses.

Brain stem death

A patient is dead when declared to be so (using accepted criteria) by a doctor. Legally this is deemed to be the time of death. Classical criteria for the diagnosis of death have been permanent cessation of breathing and of the heartbeat. With advances in medical technology, the function of organs other than the brain can be duplicated by machines. This has led to the ability to maintain vital organ function in a body with a non-functioning brain.

Therefore the nature of the criteria for diagnosing death have undergone reappraisal. The first step was the move from a classical 'cardiorespiratory' death to an understanding that a person is not dead until the brain has died. The second step was the acceptance that the permanent functional death of the brain stem constitutes brain death.

Cortical activation and consciousness depend primarily on the role of the brain stem nuclei and their global cerebral projections in the reticular activating system. All cortical sensory inputs and motor outputs traverse the brain stem. Hence the functioning brain stem is essential for meaningful function of the 'brain as a whole'. Any acute, massive, irreversible lesion of the brain stem prevents this function even if isolated parts may, for a short time, emit signals. Therefore a flat EEG is not a requirement for the diagnosis of brain stem death.

The testing of cranial nerve reflexes probes the brain stem slice by slice due to the compact arrangement of brain stem nuclei. No other area of the brain can be tested as thoroughly.

Diagnosis of brain stem death

The diagnosis of brain stem death is not made in isolation but in the context of the clinical history and examination. It is a means of confirming clinical opinion.

Preconditions
These are as follows:

- Apnoeic coma, i.e. unresponsive on a ventilator
- Irreversible structural brain damage.

The primary diagnosis must be established in every case before proceeding to testing. This is usually not difficult, as 80% of cases where brain stem death is diagnosed in the UK have suffered a head injury or intracerebral haemorrhage. It is also important that no therapeutic manoeuvres have changed the patient's condition despite an adequate period having elapsed for observation.

Exclusions
Potential causes of profound but reversible changes in brain stem function must be excluded. These include:

- drugs – intoxication, sedation, poisoning
- neuromuscular blocking agents
- hypothermia
- acid–base disturbances
- electrolyte disturbances
- endocrine disorders.

An adequate period must be allowed for the elimination of drugs (brain concentrations may lag blood concentrations) and, to ensure this, toxicological investigation may be necessary prior to testing. A simple nerve stimulator will suffice to determine whether there is any residual neuromuscular blockade.

If the preconditions and exclusions are not satisfied beyond all doubt then testing cannot take place.

Timing
The time prior to testing is the time it takes to satisfy the preconditions and exclusions, i.e. the time to establish an unequivocal diagnosis of structural brain damage and to become certain that the condition is irreversible.

The tests

Tests are carried out to prove that brain stem reflexes have been lost and to obtain precise confirmation of persistent apnoea. On examining the patient, observe for signs that the brain stem cannot be dead, e.g.

- seizure (generalised or focal)
- abnormal posturing (decorticate or decerebrate)
- the presence of doll's head eye movements

All the above require live neurones in the brain stem.

The tests are carried out by two doctors, one of whom must be a consultant; the other may be a registrar (>5 years since full registration).

Tests of five brain stem reflexes
- *No pupillary response to light.* The pupil need not necessarily be dilated; mydriasis is not a feature of brain death.
- *No corneal reflex.* Use much firmer pressure than in a conscious individual.
- *No vestibulo-ocular reflex.* The auditory canal must be wax-free (verify with an auroscope). Use at least 20 mL of ice cold water in each ear. A normal response is for both eyes to deviate towards the irrigated side; for the brain stem to be dead there must be no movement of either eye. A basal skull fracture with CSF leak precludes the test, as do extensive facial injuries.
- *No motor response within the cranial nerve distribution* in response to adequate stimulation of any somatic area, i.e. grimacing in response to firm pressure on the fingernail.
- *No gag or cough reflex.* This is assessed by bronchial stimulation with a suction catheter passed down the endotracheal tube.

Testing for apnoea
Apnoea is confirmed by not observing any respiratory effort during a period of disconnection from the ventilator. Disconnection must be for long enough to ensure that the P_aCO_2 is high enough to drive any respiratory neurons still alive. It is therefore essential to avoid hyperventilation and a prerequisite that the P_aCO_2 must be ≥ 5.3 kPa (40 mmHg) prior to testing.

Hypoxia during disconnection is avoided by pre-oxygenating the patient with 100% O_2 for 10 minutes, and on disconnection insufflating O_2 at 6 L/min via a catheter down the endotracheal tube. The P_aCO_2 will rise by at least 0.27 kPa (2 mmHg) per minute and reach 8 kPa (60 mmHg) after 10 minutes. The UK code recommends that during disconnection the P_aCO_2 should > 6.65 kPa (50 mmHg).

Patients dependent on hypoxic respiratory drive will not be able to undergo this test and will probably not be considered for a diagnosis of brain stem death.

Retesting

There is no legal requirement for a second set of tests. However, virtually all codes urge the tests to be carried out twice to rule out observer error. Retesting also ensures that the non-functioning brain stem is not just a single observation but has persisted over time. The interval between tests is left to the judgement of the doctors concerned but is usually 12–24 hours.

When applied correctly and performed precisely, the tests for brain stem function provide valid and unambiguous results.

Organ donation

If organ donation is envisaged, the 'beating heart cadaver' is reconnected to the ventilator, with organ removal then taking place at the convenience of the surgical team.

Burns

Major burns should be dealt with in a specialised unit. Only the principles of management of a severe burn will be addressed.

PATHOPHYSIOLOGY

Loss of integument and direct tissue injury lead to a generalised fluid leak into the burn area. This results in fluid loss and oedema formation. Secondary problems include myocardial depression, which usually recovers within 24 hours. There is also a degree of immuno-suppression, with the major late problem of infection (Box 10.8).

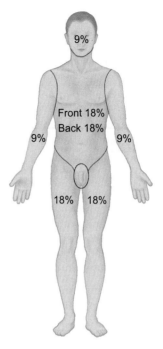

Fig 10.4 **Burn assessment.**

ASSESSMENT

The area of burn should be determined. The method used is to assess the percentage of the total body surface area which has been damaged and the depth of the injury. This can be easily done from a chart (Fig. 10.4).

MANAGEMENT

The rules of ABC – airway, breathing and circulation – apply. The airway must be assessed and, if necessary, protected by intubation. Indications for endotracheal intubation include lung injury with hypoxia from inhalational burns; in the case of head and neck burns, oedema can develop rapidly, especially during resuscitation, and can occlude the airway.

There are massive fluid losses post-burn injury due to formation of oedema fluid and loss of the cutaneous barrier. Various formulae have been produced to guide fluid management in the resuscitation period, an example of which is the Parkland formula using Ringer's lactate solution:

Volume (mL)/24 h = 4 × weight (kg) × percentage of total body surface area burnt

These formulae are rough guides and resuscitation should be more accurately guided by clinical assessment using tissue perfusion, blood pressure and urine output. It is also important to remember that burns patients may well have other injuries depending on the nature of the burn. History and full examination are very important.

> ## Box 10.8
>
> ### Problems associated with a large burn
>
> Fluid loss
>
> Myocardial depression
>
> Oedema formation – airway obstruction, compartment syndromes
>
> Airway burn – hypoxia
>
> Tissue damage – myoglobinuria
>
> Immunosuppression – infection

The other important aspect of management is the control of pain and anxiety and, as for any major injury the patient should be made as comfortable as possible. Pain may be very severe initially but anxiety becomes a growing problem as the patient becomes aware of the predicament.

Conclusion

The critically ill should be managed in an intensive care unit. It is an exciting environment where clinical signs abound. It is an area where acute medicine is managed by rapid pharmacological interventions to try to offset defined pathophysiological disturbances, and where sophisticated technology is regularly used to assist management.

FURTHER READING

Bihari D (1988) Oxygen delivery and consumption in the critically ill: their relation to the development of multiple organ failure. In: Kox WB (ed) *Shock and the Adult Respiratory Distress Syndrome*. London: Springer-Verlag, pp. 95–121.

Grant JP (1994) Nutritional support in critically ill patients. *Annals of Surgery* **220**(5): 610–616.

Hedenstierna G (1991) Mechanics of the respiratory system in ARDS. *Acta Anaesthesiol Scand* (Suppl.) **95**: 29–33

Minard G, Kudsk KA (1994) Effect of route of feeding on the incidence of septic complications in critically ill patients. *Seminars in Respiratory Infections* **9**(4): 228–231.

UK CoMRCatFit (1976) Diagnosis of death. *British Medical Journal* **ii**: 1187–1188.

Yates DW, Woodford M, Hollis S (1993) Trauma audit: clinical judgement or statistical analysis? *Annals of the Royal College of Surgeons of England* **75**(5): 321–324.

Practical procedures

Preliminaries

Informed consent

The general problem of consent is considered in Chapter 2. Should sedation be needed, the patient is then possibly unable to stop the procedure during its progress and therefore prior written consent must have been obtained. Written consent is also recommended for procedures seen to be invasive even if sedation is not always required, e.g. radiological investigation (angiography) and endoscopy.

Explanation

Alternative methods of management should be discussed before the procedure in question is carried out.

Essential information that should be given to the patient includes:

- the nature of the procedure
- what is going to be removed, cut, changed or inserted
- non-specific possible complications – haematoma, infection
- specific possible specific complications – nerve, arterial and venous injury; cosmetic effect
- explanation of type of anaesthesia (general, local, regional) and risks involved.

Additional beneficial information includes:

- the position of the scar
- what lines, drains and catheters will be in place after the procedure
- post-operative pain control
- when food and drink may be resumed
- what may happen during the hours or days after the procedure and for how long a period these matters may last
- how long before work can be resumed.

Documentation

All procedures should be recorded in the notes with comments pertinent to the individual manoeuvre, e.g. the volume of residual urine found on urethral catheterisation or, after a biopsy, the dispatch of a specimen to the pathological laboratory.

Asepsis

There are varying degrees of aseptic technique (see also Ch. 5) according to the procedure and the possible subsequent effects of sepsis.

Gloves

Gloves should be worn for every procedure that involves contact with a patient's secretions or blood. Non-sterile (but clean) gloves are indicated when there is a risk of contamination from patient to medical attendant (HIV and hepatitis B). Sterile gloves are part of the normal procedure to prevent access of organisms to the patient. The possibility of transmission of infection by the hands should always be maintained at a low level by keeping them clean, with short nails, everyday maintenance of subcuticular hygiene and washing every time a clinician is in contact with a patient – often more honoured in the breach than in the observance.

Superficial procedures

An example of such a procedure is superficial venous cannulation. An alcohol swab to the skin area and clean hands with a no-touch technique are theoretically sufficient. However, the operator requires protection against the possibility of infection from the patient. The wearing of gloves – either clean or sterile according to the circumstances – is recommended for every procedure.

Deeper and more complicated procedures

If the procedure is likely to leave a cannula, a drain or other device (pacemaker, central line) in situ, then sterile gloves, towels and handwashing and full skin preparation must be used.

Immunocompromised patients

In certain circumstances (AIDS, bone marrow transplantation, chemotherapy) immunocompromise is present and in such patients strict aseptic techniques should be used even for minor superficial procedures.

Handwashing and skin preparation

These are discussed in detail in Chapter 5.

Anaesthesia

Nearly all small procedures can be undertaken with *local anaesthesia* (LA). If general or regional anaesthesia (Ch. 6) is a possible alternative, two factors will determine which is chosen: the relative risks (regional anaesthesia usually has a marginally higher risk) and patient preference.

General features relating to the pain of administration of LA are summarised below:

- The initial needle prick is painful but, especially in children, can be lessened by the use of local anaesthetic creams or sprays (see 'Partial anaesthesia').
- Rapid injection causes pain from increased pressure in the tissues: the slower the injection, the less pain there will be; injection into dense tissue (such as the fibrous tissue of the sole of the foot) should always be slow.
- The smaller the needle (preferably 25 or 27G), the less pain the patient will feel upon insertion and also the slower will be the rate of injection; fine needles are often short but long ones are also available.
- The elderly often experience less pain on the injection of local anaesthetic, probably because of the laxity of their tissue.

Choice of local anaesthesia

Ethyl chloride spray can be used to numb the skin before a limited lance for a small abscess or for initial injections of LA. Local anaesthetic creams, e.g. EMLA cream (a mixture of the un-ionised base forms of lignocaine and prilocaine), are useful for paediatric venepuncture and for adults who have a phobia about needles, although it should be noted that they take up to an hour to become effective.

Commonly used local anaesthetics (with their maximum safe dose) are:

- lignocaine – 3 mg/kg
- bupivacaine – 2 mg/kg (it is 2–4 times more potent than lignocaine) (See Table 11.1)
- prilocaine – 5 mg/kg
- Cocaine – used in ENT surgery for its local vasoconstrictor action.

Table 11.1
Concentration of bupivicaine for local and regional anaesthesia

Procedure	Concentration
Skin infiltration	0.5%
Minor nerve block	1%
Brachial plexus	1–1.5%
Sciatic/femoral	1–1.5%
Epidural	1.5–2%
Spinal	2–5%

Addition of adrenaline

Adrenaline – a potent vasoconstrictor – added to a local anaesthetic slows the rate of absorption into the systemic circulation, reduces systemic toxicity and therefore prolongs the duration of action and may result in a more profound block. For this reason, the doses of both lignocaine and prilocaine quoted above can be increased if 1 in 200 000 adrenaline is added to the solution (e.g. lignocaine 5 mg/kg and prilocaine 8 mg/kg). The dose of bupivacaine should not be increased when adrenalin is used (see also Ch. 6).

There are, however, absolute contraindications to the use of adrenaline with local anaesthetic agents as follows:

- when the injection is close to end arteries
- ring block of the digits (fingers and toes) and of the penis
- intravenous regional anaesthesia (so-called Bier's block) which reduces venous drainage by the use of a tourniquet and so generates a high concentration of local anaesthetic; there is an unacceptable risk of ischaemia and of the escape of large concentrations of agent into the general circulation.

Principles of suturing

This is discussed in detail in Chapter 5.

Equipment

The best way to be certain that everything is available for any minor procedure is to run through the steps in your head beforehand, checking the equipment against that required for each step (see also the various procedures described throughout this chapter).

Venous access

Choosing the site

The ideal area for injection and short-term cannulation is the forearm. However, if the patient is obese, there can be difficulties with this. Sites that are not suitable and which should be avoided are as follows:

- The dominant arm is avoided.
- The arm which carries an arterio venous (AV) fistula for renal dialysis is never used.
- Poor venous or lymphatic drainage in a limb (e.g. after an axillary lymph node clearance) carries a higher incidence of infected lymphangitis and such limbs must not be used.
- Avoid foot veins whenever possible because they thrombose easily and are prone to infection.
- A skin fold which crosses a joint should be avoided, although the antecubital fossa can be used for diagnostic venepuncture.

Choice of vein (Fig. 11.1)

Look to where veins commonly occur; there is often a large vein running along the radial aspect of the forearm. Veins can sometimes only be felt rather than seen even after the application of a tourniquet. Should there be uncertainty as to whether the structure is a vein, the tourniquet should be released. If the structure becomes impalpable, it is almost certainly a patent vein – arteries or thrombosed veins do not change shape or size when a tourniquet is removed.

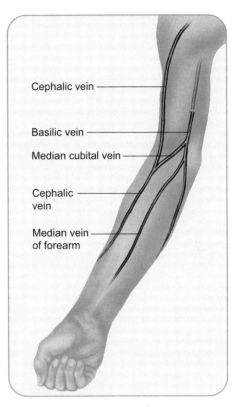

Fig 11.1 **Common sites in the arm for venous access.**

To insert a cannula the vein should be immobilised by stretching the skin, which includes positioning the adjacent joints. If the veins are extremely difficult to cannulate because of mobility, then placing the cannula at a point of junction of two veins can help. If there is substantial subcutaneous fat, then often the dorsum of the hand is the only available place; this area is not particularly convenient for the patient and can be painful during insertion. The antecubital fossa is also not particularly convenient for the patient, but for emergencies it is ideal as there are large reasonably accessible veins which can take large cannulae.

There are methods which can be used to help locate, a vein; there are listed in Box 11.1.

Choosing a needle or cannula

Intravenous cannulae available in the UK (and in many other places in the world) are shown in Table 11.2.

Venepuncture

EQUIPMENT
- Clean gloves
- Tourniquet – either a short length of latex rubber tube or, preferably, a sphygmomanometer

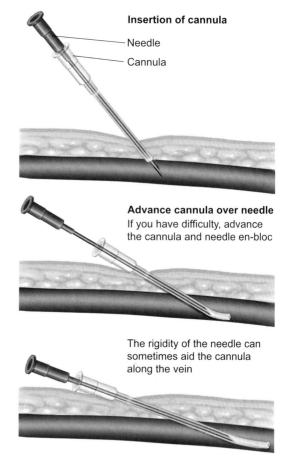

Insertion of cannula

Needle

Cannula

Advance cannula over needle
If you have difficulty, advance the cannula and needle en-bloc

The rigidity of the needle can sometimes aid the cannula along the vein

Fig 11.2 **Technique for venous cannulation.**

Box 11.1

Aids to location of a vein

- Use a sphygmomanometer and inflate it to below diastolic pressure to allow arterial inflow but not venous escape of blood

- Hang the patient's arm over the edge of the bed or couch and tap (not slap) the back of the hand to cause venodilatation

- Immerse the forearm in a bowl of warm water for 2 minutes and place the tourniquet before removing the hand from the bowl.

Additional hint
In paediatrics or for anxious adults, EMLA cream can be helpful: apply over selected veins and cover with an occlusive dressing; wipe off after 45–60 minutes; after EMLA cream has been applied, veins do not distend as easily

Table 11.2
Types of intravenous cannula

Size	Colour	Use
22G	Blue	Children, small fragile veins
20G	Pink	Low-flow intravenous infusions such as analgesia, sedation
18G	Green	Intravenous fluids and drugs
16G	Yellow	Blood transfusions
14G	Grey	Rapid fluid administration – shock, major trauma and gastrointestinal bleeding
12G	Brown	Rapid fluid administration – shock, major trauma and gastrointestinal bleeding

- Appropriate needle or cannula (see Table 11.2) but there may be need for a back-up if difficulty is encountered
- Strapping to hold a cannula in place – adhesive tape
- 5 mL syringe
- Normal saline flush
- Occasionally cotton wool and adhesive tape to secure the site of unsuccessful cannulation
- Bandage and tape for the same reason.

PROCEDURE
- Choose the preferred site.
- Place the tourniquet above the site of insertion.
- Swab the intended insertion area with antiseptic (allow alcohol to dry).
- Advance the needle or cannula-and-needle combination into the vein until a flashback of blood into the base of the cannula is seen.
- Advance the plastic cannula into the vein over the

needle to ensure that it remains in the same position and is not pushed further into the vein (Fig. 11.2).
- Remove the tourniquet.
- When venepuncture alone has been done, elevate the arm above the right atrium, remove the needle and apply a small stabilising dressing.
- For a cannulation, occlude the end or connect the infusion immediately.

COMPLICATIONS

Thrombophlebitis
Inflammation at a peripheral site of cannulation (which may be chemical irritation or infection) is manifest by pain, tenderness and a red line which spreads proximally. The cannula must be removed immediately. To prevent this complication it is best to change the site of a peripheral infusion at intervals no longer than 24 hours. There is some evidence that small amounts of heparin added to the infusion can also help.

Blockage
Sometimes patency can be restored with a flush of normal or heparinised saline (2–5 mL). The smaller the

diameter of the syringe, the higher the pressure that can be attained (use a 5 mL rather than a 10 mL syringe).

Venous cut-down

The most commonly used sites for this procedure are (Figs 11.1 and 11.3):

- medial basilic vein – approximately 2.5 cm lateral to the medial epicondyle of the humerus at the flexion crease of the elbow
- saphenous vein – either at the saphenofemoral junction (2.5 cm lateral and inferior to the pubic tubercle) or 2 cm anterior and superior to the medial malleolus at the ankle.

EQUIPMENT
- Sterile towels
- Orange needle (25G)
- Knife (10 blade)
- Fine scissors
- Artery forceps
- Two ties (4/0 vicryl)
- Cannula 12G or 14G
- Skin sutures (prolene or silk 3/0)
- Dressing.

PROCEDURE (Fig. 11.4)
- Prepare the skin with antiseptic solution.
- Drape the area.
- Infiltrate the skin over the vein with 0.5% lignocaine, but take care not to inject local anaesthetic into the vein.
- Make a transverse full-thickness skin incision (2.5 cm) through the infiltrated area.
- By blunt dissection with the tip of an artery forceps, identify the vein and release it from any fat and fibrous tissue.
- Free the vein for at least 2 cm.
- Ligate the mobilised vein at its most distal exposed part and leave the tie attached for traction.
- Place a tie around the vein proximally but do not tighten this.
- Make a small transverse incision with scissors into the vein sufficient to accept the cannula and dilate this opening with the tip of an artery forceps.
- Introduce a large plastic grey (14G) or orange (12G) cannula which has, if necessary, been separated from its needle.
- Tighten the proximal tie around the vein and the cannula firmly but be careful not to constrict the lumen of the cannula.
- Attach the intravenous apparatus and check that flow takes place.
- Close the wound with interrupted sutures and apply further antiseptic solution and a securing dressing.

COMPLICATIONS
- Perforation of the posterior wall of the vein
- Haematoma
- Phlebitis
- Cellulitis
- Venous thrombosis
- Transection of a neighbouring nerve (e.g. saphenous nerve at the medial malleolus)
- Mistake of an artery for a vein and arterial transection.

Central venous catheterisation

The objective of central venous catheterisation is to insert a hollow line into the proximal (usually superior) vena cava. The *Seldinger technique* is often used, in which a needle is placed in the vessel and an internal guide wire inserted into the vein first. The needle is then removed, the track into the vessel dilated and the cannula threaded along the wire into the lumen.

INDICATIONS
- Measurement of central venous pressure
- Infusion of certain drugs, e.g. ionotropes, high concentrations of potassium (greater than 60 mmol/L)
- Total parental nutrition (Ch. 10)
- Insertion of a Swan–Ganz catheter or cardiac pacing wires
- Inability to achieve peripheral venous access, e.g. intravenous drug abuse with extensive previous venous thrombosis.

COMMON SITES
- Internal jugular and subclavian (usually on the right)
- Femoral in the groin
- Median basilic vein at the elbow.

EQUIPMENT
- Fine scalpel blade
- Orange (25G) and green (21G) needles
- Two syringes (preferably of differing sizes, 5 and 10 mL) – one for local anaesthesia the other for heparinised saline
- Heparinised saline flush (10 mL)
- Central line infusion equipment
- Suture material (2/0 or 3/0 silk or prolene, preferably on a straight needle so that a needle holder is not required
- Transparent occlusive dressing
- One litre bag of normal saline (0.9%) and a giving set.

Prepackaged central line sets often contain not only the infusion apparatus but also many of the items mentioned above; check before looking for the rest of the materials.

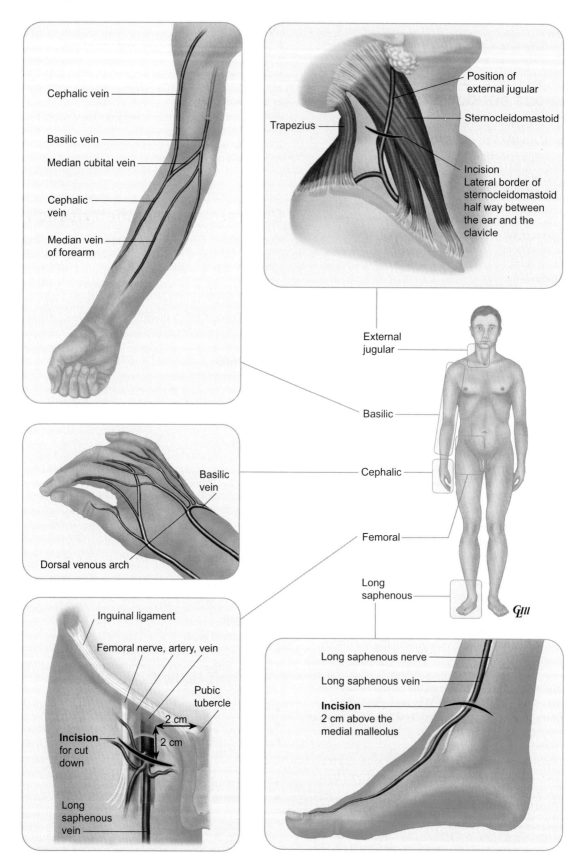

Fig 11.3 **Sites used for venous access.**

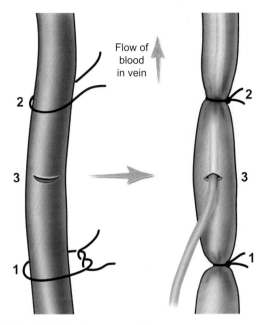

Fig 11.4 **Technique for venous cut-down.**

PROCEDURE

Many of those who require a central line are seriously ill and cannot tolerate lying flat. Therefore all the equipment must be ready before placing them in the best position for the procedure. If the patient is known to be short of intravascular volume, 500 mL of colloid or crystalline solution given through a peripheral infusion just before the procedure is often helpful to increase the diameter of the vein to be used.

The patient should be positioned in a supine position with no pillows, or with no more than one pillow. The bed should preferably be in a 15° head-down tilt at the moment of puncture of the vein. The patient's arms should be placed at the side of the trunk. For subclavian vein cannulation, an assistant holding the arm on the side of the proposed cannulation, with downward traction, opens the space between the clavicle and the first rib; again, this should be done at the moment of puncture.

The procedure for cannulation is now as follows:

- Use an orange needle (Table 11.2) to insert local anaesthetic over the proposed point of entry into the skin and infiltrate the proposed route towards the vein with a larger (green) needle.
- While allowing the anaesthetic to take effect, prepare the central line: all ports of entry on the apparatus are flushed through with heparinised saline and tested for patency; all are then closed either with a bung or a tap that is switched off, except for the distal one (usually labelled and in the centre of the cannula) which is left open.
- The guide wire should be prepared by checking that the end is hidden in the introducer and that it can be easily advanced (practise beforehand). Often the

introducer has to be released from the sheath in which the wire is coiled.
- Flush the needle and syringe to be used to identify and cannulate the vein with heparinised saline to ensure fluid runs freely.
- Make a small (5 mm) incision through the skin at the proposed entry site.
- Insert the needle and, once deep to the skin, aspirate with the syringe and advance it until venous blood is easily aspirated.
- Detach the syringe and ensure that blood flows freely out of the needle.
- Insert the wire and its introducer (if present – depends on the type of apparatus) into the end of the needle while grasping it to ensure that it does not move as the wire and introducer are advanced. The wire should be easily introduced without force (which should never be applied); sometimes rotation can help in that many of the wires have curled ends (if the wire does not have a pigtail end then the soft end of the wire should be introduced – the rigid end can perforate the vein).
- Once the wire is inserted to approximately 50% of its length, the needle is removed.
- The track is dilated by the introduction of the dilator over the wire, pushing it in until it is well inside the vein.
- Remove the dilator; this is usually associated with an increase in bleeding from the entry site – a good sign as it implies that the track is well dilated.
- The central line is introduced over the wire while this is held steady; often the wire must be pulled back slightly to allow it to come out of the end of the distal port. Again, the wire must be grasped before the cannula is further advanced, otherwise it can be lost into the right side of the heart.
- Push the central venous line in; the tip should ideally lie in the superior vena cava, judged according to the size and shape of the patient.
- Aspirate the line with a syringe to ensure that its position is truly in the vein as indicated by free flow of blood. If there is uncertainty, an infusion of normal saline can be connected and checked to see if flow is free.
- Suture the line in place, if necessary after infiltrating further local anaesthetic.

Use of the subclavian vein

There are numerous techniques for cannulation of this vessel which differ in detail, but all insertions start in the area 1 cm below the clavicle between its medial and lateral thirds (Fig. 11.5) and the aim is to cannulate the vein as it passes over the first rib. Two differing approaches are described: the lateral and the medial.

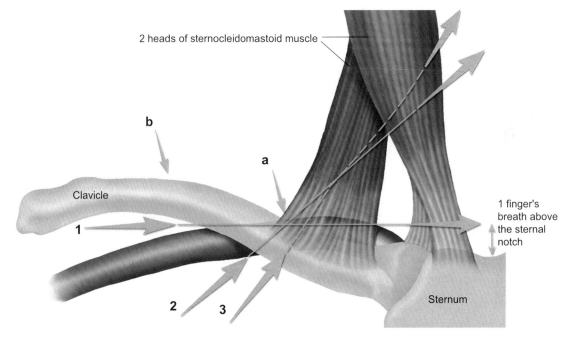

2 heads of sternocleidomastoid muscle

b

a

Clavicle

1 finger's breath above the sternal notch

1

2   **3**

Sternum

Fig 11.5 **The approach used for cannulation of the subclavian vein.**

Lateral

This is carried out at the point at which the lateral third and medial two-thirds of the clavicle intersect. The needle should be aimed at a point 2 cm above the suprasternal notch and towards the opposite shoulder; it then runs in a straight line from the insertion point, passes just inferior to the clavicle and flat to the skin; if the needle is felt to bend away from this path, the usual reason is that the tip is below the first rib and towards the apex of the pleura; in this case the advice is to withdraw and start again, using a slightly higher angle.

Medial

This is carried out at the point of intersection of the medial third and lateral two-thirds. The needle goes in initially at right angles to the clavicle, just inferior to it and towards the division of the two heads of the sternomastoid muscle (Fig 11.5). Thereafter the steps of the procedure are as outlined above.

Use of the right internal jugular vein

(Fig. 11.6)

There are two techniques: high and low.

High

- Feel for the pulse of the carotid artery on the right side with the right hand (right-handed operators) or left hand (left-handed).

- Infiltrate a small area lateral to the carotid pulse at the level of the thyroid cartilage with local anaesthetic.
- Guard the carotid artery with the left hand and insert the needle at a 45° angle to the neck and pointing towards the nipple in the male or the anterior superior iliac spine in both males and

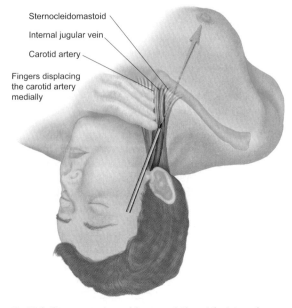

Sternocleidomastoid

Internal jugular vein

Carotid artery

Fingers displacing the carotid artery medially

Fig 11.6 **The approach used for cannulation of the internal jugular vein.**

females. Advance the needle slowly while applying negative pressure with a syringe. If there is no flashback of venous blood, release the finger from the carotid pulse and withdraw the needle slowly. This is sometimes successful because the compression had flattened the vein. Should the carotid artery be punctured, withdraw the needle immediately and apply digital pressure for at least 5 minutes.

Low

- Identify the triangle formed by the sternal and clavicular heads of insertion of the sternomastoid muscle into the sternum and clavicle.
- Infiltrate local anaesthetic at this point and along a line at 30° to the skin and just medial to the medial edge of the clavicular head of the sternomastoid. To prevent accidental intravenous injection, always apply negative pressure to the syringe before anaesthetic agent is infiltrated.
- At insertion, the needle should point towards the nipple in the male.
- Follow the same line with the needle as is used in the high technique.

Post-cannulation checks

After all central cannulations, the radial pulse should be checked. If there are frequent ectopic beats then it is likely that the line is in the right ventricle. **A chest X-ray should be performed** to verify the position of the tip of the line, which should be in the superior vena cava, and also to check for any complications (especially pneumothorax and haemothorax). If the line is not correctly placed, then adjustment is most easily performed under radiological control. Other means of ensuring that the line is within the vein are:

- easy aspiration of venous blood from all ports
- place the connected normal saline bag and tubing beneath the patient with the tap open: blood should track back easily even if the patient has a low central pressure.

Sometimes the distal opening rests on a valve and therefore blood cannot be aspirated. If the line is pulled backwards a few centimetres blood should then be easily aspirated.

Subcutaneous tunnelling

Temporary lines inserted as described above are, as time goes by, increasingly difficult to protect from the entry of bacteria. Sepsis is likely after 5–10 days, although careful care and strict asepsis decrease the incidence. However, some intensive care units judge it wise to change all central lines every 5 days. If the line is needed for long-term therapy (e.g. chemotherapy or TPN), then a subcutaneously tunnelled line should be used (Fig 11.7). An alternative for intermittent therapy is to place a port with venous access subcutaneously (Portocath).

The number of lumens available per line ranges from one to four. When placing a subcutaneous tunnelled line, two different methods can be used: one is the Seldinger technique; the other is to cut directly down onto a vein (either the cephalic vein for a subclavian approach or the internal jugular vein), then insert the cannula and create a separate exit point which lies on the anterior chest wall away from the shoulder joint.

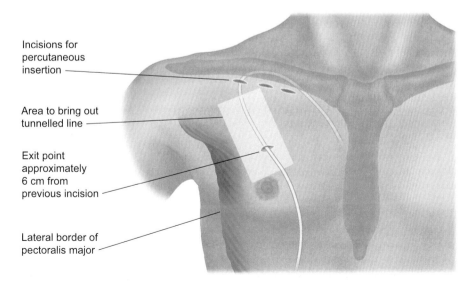

Incisions for percutaneous insertion

Area to bring out tunnelled line

Exit point approximately 6 cm from previous incision

Lateral border of pectoralis major

Fig 11.7 **Subcutaneous tunnelling of an intravenous catheter.**

Complications of central line insertion

- Haematoma
- Cellulitis
- Line infection (bacteraemia, septic shock).
- Thrombosis
- Phlebitis
- Nerve damage including transection
- Arterial puncture – more common in the internal jugular approach
- Pneumothorax – more common in thin patients and if the subclavian or low internal jugular approaches are used
- Haemothorax
- Chylothorax
- Arteriovenous fistula
- Peripheral neuropathy
- Lost wires or catheter in the venous system
- Improperly placed catheters.

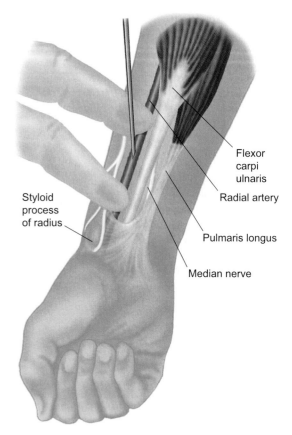

Fig 11.8 **The position of the radial artery at the wrist.**

Arterial blood sampling

Choice and localisation of arteries for puncture

Vessels of choice, in order of preference, are (unless there is a specific contraindication) the radial, femoral and brachial arteries.

Radial artery

This artery (Fig. 11.8) can be found medial to the styloid process of the radius at the wrist. Before it is used for a sample, the ulnar collateral supply should be checked (especially if there is a history of previous wrist trauma); this is done by asking the patient to repeatedly make a tight fist while occlusive pressure is applied over the radial artery and ulnar artery. The ulnar artery occlusion is then released. The hand is then relaxed and if it remains white for 10 seconds or more, collateral refill is inadequate and the other hand should be used (provided the same test is also negative).

   Isolation is best achieved between the operator's index and middle fingers of the non-dominant hand, both fingers feeling the pulse over the tips of their palmar surfaces.

Femoral artery

The artery is at the midinguinal point (a point on the inguinal ligament halfway between the pubic symphysis and the anterior superior iliac spine). It is best isolated with the index and middle fingers of the non-dominant hand on either side of the artery just

below the inguinal ligament, to prevent puncture of either the femoral vein (medially) or the femoral nerve (laterally) (Fig. 11.9).

Brachial artery

The brachial artery (Fig. 11.10) is only used if all other punctures are impossible or have failed. There is a risk of injury which could lead to peripheral ischaemia or of damage to the median nerve which lies on the medial side.

EQUIPMENT

- Syringe, 2 mL – a special syringe is often available
- Heparin 1000 U/mL (1 mL) – standard in many hospitals
- Alcohol swab
- Sterile cotton wool balls/gauze swabs
- Syringe cap
- Plastic bag full of ice.

PROCEDURE

- Draw up 0.5 mL of heparin into the 2 mL syringe, withdrawing the plunger fully to coat the syringe walls – or use a special pre-heparinised syringe.

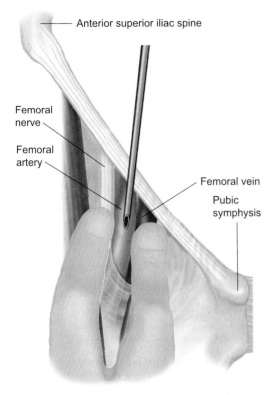

Anterior superior iliac spine

Femoral nerve

Femoral artery

Femoral vein

Pubic symphysis

Fig 11.9 **The position of the femoral artery in the groin.**

- The heparin in both the pre-prepared and self-heparinised syringes must be expelled completely to leave the plunger just moistened; large amounts of heparin in the syringe affect the pH of a

sample taken for the determination of blood gas tension.

- Hold the syringe at a 60–90° angle to the skin and slowly advance the needle, maintaining a very slight negative pressure. When a flush of blood occurs, release the negative pressure; if the syringe then fills spontaneously, the artery has been entered.
- Once 2mL of blood have been obtained, remove the syringe and needle and immediately apply pressure for at least 3 minutes.
- Tap bubbles to the needle end and expel all air that may have accumulated. Then, either take the sample immediately to the arterial blood gas analyser or place it on ice to slow down cellular use of oxygen in the sample (maximum 1 hour for reliable readings).
- If puncture fails, this may be because the artery has been transfixed: slow withdrawal of the needle sometimes yields free flow of arterial blood. If success does not follow, the arterial pulse is repalpated and a fresh attempt is made, preferably without coming out of the skin.

Understanding arterial blood gas results

Preliminaries
The percentage concentration of oxygen in the inspired air (e.g. 21% if the patient is inhaling air only) should be noted. It may take up to 20 minutes for the arterial blood gases to equilibrate after an adjustment to the oxygen supply. There may sometimes be difficulty in distinguishing between an arterial and venous sample: if the oxygen saturation (derived from the P_AO_2) is less

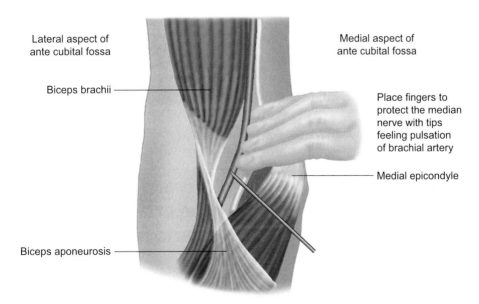

Lateral aspect of ante cubital fossa

Medial aspect of ante cubital fossa

Biceps brachii

Place fingers to protect the median nerve with tips feeling pulsation of brachial artery

Medial epicondyle

Biceps aponeurosis

Fig 11.10 **The site for puncture of the brachial artery.**

Table 11.3
Normal arterial blood gases

Measurement	Units	Level
pH	$-\log_{10}$ concentration hydrogen ion	7.35–7.45
P_{CO_2}	kPa	4.3–6.0
P_{O_2}	kPa	10.5–14
H_2CO_3	mmol/L	22–26
O_2 saturation	Percentage	95–100
Base excess	mmol/L	±2

than 50%, the blood is probably venous; 80% or above is certainly arterial. All indices should be considered together, i.e. P_AO_2, P_ACO_2, pH, base excess and H_2CO_3 (normal values are given in Table 11.3).

P_AO_2

Low values
The patient's usual level should be known – those with chronic respiratory disease can have a P_AO_2 as low as 7.5 kPa. A common cause of a truly low P_{O_2} in a surgical patient is a right-to-left shunt of blood through collapsed or consolidated lung tissue in which instance the highly diffusable CO_2 is also low because of hypoxia-induced tachypnoea and hyperventilation. However, if the associated P_ACO_2 is high, there is either chronic respiratory disease and/or acute respiratory failure (inability to ventilate). Those with known chronic respiratory disease who need oxygen to correct hypoxia must be given it carefully, starting with 24% O_2 and measuring the blood gases after 30 minutes to ensure that respiratory drive is maintained and that the P_ACO_2 does not rise. It should be noted that those with chronic respiratory disease can tolerate a much higher P_ACO_2 than normal.

Respiratory support, such as ventilation, needs to be considered in acute respiratory failure:

- if the respiratory rate is either very high (greater than 25) or very low (less than 8) on maximum supplementary oxygen from a mask
- in a previously normal patient if the P_ACO_2 is greater than 8 kPa.

High values
Hyperventilation without added oxygen cannot significantly increase the P_AO_2. The much more likely cause is that there is too high a concentration in the inspired air and this should be adjusted provided the P_ACO_2 is normal.

P_ACO_2

Low values
The patient is usually hyperventilating. The causes are:

- hypoxia
- anxiety – there is an accompanying respiratory alkalosis
- compensation for a lowered pH – metabolic acidosis.

Hyperventilation from anxiety leads to a respiratory alkalosis (increased pH). If there is obvious hyperventilation, then a paper bag over the patient's mouth and a suggestion that respiratory rate is reduced is usually effective, as may be an instruction to hold the breath.

If the clinical state is a compensation for a metabolic acidosis, then the pH will be either normal or low and there will be a negative base excess.

High values
There is retention of CO_2 because of hypoventilation from one of the following:

- chronic respiratory failure (often with an associated low P_AO_2 and normal pH – chronically compensated)
- respiratory suppression from drugs (often opiates)
- exhaustion of the respiratory muscles (associated with a low P_AO_2 and inappropriately reduced respiratory rate) – the chief cause of acute respiratory failure in surgical patients
- brain stem malfunction often with varied rates of ventilation; conscious level is decreased.

Of note when the P_AO_2 level and oxygen saturation are considered is that the O_2 saturation curve for haemoglobin is a steep one that starts around a P_{O_2} of 9.1 kPa (70 mmHg). This means that a P_AO_2 of 8.5 kPa saturation is still less than 90% because, at this point, small changes in oxygen tension are accompanied by large ones in saturation (see Ch. 6).

pH and base excess
If the pH is less than 7.35, there is acidosis, if greater than 7.45 there is an alkalosis. It is necessary to decide if either is metabolic or respiratory in origin and whether compensation is present. Compensation suggests a more chronic disease process (days or weeks), an uncompensated disorder or a more acute disease process. Compensation usually occurs by a change in the respiratory rate (e.g. in a metabolic acidosis, hyperpnoea causes increased excretion of CO_2) or by renal regulation of the amount of HCO_3 that is excreted.

Insertion of nasogastric tube or a nasogastric enteric feeding tube

INDICATIONS
- Vomiting from small bowel obstruction or pyloric stenosis

- Acute gastric dilation
- The prevention of gastro-oesophageal reflux which could cause aspiration
- Enteric feeding (a nasojejunal tube may also be used)
- Possible protection of an anastomosis distal to the pharynx – usually in the oesophagus (nasogastric tube usually positioned at operation).

EQUIPMENT
- Non-sterile gloves
- Nasogastric tube size 10 (small) to 16 (large)
- Catheter drainage bag
- Lubricant
- Glass of water.

PROCEDURE
- Inform the patient what is planned and how cooperation can help.
- Sit the patient upright with the chin on the chest; if this is not possible then the alternative is on the side with the head propped up.
- Lubricate the tube and insert into one nostril directly backward towards the occiput – a patient may be aware which side is more likely to be successful. Gently advance the tube.
- When the patient feels the tip in the pharynx, ask for a swallow and, as the tube moves, its advance is continued. Swallowing may be helped if a sip of water is given but there must not be any chance of aspiration because of an inactive gag reflex.
- Should the patient cough or becomes cyanotic, it is probably because the tube is astride the larynx or trachea. Withdraw quickly, into the hypopharynx, let the patient settle and try again (unfortunately the tube is often then pulled out completely because of a feeling of impending suffocation).
- After apparently successful insertion, check that the tube is not simply curled up in the back of the mouth. To do this, attach a 20 mL syringe to the proximal end and, with a stethoscope bell just below the left costal margin, quickly inject air; a loud borborygmus confirms that the tube is in the stomach.
- If fluid can be aspirated from the nasogastric tube. The fluid can be tested with litmus paper. It should be acidic.
- Secure the tube to the nose with strong adhesive tape.

Extra hints
- A cold tube (one that has been in a refrigerator for at least 30 minutes), is stiffer and more easy to direct down the oesophagus.
- A change in the position of the patient – as indicated above – can sometimes secure success.
- If the patient has a poor gag reflex then sometimes a laryngoscope and a Magill's forceps can be used to direct the tube into the oesophagus.

Fine-bore tubes for enteric feeding may be easier to insert because they are of smaller diameter and are equipped with guide wire. However, their rigidity may, if they are forced down against resistance, lead to an abrasion or, rarely, perforation of the oesophagus. Furthermore, in an unconscious patient, it is easy to insert them into the trachea and bronchi. **The final position should always be confirmed by a chest X-ray before use**.

Urinary catheterisation

Material
Urinary catheters are usually made of either latex or silicone rubber. Silicone is less irritant and should be used if the catheter is to be left indwelling for some days or weeks.

Special catheters
A Foley catheter is self-retaining because of an inflatable balloon (Fig. 11.11) and is usually but not invariably made of latex.

Three-way catheters are used for irrigation of the bladder, e.g. after prostatectomy.

Size
- 8–10 F: children and adults with tight urethral stricture
- 12–14 F: normal urethra or in the presence of mild prostatic hypertrophy

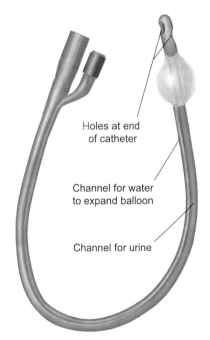

Holes at end of catheter

Channel for water to expand balloon

Channel for urine

Fig 11.11 **A Foley urinary catheter.**

- 16–18 F: moderate prostatic hypertrophy
- 20–24 F: after prostatectomy for free drainage and in other circumstances where bladder irrigation is required with the use of a three-way catheter.

The smallest size feasible should always be used.

Male catheterisation (Fig. 11.12)

INDICATIONS
- Urinary retention
- To assess hourly urinary output
- Incontinence.

EQUIPMENT
- Urinary catheter
- Sterile gloves
- Lignocaine gel 0.5%
- Bland antiseptic solution (e.g., Savlon – cetyl trimethyl ammonium bromide)
- Pre-prepared catheterisation pack – kidney dish, gauze swabs, sterile towels
- 10 mL syringe and 10 mL of sterile water
- Urine drainage bag.

PROCEDURE
- Wash hands and don sterile gloves.
- Open out everything that is needed onto a sterile towel usually on a trolley.
- Lay the patient flat – the more supine the position, the easier is the catheterisation.
- Drape the sterile towels or paper sheets to leave the penis exposed (a self-made hole in the centre of the paper sheet is often an easy way to expose just the penis).
- If right-handed, hold the penis with a sterile gauze swab with the left hand to prevent the penis from slipping; then retract the foreskin and clean the urethral opening with a swab.
- Gently squeeze the contents of a tube of lignocaine jelly into the urethra, in anyone of age less than 50, the sensitivity of the urethra often requires the content of two tubes.
- Open the plastic sheath which contains the catheter at the tip with the right hand and place a kidney bowl just below the urethral orifice of the penis.
- Hold the penis in the left hand and gently insert the catheter into the urethra using the right hand while withdrawing the plastic covering; ideally the catheter remains untouched but this almost always proves impossible and the catheter has to be advanced without its plastic covering using the clean right hand. During insertion the external end of the catheter remains in the kidney bowl because, when the bladder is entered, urine usually spills out.

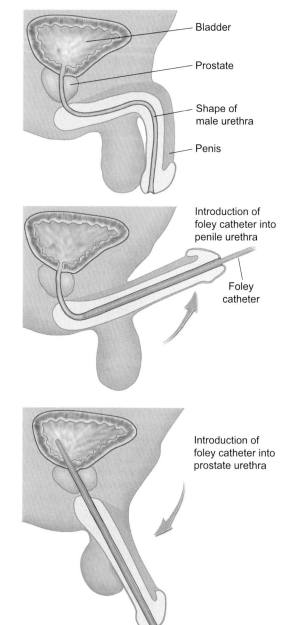

Fig 11.12 **Technique for male catheterisation.**

- If resistance is felt along the penile urethra or before the prostatic urethra has been traversed, pulling the penis gently upwards can help.
- Most often, resistance is found within the prostatic urethra and pulling the penis downwards at this point can assist. Sometimes the cause is failure of relaxation of the external sphincter and, if the tip of the catheter is held at this point of resistance for

10 seconds, this is often enough to allow the sphincter to relax spontaneously.

- Force must not be used because a false passage through the wall of the urethra can be made.
- A Foley catheter should be inserted fully to ensure that the balloon is within the bladder before inflation.
- Check the capacity of the balloon – it is usually 5–10 mL but for most three-way catheters is 30 mL. Usually only 5–10 mL capacity is needed; if the patient has just had a prostatectomy, then 20–30 mL are required so that the catheter can sit at the bladder neck and not move into the resected prostatic cavity.
- Either squeeze the already dilated water-filled area at the distal end of the catheter (after removing the clip) or insert the 5–10 mL of sterile water gently into the injection port for the balloon. If this generates pain or discomfort, stop at once, withdraw any water and advance the catheter further into the bladder.
- Once the balloon is inflated, the catheter is withdrawn until resistance is felt as the balloon lodges against the bladder neck.
- Replace the foreskin over the glans to avoid the possibility of a paraphimosis.
- Attach the catheter to the drainage apparatus.
- Send a urine sample for microscopy and culture.

If the catheter is to be in place for a considerable time – several days or more – the smallest diameter and the minimal amount of water in the balloon (5 mL) both help to decrease the likelihood of bladder spasm.

Extra hints

The catheter is in the bladder but urine does not flow. Blockage by the lubrication jelly is a possibility. Aspiration with a 50 mL catheter syringe and/or injection of sterile water or normal saline usually unblocks the catheter.

A stricture is encountered in either the penile or prostatic urethra. A narrower catheter (10–12 F) should be used.

In a patient beyond 55 years with a history suggestive of benign prostatic hypertrophy. A larger diameter catheter is paradoxically more likely to succeed.

The catheterisation fails. No more than two attempts should be made before more experienced help is sought: For the second try use a different sized catheter (depending on the probable cause of difficulty) and extra lignocaine gel. Further failure should lead to consideration of suprapubic drainage (see below).

If the patient bleeds from the urethra. Abandon the procedure and summon help to decide how to proceed which may mean the use of suprapubic catheterisation.

Phimosis makes the external meatus difficult to find. Gently dilate the narrow opening in the foreskin with the nozzle of the tube which contains the lignocaine jelly.

Removal of a urethral catheter

This is usually done by nursing staff. Failure to decompress the balloon calls for special manoeuvres.

Faulty valve

Sometimes the valve end can be cut off. If this fails, a needle inserted into the valve channel and aspirated may release obstruction.

Persistent impaction

Ultrasound identifies the balloon in the bladder, which can then be punctured with a fine spinal needle passed percutaneously under image control.

Catheterisation in relation to prostatic hypertrophy and prostatectomy

Size of catheter

As mentioned above, the prostatic urethra may, in the presence of prostatic hypertrophy, be more easily negotiated with a larger rather than a smaller catheter.

Bleeding

Initial rapid decompression of a dilated bladder may lead to rupture of distended veins at the bladder neck. A three-way irrigation system may be necessary until the condition settles, which it usually does.

Chronic retention

The presence of chronic retention with a considerably distended bladder before prostatectomy makes prolonged drainage extremely likely; a 12–14 F silicone catheter which can be left in place for 6–8 weeks allows the bladder to recover tone. Long-standing obstruction at the bladder neck without acute retention leads to back pressure on the kidney and a presentation with features of chronic renal failure and creatinine levels in excess of 1000, although the electrolyte levels are remarkably normal when there is only an obstructive cause. Catheterisation in such circumstances means that there is the likelihood of the development of a polyuric phase because of the damaged distal tubule's inability to concentrate. some 200–400 mL of urine an hour can be passed and dehydration develops quite rapidly. The most practical way to adjust fluid balance to compensate for the polyuria is to give the amount of fluid passed out in 1 hour back intravenously over the next hour. Such polyuria may be accompanied by hyponatraemia and hypokalaemia, and replacement must be adjusted accordingly. The polyuric phase usually lasts for about 12–24 hours; continuation beyond this may mean over-replacement with a vicious circle of water and electrolyte-induced diuresis The hour-on-hour replacement of urinary losses is discontinued and the situation reassessed.

Post-prostatectomy failure of micturition

Withdrawal of the initial drainage catheter after transurethral prostatectomy may not be followed by micturition. In such circumstances, first check the fluid balance chart – the bladder may not be sufficiently full to initiate micturition. Also, pain and the feeling of inability to micturate are not always caused by an overfull bladder; severe pain is often the consequence of detrusor muscle spasm within the bladder and is best treated not by catheterisation but with a smooth muscle relaxant such as oxybutynin. If the patient has been bleeding significantly and the bladder is truly distended, this may be the result of clot retention. Catheterisation with a large-bore, three-way catheter and irrigation with normal saline are necessary.

At transurethral prostatectomy it is relatively easy to dissect under the bladder neck and therefore possible to make a false passage on re-catheterisation. If the catheter easily advances its full length then this is unlikely; a check can be done by the insertion of 50 mL of water which should readily be re-aspirated.

Female catheterisation

ANATOMY

The female has a more easily traversed urinary tract than has the male. Only the muscles of the pelvic floor control access, and once the external meatus has been identified the short urethra is straight (Fig. 11.13).

EQUIPMENT

The equipment is the same as for male catheterisation except that there are some female catheters that are shorter than those used in males. Female catheterisation is often performed by the nursing staff, and doctors are asked to assist only when nursing staff have been unsuccessful.

PROCEDURE

- Collect all equipment and set up the trolley.
- Position the patient as for a vaginal examination – flat on the back with the heels together and the knees apart (hips in abduction and external rotation).
- Put on sterile gloves.
- Part the labia minora and majora with the non-dominant hand and, using the dominant hand, clean the area with a cotton wool ball soaked in Savlon.

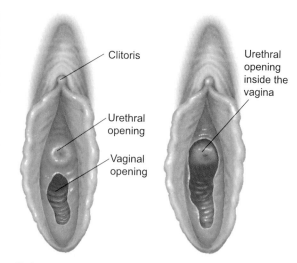

Fig 11.13 **Technique for female catheterisation.**

- Locate the urethral opening (Fig. 11.13) behind and below the clitoris and introduce a well lubricated catheter tip; a small amount of lignocaine jelly applied around the opening can aid entry.
- Successful catheterisation is followed by the procedures listed above for male catheterisation.

Difficulty

If catheterisation has not been achieved this is usually because the urethral opening has not been identified and the vagina has been catheterised instead. The labia minora must be opened generously and usually the urethral opening can be seen pouting on the anterior aspect of the vaginal wall. A focused light and lying the patient on the side can both help, as can, occasionally, a vaginal speculum.

Suprapubic bladder drainage

INDICATION

This is required when urethral catheterisation has failed and the patient has a full bladder.

EQUIPMENT

- Sterile towels
- Catheterisation pack – gauze, cotton wool balls
- Skin preparation
- Suprapubic catheter
- Needles – orange, green and white
- 1% lignocaine 10–20 mL
- 10 and 20 mL syringes
- Blade or knife
- Suture to tie the catheter to the abdominal wall – 3,0 or stronger
- Catheter bag.

PROCEDURE

- Place the patient supine and make sure that the bladder is distended by percussion from the umbilicus downwards in the midline.
- Open the pack and all the equipment; if a Foley catheter is to be used, check the balloon. Use another type only if familiar with its mechanism of insertion.
- Clean the area in the midline between the umbilicus and symphysis pubis.
- Arrange the sterile towels around this area.
- Infiltrate the skin in the midline 2 cm (approximately two finger breaths) above the pubic symphysis using the local anaesthetic and an orange needle and continue this through the layers of abdominal wall (the subcutaneous tissue and linea alba only) with the larger (green) needle.
- At the completion of infiltration, the needle is passed into the distended bladder and urine is aspirated; occasionally the longest (white) needle is required to achieve this (**urine *must* be aspirated before suprapubic catheterisation is attempted**).
- Make a stab incision in the skin large enough to take the chosen catheter.
- Insert the suprapubic trochar directly posteriorly in the same direction as that used for the final aspiration of urine.
- Once urine is obtained advance the catheter over the trochar.
- Remove the trochar and advance the catheter further to the indicated marker; ensure that easy aspiration of urine occurs and that the patient is free from pain.
- Clean and dry the entry point and then secure the catheter – preferably at more than one point.

If the catheter falls out before 2 weeks have elapsed and the patient needs recatheterisation, this must be done within 8 hours otherwise the track will have closed. After this time, the track will have become lined with epithelium and therefore a new catheter (often a simple silicone-covered urethral catheter) can be easily inserted.

Chest procedures

....

Pleural drainage (air and/or fluid)

For all chest drainage procedures:

- First check the signs and the X-rays.
- Ensure that the upper level of the pleural effusion is clearly established by percussion and mark this on the chest wall.
- Position the patient comfortably in a sitting position leaning slightly forward either in bed or on a chair. Ideally a table should be placed in front with a

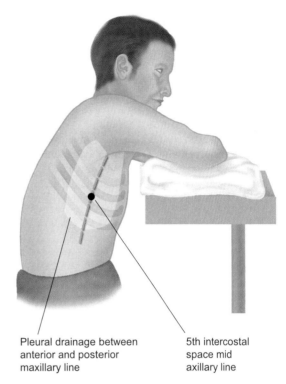

Pleural drainage between anterior and posterior maxillary line

5th intercostal space mid axillary line

Fig 11.14 **The position of a patient during pleural drainage/chest drain.**

pillow or blanket to rest on elevated to the level of the axilla (Fig. 11.14).

Diagnostic Aspiration

- Infection
- Malignancy.

EQUIPMENT

- Dressing pack
- Sterile gloves
- 10 mL syringe
- Orange (25G) and green needles (21G)
- 1% lignocaine, 10 ml
- Three sterile specimen bottles.

PROCEDURE

- Confirm the signs and X-ray findings.
- Select the insertion site by percussing out an effusion and mark the point of dullness – ideally done between the mid- and posterior axillary lines and at a point three finger breadths below the tip of the scapula.
- Infiltrate the skin over the chosen point with local anaesthetic using an orange needle and then infiltrate deeper with a green needle; the needle should pass just superior to the rib to avoid the neurovascular bundle. Always withdraw before

inserting local anaesthetic. On average fluid should be aspirated at the full depth of a green needle, but a longer needle may be required for larger or more obese individuals.

- Attach the 20 mL syringe to the appropriately sized needle and insert it through the area that has already been anaesthetised while aspirating as the needle is advanced. When flashback of fluid occurs, gently aspirate 20 mL to send for laboratory analysis: culture and sensitivity, ZN stains and TB culture; protein, glucose and amylase; cytology. When aspirating for cytological examination, the more fluid there is, the better (40 mL).

Therapeutic aspiration

INDICATIONS
- Relief of shortness of breath from a pleural effusion
- Removal of a small pneumothorax.

EQUIPMENT
Equipment is as for diagnostic aspiration plus the following additional items:

- a large-bore i.v. cannula (brown or grey)
- a three-way tap
- 50 mL syringe
- i.v. giving set and an empty sterile bowel or saline bag.

PROCEDURE
Fluid
- Larger cannulae need a small incision in the skin before their insertion.
- Attach the 50 mL syringe to the cannula and aspirate on insertion. After flashback, advance the cannula over the needle and then withdraw the needle, to leave the flexible cannula in place; as this is done the patient should breathe out and the thumb placed over the cannula hub to prevent air being sucked in.
- A closed three-way tap is quickly attached to the hub.
- Attach the 50 mL syringe to one hub of the tap and the empty saline bag to the other.
- Aspirate 50 mL at a time, switching the three-way tap settings to allow the syringe to empty into the saline bag.
- Withdraw the cannula while the patient breathes out.
- Apply an occlusive dressing to the site of puncture.

Air
- The position of insertion of the cannula should be either in the second intercostal space in the midclavicular line (Ch. 16) or in the midaxillary line in the fifth intercostal space.

- Infiltrate as already indicated just superior to the rib and ensure aspiration of air.
- Make a small incision in the skin and insert the needle/cannula through the infiltrated area. On aspiration of air through the needle, advance the cannula quickly while the patient breathes out.
- Remove the needle immediately and, with the thumb, occlude the hub until a closed three-way tap is attached.
- Air is aspirated 50 mL at a time and expelled through the spare exit on the tap. Care must be exercised to avoid the open arm coming into direct communication with the chest cavity.
- Once there is resistance to further aspiration, withdraw the cannula slightly to see if there is still residual air. It is important never to force aspiration because to do so may suck lung tissue against the end of the cannula.
- Withdraw the cannula and apply an occlusive dressing.

For a therapeutic aspiration it is advisable to halt the procedure after 1000 mL of air or fluid has been withdrawn so that the mediastinum can stabilise; procedure cardiorespiratory signs are absent, removal of air or fluid is resumed after an hour.

Failure of a chest aspiration is usually the result of a localised effusion or empyema. Ultrasound scanning and guided aspiration should be used.

Relief of tension pneumothorax

The causes and mechanisms are discussed in Chapters 3 and 16. The diagnosis is clinical rather than radiological and urgent decompression is required.

EQUIPMENT
- A large-bore needle or needle/cannula
- 20 mL syringe.

PROCEDURE
- Assess the patient's chest and respiratory function.
- Administer oxygen at 12 L/min by mask.
- Identify the second intercostal space in the midclavicular line on the side of the pneumothorax.
- If the patient is conscious and time permits, introduce local anaesthetic with an orange needle.
- Insert the needle with the 20 mL syringe attached – a small incision in the skin makes the insertion of a needle or cannula easier.
- Aspiration of air confirms the diagnosis: the syringe is removed and, in tension pneumothorax, a hissing sound is usually heard as the air is rapidly expelled; a hand held 5 cm from the needle or cannula can detect this rush of air.

The urgent procedure described converts a tension pneumothorax into an ordinary one. If air starts to enter the thorax, a three-way tap should be placed on the needle or cannula hub and sealed, which then enables further release of air before a chest drain is inserted – this is always done.

Insertion of a chest drain

INDICATIONS

- Large pneumothorax and after urgent release of a tension pneumothorax
- Spreading surgical emphysema – sometimes an X-ray shows no sign of a pneumothorax, but a chest drain should be inserted on the assumption that there is a continuing leak of air into the pleural space
- Large haemothorax with a possible continued source of bleeding
- Large pleural effusion
- Empyema.

EQUIPMENT

- Chest drain between 22 and 32 F but **without an integral trocar**
- 0.5% lignocaine, 20 mL
- Underwater seal apparatus including bottle
- Sterile water
- Surgical blade
- Small and large artery forceps

- Heavy suture, e.g. silk 0
- Adhesive tape – a waterproof variety is best.

POSITION

The position for insertion is the fifth intercostal space in the midaxillary line on the affected side – usually approximately at the level of the nipple in a male. This site is suitable for drainage of both a pneumothorax and a haemothorax and should always be used in trauma. Drainage of a pleural effusion or an empyema may need to be slightly lower but the site should be carefully checked against the available imaging, with particular attention to the possibility of the dome of the diaphragm being raised. The distance between adjacent ribs determines the size of the intercostal drain tube; the largest drain possible is advisable, particularly in trauma.

PROCEDURE

- Position the patient as for pleural aspiration.
- Make a final check of the clinical signs and the chest X-ray.
- Mark the proposed site of insertion.
- Prepare an area over two to three ribs in the mid-axillary line and drape it.
- Anaesthetise the skin and the tissues down to the upper border of the chosen rib – not all the allocated lignocaine is used because more is often needed later.
- Make a 2–3 cm transverse incision over the proposed site of insertion.

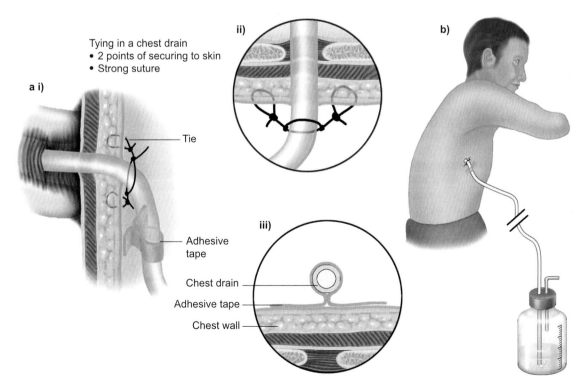

Fig 11.15 **(a) Technique for securing of a chest drain. (b) Chest drain in position with underwater drainage.**

- Use the artery forceps to dissect bluntly through the subcutaneous tissues, going down onto the superior margin of the rib and dissecting through the intercostal muscles and then the parietal pleura (Fig. 11.15a) – this is where more local anaesthetic may be required.
- When the parietal pleura is punctured with the tip of the artery forceps, there is usually the escape of fluid and/or air. Sweep the gloved index finger down the line of blunt dissection to free any adhesions within the pleural space so that injury to the lung is avoided.
- Grasp the drainage tube at its tip with artery forceps and guide it down the track with the index finger. Once the drain is within the pleural cavity, remove the forceps and advance the drain gently.
- Attach the outer end of the drain to an underwater seal drainage apparatus.
- Close the incision with interrupted sutures and a tight tie around the drain itself – there should not be leakage around the tube or through the incision.
- Insert a purse string suture around the drain or two interrupted sutures across the tube site, leaving the ends untied for final air-tight closure when the drain is removed.
- Check that the drain is working – fluid or air according to circumstances – or that the water is rising into the tube above the level in the bottle (swinging) with respiration; failure to swing may mean that the tube is misplaced.
- Secure the connection between the drain and the underwater seal with strong adhesive tape and, after wiping dry around the insertion site and applying a sterile dressing, tape the drain to the chest wall (Fig. 11.15b).
- Check the position of the drain by chest X-ray.

Complications
- Damage to an intercostal artery or vein which causes either continued bleeding at the site of insertion or a haemothorax
- Damage to an intercostal nerve which may cause later intercostal neuritis/neuralgia
- Pleural empyema
- Laceration or puncture of intrathoracic and/or abdominal organs – prevented by using blunt dissection
- Local cellulitis
- Local haematoma
- Mediastinal emphysema
- Subcutaneous emphysema.

Further hints
- Strong and long dissecting artery forceps are extremely useful.
- Do not use any trocar supplied with a drain – it is a common cause of injury to deep structures.

- The more subcutaneous fat that is present, the bigger the incision that is required; a good guide is that the incision needs to be as long as the subcutaneous fat is deep.

If the first drain does not resolve the pneumothorax or there is a large and continuing leak, further drains may well be required. The same applies if surgical emphysema continues to spread after the insertion of a chest drain.

If after pleural drainage for acute haemothorax more than 200 mL of blood (as distinct from blood-stained pleural effusion) drains every hour, thoracotomy may be indicated.

Removal of chest drain

The chest drain does not have a continued role if it fails to swing with breathing or is not draining any fluid; these are the chief indications for its removal. Before this is done the patient should be asked to cough and, if the drain does not bubble, then any leak from a hole in the lung has almost certainly been sealed; however, for certainty, the test should be repeated after 12 hours. A check X-ray before removal can be useful to confirm that the lung is completely re-expanded and that any pleural effusion has been fully drained.

Large pleural effusions should drain over several days. The maximum should be 1 L an hour and not more than 4 L a day, otherwise there is a risk of reflex pulmonary oedema.

EQUIPMENT
- Sterile gloves
- Suture cutters
- Local anaesthetic and, if occluding sutures have not been preinserted, a closure suture
- Occlusive dressing.

PROCEDURE
Ideally this should be done with two people: one to tie the suture and the other to remove the drain. Local anaesthetic and a standby suture should be available.

- Undo the adhesive dressing and check whether there is a purse string suture in situ; if there is, release the suture and place a half knot.
- Release the suture holding the drain.
- Ask the patient to take two large inhalations and then momentarily to hold the breath in expiration (Valsalva manoeuvre to raise intrathoracic pressure); now pull the drain out quickly.
- Tie the purse string immediately and cover the site with a sterile dressing and occlusive tape.
- If there is any concern after the removal of the chest drain, a chest X-ray is indicated.

- If the occluding suture is ineffective, then gauze should be available to place over the hole and prevent a sucking chest wound.

Pericardial paracentesis

INDICATIONS

This procedure is used to relieve cardiac tamponade (Ch. 17), which most commonly occurs after penetrating injuries to the chest, although a blunt injury – such as a steering wheel – can also be responsible. The removal of a small amount of blood or fluid (15–30 mL) can make a dramatic difference to the patient. Also, rarely in surgical practice, a chronic effusion may require aspiration. The pericardial sac is a fixed fibrous structure which, distended by only a small amount of blood, restricts cardiac filling. Therefore to remove 15–20 mL of effusion – blood or other fluid – can have life-saving benefits for the patient.

EQUIPMENT

- Long plastic sheathed needle 16–18 gauge – a single-lumen central line cannula is ideal; if this is unavailable then a needle is sufficient, but, if repeated aspiration is required, the procedure has to be repeated rather than re-aspirating from a cannula that remains in situ
- Three-way tap
- 20 mL syringe
- A small scalpel blade (if a cannula/needle is to be used).

PROCEDURE (Fig. 11.16)

- Continuous recording of blood pressure, pulse rate, central venous pressure and ECG throughout the procedure is ideal, but in the urgent circumstances usually encountered this can be omitted.
- If time allows, prepare the xiphoid and subxiphoid areas.
- Attach the syringe to the three-way tap and needle/cannula.
- Feel for the apex beat to ensure that there has been no marked mediastinal shift; this may be difficult or impossible when there is cardiac tamponade.
- Anaesthetise the area and incise the skin over a point 1–2 cm inferior to the left of the xiphochondral junction at a 45° angle to the skin.
- Advance a long needle and cannula (e.g. Abocath) towards the head, aiming towards the tip of the scapula or shoulder. Aspirate as the needle is advanced and watch the ECG continuously in case needling the myocardium causes any irregularities, including an injury pattern, e.g. extreme ST changes or a widened and enlarged QRS complex. Premature ventricular contractions may also occur, secondary to irritation of the myocardium.

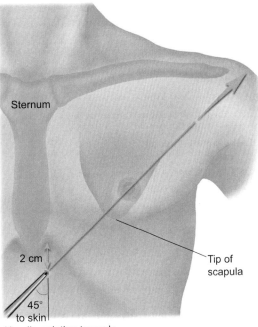

Sternum

2 cm

45° to skin

Tip of scapula

Needle pointing towards tip of scapula and shoulder

Fig 11.16 **Technique for pericardial aspiration.**

- When the needle enters the blood-filled pericardial sac, withdraw as much non-clotted blood as is possible, although it must be remembered that the epicardium will approach the inner aspect of the pericardial sac and ECG changes may then occur.
- After aspiration is complete, slide the cannula over the needle and reattach the three-way tap, closing it off. Secure a catheter in place with adhesive tape.
- If the symptoms of cardiac tamponade persist, re-aspiration or a thoracotomy may be needed.

Possible complications

- Aspiration of ventricular blood
- Laceration of coronary artery or vein
- Pericarditis
- Cardiac arrhythmias – ventricular fibrillation, tachycardia
- Puncture of aorta, inferior vena cava, oesophagus.

Peritoneal lavage

INDICATIONS

Peritoneal lavage is indicated in a patient with multiple injuries if:

- abdominal examination is equivocal because other injuries (fractures of ribs, pelvis and lumbar spine) may be obscuring physical findings

- abdominal examination is unreliable because of severe head injury, entotracheal intubation, intoxicants or paraplegia
- There is unexplained hypotension and/or blood loss.

EQUIPMENT
- Peritoneal dialysis or peritoneal lavage catheter
- 1 L of normal saline
- Intravenous giving set
- Scalpel
- Local anaesthetic – 1% lignocaine with adrenaline 10 mL
- Skin cleaner
- Dressing pack and sterile towels
- Instruments – tissue forceps, Allis clamps, arterial forceps.

PROCEDURE (Fig. 11.17)
- Decompress the bladder by the passage of a urinary catheter.
- Prepare the area around the umbilicus (15 × 15 cm).
- Infiltrate local anaesthetic just inferior to the umbilicus and along the midline for approximately 2–5 cm, depending on the amount of subcutaneous tissue. Continue dissection through the linea alba to

grasp its edges with the Allis forceps so as to provide countertraction.
- Expose the peritoneum and pick it up with arterial forceps.
- Insert the peritoneal dialysis catheter into the peritoneal cavity, advancing it towards the pelvis.
- Connect the catheter to a syringe and aspirate.
- If gross blood is not aspirated use the i.v. apparatus to instil 500–1000 mL of warmed saline.
- Given the patient is haemodynamically stable, allow the fluid to remain in the abdomen for 5–10 minutes before siphoning it off by putting the empty normal saline container on the floor and allowing the peritoneal fluid to drain from the abdomen (which can take up to 20–30 minutes). A suture secures the catheter if some time elapses before the fluid is removed and it is necessary to make sure the container is vented to allow free flow.
- After return of the fluid, remove the peritoneal catheter and repair the fascia with interrupted sutures (e.g. Prolene 0 on a J needle) and the skin (e.g. Ethilon 3,0).

Indications for laparotomy after peritoneal lavage
- Aspiration of more than 5 mL of obvious blood

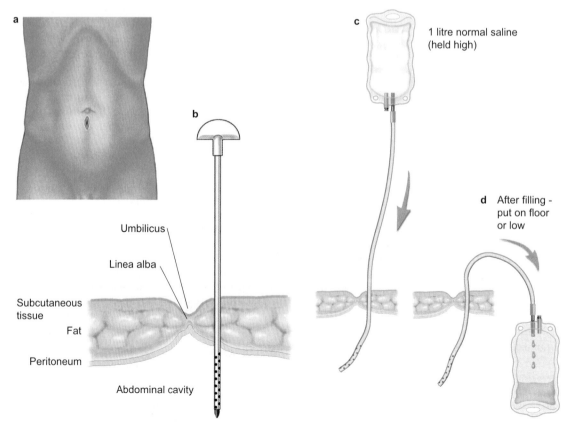

Umbilicus
Linea alba
Subcutaneous tissue
Fat
Peritoneum
Abdominal cavity

1 litre normal saline (held high)

d After filling – put on floor or low

Fig 11.17 **Technique for peritoneal lavage.**

- Aspiration of enteric contents
- Laboratory analysis of the peritoneal lavage fluid: more than 10 000 red blood cells/mm^3; more than 500 white blood cells/mm^3, bacteria and vegetable matter (usually associated with a raised WBC count).

False-negative results are obtained in 2% of peritoneal lavages, usually the consequence of isolated injury to retroperitoneal organs such as the pancreas, duodenum, diaphragm, small bowel and bladder.

Airway management

Any patient who is semi-conscious or unconscious must have an adequate assessment of the airway:

- Look for agitation, cyanosis, difficulty in respiratory effort and choking motions.
- Listen for snoring, gurgling, stridor and gargling sounds.
- Feel with the back of the hand for the exit of air with respiratory effort or see fogging of the oxygen mask on expiration.

Simple Management

Blood secretions should be removed from the nose and mouth with a rigid suction device. A cribriform plate fracture must be considered and gentleness is essential.

Chin lift

First complete clearance of the mouth, if indicated, by sweeping a finger between the tongue and the upper palate; be wary of the tendency of a semi-conscious patient to bite. Chin lift (Fig. 11.18) is a simple procedure which can be done on any patient without interfering with the cervical spine: the fingers of one hand are placed under the mandible in the midline, and are then lifted gently upwards to bring the chin forwards.

Jaw thrust

The angles of the lower jaw are grasped and the mandible displaced forwards. This is the method used with a mouth-to-face mask with a good seal.

Oropharyngeal Airway (see Ch. 6)

A semi-conscious or agitated patient may cause difficulty, but an unconscious one usually accepts an oral airway. This should be inserted upside down with the concavity directed upwards until the soft palate is encountered. Rotation through 180° is then done which places the concavity downwards and around the back of the tongue.

Nasopharyngeal Airway (see Ch. 6)

This is useful when a patient has an upper airway obstruction but is unable to tolerate an oropharyngeal airway. The nasal airway is inserted into one nostril. It needs first to be lubricated and then inserted into the less obstructed nostril (often it is easier to insert through one or other nostril). If difficulty is encountered with

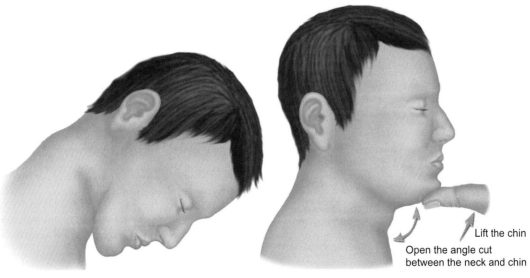

Lift the chin
Open the angle cut between the neck and chin

Before After

Fig 11.18 **Chin lift.**

one nostril, the other is used. The turbinates are often felt to fracture as the catheter is inserted, but little force is needed for this to occur and fracture is usual. **If there is a suspicion of a base of skull fracture, do not use.**

Surgical airway

INDICATIONS

An inability to intubate the trachea is the only indication for creating a surgical airway and this can occur for various reasons:

- oedema of the epiglottis
- fracture of the larynx
- severe oropharyngeal haemorrhage
- when an endotracheal tube cannot be placed through the cords.

Cricothyroidotomy

ANATOMY (Fig. 11.19)

The cricoid cartilage is the only circumferential support to the upper trachea in children and therefore surgical cricothyroidotomy is not recommended in children under 12 years. A 14 gauge needle/cannula can be used instead and is inserted through the cricothyroid

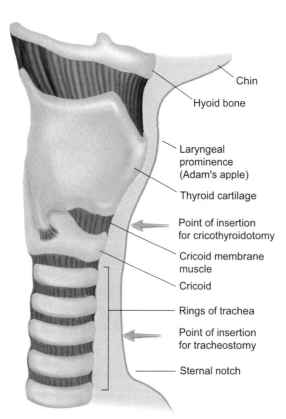

Fig 11.19 **Cricothyroidotomy and tracheostomy incision points.**

Chin
Hyoid bone
Laryngeal prominence (Adam's apple)
Thyroid cartilage
Point of insertion for cricothyroidotomy
Cricoid membrane muscle
Cricoid
Rings of trachea
Point of insertion for tracheostomy
Sternal notch

membrane with intermittent oxygen jet insufflation. This method can lead to carbon dioxide retention and therefore should not be used for more than 40 minutes.

EQUIPMENT

- Cricothyroidotomy set – often easily available in most resuscitation areas
- Surgical blade
- Curved arterial forceps and tracheal dilators
- Small endotracheal tube of internal diameter 5–7 mm; if not available, then use any type of tube – metal, rubber or plastic.

PROCEDURE

- Feel for the laryngeal prominence of the thyroid cartilage (Adam's apple) – more prominent in men than women. If it is difficult to be certain, then identify the hyoid bone and work the finger downwards; if it is still impossible to identify anything above what is thought to be the thyroid cartilage, it is possible that what was thought to be the thyroid cartilage is in fact the hyoid. As the finger descends in the midline, there is a palpable gap between the thyroid cartilage and the cricoid. It is through this window that emergency cricothyroidotomy is carried out (beneath the cricoid ring it is sometimes possible to feel the rings of the trachea but this depends on how much subcutaneous tissue is present) (Fig. 11.19).
- If time permits and the patient is conscious, insert local anaesthetic into the skin and subcutaneous tissues.
- Make a small transverse incision through the skin and extend this through the cricothyroid membrane; a hissing sound is audible once the trachea is penetrated.
- Use tracheal dilators and/or arterial forceps to expand the hole by separating the cricothyroid fibres (cricothyroidotomy set has appropriate instruments).
- Insert a small endotracheal tube (5–7 mm internal diameter) or any other appropriate tube that is available (normal tube sizes for adults are 8–8.5 mm for women and 9–10 mm for men).

Emergency tracheostomy

INDICATIONS

This is rare because cricothyroidotomy is the preferred emergency procedure. If the larynx has been completely disrupted by injury and the cricothyroid membrane is not intact, then an emergency tracheostomy is indicated.

PROCEDURE

- Ensure the patient's neck is extended as far as possible (in trauma the possibility of injury to the cervical spine must be remembered and ideally an assistant should keep the head and neck central).

- A council of perfection is to give oxygen through a mask because sometimes this gives the patient a few extra minutes without severe hypoxia.
- Make a vertical incision from the laryngeal prominence of the thyroid cartilage to the suprasternal notch and deepen it through the strap muscles.
- Find the second, third and fourth tracheal rings and, if necessary, divide the thyroid isthmus – usually avoidable and if done may result in considerable bleeding.
- Incise the trachea vertically through the second, third and fourth rings; dilate the opening with either tracheal dilators or arterial forceps and insert an endotracheal tube (ideally 7–8 mm internal diameter) and attach the oxygen supply immediately.
- Bleeding is controlled with artery forceps and ties; often the anterior jugular vein bleeds as well as the divided thyroid isthmus.
- Use a fine-bore suction tube to suck out the trachea.

Elective and semi-elective tracheostomy

It is preferable to relieve acute airways obstruction by endotracheal intubation or cricothyroidotomy and then to do an elective tracheostomy.

EQUIPMENT
- Tracheostomy set – usually obtained or used in the operating room
- An operating room scrub nurse usually comes with the set
- Tracheal tubes of internal diameter 8–8.5 mm for women and 9–10 mm for men.

PROCEDURE (Fig. 11.20)
The procedure can be done under general or local anaesthetic (preferably the latter) and should be performed by an experienced surgeon:

- Make a transverse incision halfway between the cricoid and the suprasternal notch and between the medial borders of sternomastoid muscles.
- Separate the strap muscles vertically in the midline through the investing fascia.
- Identify the thyroid isthmus, although it rarely needs to be divided in the adult and can usually be retracted upwards; in the child it is more likely to require division.
- Before the incision into the trachea is made, check the tracheostomy tube: inflate the cuff and make sure there are no leaks; deflate the cuff and then

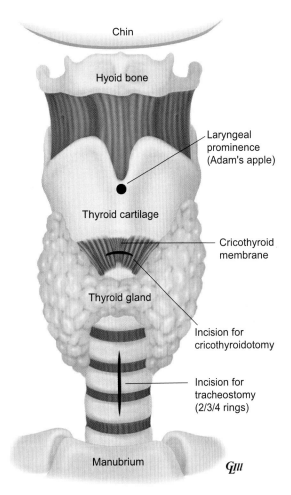

Fig 11.20 **Tracheostomy technique.**

gently lubricate the cuff and tube with lubricating jelly. Check that the connector is compatible with the anaesthetic tube and oxygen supply.
- Insert the tube at the same time as the endotracheal tube is withdrawn; make an immediate connection to the oxygen supply.
- In a child no part of the trachea should be excised as there is a high risk of subsequent stenosis. Therefore a vertical incision is made over the second, third and fourth tracheal rings and a heavy suture is inserted through each side of the tracheal incision; this aids dilatation with the tracheal dilators and allows the tube to be inserted. The ends of the sutures should be left long so that they protrude through the incision to facilitate re-intubation should the tracheostomy be accidently removed.

The same method can be used with advantage in adults. Some surgeons excise a circular piece of trachea anteriorly and others use a distally based flap. Subsequent stenosis is less likely in the adult whichever method is adopted.

Principles of surgical oncology

The management of patients with cancer frequently involves more than one specialist. Often, the initial diagnosis and treatment of a tumour may be undertaken by a surgeon (often with a special interest) who may then involve a medical oncologist, a radiotherapist and a specialist in palliative care. Oncology therefore cuts across the traditional specialities, and the development of multidisciplinary teams provides a more efficient and complete service for patients. The surgeon may be called upon to assist with diagnosis, assessment of tumour staging and removal of tumour bulk and to perform surgical procedures to deal with mechanical complications. The diverse nature of surgical intervention demands considerable familiarity with the pathological basis of malignancy and the therapeutic options available.

A further aspect of oncological practice is to detect malignancy before it has caused symptoms or to establish which patients or groups of patients are at high risk of developing malignant diseases. Both these roles are examples of screening, which is considered at the end of this chapter.

As in many other areas of medicine, the definition of terms can cause confusion. Malignancy means that a cell type has escaped normal control and is proliferating unchecked; the tissue of origin is not specified. Cancer used to mean a malignant tumour which had its origin in epithelial tissues, e.g. a squamous carcinoma of the skin or a transitional cell carcinoma of the bladder. However, this distinction has largely been lost and the terms 'cancer' and 'malignancy' are now used interchangeably.

General features of malignant disease

INCIDENCE
Figures (Table 12.1) from the Office of Population Censuses and Surveys (OPCS) show that malignant disease accounts for just under a quarter of all deaths in the UK, being second only to cardiovascular disease (approximately one-half). Table 12.1 shows the contribution of different types of malignancy to total mortality over a three-year period.

Lung cancer still causes the greatest number of deaths, although more women die of breast cancer than

Table 12.1
O.P.C causes of death

	1995
All cancers	141 297
All digestive system	38 680
Oesophagus	5780
Stomach	6900
Pancreas	5820
Colon/rectum	15 700
Lung/bronchus	33 000
Breast	12 543
Kidney	2660
Prostate	8866
Lymphatic/haemopoietic	10 000

Table 12.2
Aetiological factors associated with malignant disease

Factor	Tumour
Genetic	
Retinoblastoma (Rb) gene	Childhood retinoblastoma
Wilm's tumour gene	Nephroblastoma
p53 oncogene	Prevents malignant transformation unless mutated
FAP gene	Colonic carcinoma in patients with familial adenomatous polyposis (FAP)
Polyp-cancer sequence (multiple sequential genetic mutations)	Colorectal cancer
Environmental	
Ultraviolet light	Basal cell carinoma Malignant melanoma
Chemicals	
Benzene	Leukaemia
b-Naphthylamine	Bladder carcinoma
Vinyl chloride	Hepatic angiosarcoma
Asbestos	Mesothelioma
Tar, crude oil	Squamous carcinoma
Tobacco smoke	Lung carcinoma
Ionising radiation	Skin tumours, leukaemias
Diet	
Aflatoxins	Oesophageal carcinoma
Smoked foods	Gastric carcinoma
Alcohol	Oropharyngeal and oesophageal cancer
Drugs	
Alkylating agents (in patients treated for other malignant disease)	Leukaemias
Viral	
Hepatitis B	Hepatocellular carcinoma
Epstein-Barr virus	Burkitt's lymphoma, nasopharyngeal carcinoma
Human papilloma virus	Cervical carcinoma
Human immunodeficiency virus	Kaposi's sarcoma, B-cell lymphoma

of lung cancer. Cancer of the gastrointestinal tract is the next most common cause. Total cancer deaths continue to increase but the incidence of deaths from certain tumours is declining.

AETIOLOGY

Malignancy is of diverse and multifactorial cause. No single chemical or biological factor has been definitively shown to cause human cancer. However, combinations of individual factors, such as genetic susceptibility, chemicals, occupation, lifestyle and viruses may together induce malignant change in exposed or susceptible tissues. The assessment of a patient with suspected malignancy should include a family history and an enquiry of possible exposure to aetiological factors (Table 12.2). Their continued identification will inevitably lead to further preventative measures, comparable to the efforts being made to reduce the use of tobacco.

EPIDEMIOLOGY

Study of the population dynamics and distribution of malignancy helps in the appropriate planning of health care services and resources. In addition, detailed statistics can highlight trends in incidence that point to aetiological factors and geographical variations in the occurrence of tumours. The identification of causal occupational factors has been largely the result of epidemiological study (e.g. exposure to industrial carcinogenic chemicals). In addition, epidemiological studies can identify groups with a high risk or a poor prognosis. These can then be subject to screening or rigorous follow-up after treatment.

Biology of malignancy

Carcinogenesis and growth

Controlled cellular proliferation occurs during embryogenesis, hypertrophy, healing, regeneration, repair and during the metabolic response to trauma and sepsis. In many instances, cellular replication occurs because growth factors bind to specific receptors on the cell surface and induce intracellular signals which activate the nucleus and cause cell division. Within the nucleus, nucleoproteins ensure accurate DNA replication, DNA repair and DNA transcription to messenger RNA. However, these biochemical processes are susceptible to damage and malfunction by mutations, deletions or amplifications of the genes which code for many of the normal regulatory factors or their receptors. Mutations can occur either spontaneously or as a result of the interaction of aetiological factors with the DNA of the host. Malignancy is the consequence of escape from the normal controlling factors for cellular replication. At some point in the multi-step process of carcinogenesis, the transforming cell undergoes a number of genetic changes which result in the unchecked expression of *oncogenes*. These are constituents of the human genome which are associated with normal cellular proliferation and differentiation. They become implicated in carcinogenesis when their encoded proteins are overproduced, mutated or otherwise modified so that their function is continually expressed, rather than regulated. This unregulated expression or *neo-expression* of normal genes may be responsible for the capacity of certain tumours to secrete proteins known as *tumour markers* into the circulation, e.g. carcinoembryonic antigen (CEA) for colorectal cancer and alpha-fetoprotein (AFP) for hepatocellular carcinoma. A further genetic change may be the loss of function of tumour suppressor genes.

Unlike normal tissues where, in general, a cell divides only in order to replace one which has been lost, tumour cells fail to respond to the signals which regulate normal growth. The belief that all tumours contain cells proliferating more rapidly than those in normal tissues is false. Most tumours enlarge because either the proportion of cells in the proliferative phase of the cell cycle (growth fraction) is greater than normal, or there is decreased cell loss from apoptosis (physiological cell death). It has been estimated that up to 50% of tumour cells are lost as a consequence of hypoxia, exfoliation, metastasis and destruction by host defences. Despite

these losses, tumour cells adapt to the physiological selection pressures of their surroundings to achieve continuous advantage over the host. A further development of this adaptive nature is *progression* by which tumours become more aggressive with time and contain fewer cells which resemble their parent tissue, so producing cells with metastatic potential.

A fundamental concept is that change to malignant behaviour on the part of cells does not result in a single disease process. Tumours from the same tissue of origin may behave quite differently with respect to growth, invasion and metastases. This is frequently demonstrated by colonic tumours appearing as either bulky, locally invasive primary tumour without metastases or as small asymptomatic primary tumours with dissemination to other parts of the body. Carcinogenesis proceeds through multiple stages involving the interaction of different aetiological and host factors, each of which influences the tumour's final biological behaviour and clinical manifestations.

Influence of biology on clinical course

In general, a tumour is of sufficient size to be clinically palpable when it contains 10^9 or more cells; however, at

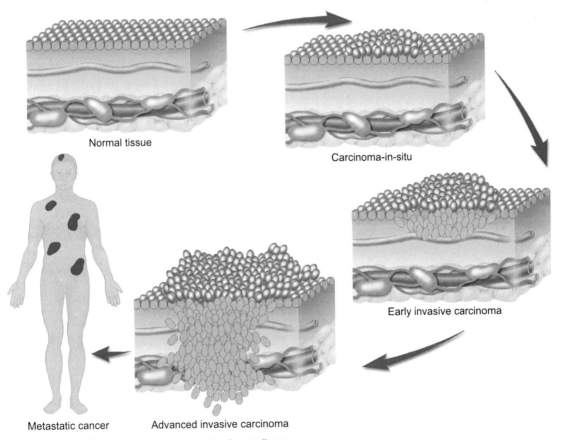

Normal tissue

Carcinoma-in-situ

Early invasive carcinoma

Metastatic cancer   Advanced invasive carcinoma

Fig 12.1 **The natural history of the development of malignant disease.**

clinical presentation most tumours have many more cells than this. Even the smallest radiologically detectable breast carcinoma contains 10^7–10^8 cells. Patients usually die when the total has reached 10^{12}. This natural history is shown diagrammatically in Figure 12.1.

Invasion and metastases

Carcinoma in situ is a collection of malignant cells confined by their normal basement membrane. This is the earliest stage at which a tumour may be histologically identified and implies that the tissue has changed under carcinogenic influences. The cells are both functionally and structurally altered – a state of *dysplasia*. This process may be multifocal, which implies that the remaining apparently normal cells are at increased risk of malignant transformation (e.g. the normal mucosa surrounding a colonic carcinoma). The advance of malignant disease is by:

● local tissue invasion through and beyond the basement membrane
● distant spread of cells (metastasis) to form autonomous tumour deposits.

Invasion occurs when tumour cells start to secrete enzymes capable of digesting intercellular stroma. Many of these enzymes are now being characterised and their physiological or pharmacological inhibitors identified. Prominent among these enzymes are the matrix metalloproteinases. Through continued growth, suitably equipped cells can encroach upon and destroy adjacent organs (e.g. duodenal and bile duct obstruction from a pancreatic carcinoma). Tissue resistance to invasion is variable: arteries and tendons are rarely destroyed, but lymphatics and veins are commonly breached.

Tumour cells have metastatic capacity when they are able to:

● invade adjacent tissues (especially veins and lymphatics)
● survive in unfamiliar tissue environments – bloodstream, peritoneal cavity
● sustain their own proliferation to form a focus of tumour cells.

Although only about 1 in 10^6 tumour cells may have metastatic potential, many thousands of cells are shed from a tumour each day. Palpation or surgical manipulation of a tumour is known to increase shedding.

Tumour metastases may themselves undergo further malignant progression and bear little pathological resemblance to the primary tumour.

Routes of metastasis

Metastasis occurs by three routes (Fig. 12.2). Invasion of the lymphatics or veins allows the transport of viable invasive tumour cells to distant sites. The pattern of

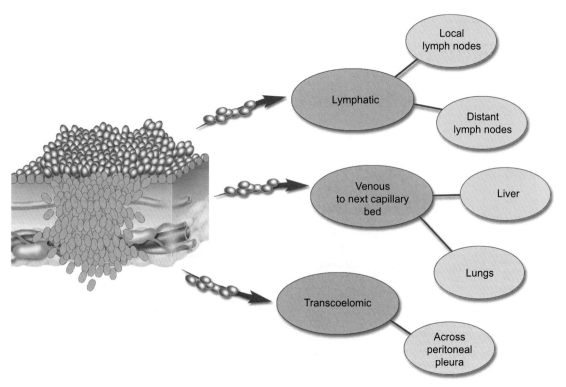

Fig 12.2 **Routes of tumour metastasis.**

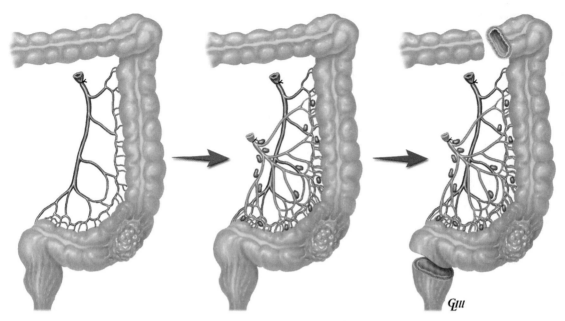

Fig 12.3 **Isolation of the tumour before surgical resection – the 'no touch' technique.**

spread can be predicted for most tumours (e.g. breast and large bowel) and may be used to plan surgical removal of the primary tumour and possible sites of distant spread. Lymphatics usually accompany the arterial supply to an organ and so, in many instances, surgical removal of an organ which contains a tumour involves dissection of the arterial supply and removal of these vessels and their associated lymphatic tissue (e.g. radical gastrectomy, colectomy). Similarly, the venous drainage of an organ is an important determinant of venous metastatic spread. Because surgical manipulation of any malignant tumour causes shedding of tumour cells into lymphatics and veins, some surgical procedures have been designed to reduce this by initially dividing the blood supply, especially the veins (e.g. ligation of the inferior mesenteric vessels before mobilising a left sided colonic tumour using a 'no-touch' technique – Fig. 12.3).

Distribution of metastases

The organ distribution of metastasis varies with the type of tumour and is related to complex interactions between the migrating tumour cell and the capillary endothelium of the organ. Metastatic deposits may become sites from which tumour cells gain access to further vessels – metastases from metastases. In this way, tumours spread from the primary to predictable local metastatic sites, and then on to other less certain places.

Some tumours have a predilection for particular metastatic sites. Gastrointestinal malignancy tends initially to metastasise to the liver via the portal venous circulation; renal and breast carcinoma to the lungs.

Bony metastases are relatively common in all terminal disease but there are five tumours that commonly metastasise to bone:

- breast
- prostate
- lung
- kidney
- thyroid.

Occult micrometastases

Microscopic tumour deposits, present at the time of original diagnosis and treatment but which escape detection, may emerge as metastases or recurrent disease some time later. They are of considerable importance in surgical oncology. Although they are often called recurrence, they are in fact the continued growth of residual tumour. Modern oncological management aims to include adequate treatment to deal with such micrometastases. This involves systemic therapy additional to local surgical measures – *adjuvant therapy*.

Clinical features of malignant disease

Most of these will be found in the individual chapters of this book devoted to regions or systems. The important clinical features of 'malignancy in general' are given in Box 12.1.

Box 12.1

Clinical features suggestive of malignant disease

Palpable swelling

This is most often painless. It is usually irregular and firm (unless bony in origin). It may be invading local structures and therefore fixed.

Anaemia

Loss of blood occurs readily from disorganised capillaries and other vessels in the tumour. Continued bleeding from a surface lesion should be viewed with suspicion. Internal bleeding (e.g. into the gut) is most often chronic and concealed; the result is iron deficiency anaemia of unknown origin.

Consequences of local invasion

Hollow tube obstruction is a sinister development in the natural history of a tumour. Examples are dysphagia (oesophageal), abdominal colic (small and large bowel), jaundice (bile duct), hydronephrosis (renal tract) and bilateral leg oedema (inferior vena cava). Perforation of a hollow tube can follow invasion with development of an acute emergency (e.g. perforation of a gastric carcinoma). Local invasion may also lead to destruction of tissue (e.g. nerves and bone) with pain.

Metastatic spread

This is common. Presentation is with a history of progressive general tiredness, weight loss and anorexia. Examination may reveal the signs of metastatic deposits: irregular hepatomegaly, lymphadenopathy, ascites, pleural effusion, pathological fracture, focal headache and epileptic fits (cerebral deposits).

Biochemical effects

This relates to the production of substances associated with clinical effects:

- *Parathyroid hormone analogue* (PTH-rp) causes malignancy-related hypercalcaemia; it is not uncommon in breast and neoplasms but may be seen in any tumour causing significant bone destruction
- *Antidiuretic hormone* in bronchogenic carcinoma
- *Adrenocorticotrophic hormone* in pituitary tumours, leading to increased corticosteroid output
- *5-Hydroxytryptamine* in carcinoid tumours
- *Adrenaline* in phaeochromocytoma.

Asymptomatic detection

During routine assessment of other conditions (e.g. preoperative check before herniorrhaphy), never overlook the possibility of malignant disease.
Do not forget: *if you do not look you cannot find.*

Management of malignant disease

Patient evaluation

The following components are involved:

HISTORY

- Duration and progression of symptoms – often symptoms last for months (rarely years) and are **progressive**
- Presence of non-specific symptoms such as fatigue, loss of appetite and weight
- Exposure to risk factors
- Family history of cancer.

EXAMINATION

- Identification of primary site (as suggested by the history)
- Evidence of local invasion (mobility or fixation, damage to local structures)
- Use of special techniques for individual circumstances – e.g. rectal examination, sigmoidoscopy
- Evidence of distant spread – palpable lymph nodes, enlargement or malfunction of organs (e.g. liver enlargement and jaundice), accumulation of effusions.

INVESTIGATION

Simple

- Full blood count — may reveal blood loss, marrow failure or infiltration
- Serum concentrations of urea and electrolytes – evidence of renal tract obstruction or dehydration

- Liver function tests – the presence of hepatic metastases or biliary tract obstruction
- Examination of urine for cytology and/or for the presence of tumour markers
- Plain X-ray, especially of the chest for primary tumour or metastases
- Measurement of serum tumour markers, e.g. CEA, CA125.

More complex

These investigations are determined by the suspected clinical diagnosis and include:

- Contrast examination of the gastrointestinal (GI) tract
- Ultrasound scan, usually of solid organs
- Computed tomography
- Magnetic resonance imaging.

Invasive

These are usually directed both towards reaching a definitive diagnosis and assessing the extent of the problem:

- Endoscopy including the upper and lower GI tracts, the biliary tree and the air passages, all of which can include biopsy
- Laparoscopy and thoracoscopy also with biopsy.

Aspiration cytology and tissue biopsy
(see also Ch. 4)

These are techniques that allow a pathological diagnosis to be reached – an **essential** preliminary to treatment. Aspiration cytology gives an assessment only of the shape and other features of individual cells. Histological examination of a tissue sample shows the pathological *architecture* (the relationship between cells and their surroundings).

Aspiration is done by passing a fine needle into the lesion and applying suction with a syringe. Small fragments are drawn back into the barrel and can be extracted and stained for examination under the microscope.

Needle biopsy uses a needle of larger calibre often equipped with a cutting device. A tissue core is extracted, processed and sectioned, so providing an histological section.

Open biopsy exposes the lesion and either removes part (incisional) or all (excisional) of it for histopathological examination. Biopsies of this nature can be processed immediately (frozen section) or by standard paraffin-embedded sections.

Guidance
All the above methods may be undertaken under some form of guidance. X-ray, ultrasonography or CT scanning may have been done previously and the site

marked; alternatively the needle biopsy or incision may be performed, under real-time image control, most commonly by ultrasound.

TUMOUR STAGING

Staging is the attempt to classify tumours into categories (stages) of their natural history by using agreed criteria which are known to be relevant to prognosis. To categorise a patient into the appropriate stage is an essential part of the decision-making process for correct treatment. Many systems have been devised for tumours of different organs or anatomical regions. Most were originally based solely upon clinical findings or sometimes upon additional findings, such as the histopathological features for an individual tumour group, e.g. the clinical staging for breast carcinoma (Ch. 27) and Duke's classification for colorectal cancer (Ch. 24). However, the more recent and widely adopted TNM (Tumour, Nodes, Metastases) system (Table 12.3) allows a single generic method to be applied to almost all tumours, which has the advantage of allowing for different biological behavior because each value of T, N and M is scored independently.

Histological grade (Table 12.4)
The histological grade, obtained either from a tumour biopsy or from the excised specimen, can be used in conjunction with the TNM stage to give a more accurate assessment of prognosis for an individual patient. This information allows more precise evaluation of the efficacy of different treatments on tumours of comparable stage. For example, a radical mastectomy (Ch. 27) for a histological grade 1 breast carcinoma of stage T1/N0/M0 may lead to cure, but the prognosis for long-term survival is more guarded in a tumour of similar stage but which is grade 3.

Table 12.3
The TNM staging system

Tumour	Nodes	Metastases
T0: primary unknown (Tis: tumour-in-situ)	N0: not involved	M0: no metastases
T1: Tumour <2 cm	N1: local nodes involved	M1: metastases present
T2: tumour > 2 cm	N2: distant nodes involved	Mx: status unknown
T3: tumour > 5 cm (or reaching serosa in GI tract)		
T4: tumour infiltrating local tissues, e.g. skin, vessels, nerves		

Postoperative
R0: no residual tumour
R1: microscopic residual disease
R2: macroscopic residual disease

Table 12.4
Histological classification

Differentiation	Features
Grade 1 – well differentiated	Forms recognisable structures of parent tissue
Grade 2 – moderately differentiated	Some attempt at organisation
Grade 3 – poorly differentiated	Architecture totally disorganised; cells not recognisable from parent tissue

Prognostic markers

Both molecular and genetic markers which give prognostic information have been identified for some tumours. In breast cancers, the presence of nuclear receptor for oestrogen indicates a good prognosis, whilst those tumours which express an excess of receptors for epidermal growth factor or the oncogene c-*erb*B2 have a worse prognosis. Many new 'markers' of prognosis are described each year.

Operative surgery for malignant disease

Histological confirmation

Before definitive elective treatment of a tumour there must be unequivocal histological confirmation of malignancy and an accurate assessment of the stage. However, some patients present with a surgical emergency (e.g. an obstructing carcinoma of the colon) which requires surgical intervention without either of the above items of information. In these cases a decision about the extent of surgical treatment is made on the operative findings, supplemented if possible by urgent pathological examination of tissue during the course of the procedure (frozen section).

Aim

The aim of surgical management is either curative or palliative. Those with obvious widespread tumours should not be treated by a surgical effort to achieve cure; a lesser procedure may be performed (e.g. bypass of a gastrointestinal tumour) to relieve distressing symptoms such as pain or gastrointestinal obstruction. Referral for non-surgical treatment or for palliative care is then appropriate.

Surgical attempt at cure involves the total excision of all tumour-bearing tissues together with the associated lymphatic and venous drainage (e.g. radical gastrectomy). Invasion of adjacent vital structures (e.g. invasion of the trachea by an oesophageal cancer) may determine the feasibility of removing a tumour (its *operability*, which is not the same as *curability*). By contrast, involvement of non-essential structures does not prevent resection of a tumour with the invaded structures (e.g. a colonic tumour that has invaded the small bowel). How far to place the resection away from the visible growth (*resection margin*) is decided by knowledge of the behaviour of the tumour and its propensity to local invasion. Both are described in the appropriate sections of this book. For most neoplasms treated by surgery the technical aim is to remove the tumour, the organ in which it is contained and the regional lymph node drainage (lymphatics and nodes) all in one piece: en-bloc.

Reconstruction after curative surgery is an important aspect of surgical technique. Most patients naturally wish to regain as near normal a lifestyle and self-perception as possible. An ileostomy (Ch. 23) requires more departures from usual habits than does a successful ileo-anal pouch (Ch. 25). Reconstruction after mastectomy (Ch. 27) restores body image and self-confidence. A careful, informed and sympathetic discussion with the patient is needed to reach a joint conclusion about the course of action.

Adjuvant therapy

One of the most challenging areas in surgical oncology is the treatment of patients with apparently early disease. Clinical experience over the last 50 years has clearly shown that curative surgery alone for tumours that seem to be localised leads to cure in only a proportion of patients. This indicates either that some patients may have undetected micrometastases at the time of presentation or that surgical intervention triggers the release and seeding of tumour cells to distant sites where their growth becomes clinically evident some time after the initial surgery. Adjuvant therapy is additional antineoplastic treatment which is used for some patients with tumours that are thought to have been completely removed by surgical excision. Adjuvant chemotherapy, local radiotherapy or hormone therapy, or sometimes various combinations of these, aim to destroy occult micrometastases. Success in this effort must always be balanced against the fact that adjuvant treatment will be given to a varying proportion of patients who do not have micrometastases and who therefore do not need it.

Accordingly, adjuvant treatments must:

- be relatively non-toxic
- have been demonstrated to have efficacy against the same tumour, usually in patients with advanced disease.

Timing of adjuvant therapy

Adjuvant therapy was traditionally used only after curative surgery. More recently, treatment has been

Table 12.5
Adjuvant and neo-adjuvant therapy

Tumour	Adjuvant protocol	Timing
Breast	Cyclophosphamide, methotrexate, 5-fluorouracil	Postoperative
	Methotrexate, mitoxantrone, mitomycin-C	Postoperative
	Radiotherapy or tamoxifen, or both	Postoperative
Oesophagus	5-Fluorouracil and other agents with or without radiotherapy	Pre- and postoperative
Colorectal	5-Fluorouracil and levamisole	Postoperative
Rectum	Radiotherapy	Pre- and postoperative
Osteosacroma	Methotrexate, epirubicin with or without radiotherapy	Pre- and postoperative

used before operation – *neo-adjuvant therapy*. Some of the protocols currently in use are shown in Table 12.5. A useful shrinkage of some tumours – oesophageal, rectal and breast – can be achieved by preoperative radiotherapy, and some of the many protocols for the treatment of breast cancer include postoperative radiotherapy.

Non-operative therapy

Radiotherapy

Knowledge of the radiotherapeutic options for a particular tumour is essential for the practising surgeon. Unfortunately, a large number of tumours are relatively radio-resistant. Examples are clear cell carcinoma of the adult kidney, adenocarcinoma of the stomach and malignant melanoma.

Principles

The unit of absorbed radiation energy is the *gray* (Gy), 1 Gy being equivalent to 1 joule per kilogram (J/kg). Radiation acts by inducing chemical changes within the nucleus of the cell that cause damage to DNA. Irradiation depopulates a tumour of its malignant cells mainly via direct effects during mitosis, and thus its efficacy is determined by:

- the number of viable cells present
- intrinsic radiosensitivity of the cells
- mitotic rate.

Because irradiation damage takes place during mitosis, it follows that normal tissues, which have a high cellular turnover (such as the bone marrow and enterocytes), will also show evidence of damage within hours of irradiation. For the same reason, it may be weeks or months before the maximum effect of radiotherapy is apparent in a more slowly proliferating tumour such as basal cell carcinoma of the skin.

Dose and fractionation

The total dose of radiotherapy for a tumour is calculated for each individual site and size. Modern therapy is now given in fractions of the total dose, because this minimises the unpleasant side-effects of treatment, i.e.:

- local soreness
- skin changes
- lethargy
- nausea and vomiting.

The spectrum of electromagnetic radiation can be adjusted to increase penetration into deep tissues. New 'super-voltage' apparatus is based on this principle. This can be used to focus treatment at a tumour site from different directions, thus enhancing the destruction of tumour cells without damaging surrounding structures. The level of expertise with this fractionated radiotherapy is now such that not only is it used as palliative therapy for certain unresectable or metastatic lesions but it is also employed as an adjuvant to surgery (e.g. following wide local excision of T1–T2 breast carcinomas or before excision of a rectal carcinoma).

Other methods of application

In addition to external beam irradiation mentioned above, radiotherapy can be applied in other ways.

Radioactive implants may be inserted into tumours to achieve maximum dose:

- endo-luminal radiation for oesophageal and rectal tumours
- iridium wires for cervical carcinoma
- yttrium implants for pituitary tumours.

Systemic administration of radioactive substances can be used if the tumour is known selectively to take up known chemicals. *Radioactive iodine* can be taken up by cells of thyroid tumours which incorporate it as they synthesise thyroxine.

Chemotherapy

Cytotoxic drugs interfere with cell division in normal and malignant cells. Therefore the success of their use depends on

- intrinsic resistance of the tumour cell to the agent
- the toxic effect on normal tissues, which limits the dose.

The gap between the two may be very narrow.

Types of chemotherapeutic agents

There are four main groups as well as additional miscellaneous agents. Many of these agents are used in varying combinations which have been developed empirically to maximise therapeutic efficacy without excessively increasing toxicity. However, their effects on normal proliferating cells result in bone marrow and intestinal toxicity.

Alkylating agents

Examples of these are the nitrosoureas and epoxide compounds – cyclophosphamide, melphalan, chlorambucil – which combine with intracellular molecules such as nucleic acids, proteins (especially enzymes) and cell membranes. Damage to the enzymes which link DNA strands, critically disrupts mitosis.

Antimetabolites

Antimetabolites – methotrexate, 5-fluorouracil, cytosine arabinoside and 6-mercaptopurine – disrupt the sequence of DNA by being incorporated instead of the normal nucleotide or by irreversibly binding to the constituting enzyme in order to render it ineffective.

Vinca alkaloids

These bind to intracellular tubulin and inhibit microtubule formation. The latter is the spindle during mitosis and in consequence this is arrested at metaphase.

Antimitotic antibiotics

These include adriamycin, epirubicin, actinomycin D, mitomycin C and bleomycin. The first two intercalate between opposing DNA strands and disturb DNA function. Actinomycin D and mitomycin C are inhibitors of DNA and RNA synthesis, respectively, and also generate free oxygen radicals which are toxic.

Miscellaneous agents

There is a further group of agents whose mechanisms of action are varied or unknown. *Cis-platinum* and its less toxic derivative *carboplatin* react with the guanine in DNA and form cross-linkages along the DNA chain as well as between DNA strands. Other agents, such as *etoposide*, are tubular poisons derived from podophylotoxin.

Biological response modification

Endocrine manipulation has been used for many years to control tumours which arise from cells that are dependent on hormones for their normal growth and division. The effect is obtained in a number of ways:

- removing the endocrine organ or organs that produce the hormone – orchidectomy for prostate cancer
- inhibiting hormone production with antagonists to releasing hormones – genetically engineered luteinising hormone release hormone (LHRH) for prostate cancer
- blocking the stimulatory action of the hormone by using the endocrine antagonist – oestrogens in large doses for prostatic cancer to exhaust testosterone production from the testis
- blocking the receptor site for the hormone on the malignant cell – tamoxifen prevents oestrogen binding in breast cancer.

The discovery of receptor sites for autocrine hormones on many different tumour cells will undoubtedly lead to the construction of synthetic analogues which block receptor binding and activation.

Assessment of response to treatment

Clinicians must assess their therapeutic performance in two ways:

- review treatment outcome in their own patients – clinical audit
- study the publications that compare current treatment with new experimental protocols.

Such periodic appraisal allows advances to be incorporated into practice and outmoded treatments to be discarded.

Methods of assessment

Five-year survival

This has been the traditional method of outcome assessment. The figure is helpful in studying groups of patients who may receive different forms of treatment, but it gives little information that is relevant to the individual patient.

Median survival time (or median time to recurrence)

This information is more useful to clinician and patient than 5-year survival and is the preferred method. For example, the 5-year survival rate for pancreatic carcinoma treated by resectional surgery is approximately 25%, but the median survival is approximately 18 months.

Serial imaging of progression

The response of inoperable or metastatic tumour to non-surgical treatment can be gauged by serial imaging (ultrasound, CT or MRI) of the tumour. In such circumstances, duration of response is of equal importance to magnitude and is measured as the median duration of response in the patients treated. Accepted grades of response are given in Table 12.6

Table 12.6
Grading of tumour response to non-surgical therapy

Grade	Assessment
Complete response	No sign of tumour
Partial response	Decrease in tumour size by more than 50%
Static disease	Less than 50% decrease or 25% increase in tumour size
Progressive disease	Greater than 25% increase in tumour size or of a deposit

---

Box 12.2

Scales for measurement of patient well-being

Karnowsky status scale provides a score eg:

This scale provides a score, e.g.:
100 Well, no complaints
 50 Requires considerable assistance and medical care
 10 Moribund

European Cooperative Oncology Group scale

ECOG 0 — asymptomatic
ECOG 1 — minor limitation
ECOG 2 — moderate limitation
ECOG 3 — severe limitation
ECOG 4 — moribund

Quality of Life score

This is obtained from a multiple field questionnaire

Patient well-being

How a patient 'feels' is a subjective marker of response to reduction in the bulk of a tumour and of the side-effects of the treatment that is being used. A number of scales have been formulated to assess this aspect of treatment (see Box 12.2).

Terminal care

Terminal care should be seen as an integral part of oncological management and of equal importance to any of the other therapeutic disciplines. Accurate assessment of the disease will enable a prediction of the likely sequence of terminal events. Some of these (e.g. nausea) can be anticipated and prophylaxis undertaken.

Informing the patient

When treatment for cure fails or when treatment for palliation begins, a full and frank discussion about the prognosis and the plan of management is essential. The patient has an absolute right to this information, which can never be justifiably withheld, even if disclosure is against the wishes of relatives. Once the patient is fully aware of the situation, referral to a team which can provide palliative care should be sought. Although not necessarily about to die at this stage, many patients are apprehensive for their the future and appreciate an introduction to those who may treat them in a later phase.

Fear of death and dying

For most patients with malignant disease, their abiding fear is of a painful, lingering death. Terminal care exists to alleviate both the psychological torment of impending death by counselling of patient and family and the physical problems posed by progressive malignant disease. Foremost in the aims of terminal care is keeping the patient in the familiar surroundings of home. Adequate facilities and the provision of satisfactory analgesia and nursing management must be available. There are a number of charity-based cancer nursing agencies in the UK for this purpose; they are staffed by nurses specially trained in the management of malignant disease and in dealing with its psychological impact on the patient and relatives.

Screening for malignant disease

Tumours might either be foreseen in those who are known to be at high risk or detected early by examining in some way or other those in the population who might be susceptible. Such activities are called screening.

Population screening. The knowledge that a large proportion of patients present with advanced disease has prompted the idea of screening the entire population. However, population screening often yields relatively few unsuspected tumours at a pathological stage which would make cure more likely. The cost of these huge projects is high.

Targeted screening of high-risk groups significantly increases the number of patients detected in relation to the cost of the procedure. The cost/benefit ratio is consequently improved.

Desirable criteria for a screening programme

For a screening programme to be effective, the following points are essential:

- The disease should be common or have defined high-risk groups.
- The natural history of the disease should be known, in order to define lesions which are truly localised and identify opportunities for curative treatment.

Table 12.7
Screening programmes

Method	Tumour
Mammography (High risk, 50–65 years)	Breast
Faecal occult blood (FOB) testing	Colorectal
Colonoscopy (genetic high-risk groups)	Colorectal
Oesophagogastroscopy (dysplasia – high-risk groups)	Oesophagus Stomach
Serum prostate-specific antigen	Prostate

Table 12.8
Tumour markers in serum

Marker	Tumour
Prostate-specific antigen (PSA)	Prostate
Carcinoembryonic antigen (CEA)	Colorectal
Alpha-fetoprotein (AFP)	Hepatocellular
Beta-human chorionic gonadotrophin (B-HCG)	Testicular, gestational
CA 19-9 (monoclonal antibody)	Colorectal, pancreatic
CA 125 (monoclonal antibody)	Ovarian

- Sensitive and specific methods of early detection must be available.
- Detection methods should be cheap, easy to use, and have a high patient compliance.
- Effective treatment for early disease should be available.
- The screening procedure must not involve significant hazard to the population tested.

Table 12.7 lists a number of tumours for which screening programmes are undergoing evaluation. However, few meet all of the above criteria.

Screening for recurrence of tumour

What is often called 'recurrence' of a tumour is in fact the development of 'residual disease'. In some cases, the latter may be amenable to further surgical treatment (e.g. excision of a metastasis in the liver after primary resection of a colorectal carcinoma).

Simple methods

In those treated with the intention of cure, clinical assessment to detect the development of residual tumour is often undertaken on a regular basis by follow-up and periodic examination. Features indicating the presence of disease, such as return of symptoms, enlargement of the liver or the development of palpable lymph nodes are sought. When such features are found, further investigation for evidence of tumour should follow. However, by this time the disease is often re-established and incurable. Earlier diagnosis of residual or recurrent disease may allow for more effective treatment. The techniques used in population screening are appropriate, because patients who have been treated for malignant disease are, by definition, a subpopulation with a high risk of recurrence, e.g. metachronous cancer of the colon or breast.

Tumour markers

These molecules (Table 12.8) are products of tumours which may be detected in body fluids or sometimes in urine in abnormally high levels. Their use in diagnostic screening is limited by the incidence of false positives in patients with benign disease.

Other methods of detection of residual disease

Monoclonal antibodies against tumour antigens can be radiolabelled. The antibodies seek out the tumour cells and can then be detected by gamma camera scanning for sites of increased uptake (e.g. colorectal tumour deposits in the liver).

FURTHER READING

Duncan W (1988) Ionising radiation and radiotherapy. In: Cuschieri A, Giles GR, Moosa AR (eds). *Essential Surgical Practice*. Bristol: Wright, pp. 190–202.

McArdle C (1990) *Surgical Oncology*. London: Butterworth.

Priestman TJ (1989) *Cancer Chemotherapy: an Introduction*, 3rd edn. New York: Springer-Verlag.

13

Organ transplanation

Over the past 30 years, organ transplantation has become a rapidly expanding and important surgical speciality. More than any other branch of surgery, organ transplantation requires the close co-operation of several disciplines – surgeons, anaesthetists, immunologists and physicians – to achieve a successful outcome. A synopsis of its historical landmarks is provided in Information Box 13.1.

---

i Information Box 13.1

Some landmarks in transplantation

Date	Event
circa 300 AD	*Cosmos and Damian*: believed to have attempted a leg transplant
1778	*John Hunter*: coined the term transplant
1863	*Bert*: observed ingrowth of vessels into skin grafts and defined autograft, allograft and xenograft
1905	*Guthrie and Carrel*: developed vascular anastomotic techniques
1933	*Voronoy*: first human renal transplant – failed because of ABO incompatibility
1945	*Hume*: first-short lived functioning renal allograft
1950	*Lawler*: first long-term survivor from renal grafting
1963	*Starzl*: first human liver allograft
1966	*Lillehei*: first human pancreas transplant – technical success
1967	*Lillehei*: first human bowel transplant – failed
1967	*Starzl*: first long-term survivor from liver transplantation
1967	*Barnard*: first successful heart transplant
1981	*Shumway*: first successful heart–lung transplant
1988	*Grant*: first long-term survivor of small bowel transplantation

Essential definitions

Autograft. Free (i.e. after disconnection of the blood supply) transplantation of tissue from one part of the body to another in the same individual.

Isograft. The transfer of tissue between genetically identical individuals – in humans this is between identical twins (*rejection is not a feature of auto- or isografts*).

Allograft. An organ or structure transplanted from an individual of the same species. Allografts are at the moment the main class of transplant in humans.

Xenograft. The transfer of organs between dissimilar species. Presently limited to tissues that have been chemically processed to make them non-antigenic, e.g. porcine heart valves. However, this is potentially the most exciting technique because, should it prove successful, the present acute shortage of organs for transplantation would be overcome. Great progress is being made in understanding the nature of the difficulties that form a barrier to xenografting.

Orthotopic graft. The donor organ is transplanted to the same site as the recipient's diseased one. The removal of the latter is first required, e.g. liver transplantation.

Heterotopic graft. The donor organ is inserted at a site different from its normal anatomical position, e.g. kidney transplantation to the iliac fossa.

Artificial (hybrid) organ implantation. The transplantation of bio-artificial organs, which are a combination of biomaterials and living cells, e.g. a hybrid artificial pancreas. At present this technique is experimental. Success would, as with xenografting, open a new chapter in transplantation.

Cadaver graft. An organ or tissue retrieved from an individual who has been pronounced dead according to criteria which differ from one culture to another (see below).

Living donors. There are two classes:

- *Related donors* – parents or siblings who may have some genetic advantages and a sense of family or social obligation
- *Unrelated donors* – those with a high philanthropic sense or, more commonly, who wish to make money; selling a kidney is outlawed in the West but there is a thriving trade in other parts of the world and the moral issues are complex.

Basic immunology of organ transplantation

Successful organ transplantation (with the exception of the cornea) requires the manipulation of the immuno-

logical defences of the recipient so as to overcome rejection. Because auto- and isografts do not elicit an immune response, it must be the genetic differences between the donor and the recipient that are of major importance in this process. These differences are expressed as *tissue* or *histocompatibility* antigens. The latter stimulate and lead the activation and proliferation of the immune cells and are also the target cells in the resultant effector mechanisms induced by the immune reaction. The key cells involved in the rejection process are *lymphocytes* and *antigen-presenting* cells.

Major histocompatibility complex (MHC)

A large group of genes is present on the short arm of human chromosome 6 (Fig. 13.1), including those that encode the class I and class II MHC molecules which are involved in the presentation of antigens to T cells. Class I molecules are integral membrane proteins found in all nucleated cells and platelets – the classical transplantation antigens. Class II molecules are expressed on B cells, macrophages, monocytes, antigen-presenting cells (APCs) and some T cells.

Human leucocyte antigen (HLA) loci

There are four of these on the short arm of chromosome 6:

- HLA-A – 20 alleles have been identified
- HLA-B – over 30 alleles have so far been characterised
- HLA-C (between A and B) – seems not to have a role in mounting the immune response

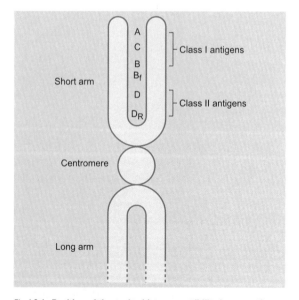

Fig 13.1 **Position of the major histocompatibility locus on the short arm of chromosome 6.**

- HLA-DR – appears to be clinically most important in that, if donor and recipient match for it, graft survival is improved.

Lymphocytes

These are the key cells controlling the immune response. They specifically recognise foreign (*non-self*) material as different from the tissues of the body. Lymphocytes are of two main types:

B cells develop in the fetal liver and subsequently in bone marrow. Mature B cells carry surface immuno-globulins which are their antigen receptor. The response to an antigenic stimulus is cell division and differ-entiation into plasma cells under the control of cytokines released by T cells.

T cells develop in the thymus which is seeded during embryonic development with lymphocytic stem cells from the bone marrow. T cells then develop their antigen receptors and differentiate into two major peripheral subsets: one expresses the CD4 marker; and the other the CD8. T cells have a number of functions, including:

- helping B cells to make antibody (CD4+)
- recognising and destroying cells infected with viruses (CD8+)
- activating phagocytes to destroy ingested pathogens (CD4+)
- controlling the level and quality of the immune response (CD8+).

Rejection

Rejection is a destructive reaction initiated by the host to foreign HLA and other non-shared antigens. The process involves:

- antigen recognition (afferent arc)
- activation of selected clones of T cells and the effector mechanisms (efferent arc).

Afferent arc

Two routes lead to activation:

- foreign antigen or donor antigen-presenting cells (e.g. dendritic cells) which are directly recognised by the recipient's T cells
- intracellular processing of foreign antigens by host antigen-presenting cells and subsequent presentation of peptides to T cells.

Class II HLA antigens activate T helper (CD4$^+$) cells and class I HLA antigens activate cytotoxic (CD8$^+$) T cells.

Efferent arc

There is proliferation and differentiation of the selected T-cell population. CD4$^+$ cells (T helper – Th cells) produce interleukin-X (IL-10) which induces macrophages to produce IL-1, which in turn stimulates Th cells to produce IL-2 and other cytokines (e.g. IL-4, IL-5, IL-6). The latter cause B cells to differentiate into plasma cells and to secrete antibody. Cytokines also stimulate CD8$^+$ cells to become cytotoxic. The coating of target cells by antibody allows K cells (large granular lymphocytes), macrophages or granulocytes to recognise and destroy them through a variety of mechanisms (release of enzymes, reactive oxygen mediators and *perforins*).

Clinical patterns of rejection

There are three patterns of rejection:

- *Hyperacute and acute accelerated rejection* – this is the result of preformed IgG antibody and occurs within hours of exposure.
- *Acute cellular rejection* – this is infiltration by activated T cells with recruitment of acute inflammatory cells; generally seen at 7–14 days post-transplant.
- *Chronic rejection* – this is a major cause of graft attrition and is probably antibody-mediated. There is intimal hyperplasia and endarteritis obliterans. In liver transplants it is associated with loss of bile duct radicles.

Chronic rejection is difficult to treat but strategies that involve the newer anti-B cell drugs (e.g., mycophenolate mofatil) may have a role in the future.

Antigen-presenting cells (APCs)

These are a group defined functionally by their ability to take up antigens and present them to lymphocytes in a form the latter can recognise. Some antigens are taken up by APCs in the periphery and transported to secondary lymphoid tissues. Others are intercepted as they arrive by APCs normally resident in lymph nodes and other lymphoid aggregates. B cell recognise antigen in its native form, but T cell recognise antigenic peptides that have been associated with self MHC molecules. In consequence, to present an antigen to a T cell, an APC must internalise it, process it into fragments and re-express these at the cell surface in association with class II MHC molecules. In addition, many APCs provide additional stimulatory signals to lymphocytes either by direct cellular interactions or via cytokines (Fig. 13.2).

Organ matching
ABO compatibility

The biological rules are the same as those which govern blood transfusion. Because ABO red cell antigens are expressed on most tissue cells, ABO-incompatible allografts undergo hyperacute rejection. However, the rhesus factor is expressed only on red blood cells and therefore a match for it is not required for successful transplantation.

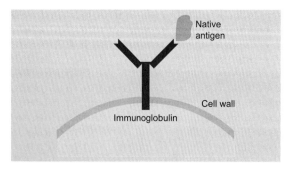

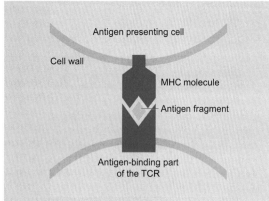

Fig 13.2 **Antigen handling by B and T cells.**

HLA-A, HLA-B and HLA-DR matching

Tissue typing (identification of the A, B and DR antigens) is carried out on the donor and the recipient by the separation of lymphocytes out of heparinised whole blood and their exposure to antibodies of known HLA-A, HLA-B and HLA-DR specificity. The technique is particularly relevant in the investigation of a family where a living donor may be available, and it also enables HLA-identical siblings to be identified. The influence of matching by tissue type on the successful outcome of organ transplantation is best established in renal transplantation, and its role in cardiac, liver and pancreatic transplantation is not yet clear.

Direct cross-matching

After a suitably matched recipient has been selected, a direct cross-match is set up because any recipient may have preformed circulating antibodies capable of reacting against donor cells. These antibodies may be the result of previous blood transfusion, pregnancy or viral infections. A direct cross-match incubates donor lymphocytes with the serum of the recipient in the presence of complement to exclude cytotoxicity from circulating antibodies.

Organ retrieval

Most organs for cadaveric transplantation come from those who have suffered irreversible structural brain

Table 13.1
Age range for donors

Organ	Range (years)
Kidney	3–75
Liver	Neonate to 70
Heart and/or lung	Neonate to 50
Pancreas	Neonate to 50

damage after road traffic accidents or cerebrovascular catastrophes and have been diagnosed brain dead by agreed criteria (See Ch. 10). In most countries that accept this practice, organs are then retrieved while the heart continues to beat and the donor receives ventilatory and other support. Such conditions are absolute requirements for transplantations of heart, heart–lung, liver, small bowel and pancreas. Contraindications to organ donation are:

● history of disease or trauma involving the organs being considered
● long-standing history of diabetes mellitus, hypertension, cardiovascular or peripheral vascular disease
● prolonged periods of ischaemia because of profound hypotension or asystole
● malignancy – other than a primary brain tumour
● untreated systemic bacterial, fungal or viral infections – however, donors who have had bacterial infections adequately treated may still be suitable.

Chronological age in donors is usually less important than biological age. The age limit for each organ is given in Table 13.1.

Organ function in donors

Function of the organ which is to be transplanted must be established. A satisfactory past medical history and physical examination are essential. A well-perfused organ – as indicated by adequate blood pressure and normal arterial blood gas tensions – is also highly desirable.

Heart
● Normal blood pressure, ECG, chest X-ray and arterial blood gas tensions.

Lung and heart–lung
● Negative Gram stain on sputum
● Absence of pathogens on sputum culture.

Liver
● Adequate liver perfusion – arterial blood pressure blood and arterial gas tensions
● Normal values for serum bilirubin, transaminase and alkaline phosphatase concentrations and a normal prothrombin time.

Kidney

- Normal urine output and urinalysis – however, oliguria may be pre-renal because of dehydration
- Normal serum creatinine and blood urea concentrations.

Pancreas

- Normal serum concentrations of amylase and glucose – hyperglycaemia often develops in acute brain stem injury because of steroid administration and intravenous crystalloid infusion which contain glucose; elevated serum glucose alone is not necessarily a contraindication.

Retrieval after cardiac arrest

The continued shortage of organ donors has provided an impetus to re-examine retrieval from donors who do not have a beating heart. Provided rapid organ perfusion with cold preservation solution can be achieved immediately after cardiac arrest, kidneys may be usable.

Live related donation

Live related donor organs can be used for kidney, liver, pancreas, lung and small bowel transplantation. Clearly the need for any organ other than the kidney must justify the operative risk of the partial resection of the relevant organ that is required.

Donor operation

Retrieval is becoming increasingly complex because many donors are now considered and consent is obtained for multi-organ donation. Frequently there is a harvest from one individual of: corneas, heart, lungs, liver, pancreas, kidneys, bone and skin. With the recent success of small bowel transplantation, the retrieval of the small bowel and the right colon may also be included. A number of transplant teams are involved and it is essential that they fully agree the order of retrieval to be used before the start of the operation.

Retrieval procedure

Currently, the local kidney/liver team starts the procedure and is followed by the heart/lung team. The procedure for the abdominal organs is illustrated in outline in Fig. 13.3. Organs are cold-perfused before removal, examined after removal to ensure they are anatomically satisfactory and then cold-preserved within double plastic bags and stored on a bed of crushed ice for transfer to the chosen transplant centre.

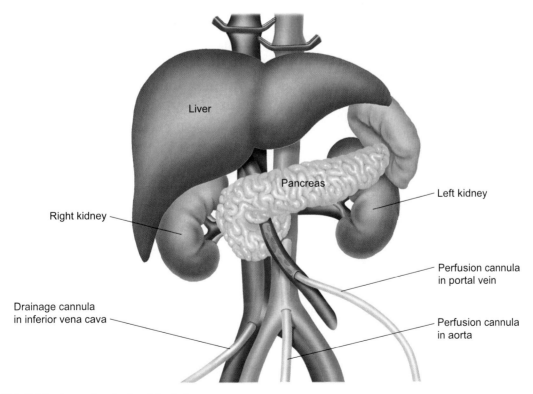

Fig 13.3 **Retrieval procedure for the abdominal organs.**

Immunosuppression in transplantation

There is a difficult balance to achieve between the prevention or reversal of rejection and the morbidity that can result from loss of host defences against infection – and also, in the long term, the development of malignant disease.

Immunosuppressive agents

Azathioprine. Metabolised in the liver to 6-mercaptopurine, this substance is a purine antagonist and reduces the synthesis of DNA and RNA in dividing cells.

Cyclosporin and tacrolimus. These act within the cell to prevent transcription of the gene for interleukin 2 (IL-2), a cytokine involved in the efferent arc of rejection.

Corticosteroids. These agents produce potent but non-specific immunosuppression and also have an anti-inflammatory action. They work by decreasing macrophage motility and phagocytic activity and also block IL-2 release from both macrophages and its generation by Th cells.

Anti-lymphocyte (ALG) and anti-thymocyte (ATG) globulins. These are derived from anti-serum to human lymphocytes or thymocytes which has been generated in another species; they are therefore polyclonal. They deplete lymphocytes in the circulation and lymphoid organs and also mask T-cell antigens non-specifically.

Monoclonal anti-T cell antibody (OKT3). This is a murine antibody to the T3 antigen of human T cells. It produces destruction of CD3-positive T cells which are associated with graft rejection. There are other similar monoclonal antibodies, but OKT3 is the one most widely used.

Mycophenolate mofetil (MMF) inhibits proliferation of T and B lymphocytes and may prove more potent than azathioprine. It may also have a role in the prevention of chronic rejection because B lymphocytes are thought to be important in this process which now accounts for the majority of renal transplants lost in the long term.

Anti-IL2 receptor antibody. This is a monoclonal antibody to human IL2 receptor on the lymphocytes. By binding the IL2 receptor it blocks the pathway of activation mediated through the release of IL2.

Rapamycin. This new drug reduces T-cell activation at a later stage in the cell cycle than cyclosporin or tacrolimus although still affecting the IL2 signal transduction pathway. One of its main advantages is that it is not nephrotoxic.

Clinical regimens

These vary greatly from centre to centre but can be approximately caegorised as follows:

Triple therapy. This is the most common standard induction and maintenance therapy, particularly in renal transplantation, and consists of:

- azathioprine – 2 mg/kg body weight reduced to 1 mg/kg at the end of the first week
- cyclosporin – 8 mg/kg body weight adjusted according to the trough (pre-dose level) of free drug in serum
- prednisolone – 0.3 mg/kg body weight.

The mainstay is cyclosporin. Measuring its trough level is important because an excess can be nephrotoxic. Further reductions in dose follow satisfactory progress over 3 months.

Another triple therapy regimen, based on tacrolimus (0.2 mg/kg) instead of cyclosporin and adjusted according to the trough level, is now being used in a number of centres and may be more effective in reducing acute rejection rates than cyclosporin.

Many American centres now also use MMF in place of azathioprine in triple therapy at a dose of 2 g/day.

Polyclonal and monoclonal agents against T cells. These agents are OKT3 and ATG. Although some use these substances for induction, they are most often reserved for acute rejection episodes which fail to respond to high-dose steroid therapy over 3–5 days.

Experimental regimens. These use FK506 and anti-B cell agents (see, for example, 'Small bowel transplantation' below).

Complications of immunosuppression

The most serious complication is an increased susceptibility to infections (see Box 13.1). Long-term immunosuppression also increase the risk of developing malignant disease, particularly squamous cell carcinoma of the skin and some forms of lymphomas. Other complications are the outcome of the specific side-effects of individual components of the suppressive regimen (see Box 13.2).

General complications of transplantation

Apart from graft rejection and problems with drug toxicity, organ transplants of most kinds share a variety of complications which are summarised in Table 13.2. Technical problems are directly related to the quality of surgery and show a steady decline with increasing experience.

Box 13.1

Infective complications of immunosuppression

Bacterial

Mycobacterium tuberculosis
Listeria monocytogenes

Fungal

Candida albicans
Aspergillus – various species

Protozoal

Pneumocystis carinii
Cryptosporidium

Viral

Cytomegalovirus
Epstein–Barr
Measles
Herpes simplex and zoster

Box 13.2

Complications of agents used in immunosuppression

Corticosteroids

Reduced growth in children
Impaired wound healing
Bone – osteoporosis and avascular necrosis
Diabetes mellitus
Peptic ulceration
Acute pancreatitis
Hypertension
Psychosis

Azathioprine

Myelosuppression
Liver – toxicity and cholestatic jaundice
Acute pancreatitis

Cyclosporin

Nephrotoxicity
Hepatotoxicity
Neurotoxicity
Gingival hypertrophy
Hypertrichosis

Monitoring the progress of a transplanted organ

The monitoring methods available are as follows:

Table 13.2
Complications of transplantation

Category	Nature	Possible effects
General surgical	Wound – infection, dehiscence, incisional hernia	Occasionally life-threatening Further surgery required
Systemic infection	From i.v. lines, especially in liver transplantation Consequent on immunosuppression (see Table 13.3)	Septicaemia
Vascular suture lines	Thrombosis Stenosis	Loss of graft In kidney – hypertension
Visceral suture lines	Leakage Stenosis	Fistula Interference with graft function (hydronephrosis obstructive jaundice)

Transplant function

- Kidney – serum urea, electrolyte and creatinine concentrations
- Liver – urea and electrolyte concentrations, liver function tests and measures of clotting activity
- Pancreas – measurement of amylase and pH in urine (the transplanted pancreas is implanted into the bladder).

Evidence of dysfunction (from the above)

- Kidney – Doppler ultrasound examination to exclude collections around it, obstruction of the ureter and arterial or venous thrombosis. In the absence of such findings, carry out percutaneous biopsy under ultrasound guidance.
- Liver – ultrasound to eliminate technical problems such as bile duct obstruction or vascular thrombosis; biliary contrast studies; biopsy if an immunological problem is suspected.
- Pancreas – the blood glucose level is not of value. Most transplants in the UK are combined kidney and pancreas and the progress of the kidney can be used to monitor the pancreas.
- Small bowel – see below.

Transplantation of individual organs

End-stage failure means that the organ is no longer able to sustain life.

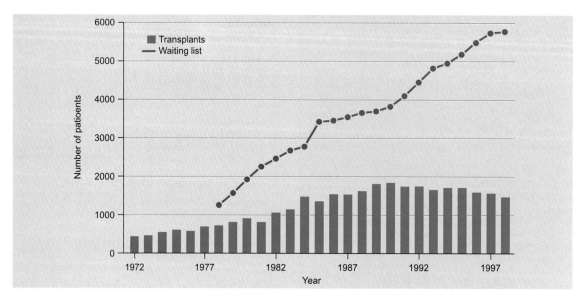

Fig 13.4 **The yearly pattern of kidney transplantations and the waiting list.**

Kidney

With increasing success, the number of allografts transplanted initially increased every year, but the numbers have now reached a plateau because of the limited availability of donors. However, more and more patients are being admitted to dialysis programmes and are subsequently added to an ever-increasing list of patients waiting for a suitable allograft (Fig. 13.4).

INDICATIONS

Indication for kidney transplantation is renal failure from the following causes:

- chronic glomerulonephritis (55%)
- chronic pyelonephritis (25%)
- polycystic disease (8%)
- diabetic nephropathy (2%)
- malignant hypertension (1%)
- Other causes, e.g. analgesic nephropathy (9%)

OPERATION

The transplant is heterotopic, with the kidney placed usually in the right iliac fossa and attached to the iliac artery and vein. The ureter is joined to the bladder to make a new ureterovesical junction (Fig. 13.5). The recipient's own kidneys are left in situ unless they are a source of recurrent urinary infection which may place the transplanted kidney at risk.

RESULTS

There is intercentre variability in graft survival, but current cadaveric graft survival rates are 80–95% at 1 year, 60–70% at 5 years and 49–56% at 10 years (Fig. 13.6).

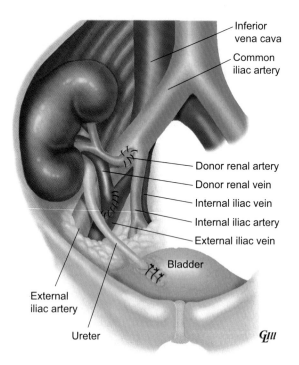

Fig 13.5 **Completed renal transplant in right iliac fossa.**

Liver

The procedure for their transplantation is more recent than kidney transplantation: However, it is now an established treatment of end-stage parenchymal liver disease, including congenital metabolic disorders. Survival figures have improved because of better patient selection and clinical support, organ preservation and

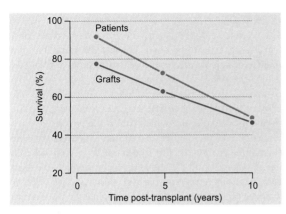

Fig 13.6 **Survival for patients and transplants after kidney transplantation.**

Table 13.3
Indications for liver transplantation

Disease process	Suitable subgroups
Cirrhosis	Primary biliary
	Post-necrotic
	Cryptogenic
	Secondary biliary
Hepatitis	Chronic active
Chlolangitis	Sclerosing
Congenital anatomical disorders	Biliary atresia
	Budd–Chiari syndrome
In born errors of metabolism	Alpha-1-antitrypsin deficiency
	Galactosaemia
	Wilson's disease
Primary liver tumours	Hepatocellular carcinoma
Rare secondary tumours, e.g. neuroendocrine	A relative indication depending on the size of the tumour and absence of extrahepatic involvement

immunosuppressive agents. In major transplant centres, a 70–90% 1-year survival is obtained and, in those transplanted for benign disease, survivors of the first year are likely to be alive at 5 years. The results of liver transplantation in the management of primary liver tumours are universally poor and its role in this situation remains controversial.

Unlike kidney transplants, the number of organs available has been better matched to the number of recipients. However, widening indications for the transplantation of the liver and the increasing awareness by clinicians of liver transplantation as a therapeutic option will undoubtedly result in a waiting list in the near future.

INDICATIONS

Transplantation is indicated by liver failure from any of the conditions shown in Table 13.3. Although these are all disorders which make the patient a candidate, many of them are rare and thus form only a small part of the liver transplant population.

OPERATION

The operation is an ultra-major one because the diseased liver may be quite difficult to remove and there are a number of vascular anastomoses to be made during which venous return to the heart must be maintained by bypass (Fig. 13.7).

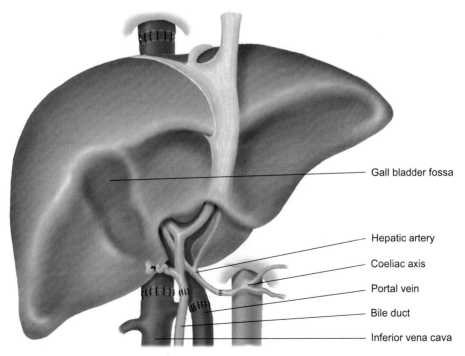

Gall bladder fossa

Hepatic artery

Coeliac axis

Portal vein

Bile duct

Inferior vena cava

Fig 13.7 **Completed liver transplant.** Note the numerous suture lines. The gall bladder is removed.

Primary failure of function may occur in up to 10% of allografts. The morbidity and mortality of this complication are high. Survival following re-transplantation for primary non-function is only half that seen when the first graft functions successfully.

RESULTS

The results of liver transplantation are rapidly improving. Currently the majority of centres report 1 year graft survival in excess of 70%. It is of note that over 85% of patients surviving more than 6 months after liver transplantation return to active life either at school or at work.

Pancreas

The large number of patients with diabetes has made transplantation of the pancreas a worthwhile goal. However, severe diabetes is often accompanied by renal disease which makes concurrent renal transplantation necessary if the patient is to be restored to health.

INDICATIONS

- Insulin-dependent diabetes with renal failure – combined pancreas and kidney transplant
- Pre-uraemic diabetic with severe complications e.g. neuropathy, retinopathy and poor control of the disease – a pancreas-only transplant is needed.

OPERATION

The technique depends on whether a *whole organ* or a *segmental* graft is to be used. The latter is removed on a pedicle of splenic artery and vein and is revascularised using the external iliac artery and vein with the pancreatic duct either occluded or drained into the urinary bladder. The whole organ is removed with the segment of duodenum which drains the pancreatic duct. Revascularisation is by a similar method to the segmental graft with the duodenal loop drained into the bladder (Fig. 13.8). The latter technique has the least complications and the highest success rate. *Enteric drainage* (anastomosis of donor pancreas or duodenum to the gastrointestinal tract) is used in some centres but complication rates are high.

RESULTS

With increasing experience, 1- and 5-year graft survivals of 70 and 40%, respectively, are being reported. However, transplantation of the whole pancreas is likely in the future to be replaced by transplantation of islet cells only.

Small bowel

Small bowel transplantation presents particular difficulties because:

- the transplant contains a large volume of lymphoid tissue (see graft-versus-host reaction below)

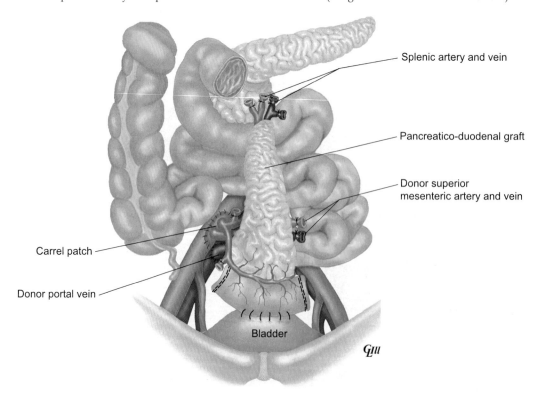

Splenic artery and vein

Pancreatico-duodenal graft

Donor superior mesenteric artery and vein

Carrel patch

Donor portal vein

Bladder

Fig 13.8 **Whole organ pancreas transplant.**

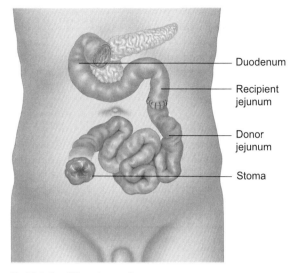

Fig 13.9 **Small bowel transplant.**

- MHC class II antigens are constitutively expressed by the bowel epithelium
- the transplanted organ is colonised with micro-organisms.

As a consequence of the last of these, there is breakdown of the intestinal barrier with the release of bacteria into the circulation (translocation), with consequent infection as well as an increased presentation of immune signals to the recipient.

INDICATIONS

The indications in adults and children are given in Box 13.3. A combined liver and bowel replacement may be necessary if there is coexistent irreversible structural damage to the liver, such as may occur with prolonged parenteral nutrition.

OPERATION

Proximal anastomosis of the graft is to the recipient's jejunum; distally the new gut is brought out as an end-ileostomy (Fig. 13.9).

RESULTS

The most encouraging results have been reported in Canada where the last five small bowel transplants have all been successful with the use of the immunosuppressive drug FK 506. In the USA, survivals are now at 65% at 1 year and 43% at 2 years.

Heart, lung and heart–lung

This is discussed in Chapter 17.

Cornea

The cornea was the first solid tissue successfully allografted in humans. In recent years, a high success rate has made corneal transplantation the most commonly performed transplant.

INDICATIONS

- Opaque cornea from any cause
- Thin or distorted cornea
- Corneal loss – necrotising ulceration or trauma.

OPERATION

A button of the recipient's cornea is removed and replaced with a corresponding graft from the donor using very fine nylon sutures. Because the cornea is avascular, rejection is not a common problem unless the recipient's cornea has undergone neovascularisation before the transplant takes place.

RESULTS

Worldwide, the survival of the graft is 95% and it may be expected to last for life. Close HLA matching correlates with an improved long-term result.

Transplantation in children

In older children with a weight in excess of 20 kg, most transplant procedures are the same as for adults, although specially skilled personnel such as paediatric anaesthetists are required to deal with the haemodynamic problems that may arise during clamping of major vessels. Such problems are greater the younger and the smaller the child.

Kidney

The results of transplanting paediatric kidneys into paediatric recipients are worse than if an adult kidney is used. Accordingly, most centres now transplant the best matched organ provided its size is not too discrepant, access may be modified to make the procedure feasible.

Other organs

For liver, heart and lung, the constraints of size are more relevant and age matching is done. However, the increasing success of using a reduced size liver graft has overcome the problem of supply in that area.

The future

Despite the great success of current multi-organ transplant programmes, further developments are required to improve the long-term outlook of recipients. It is difficult to imagine that there will be many more technical improvements in transplant surgery. Advances in immunology, formulation of new less toxic immunosuppressive drugs, xenografting and the development of cellular or biomechanical approaches to organ replacement therapy are clearly the most important areas for the future.

FURTHER READING

Morris PJ (1994) *Kidney Transplantation: Principles and Practice*, 4th edn. Philadelphia: WB Saunders.

Kapoor AS, Laks H (1994) *Atlas of Heart–Lung Transplantation*. New York: McGraw-Hill.

Cerilli JG (ed)(1988) *Organ Transplantation and Replacement*. Philadelphia: JB Lippincott.

Makowka L (1991) *The Handbook of Transplantation Management*. Austin, TX: Landes RC Co.

14

The neck and upper aerodigestive tract

Swellings in the neck

The most common cause of a neck swelling is lymph node enlargement. The majority of such swellings are secondary to infection, and the minority are the consequence of malignant disease. To make the correct diagnosis depends initially on a careful, thorough clinical assessment.

CLINICAL FEATURES

History
Important features are:

- the duration of the swelling
- progression in size
- associated pain
- other symptoms in the upper aerodigestive tract – hoarseness, dysphagia
- systemic symptoms – weight loss, night sweats
- exposure to alcohol and/or tobacco – squamous carcinoma with a cervical lymph node metastasis is rare below the age of 40 in those who have not been exposed to either of these agents.

Physical findings
Examination of a single lump must produce the following information:

- site and size
- relationship to other anatomical structures such as the great vessels
- fixation to other structures must also be assessed.
- special features such as pulsatility, the presence of a bruit or thrill, tenderness or fluctuation.

A thorough orodental examination must be carried out. The oral cavity and oropharynx can easily be examined using a tongue depressor and bright light. The nasopharynx and laryngopharynx used to require indirect examination with a mirror, but the advent of the fibreoptic nasoendoscope has made these sites much easier to view directly. However, even with this instrument there may, in some instances, not be any visible evidence of a minute focus of disease that is in fact present.

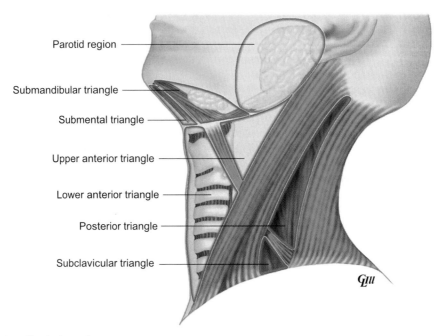

Parotid region

Submandibular triangle

Submental triangle

Upper anterior triangle

Lower anterior triangle

Posterior triangle

Subclavicular triangle

Gill

Fig 14.1 **Sites of swelling in the neck.**

CLINICAL DIAGNOSIS

After the completion of the local examination, a first attempt can often be made at a clinical diagnosis.

Site

The site often indicates a possible origin (Fig. 14.1):

Parotid swellings occur immediately in front of the tragus, over the angle of the mandible or just below the lobe of the ear. An associated facial palsy suggests a malignant tumour of the gland.

Submandibular gland swellings are sometimes indistinguishable from regional lymphadenopathy. In either case, fixation to the mandible may make it impossible to get above the mass. A submandibular swelling is more likely to be palpable bimanually (via the mouth).

Midline submental swellings are nearly always benign and, if cystic, are commonly a thyroglossal cyst, a midline dermoid cyst or a pyramidal lobe of the thyroid.

High anterior triangle swellings can be metastatic in origin with the likely primary site in the oral cavity or oropharynx. Alternatives are branchial cyst or carotid body tumour.

Low anterior triangle swellings are either related to the thyroid gland or are metastatic nodal deposits from a primary tumour in the larynx or pharynx. Such lymph node masses do not move on swallowing unless they are fixed to the thyroid gland or the larynx.

Supraclavicular swellings are more common on the left side of the neck and are commonly caused by disease below the level of the clavicle, e.g. carcinoma of the lung or stomach.

Posterior triangle swellings are rarely the result of metastatic carcinoma unless there are also palpable lymph nodes in the anterior triangle on the same side. More common causes are tuberculosis, toxoplasmosis and lymphoma. The last may occur in an otherwise fit young adult.

Multiple cervical masses

These are almost always nodal and, if accompanied by an acute systemic illness, may be caused by viral infections such as infectious mononucleosis. A more chronic presentation can be produced by tuberculosis.

Time course

The time course of the swelling may be helpful. Enlargement of a cervical lymph node(s) which has taken place over a few days, and which is tender, is almost always inflammatory. Lymphomas occasionally present in this way, but more commonly develop over a period of several weeks and are usually painless. Metastatic nodes have a similar pattern; although they may be tender on palpation, they rarely cause spontaneous pain unless there is invasion of the cervical or brachial plexus.

INVESTIGATION

Cell or tissue samples

Fine needle aspiration (FNA, Ch. 4) is the first more invasive investigation to confirm a diagnosis and is best done immediately after clinical examination has been completed unless there are clinical reasons to think that this is potentially dangerous, e.g. evidence of considerable vascularity such as a bruit or thrill. A fluctuant swelling may yield pus, which is sent for culture, or either clear or opalescent liquid which suggests a branchial or other cyst. A solid lump produces an aspirate which is examined cytologically and may give an indication of the likely pathological cause. However, confirmation must nearly always be sought by other means before treatment is undertaken.

CT scanning is valuable when the likely diagnosis is of metastatic nodal disease. The scan should extend from the base of the skull to the clavicles. Information is obtained about the relationship of the mass to other structures and other impalpable swellings may be found.

Other investigations are based on the probable clinical diagnosis, particularly if the swelling(s) is thought to be of lymph node origin. The usual procedures are indicated in Table 14.1.

Table 14.1
Supplementary investigations to be considered for a lump in the neck

Possible cause	Investigation
Acute infection	Full blood count (FBC)
Tuberculosis	Chest X-ray, Mantoux test
Infectious mononucleosis	Monospot, FBC
Reticulosis (lymphoma)	FBC, bone marrow
Malignancy in lung	Chest X-ray, CT scanning

Further diagnostic strategy

The above investigations usually provide enough information to decide whether the patient requires formal endoscopy of the upper aerodigestive tract. The diagnostic pathways are decided from the outcome of the result of FNA and endoscopy.

Cytology suggests squamous carcinoma

Regardless of whether or not the primary is apparent, a formal upper aerodigestive tract endoscopy is done, and must include examination of (Fig. 14.2):

- nasopharynx
- oral cavity/oropharynx
- hypopharynx
- larynx and trachea
- bronchi
- cervical oesophagus.

A biopsy is taken from any suspicious lesion. In approximately 2%, a second primary is found elsewhere. If the nodal mass contains squamous carcinoma but endoscopy and scanning fail to identify a primary tumour then treatment of the neck should be by radiotherapy (for nodal disease < 2 cm in diameter) or neck dissection (where nodes > 2 cm in diameter).

Cytology suggests lymphoma

Incision biopsy is necessary to obtain sufficient tissue to identify the histological type (see also below).

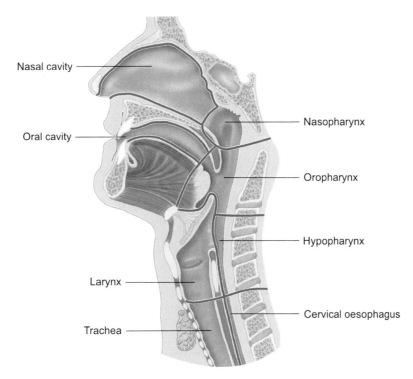

Fig 14.2 **Regions of the upper aerodigestive tract.**

Cytology is unhelpful

Lack of information from FNA and a normal endoscopy together indicate surgical excision/incision biopsy as a last resort. The reason for trying to avoid this is that local surgery for diagnosis on a lump which is malignant may lead to seeding of tumour cells at the biopsy site. Whenever feasible, excision biopsy should be performed to reduce this hazard. Furthermore, it is best to obtain a frozen section at once and, if metastatic squamous carcinoma is confirmed, to go straight on to a radical neck dissection. If fixity of the node(s) makes this unfeasible, the wound is closed and alternative treatment, usually by radiotherapy, is undertaken.

A primary tumour is found at endoscopy

If a primary tumour is found at endoscopy, the type of treatment recommended will depend on the site and size of both the primary and the cervical node metastases. A radical neck dissection should not be undertaken if the primary is known to be below the clavicle.

Benign cystic swellings

Thyroglossal cyst

AETIOLOGY

The embryonic mesoderm which ultimately develops into the thyroid gland descends from the foramen caecum of the tongue to the normal pretracheal site of the gland. The tract usually disappears, but islands of thyroid tissue may be deposited at any point along its course and develop into a cyst.

CLINICAL FEATURES

Presentation is commonly during the second or third decades of life. The mass is usually midline, between the thyroid notch and hyoid bone, and moves upwards on protrusion of the tongue.

MANAGEMENT

The cyst is removed surgically. To avoid recurrence, which may be associated with a sinus, the central portion of the hyoid bone is included in the excision because the tract can run either deep or superficial to the bone.

Branchial cyst

AETIOLOGY

The cause is uncertain. It is considered by some to be a remnant of the branchial complex which contributes so much to the development of the neck.

CLINICAL FEATURES

Presentation is typically at the age of 15–35 years with a cyst in the upper part of the anterior triangle with its posterior portion deep to the sternomastoid muscle. It is smooth, mobile and, unless infected, not tender. The diagnosis can be confirmed by FNA, which produces pale creamy fluid. Further imaging is rarely necessary. Treatment is by excision together with any sinus tract that may run from it.

Vascular tumours

Chemodectoma – carotid body tumour

AETIOLOGY

There is sometimes a family history and these tumours are more common in those who live at high altitudes. Not much else about the cause of this rare tumour is known, although the cells of origin are paraganglionic.

CLINICAL FEATURES

The patient usually presents in adult life with a history of a lump which is ovoid, non-tender and pulsatile. There is mobility in the horizontal but not the vertical plane. Auscultation reveals a bruit. A CT scan demonstrates the lesion but confirmation is best made by carotid angiography which shows a highly vascular mass. Treatment is by surgical excision, which may be difficult.

Tumours of the upper aerodigestive tract

Malignant tumours are more common than benign ones and almost all of the former are primary. Squamous carcinomas are the most common (more than 90%), followed by lymphomas, salivary gland tumours, melanomas and sarcomas.

Squamous carcinoma

AETIOLOGY

The most important predisposing factors are:

- smoking
- high alcohol intake, especially of wines and spirits
- presence of pre-malignant conditions.

Other factors include:

- chronic irritation from a jagged tooth
- chewing betel nut (common in the Indian subcontinent)
- oral syphilis (very rare).

Pre-malignant conditions

Leucoplakia

This is a descriptive term for a white patch or patches on the mucosa, usually of the oral cavity and larynx. It almost always results from chronic irritation, although in 10% it is of unknown cause. The histological picture is often one of dysplasia, but the condition may be associated with frank malignancy.

Management should be conservative, once malignancy has been excluded by biopsy. Close follow-up of the patient is essential and further biopsies may be necessary. Causative factors should be removed if possible.

Erythroplakia

These are fiery red patches in the mucosa, usually in the elderly, that bleed easily. They imply severe dysplasia and are nearly always often associated with the presence of an in situ carcinoma.

Sideropenic dysphagia

Erythroplakia may be associated with this syndrome in post menopausal women, which involves dysphagia, iron deficiency anaemia and a web in the postcricoid hypopharynx. A barium swallow demonstrates the web, which may be associated with a locally dysplastic mucosa. Endoscopy and biopsy are therefore necessary; the passage of the endoscope temporarily relieves symptoms. The condition is not, however, reversible with correction of the anaemia. Subsequent development of a postcricoid carcinoma is a distinct possibility and the patient should be kept under observation.

CLINICAL FEATURES

These are site-specific. The different regions of the upper aerodigestive tract are shown in Figure 14.2.

Symptoms

Nasal or sinus tumours can cause local problems, such as unilateral nasal obstruction and epistaxis, or can invade adjacent structures and give rise to clinical features that are misleading, such as diplopia, middle ear effusion or loosening of teeth. Oral cavity and oropharyngeal tumours commonly present with symptoms of local pain and referred otalgia but, as with tumours of the hypopharynx, the primary may be asymptomatic and it is the presence of metastases which draws attention to the lesion.

Tumours of the larynx characteristically result in hoarseness; compromise of the airway occurs only in very advanced cases. Laryngeal, hypopharyngeal and cervical oesophageal neoplasms may also cause dysphagia, initially to solid food. This is in contrast to dysphagia of neurological origin (motor neurone disease or after a cardiovascular accident), when swallowing is more difficult with liquids. Again, referred otalgia may occur and there is usually evidence of weight loss.

Clinical examination

The sequence of examination is outlined above. The primary may be readily apparent on inspection, usually as an ulcer with a raised edge. Examination is not complete without careful palpation of the neck.

INVESTIGATION

The choice of investigations depends on the known or likely site of the tumour. The principles have already been outlined.

The presence of an unexplained hoarse voice for longer than 6 weeks and inability to assess the larynx fully as an outpatient is an indication for direct laryngoscopy under general anaesthesia. A similar principle is observed for persistent dysphagia and the need for oesophagoscopy; a diagnosis of functional dysphagia (globus pharyngis or globus hystericus) should never be made until both a barium swallow and an oesophagoscopy have been shown to be normal.

MANAGEMENT

A multidisciplinary approach is required. Surgery and radiotherapy are the two principal treatments, used either alone or in planned combination. The role of chemotherapy remains unclear. Eradication of the tumour is the first priority but preservation of function (particularly of speech and swallowing) and of appearance are also important factors.

Approximately 25% of patients with head and neck cancer present with such advanced disease that it is wisest and kindest to do nothing more than provide supportive care and analgesia. Whilst this may initially be at home, hospice care usually becomes necessary later because of oral and respiratory problems.

Small tumours

In these tumours – stages T1 and T2 – radiotherapy and surgery are equally effective and, in view of the wish to preserve function, radiotherapy is often the treatment of choice. Once a full course (60–65 Gy) of radiotherapy has been given, this treatment cannot be repeated and recurrent or new tumours, however small, which occur within the irradiated field have to be treated by surgery.

Large tumours

These tumours are stage T3 or T4. The bigger the tumour, the less likely it is to be cured by radiotherapy and this is particularly so if there is invasion of bone or cartilage. Primary surgery is better. The decision as to whether or not to add planned postoperative radiotherapy may be made before surgery or may depend on histological factors revealed by study of the operative specimen: very close or positive margins of excision; and, in lymph node metastases, extracapsular penetration of tumour and involvement at multiple levels in the neck.

Given the propensity for these tumours to metastasize to the cervical nodes, these may need to be treated at the same time as the primary tumour. Small nodes can be treated by radiotherapy or surgery, and the appropriate choice may well depend on the treatment modality chosen for the primary site. Large nodes should be treated by a neck dissection. Some primary sites (e.g. tongue, bone and tonsil) carry such a high risk (50%) of microscopic nodal disease that prophylactic treatment of the ipsilateral neck should be undertaken. The modality used will usually be the same as that employed for the primary site.

PROGNOSIS

Survival rates depend on the site and size of the primary tumour, and the presence or absence of metastatic nodal disease. A patient with a tumour of the larynx is likely to fare much better than one with a tumour of the same size in the hypopharynx. This is partly the result of more ready spread of the latter to the regional lymph nodes. Once lymph node metastases have developed, the prognosis for any tumour, no matter how small the primary, worsens considerably. Overall, the 5-year survival rate for all head and neck malignancies is approximately 40%. Failure to control the disease is almost always because recurrence takes place *loco* regionally; distant metastases are unusual unless there is already advanced disease above the clavicles.

POST-SURGICAL MANAGEMENT

Reconstruction

The defect after surgery for a large tumour is often of considerable size and it may be difficult to achieve a satisfactory cosmetic and functional result by direct closure. Recent advances in plastic surgical techniques have provided a variety of options, which include:

- *Simple free grafts of split or full-thickness skin.* These are only appropriate for small defects.
- *Pedicled skin flaps.* These may be random, where there is no specific nutrient artery, or axial, where the flap has a named blood supply (e.g. the pectoralis major myocutaneous flap supplied by the thoraco-acromial artery). Axial flaps are much more reliable and are not limited by the width/length ratio of the flap.
- *Free flaps.* A piece of jejunum or of forearm skin can be dissected with its own arterial supply and venous drainage and can then be anastomosed to appropriate vessels in the neck, so restoring the graft tissues circulation. The radial forearm flap has the great advantage that it can be raised in continuity with a piece of radial bone, which will restore continuity following resection of a segment of mandible for an oral cavity carcinoma.
- *Transposed viscus.* Following a laryngopharyngo-oesophagectomy for a postcricoid carcinoma, the stomach can be mobilised and brought up through the mediastinum for anastomosis to the pharynx in the neck (stomach pull-up procedure). Another less

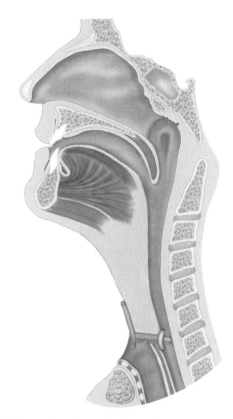

Fig 14.3 **Restoration of speech after tracheostomy.**

reliable option is to bring up a vascularised segment of transverse colon.

Restoration of speech

One of the greatest handicaps which can result from the surgical treatment of head and neck tumours is the loss of voice which follows total laryngectomy. Until recently, adequate speech after laryngectomy was often not achievable, the patient being doomed to a life of silence and a pen and paper. However, the last decade has seen the advent of surgical speech restoration.

A tracheo-oesophageal fistula is created surgically through the posterior wall of the trachea, approximately 5 mm below the mucocutaneous junction (Fig. 14.3). A one-way valve can then be introduced into the tract where it can be left for several months before replacement. By occluding the tracheostomy with a finger during expiration, the patient can divert air up through the valve into the pharynx. The air is set in vibration by the valve and speech can be produced.

Lymphoma

PATHOLOGICAL FEATURES

The majority of lymphomas in the head and neck region are non-Hodgkin's in type. They can be nodal or extranodal and those found in the tongue charac-teristically form a protruding mass, unlike squamous carcinomas.

CLINICAL FEATURES
The patient presents with a local lesion or an enlarged lymph node(s)

DIAGNOSIS
Biopsy is the only method of making an exact diagnosis.

INVESTIGATION
The studies to be done are the same as for lymphomas at other sites (Ch. 29). Surgery plays only a diagnostic role in management.

Diseases of the salivary glands

There are three paired salivary glands: the parotid, the submandibular and the sublingual glands. Scattered throughout the mucosa of the oral cavity and pharynx are numerous tiny minor salivary glands. Although tumours may arise in the latter, they are rarely a cause of inflammatory disease.

Non-neoplastic salivary gland disease

Bacterial infection

Infections in the parotid or submandibular salivary gland are relatively uncommon. Bacterial *parotitis* tends to occur in elderly debilitated patients, probably as the result of poor oral hygiene and dehydration. Bacterial infection of the submandibular gland is more common and can occur in an otherwise well patient. It is frequently due to a stone lodged in the duct.

CLINICAL FEATURES
Parotitis
The gland swells, becomes acutely tender and the overlying skin may be erythematous. A plain X-ray may demonstrate a stone in the duct but a contrast examination should not be done while there is acute inflammation.

Submandibular sialadenitis
The appearances are the same as for parotitis. A stone may be palpable on bimanual examination. Alternatively, a stone may be identified on an intraoral dental X-ray (Fig. 14.4)

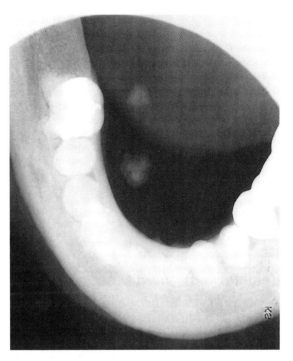

Fig 14.4 **Oblique X-ray of the floor of the mouth showing two stones in the submandibular salivary duct.**

MANAGEMENT
Parotitis
Parotitis requires energetic care of the mouth, rehydration and antibiotics. If fluctuation develops, incision and drainage of the abscess are necessary.

Submandibular saladenitis
This is treated in the same way as parotitis, but if a stone is obvious, then intraoral incision of the duct and removal of the stone under local anaesthesia may be all that is required. However, a submandibular duct stone can be very mobile and difficult to remove, particularly if it is lodged far back in the duct. An attempt to do so may cause damage to the lingual nerve. In such circum-stances, it is better to allow the infection to resolve with antibiotic treatment and then remove the entire gland.

Viral parotitis

This is a common disorder usually caused by the mumps virus. Other agents include the cytomegalovirus and Coxsackie virus. Although the gland may swell con-siderably, there is not as much pain or systemic upset as in bacterial infection.

Sialectasis

This is primarily a disease of the parotid gland and may be a forerunner to stone formation. Epithelial debris mixes with the saliva to produce sediment in the ducts, which in turns leads to stasis and poor emptying of the ducts when secretion is stimulated.

CLINICAL FEATURES AND INVESTIGATION
Painful swelling of the gland occurs at mealtimes and can last several hours. Sialography characteristically demonstrates a snowstorm appearance of the duct system, caused by patchy cystic dilatations of the ducts interspersed with areas of stricture formation.

MANAGEMENT
Salivary flow is increased by the use of sialogogues, such as lemon juice. Parotidectomy should be avoided if at all possible because of the risk of damage to the facial nerve.

Connective tissue disease

Keratoconjunctivitis sicca and rheumatoid arthritis (Sjögren's disease)
Salivary gland swelling occurs in about one-third of affected patients. Because the disease is associated with an abnormality in lymphocyte function, the patient is at significant risk of developing a lymphoma.

Benign lymphoepithelial infiltration
This causes general enlargement of the submandibular and parotid glands without any of the other features of Sjögren's disease. A sublabial biopsy of the minor salivary glands reveals a dense lymphocytic infiltrate. Again, there is an increased risk of lymphoma and any further increase in size of any of the salivary glands should be viewed with suspicion and a FNA carried out.

Drug-induced salivary gland swelling

Certain antihypertensives, monoamine oxidase inhibitors and iodide-containing drugs can cause enlargement of the parotid, as may the contraceptive pill.

Salivary gland neoplasms

Most salivary gland tumours are benign. However, the smaller the gland, the higher is the chance of a tumour being malignant. Although 70% of parotid tumours are benign, 70% of minor salivary gland tumours are malignant.

Pleomorphic adenoma

This is the most common benign tumour, so called because histologically it can mimic a variety of tissues.

If left untreated for many years, it can undergo malignant change, which is usually signalled by a sudden increase in the rate of enlargement.

CLINICAL FEATURES
The history is of a painless mass, usually in the parotid, which may enlarge very slowly over a period of several years. The lump is discrete, mobile and, if in the parotid, does not, in contrast to a malignant tumour, cause a facial palsy.

MANAGEMENT
Surgical excision is the standard treatment. The tumour has a capsule and rupture of this can lead to tumour seeding and recurrence. Most parotid adenomas are in the much bulkier superficial lobe which can be removed by superficial parotidectomy without injury to the facial nerve. A submandibular tumour is best managed by removal of the whole gland.

Cystadenoma lymphomatosum (Warthin's tumour or adenolymphoma)

This is another common benign tumour found only in the parotid gland. It is bilateral in 10%, does not undergo malignant change and bears no connection with lymphomas.

Malignant neoplasms

Malignant salivary gland tumours are rare and histologically diverse. *Muco-epidermoid carcinomas* can be high-grade (and mimic squamous carcinoma in clinical behaviour) or low-grade (when they behave in a relatively benign way). *Squamous carcinoma* is an aggressive tumour which, in the parotid gland, often produces a facial nerve palsy. It is important to differentiate this disease from metastatic squamous carcinoma in an intraparotid lymph node. *Adenocarcinomas* and *adenoid cystic carcinomas* can also develop in the salivary glands. The latter has a tendency to infiltrate along nerves for considerable distances.

MANAGEMENT
Surgical removal is the main treatment. If a malignant parotid tumour is found to directly involve the facial nerve, then that structure must be sacrificed and continuity of the nerve re-established using a segment of greater auricular or sural nerve.

Lymphomas

These tumours may develop in any of the larger salivary glands. Once the diagnosis has been made by either FNA or biopsy, treatment is by conventional methods (see Ch. 29).

Neck space infections

Peritonsillar abscess (Quinsy)

ANATOMY AND PATHOLOGICAL FEATURES

The faucial tonsil lies medial to the pharyngeal constrictor muscle and has a pseudocapsule of fibrous tissue around its deep surface. A peritonsillar abscess develops when this potential space becomes infected by direct spread from acute tonsillitis. The problem is usually unilateral, and in the early stages there is a local cellulitis rather than overt abscess formation.

CLINICAL FEATURES

History

There is a background of acute tonsillitis which suddenly progresses with increasing unilateral pain and dysphagia. The patient may be unable to swallow saliva and usually has marked trismus because of reflex spasm in the adjacent pterygoid muscles.

Physical findings

A fluctuating pyrexia is invariable. The tonsil is displaced downwards and medially. There may be obvious cervical lymphadenopathy or just a vague fullness on that side of the neck.

MANAGEMENT

In the early stages, intravenous antibiotics (penicillin and metronidazole) are given. However, if there is any suspicion of a local collection of pus, then the inflammatory mass should be incised. This is best performed with a fine blade on a long-handled scalpel, having sprayed the palate with lignocaine. The site is shown in Figure 14.5.

Parapharyngeal abscess

ANATOMY AND PATHOLOGICAL CONSIDERATIONS

The parapharyngeal space is a potential one that is triangular in cross-section (Fig. 14.6). It lies lateral to the pharyngeal constrictors, anterior to the prevertebral fascia and deep to the deep cervical fascia. Its chief contents are the carotid tree, the internal jugular vein and the last four cranial nerves. Infection of this space is usually the consequence of dental sepsis or uncontrolled tonsillitis. Two dangerous complications may result:

- spread of the infection inferiorly into the mediastinum

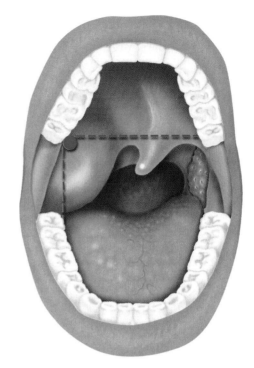

Fig 14.5 **The site of a right-sided peritonsillar abscess with the point of incision.**

- mucosal oedema in the adjacent larynx and pharynx with airways obstruction.

CLINICAL FEATURES

There is fever with diffuse swelling of the affected side of the neck and loss of the normal gutter anterior to the sternomastoid muscle.

MANAGEMENT

Prompt treatment is essential because of the risk of complications. Intravenous antibiotics should be administered and a CT scan obtained to ascertain whether or not there is a collection of pus. When present, pus is drained through an incision running down the anterior border of the sternomastoid muscle.

Ludwig's angina

ANATOMY AND PATHOLOGICAL CONSIDERATIONS

Soft tissue infection of the floor of the mouth on both sides of the mylohyoid muscle usually results from gross dental sepsis. A combination of bacteria is often involved, which includes anaerobes. A brawny swelling of the submandibular and submental triangles results.

CLINICAL FEATURES

On intraoral inspection, there is gross oedema of the mucosa of the floor of the mouth with upward and

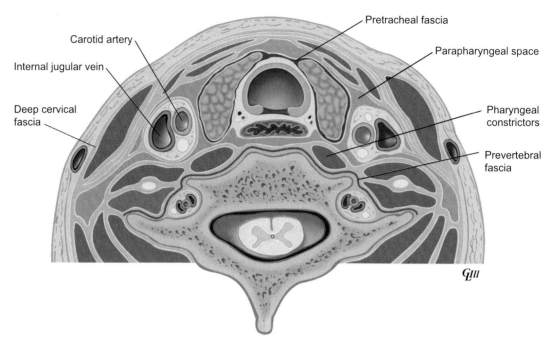

Fig 14.6 **The parapharyngeal space.**

posterior displacement of the tongue. The latter is potentially fatal, in that the tongue may obstruct the airway.

MANAGEMENT
Treatment is initially with antibiotics, which should be chosen to include cover for anaerobic infection. Any collection of pus should be drained, if necessary using *through-and-through incisions* running from the floor of the mouth medial to the mandible and out into the neck. It may be necessary to maintain the airway by nasopharyngeal or nasotracheal intubation. If this is unsatisfactory, a tracheostomy is required.

Tonsillar swelling from infectious mononucleosis

Alarming swelling of both tonsils may occur and, in extreme cases, compromise the pharyngeal airway. However, peritonsillar abscess does not occur unless a bacterial tonsillitis supervenes. Impending airways obstruction can often be prevented by using steroids.

Vocal cord paralysis and upper airways obstruction

Paralysis of a vocal cord is usually the consequence of

damage to the ipsilateral recurrent laryngeal nerve, which is a branch of the vagus nerve.

ANATOMY AND PHYSIOLOGICAL FEATURES
The left nerve runs a significantly longer course than the right, down into the superior mediastinum and around the arch of the aorta. Therefore it is three times more likely to be affected. When the recurrent laryngeal nerve is damaged or divided, the cord assumes a paramedian position. This may be asymptomatic or result in hoarseness; however, if both recurrent nerves are affected then acute airways obstruction is almost inevitable. Damage to or division of the main vagus nerve at the base of the skull causes the ipsilateral cord to assume a more lateralised position. Although this does not threaten the airway, it results in a very poor breathy voice and serious problems with aspiration of the saliva and food.

AETIOLOGY
Common causes of distal disruption of the recurrent laryngeal nerve are:

- thyroid surgery (Ch. 31)
- cardiac (aortic arch) surgery
- carcinoma of the bronchus
- carcinoma of the thyroid
- carcinoma of the oesophagus.

There is, in addition, a large idiopathic group in which the cause is never found and where spontaneous recovery is relatively common.

DIAGNOSIS

The development of a recurrent laryngeal palsy should lead to a detailed search for the cause, which may require a variety of special investigations to find or exclude an intrathoracic cause.

MANAGEMENT

The frequency with which idiopathic palsy occurs and its spontaneous recovery mean that surgery for hoarseness, airways obstruction or aspiration should only be undertaken in those patients who have an identifiable, non-reversible cause or who have had symptoms for at least 9 months and are therefore very unlikely to recover.

Surgical treatment

There are two categories:

- medialisation of the vocal cord
- lateralisation of the vocal cord.

Medialisation is used when one cord is paralysed and the other unable to provide complete closure of the glottis. The affected cord is moved medially to improve the voice and reduce aspiration. Either polytetrafluoroethylene (Teflon) paste is injected endoscopically at two or three sites immediately lateral to the cord, or a piece of thyroid cartilage is wedged between it and the thyroid ala (thyroplasty).

Lateralisation is used in an attempt to improve the airway in bilateral palsy with the cords lying in the paramedian position. Relatively complicated techniques are required and treatment is inevitably a compromise: as the gap between the cords is increased, the airways improve but the voice deteriorates and aspiration becomes an increasing problem.

In bilateral paralysis, permanent tracheostomy is usually the best management.

Common surgical procedures on the neck

Tonsillectomy

The indications for tonsillectomy are given in Box 14.1. Although this is one of the most commonly performed operations, it is not without complications. Haemorrhage is the most important and may be primary (within 24 hours of surgery) or secondary (days 5–10), when it is usually the result of infection at the site of excision. A bleeding diathesis, such as von Willebrand's disease, may present with bleeding during or after tonsillectomy.

Tracheostomy

There are two types of tracheostomy (Fig. 14.7):

Box 14.1

Indications for tonsillectomy

- Recurrent tonsillitis with more than four attacks per year
- Obstructive sleep apnoea with tonsillar hypertrophy in children
- Peritonsillar abscess with a past history of recurrent tonsillitis
- Persistent sore throat after glandular fever
- Unilaterally enlarged tonsil with lymphoma a possibility

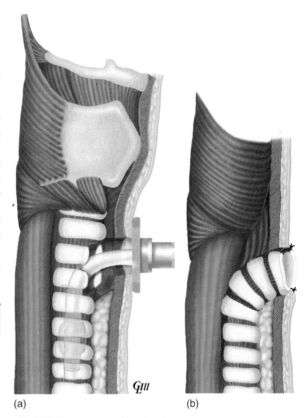

(a)   (b)

Fig 14.7 **The two types of tracheostomy.**

- After a laryngectomy, the divided trachea is brought out and sutured to the skin.
- More frequently a side opening is made with the larynx still in situ. It may be a temporary or permanent, elective or emergency procedure.

Whenever possible, a tracheostomy should be performed with an endotracheal tube in situ. This way, the airway remains secure throughout the procedure. In adults, a window should be excised from the anterior tracheal wall: a trap door flap is dangerous. In children, a vertical slit controlled by stay sutures should be employed.

The indications for tracheostomy are given in Box 14.2.

One of the fallacies about a tracheostomy is that the patient is unable to speak afterwards. This is not usually true. Once the operation site has healed, the initial tube is replaced by a silver or plastic one without a cuff. A speaking valve can then be attached: during quiet respiration, air travels back and forth through the tube, but on forced expiration the valve will shut, diverting the air up through the glottis where it can be set into vibration and used for phonation.

Box 14.2

Indications for tracheostomy

Supralaryngeal obstruction
Ludwig's angina
Severe facial fractures
Glandular fever

Laryngeal obstruction
Epiglottitis
Laryngeal tumour
Bilateral vocal cord palsy

Recurrent aspiration
Coma
Myasthenia gravis
Bulbar or pseudobulbar palsy

Respiratory support
Injury to the chest wall
Seriously ill or injured patients (ARDS)
Prolonged endotracheal intubation

Ear and nose

The ear

ANATOMY

External ear

This is merely the pinna and the auditory meatus. (Fig. 15.1)

Middle ear (tympanic cavity)

The tympanic membrane separates the external from the middle ear. The middle ear cleft comprises the Eustachian (auditory) tube and middle ear cavity which communicates with the mastoid air cells. The bony roof of the attic of the middle ear separates it from the middle cranial fossa. The middle ear cavity is in contact with the external atmosphere through the Eustachian tube, which opens into the postnasal space and contains three articulating ossicles (Fig. 15.1) – the malleus, incus and stapes – which are supported by ligaments. The annular ligament surrounds the footplate of the stapes (3.5 mm^2 in area) and restrains this to movement in the oval window. The second, round window, below the oval window, is covered only with a membrane, which allows the transmission of pressure and movement of fluids in the inner ear.

There are two muscles in the middle ear: tensor tympani and stapedius; these pull in opposite directions and modify the motion of the ossicles, increasing their stiffness and protecting the delicate inner ear from excessive oscillation of the chain of small bones.

Inner ear

There are three parts to the inner ear:

- anteriorly, the cochlea with the organ of Corti, for hearing
- in the middle, the vestibule with the utricle and saccule, which are concerned with static balance and linear acceleration
- posteriorly, three semicircular canals in different planes – the organ of balance, which is concerned with angular acceleration.

The otic capsule of the inner ear contains perilymph and has connection with the subarachnoid space. Inside the capsule is the membranous labyrinth with sensory cells and containing the endolymph, which is produced by stria vascularis. Endolymph is absorbed mainly by

Ear and nose

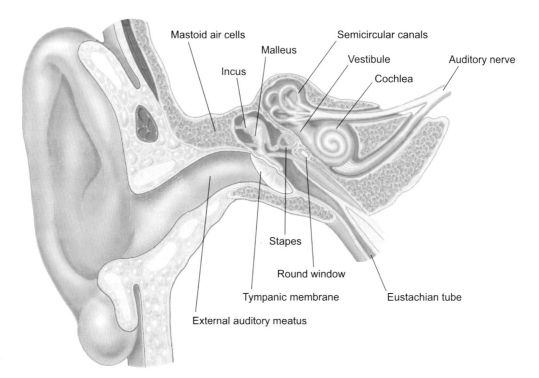

Fig 15.1 **Anatomy of the ear.**

the endolymphatic sac which lies in the posterior cranial fossa between the petrous bone and the dura. The cochlear and vestibular divisions of the VIIIth nerve join and travel through the internal auditory meatus to the brain stem. The VIIth (facial) nerve also travels through the internal auditory canal and traverses the medial and posterior walls of the middle ear cavity to emerge through the stylomastoid foramen.

PHYSIOLOGY

Hearing

The eardrum and the ossicles amplify sound waves through the lever effect of the ossicles and because the area of the eardrum is more than 20 times that of the footplate of the stapes. This allows reduction of acoustic impedence when sound energy is passed from air into liquid in the labyrinth.

Micromechanical oscillations of the stapes result in movement of liquid in the cochlea and motion of the basilar membrane with the sensory hair cells. The point of maximum movement of the basilar membrane is determined by the frequency of the introduced tone: high-frequency tones correspond to a place in the basal turn of the cochlea; and low-frequency tones to one in the apical turn. The movement of the cilia of the receptor hair cells generates electric impulses in the cells, and bioelectric events then follow in the auditory nerve.

Sound frequency is measured in hertz (Hz) where 1 Hz is equal to 1 cycle per second. The range of frequencies which can be appreciated as sound by humans is approximately 20–18 000 Hz. The ear can discriminate an enormous intensity range of 100 000:1, and for practical measurement it can be compressed into a logarithmic decibel scale of O to 120 dB.

Balance

Movement and acceleration in any of the three planes of the semicircular canals cause movement of the endolymph with deviation of the gelatinous cupola with the embedded sensory hair cells in the semicircular canals. In the saccule and utricle, there is displacement of the sensory hair cells, which are embedded in the gelatinous otolith membrane containing particles of calcium carbonate, and respond to changes in linear acceleration or gravity force. The stimulus triggers the action potential of the vestibular nerve. All of the imputs from the labyrinth, the eyes and somatosensors relay to the brain. Central processing takes place and responses return to the muscles to maintain posture and eye position, with the cerebellum ensuring a smooth, coordinated response. An alteration in vestibular response on one side as opposed to the other, results in imbalance in the central response which affects control of the eyes, causing them to oscillate – *vestibular nystagmus*.

COMMON SYMPTOMS

● Hearing loss – congenital or acquired (sudden or progressive)
● Aural discharge

- Otalgia – pain in the ear
- Tinnitus – variable noises in the ear
- Vertigo.

Otalgia
Pain in the ear may arise from pain receptors supplied by the afferent fibres of:

- the Vth and Xth cranial nerves
- C2 and 3 which supply the external ear
- the IXth cranial nerve supplying the middle ear.

When otalgia is a presenting symptom and no local disease is found in the ear, a referred otalgia is possible from a distant area innervated by any of the above nerves. Usual causes are:

- dental disease
- temporomandibular joint disorders
- maxillary sinusitis (Ch. 14)
- inflammatory and malignant lesions of the pharynx, posterior tongue and larynx
- conditions in the back of the neck and cervical spine.

Tinnitus
The subjective perception of tinnitus, which is characterised by rushing, hissing or ringing sounds of varying intensity in the ear or head, may be associated with dysfunction in the cochlea and the auditory pathway. A rhythmic pulsatile tinnitus is suggestive of vascular lesions such as:

- arteriovenous malformations
- arterial aneurysms
- glomus tumour in the middle ear
- sound transmission from major vessels in the neck.

Tinnitus can sometimes be detected objectively on auscultation of the ear and the mastoid. Crackling sounds can be associated with dysfunction of the Eustachian tube and rhythmic myoclonus of the muscles attached to it.

Vertigo
Vertigo associated with a peripheral vestibular lesion is most commonly rotatory but can be experienced as a swaying or tilting of either the patient or the surroundings. Movement and positional changes tend to make the vertigo worse. Central vestibular lesions tend to produce less intense vertigo, positional changes have less effect and the patient may experience disturbance of gait and other neurological symptoms and signs.

CLINICAL EXAMINATION
Examination of the auricle and the mastoid precedes otoscopic examination. Wax should be removed if it obstructs the view, but this should not be done by syringing if a perforation of the tympanic membrane is suspected because of a risk of introducing infection. The normal tympanic membrane reflects the directed light in the shape of a cone which is seen in the anteroinferior part of the membrane. The prominent landmark is the handle of the malleus (Fig. 15.2). The tympanic membrane is divided into the pars tensa and the pars flaccida (the upper area). It is very useful to use examination with a microscope to evaluate scars, retractions and types of perforation. The presence of perforation may allow damage to the ossicles, granulations and cholesteatoma to be seen. The nasal cavities and posterior nasal space must be examined in order to exclude infection or tumour which may cause Eustachian

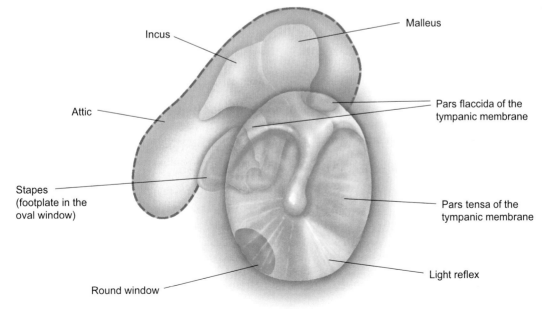

Fig 15.2 **The external aspect of the tympanic membrane.**

tube insufficiency or blockage and consequent failure of air circulation to the middle ear. A full assessment of the head and neck is performed to exclude referred otalgia.

INVESTIGATIONS

Auditory function
There are different types of hearing loss, as follows:

- conductive – from lesions in the external auditory meatus and the middle ear
- sensorineural – from cochlear and and retrocochlear lesions
- mixed – when both types of hearing loss are present.

Tuning fork tests
Rinne test. A vibrating tuning fork which generates sound at 512 Hz is placed near the external meatus (air conduction, AC) and then firmly on the mastoid process (bone conduction [BC], a measure of sensorineural function of the cochlea). Normally sound is detected better by AC than by BC. Conductive loss means that sound conduction through the middle ear apparatus is reduced. The convention is as follows:

- normal – AC better than BC → Rinne test positive
- conductive loss – BC better than AC → Rinne test negative
- sensorineural loss – AC better than BC but both reduced compared with normal → Rinne test positive and reduced.

Weber test. A vibrating tuning fork is placed either on the vertex of the skull or on the forehead midway between the ears. The patient indicates on which side the sound is better lateralised by bone conduction. The interpretation is as follows:

- conductive loss – sound lateralised to the affected side
- sensorineural loss – sound lateralised to the side with better cochlear function.

Pure tone audiometry
The hearing threshold can be measured in decibels of hearing level (dBHL) for air and bone conduction at each frequency between 250 and 8000 Hz (Figs 15.3a and b).

Impedance audiometry
The middle ear compliance (i.e. how much of the applied sound energy is reflected from the tympanic membrane) and middle ear pressure (the difference, if any, between pressure externally and in the cavity) can be measured with an instrument applied to the ear canal. A very low compliance could be the result of a middle ear effusion. A lower or negative pressure within the middle ear than without indicates insufficiency of the Eustachian tube.

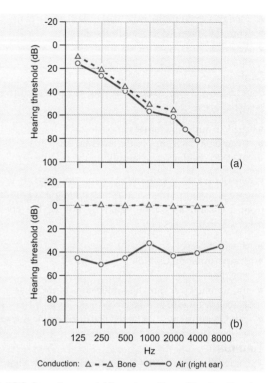

Fig 15.3 **An audiogram.** (**a**) Sensorineural loss with reduced hearing levels by both air and bone conduction. (**b**) Conductive hearing loss with reduced hearing level by air conduction and normal bone conduction.

Electric response audiometry
Electrical responses to sound stimuli can be recorded from the cochlea, brain stem and cortex. Auditory-evoked potentials of a few microvolts can be recorded from the scalp as the 'auditory brain stem response' which occurs within 10 ms. This has become a useful objective test in children and in patients in whom reliability of subjective audiometric tests is doubtful. It also has wide-ranging application in neuro-otological diagnosis and detection of acoustic tumours.

Vestibular function

Clinical
Spontaneous and positional nystagmus, eye movements, stance, gait and limbs are all tested.

Nystagmus. This condition is defined as involuntary (usually rapid) rhythmic, transverse (although occasionally vertical – see below) eye movements:

- *Vestibular nystagmus* is a rhythmic oscillating movement of the eyes resulting from either induced stimulation of the labyrinth or vestibular disease; it has a slow vestibular and a fast cerebral correcting component trying to restore the eye position in the direction of gaze.
- *Labyrinthine nystagmus* is always horizontal-rotatory or horizontal.

- *Vertical nystagmus* and multiple other forms occur only in central vestibular lesions.

Head positional testing

This can induce benign positional vertigo (BPV) and nystagmus when the defect is thought to be in the labyrinth. BPV occurs with a short latency, lasts a few seconds and fatigues on repetition; usually it is a self-limiting condition which resolves within a few months.

Electronystagmography

The velocity of nystagmus can be assessed by graphic recording. Labyrinthine nystagmus is enhanced when visual input is abolished by closing the eyes or by darkness.

Caloric test

This test is based on the principle of cooling or heating the labyrinth by a flow of water in the external ear canal. A convection current is set up in the semicircular canal which in turn induces vertigo and nystagmus. In vestibular hypofunction these may be reduced or absent.

Diseases of the external ear

Foreign bodies

In these cases, there is always a danger of forcing the foreign body further into the ear canal where it may damage the drum and the middle ear. Extraction of foreign bodies should therefore be done by skilled ear, nose and throat (ENT) personnel.

Trauma to the auricle

AETIOLOGY AND PATHOLOGICAL FEATURES

Haematoma of the auricle occurs in boxers and those who take part in other contact sports such rugby football. The blood extravasates between the cartilage and perichondrium. If untreated, the blood becomes organised, causing a cauliflower deformity composed of fibrous tissues. Perichondritis and abscess may develop as a consequence of secondary infection. The cartilage deprived of vascular supply may undergo necrosis and lead to marked deformity of the auricle.

MANAGEMENT

Prevention

Suitable headgear should be worn by those engaged in contact sports.

Treatment

The haematoma is evacuated through a wide-bore needle or by incision of the skin. A firm dressing must be applied in order to prevent further bleeding. If a subperichondrial abscess forms, it should be incised and drained. *Pseudomonas aeruginosa* is not uncommonly cultured in these patients and broad-spectrum antibiotics are indicated.

Furuncle

AETIOLOGY AND PATHOLOGICAL FEATURES

This is an infection of hair follicles and is usually caused by *Staphylococcus aureus*. Recurrent infection may have diabetes as the underlying cause.

CLINICAL FEATURES

There may be severe earache, and any movement of the auricle (and thus of the auditory canal) or pressure on the tragus causes considerable pain. Mild hearing deficit may occur in cases of complete obturation of the ear canal. The external canal will be oedematous with swelling in front of or behind the auricle.

MANAGEMENT

Furuncle is treated by a combination of the insertion of an antiseptic wick and systemic antibiotics.

Otitis external

AETIOLOGY AND PATHOLOGICAL FEATURES

Environmental factors which predispose to otitis externa are:

- heat
- humidity
- swimming
- any irritation which predisposes to scratching.

Specific causes are:

- infection – bacterial, fungal, viral
- reactive inflammation – eczema, seborrhoeic dermatitis, neurodermatitis.

A spreading necrotising type with osteomyelitis of the base of the skull may develop in immuno-compromised or elderly diabetic patients. *Pseudomonas aeroginosa* and anaerobic organisms are often found.

CLINICAL FEATURES

In the common irritative type, discharge from the ear and, sometimes, mild pain are present. In the spreading, necrotising variant, there is systemic disturbance, more severe local symptoms and signs of spread which may include the development of a VIIth nerve palsy.

MANAGEMENT

In the *mild* type, treatment is by a combination of topical antiseptics or antibiotics incorporated into steroid-containing ear drops; if the condition is particularly troublesome, this is supplemented by systemic antibiotics after culture has been obtained. Aural toilet is essential and infected debris is removed by mopping with a cotton wool carrier or by microsuction. Fungal infection may follow after prolonged treatment with antibacterial drops. In the *severe necrotising* form, therapy should consist of intensive local treatment with excision of dead tissue, the administration of systemic antibiotics and control of diabetes if this is present.

Diseases of the middle ear

Acute otitis media

AETIOLOGY AND PATHOLOGICAL FEATURES

The incidence is highest in the first 5 years of life and thereafter it becomes infrequent. Most children have a history of preceding viral upper respiratory tract infection. Inflammation of the postnasal space and adenoids may spread via the Eustachian tube to the middle ear. Oedematous mucosa in the tube causes blockage and, if secondary bacterial infection spreads along the tube, a middle ear abscess will result. Under the age of 5 years, *Haemophilus influenzae* is isolated in about 30% of cases.

As tension rises, rupture of the tympanic membrane occurs usually in the pars tensa. In the majority, the inflammation resolves and the tympanic membrane heals without any sequelae. However, in a small proportion, complications develop and there is loss of hearing. Other problems are:

- a chronic middle ear effusion in about 5%
- scarring of the tympanic membrane and the middle ear (tympanosclerosis)
- chronic suppurative otitis media consequent to a non-healing perforation
- progression to acute mastoiditis.

CLINICAL FEATURES

Symptoms

Pain and hearing loss are early symptoms; if the drum perforates, a purulent discharge develops and the pain usually subsides.

Signs

There is malaise and pyrexia. The drum is reddened and tense. A perforation may be visible with discharge emerging through it.

MANAGEMENT

Amoxycillin is the preferred drug in children and should be administered for 10 days.

Acute mastoiditis

AETIOLOGY AND PATHOLOGICAL FEATURES

Mastoiditis is the consequence of a preceding otitis media and with the advent of powerful antibiotics the incidence has diminished considerably. Nevertheless, silent or masked mastoiditis can develop. There is cellulitis and osteitis in the air spaces which may go on to abscess formation. Spread can take place through the temporal bone to cause subperiosteal abscess or intracranial complications – an extradural abscess.

CLINICAL FEATURES

Symptoms
- Pain
- Fever
- Aural discharge
- Hearing loss.

Signs
- Erythematous swollen mastoid and external canal
- The ear is pushed outward and forward if subperiosteal abscess develops.

INVESTIGATION

Sometimes, because of swelling in the canal, it is difficult to visualise the inflamed drum. Mastoid X-ray shows clouding of the air cells and sometimes formation of an abscess with erosion of bone.

MANAGEMENT

Very early stages are treated with intensive parenteral antibiotics. If resolution fails to occur, the inflammatory process is decompressed by a simple cortical mastoidectomy, preserving the posterior meatal wall and the middle ear ossicles.

Otitis media with effusion

The alternative names for this condition are *chronic serous otitis media* and *glue ear*.

AETIOLOGY AND PATHOGENESIS

Accumulation of non-purulent fluid in the middle ear is common in children aged between 2 and 6 years. Many causative factors have been suggested, but the most probable is low-grade inflammation with partial block and dysfunction of the Eustachian tube and interference with the free flow of air in and out of the middle ear so that negative pressure develops in the middle ear.

CLINICAL FEATURES

Symptoms

- Impaired hearing
- Delay in learning to speak and acquiring a vocabulary
- Other learning difficulties
- Inattentiveness
- Recurrent earaches.

Signs

Many children with this condition are discovered during routine audiometric screening. Otoscopic examination reveals a lustreless immobile tympanic membrane. Sometimes fluid levels can be seen in the middle ear. In longstanding disease the drum may become thin, atrophic and retracted.

MANAGEMENT

In many instances, reassessment after 3 months is advisable because in more than 90% the effusion will resolve spontaneously. Unresolved middle ear effusion with hearing loss requires anterior–inferior myringotomy, aspiration of the liquid and a ventilation tube (*grommet*) inserted into the tympanic membrane. If there are associated features of nasal obstruction, the adenoids are curetted. The ventilation tube remains in the tympanic membrane for about 12 months, helping to restore to normal the mucus-producing mucosa of the middle ear, and is then spontaneously extruded from the tympanic membrane.

Middle ear effusion in adults

AETIOLOGY AND PATHOGENESIS

Serous middle ear effusion may develop after:

- an upper respiratory tract infection
- allergic or vasomotor rhinitis
- exposure to changes in ambient pressure such as flying or diving (barotrauma) when the Eustachian tube does not equalise pressure.

In adults, carcinoma of the postnasal space invading the Eustachian tube is a rare precipitating cause.

Chronic suppurative otitis media

AETIOLOGY AND PATHOLOGICAL FEATURES

This condition usually follows acute otitis media and has the same underlying causes. However, it may be chronic from the outset. There are two types:

- *tubotympanic suppuration*, which is limited to inflammation of the mucosa
- *attico-antral disease* with destruction involving the mastoid bone.

The former is regarded as safe in that complications are unlikely, while the latter is unsafe.

CLINICAL FEATURES

Tubotympanic disease

The discharge is mucopurulent but it may cease and reappear after an upper respiratory tract infection or if water passes through the perforation in the tympanic membrane. This opening is central in the pars tensa and does not involve the bony margins. An audiogram shows conductive hearing loss.

Attico-antral disease

This presents as suppuration with or without cholesteatoma. The latter is a mass of keratinised squamous epithelium which increases in size as skin desquamates. Initially it forms in the developed retraction pocket of a perforated tympanic membrane in the attic. Spread then occurs, so destroying the middle ear ossicles and the temporal bone. Hearing loss can be marked. Vertigo may be present if the cholesteatoma has eroded the bony wall of the most prominent lateral semicircular canal. Otoscopy reveals a superior perforation leading into the attic or a posterior marginal type perforation involving the bony margin. With bony involvement, granulations are common. Flakes of cholesteatoma can be seen in the area of the attic. CT may sometimes be helpful to reveal the extent of the bony erosion.

MANAGEMENT

Tubotympanic disease

Active suppurative tubotympanic disease is treated with combined antibiotic and corticosteroid ear drops. For those who do not wish to wear a hearing aid or who want to swim, repair of the tympanic membrane (*myringoplasty*) can be done when the perforation is dry. The tympanic membrane can be supplemented by a graft of fascia from the temporalis muscle.

Attico-antral disease

Conservative treatment is ineffective in the presence of cholesteatoma. Classical radical mastoidectomy lays open the mastoid and excises the posterior meatal wall and the contents of the tympanic cavity (apart from the stapes) to create one safe cavity. Reconstruction of the tympanic membrane with a fascial graft and artificial ossicles (tympanoplasty), with the aim of improving hearing, may then be considered.

Complications of otitis media

PATHOLOGICAL FEATURES

The infective process in both acute and chronic otitis media may cause bone destruction and may also spread along veins so leading to intracranial sepsis and the complications listed in Information Box 15.1.

Information Box 15.1

Complications of otitis media

Intratemporal

Mastoiditis

Labyrinthitis

Facial nerve palsy

Intracranial

Extradural abscess

Meningitis

Lateral sinus thrombosis

Temporal lobe abscess

Cerebellar abscess

CLINICAL FEATURES

In chronic otitis media, the development of pain in the ear and headache are a warning of a possible intracranial complication. Vertigo occurs in labyrinthitis and suppuration will lead to complete destruction of the hearing and balance organs. In developed intracranial complications the symptoms and signs are those of:

- systemic infection
- meningitis
- raised intracranial pressure (Ch. 30)
- focal neurological abnormalities.

CT and MRI of the head are essential for accurate diagnosis.

MANAGEMENT

Joint management with the neurosurgeon is essential. The underlying disease in the mastoid is explored as described above.

Otosclerosis

AETIOLOGY AND PATHOLOGICAL FEATURES

Otosclerosis is a localised disease of bone which affects the otic capsule. It is inherited as an autosomal dominant trait with incomplete penetrance. New spongy bone forms and, if this is in the area of the stapes, there may be ankylosis and conductive deafness.

CLINICAL FEATURES

History

There is a strong family history and both ears are affected in 90% of patients. The first manifestations are in the second decade and are progressive. Pregnancy and lactation aggravate the condition.

Physical findings

The tympanic membrane is normal and mobile in the presence of conductive hearing loss on an audiogram.

MANAGEMENT

If the patient does not wish to have a hearing aid, then stapedectomy is advised. The operation restores the mobility of the ossicular chain by perforating the stapes footplate, removing the arch of the stapes and replacing this with a piston prosthesis.

Diseases of the inner ear

Sensorineural hearing loss

The causes of this kind of loss are:

- genetic abnormalities of the cochlea
- maternal infections during pregnancy – rubella, cytomegalovirus, syphilis
- perinatal hypoxia
- viral and bacterial labyrinthitis
- meningitis
- ototoxic drugs – gentamicin, neomycin, frusemide, salicylates
- sudden idiopathic hearing loss (possibly viral or vascular)
- noise-induced hearing loss
- fracture of the temporal bone and trauma to the ear
- barotrauma, rupture of the round window membrane, perilymph leak.

In acquired hearing loss, the high audiometric frequencies are usually affected first and this type of loss is associated with the hair cell loss in the basal turn of the cochlea. Tinnitus is often associated with sensorineural loss. Presbycusis is sensorineural hearing loss with ageing; an audiogram reveals bilateral symmetrical high-frequency loss. Exposure to high-intensity noise causes characteristic bilateral hearing loss on the audiogram with a dip at 4000 Hz as the earliest change with depletion of hair cells at the basal turn of the cochlea.

MANAGEMENT

Hearing aids

Normal speech is at an intensity of between 40 and 70dB and some form of amplification is required if the audiogram shows a hearing loss of more than 40 dB. An aid may also have a masking effect on tinnitus which is often associated with sensorineural hearing loss.

Air conduction aids consist of a miniature microphone, an amplifier and a receiver which feed the sound into the ear and a mould in the auditory canal. The apparatus is usually mounted behind the ear, but the advent of microelectronics means that a more cosmetically acceptable aid can, in mild to moderate loss, be placed entirely within the auditory canal. Improved signal processing and programmable digital multichannel aids work more selectively to amplify various speech frequencies and reduce interference from ambient noise.

Bone conduction aids are used when there is a congenital absence of the pinna and atresia of the canal. The aid is anchored to a titanium screw in the mastoid that has become osseo-integrated by ingrowth of bone.

Sound waves are transfered into the cochlea by bone conduction.

Cochlear implant

Those who do not benefit from even the most powerful hearing aid and have profound bilateral deafness usually have a destroyed receptor organ and may be considered for a cochlear implant. In this procedure, electrodes are inserted into the spiral of the cochlea to

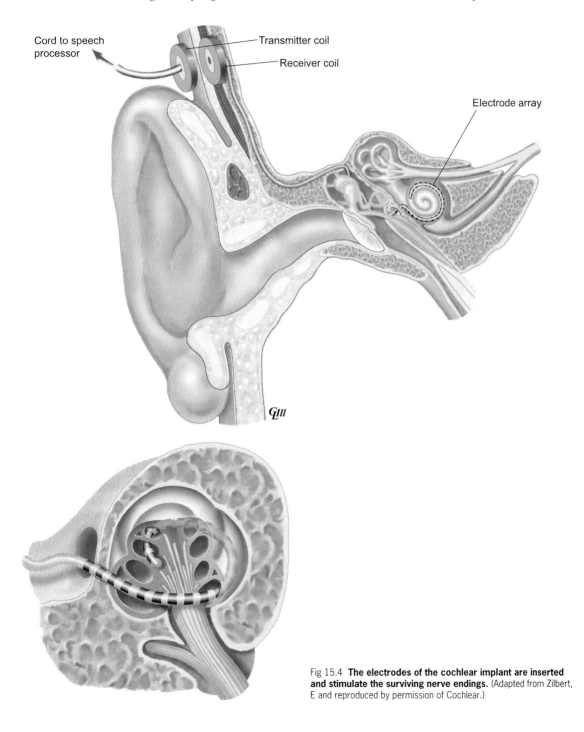

Cord to speech processor

Transmitter coil

Receiver coil

Electrode array

Fig 15.4 **The electrodes of the cochlear implant are inserted and stimulate the surviving nerve endings.** (Adapted from Zilbert, E and reproduced by permission of Cochlear.)

stimulate the surviving neurones electrically (Fig. 15.4). Speech is coded in a small speech processor worn externally and transmitted across the skin behind the ear into the implant. The patient hears the sound (about 50% can discriminate speech without having to lip read) and their speech production improves.

Acoustic neuroma

CLINICAL FEATURES
The early symptoms are unilateral or markedly asymmetric sensorineural hearing loss and tinnitus. Such patients should be suspected of having an acoustic tumour unless there is a clear association with trauma or acute infection. Vertigo is rare but patients with large tumours may have ataxia. Numbness of the side of the face (Vth nerve) follows.

INVESTIGATION
The audiogram reveals unilateral sensorineural hearing loss. MRI scan of the internal auditory meatus and the posterior cranial fossa reveals even the smallest tumour.

MANAGEMENT
The tumour is removed by neurosurgery. The smaller the tumour, the easier the operation and the less the likelihood there is of damage to the facial nerve.

Ménière's disease

PATHOLOGICAL FEATURES
Endolymphatic hydrops which causes distension of the membranous labyrinthine spaces is thought to be a pathological feature of Ménière's disease but the reason for this is unknown.

CLINICAL FEATURES
Symptoms
There is a characteristic triad of symptoms which recur:

- attacks of vertigo
- fluctuating sensory hearing loss at low audiometric frequencies
- tinnitus.

Some patients also experience a sensation of fullness and pressure in the ear during the attack. Over years the hearing gradually deteriorates in the affected ear and occasionally the disease is bilateral.

Signs
There are no specific physical findings.

MANAGEMENT
Attacks of vertigo are treated with vestibular sedatives

(diazepam, cinnarizine, prochlorperazine) A salt-restricted diet is advised in an endeavour to reduce the frequency of attacks. It is thought that betahistine may have a positive prophylactic effect on the micro-circulation in the cochlea, and it also has a positive effect on balance by reducing vestibular receptor resting firing rate. Surgery is indicated if medical treatment fails. Decompression of the endolymphatic sac and vestibular neurectomy does not destroy hearing and therefore is preferred to labyrinthectomy which destroys the inner ear completely. Injections of gentamicin into the middle ear and delivery to the membranous round window are effective in alleviating vertigo by reducing vestibular function.

Ear trauma and fracture of the skull base

PATHOLOGICAL AND CLINICAL FEATURES
Fractures of the temporal bone are associated with a severe head injury. Haematoma over the mastoid and blood in the external canal are important signs easily detected on simple clinical examination. A leak of cerebrospinal fluid (CSF) into the middle ear and through the auditory canal is a complication of fracture of the middle cranial fossa. CSF may also escape from the middle ear through the Eustachian tube – *CSF rhinorrhoea*. Conductive hearing loss is the result of blood in the middle ear (haemotympanum) or disruption of the ossicular chain. Vertigo or imbalance may suggest rupture of the round or oval windows. Profound deafness occurs if the fracture extends into the inner ear and may be associated with the above symptoms and also tinnitus. Fractures which involve the facial canal may produce a VIIth nerve palsy.

MANAGEMENT
The ear canal should not be syringed nor should drops be instilled because of the risk of introducing infection. Antibiotics are given and any CSF leak usually settles spontaneously. At a later stage, reconstruction of the ossicle chain (ossiculoplasty) may be needed to improve hearing. Very occasionally, exploration of the facial nerve is indicated with neural repair. Compensation for vestibular dysfunction can take several months.

The nose and paranasal sinuses

ANATOMY
A central septum divides the nasal cavity into two halves and supports the cartilaginous part of the nose. The anterior part is cartilage and the posterior bone.

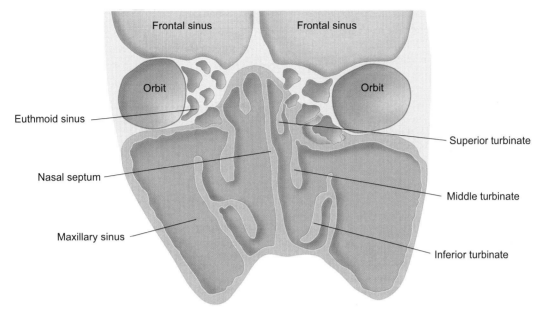

Fig 15.5 **Coronal section to show the sinuses and particularly the ethomoid air cells.**

The lateral wall has three turbinates – inferior, middle and superior – with a corresponding meatus under each turbinate (Fig. 15.5). The anterior ethmoidal cells and the maxillary and frontal sinuses open into the middle meatus, and their ostia, which are close together, form the ostiomeatal complex. The posterior ethmoidal cells and the sphenoid sinus open into the superior meatus. The nasolacrimal duct opens into the inferior meatus.

The relationships between the sinuses and other structures have clinical importance in the spread of infection and tumours and in trauma. The maxillary, ethmoidal and frontal sinuses are related to the orbit, and the ethmoidal and frontal sinuses to the anterior cranial fossa. The sphenoid sinus is concealed by its position. On the lateral sides of the sinus lie the cavernous venous sinus, the internal carotid artery and the IIIrd, IVth and Vth cranial nerves. The pituitary fossa intrudes into the roof.

The arterial supply of the nose is provided from branches of both external and internal carotid arteries. The venous drainage is extracranial but there are intra-cranial communications. The nerve supply to the nose and its sinuses is from the trigeminal nerve. The olfactory epithelium is in the branches of the superior part of the nose and the filaments of the olfactory nerve pass through the cribriform plate. Autonomic sympathetic and parasympathetic fibres provide vasomotor inner-vation to the cavernous tissue in the nasal mucosa and also secretomotor control. The parasympathetic fibres relay in the pterygopalatine ganglion and their stimu-lation causes swelling and increased secretion from the mucosa.

PHYSIOLOGY

The functions of the nose and sinuses are:

- air passage to and from the lungs
- warming, humidification and cleaning of incoming air (air conditioning)
- protection by mucociliary transport and immunological factors
- sense of smell
- resonators for speech production
- initiation of nasal reflexes – sneezing

General features of nasal and sinus disease

CLINICAL FEATURES

Symptoms
These include:

- Nasal obstruction – which can be unilateral or bilateral, intermittent or permanent.
- Mouth breathing – because of nasal obstruction, which in turn leads to dryness in the throat.
- Discharge and postnasal drip – clear serous discharge is common in allergic conditions and mucous or purulent discharge is associated with rhinosinusitis. A unilateral discharge in a child probably originates from a foreign body. A bloodstained discharge with unilateral symptoms may be associated with tumour. Unilateral copious watery discharge suggests CSF rhinorrhoea.

- Facial pain – dull and well-localised, although it sometimes may radiate into the teeth and around the eyes or ear.
- Headaches, especially in sphenoiditis.
- Loss of smell
- Bleeding
- Cosmetic nasal deformity.

It is important to distinguish sinus pain from neuralgia, and referred pain from the teeth, temporomandibular joint or cervical spine.

Signs

The anterior part of the nose can be examined using a nasal speculum and a head light. Deformities of the septum, mucosal changes, prominent vessels and inferior and middle turbinates can be seen. Nasal polyps, tumours, ulcerations and foreign bodies can be identified. The posterior nasal space with the choanae and openings of the Eustachian tubes can be examined through the mouth by introducing a small mirror behind the soft palate.

Application of decongestant drops or 10% cocaine spray causes vasoconstriction and, by reducing the swelling of the mucosa, improves visibility. Cocaine also has a topical anaesthetic effect, and rigid or flexible nasal endoscopes can be used to examine the ostiomeatal complex and the posterior part of the nose and the postnasal space.

INVESTIGATION

Imaging
Plain X-ray will show if there is gross disease. CT scanning of the sinuses gives percise images and shows mucosal swelling, fluid levels or opacity as well as bony erosion by tumours. MRI is especially useful for delineating tumour spread.

Rhinomanometry
Nasal resistance to airflow can be calculated from measurements of flow and transnasal pressure. However, the results do not always correspond to the subjective feeling of nasal obstruction.

Immunological
Skin prick tests may identify a possible allergen. A weal of at least 2 mm diameter and greater than the reaction to the control solution is considered positive. The serum-specific IgE and the radio allergosorbent test (RAST) quantify an allergic response.

Mucociliary clearance
Saccharin is placed in the front of the nose and the time (normally 20 min.) is measured for a sensation of sweetness to be recognised as the substance reaches the pharynx on the mucous blanket.

Smell
A short exposure to various bottles containing pungent substances establishes whether smell is reduced or distorted.

Common conditions of the nose and paranasal sinuses

Nasal foreign bodies

It is not unusual for children to insert foreign bodies into a nostril. The object may go undetected for some time and presentation is with symptoms of unilateral purulent and sometimes offensive discharge. A radio-opaque concealed foreign body may be seen on X-ray. It should be removed with forceps or a hook, a procedure which may require a general anaesthetic.

Fractures of the nose

A nasal injury may be associated with other fractures of the face, including those of the zygoma, bony orbit and middle third of the face.

CLINICAL FEATURES
The symptoms are:

- nasal deformity
- obstruction
- bleeding.

Examination of the nasal cavity may reveal:

- deviated septum
- septal haematoma.

MANAGEMENT
Displaced nasal fractures may be reduced immediately or in 7–10 days after swelling has subsided. For old nasal injuries, the nasal deformity may be corrected by mobilising the external nasal pyramid by performing osteotomies of the nasal bones and rhinoplasty. A plaster of Paris splint is applied for 2 weeks to stabilise the nasal bones.

Septal haematoma and abscess
PATHOLOGICAL FEATURES
After nasal trauma a haematoma may develop between the mucoperichondrial flaps of the septum. The outcome may be that the septal cartilage is deprived of its blood supply. Secondary infection can develop and an abscess may form. If untreated, the cartilage may

undergo necrosis and the nasal bridge lose its support, leading to a saddle-type nasal deformity.

Upon examination, the septum will be very swollen and fluctuant to palpation with a probe.

MANAGEMENT
The haematoma must be incised and drained. Nasal packing should be applied so as to allow the perichondrium to adhere to the cartilage. Antibiotics should be given.

Deviated nasal septum

A septal deviation can be either traumatic or developmental. In either event, nasal obstruction results. The patient will complain of such obstruction and the deviation will be apparent on clinical examination.

TREATMENT
Submucous resection (SMR) of the septum is done by elevating the mucoperichondrial flaps and resecting the deviated part of the septal cartilage and bone. In septoplasty, the cartilage is mobilised and the excision is more conservative. Excessive resection of the cartilage may lead to collapse of the nasal dorsum and tip. A septal perforation may occur if the mucoperichondrial flaps are perforated on both sides.

Epistaxis

PATHOLOGICAL FEATURES
Bleeding from the anterior part of the nose is more common and less severe than that from the posterior part, where the arteries are larger and have undergone degenerative change in older patients. Several vessels anastomose in the anterior septum, known as Little's area, which is a frequent site of origin of bleeding.

Bleeding can be the consequence of local or systemic causes, which include:

- trauma: – nose-picking, fracture, surgery
- tumours – angioma, angiofibroma of postnasal space, carcinoma of the nose, postnasal space or sinuses
- local infection with ulceration
- prominent vessels in Little's area
- atherosclerotic degeneration of greater nasal arteries
- haematological – blood disease, bleeding diatheses, hereditary telangectasia, coagulation defects, treatment with anticoagulants.

MANAGEMENT
The nose is anaesthetised and decongested with 10% cocaine. The bleeding vessel can be cauterised chemically with silver nitrate or by electrocautery. More accurate cauterisation of the bleeding vessels may be achieved by using a fibreoptic naso-endoscope, particularly in the posterior aspect of the nasal cavity. If the bleeding point cannot be identified or is not controlled with cautery, ribbon gauze impregnated in bismuth iodoform paraffin paste (BIPP) is packed into the anterior nasal cavity. When the bleeding is from the back of the nose and anterior packing is ineffective, an epistaxis balloon is introduced through the nose into the postnasal space to occlude the posterior nares and choanae; it is then drawn forward through the nose and secured.

When even a balloon is ineffective, re-insertion of a postnasal pack through the mouth and securing this in front of the nose is required and is combined with anterior packing usually under general anaesthesia. The packs remain for 48 hours during which time antibiotics are necessary. Frequently repeated haemorrhage may require ligation of the appropriate vessel. The external carotid artery can be ligated in the neck or, alternatively, the maxillary artery can be clipped by an approach through the maxillary sinus. If the bleeding arises from the upper part, the ethmoidal arteries are ligated by gaining access through the medial wall of the orbit.

Rhinosinusitis

AETIOLOGY AND PATHOLOGICAL FEATURES
Pathological changes in the nasal cavities are usually accompanied by similar mucosal changes in the sinuses. The causes are:

- allergy
- idiopathic/vasomotor
- infective.

In *allergic rhinitis*, inhaled substances are the most common allergens. Pollens from grass, trees and flowers are responsible for seasonal symptoms. House dust, the house dust mite, dog and cat fur cause more perennial symptoms.

Vasomotor rhinitis is a disorder of the autonomic nervous system in which a predominance of parasympathetic stimulation causes swelling of the nasal mucosa and hypersecretion.

Acute *infective rhinitis* is that which occurs in the common cold as a result of viral infection. Secondary bacterial infection may supervene and the common microorganisms are *Haemophilus influenzae* and *Streptococcus pneumoniae*. Sinusitis is usually an extension from the nasal infection. Any condition which interferes with mucociliary transport, drainage and ventilation, including mechanical factors such as a deviated septum, polyps, hypertrophy of the turbinates and swollen mucosa, especially around the ostiomeatal complex, predisposes to the development of infective sinusitis. Swollen mucosa blocks the natural ostia of the sinuses. Pus reduces the activity of cilia, thus leading to stasis in the sinuses. In chronic infection, the mucosa may be damaged and granulations may develop. Infections of the maxillary sinus can also develop from a dental abscess. Mycotic infections occasionally occur in immunosuppressed and diabetic patients.

CLINICAL FEATURES

Allergic rhinitis

Symptoms. These include:

- nasal itching
- bouts of sneezing
- profuse watery discharge
- postnasal drip.

In chronic allergic rhinitis, nasal stuffiness is a prominent symptom.

Signs. The mucosa will look oedematous and wet and the turbinates can become hypertrophic.

Infective rhinosinusitis

Symptoms. These are usually unilateral and include:

- pain over the affected sinus and around the eye
- headache
- mucopurulent discharge
- nasal obstruction
- loss of smell.

In chronic infection, pain may not be present.

Signs. The mucosa will be congested and the turbinates swollen with muco-pus in the nasal cavity. The sinus can be tender to palpation.

Sinus X-ray and CT may reveal opaque sinuses or a fluid level. Bacteriological studies should be carried out on the muco-pus.

MANAGEMENT

Allergic rhinitis

Once the allergen is known, appropriate advice should be offered on how best to avoid it. Desensitisation is possible, but carries a small risk of anaphylaxis.

The prophylactic use of a mast cell stabiliser (sodium chromoglycolate) and steroid sprays (flixonase) is effective in allergic and sometimes vasomotor rhinitis, and they do not seem to have any adverse systemic effects. If the symptoms are not controlled by sprays, non-sedating oral antihistamines can be added. If medical treatment fails to relieve the nasal obstruction, the enlarged hypertrophic turbinates can be reduced by diathermy to the inferior turbinates.

Infective rhinosinusitis

Initially acute sinusitis is treated with antibiotics (amoxicillin) and decongestant drops (0.5% ephedrine, xylometazoline) which reduce the swelling of the mucosa and may improve ventilation and drainage through the natural ostia. Surgery of varying extent is required to re-establish air flow, drainage and mucociliary clearance when medical treatment has proved ineffective.

Sinus washout is done under local anaesthesia with 10% cocaine in acute sinusitis if the pain and infection do not resolve. A trocar and cannula are passed through the thin medial wall of the sinus under the inferior turbinate. The washout is examined bacteriologically.

Intranasal antrostomy is a permanent large opening made under the inferior turbinate or usually by expanding the natural ostium in the middle meatus.

Radical antrostomy (Caldwell–Luc operation) removes the anterior wall of the maxillary sinus above the gum. The irreversibly changed granulating mucosa is then removed.

Operations on the ostiomeatal complex open the maxillary ostia, the ethmoidal air cells and fronto-ethmoidal duct, and the maxillary and sphenoid ostia, so enabling their ostia to be expanded intranasally under direct vision through a fiberoptic endoscope – endoscopic sinus surgery.

External ethmoidectomy decompresses the orbit where there are orbital complications due to unresolving ethmoiditis and abscess formation. The incision is made between the medial canthus of the eye and the bridge of the nose, and after it has healed the scar is invisible.

Frontal sinus trephine is indicated when the frontonasal duct remains blocked and serious complications are imminent. The incision is made below the lower margin of the eyebrow and a hole drilled through the orbital wall of the sinus. A plastic tube is left in situ to permit irrigation of the sinus.

Fronto-ethmoidectomy is carried out for complications of sinus infection and when there is permanent change to the mucosa which requires its removal. It is also undertaken for mucoceles of the sinus. A large frontonasal opening is created for drainage and a plastic tube left in for several months.

COMPLICATIONS OF INFECTIVE SINUSITIS

The following may occur in acute or chronic sinusitis:

- *Orbital complications* – periorbital cellulitis, subperiosteal abscess, blindness, suppuration of orbital contents.
- *Osteomyelitis complications* – in the frontal bone and maxilla; a discharging sinus may follow.
- *Intracranial complications* – meningitis, extradural, subdural and brain abscesses, cavernous sinus thrombosis.

Orbital and intracranial complications more often follow infection in the adjacent ethmoidal, frontal and sphenoid sinuses.

Infection spreads:

- along veins

- by rupture of an abscess through eroded thin bone and then periosteum
- through a bony defect after injury.

Clinical features

Orbital complications
Symptoms are:

- diplopia and restricted eye movement
- reduction of visual acuity.

Signs are:

- swollen eyelids
- proptosis with displacement of the orbit outwards and downwards.

Intracranial complications
Symptoms are:

- headache
- drowsiness
- photophobia.

Signs are:

- pyrexia and rigors
- personality changes (frontal abscess)
- fits and neurological localising signs.

Cavernous sinus thrombosis occurs rarely and is characterised by:

- proptosis
- swelling of the eyelids and conjunctiva
- ophthalmoplegia.

Investigation of complications
CT scan demonstrates opaque sinuses, bony defect, abscess formation in the ethmoidal and orbital areas with displacement of the eye, and brain abscess.

Nasal polyps

AETIOLOGY AND PATHOLOGICAL FEATURES
Nasal polyps are pale greyish pedunculated oedematous mucosal tissue masses which project into the nasal cavity. Usually they originate in the region of the ethmoids but can arise from any part of the nose or sinuses, and usually they are multiple and bilateral. Their cause is not fully understood. They are rare in children and, if found, the possibility of muco-viscoidosis should be considered. Confusion may also occur with a congenital meningocele. In about 25% of cases, they are associated with asthma and in 8% there is a linkage with both asthma and aspirin sensitivity. Polyps have a tendency to recur following treatment.

CLINICAL FEATURES
Symptoms
Nasal obstruction is the main complaint. Loss of smell and sneezing are common. Nasal polyps may block the ostia of a sinus and predispose to development of secondary sinus infection and a mucopurulent discharge.

Signs
The lesions are visible on endonasal examinational, although a polyp may develop in the maxillary sinus and protrude through the ostium into the back of the nasal cavity and the postnasal space (*antrochoanal polyp*).

INVESTIGATION
A sinus X-ray may show swollen mucosa but is not of particular help.

Unilateral nasal polypoidal swellings should always be subject to biopsy and histological examination to exclude a tumour.

MANAGEMENT
Medical treatment with topical steroid sprays can be employed if the symptoms are not severe, the polyps are small and there is no associated infection. However, in the majority, surgical removal is required. A snare or forceps is used close to the stalk and sometimes the ethmoidal air cells are also cleared. The postoperative use of a steroid spray can reduce recurrence. A short course of systemic steroids could be considered in severe recurrent polyposis.

Tumours of the nasal cavity and sinuses

Both benign and malignant tumours in the nasal cavity and sinuses are rare.

Benign tumours

Inverting papilloma
The presentation is with unilateral nasal symptoms, usually of obstruction. The examination will reveal a unilateral polypoidal swelling, biopsy or removal of which will reveal the benign nature of the tumour. It has a tendency to recur and there is a small risk of malignant change. A CT scan indicates the extent of the tumour. The tumour is removed using the lateral rhinotomy approach, with the incision on the side of the nose.

Osteomas
An osteoma may be an accidental finding on sinus X-ray and is more common in the frontal sinus. The

frontonasal duct may be obstructed and be responsible for sinusitis or mucocele. Sometimes osteomas expand in all directions causing pressure erosion of the bony walls of a sinus. In the presence of symptoms, they are removed using a frontoethmoidectomy or sometimes an osteoplastic frontal flap operation which lifts the anterior wall of the sinus.

Angiofibroma

Found only in adolescent males, this tumour occurs in the posterior part of the nose and the postnasal space and expands towards the base of the skull. Patients present with frequent severe nose bleeds. Embolisation to reduce vascularity is carried out before removal by surgery. Radiotherapy is used in some centres.

Malignant tumours

The majority of malignant tumours are of squamous cell origin. An increased occurrence of adenocarcinoma has been described in workers with wood.

Tumours arising in the nasal cavity and the ethmoids present with nasal and eye symptoms when they expand towards the orbit. Maxillary tumours present late with dental, orbital and nasal symptoms and facial swelling. Sometimes the first feature is a lymph node in the neck.

Treatment in most cases is by a combination of radiotherapy and surgery. Maxillectomy may need to be combined with exenteration of the orbital contents. Cranio-facial resection may be required when there is an extension of tumour into the anterior cranial fossa.

FURTHER READING

Abramovich S (1990) *Electrical Response Audiometry in Clinical Practice*. Edinburgh: Churchill Livingstone

Alberti P, Ruben P (eds) (1988) *Otologic Medicine and Surgery*, vols 1 and 2. New York: Chuchill Livingstone.

Colman B (ed.) (1992) *Hall and Colman's Diseases of the Nose, Throat and Ear and Head and Neck*. 14th edn Edinburgh: Churchill Livingstone.

Kerr A (ed.) (1997) *Scott-Brown's Otolaryngology*, vols 3 and 4. 6th edn London: Butterworth Heinemann.

Ludman H, Wright T (1997). *Diseases of the Ear*. Arnold: London

16

Chest and lungs

Carcinoma of the bronchus

EPIDEMIOLOGY
Carcinoma of the lung is the most common form of death from tumour in the world (900 000 deaths per year) and the third most common cause of death overall. The incidence is rising in women, sufficient for this condition to be the second most important cause of death in women, after that of the breast.

AETIOLOGY

Tobacco
There is a very clear association between lung cancer and tobacco with a latent period of 10–30 years; the primary determinants are:

- number of cigarettes consumed
- age of onset of smoking; those under 16 years of age· at start have irreversible damage to their bronchial genetic make up
- length of time of smoking
- type of tobacco – cigarettes or pipe, filter or non-filter
- *passive* exposure to tobacco smoke.

Other factors

- Exposure to asbestos
- Certain chemicals, toxic metals and irradiation.

PATHOLOGICAL FEATURES

Squamous cell carcinoma
This is the commonest type and accounts for 60% of lung tumours. It is associated with smoking and is rare in non-smokers. The growth starts as squamous meta-plasia and converts first to carcinoma in situ and then invasive carcinoma. Although usually solitary, there may be more than one area of primary squamous carcinoma occurring in the lung at one time. Continuing to smoke after treatment encourages further development of squamous carcinoma.

Adenocarcinoma
This accounts for 15% of lung tumours, increasing in frequency in the USA and Japan. It has a tendency to be more peripheral, arising in the small bronchial glands, which may reflect deeper penetration from inhalation

233

of filtered low tar cigarettes. It is most common in women and is the type seen in those who do not smoke.

Small cell carcinoma (oat cell)

This type of carcinoma arises from the Kulchitsky chromaffin cells and represents 20% of lung tumours. Histologically the cells are very small and round. This is an anaplastic tumour, which may occur in multiple lung sites and is highly malignant. Hormone production is common because its cells produce amine precursors. A benign form of small cell carcinoma is a *carcinoid tumour*.

Alveolar cell or bronchoalveolar carcinoma

This is relatively rare, comprising 5% of lung tumours. It arises in the distal airways, often diffuse, multifocal and bilateral. They are resistant to radiotherapy and chemotherapy. Prognosis is poor.

CLINICAL FEATURES

Symptoms

- *Cough* is the most common symptom, occurring in nearly half of patients
- *Haemoptysis* on at least one occasion is frequent but rarely persistent
- *Chest pain* is also quite common, usually a diffuse chest wall heaviness; specific local pain may be associated with the tumour's local spread
- *Pain or numbness* in the arm occurs from brachial plexus invasion
- *Shortness of breath* is the consequence of loss of lung volume from consolidation distal to an occluded bronchus
- *Hoarseness* occurs from involvement of a recurrent laryngeal nerve.
- *Dysphagia* is the consequence of involvement of the oesophagus by direct spread
- *General features* of malignancy are weight loss, malaise and fatigue.

Signs

General

Clubbing of the fingers may occur in 30% and hypertrophic pulmonary osteoarthropathy in 3% with painful swelling of the wrists and ankles. A marked increase in jugular venous pressure occurs with superior vena caval obstruction and distended veins may be visible over the upper arms and chest.

Signs of metastases are:

- tender areas in bones
- palpable supraclavicular lymph nodes
- An enlarged irregular liver
- Anaemia.

Respiratory

Patients are frequently smokers and therefore have some form of obstructive airways disease with ausculatory crackles and localised wheeze indicating a partially obstructed bronchus. Decreased air entry to a zone may occur from an obstructed bronchus or pleural effusion, the latter being common in extensive disease. Pleural rubs are rare.

INVESTIGATION

Chest X-ray

The standard postero-anterior (PA) and lateral projections define the lobar position of any mass and reveal pleural effusions, elevation of the hemidiaphragm (an indication of phrenic nerve involvement), erosion of ribs and secondary pulmonary sites of tumour.

CT or MRI of the thorax

Better assessment of the lesion is achieved with either of these methods than with chest X-rays in regard to position, nature and relationship with other structures. The examination should include inferior cuts to examine the liver and adrenals. In particular, CT defines:

- additional small lung lesions
- involvement of the pericardium, diaphragm, chest wall and oesophagus, all of which may indicate inoperability
- enlarged mediastinal glands, which suggest malignant involvement, if greater than 1 cm
- the anatomy of the liver and adrenals; both are frequent sites of secondary spread.

CT scans must be interpreted with caution. There is a small technical over-enlargement so that *abutment* does not necessarily mean *invasion*. This applies to lesions adjacent to the aorta, pericardium and chest wall.

Mediastinoscopy

The aim is to obtain tissue from the mediastinal lymph nodes around the lower trachea. It is the most important staging procedure for inoperability (N2 disease). A transverse incision is made just above the sternal notch. The lymphatic drainage of the right lung and of the lower lobe of the left lung is to the right paratracheal region. Sampling of tumour here reflects N2 disease with a poor prognosis and operation is usually contraindicated unless associated with neo-adjuvant therapy.

Biopsy of mediastinal glands is useful in the diagnosis of conditions other than carcinoma, in particular sarcoid, lymphoma, including Hodgkins, and tuberculosis.

Bone scan

Carcinoma of the bronchus frequently spreads to bone. Bone scans should be carried out if there is any clinical suggestion that there might be bone involvement. These include:

- bone pain
- tenderness over the spine and other bony areas
- raised alkaline phosphatase or serum calcium.

A single solitary hot spot on a bone scan can cause difficulty and should not be used as the sole criterion of inoperability. An MRI scan may be helpful to establish the nature of a single problematic lesion. Multiple secondaries, however, are an absolute contraindication to surgery.

Liver ultrasound examination

Bronchial carcinoma frequently spreads to the liver. Involvement of the liver can be detected by many forms of imaging – ultrasound, MRI, CT scan and radio-isotope scan. Ultrasound is the easiest and has a good chance of detecting secondaries. Scanning should definitely be done if there are abnormalities of liver function or if there is hepatic tenderness or enlargement.

Brain isotope scan

This investigation is indicated if neurological abnormalities are features of the clinical assessment, e.g.:

- severe persistent headache
- syncope
- ataxia or falls
- stroke
- behavioural change
- neuropathy which is more common than cerebral metastases.

DECISION-MAKING

An algorithmic guideline to the assessment of operability of carcinoma of the bronchus is shown in Figure 16.1. The essential items of information are:

- *a histological diagnosis* – oat cell carcinoma is usually inoperable
- *precise definition of the site* and of the amount of lung that must be removed – e.g. a wedge, a lobe or a whole lung
- *assessment of respiratory function*, which is balanced against the amount of lung that is to be removed
- *evidence of lymphatic spread* – mediastinal enlargement on CT and positive mediastinal biopsy; supraclavicular node involvement
- *presence of malignant cells in pleural effusion or heavy blood-stained effusions*
- *evidence of distant spread* – e.g. in bone, liver, adrenal gland and brain.

In practice, all patients being considered for lung resection receive a CT scan covering the thorax, mediastinal glands, liver and adrenals. But judgement is required in selecting additional diagnostic techniques and in correlation of the findings with suitability for surgery.

Respiratory function tests

Formal evaluation of respiratory function is necessary before surgery to determine the reserve of the remaining lung. Simple spirometry gives the following data:

- forced expiratory volume in 1 second (FEV_1)
- forced vital capacity (FVC)
- forced expiratory ratio (FER: the ratio of FEV_1/FVC).

These vary with the patient's age, height and sex but norms are available against which the figures for an individual patient can be assessed. There is not an absolute figure for inoperability. However, when FEV_1 is less than 1.2 L in a reasonably sized adult, resection is likely to mean a high risk of ventilatory insufficiency. When the FER is less than 50, lobectomy is not recommended and, when it is less than 55, pneumonectomy is not likely to be compatible with respiratory health.

As an adjunct to the above measurements, clinical assessment can be made by exercising the patient up and down two flights of stairs, assessing pulse and respiration and the return of these to normal, i.e. within 3 minutes. There should be no obvious subjective distress. This is a useful combined haemodynamic and pulmonary function test in patients with borderline respiratory function. Ventilation perfusion scans are used in some centres to give detailed respiratory analysis.

SURGICAL MANAGEMENT

Thoracotomy and lung resection are done whenever the tumour is assessed as operable. Early ligation of the pulmonary vein may help to prevent metastatic spread from tumour manipulation. An extrapleural dissection may be both useful and necessary when the tumour is adherent to the pleura. Intrapericardial resection may be carried out when the tumour is close to or involving the pericardium.

Surgical mortality depends on patient-related risk factors and the extent of resection: with pneumonectomy average mortality 6–12% and for lobectomy 3–6%. Specific risk factors are:

- age
- extent of resection
- chronic lung disease
- coronary artery disease/previous myocardial infarction
- concommittant disease of the liver, kidney and diabetes
- the work load, volume and experience of the surgical unit.

OUTCOME IN MALIGNANT DISEASE

Squamous carcinoma

The overall 5-year survival of primary lung cancers treated by surgical resection is about 45% and this figure

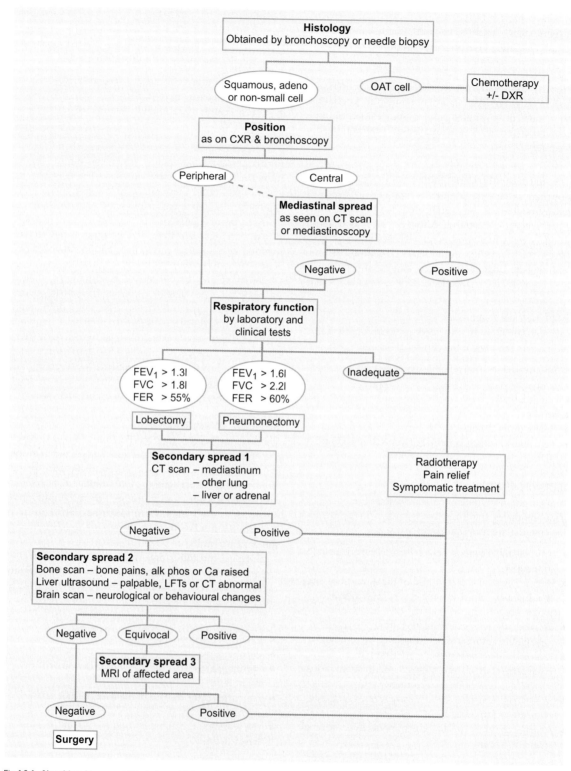

Fig 16.1 **Algorithm for operability in bronchial carcinoma.**

has not changed dramatically over many years. Survival depends on:

- *Histological type.* Squamous cell tumours do better than:
    - adenocarcinoma
    - undifferentiated tumours
    - small cell tumours.
- *Tumour size*: Stages T1–T4.
- *Lymph node spread*: Stages N0–N3.

Five-year survival[*] TNM classification (simplified) for squamous carcinoma is shown below:

- Stage 1 & N0 = 50–60%
- Stage 2 & N1 = 30–55%
- Stage 3a & N2 = 10–25%
- Stage 4 or N3 = 0–2%.

Small cell (oat cell) carcinoma

The outcome is particularly poor with resection alone – less than 5% survival at 5 years. Chemotherapy with cytotoxic combinations is now the preferred method of treatment and trials have shown an improved life expectancy, although still very poor.

Benign tumours

Benign tumours are far less common as a cause of masses detected on X-ray than are malignant tumours. They tend to be small, well-circumscribed nodules. Diagnosis between benign and small malignant tumours is very difficult. The rate of growth of a benign lesion is relatively slow – an important diagnostic point. If a previous chest X-ray has been taken, it is important to obtain it for comparison. Calcification is often an important sign of benign disease. CT may show calcification and absence of spiky projections into the lung. A percutaneous needle biopsy, under X-ray or CT guided control, is frequently done. However, small lesions are difficult to target so a negative result does not exclude malignancy. Because of this uncertainty, decisions regarding surgery often require clinical experience and judgement.

MANAGEMENT

The most important matter is to exclude malignancy. To make an extensive excision of a lesion that proves to be benign is better than to risk leaving one which ultimately proves to be malignant.

Hamartoma

This is the most frequent benign lung tumour; the lesion is nearly always smooth, round and coin-shaped on X-ray appearance. Its gradual growth is noted on serial X-rays. Surgery requires wedge resection of the tumour only and this is now possible by thoracoscopy or limited access video-assisted thoracotomy.

Carcinoid tumours

These are varieties of bronchial adenomas which arise from neuroendocrine cells (Kulchitsky) in the bronchi. They are relatively slow-growing and frequently cause complete occlusion of the bronchus in which they arise. In their clinical presentation, haemoptysis is frequent. An irritating cough, wheeze or dyspnoea from obstruction of the bronchus may also be present. Chest X-ray shows a small hilar mass or a smooth round peripheral one. These tumours can secrete substances such as adrenocorticotrophic hormone (ACTH), melanocyte-stimulating hormone (MSH) and insulin. The carcinoid syndrome with secretion of 5-hydroxy-tryptamine is not seen in bronchial carcinoids. The tumours can have considerable local growth and occlude major airways; there may be some local invasion of tissues even though they are benign. Malignant change is very rare.

Infections

Infective bronchiectasis

Bronchiectasis is a gross dilatation of the structure of the terminal bronchioles caused by infection, typically following measles and tuberculosis. Long-term antibiotics and physiotherapy with postural drainage are the standard treatments of this now uncommon condition. Surgery is occasionally needed. The clinical features which indicate a need for operation are severe haemoptysis or excessive sputum production (a cupful a day) not relieved by medical therapy and a demonstration of severe localised disease suitable for lobar or segmental resection. The diagnosis can be confirmed by bronchogram or, now more easily, with CT of the thorax. Local highly symptomatic bronchiectasis responds well to surgery.

Tuberculosis

Surgery is rarely required for this condition. In the pre-antibiotic era, thoracoplasty was very frequently done to collapse the lung. The only indications for surgery now are:

- persistent bronchopleural fistulae
- life-threatening or recurrent severe haemoptysis
- severe pleural thickening and scar which requires decortication
- gross destruction of the lung which prevents penetration of antibiotics

- large cavities or disease totally resistant to antibiotics.

Lung resection carries a high risk of complications, including haemorrhage from excessive vascular adhesions and late bronchopleural fistula.

Congenital lung cysts

Congenital lung cysts may be intrapulmonary, bronchogenic or related to a sequestrated pulmonary segment. Patients with any of these cysts may be asymptomatic or become secondarily infected, producing copious sputum with cough and occasional haemoptysis, which can be severe. Cysts may also be secondarily infected by aspergillosis, especially when they are associated with asthma or allergic alveolitis. Distinction may need to be made from primarily infective conditions, such as hydatid disease, paragonomiasis (Chinese liver fluke) and tuberculosis. Malignancy in lung cysts is rare.

Pneumothorax

The commonest problem in the pleura that the surgeon encounters is pneumothorax.

AETIOLOGY

There are three underlying causes:

- Rupture of a pleural bleb – often called simple or spontaneous pneumothorax – commonly occurring in those under 40 years of age
- Cystic disease of the lung – alpha-1-trypsin deficiency – in the young and chronic emphysema in the middle-aged or elderly
- Opportunist infections – such as *Pneumocystis carinii* – in immunodeficient states.

PATHOPHYSIOLOGICAL FEATURES

As air enters the pleural space, the lung collapses. Blood continues to flow through it so there is a right-to-left shunt of unoxygenated blood. However, if the contralateral lung is normal, there is rarely any change in the composition of arterial blood: any rise in $P_A\text{CO}_2$ is corrected by an increase in ventilation. If air continues to enter the hemithorax once the collapse is complete and cannot escape, tension pneumothorax may develop (Fig. 16.2) which has two effects:

- mediastinal shift and interference with venous return
- compression of the contralateral lung which reduces ventilation and, in consequence, gas exchange.

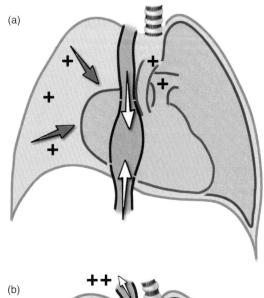

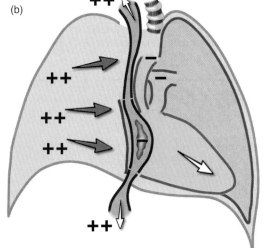

Fig 16.2 **Mechanisms in tension pneumothorax.**

Tension pneumothorax is thus accompanied by cardiorespiratory changes with a diminished cardiac output and reduction in the arterial partial pressure of oxygen.

CLINICAL FEATURES

Symptoms
Presentation is usually with sharp pain in the chest often associated with breathlessness. Unless the condition is bilateral or tension develops, severe dyspnoea is not present.

Signs
These are few and if the amount of air in the pleural space is only 25% of the capacity of the hemithorax, they may be absent. Unless there is a complication or the patient's lung

function is already much reduced, cyanosis is absent and only mild dyspnoea is seen. Local features are:

- decreased movement of the affected hemithorax
- hyperresonant percussion note over the same side
- absent breath sounds
- subcutaneous surgical emphysema is not usual in non-traumatic pneumothorax, but if it occurs it may indicate more aggressive management (see below).

In tension pneumothorax (which is relatively rare), breathlessness is more severe for the reasons given and signs of compression are evident, including:

- engorged neck veins
- cyanosis
- tachycardia and hypotension
- tracheal displacement in the suprasternal notch away from the affected side.

A tension pneumothorax is frequently a surgical emergency and treatment may be of such urgency that time should not be wasted in confirming the diagnosis by chest X-ray.

MANAGEMENT

Spontaneous pneumothorax

Management options include:

- *No intervention with observation only* – this is applicable where the pneumothorax is 10–20% of the capacity of the hemithorax (a rule of thumb is two finger-breadths in width on a chest X-ray) and symptoms are absent
- *Needle aspiration followed by daily X-ray* and, if necessary, repeat aspiration
- *Intercostal drainage with suction* – appropriate for a 50% pneumothorax or one associated with respiratory distress or subcutaneous emphysema.

Tension pneumothorax

Emergency treatment is necessary by immediate insertion of a large-bore needle into the thoracic space followed by an intercostal drain (see also Chs 3 and 11).

Intercostal drainage

The drain should be placed as near as possible to the apex of the thorax. The larger the tube the better, because there is always a small pleural effusion and fibrinous exudate associated with a pneumothorax which blocks a small-sized drain. The recommended size is 24 French.

Access routes are:

- second intercostal space anteriorly – access is simple and good for apical placement
- first or second intercostal space posteriorly – specialised access but provides excellent apical placement

- mid-axillary line bilaterally – cosmetic access but more prone to infection and very often fails to produce an apically sited drain.

Negative pressure (5–10 mmHg) should always be applied and must be sufficient to maintain negative pressure during maximum expiration.

Criteria of satisfactory management of intercostal drainage

- Elimination of any air space between lung and pleura
- Maximum inflation of lung
- Adherence of lung to chest wall by natural fibrin adhesions which maintains expansion and seals the air leak.

Removal of the drain

Before this is done it is essential to ensure that the air leak has ceased. Clamping a drain in the presence of a continued leak of air collapses the lung and delays resolution. Therefore this should not be done in an attempt to find out if leakage has ceased. Confirmation is obtained from the following:

- bubbling is absent on suction
- bubbling does not occur when suction is turned off or when the patient coughs
- full expansion on chest X-ray
- surgical emphysema is decreasing or has disappeared.

When the above conditions have applied for at least 24 hours, the drain may safely be removed.

Surgical treatment of recurrent or persistent pneumothorax

There are two methods: obliteration of the pleura (pleurectomy); and irritation of the pleura, usually with chemicals (pleurodesis).

Pleurectomy

The parietal pleura is stripped as fully as possible from the chest wall, including the apex, and anteriorly down to the diaphragm. Additional ligation or stapling of large lung bullae may be carried out at the same time. There is close to 100% success. Complications are Horner's syndrome and bleeding. Pleurectomy can be achieved by video-assisted thoracoscopy or video-assisted mini-thoracotomy.

Pleurodesis

The pleura is inflamed by the use of chemical agents or abrasion but not excised. Agents used are iodised talc, tetracycline and blood. The success rate is not as good as open pleurectomy. Pleurodesis is particularly indicated for elderly patients with chronic obstructive airways disease in whom a thoracotomy may be hazardous. Video-assisted thoracoscopy provides the ability to place the chosen irritant over a wide area of pleura with better results than by closed blind instillation; in addition bullae can be stapled. A rare potential complication of talc pleurodesis is late malignant change. A combination of talc pleurodesis with apical stapling under VATS is favoured by many.

Diagnostic and therapeutic thoracoscopy

With advancing technology, video-assisted thorascopy has become both a valuable diagnostic and therapeutic tool. It produces only minor trauma to the patient through tiny incisions. It may be used as a closed procedure or open, combined with a mini-incision. When the incision is increased to 10 cm, lung resection can be performed. The main indications for diagnostic and therapeutic endoscopy are shown in Tables 16.1 and 16.2

Table 16.1
Diagnostic thoracoscopy

Problem	Possible diagnosis
Pleural effusions	Malignancy, tuberculosis, lymphoma
Pleural nodules/thickening	Mesothelioma, tuberculosis, malignancy, fibromas
Diffuse parenchymal lung disease	Sarcoid, lymphoma, HIV-related conditions, opportunistic infections, granulomata
Staging of lung cancer	Mediastinal and hilar node sampling
Lung nodules	Primary or secondary tumours, granuloma, including tuberculosis

Table 16.2
Therapeutic thorocoscopy

Indication	Procedure
Empyema	Drainage and breakdown loculi
Recurrent pneumothorax	Pleurectomy or pleural abrasion (talc) Stapling of opical bullae
Pericardial effusion	Creation of pericardial to pleural window
Malignant effusion	Pleurectomy or talc or tetracycline pleurodesis
Lung masses	Resection as wedge or lobectomy

17

Cardiac surgery

There are two groups of conditions in which surgery is undertaken – coronary artery disease and diseases of the heart valves.

Coronary artery disease

Coronary artery disease (CAD) is the term used to include all the manifestations of narrowing or occlusion of the coronary arteries by atherosclerosis. Surgery is now involved in management because it is possible to restore flow around narrow involved segments by coronary artery bypass grafting (CABG). This surgical technique is now complemented by percutaneous transluminal coronary angioplasty (PTCA) in which the stenosis is dilated by a balloon at the tip of a catheter. The requirement for surgery in the United Kingdom (UK) and similar Western countries is based on epidemiological studies which suggest a need for between 300 and 450 operations per million of the population per year. In the UK this means between 17000 and 25000 operations annually. The current male:female ratio of both incidence and procedures is 4:1, but the number of operations in women is rising. The need for PTCA in those with lesser indications for therapy of CAD is about the same.

ANATOMY
The terms used by surgeons vary somewhat from those of the anatomists and additionally there are differences between surgeons. In practice the anatomical description for an individual patient is based on the radiological appearances at coronary angiography, a procedure which is undertaken by passing a catheter into a major artery and injecting contrast medium into the root of the aorta and selectively into the ostia of the coronary vessels. Video X-rays are taken in two planes.

In terms of a *normal anatomy* (Fig. 17.1) the heart is supplied by a left artery which arises posteriorly from the aorta and a right artery with an anterior origin. The left has a main stem 1 cm in length and then divides into:

- *The left anterior descending (anterior intraventricularis)* artery, which descends over the anterior part of the heart, above the septum and between the right and the left ventricles to supply the anterior part of both ventricles as well as the anterior part of the septum.

241

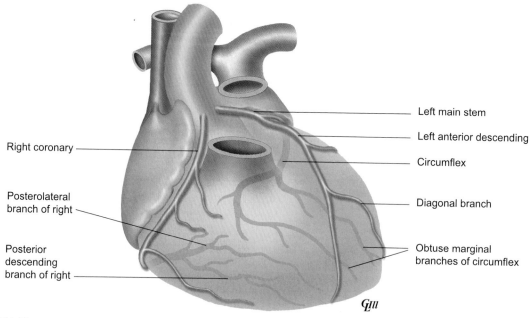

Fig 17.1 **The anatomy of the coronary arteries.**

It is considered the most important of the three major coronary arteries because of its additional supply of the interventricular septum. The main branch of the left anterior descending is called the diagonal.

- *The circumflex*, which runs around the back of the heart between the left atrium and the left ventricle in the atrioventricular groove and supplies the lateral and posterior walls of the left ventricle. The vessels of the circumflex supplying the lateral and posterior walls are termed the obtuse marginal branches.

The right artery supplies both the right and left ventricles. It runs anteriorly between the right atrium and right ventricle and divides at the lower border of the right ventricle into two branches, both of which supply part of the inferior aspect of the left ventricle:

- *The posterior descending artery (posterior intraventricular)*, which runs along the posterior intraventricular groove, between the right and left ventricles, and supplies the posterior part of the septum and inferior parts of both right and left ventricles.
- *The right posterolateral artery*, which supplies the inferior aspect of the left ventricle.

Pathological effects of occlusion

The effects of obstruction of an individual artery are modified by the degree of anastomosis between it and other vessels. However, occlusions generally cause the following:

- Left anterior descending artery – an anterior or anterolateral infarction of the wall of the left ventricle

- Circumflex artery – a posterolateral infarction
- Right coronary – likely to produce inferior myocardial infarction.

EPIDEMIOLOGY
CAD is widespread throughout the world, especially in temperate zones, including the USA, most of Europe, the Middle East and the Indian subcontinent. There is a low incidence in China and Japan as well as in most of Africa. It is less common in France than in most other European countries.

AETIOLOGY AND PATHOLOGICAL FEATURES
Atherosclerotic disease in the coronary arteries is only one manifestation of a general metabolic abnormality in the arterial wall in which lipid and cholesterol accumulate in the media. There are also some features of inflammation which lead to fibrosis, and infective agents are being intensively investigated as a cause. The intima overlying the lesions in the media may become elevated (plaques) or be shed (ulceration). Turbulent blood flow in such areas predisposes to platelet deposition and thrombosis. The outcome of clinical importance is narrowing (stenosis) or occlusion (thrombosis) of the artery or its branches. Both may produce insufficient supply of blood to the myocardium, which in turn produce:

- exercise-induced myocardial pain (angina)
- death of the area of myocardium supplied – usually referred to as coronary thrombosis or acute coronary occlusion
- ischaemia and consequent malfunction of the neural conduction system with arrhythmias

- reduction in the efficiency of ventricular contraction
- attenuation of the ventricular wall with the development of an aneurysm.

Risk factors

Age. The incidence increases with age.

Genetic. The condition runs in families but a specific gene has not been identified. The family history may be sufficiently strong to produce major cardiac events at a similar age in each generation.

Cholesterol and triglyceride levels. Familial hyper-lipidaemia results in a higher and earlier incidence of CAD and accounts for some of the patients with a family history. It is also associated with arterial fibrosclerosis, which affects the root of the ascending aorta and leads to narrowing of the origins of both coronary arteries. Apart from this condition, there is also a direct relationship between levels of cholesterol and triglyceride in blood above the population normal, the incidence of atherosclerotic plaques and the likelihood of coronary artery disease occurring at a young (30–40) age. Further, low population or regional levels correlate with low incidences of CAD. Recent evidence suggests that reduction in cholesterol levels slows the rate of advance of coronary atheroma.

Smoking is the single most important risk factor. One possible explanation is that high levels of carbon monoxide are produced by filter-tipped cigarettes; this is supported by the fact that their introduction was followed 40 years later by an increased incidence of coronary artery disease. However, the pathological effects of tobacco are complex and not well understood.

Arterial hypertension and CAD are related but not in a simple way. On the one hand, there is a close correlation between high blood pressure and the occurrence of atherosclerosis; on the other hand, in many hypertensive groups (Africans, West Indians), hypertension does not result in an increased incidence of CAD. However, hypertensive patients with widespread vascular disease represent a special and complex subgroup in terms of operative risk and tactics.

Diabetes mellitus. There is an increased incidence of coronary artery and peripheral vascular disease in both insulin-dependent and non-insulin dependent diabetics.

Risk table. A risk analysis table of the percentage liklihood of developing a coronary event over 10 years has been produced by the British Heart Association and accepted by the Department of Health, linking all these factors for an individual's risk.

CAD and atherosclerotic disease elsewhere in the body

In view of the systemic nature of atherosclerosis, it is not surprising that patients with CAD often have pathological or clinical manifestations of arterial disease in other parts of the body. For example there is an association between stenosis of the main stem of the left coronary artery and stenosis at the bifurcation of the common carotid artery; and patients who present for repair of abdominal aortic aneurysms have a 35% incidence of significant coronary artery disease.

INVESTIGATION

Angiography

The definitive investigation of patients suspected of having CAD is the coronary angiogram. Coronary disease is present when there is **significant narrowing** of a coronary artery as defined as a reduction in diameter of 50% or more in a vessel as shown on two different projections (preferably at 90% to each other). The use of the term *haemodynamically significant* is the consequence of Poiseuille's formula which states that the reduction of flow across a narrowed vessel is proportional to the:

- length of narrowing
- fourth power of the radius at the point of narrowing.

The second of these is more important and the greater the narrowing, the greater is the exponential reduction in flow.

Radiological classification

Three vessel coronary disease is significant narrowing in all three major coronary vessels:

- right artery
- left anterior descending artery
- circumflex artery.

Left main stem disease is the presence of a significant narrowing in the first common part of the left coronary artery before it divides into the anterior descending and the circumflex.

Single vessel disease is significant narrowing in just one of the three vessesls excluding the main stem.

It should be noted that these radiological classifications are used as a basis for defining treatment options based on prognosis. They do not limit the actual revascularisation procedures to just three vessels as each of these carry important branches which may themselves require therapy; thus it is possible and common for patients to have 4 or 5 coronary grafts.

Intravascular ultrasound probe catheters IVUS are a new device available to clarify stenoses difficult to interpret from the angiogram.

Ventricular function

Assessment of ventricular function is done in two ways:

Ventricular contraction is observed at angiography, by echocardiography or by the use of an isotope scan. The movement of each of several segments of the ventricle can be quantified (regional wall motion) and the overall contraction measured by calculating the following ratio:

Table 17.1
Classification of left ventricular function and prognosis in CAD

Category	Ejection fraction (%)	5-year survival (%) after surgery for three-vessel disease
Good	70–50	90
Moderate	50–30	
Poor	30–15	45

$$\frac{\text{Ejection}}{\text{fraction}} = \frac{\text{diastolic volume} - \text{systolic volume}}{\text{diastolic volume}} \times 100$$

The normal value is 70%.

The use of ejection fraction to categorise left ventricular function and prognosis in CAD is shown in Table 17.1.

Left ventricular pressure is directly measured by catheterisation. Pressure at the end of diastole reflects tension in the cardiac muscle. The higher this end-diastolic pressure (LVEDP) the poorer is ventricular function. Normal values are 8–12 mmHg, and these rise to 25–35 mmHg in left ventricular failure. The rise is reflected back through the left atrium, pulmonary veins and capillaries, ultimately to cause a rise in pulmonary artery pressure.

MANAGEMENT

Comparisons between surgical and medical management

Prospective randomised trials of medical versus surgical management on the mortality at 5 years were carried out both in Europe and in the USA during the mid-1970s. Three results are important:

- *Left main stem disease* was studied in the first trial, that of the Veterans Administration (VA) in the USA: survival was better with surgical management.
- *Three-vessel disease* was the subject of a European multicentre study: survival was better with surgical management.
- *Subset information* on the importance of individual arteries came from the American Coronary Artery Surgery Study (CASS): restoration of flow in the left anterior descending artery is more important than in the circumflex and right coronary; and surgical management is better than medical management in two-vessel disease if the left anterior descending artery is narrowed by 70% or more.

Medical management has altered since the mid 1970s and several trials have been undertaken comparing angioplasty to surgery in specific situations. These tend to show equal survival and freedom from myocardial infarction rates in the very long term but much greater reintervention rates in the short term. Cost differentials are nearly even.

Coronary artery bypass grafting

Clear indications for CABG

These indications follow from the results of the trials described above:

- left main stem disease.
- three-vessel disease, with or without angina pectoris and/or moderate left ventricular damage.

In addition, it is accepted that surgery may be urgently required in:

- complete occlusion or dissection of a coronary artery after percutaneous coronary angioplasty
- rupture of an ischaemic ventricular septal defect or of the mitral papillary muscle apparatus; in these conditions, surgery is directed primarily to repair of the defect and only secondarily to grafting of arteries.

Relative indications for CABG

- Three-vessel coronary disease without angina pectoris, especially if there is:
  - a highly significant haemodynamic lesion
  - silent ischaemia, as shown in strongly positive exercise tests without angina or positive thallium isotope scan
  - accelerated atherosclerosis in immunosuppressed renal or cardiac transplant patients
  - reduction of the risk of myocardial infarction when surgical treatment is required for a coexistent disease.
- Three-vessel disease with poor ventricular function, especially if there is evidence of reversible ischaemia or of a ventricular aneurysm
- Large left ventricular aneurysm associated with dyspnoea or signs of significant ventricular dysfunction
- Two-vessel coronary disease with highly significant lesions, particularly when these involve the left anterior descending artery
- Angina pectoris, not remedial to medical therapy (including PTCA) and irrespective of the number of vessels involved.

Risk in CABG

A *first elective operation* has a mortality of 0.5–2.5%. Current determinants of risk include:

- age greater than 75 years
- poor ventricular function, especially with an ejection fraction under 25% and left ventricular end-diastolic pressure greater than 25 mmHg
- female – probably related to the smaller and finer condition of the coronary arteries and therefore a technical factor
- hypertension, renal disease and obesity

- additional simultaneous procedures such as:
  - aortic or mitral valve surgery, particularly in the elderly and if the mitral disease is ischaemic in origin
  - other vascular procedures, e.g. carotid endarterectomy
  - severe atheroma of the ascending aorta; both this and carotid artery disease cause an increased risk of stroke.

Second or subsequent operations have greater risks mainly because of technical factors, such as:

- potential damage to the heart when the incision is reopened
- difficulty with aortic cannulation for connection of the heart–lung machine
- technical problems with grafting
- damage to an existing patent graft
- emboli detached from partially thrombosed but patent grafts which cause occlusions in the distal coronary vessels.

Emergency procedures which involve impending or developed acute myocardial infarction can carry a mortality as high as 20%.

Choice of graft

Arteries

The internal mammary (internal thoracic) artery is the first choice conduit as it has excellent 10-year patency results, greatly better than saphenous vein. The vessel is mobilised in continuity from the subclavian artery by dividing its intercostal branches to the chest wall. The most frequent site for anastomosis is to the left anterior descending artery but it can be used for the circumflex. Jump grafts to more than one branch can be done. It can also be used as the base for Y grafts to other vessels utilising other arterial conduits. Bilateral internal mammary grafts have now been shown to provide better long-term (10-year plus) survival than the use of only one mammary graft with additional veins.

The radial artery is harvested from the forearm and used as a free graft; it has also recently been shown to perform well over many years and is becoming popular because it maintains the consistency of an artery rather than that of a vein. The gastro-epiploic artery can be mobilised from the greater curvature of the stomach to reach the posterior descending artery as a pedicle. It may be more prone to spasm and is not used frequently.

Vein

A free graft of the long saphenous vein has been used for the longest time and has given good results over 10 years after insertion. Arm veins can be substituted if necessary. However, at 10 years, some 30% veins will be occluded and others stenosed.

Choice of by pass

Recent advances in technology have allowed coronary artery grafting to be carried out without the use of the heart-lung machine (bypass machine or pump). Early results indicate benefits in reduction of general inflammatory markets of body damage and perservation of previously impaired organs such as the kidney and brain. The method (called off pump or beating heart surgery) uses a mechanical stabiliser to lift and hold steady the heart whilst the coronary anastomoses are carried out with the remaining heart beating and maintaining a good blood pressure and circulation. In some hands, 90% of first-time coronary grafting can be performed this way.

Complications of CABG

Preoperative

- Myocardial infarction from stress/anxiety or critical ischaemia.

Intraoperative

- Myocardial failure and lack of adequate myocardial contraction at the end of bypass which requires additional cardiac support
- Catecholamine infusion, intra-aortic balloon pumping, ventricular assist devices or even transplantation
- Embolic infarction from detached fragments released by manipulation of a thrombosed graft during a repeat CABG.

Postoperative

The specific complications of CABG are:

- Myocardial failure – infarction, inadequate myocardial protection or excess fluid load
- Stroke – which may have occurred intraoperatively or become manifest some hours later; causes are shown in Table 17.2.

Other surgery in CAD

Ischaemic ventricular arrhythmias may require electrical mapping at open surgery and treatment by destruction

Table 17.2
Causes of stroke in open heart surgery

Event	Origin
Solid emboli	From any left-sided site where thrombosis may have occurred – left atrial appendage, suture lines. Disruption of atheromatous plaques
Air emboli	Technical in cardiopulmonary bypass
Hypoxic infarction	Low bypass pressure or flow
Hypertension	Uncontrolled during operation or soon thereafter. Both hypoxic and hypertensive events may have intra- or extracranial atherosclerosis as coexistent and associated cause
Intracranial haemorrhage (rare)	Poorly controlled anticoagulation Rupture of a cerebral aneurysm

of the focus with or without CABG. A left ventricular aneurysm may need to be excised.

Congenital disorders of the heart and great vessels

Congenital heart disease has an incidence which is fairly steady at 1 per 100 births and results in about 40 operations per million of the population being carried out each year in the UK. Lesions are either valvular, septal or a combination. Some of the latter are so complex that they are no longer known by any particular name and the abnormalities are described as a long sequence of anatomical diagnoses based on the details of the connections. The commonest lesion is a ventricular septal defect (1:500 births). Other disorders are listed in Box 17.1.

AETIOLOGY AND ANATOMICO-PATHOLOGICAL FEATURES

The cause of congenital defects is multifactorial (Table 17.3).

Congenital disorders of valves

These are preferably treated by surgical repair rather

Table 17.3
Aetiology and nature of congenital cardiac defects

Factor	Outcome
Maternal virus infection (rubella)	Persistent ductus arteriosus
	Pulmonary valve stenosis
	Pulmonary artery stenosis
Maternal alcohol abuse	Septal defects
Maternal drug and radiation treatment	Various
Genetic abnormalities	Down's syndrome
	Septal defects
	Tricuspid and mitral valve abnormalities
	Turner's syndrome
	Coarctation of aorta
	Marfan's syndrome
	Dilatation of aortic ring
	Aortic incompetence
	Aortic aneurysm
Uncertain	Congenital aortic stenosis

---

than by replacement to allow for growth. The requirement for these operations in the UK is constant at about 40 per million per year, giving a total of about 2300.

PATHOLOGICAL ANATOMY

- Valves commonly involved are the aortic and the pulmonary
- A pinhole in a domed valve without clear leaflet development
- Marked hypoplasia
- Two rather than three cusps (bicuspid valve), congenital narrowing of the mitral valve is rare.

Other congenital cardiovascular disorders

Patent ductus arteriosus is the most common disorder. Other and more complicated disorders are shown in Box 17.1. The more severe types require very early correction during childhood. Aortic valve stenosis which presents in childhood usually means that the valve is bicuspid, but milder forms of aortic bicuspid stenosis may not present for surgery until between the third and fifth decade of life.

Acquired disorders of valves

AETIOLOGY AND PATHOLOGICAL FEATURES

Infective

Subacute bacterial endocarditis (SBE)

This is common and usually affects the aortic or mitral

Box 17.1

Disorders in congenital heart disease

Common

Atrial septal defect
Pulmonary valve stenosis
Aortic stenosis
Patent ductus arteriosus
Coarctation of the aorta
Fallot's tetralogy
    Ventricular septal defect
    Right ventricular outflow obstruction
    Overriding aorta
    Right ventricular hypertrophy

Rare

Pulmonary artery atresia
Tricuspid valve stenosis
Atrioventricular canal
Left heart hypoplasia
Ventricular septal defect and transposition
    (venous input into left heart, arterial output from
    right heart)
Single ventricle
Double outlet ventricles

Table 17.4
Abnormalities associated with subacute bacterial endocarditis

Site	Abnormality
Aortic valve	Congenital bicuspid
	Rheumatic disease
	Degenerative disease
Mitral valve	Rheumatic disease
Prosthetic valve	Clot formation
Cardiac abnormalities	Patent ductus arteriosus
	Ventricular septal defect

Table 17.5
Organisms involved in subacute bacterial endocarditis

Bacterium	Antecedents	Pathological features
Streptococus viridans	Dental extraction	Often congenital abnormality of valve
	Other instrumentation	
	GI endoscopy	
	Cystoscopy	
	Bronchoscopy	
Enterococcus	Prostatic disease	Older patients
	Pelvic surgery	
Staphylococcus aureus	Intravenous prostheses	Acute ulcerative disease
	Drug addicts	Abscess formation
Streptococus epidermides	Intravenous prostheses	Low-grade disease
	Drug addicts	
	Artificial heart valves	
Fungal infection	Immunosuppression	Indolent disease

Table 17.6
Connective tissue disorders and degenerative cardiovascular disease

Disease	Pathological effects	Outcome
Marfan's syndrome	Cystic medial necrosis	Mitral and aortic valve degeneration
		Aortic dilatation with aortic regurgitation
Ankylosing spondylitis	Inflammatory infiltration	Dilated aortic root
		Aortic regurgitation

valves. The tricuspid is often involved in patients who abuse drugs. Valves affected are not often normal unless there is some other factor such as immunosuppression or drug abuse; more often there is a congenital or acquired abnormality or the valve is a replacement one (Table 17.4). The organisms responsible are indicated in Table 17.5.

The pathological findings are of destruction of the valve and clumps of infected fibrin and platelets (vegetations), particularly on the underside of the valve cusps, which may go on to cause circular erosions or abscess formation at the valve annulus. There is accompanying bacteraemia.

Rheumatic fever

This usually occurs in childhood between the ages of 5 and 12. The cause is thought to be an autoimmune reaction set in motion by an infection with group A *Streptococcus*. The effects are infiltration of the myocardium with *Aschoff bodies* – granulomatous lesions with central necrosis – which progress to fibrosis. The valves develop sterile vegetations which interfere with their function, and as fibrosis progresses they may become incompetent or fibrotic, or both. Severe damage to the valve may occur within 10 years, but more commonly change sufficient to cause presentation for

surgery does not occur until patients are between 30 and 50 years old. There is continuing damage both to the valves and to the myocardium throughout this period which may continue after surgical treatment.

Degenerative

Degenerative valve disease: is age-related in the aortic valve, may be associated with hypertension and produces aortic stenosis. Myxomatous degeneration of the mitral valve is common and 3% of the population have mild asymptomatic prolapse. Clinically significant prolapse with significant mitral regurgitation is less common although excessive valve tissue, particularly of the anterior mitral cusp (Barlow syndrome), may lead to regurgitation. More common is simple degeneration and elongation of the papillary cords, which is associated with cusp prolapse, annular dilatation and eventual cord rupture with staged increases in the amount of regurgitation and therefore of symptoms.

Connective tissue disorders associated with degenerative valve disease are listed in Table 17.6

- Ischaemia may affect the papillary muscles and their support from the ventricular wall and may cause mitral regurgitation.

HAEMODYNAMIC EFFECTS

Stenosis and/or *regurgitation* at any valve create a haemodynamic effect on the adjacent heart chambers and the lungs, according to the position and nature of the lesion. Stenosis produces a proximal pressure overload. A simple example is aortic stenosis with left ventricular hypertrophy. Also, reduction of flow means a reduced cardiac output either on exercise or at rest. Regurgitation causes volume overload of the proximal chamber, usually with dilatation, e.g. mitral stenosis with left atrial enlargement.

Stenosis and regurgitation in combination cause both volume and pressure overload and may lead to secondary effects. On the left side, these are pulmonary congestion and hypertension. The latter causes irreversible damage to the pulmonary arterioles (similar in nature to the effect of arterial hypertension on the systemic arterioles) and tertiary effects follow. Pulmonary hypertension leads to right ventricular hypertrophy and distension with tricuspid regurgitation and ultimately congestion of the liver and periphery.

CLINICAL FEATURES

Symptoms

Symptoms are a result of the haemodynamic effects:

- *Low cardiac output* is associated with fatigue and lethargy.
- *In aortic stenosis*, syncope and angina may occur because of low output, the latter even if the coronary arteries are normal.
- *Pulmonary congestion* in any combination of disease of the left side of the heart, but particularly from mitral stenosis or mitral regurgitation, gives rise to breathlessness on exertion, orthopnoea, paroxysmal nocturnal dyspnoea, cough, frothy sputum and haemoptysis. A combination of the last two implies that congestion is severe.
- *Right-sided congestion* causes fatigue, headaches, high skin colour, right hypochondrial pain (liver enlargement), abdominal swelling (ascites) and ankle swelling (peripheral oedema).

Examination and physical findings

Examination should be methodical; attention to detail greatly facilitates the task of reaching the correct diagnosis.

General examination can reveal some of the systemic features of heart disease particularly of right heart failure (Table 17.7) The visible and palpable aspects of the peripheral circulation also provide provisional diagnostic information (Table 17.8).

Jugular venous pulsation is best seen with the patient at 45°, but it may be necessary to change this to 90° to detect gross elevation of the jugular venous waveform. Observation of movement as high as the lobes of the ear may be required. The A, C and V aspects of the waveform should be assessed (Fig. 17.2). The jugular venous pressure (JVP) normally falls during inspiration: the opposite indicates tamponade (Fig. 17.3).

Examination of the precordium is summarised in Table 17.9.

Table 17.7
Systemic signs of right heart failure

Site	Finding	Significance
Skin colour	Dusky; blue	Pulmonary congestion CCF
Liver	Smooth general enlargement	Right heart failure
	Pulsation	Tricuspid incompetence
Ankles	Bilateral pitting oedema	Possible right heart failure
Lungs	Pleural effusion	Possible left heart failure
	Crackles	Pulmonary oedema

Table 17.8
Features of physical examination of peripheral circulation in heart disease

Feature	Findings	Significance
Fingers and hands	Cool	Low cardiac output
	Capillary pulsation	Aortic regurgitation
	Splinter haemorrhages	Bacterial endocarditis
	Clubbing	Cyanotic heart disease
Arm pulse	Low amplitude	Low cardiac output
	High amplitude	Aortic regurgitation Aortopulmonary shunt CO_2 retention
	Jerking	Cardiomyopathy
	Double pulse	Mixed aortic stenosis/ aortic regurgitation
	Locomotor brachialis	Hypertension
Carotid pulse	Slow rising; low amplitude	Aortic stenosis
	Bouncing full	Aortic regurgitation
	Head nods	Aortic regurgitation
	Systolic murmur	Referred from aortic stenosis Carotid artery stenosis
	Systolic thrill	Carotid artery stenosis
Neck veins	High jugular pressure (JVP)	Congestive heart failure Right ventricular failure Tricuspid regurgitation Tamponade (JVP rises on inspiration) Constrictive pericarditis

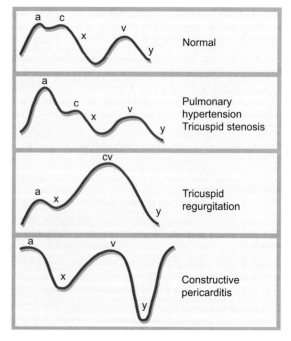

Fig 17.2 **Various jugular venous waveforms.**

Mechanism of Cardiac Tamponade

- Blood and thrombus accumulate in pericardium

- Pressure is exerted on vena cavae, right atrium and on the ventricle

- Venous return is reduced, diastolic filling of ventricles is reduced

- Cardiac input is reduced by both mechanisms

- Venous pressure outside the pericardium rises, heart rate rises, cardiac output falls, urine output falls, blood pressure falls

- No cardiac input = no cardiac output

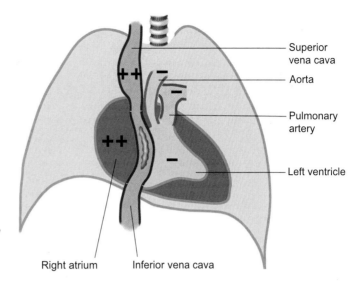

Fig 17.3 **Sequence of events in cardiac tamponade.** As effusion develops, both atria and ventricles are compressed. Inflow pressure in the superior and inferior vena cavae and right atrium rises, but inspite of this ventricular volume falls and arterial pressure is reduced.

Table 17.9
Precordial examination

Site	Finding	Significance
General	Thrills	Aortic area: aortic stenosis LSE 3: VSD Apex: mitral regurgitation
Apex	Heavy displacement	Large hypertrophied or dilated left ventricle
Apex	Local tap not displaced	Mitral stenosis
Sternum	Lifting	Right ventricular hypertrophy and dilatation

Auscultation. It is necessary to concentrate on each area separately. Ejection systolic murmurs in the *aortic area* indicate aortic stenosis but may also occur in subaortic stenosis and sclerosis of the ascending aorta. In aortic regurgitation, a soft systolic murmur is most common from mild thickening of the aortic valve but does not in fact imply aortic stenosis. Aortic regurgitation can only be excluded when the patient is sitting forward with the breath held in expiration, while auscultation is done at the left sternal edge at the level of the third or fourth costal cartilages.

Auscultation at the *pulmonary area* in pulmonary hypertension reveals a loud pulmonary second sound and in the presence of an atrial septal defect a fixed, widely split, second sound. In both these disorders there may be an associated pulmonary flow murmur.

Auscultation at the *lower left sternal* edge is a good site to hear the heart sounds and when they are present, the third and fourth sounds are best heard here. The opening snap of mitral valve disease can be as well heard at the left sternal edge as at the apex, and as well

or better with the diaphragm of the stethoscope as with the bell. The opening snap is a medium-pitched noise, similar to a very widely split second sound. The apex is the best site to hear the mid-diastolic rumble of mitral stenosis which is low-pitched and best heard with the bell and with the patient turned towards the left. The pansystolic murmur of mitral regurgitation is loudest at the apex and radiates widely laterally as well as across the midline, occasionally reaching up to the aortic area.

INVESTIGATION

Haematological

Haematological changes are relevant in valve disease. Anaemia accentuates or creates systolic murmurs. Haemolysis, created by flow at high velocity through a small orifice in or around a valve, is associated with a high reticulocyte count. Although haemolysis may occur de novo in valve disease, it is more common after artificial valve implantation or valve repair. Elevation of the sedimentation rate (ESR) to 50 mm/h or more suggests endocarditis. Other abnormalities in this condition are raised serum immunoglobulins and lowered C3 and total complement. The last two changes are a result of the formation of immune complexes, but these are not routinely measured. Elevated titres of antisteptolysin-O (ASO) antibody are associated with recent post-streptococcal infection which may be relevant to the diagnosis of recent rheumatic fever.

Electrocardiogram (ECG)

Left ventricular hypertrophy is commonly present in significant aortic valve disease, mitral regurgitation and coarctation of the aorta. Associated T-wave inversion (grade 2) and ST depression with T-wave inversion (grade 3) indicate advancing damage to the myocardium as well as increasing strain on the heart.

Rhythm. Atrial fibrillation is commonly seen in conditions in which the atria are grossly dilated, of which mitral valve stenosis is the most common. A pattern of bundle branch block often indicates ischaemia but can result from aortic stenosis. In acute aortic endocarditis, the presence of bundle branch block strongly suggests an abscess at the aortic root. An enlarged P-wave with sinus rhythm is of two types: a bifid M pattern in mitral valve disease; and a single peak pattern (p-pulmonale) in pulmonary hypertension.

Chest X-ray

The overall size of the heart is shown and it is important to realise that this is a combination of both the atrial and the ventricular size. In mitral stenosis, the double outline of the left and right atrium can be separated along the right heart border; these are important features whose change can be measured over a period of time. The pulmonary artery knuckle is a reflection of the size of the pulmonary artery; size is increased in pulmonary valve stenosis with post-stenotic dilatation, in atrial or ventricular septal defects and in pulmonary hypertension. The aortic knuckle may be wide in aortic valve stenosis with post-stenotic dilatation and in degenerative or collagen conditions which cause aortic regurgitation. A double aortic knuckle is seen in coarctation.

Other features of the X-ray which are typical of mitral stenosis are:

- splayed left bronchus with enlargement of the left atrium
- distended lymphatics at the lung bases
- pulmonary calcification
- pleural effusion
- increase in vascularity (plethora).

Upper lobe venous diversion, particularly in the right upper lobe, is a sign of high pulmonary blood flow or congestion from high left atrial pressure.

Echocardiography

Echocardiography is assuming an increasingly important role in the assessment of valve disease and can be done by either a surface probe (transthoracic) or one passed into the oesophagus (transoesophageal). Transoesophageal echoes are particularly valuable in looking at the back of the heart – the left atrium and the mitral valve – whereas transthoracic anterior echocardiography provides better views of aortic and tricuspid valve conditions. Both approaches show ventricular movement and left ventricular function. In each, echocardiographic study combines two-dimensional echoes, M-mode echoes, duplex colour Doppler, all coordinated with ECG waveforms and measurements of blood transit times through valves, from which pressure gradients can be measured. Echocardiography alone may be sufficient for the diagnosis of many valve conditions and angiography is only required for the exclusion of coronary artery disease.

Angiography

Catheterisation of both the right and left heart chambers with left ventricular angiography remains an important technique for determining the severity of valve disease. The pressure gradient across each valve and an assessment of ventricular function are made. The gradients measured directly at angiography tend to vary from those obtained from Doppler echocardiography. The latter is usually 20% higher because of a difference in the point in the cardiac cycle at which the two are measured. Definitive reference is made to mmHg measured at angiography.

SURGICAL MANAGEMENT

Indications for operation

Pressure gradients
- In excess of 50 mmHg (catheter) or 65 mmHg (Doppler) across the aortic valve
- In excess of 10 mmHg (catheter) or 13 mmHg (Doppler) across the mitral valve.

Size of valve orifice
- Less than 1.3 cm^2 in the mitral valve as measured by planimetry or velocity half-time at echocardiography.

Ventricular decompensation
- Progressive decompensation of left or right ventricle shown by dilatation or hypertrophy on serial studies of ECG, chest X-ray echocardiogram or angiogram.

Development of low cardiac output or lung congestion
- New or increasing symptoms.

Infection of a valve
- Lack of response to intensive antibacterial therapy
- Impending or actual major complications, such as abscess formation, increasing size of vegetations, embolisation or increasing functional cardiac deterioration with ventricular failure.

Age
Age may not necessarily be a contraindication to surgery, particularly with tight aortic valve stenosis, for which successful operations are not uncommonly carried out in patients up to 85 years of age, provided they are otherwise fit. Conversely, valve replacement is avoided in children and adolescents in order to achieve maximum growth of the annulus of a valve. Conservative procedures rather than replacement are preferred in

Table 17.10
Choice of operation on heart valves

Technique	Indication
Mechanical valve replacement	Up to age 65
Tissue valve replacement	Beyond age 65 Women of child-bearing age
Homograft replacement	Some complex problems; for other groups if freely available
Valve repair	Mitral or tricuspid stenosis treated by valvotomy, but with persistent regurgitation

children and there is also an increasing tendency in adults to conserve the mitral and tricuspid valves.

Choice of procedure

There are three options: replacement with either a mechanical or a tissue valve, the latter being a homograft (human) or a xenograft (animal – usually pig); and repair of the damaged tissue perhaps supplemented by prosthetic material (see Table 17.10).

The advantages and disadvantages of the three methods are given in Information Box 17.1.

Mechanical valves

These have been used unchanged for up to 24 years and include the Starr–Edwards silastic ball valve and the St Jude bi-leaflet pyrolytic carbon valve.

Tissue valves

Xenografts are currently mounted on a cloth-covered

mechanical stent and have opening characteristics more like those of human valves. Those manufactured recently have a cloth-covered support – a semi-rigid framework – without a stent (stentless).

Homografts are harvested at death and maintained sterile by antibiotics in a tissue bank until used. They are not mounted on a stent and in theory have satisfactory opening characteristics.

Repair

This technique is being increasingly developed and is becoming more effective particularly in the mitral and tricuspid valves. Conservation of the mitral valve by open valvotomy for mitral stenosis gives good long-term results. Mitral valve prolapse may be excised with subsequent reconstruction of the valve apparatus, including either cordal shortening or lengthening, cordal transfer or the creation of a new cord from PTFE (Goretex). Repair often requires an additional prosthetic annular ring both to narrow the dilated annulus and to prevent excess strain on the subvalvular mechanism. Conservation procedures on the aortic valve are under development.

ANTIBIOTIC MANAGEMENT

Prophylactic antibiotics are used during the insertion of valves and are essential for all subsequent operations of whatever nature, including dental and endoscopic procedures, particularly those which involve the lower bowel. Failure to use prophylaxis can lead to organisms released from operation sites into the blood lodging on

---

i Information Box 17.1

Advantages and disadvantages of different types of valve surgery

Procedure	Advantages	Disadvantages
Mechanical valve replacement	Should last for life Good haemodynamics Low incidence of infection Low incidence of re-operation	Absolute need for long-term anticoagulation Slightly increased risk of thromboembolic complications High risk of anticoagulant complications
Xenograft replacement	Anticoagulation not required after 3 months	Deterioration after 7–12 years – high re-operation rate (up to 30% at 10 years) Not to be used in children Increased risk of infection
Homograft	Anticoagulation not required	Difficult to obtain and often in short supply Prone to fungal infection Deteriorate over 20 years
Reconstruction	Most suitable for complex congenital problems and recurrent valve infection Low embolism incidence Long-term anticoagulation not required Low infection rate Improved ventricular contraction	Technically demanding Risk of rupture early postoperatively Inadequate repair may give poor results Long-term possibility of degeneration

a valve and initiating endocarditis. Common regimens are 1 g vincomycin or 1g ampicillin given 1 hour before operation and repeated 1 hour after the procedure is complete.

ANTICOAGULANT MANAGEMENT

Mechanical valves
Full anticoagulation with warfarin to an INR of 3.0 (range 2.8–3.6) is essential and must be continued for life. Aspirin and dipyridamole are not suitable substitutes for anticoagulation of mechanical valves. Dental treatment and other operations mean anticoagulants must be stopped 48–72 hours before and restarted 24 hours after the procedure – or earlier if there is no bleeding.

Xenografts and homografts with prosthetic rings
For the first 3 months, full anticoagulation to an INR of 2.5–3 is advised.

COMPLICATIONS OF OPEN HEART SURGERY
These are shown in Information box 17.2.

Cardiomyopathy

DEFINITION AND GENERAL FEATURES
The term cardiomyopathy refers to more than one type of muscle abnormality. The commonest is *hypertrophic obstructive cardiomyopathy* (hocum) – massive hypertrophy of the septum and muscle of the left ventricle leading to left outflow tract obstruction. Half of the cases are the result of a genetic disorder; the remainder are of unknown cause. There is associated abnormal movement of the mitral valve – systolic anterior movement of the posterior leaflet (SAM) which makes the outflow tract obstruction worse.

Dilated or congestive cardiomyopathy is failure of good myocardial contraction with a dilated left ventricular cavity without severe muscular hypertrophy. It may be of unknown cause or secondary to other conditions, which include amyloidosis, alcoholism, sarcoidosis, systemic lupus myocarditis and thyrotoxicosis.

Restrictive cardiomyopathies occur when the ventricles are of small size without muscular hypertrophy and with no ability to relax to provide an adequate filling volume. The cause is usually unknown although some of the above systemic causes may be present. One specific cause is eosinophilic myopathy in which eosinophils infiltrate into the endocardium producing fibrosis and restriction. This can be mistaken for constrictive pericarditis of tuberculous origin.

MANAGEMENT
In restrictive cardiomyopathy, endomyocardial de-

cortication with valve replacements for both and right and left ventricles may be required.

In cardiomyopathy with severe symptoms and cardiac failure and when medical management has nothing more to offer, transplantation may be indicated.

Transplantation

For details of organ retrieval and matching for transplantation see Chapter 13. Because the heart and lung are so intimately related, heart, lung and heart–lung transplants are considered here.

Heart transplantation
The results of cardiac transplantation are now good

enough for this to be used for patients with very severe cardiac conditions for which medical management can achieve nothing further.

INDICATIONS
- Severe cardiomyopathy
- Severe ischaemic heart disease, unsuitable for coronary bypass grafting or after repeated failure of that procedure
- Untreatable ventricular aneurysm
- End-stage valve disease
- Severe congenital cardiac abnormalities but normal lungs.

Positive criteria
- Age under 50
- Absence of generalised organ deterioration or failure
- No persistent causative problems (e.g. alcohol)
- No major psychological difficulties.

In patients who fall into the above groups, transplantation should be considered early. There is a significant mortality for those who have to wait for a transplant until their disease is in its end stages.

OPERATION
The heart, including the pulmonary and aortic valves, is removed, leaving atrial cuffs to which the atria of the donor heart are then anastomosed (Fig. 17.4a). The operation is completed by joining the pulmonary vessels and the supravalvular aorta of the recipient to the transplant (Fig. 17.4b).

RESULTS
These vary according to the selection of patients and also between different centres. In general in the UK, survivals are:

- 1 year – 72%
- 3 years – 67%
- 5 years – 62%.

Heart–lung transplantation

INDICATIONS

- Severe pulmonary hypertension
- End-stage mucoviscidosis (cystic fibrosis)
- Severe congenital cardiac abnormality.

A *domino* procedure can sometimes be used in which a patient with a normal heart but diseased lungs receives a heart–lung transplant and donates the heart to a second recipient. However, as success rates of lung transplantation improve, the procedure is less commonly used.

RESULTS
Results are not sufficiently encouraging for the procedure to be used widely, but special centres should continue to undertake it under carefully controlled conditions.

Single lung transplantation

INDICATIONS
The main indication is severe lung disease in young patients, particularly severe emphysema or obstructive airways disease. Freedom from current active infection is important.

RESULTS
These are a little more encouraging, although there are severe problems with infection in the lungs and with the breakdown of bronchial anastomoses. Current survival figures are:

- 1 year – 62%
- 3 years – 46%
- 5 years – 38%.

Conduct of thoracic and open heart operations

General
Nearly all procedures, and particularly those for infection or heart valve replacement, are done under peri-operative antibiotic prophylaxis (Ch. 9) and prophylaxis against deep vein thrombosis (Ch. 29).

Access
For cardiac surgery and transplantation this is nearly always by a median sternotomy, although more limited (minimal access) approaches are being developed for all types of cardiac procedures. Operations on the lungs are usually done through a thoracotomy, which is made by entering the chest through an intercostal space on one side below the scapula. Limited access incisions with video assistance are being developed.

Preoperative patient briefing
Patients should be introduced to the fast track or intensive care unit and have its environment made familiar. Any special problems relating to individual operations should, as far as possible, be explained. Physiotherapy is begun and the need for cooperation is emphasised.

Types of surgical procedure

Open heart surgery
The following apply:

- Intensive monitoring of cardiovascular function.

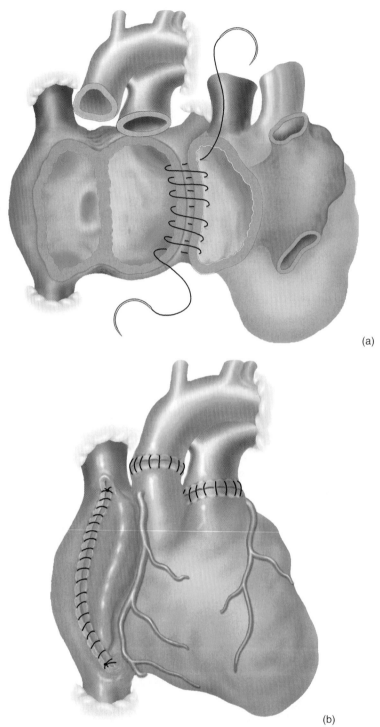

(a)

(b)

Fig 17.4 **The technique of cardiac transplantation.**

- *Heart–lung bypass* which means diverting the blood from the patients right atrium through a cannula to the heart-lung machine and returning the blood cooled (as required) and oxygenated via a cannula in the aorta under full heparinisation with heparin. The heart is usually stopped in asystole by infusing cold blood solutions containing rich potassium heart-stopping agents (cardioplegia) into the coronary arteries whilst the aorta is clamped, or its ejection may be prevented by inducing ventricular fibrillation electrically.

- *Beating heart surgery* in which the heart is allowed to beat normally without the use of the heart-lung bypass or cardioplegia but that part of the heart being operated on (coronary artery) is kept steady by the use of a mechanical stabiliser.

Pulmonary procedures

These are nearly all major operations and require assisted ventilation, often with a double lumen endotracheal tube to allow one lung to be let down whilst it is operated upon, and careful cardiovascular control.

POSTOPERATIVE MANAGEMENT

ITU/Fast track

Most cardiac surgical patients now go through a specialised cardiac surgical unit outside the ITU with less than a 24-hour stay (fast track unit): the most complex patients may still require intensive care unit stay. On return to the ward all patients are further monitored in a high-dependency area and early mobilisation and physiotherapy are essential in helping patients become able to be discharged home within one week of operation.

ITU/fast track monitoring involves:

- continuous ECG, pulse and arterial and central venous pressure monitoring
- digital oxygenation saturation probe
- hourly measure of urine output (patient catherised)
- hourly measure of peripheral and central temperature
- quarter hourly, later hourly, measure of blood loss from chest drains
- frequent arterial blood gas measurements for PO_2, PCO_2, pH and acid-base balance
- controlled infusion pumps for fluid and drug administration
- general neurological assessment.

Ventilation

Cardiac patients are ventilated until they are stable, rewarmed and are making good respiratory efforts with appropriately good arterial gases (usually 4–6 hours post operatively). Thoracic patients are extubated in theatre and sat up early to encourage better respiratory mechanics. They are usually managed in a general recovery area rather than fast track or ITU.

Pain control

Effective prevention of pain is of importance in all cardiothoracic surgery because it lessens the risk of postoperative myocardial events, improves postoperative respiratory movements and increases the value of physiotherapy.

Epidural analgesia and continuous opioid infusion controlled by the patient (patient-controlled analgesia, PCA) are common methods which may be combined with local analgesia block of intercostal nerves at the time of thoracotomy.

Chest drainage

All thoracic and cardiac drains are connected to a closed underwater system to prevent an open pneumothorax occuring and allow the lungs to maintain the normal negative intrathoracic pressure. Aditionally, low pressure suction is applied to encourage the release of air or blood from the operated site; this is particularly valuable after lung resection as suction helps the lung to seal its leaks by sticking to the chest wall.

Antithrombotic therapy

For CABG, aspirin (150 mg) is commenced on day 1 and continued long term. For valve patients, warfarin is commenced on day 1 and monitored to give an INR of 2.8–3.5. Mechanical valve replacement patients require warfarin for life. Tissue valve replacement and valve–repair patients often require warfarin for only 3 months. Subcutaneous heparin is given in hospital for embolism prophylaxis.

Long-term anti-thrombotic treatment depends on the procedure. After CABG with vein grafts, soluble aspirin 150 mg daily is combined in some centres with either dipyridamole or short-term warfarin. Heart valve replacement usually requires permanent oral anti-coagulation.

Return to full activities

Most patients are able to return to work or full activities 2–3 months after a CABG. Convalescence after thoracic procedures may be shorter but this depends on the degree of respiratory reserve available.

Secondary control of coronary risk factors is important long term. A statin drug is given to all hyperlipidaemic patients: hypertension and diabetes medication should be continued. Smoking must cease.

COMPLICATIONS

Patients who undergo cardiothoracic operations are subject to the same general complications as occur in all surgical procedures (Ch. 7). However, some complications are specific to the region or to the procedures involved.

Open heart surgery

Complications specific to open heart procedures are discussed in Chapter 17.

Pulmonary procedures

The common complications encountered are shown in Table 17.11.

Cardiac surgery

Table 17.11
Complications of pulmonary procedures

Nature	Cause	Effects	Management
Intraoperative haemorrhage	Injury to a major artery or vein – sometimes from vascular invasion by a tumour	Shock	Urgent control Transfusion
Postoperative haemorrhage	Slipped ligature Oozing from extensive raw surfaces Inadequate haemostasis	Shock	Urgent re-exploration Transfusion
Retained bronchial secretions	Poor respiratory reserve Poor pain control Inadequate respiratory effort	Respiratory failure Hypoxia Fatigue	Bronchoscopy Physiotherapy Mini-tracheostomy Tracheostomy Assisted ventilation
Pneumonia	Infected retained secretions Aspiration	Hypoxia Toxaemia	Antibiotics Physiotherapy Assisted ventilation
Bronchopleural fistula (after pneumonectomy)	Rupture of main bronchial suture line with severe breathlessness Shock	Aspiration of contents thoracic space	Urgent drainage of pneumonectomy space Bronchoscopy and operative repair Antibiotics Assisted ventilation
Other bronchopleural fistula	Persistent open distal bronchus	Excessive air bubbling from chest drain	Prolonged chest drainage with or without suction
Excess air leak	Damaged lung surface	Pneumothorax Inability to remove drain Prolonged hospital stay	Possible re-exploration
Other Wound infection Arrhythmias	Surgical technique Usually atrial fibrillation	Risk of cross-infection Low cardiac output	Antibiotics Drainage Digoxin, amiodarone Search for possible cause

Oesophagus, stomach and duodenum

Oesophagus

ANATOMICAL AND PHYSIOLOGICAL CONSIDERATIONS

The oesophagus is a muscular tube connecting the pharynx to the stomach lined predominantly by squamous epithelium and guarded at both ends by sphincters. It lies anterior to the cervical vertebrae in the neck and in the posterior mediastinum in the chest and enters the abdomen through the oesophageal hiatus in the diaphragm. The last 2–3 cm are within the abdomen above the gastro-oesophageal junction with the stomach. The anatomical relationships between the oesophagus and the other mediastinal structures are illustrated in Figure 18.1. The mucosal lining of the oesophagus is pale grey and consists of squamous epithelium. The musculature of the upper two-thirds of the oesophagus

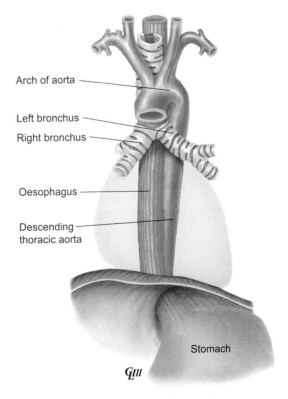

Arch of aorta

Left bronchus

Right bronchus

Oesophagus

Descending thoracic aorta

Stomach

Fig 18.1 **Anatomical relationships of the oesophagus.**

257

is striated (though not under voluntary control) and that of the distal third is smooth. In contrast to the majority of the intraperitoneal gastrointestinal tract, the oesophagus is devoid of a serosal layer – a matter of some importance to the spread of malignant disease. For descriptive purposes, tumours are usually classified as occurring in the upper, middle and lower thirds.

The two sphincters are at the pharyngo-oesophageal junction (upper) and in the region of the oesophageal opening (hiatus) in the diaphragm. Both have intrinsic and extrinsic components. The upper intrinsic sphincter has the main function of preventing access of air to the oesophagus and working in conjunction with laryngeal closure during swallowing. It relaxes on initiation of the swallowing reflex and the superior constrictor extrinsic component contracts to expel food or liquid into the oesophagus where a wave of peristalsis carries it downwards. Disorders of the upper sphincter are considered in Chapter 10.

The lower intrinsic sphincter is the circular smooth muscle of the oesophagus, although anatomical as distinct from physiological identification of a specific sphincter zone has proved difficult. Its role is to prevent gastro-oesophageal regurgitation and it is normally closed but relaxes in response to the swallowing wave. Relaxation may fail in oesophageal motility disorders or may be disordered in gastro-oesophageal reflux disease (GORD). The intrinsic sphincter is supplemented by the striated muscle of the right crus which splits to embrace the lower end of the oesophagus, but it is probably involved only in keeping the gastro-oesophageal junction closed when intra-abdominal pressure is significantly increased as in straining. Another factor which prevents reflux from the stomach is the acute angle of insertion of the oesophagus into the stomach which brings the gastric and oesophageal walls in contact when intra-abdominal pressure rises. Anatomical disorders at the diaphragmatic hiatus reduce the efficacy of the intrinsic sphincter (see 'Hiatus hernia').

CLINICAL FEATURES OF OESOPHAGEAL DISEASE

Symptoms

Dysphagia (difficulty in swallowing) may be:

- *progressive* when a lesion such as a malignant growth or a stricture reduces the size of the oesophageal lumen
- *non-progressive* in disorders of function either of the whole oesophagus or at the lower sphincter.

Progressive difficulty eventually goes on to total dysphagia when neither food, liquid nor the patient's own saliva can be swallowed. This circumstance is an emergency.

High grades of dysphagia are often associated with *regurgitation* into the pharynx and upper air passages and therefore with respiratory infection.

Pain is ill-localised in the chest (often called substernal but more correctly retrosternal) and may accompany partial dysphagia from obstruction. It also occurs in motility disorders. Confusion with pain originating in heart muscle is common.

Heartburn is a retrosternal sensation of discomfort and burning and may be a minor form of pain. It is the consequence of regurgitation from the stomach into the normally empty oesophagus. If there is considerable reflux, the patient may be conscious of the presence of liquid in the pharynx.

Signs

The deep situation of the oesophagus usually makes specific clinical features entirely absent. Those which may accompany individual disorders are considered below.

INVESTIGATION

Radiology

Anteroposterior plain X-ray may occasionally show a broadening of the mediastinal shadow by a dilated oesophagus but the finding is non-specific. An air–fluid level may be seen behind the heart if there is distal oesophageal obstruction.

Contrast radiology usually with barium sulphate but in special circumstances with a water-soluble contrast medium is the standard method of establishing both anatomical and functional abnormality.

Endoscopy

The flexible oesophago-gastroduodenoscope (see Ch. 4) is now often used as an alternative or complement to contrast radiology to achieve a diagnosis and has the advantage of being able to take tissue for histological examination.

Manometry

This investigation has an increasing role in the analysis of disorders of motility. In addition, similar equipment can be used for monitoring the acid level in the oesophagus in patients with suspected reflux and this is now an essential preliminary before attributing symptoms to gastro-oesophageal reflux. The technique is to place a pH sensor at the end of a tube in the lower oesophagus and to make continuous recordings over 24 hours. In normals there should be little change; however, in those with reflux of acid contents, the pH falls sporadically, particularly at night.

Motility disorders

Much has still to be learnt about these disorders, but a working classification is into those which involve:

- *hypermotility* – chiefly diffuse spasm
- *hypomotility* – usually secondary to systemic sclerosis (scleroderma)
- *sphincter dysfunction* – especially the inability of the lower sphincter to relax (achalasia).

Hypermotility
Diffuse oesophageal spasm

AETIOLOGY
The cause is unknown and the condition is rare – or at least rarely recognised. There may well be a physiological link between this condition and achalasia (see below).

CLINICAL FEATURES
The combination of intermittent, often quite severe, chest pain with dysphagia is characteristic. The condition may lead to investigation under a provisional diagnosis of angina pectoris.

INVESTIGATION AND MANAGEMENT
A contrast study shows exaggerated oesophageal contractions which may outline the gullet as a corkscrew. Oesophagoscopy is usually normal but manometry shows exaggerated contractions.

Drugs that reduce smooth muscle contraction (nitrates and calcium channel blockers such as nifedipine) occasionally help. Balloon dilatation is also an option, but in those with severe symptoms, a long oesophageal myotomy in which all layers of muscle down to mucosa are divided may be required.

Nutcracker (super-squeeze) oesophagus

It is uncertain whether this condition is a distinct entity. It is a common manometric finding in patients who present with chest pain which is of non-cardiac origin. The symptoms are the same as those for diffuse spasm, as is the management. However, surgical treatment is rarely required.

Hypomotility

The only well recognised disorder that causes hypomotility is *systemic sclerosis* – a condition of unknown cause. The muscle layer is replaced by fibrous tissue. The presence of the disease may be suspected from other features such as loss of mobility of the face and microvascular features, e.g. digital ischaemia.

INVESTIGATION AND MANAGEMENT
Contrast radiology shows diminished peristalsis and this can be confirmed by manometry. The treatment of hypomotility is that of the complications such as gastro-oesophageal reflux (see 'Hiatus hernia').

Achalasia

This is commonly known as *cardiospasm*

AETIOLOGY
In the great majority of patients the cause is unknown but a similar clinical condition is found in South America as a result of infection with a protozoan organism *Trypanosoma cruzi*. The lower sphincter fails to relax in response to the normal peristaltic wave and the bolus is partially retained in the oesophagus.

CLINICOPATHOLOGICAL FEATURES
Dilatation and muscular hypertrophy occur above the lower sphincter. Histological examination shows loss of ganglion cells (see also 'Hirchsprung's disease'). In long-standing cases the oesophagus becomes elongated and its mucosa inflamed from stasis of food. The latter finding is a probable cause of the development of malignant change.

There is not initially frank dysphagia but rather a slowing down of the normal rate of ingestion of food, so that at a meal the patient gets 'left behind.' Obvious dysphagia ultimately develops with retrosternal discomfort, regurgitation and weight loss. Onset of these symptoms in later life may lead to confusion between achalasia and carcinoma.

INVESTIGATION
Endoscopy is essential and in older patients may show a secondary cause such as infiltration of the distal oesophagus by malignant disease. Contrast study confirms delay at the lower sphincter, although in early symptomatic patients the abnormality may be difficult to identify. Manometry shows incomplete relaxation of the lower sphincter in response to a swallow.

MANAGEMENT
Medical treatment with muscle relaxants is usually unrewarding. The two effective methods are:

- *balloon dilatation*, which leads to resolution of symptoms in 80% although it may have to be repeated and carries a small risk of oesophageal perforation
- *Longitudinal myotomy* of the gastro-oesophageal junction (known to surgeons as Heller's operation) which can be done either at open operation or via a laparoscope or thoracoscope; some surgeons combine myotomy with an anti-reflux procedure.

Surgical myotomy is associated with a small risk of gastro-oesophageal reflux but is otherwise a very satisfactory procedure.

Endoscopic injection of botulinum toxin into the oesophageal wall to paralyse the lower oesophageal sphincter is currently being evaluated and may have a role in the treatment of achalasia.

Gastro-oesophageal reflux disorders (GORD)

Features of reflux occur in association with many different oesophageal conditions including most of the motility disturbances described above. However, reflux is particularly a symptom of abnormalities at the diaphragmatic hiatus.

PATHOPHYSIOLOGICAL FEATURES
If either acid or strongly alkaline (as may occur if there are large amounts of reflux from the duodenum) secretions reach the lower oesophagus, mucosal inflammation follows. Although this is mostly a superficial oesophagitis, there may be two consequences:

- *Stricture* – this is usually predominantly an inflammatory reaction in the mucosa and submucosa, but it can, if inflammation takes place, become a fibrous narrowing.
- *Metaplastic change* – this leads to the development of gastric-type columnar epithelium in the lower oesophagus. This was first described by a British surgeon (Norman Barrett) and is, in consequence, often known as 'Barrett's oesophagus'. Its significance is that it is a premalignant lesion: adeno-carcinoma of the lower oesophagus may follow.

CLINICAL SYNDROMES
There are two main causes:

- hiatus hernia with reflux
- reflux without abnormal anatomy.

Hiatus hernia

There are two types of hiatus hernia – sliding and para-oesophageal. Although only the first is usually associated with reflux, both will be considered here.

Sliding hernia

The proximal stomach ascends into the chest through a lax or enlarged diaphragmatic opening, taking a circum-

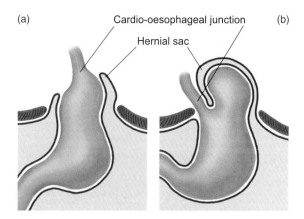

Fig 18.2 **(a) The oesophagastric anatomy in a sliding hiatus hernia. (b) The anatomy in a para-oesophageal hernia.**

ferential cuff of peritoneum with it. The normally acute oesophagogastric angle is reduced so that reflux is common even though the intrinsic lower sphincter is normal (Fig. 18.2a)

AETIOLOGY
Some examples of sliding hernia may be congenital but in most the cause is not established. Obesity, increase in abdominal contents (pregnancy) and ageing may be contributory factors.

CLINICAL FEATURES
There is postural reflux, heartburn and occasionally some lower left chest pain. However, the latter should only be ascribed to a postulated or actual hiatus hernia with caution. Vague indigestion is rarely caused by a sliding hernia and must be explored clinically and by investigation for an underlying cause.

INVESTIGATION
Patients with the recent onset of symptoms, particularly if they are elderly, should be investigated for possible oesophagogastric cancer.

Contrast radiography
The standard method of making the diagnosis is by barium swallow and meal although some cynics say that a determined radiologist can identify a hiatus hernia in almost anyone.

Endoscopy
Although it is not always easy to identify the oesophagogastric junction, this examination allows assessment of the severity of oesophagitis and a tissue diagnosis by examination of a biopsy may be made in a doubtful instance of Barrett's oesophagus.

pH Monitoring
As mentioned above, this is an essential preliminary to a decision about control of symptoms. Considerable

reflux which is difficult to control by posture is a relative indication for surgery.

MANAGEMENT

The great majority of patients can be managed by medical measures for the control of reflux, including:

- weight loss in the obese
- sleeping with the head of the bed raised to avoid nocturnal reflux
- alginate-containing antacids which are thought to reduce free liquid in the stomach and thus reduce the volume of reflux
- acid reduction by H_2-receptor antagonists (cimetidine or ranitidine) or proton pump inhibitors (omeprazole or lansoprazole)

If these measures fail and reflux and oesophagitis persist, surgery is indicated. However, it must be absolutely clear that the symptoms of which the patient complains are the consequence of the presence of the hernia, otherwise a dissatisfied patient will be the outcome. A surgical repair may be carried out at open operation, but is now usually carried out at laparoscopy. This involves:

- reduction of the herniated stomach below the diaphragm
- removal of the circumferential peritoneal sac
- re-establishment of the oesophagogastric angle
- an anti-reflux procedure – often loosely called a *fundoplication*.

The last procedure is increasingly used although it may not always be justified. The fundus of the stomach is wrapped around the terminal oesophagus so that, as intra-abdominal pressure rises, the oesophagus is compressed (Fig. 18.3). One complication of such a procedure may occasionally be the inability to belch and, in consequence, bloating – a sensation of unrelieved fullness of the stomach. In addition, some patients experience postoperative dysphagia which is usually transient. However, the outcome is usually satisfactory and surgery should not be withheld provided the gastro-enterologist and surgeon are satisfied with the relationship between the symptoms and the hernia – particularly given evidence from pH monitoring.

Para-oesophageal hernia

AETIOLOGY

A discrete peritoneal sac occurs at the left lateral border of the oesophagus and the fundus of the stomach rolls into this, sometimes carrying the oesophagogastric junction into the chest (Fig. 18.2b). More complicated examples may cause a twist of the whole stomach – a gastric volvulus.

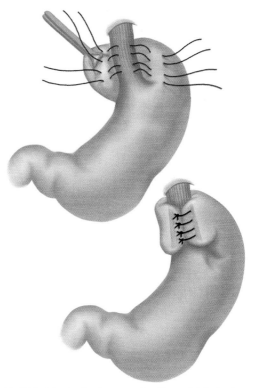

Fig 18.3 **A fundoplication operation.** The gastric fundus is wrapped around the abdominal oesophagus.

CLINICAL FEATURES

These patients are usually asymptomatic, although vague upper abdominal pain may occur. Incarceration going on to strangulation is not common but causes acute upper abdominal pain and what appears to be vomiting but is in fact total dysphagia. This occurrence – usually in elderly frail individuals – is a surgical emergency.

MANAGEMENT

Unless the patient is unfit, para-oesophageal hernias should be repaired surgically because of the risk of strangulation.

Reflux without abnormal anatomy

AETIOLOGY AND CLINICAL FEATURES

Many patients have symptoms of reflux without any demonstrable anatomical abnormality. In some, obesity is a factor; others may have hyperchlorhydria with or without a demonstrable peptic ulcer. In the majority a definite cause is not identified.

Features of heartburn and dyspepsia are universal, with regurgitation of gastric contents in some.

INVESTIGATION

Many patients are probably treated symptomatically in general practice without investigation. However, those with troublesome features should have a barium swallow and endoscopy. Ambulatory monitoring of lower oesophageal pH may establish that there is persistent reflux, and oesophageal manometry identifies those with a motility disorder.

MANAGEMENT

Medical management as described above is often sufficient. For those with oesophagitis which is unresponsive to treatment, an anti-reflux operation should be considered but only after careful assessment of the benefit that is likely to be achieved.

Oesophageal diverticula

Hypopharyngeal pouch is the most common of these. Other diverticula in lower parts of the oesophagus are rare.

Oesophageal rupture and mucosal tear (Mallory-Weiss syndrome)

AETIOLOGY

Vomiting is usually a coordinated event. The stomach and diaphragm contract so that intragastric pressure is raised; the oesophageal sphincters then relax, as does the oesophagus as a whole, and the stomach content is ejected. However, this orderly course may not take place if:

- voluntary inhibition is necessary
- vomiting is artificially induced
- the individual is confused – usually from excessive consumption of alcohol.

In such circumstances, intragastric pressure forces stomach contents into the distal oesophagus, dilating it. The oesophagus may rupture with emptying of stomach contents into the left pleural cavity or, because the relatively elastic muscle has a greater capacity for stretch than does the folded mucosa and submucosa, only these are split to produce a longitudinal tear at the oesophagogastric junction.

Oesophageal rupture

CLINICAL FEATURES

History

Forceful vomiting may be recalled, but if there has been much intake of alcohol it is sometimes forgotten. Vomiting may also have been induced either in a glutton or in someone who is mentally disturbed with a history of excessive eating but with the paradoxical desire not to gain weight (*bulimia*). There will be sharp left-sided pleuritic pain.

Physical findings

The effect of gastric content within the chest is to rapidly produce signs of severe sepsis with fever and circulatory disturbance. A left pleural effusion is present. The course is downhill with all the features of systemic inflammatory response syndrome. Occasionally, however, the rupture is localised and the patient is less ill with localised pleural signs and features of sepsis which are less severe. Nevertheless these are usually progressive.

MANAGEMENT

In early rupture, the oesophagus is exposed and repaired. Gastrostomy is often done to drain gastric secretions, although whether it is effective is not established. Parenteral or enteral (jejunostomy) nutrition is used until healing is assured.

Mucosal tear

The presentation of this condition is with haematemesis and it is therefore considered in Chapter 23.

Cancer of the oesophagus

EPIDEMIOLOGY

This condition is relatively rare in the Western world. However, studies have revealed a wide geographical variation with pockets of high incidence. For example, although the incidence in Europe overall is between 2 and 8 cases per 100 000 population, in some areas of northern France this figure may be as high as 30/100 000. In the Far East the incidence is in general much higher and may be between 100 and 150/100 000 in some provinces of China. Such a level warrants screening programmes within populations at high risk. Overall, the incidence is rising worldwide.

AETIOLOGY

Squamous carcinoma

The wide geographical variation in incidence has been

attributed to social and environmental factors. There appears to be a strong association between cigarette and alcohol consumption and the incidence of the disease. However, diet is probably of greatest importance. Three factors are recognised:

- high intake of nitrosamines derived from nitrates used in food preservatives
- low intake of both vitamin A and nicotinic acid
- iron deficiency anaemia is a known associate of hypopharyngeal cancer but is probably also a factor in cancer of the body of the oesophagus.

Long-standing achalasia may lead to cancer, presumably because of stasis and mucosal irritation. The reported incidence is highly variable but may reach 2%.

Adenocarcinoma

Metaplastic change in the oesophageal mucosa from squamous to columnar epithelium as a result of reflux predisposes to the development of adenocarcinoma. The magnitude of this risk is unknown; however, regular endoscopic biopsy in such patients, particularly if the reflux remains uncorrected, is indicated in an effort to detect malignant change early.

PATHOLOGICAL FEATURES

Nearly all lesions are a combination of *narrowing* and *ulceration*, although the extent of each varies. Spread takes place by:

- *Direct invasion* first through the full thickness of the oesophageal wall and thence into adjacent structures such as the trachea or bronchi, the pericardium, chest wall and diaphragm. Once a fistula into the air passages has occurred, the condition is incurable and life expectation is short.
- *Submucosal infiltration* both proximally and distally so that if mucosal destruction is used as an indication of the extent of spread there may be an underestimate of the extent of the growth.
- *Lymph node involvement* in the mediastinum and, in distal lesions, around the stomach – the pattern is often not sequential. Upward spread in the mediastinum may produce a sentinel node in the supraclavicular fossa.
- *The bloodstream* – this is unusual in the early stages, but by the time of death up to 90% of patients may have distant metastases (liver, lung and brain).

CLINICAL FEATURES

Symptoms

The mean duration of symptoms is 4–6 months but may be up to 3 years. To compound this, as is explained below, the average delay in presentation after their onset is 3–4 months.

Early ill-defined symptoms. The lack of well-defined symptoms while the disease is developing is one reason why so few cases of oesophageal cancer are diagnosed while the condition is still in a pathologically early stage. There may be a feeling of something stuck in the oesophagus, although not necessarily after eating. Retrosternal discomfort, belching and dyspepsia are often elicited on detailed questioning but may have been discounted by the patient.

Progressive dysphagia is the most common and important presenting symptom but may not be noticed until the oesophageal diameter is reduced by two-thirds. In the early stages, dysphagia is for solids only – particularly bulky foods such as meat and bread; only later is there difficulty with liquids. In the interim, most patients have simply accommodated to their symptoms by dietary alteration such as avoiding solids. Regurgitation after eating may be misinterpreted as vomiting and in consequence there may be delay until dysphagia is total (inability to swallow saliva).

Weight loss. As dysphagia develops there is usually an associated dramatic decline in weight. More than 10–15% of the pre-illness weight may be lost over 4–6 weeks.

Acute obstruction. A sudden acute obstruction may occasionally be precipitated in a symptomless patient by the impaction of a large (usually inadequately chewed) food bolus.

Miscellaneous. For those patients who have developed an adenocarcinoma in an area of columnar metaplasia, a long history of *heartburn* suggestive of acid reflux may be elicited but is rarely volunteered. *Pain* is ominous and may indicate penetration of the tumour outside the wall of the oesophagus. *Productive cough*, particularly at night, may be produced either by aspiration of retained material into the respiratory tract or by the development of a malignant oesophagotracheal fistula. *Hoarseness* may mean involvement of the recurrent laryngeal nerve. Features of *distant metastases* can be the cause of presentation of a few patients.

Signs

Clinical examination of a patient with localised oesophageal cancer usually does not reveal any abnormalities other than evidence of recent weight loss. Total dysphagia is associated with signs of lack of water – reduced skin turgor and a coated furred tongue. A quarter of patients have palpable lymphadenopathy, which is usually in the supraclavicular region and is an indication of metastatic disease. Other signs of dissemination include hepatomegaly, jaundice, ascites, cardiac arrhythmias and features of pulmonary consolidation. Although the last may indicate advanced disease, respiratory infection may develop because of aspiration of oesophageal content.

INVESTIGATION

Every patient with the suspicion of oesophageal malignancy must have a contrast radiographic study and an endoscopy.

Radiography

Barium swallow has the advantages of:

- simplicity
- relative lack of expense
- high sensitivity in diagnosis of a stricture although this does not necessarily indicate that it is malignant
- Accurate determination of the anatomical site
- Definition of the anatomy of the stomach and duodenum – important for surgical planning
- Creation of a 'road map' for endoscopy and thus a reduction in the risk of perforation, as well as indicating the level at which a lesion is likely to be found.

For several of these reasons, imaging by contrast study is the preferred first investigation.

Endoscopy

This procedure is now usually done with a flexible instrument under local anaesthesia. It allows:

- biopsy and brush cytology
- assessment (partial) of the extent of the lesion
- concurrent dilatation and temporary relief of obstruction.

However, it has some dangers, such as:

- failure to detect a small lesion – though in experienced hands this is rare
- perforation of a growth – flexible instruments make this unlikely.

Further investigation

Once the diagnosis is confirmed, further study is required to assess the stage of the disease and determine the suitability of the patient for operative treatment.

Ultrasound examination

This may demonstrate liver metastases and also enlarged lymph nodes. Recently it has become possible to obtain images from an ultrasound probe attached to an endoscope within the oesophagus (endoscopic ultrasound), which can measure the depth of penetration of the growth into the oesophageal wall and assess enlargement of mediastinal lymph nodes.

Computerised tomography

CT scan of both chest and abdomen may also detect metastases but is also helpful in determining the size of the primary and whether it is attached to surrounding structures. A fistula into the air passages may also be detected in which case a bronchoscopy should be done for confirmation.

SCREENING

The relative rarity of the condition in the Western societies makes screening economically inappropriate.

However, in places where the incidence is high (such as China and Japan), routine flexible oesophagoscopy and/or obtaining oesophageal specimens for cytology are increasingly being recommended to detect early asymptomatic disease. The efficacy of this approach is still under evaluation.

MANAGEMENT

The only treatment option that presents any prospect for cure is surgical resection. The majority of patients in the Western world have advanced tumours and palliation – usually of dysphagia – is the chief objective. Surgical resection for this purpose is still an option and gives good quality of life at the expense of a major procedure.

Surgical resection

The use of resection is still controversial in that a major operation is required (but see below) and that, except for tumours confined to the mucosa, the long-term outcome is poor. Indeed some believe that all resections should be regarded as palliative rather than curative; however, the contrary view is that there is a possibility of long-term survival and that this slim chance justifies the high risk of operation. The current compromise is that surgical removal gives good palliation with the occasional bonus of permanent cure and this attitude makes a decision relatively simple.

The procedure is offered to patients who are in good condition and where investigation has shown that there is a chance of removing all local tumour. Contraindications are:

- poor cardiovascular, pulmonary or renal function
- tracheo-oesophageal fistula
- other evidence of advanced local disease
- irremovable or multiple metastatic disease.

Asymptomatic and small metastases may, on occasion, not be a contraindication to the restoration of satisfactory swallowing by resection but other methods should be considered (see below).

The principles of resection with cure in mind are:

- wide resection margins
- radical lymph node clearance within the chest and for distal growths at the oesophagogastric junction also in the upper abdomen.

The conventional method of resection is by open operation which may involve opening both the abdomen and thorax. However two alternatives are now available:

Trans-hiatal removal. The abdomen alone is opened and the oesophagus freed in the chest by blunt dissection through the diaphragmatic hiatus. Stomach or colon for reconstruction is then passed through the posterior mediastinum to the neck where it is anastomosed to the upper oesophagus through a cervical incision.

Endoscopic removal. The whole procedure can now be done endoscopically by dissection within the chest (thorascopy) and abdomen (laparoscopy), although there is no evidence that this method is better than open operation.

Other methods of restoring swallowing

In patients unsuitable for surgical treatment other methods can be used to relieve dysphagia:

Radiotherapy for squamous carcinoma. Relief is not immediate, is usually temporary and up to one-third of patients develop a fibrous stricture.

Chemotherapy (5-fluouracil [5-FU] and cisplatin) either alone or preferably in combination with radiotherapy may lead to total disappearance of the local tumour in one quarter of patients. However, recurrence after some months is inevitable.

Dilatation and intubation with a large specially designed tube were formerly popular. However, fracture of the growth with later perforation was not uncommon and often fatal; the quality of swallowing was not very good; regurgitation and aspiration could occur and, in distal tumours, migration of the tube into the stomach frequently took place. Such tubes have now been replaced by expanding metal endoprostheses – some of which are covered with a plastic membrane and carry less problems of insertion and the possibility of better palliation.

Local endoscopic destruction of the tumour by laser which can be repeated.

Local injection of absolute alcohol via the endoscope is cheaper than the use of a laser and appears to be almost equally effective but usually requires repeated treatments.

PROGNOSIS

The outcome of resection depends on the stage of the growth. When tumour is confined to the mucosa, a 5-year survival of 60% is possible, but any further spread means a fall-off to less than 5% in growths that have penetrated the full thickness of the gullet. Combined regimens of resection and neoadjuvant combinations of radiotherapy and chemotherapy have yielded marginally better results.

Stomach and duodenum

Peptic ulcer disease

Surgeons are now mainly called on to treat the complications of this condition (see Box 18.1), but to do so they require some understanding of the causative mechanisms responsible, the pathological changes and their effects.

> **Box 18.1**
>
> *Indications for surgical intervention in peptic ulcer*
>
> **Urgent complications**
>
> Bleeding (Ch. 22)
>
> Perforation (Ch. 22)
>
> **Obstruction** – usually by inflammation and fibrosis at the outflow of the stomach
>
> **Failure of non-operative treatment (now rare)** – persistent intractable symptoms; need to take non-steroidal anti-inflammatory drugs (NSAIDs)
>
> **Possible malignancy** – gastric 'ulcer' (always a primary cancer which has been partially digested)

EPIDEMIOLOGY

There is a close association between peptic ulcer disease and poor socioeconomic conditions and their consequences. Hence the condition is more common in the developing rather than the developed world: relevant factors may be tobacco and alcohol consumption, which tend to be higher amongst the poor and deprived; however, *Helicobacter pylori* infection is probably the most important reason.

In duodenal ulcer, males outnumber females by a factor of 4, but gastric ulcer is equally distributed and its incidence increases with age.

AETIOLOGY

The classical hypothesis for the occurrence of most duodenal ulcers was that acid secretion is increased, so exposing the first part of the duodenum to greater acid-pepsin digestion. Gastric ulceration was looked upon as an outcome of gastritis of unknown cause with secondary acid-peptic digestion. However, these simple views have been greatly modified by the discovery of Helicobacter pylori as a strong associate of peptic ulceration in both the stomach and duodenum, and the additional observation that its eradication can lead to cure. The mechanisms by which the organism exerts it effects, and particularly the way in which it causes the acid hypersecretion commonly seen in duodenal ulcer, are still uncertain.

A relationship is also apparent between acute peptic ulceration and the consumption of non-steroidal anti-inflammatory agents (NSAIDs). Patients, particularly those who are elderly, are increasingly being prescribed these drugs and therefore there is a rising incidence of acute ulceration with complications such as perforation and haemorrhage. It is not clear whether the relationship implies a cause of peptic ulceration, but it seems more

Table 18.1
Contributing factors in the cause of peptic ulcer

Factor	Site of ulcer	Presumed mechanism
Genetic susceptibility	Duodenum	Non-secretors of blood Group O into gastric secretions
Hyperchlorhydria	Duodenum	Increased number of acid secreting cells in stomach (increased parietal cell mass-? also genetic)
Hyperparathyroidism	Duodenum	Hypercalcaemic stimulation of acid secretion
Benign or malignant gastrinoma (Zollinger–Ellison syndrome)	Stomach and duodenum	Unchecked gastrin hypersecretion
Non-steroidal anti-inflammatory drugs (NSAIDs)	Stomach and duodenum (usually acute)	Imbalance between mucosal regeneration and acid-pepsin digestion (speculative)

likely that NSAIDs upset the balance between mucosal regeneration and repair and therefore present a hazard for anyone who also has a peptic ulcer.

Other antecedents of peptic ulcer which can have a bearing on management are shown in Table 18.1.

ANATOMICAL AND PATHOLOGICAL FEATURES

These features are of mucosal loss accompanied by chronic inflammation with varying amounts of fibrosis. An ulcer penetrates to a varying depth in the gastric or duodenal wall and may involve neighbouring organs such as the pancreas. Free perforation into the peritoneal cavity takes place when the rate of ulceration exceeds that of repair and the final event is that the base of the ulcer becomes necrotic and gives way. An artery in the base may undergo fibrinoid necrosis of its media so that it becomes rigid and therefore more difficult for natural processes to close should bleeding take place; this is a more likely explanation of continued bleeding than the presence of atherosclerosis in the arteries of the gastric or duodenal wall, which is almost unknown.

Gastric ulcers can occur anywhere but are most commonly found on the lesser curvature at the junction of antral and acid-secreting mucosa. It used to be thought that a benign gastric ulcer could undergo malignant change, but what appear to be instances of this are merely partial peptic digestion of a primary malignant tumour.

CLINICAL FEATURES

Symptoms

Both gastric and duodenal ulcer cause epigastric pain and it is often difficult to distinguish one from the other, although it is often stated that patients with gastric ulcer have pain on eating and those with duodenal ulcer complain when they are hungry. Pain felt in or going through to the back can mean that the ulcer has penetrated into retroperitoneal structures such as the pancreas. Indigestion is often associated with the pain. Heartburn from acid-peptic reflux is common. Symptomatic episodes with temporary remissions which can last weeks or months are more characteristic of duodenal than gastric ulcer. In both, the symptoms are relieved by antacids.

Vomiting is seen in gastric outflow obstruction (usually from a duodenal ulcer, although a pyloric channel gastric ulcer can also be the cause). Obstruction is the consequence of inflammatory oedema and/or fibrosis. In the first it subsides with effective anti-ulcer treatment; in the second it persists. The vomitus is usually free from bile and may contain partially digested food, recognisable as a meal taken a day or more before. Patients with gastric outflow obstruction often lose weight, but unless the obstruction is complete and vomiting profuse, they do not become dehydrated in that absorption of water and electrolyte still takes place across the gastric wall.

Signs

In uncomplicated peptic ulcer, epigastric tenderness is the only feature and even this is non-specific as a mild degree of tenderness can be present in normal people. Obstruction is associated with a succussion splash – a splashing sound heard upon gently rocking the patient's abdomen to and fro. When obstruction is present, there may be signs of weight loss and of extracellular fluid volume deficiency with a lax dry skin and empty collapsed veins. Features of hypokalaemia such as drowsiness are the consequence of:

- loss of hydrogen ion from the stomach
- compensatory renal excretion first of sodium ions but later, and more importantly, of potassium ions.

INVESTIGATION

Endoscopy

The current initial investigation of the patient with indigestion which suggests peptic ulceration is by this means, although, if this is the first episode, young patients (< 40 years) may be treated symptomatically in the first instance. The whole of the upper GI tract, from the oesophagus to at least the junction of the first and second parts of the duodenum, is examined. All gastric ulcers are subjected to biopsy and brush cytological examination. Duodenal ulcers are assessed for their depth and degree of obstruction and for any stigmata which suggest bleeding. Repeat endoscopy may be used to follow the success or otherwise of treatment but is essential for those with a gastric ulcer.

Contrast radiography

Before the development of flexible endoscopy, a double contrast barium meal was the usual method of investigation in suspected ulcer disease and it is still widely used. Ulcers are identified as craters which retain a fleck of barium and the surrounding mucosal oedema can also often be shown.

Biochemical investigations

Measurement of gastric acid secretion is no longer done routinely, although in those with duodenal ulcer, acid output is usually raised. Such investigation may have a small place in assessment of:

- suspected gastrin-induced hyperchlorhydria (Zollinger–Ellison syndrome)
- peptic ulcer recurrence after surgical treatment (see below).

Gastric outflow obstruction. If this is suspected, serum concentrations of sodium, potassium and chloride and the arterial $P\text{CO}_2$ level should be measured, especially if operation is contemplated.

MANAGEMENT

Uncomplicated peptic ulcer is treated by:

- *Regimens to eradicate H. pylori* using antibiotics such as amoxycillin and metronidazole or clarithromycin in combination with acid-reducing proton pump inhibitors (omeprazole or lansoprazole).
- *Reduction of acid secretion* with H_2-receptor antagonists such as cimetidine and ranitidine; or with proton pump inhibitors, which block the hydrogen– potassium adenosine triphosphate enzyme system in the gastric (parietal) cells that secrete acid.

The place of surgery

There is no doubt that surgical procedures can reduce acid output and, because the final common pathway to peptic ulcer is the action of acid-pepsin on the gastroduodenal mucosa, they may prevent ulceration. However, as more effective agents for treatment have been developed, and particularly as the elimination of *H. pylori* seems to be able to produce permanent cure, elective operation is hardly ever used, at least in developed countries. The indications that remain are given in Box 18.1 and usually necessitate an additional procedure in association with an acid reduction operation. Two principles are used:

- reduction of the parietal cell mass by removal of part of the stomach – *partial gastrectomy* (Figs 18.4a and b)
- elimination of the *cephalic phase* of acid secretion by division of the vagus nerve (*total, selective or highly selective vagotomy*) (Fig. 18.4c).

Both methods are effective in healing ulcers but both have disadvantages, which are summarised in Table 18.2.

COMPLICATIONS

Perforation. See Chapter 22..

Bleeding. See Chapter 22.

Gastric outflow obstruction. A trial of non-operative treatment is undertaken because the features of obstruction may stem from inflammation and oedema. If this fails, then fibrosis is present and a bypass (gastroenterostomy) is necessary. Rarely the anatomy at the pyloroduodenal junction necessitates a partial gastrectomy.

Gastrocolic fistula. In Zollinger–Ellison syndrome and, in the past, after simple gastroenterostomy, an ulcer may penetrate from stomach to colon and cause faecal contamination of the stomach and small bowel. The result is intractable diarrhoea. Complicated surgical procedures are then required after acid secretion has been brought under control.

Gastroduodenal tumours

The only common tumour of the stomach is cancer. Occasionally benign *leiomyomata* are found in the stomach and duodenum, as are *polyps*. Cancer arising in the duodenum is very rare and probably originates from the periampullary mucosa at the lower end of the common bile duct.

Gastric cancer

EPIDEMIOLOGY

After cancer of the colon, rectum and pancreas, carcinoma of the stomach is the most common cause of death from gastrointestinal cancer, and also the third most common cause of cancer death in men and the fourth in women. However, in the Western world, the incidence of this condition has diminished: in England and Wales in 1960 there were around 14000 recorded deaths compared with just over 10 000 in the mid 1980s. However, over the last decade there has been a marked rise in the incidence of adenocarcinoma around the oesophagogastric junction including the gastric cardia.

As with oesophageal cancer, there is a worldwide variation in incidence: more common in the East (China and Japan) than the West. Even in the West, racial differences occur: proximal tumours are more commonly seen in whites. The peak age distribution is 50–70 years, but the disease can occur at any age from early adulthood; 5% of patients are less than 35 years of age. Gastric cancer is predominantly a male disease (M:F ratio = 3:1).

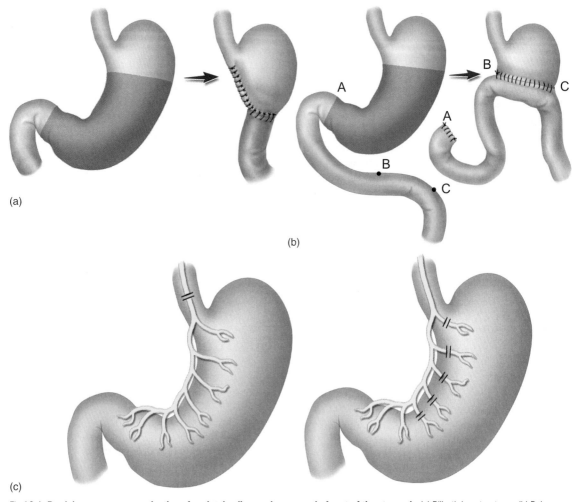

Fig 18.4 **Partiel gastrectomy – reduction of parietal cell mass by removal of part of the stomach.** (a) Billroth I gastrectomy. (b) Polya (or Billroth II) gastrectomy. (c) Vagotomy – can be either (i) truncal, or (ii) highly selective with preservation of the antral and pyloric innervation.

Table 18.2
Operative procedures to reduce acid-pepsin secretion

Operation	Mechanism	Severity	After Effects
Partial gastrectomy	Reduces parietal cell mass and antral gastrin secreting cells	Major procedure	Destroys pylorus and may result in dumping syndrome with weight loss and diarrhoea. Gastric atrophy may predispose to late gastric cancer
Total vagal pyloric section (vagotomy)	Removes cephalic phase of acid secretion	Less severe procedure than gastrectomy	Requires destruction (pyloroplashy) or bypass (gastroenterostomy): dumping may result
Highly selective vagotomy	As total vagotomy	Benign procedure. Possible by laparoscope	Minimal side effects; procedure of choice

AETIOLOGY

The cause is largely unknown. The most likely proximate pathological event is gastric atrophy which causes hypochlorhydria and is a consequence of:

- prolonged *H. pylori* infection after initial active chronic gastritis

- pernicious anaemia
- gastric operations for peptic ulcer, particularly partial gastrectomy; the *lead time* is long – up to 25 years – but the widespread use of this type of operation in the 1950s and 1960s has led to the suggestion that those who have been subjected to it

should have routine endoscopic follow-up (see 'Screening').

Contributory factors may be:

- nitrate intake (see 'Oesophageal cancer')
- smoking

A few tumours may originate in adenomatous polyps or dysplastic mucosa but this is rare in contrast to the colon (see Ch. 12).

PATHOLOGICAL FEATURES

At the time of clinical presentation, most cancers of the stomach are microscopically if not macroscopically advanced. The gross disease is of four types (Fig. 18.5). Microscopically, the great majority of tumours are adenocarcinomas of columnar or cuboidal type, but classifications based on cellular patterns are not of value in prognosis. Adenocarcinoma is a locally invasive tumour which directly infiltrates the full thickness of the gastric wall to involve the serosal layer and contiguous structures such as the pancreas, transverse mesocolon, or left lobe of the liver (free perforation into the peritoneal cavity occurs in only 1%). Peritoneal seeding (transcoelomic spread) may then take place with either diffuse nodules and ascites or deposits on the ovaries in the female (Krukenburg tumours) or in the rectovesical or rectovaginal pouch (Fig. 18.6). In addition gastric cancer is a good example of a tumour which spreads via lymphatic channels to local and regional lymphnodes (Fig. 18.7). These two features – serosal and lymphatic involvement – are the most important determinants of long-term survival

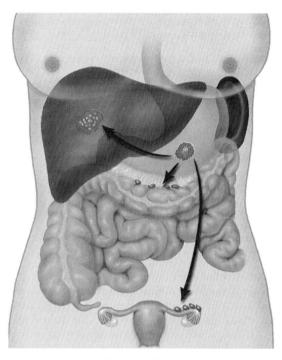

Fig 18.6 **Peritoneal seeding in a patient with gastric carcinoma.**

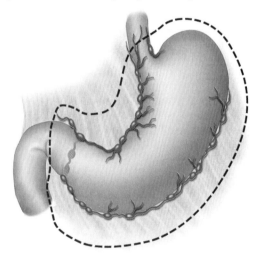

Fig 18.7 **The local and regional lymph nodes surrounding the carcinoma.**

following surgical resection. Liver metastases are, unlike colon cancer, a late feature.

STAGING

Rather than histological classification of the primary tumour, pathological staging (see Ch. 5) is a more useful indicator of prognosis. A number of staging systems have been devised, the most popular of which are the Union International Contra Cancer (UICC) stage and the TNM system. Comparison of the two for gastric cancer are given in Table 18.3 together with 5-year

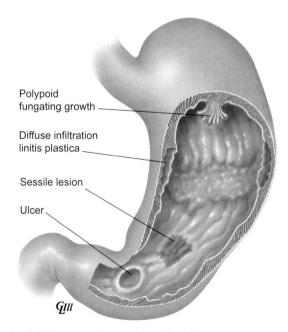

Polypoid fungating growth

Diffuse infiltration linitis plastica

Sessile lesion

Ulcer

Fig 18.5 **Macroscopic types of gastric carcinoma.**

Table 18.3
Staging, treatment and survival in carcinoma of the stomach

UICC Stage	TNM Stage	Method of treatment	5-year survival (%)
I	$T_1N_0M_0$	Radical resection	70
II	$T_2N_0M_0$	Radical resection	30
III	$T_{0-4}N_{1-3}M_0$	Radical resection	10
IV	$T_4N_3M_{0-1}$	Palliation	1–2

survivals after radical resection. UICC stage I ($T_1N_0M_0$) is often called 'early gastric cancer' and implies that the disease has not spread beyond the submucosa. At this stage, there is a high possibility of a cure (see 'Prognosis', below).

CLINICAL FEATURES

Failure to recognise the early features (chiefly symptoms) and to submit the patient to appropriate investigation and biopsy as soon as possible is an all too common occurrence in patients with gastric cancer. As with all gastrointestinal cancer, it cannot be sufficiently emphasised that early diagnosis is the key to cure.

Symptoms

Early tumours are usually without symptoms and are only detected by screening endoscopy. The nature and frequency of symptoms are shown in Box 18.2 and lead to some general principles:

- Any feature of dyspepsia in a previously asymptomatic individual over the age of 40 should always be viewed with the gravest suspicion and presumed to be caused by carcinoma of the stomach until proven otherwise.
- Anorexia is common and rarely is the only symptom of an early lesion.
- Dysphagia is usually associated with proximal lesions.
- Weight loss and abdominal pain are the most common symptoms, and the frequent occurrence of the first is a reflection of the advanced nature of the majority of tumours.
- Significant bleeding – haematemesis and/or melaena – is not all that common, but all gastric cancers cause some oozing and this may be sufficient to produce microcytic hypochromic anaemia with the non-specific symptoms of lassitude and fatigue (see below)
- Tumours within the antrum and pylorus present with the symptoms of gastric outflow obstruction – fullness, nausea and vomiting.

Physical findings

The best circumstance is not to find any abnormalities. The frequency of occurrence of individual signs is

Box 18.2

Symptoms and signs of carcinoma of the stomach

Symptoms

Weight loss (72%)

Pain (51%)

Nausea/vomiting (40%)

Anorexia (35%)

Abdominal discomfort (22%)

Dysphagia (22%)

Melaena (20%)

Upper gastrointestinal bleeding (11%)

Signs

Weight loss (26%)

Abdominal mass (17%)

Abdominal tenderness (15%)

Hepatomegaly (13%)

Rectal 'shelf' (4%)

Cervical lymphadenopathy (4%)

Ascites (3%)

given in Box 18.2. Signs of gastric outflow obstruction may be present. The presence of metastatic spread is indicated clinically by:

- a hard lymph node in the left supraclavicular fossa at the junction of the thoracic duct with the subclavian and internal jugular veins
- ascites
- irregular hepatomegaly
- a hard 'shelf' anteriorly on rectal examination.

SCREENING

Routine endoscopic screening has been widely adopted in Japan where the disease is much more common than in Europe. Because the disease occurs less frequently in the West, screening is not cost-effective. Screening of those at high risk (pernicious anaemia and after gastric surgery) has also been suggested but not uniformly applied, and in consequence there is little information on its value.

INVESTIGATION

In a patient suspected of having a carcinoma of the stomach, the following investigations are appropriate.

Faecal occult blood analysis

This is positive in 80% but the investigation is non-specific.

Oesophagogastroscopy

This is the most sensitive procedure for determining the presence or absence of a gastric neoplasm. It provides information on the anatomical site and enables multiple biopsies and brush cytology to be taken. However, if the histological and cytological reports on a gastric ulcer fail to show malignant cells, this must not be taken as absolute proof that the condition is benign. A short period (6–8 weeks at the most) of appropriate treatment for peptic ulcer is given and the examination repeated. Even if there are signs of healing, this does not mean the lesion is benign and careful examination of further biopsies is necessary.

Imaging

Double contrast barium meal. This examination can provide similar information to that of endoscopy but cannot reliably detect early cancer or give pathological confirmation of the disease.

Computerised axial tomography and ultrasound may be helpful by their ability to demonstrate the presence of unsuspected liver or other distant metastases. Both may also help to decide on resectability (sometimes called 'operability', which is distinct from 'curability').

Haemoglobin level and red cell morphology

It is important to recognise that to discover microcytic hypochromic anaemia in a patient with gastrointestinal symptoms is not to have made a diagnosis which initiates a course of treatment but only to have elicited a sign, which should lead to an urgent search for a source of blood loss within the gastrointestinal tract.

Almost half of those with gastric cancer are anaemic and this may require correction by transfusion. In some with unresectable tumours, repeated blood transfusions may be the only palliative procedure possible.

Laparoscopy

This procedure has contributed considerably to identifying irresectability, particularly by the detection of small liver or peritoneal metastases. Laparoscopy is now usually done before a laparatomy is undertaken.

MANAGEMENT

Cure

The only curative treatment is surgical resection. In the UK, only 30–40% of patients are suitable for an attempt at cure, although up to 70% of growths may be resectable. Resection for cure means removal of the growth, the stomach or a large proportion of it and the regional lymph nodes as a single anatomical block. The extent of resection is a subject of debate. In Japan, where the best results are obtained the stomach is removed together with the nodes within 3 cm of the tumour (N1) and the regional nodes (N2), sometimes with even more radical node resections (N3). In the West, many surgeons question the use of such radical resections because of a higher operative mortality and morbidity and the lack of randomised controlled trials which show a survival benefit; they prefer partial resections of the stomach and the N1/N2 nodes only. The methods of reconstruction after resection are shown in Figure 18.8.

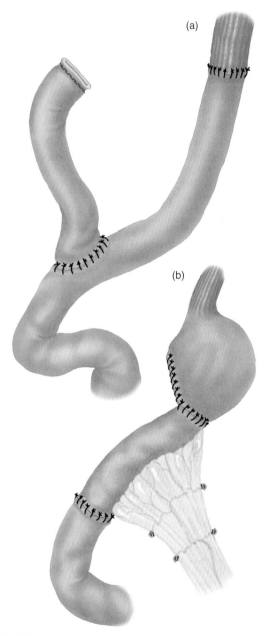

(a)

(b)

Fig 18.8 **Types of reconstruction after gastrectomy.**

Preoperative total parenteral nutrition (TPN) is indicated only in those patients with objective criteria of malnutrition. In this group, postoperative infections are diminished by nutritional support, but TPN has no other impact on mortality and morbidity.

Palliation

Surgical resection

This may be done in spite of nodal or metastatic disease that makes cure impossible. Such treatment often alleviates troublesome symptoms such as abdominal pain, dysphagia, blood loss and vomiting. However, because of late diagnosis and advanced disease, bypass of an obstructing lesion in the distal part of the stomach may be all that is possible.

Laser ablation

For unresectable tumours at the cardia, considerable improvement in swallowing may be obtained by the use of a laser through the endoscope so as to core out a passage through an obstruction. Repeated treatments throughout the remaining life of the individual are required and can occasionally be supplemented by the endoscopic insertion of a tube across the malignant stricture.

Chemotherapy

Until recently, chemotherapy has been relatively ineffective, and even now probably should not be used other than in clinical trials. However, there is recent evidence that a considerable proportion of patients respond to chemotherapy with carboplatin-based regimens. This may be at the cost of myelotoxicity and alopecia. Measurement of tumour markers such as plasma CEA or CA-50 may be useful in assessing response.

PROGNOSIS

The relationship between stage and prognosis has been given in Table 18.3. In consequence, in the West the outlook for most patients is poor and is rather worse for patients with tumours of the cardia and fundus than for those with antral lesions. Increasing the public and general practitioner awareness of the importance of prompt investigation of new dyspeptic symptoms should result in more patients being identified who are suitable for curative resection.

FURTHER READING

Oesophagus

De Vita VT, Hellmann S, Rosenbergy SA (eds) (1993) *Cancer: Principles and Practice of Oncology*, 4th edn. Philadelphia: Lippincott.

Hennessy TPJ, Cuschieri A (1986) *Surgery of the Oesophagus*. London: Baillière Tindall.

Jamieson GG (ed.) (1988) *Surgery of the Oesophagus*. Edinburgh: Churchill Livingstone.

19

Liver and biliary tree

Hepatic and biliary anatomy

Liver

The liver is adherent at the bare area below the under-surface of the diaphragm surrounded by the peritoneal reflections which form the coronary and triangular ligaments (Fig. 19.1). It is also supported by the falciform ligament.

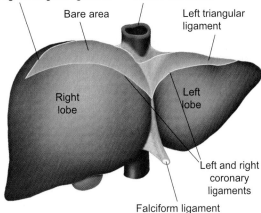

Superior view

Right triangular ligament

Inferior vena cava

Bare area

Left triangular ligament

Right lobe

Left lobe

Left and right coronary ligaments

Falciform ligament

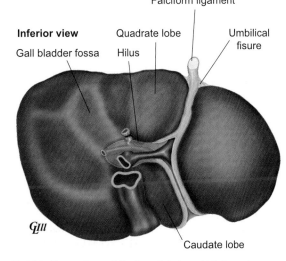

Inferior view

Quadrate lobe

Umbilical fisure

Gall bladder fossa

Hilus

Caudate lobe

Fig 19.1 **The anatomy of the liver.** Anterior and inferior surface view.

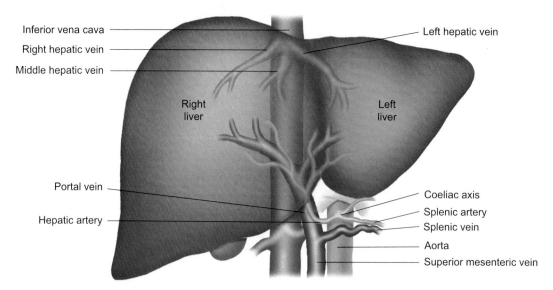

Fig 19.2 **The blood supply to and drainage from the liver.**

Blood supply (Fig. 19.2)

The liver derives blood from the hepatic artery (25%) and the portal vein (75%). The hepatic artery usually arises from the aorta at the coeliac axis and divides into the right and left branches at the hilus. The portal vein is formed behind the pancreas from the superior mesenteric and splenic veins and runs at the back of the free edge of the lesser omentum; at the hilus it divides into right and left branches.

The venous drainage from the liver is by three large hepatic veins – right, middle and left – into the inferior vena cava (IVC), just below the diaphragm. Their confluence with the IVC can be obstructed to produce one form of portal hypertension – the Budd–Chiari syndrome.

Anatomical sectors

These have recently become of more importance as technical advances have made removal of diseased segments feasible.

The organ is divided into two units of function with separate blood supply and biliary drainage, either of which can sustain life if the other is removed. The plane between them extends between the gall bladder fossa anteriorly and the inferior vena cava posteriorly (Fig. 19.3). Surgical removal is described as a right or left hemihepatectomy. The right and left sides of the liver can be further divided into medial and lateral sectors (Fig. 19.4). The falciform ligament provides the surface landmark for the division between left medial and lateral sectors. On the right, the two sectors (medial and lateral) are delineated by an imaginary plane which passes from a point equidistant between the gall bladder fossa and the antero-inferior angle of the liver anteriorly to the IVC posteriorly. Within the liver, the middle

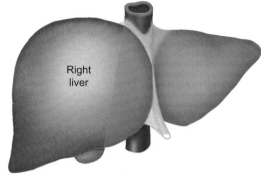

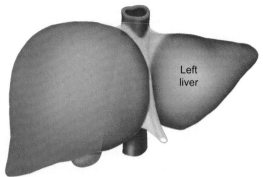

Fig 19.3 **The right and left liver.**

hepatic vein runs between the right and left sides of the liver, the right vein between the right medial and lateral sectors and the left vein between the left medial and lateral sectors. The liver can be divided into eight smaller functional segments each with its own vascular supply and bile drainage, two of the segments forming each

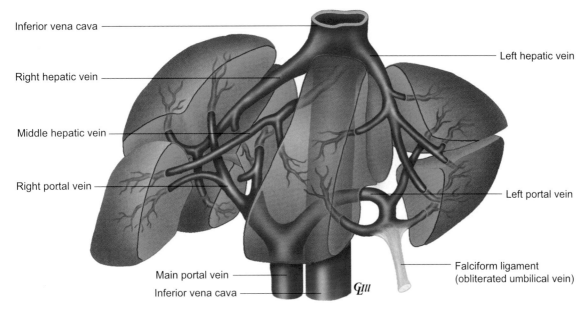

Inferior vena cava

Right hepatic vein

Middle hepatic vein

Right portal vein

Left hepatic vein

Left portal vein

Main portal vein

Inferior vena cava

Falciform ligament
(obliterated umbilical vein)

Fig 19.4 **The segments of the liver.**

sector. These segments are now of surgical importance in that they can be resected separately.

Bile collecting system – ducts and gall bladder

Bile canaliculi are found as a meshwork surrounding liver cells and unite to form intralobular and ultimately interlobular ductules. These converge to form intra-hepatic ducts which unite to form the two main (right and left) hepatic ducts; these leave the liver at the porta hepatis and join to form the common hepatic duct which is the most superficially placed structure in the free edge of the lesser omentum (Fig. 19.5). The cystic duct from the gall bladder (see below) unites with this to make the common bile duct which passes down behind the duodenum and through the posterior substance of the pancreas where it is joined by the pancreatic duct to finally open into the posteromedial aspect of the duodenum at the papilla. Surgeons often refer to the confluence of common bile and pancreatic ducts as the *ampulla of Vater* but it is rare to find the flask-shaped dilatation that characterises such a description. The opening is surrounded by the circular *sphincter of Oddi* which, in conjunction with the villous folds of the mucosa, normally prevents reflux of duodenal content into the bile or pancreatic ducts (see 'Pancreatitis', Ch. 21).

The gall bladder

The gall bladder is a pear-shaped reservoir which lies in a fossa on the inferior surface of the right lobe of the liver. Its capacity is normally 50 mL but in certain

pathological conditions it can swell to enormous proportions. Anatomically, the gall bladder is subdivided into a fundus, a body and a neck which opens into the cystic duct (Fig. 19.5). Many gall bladders develop a

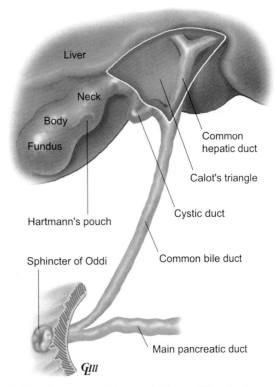

Liver

Neck

Body

Fundus

Common
hepatic duct

Calot's triangle

Hartmann's pouch

Cystic duct

Sphincter of Oddi

Common bile duct

Main pancreatic duct

Fig 19.5 **The anatomy of the gall bladder and biliary tract.**

pouch (Hartmann's) on the ventral aspect of the body, immediately proximal to the neck, where gallstones may lodge. The cystic duct is usually about 2.5 cm in length and contains a spiral mucosal valve (*valve of Heister*).

Calot's triangle

This is an important surgical landmark in operations on the gall bladder and biliary tree; being made up of the following (Fig. 19.5):

* common hepatic duct – medial
* cystic duct – inferior
* liver substance – superior

It is usually crossed by the cystic artery.

Anatomical variations

In 10%, the biliary collecting system has variations in its anatomy as a result of its complex development (Box 19.1). Such variations may be a cause of injury to the bile ducts during surgical operations.

Hepatobiliary physiology

Reticuloendothelial

Sixty-five per cent of the reticuloendothelial system is within the liver and it is responsible for filtering and destroying bacteria and their products which have been absorbed from the gut and for the removal of debris which results from the breakdown of intestinal cells. The hepatic reticuloendothelial cells also have similar functions in filtering blood which reaches them via the

hepatic artery but in this they are of less quantitative importance than the spleen (see Ch. 20).

Detoxification

The liver detoxifies a variety of endogenous and exogenous substances (chiefly drugs) mainly by conjugating them into less active forms.

Intermediary metabolism

Hepatocytes play a dominant role in metabolism and storage of basic foodstuffs:

* *Carbohydrates* are stored as glycogen and released in response to changes in blood sugar concentration to meet urgent energy needs.
* *Fats* are metabolised – to ketone bodies – for energy transfer and release. Some special products, such as cholesterol, are synthesised.
* *Storage.* Fat-soluble vitamins (A, D and K) are principally or exclusively stored in the liver.
* *Protein.* The liver is the only source of albumin and alpha-globulin. Many specialised proteins, such as clotting factors, are synthesised there. Operations on patients with liver disease and defective protein synthesis require management of deficiency states.

Excretory

The production, storage and release of bile into the duodenum is a fundamental function of the liver and has an impact on surgical practice because of:

* gallstone formation
* the enterohepatic circulation of bile acids which is of importance in the digestion and absorption of fat.

Bilirubin is a breakdown product of the cleavage of haem from red blood cells by the reticuloendothelial system. On release into the circulation it is unconjugated (fat-soluble) and transported in the plasma bound to albumin. On extraction from the plasma by the hepatocyte it is conjugated with glucuronide by the enzyme glucuronyl transferase to become water-soluble and is excreted continuously in the bile. Bacterial deconjugation in the colon produces stercobilin which colours the faeces brown. If there is infection in the biliary tree, deconjugation may take place within it and the bilirubin aggregates to form stones (see 'Oriental cholangiohepatitis').

Although bile is secreted continuously by the liver cells, one of its main functions is assisting in digestion, and therefore it is only intermittently released into the duodenum. In the interim, the gall bladder acts as a reservoir in which bile is concentrated from five to 20 times by removal of sodium and water. Release of bile into the duodenum begins shortly after the ingestion of food – in response to stimulation of the vagus. The main flow, which is accompanied by gall bladder

---

Box 19.1

Congenital abnormalities of the biliary tree

Gall bladder
Absence
Reduplication
Mesentery (floating gall bladder)
Phyrgian cap (fundus of gall bladder folded or kinked upon body)

Bile ducts
Obliteration
Low or otherwise abnormal entry of cystic duct into the common bile duct
Low junction of a right sectoral duct with common hepatic duct
Direct drainage of a bile duct into the gall bladder via the liver bed

contraction and relaxation of the sphincter of Oddi, takes place as the result of the secretion of chole-cystokinin from the duodenal wall in response to the presence of fat in the lumen. Contraction of the gall bladder in this manner against an obstruction causes pain.

In addition to concentrating bile, mucin is secreted from the gall bladder mucosa and is believed to have a role in preventing stone formation.

Jaundice

Jaundice is an increased concentration of bilrubin in plasma the normal upper limit of which is 17 μmol/L. When hepatic uptake and excretion are decreased, the excess bilirubin in plasma spills over into the interstitial space so that the tissues become stained yellow. A symptom that often accompanies jaundice is itching but this is probably caused by bile salts rather than bilirubin. A bilirubin level of 35 μmol/L or more in plasma is usually associated with clinically detectable jaundice, but between 17 and 35 μmol/L the patient is said to be biochemically jaundiced. To distinguish between jaundice that occurs because of increased bilirubin production or because of a block to excretion at the hepatocyte or canaliculus (which usually requires medical management) and that caused by extrahepatic obstruction to bile drainage (which may need surgical management) requires close cooperation between gastroenterological physicians and surgeons.

CLASSIFICATION OF JAUNDICE

Prehepatic

This is a sequel to increased breakdown of red cells – haemolysis. The rate of production of bilirubin is sufficiently fast to saturate the uptake–conjugation mechanisms in the liver. The bilirubin in plasma is unconjugated and therefore is not excreted by the kidney (*acholuric jaundice*).

Hepatic (or hepatocellular)

This, as its name implies, is caused by some disorder of the liver cell at the stages of uptake, conjugation or secretion of bilirubin, including also malfunction of the cells which line the bile canaliculi. For example:

- *defective uptake* occurs with mild intermittent jaundice in otherwise healthy individuals (Gilbert's disease)
- *congenital absence of glucuronyl transferase* is associated with severe jaundice and early death (Crigler–Najjar syndrome)
- *congenital impairment of excretion* of conjugated bilirubin into the bile is known as the Dubin–Johnson–Rotor syndrome.

All the above conditions are rare, apart from Gilbert's disease, and the commonest causes of hepato-cellular jaundice are:

- viral diseases of the liver cell – hepatitis A, B, C, D and E
- other hepatic infections
- hepatotoxic drugs, such as the chlorpromazines, which act mainly on the canalicular cells, but including many others with varied actions within cells.

Posthepatic

This type of jaundice is often called *obstructive* or *surgical* jaundice, which implies that the cause is a mechanical obstruction in the extrahepatic biliary tree. The term identifies those patients whose jaundice may be capable of relief by some form of mechanical inter-vention – either by surgery or by endoscopy. In these patients, the relatively intact hepatocyte conjugates bilirubin which is then released back into the plasma and excreted by the kidney so that the urine is dark and the stools pale. Causes include:

- in the lumen of the biliary tree – gallstones
- in the wall of the ducts – biliary atresia; bile duct carcinoma (cholangiocarcinoma); postoperative stricture
- extrinsic compression – pancreatitis; pancreatic tumour; secondary deposits in the hilar lymph nodes of the liver.

INVESTIGATION

Biochemical

The three most useful measurements in blood are of the concentration of bilirubin, alkaline phosphatase and the transaminases.

Bilirubin. A raised level of plasma bilirubin indicates disruption of its normal passage from blood, through the hepatocyte and down the biliary collecting system into the duodenum. Serial measurements are helpful in following the course of hepatic or biliary disease.

Alkaline phosphatase. This substance is secreted predominantly from the cells of the collecting system which proliferate in the presence of obstruction. A raised level in the blood is therefore a good indicator of extrahepatic obstruction, although elevations also occur in jaundice caused by some drugs such as chlor-promazine and its derivatives and also in the later stages of viral hepatitis (intrahepatic cholestasis).

Transaminases. These enzymes are constituents of the hepatocyte and, if their level is raised in the blood, the implication is that there is hepatocellular damage. Usually this is primary within the hepatocyte but, in long-standing extrahepatic obstruction, secondary inter-ference with hepatocellular function may take place.

Table 19.1
Biochemical patterns of jaundice

	Alkaline phosphatase	Aspartate and alanine transaminases
Hepatocellular damage	↑	↑↑↑
Extrahepatic biliary obstruction	↑↑↑	↑

The biochemical patterns of jaundice in hepatocellular and extrahepatic obstruction are shown in Table 19.1 although there can often be some overlap. Other measurements that may be of value in jaundice are

Albumin concentration. This gives a guide to the synthetic capacity of the liver and the nutritional state of the patient.

Clotting factors are synthesised in the liver. The most easily assessed is prothrombin. Vitamin K is a cofactor in its synthesis. Because the vitamin is fat-soluble and is therefore not well absorbed from the intestine in the absence of bile, its limited hepatic stores soon become exhausted. The hypoprothrombinaemia of jaundice responds to the administration of parenteral vitamin K provided hepatocyte function is preserved, as is nearly always the case when the jaundice is caused by obstruction. Measurement of the prothrombin time is therefore an essential preliminary before operation in a jaundiced patient.

Alpha-fetoprotein (AFP). See hepatocellular carcinoma.

Imaging

Ultrasound is undoubtedly the most useful initial investigation because it is:

- non-invasive
- inexpensive
- repeatable.

Ultrasound scanning reliably detects a dilated duct system and so helps to distinguish parenchymal liver disease from extrahepatic bile duct obstruction. The characteristic texture of the cirrhotic liver can also be identified. In addition, cysts, abscesses and tumours can be delineated, and guided fine-needle aspiration and biopsy (Ch. 4) are possible.

CT Scan has the advantage over ultrasound of providing more precise anatomical information and, unlike ultrasound, is unaffected by the presence of obesity or bowel gas. The image is enhanced with oral contrast medium to delineate the bowel and with an intravenous contrast agent to show vascular structures.

Cholangiography. In *oral cholecystography* the patient ingests contrast medium which, after absorption from the gastrointestinal tract, is excreted in the bile and concentrated in the gall bladder. Given that the gall bladder is functioning, stones may be seen as filling defects and the function of the gall bladder assessed by feeding a fatty meal which causes a normal organ to contract and empty. Oral cholecystography is now much less commonly used because the same – and often additional information – can be obtained on ultrasound.

Intravenous or *excretion cholangiography* (IVC) by the injection of a contrast agent into the bloodstream, which is then taken up by the liver and excreted into the bile, is only possible when bile production and excretion are also taking place, i.e. in the absence of jaundice. The technique is now seldom used.

Percutaneous transhepatic cholangiography (PTC – Fig. 19.6) is achieved by introducing a fine needle (usually called a skinny or Chiba needle) through the substance of the liver into a bile duct. Success rates are reduced if the biliary system is not dilated. PTC is of particular value in determining the anatomical level and the nature of an obstructing lesion.

Endoscopic retrograde cholangiopancreatography (ERCP – Fig. 19.7) similarly delineates the biliary tract but also can show the pancreatic ductal system.

At both ERCP and PTC, bile may be aspirated for microbiological examination and cells may also be obtained for cytological assessment. Both procedures may also be the gateway to treatment such as the placement of biliary stents to relieve obstruction or the removal of biliary stones by endoscopic sphincterotomy or dilatation of the sphincter of Oddi.

Magnetic resonance imaging (MRI). Demonstration of the biliary and pancreatic ductal system (MRCP)

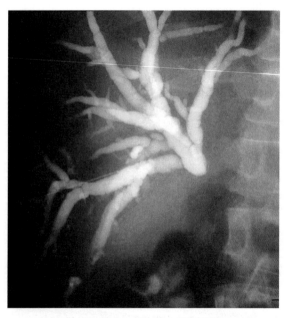

Fig 19.6 **A percutaneous transhepatic cholangiogram.** The needle is seen coming from the patient's rightside. The common hepatic duct is obstructed by a tumour.

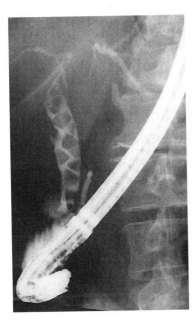

Fig 19.7 **An ERCP showing the biliary ductal system with multiple bile duct stones.**

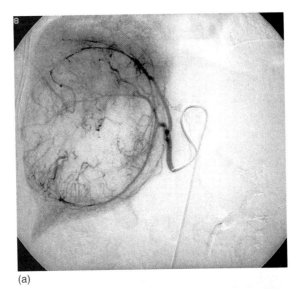

(a)

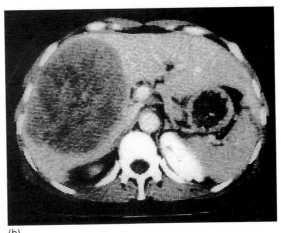

(b)

Fig 19.8 **A tumour blush seen on hepatic angiography (a) with the corresponding CT scan (b).** Note that the arteries are displaced around the tumour.

now provide good images and this non-invasive method is likely to replace diagnostic ERCP and PTC.

Arteriography. Selective coeliac and superior mesenteric angiograms can show the abnormal circulation of a tumour (tumour blush – Fig. 19.8). The late-phase images of an angiogram demonstrate the portal vein, and therefore neoplastic involvement of both arterial and venous vessels can be assessed.

Laparoscopy permits direct visualisation of the liver and may be combined with endoscopic ultrasound to provide both accurate staging and biopsy of diseased liver tissue.

Percutaneous liver biopsy is an invasive procedure which is particularly valuable in the diagnosis of diffuse liver disease or for confirmation of metastatic malignancy. Accuracy is increased when insertion of the needle for biopsy or liver cytology is guided by ultrasound, CT or at laparoscopy.

GENERAL MANAGEMENT

Preparation for liver surgery

Surgical operations are usually major and the preparations outlined in Chapter 5 must be followed in detail. Major resections may require specialised support for abnormalities in the clotting system and for postoperative nutrition by either the enteral or parenteral route (see Ch. 5).

The jaundiced patient

Clotting. The most likely problem is vitamin K deficiency which can be corrected by parenteral administration of the synthetic derivatives menadione or phytomenadione (K_1). The synthesis of prothrombin, set in motion by restoring supplies of vitamin K, takes some hours so that the prothrombin time must, except in dire emergencies, be rechecked before operation is undertaken.

Antibiotic prophylaxis. Sepsis from organisms that originate in the gastrointestinal tract is a major cause of death in the surgical management of jaundice, partly because of interference with hepatic reticulo-endothelial function. Prophylactic antibiotics against enteric organisms are used routinely and also in invasive diagnostic procedures such as PTC and ERCP.

Preliminary biliary decompression. In a patient who will subsequently require an operation, liver function may be improved by biliary decompression which is done by one of the following methods.

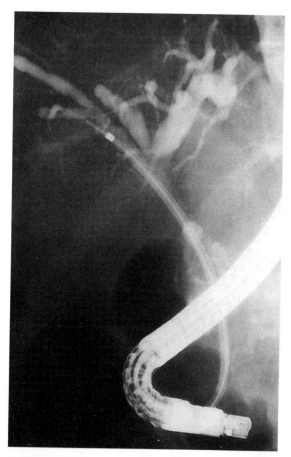

Fig 19.9 **Endoscopic insertion of a biliary stent over a guide wire.**

- passing a catheter percutaneously into the liver substance and then into a bile duct as for cholangiography
- ERCP with or without dilatation of an obstructing lesion and insertion of a nasobiliary drainage catheter or a stent (Fig. 19.9).

Hepatorenal syndrome. This condition is probably one variant of the systemic inflammatory response syndrome (SIRS) in which renal and hepatic failure develop in response to severe injury or sepsis, especially if there is depression of the immune system. A patient with jaundice is particularly liable to develop renal failure and measures to prevent this include:

- adequate preoperative hydration
- avoidance of intraoperative hypotension
- maintenance of high urine flow by the use of an osmotic diuretic (mannitol) which opposes the action of increased secretion of antidiuretic hormone on the distal tubule after operation; and also by administration of a low dose of dopamine which increases renal plasma flow and glomerular filtration rate

Non-neoplastic conditions of the liver

Congenital conditions
Biliary atresia
AETIOLOGY AND PATHOLOGICAL FEATURES
The commonest cause of prolonged neonatal jaundice is extrahepatic biliary atresia. The cause is not known. There may be single or multiple points of obstruction and the proximal ducts may dilate considerably. If not relieved, liver failure ultimately ensues with death in the first year of life; only a few infants surviving beyond 6 months.

CLINICAL FEATURES
Mild jaundice is not uncommon in the neonatal period. However, persistence and progression beyond 2 weeks is definitely abnormal and then the distinction has to be made between obstruction and hepatitis. This can usually be achieved by the biochemical profile (Ch. 4) and ultrasound.

MANAGEMENT
There are two management options:

- For the majority, hepatic portoenterostomy (Kasai operation – Fig. 19.10) should be attempted within 60 days of birth; delay beyond this time is associated with the rapid development of intrahepatic fibrosis and a reduced chance of success.
- When evidence of deteriorating liver function is apparent, liver transplantation should be considered (see Ch. 13).

Congenital cystic disease

Cysts may be solitary or multiple. Multiple cysts are frequently associated with polycystic disease of the kidney (see Ch. 32).

CLINICAL FEATURES
The cysts are often small, asymptomatic and found only incidentally either at laparotomy, during investigation of other problems, or at postmortem examination. Large cysts may present with pain in the right upper abdomen, which may radiate to the right shoulder and is believed to be caused by stretching of the liver capsule.

MANAGEMENT
In a few instances, percutaneous aspiration under

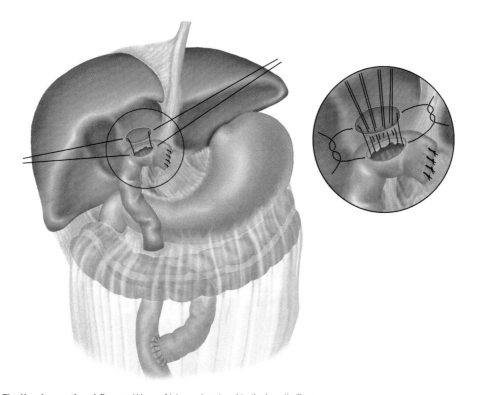

Fig 19.10 **The Kasai operation.** A Roux en Y loop of jejunum is sutured to the hepatic ilium.

image control or occasionally surgical decompression is required for the relief of symptoms.

Congenital cystic dilatation of the intrahepatic ducts (Caroli's disease)

This is a rare congenital but non-familial disorder with saccular dilatation of the intrahepatic ducts. The cause is not known. The disease is usually diffuse but is occasionally confined to one segment or liver lobe. Clinical features are of recurrent upper abdominal pain and cholangitis in childhood or early adult life.

Cholangitis is treated with systemic antibiotics. Localised disease is susceptible to resection.

Inborn errors of metabolism

These are discussed in detail in Chapter 13 (see 'Liver transplantation').

Hepatic trauma

In the UK, liver injury is usually the result of blunt trauma such as a road traffic accident and is frequently accompanied by other serious head, skeletal, thoracic or abdominal injuries. Penetrating trauma from knives or missiles is uncommon but the incidence is rising.

PATHOLOGICAL FEATURES

Blunt injury varies widely in severity. Small haematomas resolve spontaneously but there may be extensive bruising and devitalisation of liver tissue and sometimes detachment of one or more hepatic veins with formation of a large retroperitoneal haematoma. In penetrating injury there is usually an obvious track which, in knife and low-velocity missile wounds, leads to a localised area of bleeding without much hepatic damage. High-velocity injury is usually associated with extensive damage caused by shock waves around the missile track.

CLINICAL FEATURES

Other injuries (particularly to the head) may call attention to themselves while the liver injury is initially unapparent. The usual presentation is with intra-abdominal haemorrhage. An extensive haematoma which has remained undetected may present later with jaundice, biliary colic and gastrointestinal haemorrhage caused by bleeding into the biliary tree (haemobilia).

MANAGEMENT

This is a highly specialised subject and patients with major liver injuries should be transferred to an expert centre provided he or she can be stabilised. Stab wounds usually stop bleeding spontaneously and the same may be true of low-velocity missile injuries. Low-velocity bullet wounds only need removal of the foreign body (if possible) and any devitalised tissue.

Parenchymal shattering after a high-velocity injury is often best treated by hepatic resection. Blunt injuries may also require resection but are often manageable by removal of dead and damaged tissue and control of haemorrhage. Haemobilia can usually be treated by embolising the bleeding vessel after selective hepatic angiography.

Liver infections

Pyogenic liver abscess

AETIOLOGY

This condition is rare in the UK, usually affecting the elderly or debilitated. In 25–50% of sufferers, the abscess is cryptogenic, i.e. the primary site of infection remains undiscovered. Biliary infection (cholangitis) is the commonest source; the other main cause is bacterial seeding via the portal vein (portal pyaemia) from an intra-abdominal site – an abscess related to appendicitis, pancreatitis, diverticular disease or perforation of the gastrointestinal tract. Other causes are direct liver trauma and haematogenous spread from an extra-abdominal focus.

PATHOLOGICAL FEATURES

About half of all liver abscesses are multiple. Solitary abscesses are usually found in the right lobe of the liver directly under the diaphragm. Common organisms are:

- *Streptococcus milleri*
- *Escherichia coli*
- *Streptococcus faecalis* (*enterococcus*)
- *Staphylococcus aureus*
- Anaerobes such as *Bacteroides* spp.

CLINICAL FEATURES

Presenting symptoms are variable but there is often fever, malaise, anorexia and upper abdominal pain. Less than 50% have a swinging pyrexia and only 10% have positive blood cultures. Jaundice is rare.

INVESTIGATION

Laboratory investigation

There may be a neutrophil leucocytosis, secondary anaemia and hypoalbuminaemia. The concentration of alkaline phosphatase is sometimes raised.

Imaging

Abdominal X-rays may show a raised right hemidiaphragm, right basal pleural effusion, or an air–fluid level within the liver.

Ultrasound and CT are the best methods with which to establish the diagnosis and, with prophylactic antibiotics, may be used to guide aspiration to obtain pus for microbiological analysis.

MANAGEMENT

All patients are treated with systemic antibiotics which, in multiple abscesses, may be the only form of treatment feasible. Those large enough to be readily detected on imaging rarely respond to antibiotics alone and require drainage. Under ultrasound or CT guidance, the abscess may be aspirated and, if necessary, a drain inserted percutaneously. Follow-up scans are required to assess the response to treatment.

The treatment of liver abscesses by aspiration under imaging control has the disadvantage of not dealing with the primary site and may not be successful if there is marked loculation within a chronic cavity. Open surgical drainage may 'therefore' be required. The morbidity and mortality are high if abscesses are multiple or inadequately drained.

Hydatid disease

This is a common condition, particularly in rural communities in the Mediterranean, Middle East and, until recently, Australasia.

AETIOLOGY

The most common cause is the parasite *Echinococcus granulosus*. The main host is the dog which becomes infested by eating contaminated bovine or sheep offal. The parasite lives in the canine small bowel as a worm about 4–6 mm in length. These produce ova which are passed in the faeces. Close handling of dogs or work or play in a contaminated environment can lead to oral ingestion of ova. There are other, much rarer echinococcal infections which are not considered here.

PATHOLOGICAL FEATURES

The ingested ovum is partially digested in the upper gastrointestinal tract and the embryo can then penetrate the bowel wall and enter the portal circulation. Most are trapped in the sinusoids of the liver – hence the frequency with which this organ is involved. The hydatid cyst has an outer fibrous adventitia, a gelatinous laminated membrane and an inner germinal epithelium from which the infective brood capsules – containing potential worm heads – are derived. The cysts usually occupy the upper pole of the right lobe and are slow-growing so that disease acquired as a child may not be manifest until adulthood is reached. Cysts frequently become inactive (dead) and calcified.

CLINICAL FEATURES

History

The common presentation is with right upper quadrant pain. Occasionally, rupture of a cyst into the biliary tree releases brood capsules that cause obstructive jaundice and features of cholangitis. Spread through the diaphragm may lead to respiratory symptoms.

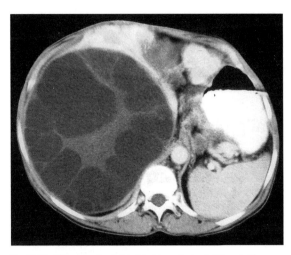

Fig 19.11 **CT scan of a right-sided hepatic hydatid cyst.** The daughter cysts can be easily seen.

Physical findings

Hepatomegaly may be present which, if the cyst is active or infected, is associated with tenderness.

INVESTIGATION

Imaging

Plain X-ray of the upper abdomen may show calcification.

Ultrasound and CT (Fig 19.11) will show whether a cyst is single or multiple. Both also detect calcification.

Serological testing

A number of tests are available which vary in their sensitivity and specificity. Complement fixation is widely used but is relatively insensitive, although it has the advantage that it becomes negative after successful treatment.

MANAGEMENT

Calcified cysts are usually dead and therefore do not require treatment. Small and deeply situated cysts are managed non-operatively and their course followed by serial ultrasound examinations.

Drug therapy has been more effective since the introduction of albendazole but is not yet proven as the sole treatment for liver cysts. Obstructive jaundice or cholangitis by daughter cysts obstructing the common bile duct is managed initially by endoscopic sphincterotomy. Large, superficially placed and symptomatic cysts require surgical evacuation with special precautions being taken to kill the brood capsules before the contents are released.

Amoebic liver abscess

Amoebic liver infection and abscess is a complication of *Entamoebic histolytica* colitis (Ch. 24). The amoebae enter the portal circulation through an ulcer in the colonic mucosa.

PATHOLOGICAL FEATURES

The amoebae establish a colony which first leads to hepatitis and then to necrosis and abscess formation most commonly in the upper part of the liver. The pus formed is thick and contains a small amount of blood from erosion of small vessels; hence the often used description that it resembles anchovy sauce – creamy with a tinge of red caused by the phagocytosis of red blood cells by the amoebae. Extention of the focus may lead to pleural effusion, bronchopleural fistula and lung abscess. Rupture into the peritoneal cavity may also occur.

CLINICAL FEATURES

History

There may or may not have been a background of colitis. There is progressive painful right upper quadrant pain with sweating, rigors and a swinging pyrexia. Involvement of diaphragm and lung may lead to respiratory symptoms. Shoulder pain is not uncommon.

Physical findings

Right upper quadrant tenderness, hepatomegaly and jaundice are common findings.

INVESTIGATION

Ultrasound or CT delineates the abscess and. with guidance allows a specimen to be obtained for microscopy and bacteriological culture because secondary contamination is not uncommon.

Stool examination is routine. In serological testing, the amoebic flourescent antibody titre is raised in 90% of patients.

MANAGEMENT

Metronidazole is specific for amoebic infection although resistance is increasing. Therapy is given once the diagnosis is suspected or established, first by the intravenous route and thereafter orally. Consideration should be given to administering another antibiotic that is effective against enteric organisms because of the frequency of secondary infection. Abscesses may need to be aspirated percutaneously, but only occasionally is open operation required.

Neoplasms of the liver

Benign tumours

These are relatively common, often presenting incidentally or by mimicking biliary disease.

AETIOLOGY AND CLINICAL FEATURES

The usual growths are haemangioma (Fig. 19.12), focal nodular hyperpalsia and hepatic adenoma (Fig. 19.13). Some adenomas are associated with the use of oral contraceptives and may regress when the agent is withdrawn.

Identification may be by chance during imaging for other conditions or because of non-specific abdominal pain. Rarely, benign tumours (particularly adenomas) present with intraperitoneal rupture and haemorrhage, which has a mortality of at least 20%.

INVESTIGATION

The imaging techniques described above are used to delineate, and if possible identify, the tumour and also in some patients to determine feasibility for surgical excision. The diagnosis of haemangioma relies on complete filling of the lesion with contrast during dynamic CT scan. Percutaneous biopsy is contra-indicated for haemangioma but may be used to establish a histological diagnosis and assist in making a decision on treatment.

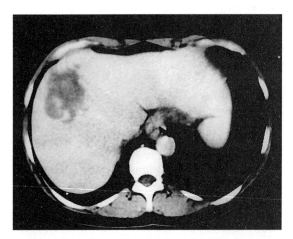

Fig 19.12 **A CT scan of the liver showing a haemangioma.**

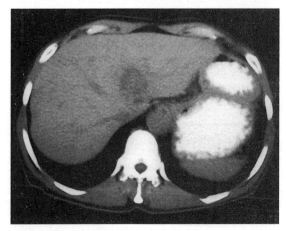

Fig 19.13 **A hepatic adenoma seen on CT scanning.**

MANAGEMENT

Most haemangiomas do not require treatment. For other tumours, surgical excision is usually advised although the risks of operation must be balanced against the potential benefits of excision.

Malignant tumours

Hepatocellular carcinoma (HCC)

This condition is rare in the UK – fewer than 2 cases per 100 000 of the population per annum. However, it is very common in Africa and the Far East around the Pacific rim.

AETIOLOGY AND PATHOLOGICAL FEATURES

Known predisposing factors are:

- chronic liver disease – usually hepatitis B or C virus infection
- alcoholic cirrhosis

The disease is frequently multifocal especially if it arises in a cirrhotic liver. Local invasion of the remaining organ is the rule and metastatic spread to the lungs and elsewhere is common.

CLINICAL FEATURES

The presenting features are often vague, especially if they are superimposed on ill health from chronic liver disease. Common complaints are of malaise, weight loss, abdominal discomfort, unexplained fever or jaundice.

The liver may be enlarged, slightly tender and often contains a palpable mass. Signs of metastatic disease may be obvious.

INVESTIGATION

Biochemical

Tests of liver function may be disordered but are non-specific. However, more than 70% have increased levels of the tumour marker alpha-fetoprotein (AFP).

Imaging

CT is the most commonly used method to confirm the presence of a tumour and to define the extent of the growth and invasion of neighbouring structures. ·

Angiography is useful in showing the vascular anatomy of the liver in patients who are to undergo resection.

MANAGEMENT

Resection

Surgical removal offers the only hope of cure. Unfortunately in many instances the disease is extensive, multifocal or the remaining organ is so diseased that resection is not safe. Patients who undergo a potentially curative resection have a 45% 5-year survival.

Palliation

There are many approaches to palliation in hepatocellular carcinoma. They include:

- *Hepatic de-arterialisation* – based on the fact that tumours obtain most of their blood supply from the hepatic artery rather than the portal vein; interruption may be achieved by radiological embolisation or at operation.
- *Chemotherapy* – either by the systemic or intra-arterial routes; attachment of the chemotherapeutic agent to lipiodol which is retained by the liver has shown promising results.
- *Direct absolute alcohol injection* into the hepatic mass which may be useful to arrest bleeding from a ruptured tumour.
- *Ablation by cryotherapy or laser* either at operation or under CT or ultrasound guidance.

Cholangiocarcinoma

AETIOLOGY AND PATHOLOGICAL FEATURES

Cholangiocarcinoma may be either intra- or extra-hepatic. Liver flukes, which are common on the Pacific rim, are known to excite an intense inflammatory reaction within the bile ducts and have been linked with intrahepatic tumours. Choledochal cysts and Caroli's disease are associated with the development of cholangiocarcinoma. Intrahepatic lesions are typically solitary space-occupying lesions which mimic hepato-cellular carcinoma. Extrahepatic tumours produce either a fibrous stricture (usual) or a spongiform mass (rare).

CLINICAL FEATURES

Progressive jaundice and weight loss are usual present-ing features, sometimes associated with prodromal itching. Rarely, extrahepatic tumours may cause cholangitis. Physical findings are of jaundice and occasionally a mass in the right upper quadrant.

INVESTIGATION

A combination of ultrasonography and CT or MRI with PTC or ERCP usually demonstrates the site and extent of the lesion. However, differentiation between cholangiocarcinoma and sclerosing cholangitis may be difficult. CT or ultrasound guided percutaneous fine-needle aspiration cytology (FNAC) of a mass or exfoliative cytology of bile specimens (obtained at PTC or ERCP) may provide confirmation. Arteriography, including venous phase studies, is important to deter-mine arterial or venous encasement, which implies irresectability of the tumour.

MANAGEMENT

Resection with reconstruction to restore bile flow into the intestine is the treatment of choice. Up to 40% 5-year survival can be obtained with appropriate selection of patients based on:

- fitness for a major surgical procedure
- an uninvolved bile duct, hepatic artery and portal vein on one side of the liver.

Resection may provide good palliation. Other palliative options include:

- insertion of a stent (endoprosthesis) either percutaneously. under radiological control or endoscopically
- biliary-enteric bypass.

Although an endoprosthesis provides good relief of obstructive jaundice, in 25–30% it becomes occluded by biliary sludge or tumour to produce recurrence of jaundice or cholangitis. Reinsertion is then required.

Metastatic cancer

In the Western world, this is by far the commonest form of malignant liver tumour

AETIOLOGY

Common primary cancers that metastasise to the liver are those of the colon, breast, lung, pancreas and stomach. However, there is a less common group of metastatic tumours that arise from the intestine – carcinoid tumours. Their clinical course may be improved by hepatic resection.

CLINICAL FEATURES

Most metastases are asymptomatic. Large or multiple lesions cause right upper quadrant pain, ascites, jaundice and anorexia. The liver may be enlarged or contain a palpable mass which is discrete and hard.

INVESTIGATION

Assessment for possible resection is by standard imaging. Serial assays of carcinoembryonic antigen (CEA) after removal of a primary large bowel cancer may detect early metastatic disease and lead to investi-gation of the liver as a possible site.

MANAGEMENT

Untreated metastatic disease has a poor prognosis. The mean survival rate is less than 3 months and 1-year survival is less than 7%.

Surgical removal

About 10% of metastatic deposits are solitary or, if multiple, are confined to a single hepatic segment. The malignant deposit is then suitable, in the absence of detectable tumour elsewhere, for a potentially curative resection. The ultimate outcome will depend on whether undetected micrometastases are present. The operative mortality is about 5% and 5-year survival is 30% for patients with resected colorectal liver metastases.

Liver transplantation
This is discussed in Chapter 13.

Gallstones (cholelithiasis)

EPIDEMIOLOGY
Gallstones are very common, with a prevalence of 10%. Although the aphorism that gallstones arise in 'fair, fat and fertile females in their fifties' often holds true, stones can affect patients of all ages and both sexes. However, they are 2–4 times more common in women. Cholesterol is the principal constituent of the great majority of stones, either as a pure cholesterol stone (20%) or as a mixed one combined with deconjugated bile pigment, especially bilirubin (75%). Stones composed of pigment alone account for the remaining 5%.

AETIOLOGY
Three predisposing factors to gallstone formation act in concert.

Cholesterol supersaturation
Although cholesterol is insoluble in water, in bile it is normally solubilised in lecithin-bile acid aggregates (known as micelles). If the concentration in bile is high, the capacity of this mechanism may be exceeded (cholesterol supersaturation). Nucleation may occur and leads to crystal formation followed by agglomeration and the formation of stones. Pro-nucleating factors include calcium bilirubinate and non-mucous glycoproteins. Cholesterol supersaturation occurs when:

- plasma oestrogen levels are increased – e.g. obesity, pregnancy and in women taking oral contraceptives
- there is depletion of the bile acid pool – e.g. in resection or disease of the terminal ileum which interrupts the enterohepatic circulation.

Stasis
Stone formation is enhanced by a reduced rate of bile flow (stasis) which occurs particularly in:

- fasting – lack of food stimulus to gall bladder emptying
- total parenteral nutrition – for the same reason as fasting

- truncal vagotomy – loss of neural stimulus to gall bladder emptying.

Increased bilirubin secretion in bile or deconjugation
Bilirubin is kept in solution in bile by conjugation with glucuronide. Pigment stones are encountered when there is:

- increased breakdown of red blood cells – haemolytic disorders such as spherocytosis, sickle cell disease and malaria
- failure of conjugation – hepatocyte insufficiency in the formation of glucuronide or excess glucuronidase; the latter may be the consequence of bacterial activity but the role of infection in stone formation remains uncertain and bacteria may be a consequence of stones rather than their cause.

CLINICAL FEATURES
Asymptomatic stones
Gallstones anywhere in the biliary tree may remain asymptomatic (silent) and therefore undetected for many years. Ultrasound scanning done on patients with vague abdominal symptoms has resulted in more frequent discovery of such incidental stones.

Symptomatic stones
Stones become clinically evident by the complications they cause, which are classified according to their anatomical site (Box 19.2).

Box 19.2

Complications of gallstones

Gall bladder
Biliary colic
Acute cholecystitis
Empyema
Mucocele
Chronic cholecystitis

Common bile duct
Obstructive jaundice
Cholangitis
Pancreatitis

Small intestine
Gallstone ileus

Stones in the gall bladder: urgent management

Biliary colic

CLINICAL FEATURES

History

A stone impacted within the gall bladder – usually in Hartmann's pouch or the cystic duct – causes pain. Although often referred to as colic, the pain is usually constant in the epigastrium and right upper quadrant and may radiate through to the back in the region of the inferior angle of the scapula. Such pain is better called obstructive (see also 'Renal colic', Ch. 32). Attacks last for a few minutes to half an hour and may be exacerbated by ingestion of fatty food which stimulates the release of cholecystokinin (CCK) and consequent gall bladder contraction. Vomiting is common. Fever is absent. The pain spontaneously settles when the stone either becomes disimpacted or, less commonly, is passed into the common bile duct.

Physical findings

The patient is apyrexial. Abdominal tenderness is absent, although a gall bladder that has become distended may cause slight signs of peritoneal irritation.

INVESTIGATION

Blood examination

The white cell count and liver function tests are usually normal.

Imaging (see Table 19.2)

Plain radiography reveals only 10% of gallstones; the remainder do not have sufficient radiodensity.

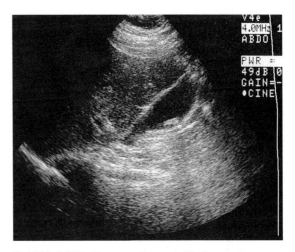
Fig 19.14 **Gall bladder stones detected with ultrasound.**

Ultrasound reliably detects 98% of gall bladder stones (Fig. 19.14) but is less reliable in identifying those that are within the bile ducts. In addition, ultrasound can also provide information about the:

- thickness of the gall bladder wall, an increase above normal being indicative of past or present inflammation
- diameter of the common bile duct
- architecture of the liver and pancreas.

MANAGEMENT

The initial administration of a parenteral analgesic such as morphine or pethidine relieves the acute exacerbations of pain, and over a few hours the condition nearly always resolves. If the diagnosis is confirmed by imaging, subsequent cholecystectomy is usually indicated.

Acute cholecystitis

When a stone impacts at the outlet of the gall bladder, water continues to be absorbed through the gall bladder wall and the concentrated bile can initiate a chemical cholecystitis. Secondary infection superimposed on this generates acute bacterial cholecystitis.

CLINICAL FEATURES

History

The symptoms are similar to biliary colic but the pain is more severe and persistent. Nausea and vomiting are not uncommon and fever is usually present.

Physical findings

Tenderness and guarding are often present in the right upper quadrant. In less severe instances, laying the hand lightly on the upper right abdomen and asking

Table 19.2
Imaging in gallstone disease

Investigation	Information	Comments
Plain X-ray	10% of gall bladder stones	Not a useful investigation
Ultrasound	98% of gall bladder stones	Unreliable for duct stones
Oral cholecystogram	50% of gall bladder stones Assesses function of gall bladder	Ducts rarely seen
Intravenous cholangiogram (i.v. cholangiography)	Common duct usually seen Gall bladder may fill	Occasional reaction to i.v. contrast medium Interpretative errors in ducts not uncommon
Radionucleide biliary (e.g. HIDA)	Bile ducts seen Helpful for fistulas	Poor anatomical detail Not useful for detection of stones

the patient to take a deep breath cause a catch in breath because of pain when the inflamed gall bladder impacts on the examining hand – Murphy's sign. Hyperaesthesia of skin over the right ribs 9–11 posteriorly (Boas's sign) may also be present. If inflammation spreads beyond the gall bladder, a mass, composed of the enlarged gall bladder and adherent omentum and bowel, may be palpated under the right costal margin.

INVESTIGATION

Blood examination

There is leucocytosis and the bilirubin concentration may be raised either as a result of partial obstruction of the common hepatic duct by a stone lodged in Hartmann's pouch or because of local inflammation. The serum amylase concentration may be moderately elevated but not to the levels seen in acute pancreatitis (Ch. 21).

Imaging

Ultrasound shows the enlarged gall bladder with stone(s), a thickened wall and a surrounding rim of fluid from local oedema (Fig. 19.15).

MANAGEMENT

Initial treatment is non-operative with pain relief and systemic antibiotics. Intravenous fluids may be required initially. Most attacks resolve and definitive treatment by cholecystectomy can be done later. However, a few do not and, unless operation is done, go on to either perforation or the formation of an empyema. If progression is thought to be taking place, as judged by failure of symptoms to subside and the persistence of local signs, exploration by either laparotomy or laparoscopy should be undertaken. Alternatively, the gall

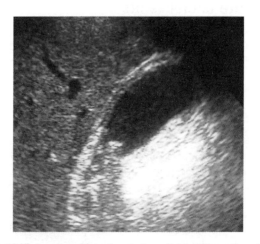

Fig 19.15 **A patient with acute calculous cholecystitis confirmed on ultrasound scanning.**

bladder may be decompressed by percutaneous insertion of a drain under ultrasound guidance.

Free perforation

This is caused by a progressive rise in tension in the gall bladder; the blood supply of the wall is reduced and gangrene occurs, usually at the fundus. Abdominal pain becomes increasingly severe and more generalised. Perforation may lead to diffuse peritonitis which demands urgent exploration and, if possible, cholecystectomy. A variant is local perforation with abscess formation.

Empyema and pericholecystic abscess

The infection remains localised with the accumulation of pus within the gall bladder. There is a swinging pyrexia, tachycardia and a tender mass in the right upper quadrant. Ultrasound confirms the diagnosis. Treatment is often best limited to drainage of the gall bladder (cholecystostomy) which may be done either at open operation or percutaneously under ultrasound guidance. Once the inflammation has resolved, a cholecystectomy should be considered.

Mucocele

A stone may impact in the neck of the gall bladder without causing inflammation either from the concentrated bile or from secondary infection. The result is a mucocele – a distended gall bladder full of clear mucus. Cholecystectomy is usually indicated.

Chronic cholecystitis

This pathological entity is the outcome of recurrent attacks of obstruction and inflammation which result in the changes of chronic inflammation in the gall bladder wall and often in the adjacent liver.

CLINICAL FEATURES

There may be a past history of attacks of acute cholecystitis. Frequently there is chronic discomfort in the right upper quadrant which is often punctuated by intermittent acute exacerbations. A history of intolerance to fatty foods may be elicited but is non-specific.

Unless an acute attack is in progress, signs are minimal – some tenderness in the right upper quadrant may be found.

INVESTIGATION AND MANAGEMENT

Gallstones are detected on ultrasound.

Provided the cause of the symptoms can be confidently ascribed to the disease in the gall bladder, cholecystectomy, which typically reveals a shrunken organ with a thick fibrotic wall, can be expected to result in cure.

Common bile duct stones (choledocholithiasis): urgent management

The majority of common bile duct stones originate in the gall bladder but some may form within the duct system. Between 10 and 14% of patients with gallstones also have stones in the common bile duct.

Ductal stones are responsible for three clinical entities:

- obstructive jaundice
- acute cholangitis
- acute pancreatitis (see Ch. 21).

Obstructive jaundice

Impaction of a stone in the common bile duct, usually at the duodenal papilla, causes obstructive jaundice. There may have been preceding biliary colic but the main presenting complaints are jaundice, pruritis, dark urine and pale bulky stools. Little is to be found on clinical examination and, in particular, the gall bladder is impalpable because it is likely to have undergone inflammation and fibrosis.

INVESTIGATION

Ultrasound usually shows dilatation of the bile ducts and may identify ductal stones. ERCP confirms the diagnosis and makes the distinction between a stone and other causes of obstructive jaundice.

MANAGEMENT

ERCP and extraction of the ductal stone(s) after division or dilatation of the sphincter of Oddi comprise the treatment of choice. Subsequently, if it has not already been done, the gall bladder should be removed unless the patient is elderly or at high operative risk.

Acute cholangitis

AETIOLOGY AND PATHOLOGICAL FEATURES

Organisms enter the biliary tree either from the gastro-intestinal tract via the duodenal papilla or by excretion in the bile after reaching the liver via the bloodstream. In the bile they multiply in the presence of obstruction to cause inflammation, Ductal stones are the cause in the western world. On the Pacific rim, parasitic infection with liver flukes (clonorchis sinensis) and ascariasis are associated with secondary bacterial cholangitis. The causative organism is usually a Gram-negative enteric bacterium, typically *Escherica coli*.

Infected bile in the biliary tree is potentially fatal because it may lead to septicaemia and hepatorenal failure. Long-term sequelae of repeated attacks of cholangitis include liver abscesses, secondary biliary cirrhosis, liver failure and portal hypertension.

CLINICAL FEATURES

A past history of biliary disease may be obtained. Presentation is with abdominal pain, high fever with rigors and jaundice (sometimes termed Charcot's triad). The liver may be somewhat enlarged and tender. The gall bladder is impalpable.

INVESTIGATION

The white cell count will usually reveal leucocytosis, while liver function tests will show cholestasis. There is a positive blood culture in most instances.

Ultrasound may show gall bladder stones, a dilated duct and sometimes a ductal stone.

MANAGEMENT

Resuscitation with intravenous fluids and parenteral antibiotics are begun on a best guess basis. A prompt response, will result in:

- relief of symptoms
- resolution of fever
- rapid reduction in jaundice

Failure to achieve this indicates the need for bile duct drainage by urgent ERCP. If possible, stones should be extracted, but effective biliary drainage is the first essential requirement. Definitive treatment of cholelithiasis can be deferred until the acute episode has settled.

Stones in the small intestine: urgent management

Gallstone ileus

AETIOLOGY

A gall bladder which contains stones erodes into adjacent small bowel, usually the duodenum. Stones can then be shed through this cholecystenteric fistula into the gut. A stone that has a diameter greater than the narrowest part of the small bowel (terminal ileum) may impact to produce lower small bowel obstruction (Ch. 23).

CLINICAL FEATURES

The biliary tract disorder is usually silent, particularly, as is often so, when the patient is elderly. Vague attacks of colic may have occurred as the stone passes down the gut. Eventually the history is of low small bowel obstruction.

Physical findings are discussed in Chapter 23.

INVESTIGATION

In addition to the characteristic features of small bowel obstruction on a straight film, it may be possible to see:

- air in the biliary tract (aerobilia)
- a gallstone in the right lower quadrant.

MANAGEMENT

The condition is usually found at operation for small bowel obstruction without a clear cause. A soft stone is crushed from without; a harder one is milked retrogradely and extracted via a small enterotomy. The small bowel proximal to the obstruction is carefully examined to exclude other stones. Treatment of the fistula should usually be undertaken later.

General management of gall stones

Stones in the gall bladder

As described above, there are a number of complications of cholelithiasis which demand relatively urgent intervention, whether this is by operation or endoscopic means. However, the approach in the case of the patient with silent or with relatively uncomplicated gallstones which cause symptoms such as recurrent biliary colic is still subject to some controversy.

Asymptomatic stones

Only a minority (about 10%) will become symptomatic. Therefore, for most patients operation is not advised. Operation may be considered in the following cases:

- there is a non-functioning gall bladder which is thought to render an attack of acute cholecystitis more likely
- in diabetics, because this condition carries a greater risk of complications following the development of such features as biliary colic or cholecystitis; elective operations for silent stones may pre-empt this risk
- a cholecyst-enteric fistula has been identified
- the patient is young and has a large stone.

Symptomatic stones

The common presentation is with acute episodes of biliary colic, acute cholecystitis or obstructive jaundice. Occurrence of one of these is an indication for operation unless:

- the patient refuses, in which case non-operative management is attempted
- there are strong medical contraindications such as cardiorespiratory disease, although it must be remembered that a further acute attack may lead to disastrous decompensation.

Non-operative management

A number of non-operative methods are available for the treatment of gall bladder stones, but they are infrequently used.

Pharmacological dissolution therapy

Improved understanding of the mechanisms of bile production and storage (see p. 000) has led to the development of oral dissolution therapy. Cholesterol stones may dissolve if the concentration of bile salts is increased; ursodeoxycholic and chenodeoxycholic acid are the usual agents. For a high degree of success, the stones must be:

- less than 1 cm in diameter
- radiolucent, i.e. almost completely composed of cholesterol and non-calcified.

In addition, the gall bladder must be functioning so that high concentrations of bile salts can be achieved within it.

These criteria are met by only 30% of candidates and treatment for between 6 months and 2 years is required for success. Half the patients develop recurrent stones within 5 years.

Mechanical fragmentation and dissolution

Extracorporeal shock wave lithotripsy focuses ultrasonic shock waves on the stones and can successfully fragment some of them. The technique is painless, does not require anaesthesia and can be undergone as an outpatient. Adjuvant oral dissolution therapy is required for dissolution of stone fragments that are left behind. Selection criteria include no more than three radiolucent stones less than 3 cm in diameter in a functioning gall bladder with a patent cystic duct. Best results are achieved from the minority of patients with a solitary stone (over 90% stone clearance).

Surgical management of symptomatic stones

Cholecystectomy and methods to establish that the bile ducts are free from stones form the treatment of choice in patients who have had biliary colic, acute cholecystitis or an episode of obstructive jaundice. However, it is unwise to remove the gall bladder for vague upper abdominal pain or doubtful findings on ultrasound, because symptoms often persist.

Before operation, consideration should always be given to the possibility of choledocholithiasis. Common bile duct stones are only reliably detected by cholangiography. There are many permutations and combinations regarding the diagnosis, timing and method of extraction of common bile duct stones. Some surgeons perform cholangiography (operative or otherwise) on all patients, whereas others opt for a selective policy. Factors which alert the surgeon to the possibility of choledocholithiasis include:

- history of jaundice or pancreatitis in the preceding 6 months
- elevation of serum bilirubin or alkaline phosphatase concentrations
- dilatation of the common bile duct beyond 10 mm on ultrasound scanning.

Cholecystectomy is a procedure now commonly done by laparoscopic means (see Ch. 5) and with a mortality well below 1%. In acute cholecystitis, cholecystectomy may be done early (within 48 hours of the onset of symptoms) either as a standard policy to avoid recurrent attacks of cholecystitis or because symptoms and signs have failed to resolve. Other surgeons routinely operate later (some 4 weeks after an attack). Operation in the interim period may be difficult because of inflammatory adhesions.

Complications include:

- leak of bile from the the gall bladder bed, the stump of the cystic duct or injured bile duct, which leads either to a biliary fistula, usually through a drain inserted at operation, or to an intraperitoneal accumulation which may require drainage
- bleeding from a ligature that has slipped off the cystic artery
- operative damage to the bile ducts.

The last of these is the most serious and its occurrence temporarily increased after the introduction of laparoscopic cholecystectomy. It is prevented by a sound understanding of the possible ductal anatomical variations, by careful preoperative investigation and by careful operative technique. If it occurs, it may be recognised at once and repaired (although a stricture may still subsequently result) or it may present postoperatively with a bile leak, recurrent attacks of cholangitis or obstructive jaundice.

Late complications of damage to the bile ducts are best dealt with at specialised hepatobiliary centres by dissection and anastomosis of the dilated ducts above the site of obstruction to the small intestine usually via an isolated loop.

Stones in the bile ducts

These may be the prime cause of symptoms or be present along with gall bladder stones and identified either pre-operatively or by cholangiography during operation. In either event they should be removed. The choice for ductal stone extraction lies between the following:

- pre-or postoperative ERCP in combination with laparoscopic cholecystectomy
- cholecystectomy and exploration of the common bile duct either at open operation or laparoscopically.

Acalculous cholecystitis

AETIOLOGY AND PATHOLOGICAL FEATURES
Acute cholecystitis may develop in the absence of gallstones. This primary (or acalculous) cholecystitis usually afflicts very ill, often diabetic, patients on an intensive therapy unit, suffering from burns or the septic complications of major surgery. Predisposing factors include gall bladder stasis secondary to parenteral nutrition and opiate analgesia. The hypothesis is that there is bacteraemia with trapping of organisms by the liver and their secretion into stagnant bile.

The condition is a severe form of acute cholecystitis which often progresses to gangrene and performation. The mortality may approach 15%.

CLINICAL FEATURES
The coexistence of other serious illnesses in a patient who may be unconscious often masks the diagnosis. It is important to remember the possibility in a critically ill patient who develops signs of an acute abdomen.

INVESTIGATION
Diagnostic features on ultrasound scanning are those of gall bladder dilatation with oedema in the wall.

MANAGEMENT
Percutaneous cholecystostomy under ultrasound guidance with gall bladder drainage and parenteral antibiotics may suffice unless perforation has occurred when operation is required.

Gall bladder tumours

Benign

Adenoma
This is an uncommon tumour which predisposes to gall bladder carcinoma. It is usually an incidental finding on ultrasound scanning. Adenomas less than 1 cm in diameter can be observed but larger ones should be removed by cholecystectomy.

Two other conditions can mimic the appearance of an adenoma on ultrasound:

- *Cholesterosis* in which plaques of cholesterol are laid down in the gall bladder mucosa and cause a thickened irregular mucosal appearance which is sometimes known as *strawberry gall bladder*. Cholecystectomy is indicated in patients with symptoms provided these are clearly related to the biliary tree.
- *Adenomyoma* is a localised collection of cystic spaces in the gall bladder wall; it is a benign condition and, in its generalised form, is known as *adenomyomatosis*.

Malignant

EPIDEMIOLOGY AND AETIOLOGY
Cancer of the gall bladder is rare. Careful examination of cholecystectomy specimens suggests an incidence of

1%. The peak incidence is in the 60–80 year age range. Ninety-five per cent are associated with gallstones and this is reflected in the male:female ratio of 1:4. Ninety per cent of the growths are adenocarcinomas and the remaining 10% are squamous carcinomas which are believed to arise from areas of mucosal squamous metaplasia.

PATHOLOGICAL FEATURES

Gall bladder cancers tend to invade locally into the adjacent liver. They have a dismal prognosis because the great majority have invaded the liver beyond resectability at the time of presentation. The overall 5-year survival is 2–5%. The only tumours with a favourable prognosis are those early cancers found during pathological examination of a gall bladder removed for biliary symptoms.

FURTHER READING

Blumgart LH (1994). *Surgery of the Liver and Biliary Tract.* Edinburgh: Churchill Livingstone.

Broelsch CE (1993). *Atlas of Liver Surgery.* New York Churchill Livingstone

Launois B (1993). *Modern Operative Techniques in Liver Surgery.* Edinburgh: Churchill Livingstone

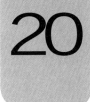

20

The spleen

Structure and function of the spleen

ANATOMY

The spleen lies in the left hypochondrium within the protection of the rib cage, weighs 150 g in the adult and is impalpable; threefold enlargement is required for the organ to become palpable. Its surface marking is the left ninth, 10th and 11th ribs in the mid-axillary line. The organ is friable and highly vascular, being supplied primarily by the splenic artery. Ligation of the splenic artery away from the hilum does not usually cause infarction because of collateral flow via the left gastro-epiploic and short gastric arteries. The artery usually divides before it enters the spleen so that each major branch supplies a segment. Thus the organ can be divided into transverse segments each supplied by an end artery, with relatively little blood flow between them; partial resection is thus possible, particularly in trauma. Blood enters the red pulp of the spleen, percolates along the splenic cords and is then filtered through tiny pores into the venous sinuses. Segmental veins leave the hilum and unite to form the splenic vein behind the tail of the pancreas. The vein contributes up to 40% of portal venous blood flow.

The spleen lies against the undersurface of the diaphragm, and in certain pathological states adhesions can develop between the diaphragmatic peritoneum and the splenic capsule. Embryologically the organ grows within the dorsal mesogastrium. Thus in adult life it is connected to the greater curvature of the stomach and to the left kidney by double peritoneal folds usually known (loosely) as ligaments: the gastrosplenic ligament contains the short gastric vessels (vasa brevia), but the lienorenal ligament is relatively bloodless. The medial or visceral surface of the spleen is related to the greater curve and fundus of the stomach, tail of pancreas and colon at the left colic (splenic) flexure and to the left kidney and adrenal gland. Because of these arrangements, the stomach or pancreatic tail may be injured during splenectomy, and the spleen can also be damaged during mobilisation of the stomach or left colon, operations on the distal pancreas or sometimes during a transabdominal approach to the left kidney and adrenal gland.

The spleen contains a higher proportion of fibrous tissue in the young and appears to become softer with age; this feature has a bearing on attempts to conserve the spleen after injury.

PHYSIOLOGICAL CONSIDERATIONS

Haematological functions

Haemopoiesis

In fetal life the spleen makes red cells, but in adults this function is reactivated only in myeloproliferative disorders that impair the ability of the bone marrow to produce sufficient red blood cells.

Red cell maturation and destruction

The spleen moulds reticulocytes into biconcave discs and also removes effete and damaged red cells from the circulation. After splenectomy, abnormal erythrocytes, which would have been destroyed by the organ, appear in the peripheral blood. They include *target cells* and some which contain intracellular inclusions such as *Howell–Jolly bodies* (nuclear remnants), *Heinz bodies* (denatured haemoglobin) and *Pappenheimer bodies* (iron granules). Although the human spleen has little or no function as a red cell reservoir, it is a major storage site for iron and holds a proportion of the platelets and macrophages that are available to the circulation.

Immunological functions

An increased susceptibility to severe infection after splenectomy (overwhelming postsplenectomy infection, OPSI) was reported 70 years ago but remained virtually unknown until 1952. It is now realised that the spleen plays a major role in both humoral and cell-mediated immunity.

Antigens are filtered from the circulating blood and are transported to the germinal centres of the organ, where IgM is synthesised. The spleen is a crucial site for production of the opsonins tuftsin and properdin, which are important in the phagocytosis of encapsulated bacteria.

Disorders of the spleen

Hyposplenism

Splenic agenesis

This is occasionally seen as a congenital anomaly, and splenic atrophy can develop in conditions such as coeliac disease and sickle cell anaemia. However, most patients become hyposplenic as an outcome of splenectomy. The haematological consequences are mostly short-lived. Persistence of abnormal red blood cells is accompanied by leucocytosis and thrombocythaemia, with peak values 1–2 weeks after operation; the platelet count can remain

elevated for months or years. The raised count probably does not mean a greater tendency to thrombosis.

Immunological consequences of splenectomy

Such consequences depend on the age of the patient and are greatest in infants. Reduced ability to opsonise and then phagocytose encapsulated bacteria leads to an increased incidence of infection by *Streptococcus pneumoniae* (pneumococcus) but also by *Neisseria meningitidis*, *Haemophilus influenzae* and *Escherichia coli*. The lifetime risk of developing OPSI is estimated at between 2 and 4% and is higher in children than in adults; the risk is also greater if the spleen is removed because of a haematological disease (thalassaemia, lymphoma) rather than for trauma.

Hypersplenism and splenomegaly

Hypersplenism is defined as overactivity of the spleen in one or more of its functions in relation to destruction of formed elements in the blood with or without splenomegaly. The consequences may be anaemia, leucopenia, thrombocytopenia or a combination of all three – *pancytopenia*. In spite of increased production of cells in the bone marrow, pooling and increased destruction in the spleen explains the pancytopenia. Causes of hypersplenism are listed in Table 20.1.

Splenomegaly is enlargement of the spleen and can be either primary (of unknown cause) or secondary to other splenic disorders. Hypersplenism and splenomegaly may occur together or separately.

AETIOLOGY

Infections

Infectious causes, other than the mild enlargement which may be seen with any acute and prolonged infection, include viruses (such as Epstein–Barr) and tuberculosis.

Tropical diseases

Diseases such as malaria, kala-azar (leishmaniasis) and schistosomiasis can lead to massive enlargement of the spleen, which is then susceptible to minor trauma. There is also an idiopathic form of tropical splenomegaly.

Splenic abscess

This is an uncommon lesion usually associated with severe systemic infection and a high mortality rate.

Portal hypertension

Whatever the underlying cause, the spleen enlarges but seldom to a great extent. Features of liver disease and of hypersplenism may be present. Splenic vein thrombosis without occlusion of the portal vein may

Table 20.1
Causes of hypersplenism; possible indications for splenectomy

Condition	Mechanism	Blood disorder	Splenomegaly
Inherited haemolytic anaemias			
Spherocytosis	Increased red cell fragility	Anaemia	Variable but rarely large
Elliptocytosis			
Thalassaemia	Abnormal Haemoglobins	Anaemia	Variable
Sickle cell disease			
Autoimmune haemolytic anaemias	Antibodies to red cells	Anaemia	Usual
Immune thrombocytopenic purpura (primary or secondary)	Antibodies to platelets	Thrombocytopenia	Rare
Portal hypertension	Raised splenic venous pressure with delayed transit of blood	Pancytopenia	Always
Rheumatoid arthritis (Felty's syndrome)	Uncertain	Leucopenia or pancytopenia	Always

produce segmental or left-sided portal hypertension with splenomegaly and oesophageal varices, for which splenectomy alone is curative.

Blood disorders

Haemolytic anaemias
Haemolytic anaemias of all types increase the workload of the spleen in removing defective red cells. The organ progressively enlarges and may eventually become too active in red cell destruction and exacerbate the anaemia.

Hereditary spherocytosis
This is the commonest type of congenital haemolytic anaemia. The erythrocytes have a typical spherical shape on a peripheral blood film and demonstrate increased osmotic fragility; periodic crises of anaemia occur, especially if the patient develops a viral illness. Hereditary elliptocytosis is a rare variant. Thalassaemia is common in those from the Mediterranean littoral and sub-Saharan Africa, and is characterised by persistence of fetal haemoglobin into adult life. Heterozygotes have a mild form of anaemia, whereas homozygotes have severe chronic anaemia and retardation of growth (thalassaemia major). The characteristic molar hypertrophy is due to overactive haemopoiesis in the upper jaw.

Acquired haemolytic anaemia
This is an autoimmune disease, which occurs either in a primary (idiopathic) form or secondary to an underlying disorder such as a collagen disease or to the administration of certain drugs (e.g. penicillin); it is commonest in older women. Splenomegaly is generally associated with mild fever and jaundice. The Coombs' test is positive because the red cells are coated with immunoglobulins or complement; the reaction occurs at different temperatures according to the presence of warm or cold antibodies.

Sickle cell disease
Another common haemoglobinopathy, sickle cell disease is more likely, because of repeated minor splenic infarctions, to cause hypo- rather than hypersplenism.

Immune thrombocytopenic purpura (ITP).
Although this disorder involves splenic destruction of platelets, the organ is rarely enlarged. Splenomegaly can, however, be a feature of the secondary type that develops as a consequence of lymphoproliferative disease, infection or drugs. Both types of IPT are associated with circulating antiplatelet antibodies. ITP can develop acutely in children, often after a viral illness. The chronic form tends to be seen in adult females and is characterised by a history of heavy periods.

Splenic cyst
This is a rare condition. Cysts can be either congenital in origin or parasitic from echinococcal (hydatid) infestation. Occasionally a traumatic pseudocyst results from liquefaction of a previous splenic haematoma.

Myeloproliferative diseases
Many types of myeloproliferative disease are characterised by splenomegaly, including:

- myeloid and lymphocytic leukaemia
- polycythaemia rubra vera
- myelofibrosis (also called myelosclerosis).

In myeloid leukaemia there is enlargement of the red pulp, whereas in myelofibrosis extramedullary haemopoiesis develops in the liver and spleen as a result of obliteration of the bone marrow by fibrous tissue. Massive splenomegaly and secondary hypersplenism may result. The huge spleen causes dragging abdominal discomfort, which may be exacerbated by the pain of recurrent splenic infarcts. Hypersplenism predisposes to fatigue and dyspnoea (anaemia), spontaneous bleeding (thrombocytopenia) and opportunist infection (neutropenia).

Lymphatic malignancy
The spleen is very frequently enlarged in patients with tumours of the lymphoid system, e.g. lymphoma, Hodgkin's disease and other, rarer disorders which are more difficult to classify.

CLINICAL FEATURES

History

Splenomegaly is generally painless unless the organ undergoes patchy infarction, as can occur in chronic myeloid leukaemia, when there may be both pleuritic and shoulder pain. Otherwise the history is that of the disease causing the splenic enlargement or hypersplenism.

Features include recurrent anaemia, purpura and respiratory infections, which are the consequences of the neutropenia. Specific symptoms related to the underlying condition may be present.

Physical findings

These vary with the cause. Splenomegaly is frequent but, as indicated in Table 20.1, may not be present when the condition involves destruction of only one cellular element of the blood. Thrombocytopenia is associated with purpuric skin lesions and a risk of intracranial haemorrhage. Leucopenia occurs with a variable increase in bacterial infections.

There can be mild tenderness if the spleen is enlarged secondary to an acute infection. A mass in the left upper quadrant of splenic origin has the following characteristics:

- it is dull on percussion
- it moves downwards with respiration
- it can sometimes be notched on palpation
- it cannot have its upper margin defined on palpation.

In addition, care must be taken to ensure that the examining hand can get below a very large spleen; palpation is begun low down in the right iliac fossa. Difficulty may be experienced in differentiating splenomegaly from the following:

- *an enlarged left kidney*, which also moves on respiration but should be palpable in the loin and have a band of resonant gas-containing colon in front of it
- *gastric or colonic tumours* – these scarcely move on respiration, and the examining hand can generally interpose between the mass and the costal margin
- *mass arising from the pancreatic tail*, such as a large pseudocyst; this is typically deeply placed and less discrete on palpation.

When there is doubt, imaging by either plain X-ray, ultrasonography, isotope scan (scintigraphy) or CT shows the size of the spleen and whether it is indeed the cause of the mass.

INVESTIGATION OF HYPERSPLENISM

Marrow function

A precise diagnosis is essential before proceeding to splenectomy because splenomegaly may, in such circum-

stances as infiltration of the bone marrow (malignancy, myelofibrosis), indicate that the spleen has taken over the marrow's function in producing formed elements of the blood. Bone marrow biopsy should therefore be performed to confirm that the marrow is still active.

Red cell dynamics

Production can be studied by giving radiolabelled iron and destruction by ^{51}Cr labelling. External scanning over the spleen demonstrates its activity in each regard. If splenectomy is undertaken for hypersplenism, a pre-operative search by imaging, supplemented by a wide exploration at operation, must be made for accessory spleens (splenunculi) which could otherwise enlarge and lead to recurrence of the original condition.

MANAGEMENT

Infections

Splenomegaly during the course of an acute infectious illness is treated with the appropriate antimicrobial agents. The massive enlargements seen in the tropics because of specific infections may require splenectomy because of pain and/or secondary hypersplenism. Splenic abscesses are drained as part of the overall management of severe septic states.

Blood disorders

Many of the congenital red cell and haemoglobin disorders respond to splenectomy (which must include the removal of any accessory spleens), especially if there is a high rate of haemolysis. In diminishing order, the operation is indicated for:

- spherocytosis
- thalassaemia major
- sickle cell disease
- elliptocytosis.

In ITP, corticosteroid therapy will often (75%) improve the platelet count, but splenectomy is indicated for patients who fail to respond or relapse when steroids are withdrawn. Steroids have a similar response rate in acquired haemolytic anaemia, but again splenectomy is indicated for treatment failures; generally only those patients with warm antibodies respond to the operation.

Lymphatic malignancy

The role of operative treatment in these disorders is:

- establishment of the diagnosis by node biopsy usually from the neck but occasionally from the axilla
- staging of disease by laparotomy, splenectomy and multiple lymph node biopsies, although better techniques of imaging and concern about OSPI have reduced the use of this method
- very occasionally to remove a massive spleen that is causing symptoms.

Ruptured spleen

AETIOLOGY

In *blunt abdominal trauma*, the spleen is the most vulnerable organ despite its relatively protected site. The mechanism is a direct blow or fall. Road traffic accidents and sports injuries are common causes. Rupture is often associated with fractures of the overlying ribs. Other injuries – particularly to the head – may also occur and appear to dominate the damage profile. In most patients the spleen is healthy and of normal size, but if there is splenomegaly, relatively minor trauma can cause bleeding (e.g. infectious mononucleosis and malaria). *Spontaneous rupture* can occasionally occur, although in such circumstances very minor trauma may have been forgotten. The spleen can also be damaged inadvertently during the course of an abdominal operation which involves procedures in the left upper quadrant, when a relatively minor capsular tear may cause persistent bleeding.

PATHOLOGICAL FEATURES

Elaborate classification of the extent and nature of splenic rupture has been devised and can assist the surgeon in deciding whether to attempt splenic conservation.

The important practical distinction is between *immediate* and *delayed* rupture. In the first, the capsule and, to a greater or lesser extent, the underlying organ are torn and bruised, bleeding is extensive and the clinical presentation is prompt. The most extreme example is when the spleen is completely avulsed from its artery or vein. In delayed rupture, the capsule remains initially intact or, on occasion, the leak of blood is local and only into the left upper quadrant. Presentation may then be delayed for hours, days or even weeks.

CLINICAL FEATURES

History

An obvious injury to the left chest wall or the abdomen may have been sustained. Conscious patients complain of *abdominal pain* that is generalised but usually most severe in the left upper quadrant. Pain may also be felt in the tip of the left shoulder because irritation of the undersurface of the diaphragm stimulates the phrenic nerve (C4 dermatome: Kehr's sign). An unconscious patient cannot report these symptoms, and there is danger that the abdominal condition may be overlooked unless very careful attention is paid to the clinical findings. Head injuries do not cause circulatory collapse.

Physical findings

Hypovolaemia. In frank rupture there is considerable rapid blood loss into the peritoneal cavity, and pallor, low blood pressure, rapid pulse and restlessness develop.

Abdominal signs. There may be external bruising and tenderness over the upper left abdomen and lower left ribs – the second suggesting fracture. Typically there is abdominal tenderness, guarding and rigidity. Occasionally a splenic mass is felt.

Delayed rupture

This has an insidious presentation with anaemia, vague left upper quadrant and left shoulder pain and mild tenderness in the left upper quadrant. The signs may become acute if free rupture eventually takes place.

INVESTIGATION

Few tests are required when frank rupture of the spleen causes a haemoperitoneum. In other patients, imaging may be required to confirm the diagnosis of rupture or a subcapsular haematoma.

Blood examination

Haematocrit is normal at first until haemodilution occurs over some hours.

Leucocyte count is raised (as in other forms of trauma).

Imaging

X-ray. Chest X-ray often shows fractured ribs, and the left hemidiaphragm may be elevated by the underlying haematoma. Abdominal X-ray may show splenomegaly or a subdiaphragmatic soft tissue mass.

Ultrasound and CT may demonstrate the rupture of the splenic capsule and show free blood in the peritoneal cavity. A subcapsular haematoma can be demonstrated (Fig. 20.1). In a haemodynamically stable

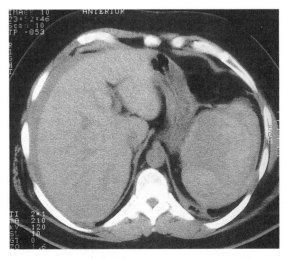

Fig 20.1 **Abdominal CT showing a large splenic mass of mixed attenuation in a patient who has recently undergone blunt abdominal trauma.** Increasing pain and anaemia led to laparotomy and splenectomy. The spleen was lacerated and surrounded by a large quantity of blood and fresh clot.

patient, the progress or resolution of a haematoma may be assessed by repeated scanning (see below).

Specific procedures

Needle aspiration of the peritoneal cavity may reveal blood, but the technique is much less sensitive than peritoneal lavage.

Peritoneal lavage (see Ch. 11). This procedure is particularly valuable to confirm or exclude serious abdominal injury in an unconscious patient with head injury and unexplained signs that suggest loss of blood. Laparoscopy can also be useful to determine the extent and site of bleeding.

MANAGEMENT

Until recently, any but the most trivial splenic injury was regarded as an indication for splenectomy. Nowadays, because of better recognition of the risk of postsplenectomy sepsis, an attempt is made to preserve splenic tissue. Splenic salvage is particularly desirable in children, who are at grater risk. However, the prime goal is to save the patient's life, and attempts at splenic preservation should not be continued if there is continuous bleeding.

Management may follow three main courses:

- *Non-operative* – splenic injury is suspected, but there are few clinical signs and imaging shows a limited haematoma; the patient is admitted for a few days to ensure that the haematocrit does not decrease and repeated imaging does not show enlargement or that there is resolution.
- *Initial non-operative followed by operation* – indicated by increasing physical findings and decline in haematocrit which mean continued bleeding. As a rough guide, the need for more than two units of blood to be transfused indicates laparotomy.
- *Emergency operation* – a patient in hypovolaemic shock is, if possible, resuscitated immediately and then proceeds to laparotomy; sometimes it may be necessary to operate in the presence of hypotension in order to control bleeding.

At operation, a rapid search is made for other sites of bleeding, notably from the liver and tears in the mesentery. Unless the organ is extensively shattered or bleeding is uncontrollable, an attempt is made to preserve it. Simple manoeuvres may suffice, such as topical haemostatic agents (e.g. oxidised regenerated cellulose: Surgicel) applied with gentle pressure over a swab. Alternatively, the organ is mobilised and accurate suture is performed with or without ligation of the splenic artery to reduce blood flow. Enclosing the spleen in a bag of absorbable mesh may also control bleeding. Finally segmental resection may be feasible. If splenectomy proves unavoidable, some surgeons leave splenic tissue behind within an omental pocket, but the function of such autotransplants is doubtful.

Operation is also indicated for a delayed rupture that presents with late haemoperitoneum or (rarely) an expanding traumatic pseudocyst.

Splenectomy

PREOPERATIVE MANAGEMENT

Hypersplenism

Before removing the spleen it is necessary to show that there is excessive destruction of blood elements in the spleen and that there is adequate bone marrow function to cope should the spleen have become an important site of erythropoiesis.

Prophylaxis against OPSI

This should be undertaken in all patients who are to undergo an elective operation which could involve splenectomy. Immunisation is required not only when splenectomy is planned but also in operations on adjacent organs in which the spleen may form part of the dissection – e.g. total gastrectomy and operations on the distal pancreas. The regimen is considered in Information Box 20.1.

Correction of cytopenia

Specific correction includes that of anaemia and occasionally of thrombocytopenia (steroid therapy and platelet transfusion, although platelets are better infused only after the spleen has been isolated by ligation of its artery).

Risk of infection

Patients with leucopenia should receive antibiotic prophylaxis against Gram-positive organisms. Immunoglobulin therapy may also have a role.

OPERATION

The spleen can be safely removed via a subcostal or midline laparotomy, but extension into the chest is occasionally needed if the organ is massive. A search should be made for (pigment) gallstones in patients with haemolytic anaemia and for accessory spleens which can cause recurrence of haemolytic and thrombocytopenic disorders. If the organ is enormous and adherent, it may be advisable to expose and ligate the splenic artery at an early stage. Adhesions to the diaphragm and mesocolon need to be divided before the peritoneal attachments of the spleen are incised and the organ is mobilised into the wound. Care must be taken when dividing the short gastic vessels not to injure the stomach and, when the splenic vessels are ligated, to avoid injury to the tail of the pancreas.

COMPLICATIONS

Bleeding

This may result from persistent oozing in the splenic bed, and this is the commonest cause of subphrenic haematoma and abscess. These complications are more frequent in patients with preoperative thrombocytopenia.

Gastric and pancreatic fistulae

These may follow injury to the stomach, but with good technique they are very rare.

Thrombocytosis

This is the rule after splenectomy, but venous thrombo-embolism is not especially common; antiplatelet agents or subcutaneous heparin may be given if the platelet count rises above $100 \times 10^9/L$.

Overwhelming postsplenectomy infection (OPSI)

This is the most serious late complication of splenectomy.

Pathological features

The functional role of the spleen in protection from infection has been discussed above and, although much remains to be discovered, it is apparent that it plays a major part in dealing with bloodstream invasion by encapsulated organisms such as pneumococci and meningococci. The commonest form of OPSI is therefore pneumoccoccal or meningococcal septicaemia. Adrenal haemorrhage may occur and contribute to death by adding an element of acute adrenal insufficiency. In addition, infections with *H. influenzae* are an important risk. In tropical regions, tick-borne infections and malaria are also common.

Clinical features

Postsplenectomy sepsis often starts insidiously but can rapidly develop into a fulminant infection. There is fever, vomiting, dehydration and circulatory collapse often without specific features that alert the clinician to the diagnosis. An upper abdominal scar may be indicative even in the absence of a definite history of splenectomy.

Investigation

Evidence of acute infection should be sought by:

- leucocytosis
- blood smear examination for organisms
- blood culture
- CSF examination and culture in the presence of neurological clinical features.

Management

The intravenous administration of fluids and anti-biotics should be started on a best guess basis without waiting for the results of culture and organism

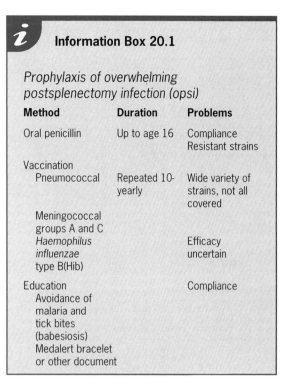

Information Box 20.1

Prophylaxis of overwhelming postsplenectomy infection (opsi)

Method	Duration	Problems
Oral penicillin	Up to age 16	Compliance Resistant strains
Vaccination Pneumococcal	Repeated 10-yearly	Wide variety of strains, not all covered
Meningococcal groups A and C *Haemophilus influenzae* type B(Hib)		Efficacy uncertain
Education Avoidance of malaria and tick bites (babesiosis) Medalert bracelet or other document		Compliance

sensitivities. The mortality rate is at least 50%, which emphasises the need for prophylaxis.

Prophylaxis

The occurrence of OPSI could be much reduced (although exactly by how much is not known) if vigorous preventive measures were used in those at risk. Although the condition was originally thought to be limited to infants and children, it is now known to occur at all ages, which justifies universal prophylaxis after splenectomy.

There is no absolute agreement on regimens, but guidelines have been issued and are summarised in Information Box 20.1. Patients should not leave hospital without prophylaxis having begun.

FURTHER READING

Spleen

Cooper MJ (1991) Spleen. In: O'Higgins NJ, Chisholm GD, Williams RCN (eds) *Surgical Management*, 2nd edn. Oxford: Butterworth Heinemann, pp. 552–561.

Cooper MJ, Williamson RCN (1984) Splenectomy: indications, hazards and alternatives. *British Journal of Surgery* 71, 173–180.

Williamson RCN (1994) Spleen, In: Kirk RM (ed.) *General Surgical Operations*, 3rd edn. Edinburgh: Churchill Livingstone, pp. 395–399.

21

Surgical aspects of pancreatic disease

The pancreas

EMBRYOLOGY

The pancreas begins in fetal life as ventral and dorsal buds of the foregut, each with its own drainage duct. As the foregut rotates and develops, the two buds fuse to surround the superior mesenteric vessels. The larger dorsal pancreas forms the adult body, tail and upper part of the head and the ventral pancreas the rest of the head and the uncinate process. Fusion of the duct system results in the duct of the ventral bud becoming the main duct (of Wirsung) which drains into the duodenum through a shared opening with the common bile duct at the so-called major papilla (Ampulla of Vater). The duct of the dorsal bud duct persists as the smaller accessory duct of Santorini which drains through the minor papilla.

ANATOMY

In adult life the pancreas lies across the posterior abdominal wall at the level of L1. The head is surrounded by the concavity of the duodenum.

The uncinate process and lower part of the head (ventral duct derivatives) pass posteriorly and to the left of the superior mesenteric vessels. The body of the pancreas forms the main bulk of the gland and extends across the midline ending in a tail lying close to the splenic hilum (Fig. 21.1). The main pancreatic duct leads from the tail to the head of the organ, gradually increasing in size as it drains ductules from the pancreatic substance. It usually joins the common bile duct to open into the second part of the duodenum through a common channel and single orifice. This opening is visible from the luminal surface of the duodenum as a small nipple – the major papilla.

Developmental anomalies of the pancreas

Pancreas divisum

This is an anatomical variation in which most of the pancreas drains into the duodenum through the accessory duct of Santorini, usually about 2 cm proximal to the duodenal papilla.

Annular pancreas

This is a rare cause of extrinsic compression of the second part of the duodenum from failure of the two

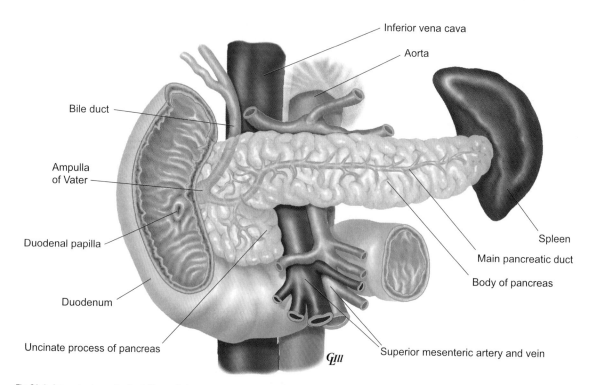

Fig 21.1 **Important surgical relations of the pancreas.** Note the intimate relationship of the uncinate process and neck of the pancreas with the superior mesenteric vessels.

developing pancreatic buds to fuse. A cuff of pancreatic tissue surrounds the duodenum.

Both pancreas divisum and annular pancreas may be associated with drainage abnormalities and pancreatitis (see p. 000).

Heterotopic pancreas
Accessory budding of the primitive duodenum results in nodules of pancreatic tissue in abnormal positions such as the stomach, duodenal wall or jejunum. Heterotopic nodules are present in 20% of the population and occasionally produce obstructive or dyspeptic symptoms.

PHYSIOLOGY

The human pancreas is both an endocrine and exocrine organ and these two functions are performed by different cell populations. By far the majority of the gland (up to 98% by weight) consists of acinar cells which synthesise the exocrine pancreatic enzymes and drain into the intraglandular ductules which are tributaries of the main pancreatic duct. The principal hormones that control release of exocrine secretions are secretin and cholecystokinin (CCK), which are produced from the APUD group of cells in the duodenum and upper jejunum.

Secretin is released into the bloodstream when acidic gastric contents enter the first part of the duodenum. It stimulates secretion of a watery, alkaline pancreatic juice rich in electrolytes.

CCK is released when fatty acids and amino acids enter the duodenum; it stimulates contraction of the gall bladder and bile ducts as well as secretion of a pancreatic juice rich in enzymes. These are involved in the breakdown of carbohydrates, fats and proteins, the most important of which are pancreatic amylase, lipase, colipase, phospholipase and a family of proteases (trypsinogen, chymotrypsinogen and elastase). The proteases are secreted in inactive forms (pro-enzymes – zymogens) which are subsequently activated in the lumen of the duodenum by enterokinase, which is probably secreted from the same source as secretin and CCK. Intrapancreatic enzyme activation can cause autolysis of the pancreas and may be one of the pathophysiological mechanisms of pancreatits.

The endocrine portion of the human pancreas is arranged as islands (the islets of Langerhans) of endocrine tissue within the exocrine gland. The islets have a rich vascular supply and the endocrine cells secrete hormones directly into the portal blood rather than by drainage into the duct system. Surgical disorders that affect the islets are considered below.

Measurement of function

A large number of physiological tests have been devised to measure both the exocrine and endocrine functions of the pancreas. Some of the most important are shown in Box 21.1.

standardised diet. Elevated faecal fat content (greater than 5 g/day) indicates malabsorption of triglycerides, although the spread of results is wide.

$^{14}CO_2$ **breath test.** The amount of $^{14}CO_2$ in expired air is measured following oral ingestion of a ^{14}C-labelled fatty acid (^{14}C-oleic acid) compared with that after ingestion of labelled triglyceride (^{14}C-itrolein). Impaired triglyceride absorption with normal fatty acid absorption indicates that pancreatic disease is the cause of the steatorrhoea.

Serum amylase measurement is used in acute pancreatic disease but is of no value in chronic disease.

Endocrine function

Measurement of pancreatic endocrine function may be required if a functioning endocrine tumour is suspected.

IMAGING (see also Table 21.1)

Plain X-ray

This is discussed in detail in Chapter 4.

Ultrasound and CT

These techniques are the mainstays of modern imaging. Both can be used to detect abnormalities of pancreatic size and shape and the presence of cysts or tumours. In combination with guided needle cytology and biopsy, they are powerful diagnostic tools. Ultrasound is commonly used as a first-line investigation because it is cheap, non-invasive and relatively easy to perform. CT gives more precise anatomical definition (see Fig. 21.3)

Box 21.1

Investigation of pancreatic function

Exocrine

Serum amylase concentration

Duodenal enzyme concentrations after:
— stimulation with CCK and/or secretin
— food stimulation (Lundh meal)

PABA test

Faecal fat

$^{14}CO_2$ breath test

Endocrine

Glucose tolerance test
Plasma levels of:
  insulin
  glucagon
  pancreatic polypeptide

Exocrine function

Direct tests

Direct tests of exocrine function rely on measurements of secreted enzymes into the gut. The Lundh meal and its variants involve the collection of pancreatic secretion through a nasogastric tube first at rest and then after the administration of a standard meal. Alternatively the gland may be stimulated by secretin or CCK. Bicarbonate concentration and trypsin and lipase levels are the most common measurements made. Pancreatic insufficiency results in low post-stimulation secretion of enzymes. However, enzyme secretion has a large reserve capacity and measurement of secretion in this manner is rarely helpful in the diagnosis of mild to moderate insufficiency such as may occur in the early stages of chronic pancreatitis.

Indirect tests

Indirect tests that may be of value include:

- the PABA test
- faecal fat estimation
- $^{14}CO_2$ breath test
- concentration of amylase in the serum.

PABA test. N-benzoyl-l-tryosyl *p*-aminobenzoic acid is a synthetic peptide which is hydrolysed by pancreatic chymotrypsin to release free *p*-aminobenzoic acid (PABA) which is absorbed, metabolised and excreted in the urine. Reduction in the absorption of PABA occurs if pancreatic chymotrypsin secretion is low.

Faecal fat estimation is useful to confirm steatorrhoea. Faeces are collected for 3 days with the patient on a

---

Table 21.1
Methods of visualisation of the pancreas

Technique	Purpose
Abdominal X-ray	Calcification
	Sentinel loop in acute pancreatitis
Ultrasound	Gland size
	Presence of gall stones
	Cysts
	Calcification
	Tumour
	Duct dilatation
CT	As for ultrasound and may define vascular involvement in malignant disease
MRI	Similar to CT and can give good images of the ducts
ERCP	Duct and ductular anatomy
Angiography	Tumour detection
	Anatomical definition and vascular involvement
Endoscopic ultrasound	In experienced units may give additional information
Laparoscopy with or without ultrasound	Valuable for detection of small liver and peritoneal metastases

Note: percutaneous biopsy under image control can be done to determine the nature of pancreatic swellings.

but is more costly. Rapid sequence spiral CT (Ch. 4) accompanied by intravenous injection of contrast can now provide high-definition images of pancreatic tumours and show their relationship to major vessels such as the superior mesenteric and portal veins and the superior mesenteric artery. In many subjects this is as accurate as the more invasive visceral angiography. MRI is still under development but impressive images of the pancreatic and biliary ductal systems are currently being obtained and so-called magnetic resonance cholangiopancreatography (MRCP) is likely to replace diagnostic ERCP.

Endoscopic retrograde cholangiopancreatography (ERCP)

Involves passage of a flexible, side-viewing endoscope into the duodenum and cannulation of the duodenal papilla. Contrast medium is injected to outline the pancreatic duct (pancreatography) and the bile ducts (cholangiography). The procedure is described as retrograde because the contrast medium flows in the opposite direction to normal biliary and pancreatic juices. The technique produces good images of the pancreatic duct and is useful in the diagnosis of pancreatic duct strictures and their cause, for the identification of bile duct and pancreatic duct stones and for defining congenital abnormalities and leaks from the biliary system. Transient asymptomatic hyperamylasaemia after ERCP is common. Complications of diagnostic ERCP occur in 2–3% of patients and include acute pancreatitis and cholangitis.

ERCP also permits treatment, e.g. the removal of bile duct stones after diathermy cutting of the sphincter at the major papilla (sphincterotomy) or balloon dilatation. Plastic or expanding metal tubes (stents) can be placed through strictures of the bile and pancreatic ducts to relieve obstruction. Additional complications of therapeutic ERCP include bleeding and duodenal perforation.

Visceral angiography

This technique is reserved for use only when surgical resection for pancreatic disease is under consideration. Angiograms show abnormal tumour circulation, aberrant blood vessels and the anatomy of arteries supplying surrounding viscera. Selective catheterisation may show irregularity, encasement or occlusion of arteries or the superior mesenteric or portal veins. All these are indications of unresectability of a malignant lesion.

Endoscopic ultrasonography

In expert hands, an ultrasound probe attached to the end of a flexible endoscope can give additional information about pancreatic disease. The body of the gland is well visualised because of its close proximity to the posterior aspect of the stomach and the head is within the duodenal loop and also easily seen.

Laparoscopy and laparoscopic ultrasonography

Laparoscopy is useful as a final staging investigation in those under consideration for resection of a pancreatic tumour. Small, undetected liver or peritoneal metastases are discovered in up to a third of instances. The addition of ultrasound may also allow more precise assessment of lymph node and vascular involvement.

DIAGNOSIS OF A PANCREATIC MASS

A common clinical situation in the pancreas is a mass which may or may not be causing jaundice. Differentiation between a benign and malignant condition is vital. Any combination of the above imaging techniques may be used but none is error-free. Elevated levels of tumour markers in the blood, particularly CA 19-9, suggest malignancy, but raised levels also occur in inflammatory conditions. Percutaneous needle aspiration for cytology, or needle biopsy under ultrasound or CT or at laparoscopy may confirm malignancy but this is technically demanding and the lesion may not be accurately targeted. False-negative results are common.

Pancreatitis

CLASSIFICATION

Pancreatitis is by far the most important benign condition of the pancreas. There are a number of methods of classification based on presentation (acute and chronic pancreatitis), aetiology (e.g. gallstone pancreatitis, alcoholic pancreatitis) or pathological events (e.g. oedematous pancreatitis, necrotising pancreatitis).

These different classification systems have caused confusion for many years. The essential distinction is between acute and chronic pancreatitis. In acute disease, endocrine and exocrine function, as well as the gross structure of the gland, return completely to normal after resolution of the attack unless complications occur. In chronic pancreatitis, there are permanent structural changes which can lead to a small, fibrotic gland with either exocrine or endocrine functional impairment or both. Other changes seen in chronic pancreatitis include:

- calcification
- ductal strictures and dilatation
- ductal stones
- intrapancreatic cysts.

The classification of a patient presenting with an attack of pancreatitis thus depends on the underlying structural changes in the gland. As this may not be evident unless more extensive visualisation of the pancreas is performed, such a patient is classified as having acute pancreatitis. Once structural changes are confirmed (in the same or subsequent attacks) the diagnosis of chronic pancreatitis can be made. Patients with chronic pancreatitis may have pain-free intervals and acute exacerbations of their chronic condition.

AETIOLOGY

A number of conditions are known to predispose to pancreatitis (Table 21.2). The commonest (60–70%) are gallstone disease and alcohol consumption. The mechanism by which these aetiological factors trigger pancreatitis is not clear and may differ between patients. Intraglandular activation of pancreatic juice, obstruction to drainage of secretions, metabolic intralobular changes and ischaemia have all been implicated.

Gallstones

The mechanisms by which gallstones cause acute pancreatitis are not fully understood. However, it is known that patients with multiple small stones in the gall bladder are more likely to develop pancreatitis than those with large or solitary stones; small gallstones can be detected in the faeces of patients soon after an attack of stone-related pancreatitis. It has therefore been postulated that acute pancreatitis may follow passage of a stone through the major papilla; less commonly, a stone may be identified impacted in the papilla during an attack. In either circumstance, reflux of bile or duodenal contents along the pancreatic

Table 21.2
Known and suspected causes of pancreatitis

Cause	Possible mechanism
Gallstones	Duodenopancreatic reflux
	Infection
Alcohol	Unknown
Iatrogenic	ERCP
	Operation at or around the papilla
Obstruction	Neoplasm, pancreas divisum, choledochocele, duodenal cysts
Viral infections	Coxsackie B
	Mumps
	ECHO
	Epstein–Barr
	Hepatitis A and B
Bacterial infections	*Mycoplasma pneumoniae*
Trauma	Usually ruptured duct
Hypercalcaemia	Hyperparathyroidism
	Sarcoidosis
	Malignancy
Hyperlipidaemia	Unknown but occurs in Fredrikson's types I, III, IV, V
Drugs	Corticosteroids
	Azathioprine
	Thiazides
	Tetracycline
	Valproate
	Frusemide
	Sulphonamides
Cushing's syndrome	
Hypothermia	
Miscellaneous	Hereditary
	Pregnancy

duct may follow with intraductal activation of pro-enzymes by enterokinase or possibly infected bile. Autodigestion of the pancreas (particularly by trypsin and phospholipase A) then occurs. Once enzymes are activated, cell membranes are digested and oedema, proteolysis, vascular damage and necrosis may follow. Gallstones rarely lead to chronic pancreatitis but are often associated with recurrent attack of acute pancreatic inflammation unless they are surgically removed.

Alcohol

Alcohol alone can damage the pancreas and excessive drinking can precipitate an acute episode of pancreatitis. Often the gland has been previously damaged by alcohol, so that it may be more correct to use the term acute-on-chronic pancreatitis for the acute episodes seen in heavy consumers of alcohol. The precise mechanism of action is not known. Alcohol is the usual cause of chronic pancreatitis (80% in developed societies).

Other causes (Table 21.2)

Pancreatitis can also occur in other conditions where free drainage of the pancreatic duct is impeded (e.g. pancreas divisum, papillary or pancreatic tumours, biliary stents). In these conditions, the pancreatitis may be acute, or structural changes may develop, leading to chronic pancreatitis. Other causes of chronic disease include:

- familial
- nutritional in tropical countries probably of toxic origin
- trauma.

PATHOLOGICAL FEATURES

The mildest form of pancreatitis is characterised by interstitial oedema with inflammatory exudate (oedematous pancreatitis). In more severe forms, there is glandular necrosis (necrotising pancreatitis) which results from microcirculatory stasis within the gland leading to infarction. Surrounding peripancreatic tissues may also develop necrotic changes (peripancreatic necrosis). Infection may supervene in necrotic tissue (infected necrosis) possibly by translocation of organisms from adjacent bowel.

In chronic pancreatitis, glandular structure is lost with areas of obstructive changes and fibrosis. A chronic inflammatory infiltrate and extensive fibrosis are seen. Calcification, duct and ductular dilatation and cyst formation frequently take place.

Acute pancreatitis

Acute pancreatitis exhibits a broad spectrum of clinical severity, ranging from mild and self-limiting (in most cases), to a rapidly fatal disorder associated with multi-organ failure and death.

CLINICAL FEATURES

These vary with the severity of the attack.

History

The principal symptom is abdominal pain, usually localised to the epigastrium or upper abdomen but which may radiate to the back in the upper lumbar region between the scapulae. Pain ranges from mild discomfort to an excruciating level in severe cases. Rarely, acute pancreatitis can occur in the absence of pain. Nausea and repeated vomiting are present in most instances.

Physical findings

General findings may be of an acutely ill patient with signs of circulatory insufficiency. In the abdomen, the degree of tenderness, guarding and rigidity found depends on the amount and nature of the inflammatory process. Rarely, body wall ecchymoses occur, around the umbilicus (Cullen's sign) or in the flanks (Grey Turner's sign – Fig. 21.2). Both are a consequence of haemorrhagic fluid tracking from the retroperitoneum. The remaining clinical features depend on the local and systemic complications that occur.

DIAGNOSIS

The clinical manifestations of acute pancreatitis are so varied that the condition must be considered in the differential diagnosis of all instances of upper abdominal pain until the serum amylase concentration (see below) has been demonstrated as being within the normal range. Hyperamylasaemia, however, cannot be relied upon alone and must be evaluated in conjunction with the history and physical signs.

INVESTIGATION

Serum amylase concentration

Elevation of the serum amylase level occurs in a number of acute abdominal emergencies such as acute cholecystitis, bowel ischaemia and perforated peptic ulcer, but a concentration in excess of 1000 IU/L is highly suggestive of acute pancreatitis. Very rarely, other causes of hyperamylasaemia (such as macroamylasaemia – a benign condition associated with abnormally large molecular weight amylase molecules which are not adequately cleared by the renal tubules) may confuse the diagnosis.

Imaging

Plain abdominal and chest X-rays are useful in two respects. A sentinel dilated loop of small bowel may be seen overlying the pancreatic region (Fig. 21.3). If an upright chest X-ray shows air under the diaphragm, then the cause of the acute abdomen is not pancreatitis but a gastrointestinal perforation.

Ultrasound and CT may be useful in clinching the diagnosis by demonstrating a swollen gland (Fig. 21.4) and identifying underlying causes such as gallstones. They are also used for the assessment of progress and the detection of necrosis (see below). Dynamic CT need only be performed in patients predicted as severe.

Peritoneal lavage

This procedure may be used if the diagnosis remains unclear. Amylase concentration is measured in the lavage fluid which is also often haemorrhagic in severe disease.

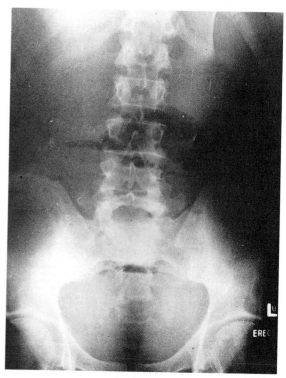

Fig 21.3 **Plain abdominal X-ray showing a dilated loop of small bowel in the epigastrium in acute pancreatitis – the sentinel loop.**

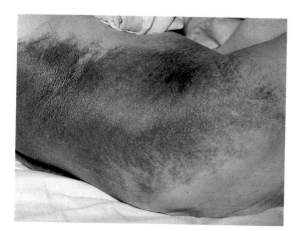

Fig 21.2 **Extensive flank bruising in acute pancreatitis – Grey Turner's sign.**

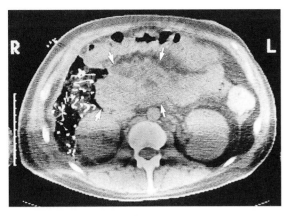

Fig 21.4 **CT of acute pancreatitis.**

recently the APACHE II score has been applied and gives a semi-continuous assessment of severity of pancreatitis, as it does of any acute surgical illness.

MORTALITY RATES

The overall mortality is 8–10%. Most patients (70%) have a mild attack with less than three positive prognostic criteria and a low mortality (0–2%). A severe attack carries a higher mortality (20–30%). Death occurs for three principal reasons:

- *Early* – from multisystem organ failure (p. 000) in fulminant attacks
- *From comorbid conditions* – mainly cardiorespiratory problems, particularly in the aged
- *Late* – from local complications, mainly infected necrosis but more rarely colonic necrosis or haemorrhage from eroded vessels on the posterior abdominal wall.

MANAGEMENT

Specific treatment for pancreatitis is not available. Therapy is supportive, with management of complications if and when they develop. Mild pancreatitis usually resolves with parenteral fluid replacement, bowel rest (nothing by mouth and occasionally nasogastric intubation because of ileus and distension) and analgesia. Opiate analgesia is often necessary but morphine is avoided because it is associated with contraction of the sphincter of Oddi. A severe episode requires more intensive support (based on standard assessment), replacement of large amounts of fluid lost into the retroperitoneum, respiratory management, which may include endotracheal ventilation, and the treatment of renal failure. Paralytic ileus may be prolonged for several weeks and intravenous nutrition is then necessary.

COMPLICATIONS

The more severe the attack, the more likely it is that complications will develop (Table 21.4).

Systemic complications usually occur soon after the onset of the acute attack (within 0–7 days), although they can still take place after this time. They include:

- cardiovascular collapse because of hypovolaemia from massive exudation of fluid into the retroperitoneal tissues and the release of inflammatory cytokines; cardiac function may also be directly depressed
- hypoxia is common and of multifactorial origin – abdominal distension, cytokine release and bacterial translocation from the gut; ARDS (Ch. 10) may develop
- hypocalcaemia – thought to be the result of calcium deposition in areas of fat necrosis
- hyperglycaemia – from disturbances of insulin metabolism
- acute coagulopathies.

Laparotomy

Before the advent and widespread use of the above investigations, patients were not infrequently submitted to laparotomy for the diagnosis of acute abdominal pain. However, this is now a rare occurrence.

PROGNOSIS

The severity of an attack of acute pancreatitis can be assessed in a number of ways, including:

- initial clinical state
- single prognostic factor measurements such as CRP
- Multiple prognostic factor scoring systems.

The Ranson and Glasgow scoring systems are widely used (Table 21.3).

Measurements are made at presentation or within 48 hours. The presence of three or more positive factors indicates a severe attack of acute pancreatitis with an increased mortality correlated with the number of positive factors. It is worth emphasising that hyperamylasaemia is not one of the predictive criteria. More

Table 21.3
Factors which predict the severity of pancreatitis (Glasgow system)

Factor	Level
Age	> 55 years
Leucocytosis	$> 15 \times 10^9/L$
Blood urea concentration	> 16 mmolo/L (no response to fluid administration)
Blood glucose concentration	> 10 mmol/L in the non-diabetic
Serum albumin concentration	< 32 g/L
Serum calcium concentration	< 2.0 mmol/L
Lactate dehydrogenase	> 600 IV/L
Aspartate aminotransferase	100 IV/L
Arterial P_{O_2}	< 60 mmHg (8.0 kPa)

If more than three of the above are positive the attack is severe.

Table 21.4
Complications of acute pancreatitis

System or site	Nature and cause
Cardiovascular	Circulatory failure Hypovolaemia Cytokine release
Respiratory	Hypoxia and respiratory failure (adult respiratory distress syndrome, ARDS) Abdominal distension Cytokine release Bacterial translocation
Renal	Acute renal failure – hypovolaemia
Haematological	Disseminated intravascular coagulation
Metabolic	Hypocalcaemia – calcium deposition in areas of fat necrosis Hyperglycaemia – islet cell dysfunction Acid–base disturbance from tissue necrosis
Nutritional	Muscle wasting/catabolism SIRS
Sepsis in damaged tissue	Infected retroperitoneal slough – bacterial translocation
Retroperitoneum	Fat necrosis – enzyme release
Pseudocyst	Effusion with or without duct damage
Gastrointestinal	Prolonged paralytic ileus – retroperitoneal inflammation GI bleeding – necrosis of gut wall Colonic necrosis Duodenal obstruction
Hepatobiliary	Jaundice/obstruction of CBD
Vascular	Portal vein thrombosis

Local complications usually occur more than a week after onset. Pancreatic and peripancreatic inflammation may lead to tissue necrosis and collections of inflammatory fluid. Secondary infection of these may follow, probably by bacterial translocation from the gut, and lead on to infected slough, abscess, bacteraemia and a secondary systemic response (SIRS – Ch. 9). Biliary obstruction may be caused by inflammation or fluid collections around the head of the gland. Inflammation may also cause portal or, more commonly, splenic vein thrombosis. CT changes in the early stages of the disease (multiple fluid collections, extensive pancreatic necrosis as indicated by non-enhancement of necrotic areas on contrast enhancement) may also give an additional indication of and identify local complications early.

Necrosis and infection

Dead areas within the gland or surrounding tissues may, if they remain sterile, resolve over time and whether they should be removed is a matter of controversy. However, when these areas are infected and there is a systemic response, they should be removed by surgical debridement. Some surgical teams add postoperative retroperitoneal irrigation with multiple drains.

Active fluid collections/pseudocysts

Active fluid collections are relatively common and many will resolve spontaneously. They may mature into pseudocysts after four weeks as a wall of granulation and fibrosis is formed. They start either as sympathetic inflammatory collections (usually in the lesser sac of the peritoneum) or as the consequence of rupture of the pancreatic duct or one of its tributaries. When a peripancreatic fluid collection is of the first kind, it usually resolves spontaneously and is managed expectantly. Pseudocysts larger than 6 cm diameter that persist for longer than 6 weeks are more often in communication with the duct and require internal draining by cyst gastrostomy or cyst jejunostomy. Percutaneous or endoscopic drainage is applicable in a small number of pseudocysts.

Pseudocysts are also a feature of chronic pancreatitis.

Chronic pancreatitis

AETIOLOGY AND PATHOLOGICAL FEATURES

Aetiological factors associated with the development of pancreatitis have been outlined above. As with acute pancreatitis, the precise underlying mechanisms leading to the development of chronic pancreatitis are not fully understood. Heavy consumption of alcohol is a common association and it is in such circumstances that the morphological changes have been most studied. The earliest change appears to be deposition of plugs of protein within the smaller pancreatic ducts. The lumen becomes obstructed and dilatation follows. Atrophy of the acini then occurs. There may be an accompanying inflammatory infiltrate but this is variable. Fibrosis takes place around the affected ducts. Eventually only a few acinar and islet cells remain, with widely dilated pancreatic ducts. Intraluminal calcification of the protein plugs also occurs, so that stones form.

Chronic pancreatitis is not reversible but it is possible that progress can be arrested if the causative factor, such as alcohol, is withdrawn. However, this is an uncommon outcome in the alcoholic so that the disease is most often progressive.

CLINICAL FEATURES

History

The predominant symptom is chronic abdominal pain, mainly in the epigastrium or upper abdomen. It may radiate to the back, can be continuous and relentless and may reach a level of severity comparable to that in acute pancreatitis. An alternative course is chronic pain punctuated by acute exacerbations which resemble acute pancreatitis. Such episodes are usually mild and of brief duration; their relationship to alcohol is variable but some seem to be precipitated by a bout of heavy alcohol consumption. Chronic pain may be accompanied by severe weight loss caused by anorexia.

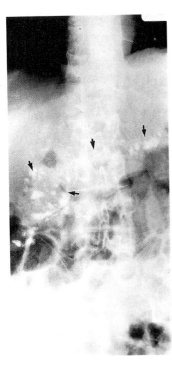

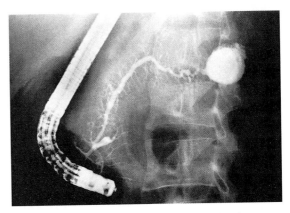

Fig 21.6 **Endoscopic retrograde pancreatogram showing a pancreatic duct of irregular calibre with blunted side branches.** Distally the duct has a large cystic dilatation. The endoscope and cannula can be clearly seen.

Fig 21.5 **Plain abdominal X-ray showing scattered calcification throughout the pancreas (arrowed) in a case of chronic pancreatitis.**

Regular analgesic consumption frequently leads to opiate addiction.

Steatorrhoea occurs when the secretion of pancreatic lipase is reduced by 90% and is present in about half the patients. The development of diabetes is more common. Both occur more often when the pancreas is calcified (Fig. 21.5).

A relatively short clinical presentation suggestive of chronic pancreatic inflammation should always raise the suspicion of cancer of the gland (see below). Conversely, chronic pancreatitis carries an increased risk for the development of cancer. Less commonly, there is obstructive jaundice and occasionally cholangitis. Obstruction or thrombosis of the splenic vein can lead to segmental portal hypertension.

Physical findings

Evidence of malnourishment may be obvious and features of mental depression may be present. Other signs may be few, but some of these are likely to be characteristic of alcoholic liver disease.

INVESTIGATION

Endocrine function

If frank clinical diabetes is not present, the glucose tolerance test may still be abnormal although this is also true in pancreatic carcinoma.

Exocrine function

Tests have been outlined above but are not often used for diagnostic purposes as distinct from planning therapy.

Concentration of serum amylase

In the diagnosis of chronic disease this is not of value, although the level may be increased during an acute episode of pain.

Imaging

Plain X-ray can show a characteristic transverse outline of the calcified gland.

Ultrasound and CT can demonstrate both a reduction and an increase in the size of the gland, duct dilatation or the presence of calcification that is not obvious on a plain X-ray.

ERCP (Fig. 21.6) and MRCP are also useful to confirm the anatomical abnormality – a dilated and/or strictured main (chain of lakes), blunted side branches and sometimes associated stones.

Pancreatic imaging combined with percutaneous biopsy may be helpful although occasionally laparotomy may be necessary to distinguish between chronic pancreatitis and carcinoma. A needle biopsy which shows chronic pancreatitis does not exclude carcinoma and inflammation is often found adjacent to a carcinoma.

MANAGEMENT

Measures for control

In alcohol-induced chronic pancreatitis, absolute cessation of drinking is advised but rarely achieved. Control of pain may require long-term use of opiates which, together with the misery of the disease, may lead to addiction.

Steatorrhoea is treated with a low-fat diet and pancreatic supplements, usually with acid suppression therapy. Diabetes mellitus may be unstable and difficult to control. The insulin requirement is often greater than in idiopathic diabetes, perhaps because pancreatic glucagon is lacking.

Surgical intervention
The indications for operation are:

- correctable anatomical complications which are considered to be associated with either pain or recurrent exacerbations of pancreatitis – e.g. an obstructed pancreatic duct, or a pseudocyst
- obstructive jaundice
- rarely, intractable pain with a diffusely damaged gland.

Surgical management is controversial. Good results are only obtained if other factors, such as alcohol, are controlled and patients are well motivated and highly selected.

COMPLICATIONS
Pancreatic cysts
These are the commonest complication found, especially if careful ultrasound examinations are performed, and they usually arise from within pancreatic tissue. Small cysts do not usually require drainage. Larger ones can give rise to localised pain, nausea and vomiting or biliary obstruction. A smooth, tender mass is occasionally palpable in the epigastrium but a cyst can be easily identified on ultrasound or CT scan. Surgical treatment has been used for most large pseudocysts but a non-operative policy with aspiration and close follow-up by ultrasound examination, is now advocated by some centres.

Pancreatic ascites
Alcoholic pancreatitis with a communication between the pancreatic duct and the peritoneal cavity is the usual cause of this rare complication. The amylase content of the ascitic fluid is very high. Treatment is by temporary endoscopic insertion of a stent into the pancreatic duct, operative drainage of the duct fistula into a jejunal loop or resection of the portion of the gland that contains the fistula.

Pancreatic tumours

Pancreatic carcinoma

Cancer of the exocrine pancreas is an aggressive disease with a poor prognosis; the median survival from the time of diagnosis barely exceeds 5 months. Even with recent advances in surgery, anaesthesia, intensive care, cytotoxic chemotherapy and radiotherapy, there have

been only modest improvements in outcome over the last 50 years.

EPIDEMIOLOGY
Pancreatic cancer has now overtaken gastric cancer to become the fourth leading cause of death from malignant disease in Western society. In the UK, this amounts to some 5000 deaths a year and is continuing to increase steadily. Across western Europe the disease causes some 30 000 deaths a year and in North America over 27 000. The peak incidence occurs between the ages of 50 and 70 years, although it occasionally occurs in those as young as 30. Pancreatic cancer is a disease of Western society; for example, the prevalence of the disease in Afro-Caribbeans in the Bay Area around San Francisco is twice as high as that seen in Western Africa and there is a 10-fold difference in incidence between the USA and India. Within the USA, the incidence of pancreatic cancer in Blacks is five times greater than that in Japanese Americans and Hispanics from Puerto Rico.

AETIOLOGY
Putative factors are shown in Information Box 21.2. However, their exact contribution is unclear. All studies show the disease to be commoner in men than in women, with a ratio ranging from 1.5:1 to 2:1. The difference may be hormonal but men are also on the whole more exposed to other risk factors for the disease. Because women in Western society are now also increasingly exposed to these same influences, there is a rising incidence in women.

There is an established link between pancreatic cancer and cigarette smoking, perhaps through nitrosamine inhalation. Smoking also raises serum lipids, which in turn may predispose to pancreatic cancer, because high-fat diets are also related to an increased incidence of the disease. Other factors are contact through employment in industry with:

- beta-napthylamines
- benzidine
- petroleum

---

i | **Information Box 21.2**

Putative aetiological factors in exocrine pancreatic cancer

- 'Western' lifestyle
- Cigarette smoking
- High-fat diet
- Working in chemical industries

- coke and coal gas
- dry cleaning
- radioactive materials for nuclear fuels and warheads.

An unsubstantiated risk is urban living; early studies which suggested this link have subsequently been disproved by careful and large-scale investigation.

Coffee and caffeine have been linked to pancreatic cancer, but the connection remains uncertain in that beverage habits are often confounded with other risks such as cigarette smoking.

The role of alcohol consumption is also unclear, although chronic pancreatitis has been linked to the development of pancreatic cancer. A causal relationship with diabetes mellitus has been confused by the fact that up to 15% of patients with pancreatic cancer develop diabetes in the period before presentation.

PATHOLOGICAL FEATURES

All but 5% of cancers are adenocarcinomas which originate from the pancreatic ducts; the remainder are of acinar origin and said to be less aggressive. Seventy per cent of tumours occur in the pancreatic head. Only 1% have a cystic component (cystadenocarcinomas). The solid tumours are white in appearance and woody on palpation; at operation their gross appearance can mimic chronic pancreatitis, making histological diagnosis essential either by biopsy or by resection. Spread of the growth is by the four typical routes:

- direct invasion of neighbouring tissues
- lymph node involvement
- blood-borne metastases to the liver and beyond
- within the peritoneal cavity – transcoelomic spread.

Direct invasion

Cancers arising in the pancreatic head invade and obstruct the lower end of the common bile duct to produce extrahepatic obstructive jaundice. The development of obstruction causes the biliary tract to dilate and if, as is usually the case, the gall bladder is not diseased, then it shares in the distension (see Courvoisier's law below).

Further, in 15–20% of those with a carcinoma in the pancreatic head, direct invasion of the duodenum results in gastric outflow obstruction and vomiting. Local infiltration of retroperitoneal tissues – the coeliac plexus, splenic and portal veins – may be responsible for some of the symptoms and may also determine irresectability.

Lymphatic

The nodes adjacent to the gland, the pre-aortic coeliac glands and the nodes at the porta hepatis are all frequently involved.

Vascular

The tumour drains into the portal vein and liver metastases are most common.

Transcoelomic

Spread across the peritoneal cavity resulting in peritoneal seedlings and ascites.

CLINICAL FEATURES

History

The typical presenting history is of a middle-aged patient with obstructive jaundice and pruritis. There may be associated weight loss and epigastric pain which radiates through to the back and can sometimes be alleviated by sitting crouched forward. A recent diagnosis of diabetes mellitus may have been made. If duodenal invasion has occurred, vomiting is present and is usually indicative of an advanced tumour.

A carcinoma of the body or tail inevitably presents late because of the insidious progression of the tumour before symptoms occur. However, in retrospect there is often a non-specific prodromal phase of vague symptoms of malaise, weight loss and epigastric pain radiating to the back. Very few such patients have surgically resectable tumours by the time these symptoms occur.

The major clinical diagnostic problem is that early symptoms mimic other commoner disorders such as peptic ulcer, oesophagitis with heartburn, angina and biliary colic. Many will have spent several months undergoing investigation for these disorders before the correct diagnosis is established or jaundice develops.

Physical findings

Examination may reveal only jaundice. There may be scratch marks over the trunk and limbs as a consequence of bile salt-induced pruritus. Features of weight loss, such as ill-fitting clothes, are often present. Possible other findings are:

- a palpable hard left supraclavicular lymph node (Virchow's gland)
- abdominal distension and ascites
- a palpable enlarged gall bladder – two-thirds of those with pancreatic cancer and obstructive jaundice exemplify Courvoisier's law, which states that this finding indicates a distal biliary obstruction, often malignant; however, the reverse is not true because previous biliary tract disease may have produced fibrosis and rendered the gall bladder non-distensible
- a palpable mass in the epigastrium which characteristically transmits aortic pulsation.

DIAGNOSIS

The other condition that frequently produces a similar clinical picture is an uninfected gallstone in the common bile duct, usually impacted at the lower end and causing progressive obstructive jaundice but not infection.

Less common causes are:

- malignant compression of the bile duct by metastases in portal lymph nodes
- drug-induced cholestatic jaundice
- a carcinoma of the duodenum or papilla at the lower end of the common bile duct
- carcinoma of the bile duc
- Mirizzi's syndrome – cholecystitis and a gallstone in Hartmann's pouch with local inflammation and oedema and sometimes erosion into the common hepatic duct
- sclerosing cholangitis.

INVESTIGATION

Biochemical

Liver function shows an obstructive pattern. The commonest difficulty is with intrahepatic cholestatic jaundice where the pattern may overlap with extra-hepatic obstruction.

Glucose tolerance is impaired in many patients.

Coagulation studies

In the presence of jaundice, prothrombin time is pro-longed (see the International Normalised Ratio).

Imaging

Ultrasound excludes gallstones in the gall bladder and may show a normal common bile duct and demon-strate a dilated intra- and extrahepatic biliary tree, a mass in the head of the pancreas and possible liver metastases.

Endoscopy can demonstrate a malignant mass infiltrating the medial wall of the second part of the duodenum from which a biopsy may be obtained. Retrograde cholangiogram and pancreatogram (ERCP) may indicate a malignant stricture of the common bile duct or pancreatic duct, the appearances of which are shouldered, abrupt and tight. Bile and pancreatic juice can be collected or ductal brushings or biopsy taken for cytological or histopathological analysis.

Percutaneous transhepatic cholangiography (PTC) is done by direct puncture of the bile duct through the liver substance, but in pancreatic cancer is a less useful investigation than an ERCP and is reserved for patients in whom ERCP has failed. MRC is increasingly being used.

CT Scan is valuable in demonstrating the relation-ship of the tumour to the superior mesenteric vessels and portal vein. In addition, it may show lymphatic and hepatic metastases.

Selective visceral angiography gives a dynamic view of the vascular anatomy of the head of the pancreas and may be indicated if an attempt at removal of the tumour is under consideration. Variations in the hepatic artery which may influence the operation are identified (particularly the origin of the right hepatic artery from the superior mesenteric artery in 25%). In addition, during the venous phase, encasement of the portal vein by tumour may suggest irresectability.

Endoscopic ultrasound is occasionally useful in the detection and evaluation of small pancreatic tumours, ductal stones and cholangiocarcinoma of the biliary ducts.

Laparoscopy is used to exclude peritoneal or liver metastases before an attempt at resection.

Specific serum tumour markers

Both carcinoembryonic antigen (CEA) and carbohydrate antigen 19-9 (CA 19-9) are elevated in pancreatic cancer. CA 19-9 is 90% specific for pancreatic cancer but is excreted in bile so estimations are inaccurate in patients with unrelieved jaundice. Although these markers are not usually at a high enough level to be diagnostic, they often support a clinical diagnosis, particularly if there is a progressive rise on repeated estimations.

MANAGEMENT

The objectives and methods of intervention are:

- resection of the primary lesion for cure (feasible in less than 20%)
- alleviation of obstructive jaundice
- pain control
- treatment of exocrine failure and of diabetes
- radiation and chemotherapeutic palliation.

Surgical resection

Less than 20% of pancreatic cancers are resectable at the time of presentation and these are predominantly lesions in the pancreatic head.

The modern one-stage operation is still often named a Whipple's operation after the originator of the previous two-stage procedure. Whipple first drained the biliary tree into the small intestine and secondly resected the tumour. Preliminary decompression of an obstructed biliary tree is now usually achieved by ERCP (see below). The operation is a major *tour de force* and should only be carried out in specialist centres by surgeons with exten-sive experience of pancreatic surgery. In such expert hands, the operative (30 day) mortality is less than 5%.

Tumours found at operation to be irresectable are palliatively treated by biliary and usually duodenal bypass.

Alleviation of obstructive jaundice

Endoscopic percutaneous radiological or surgical methods can be used to achieve this.

Stenting

In frail, elderly patients, the bile duct can be decompressed safely at the time of ERCP. The major papilla is cannulated via the endoscope and a silicone or expanding metal stent placed through the obstructing tumour. However, the procedure is not free from hazard:

- the mortality is 1–2%, usually related to the introduction of infection into an obstructed biliary system
- silicone stents shave a median survival of 14 weeks before silting up with biliary debris and, should the patient survive beyond this time, a replacement is necessary; expanding metal inserts last longer but may occlude from tumour ingrowth.
- duodenal obstruction may develop because of progression of the tumour.

In some patients ERCP stenting is unsuccessful. A percutaneous cholangiogram (PTC) can be performed and a plastic or metal stent inserted along the track.

Palliative surgical decompression

This can be undertaken by either anastomosis of the gall bladder to the jejunum (cholecystojejunostomy) or direct anastomosis of a loop of isolated jejunum to the dilated hepatic duct (hepaticojejunostomy). Both can be combined with a gastroenterostomy to manage duodenal obstruction – currently the most frequent indication for operative palliation. Although cholecystojejunostomy is quick and easy for both the patient and the surgeon, early failure may follow from occlusion of a low insertion of the cystic duct into the common hepatic and the slightly more demanding heapticojejunostomy is preferred.

Pain relief

Many patients with pancreatic cancer die with a significantly smaller tumour burden than those with gastric or colorectal dissemination. One reason is the heavy analgesic (usually opioid) requirement to deal with intractable pain caused by invasion of the coeliac plexus. Relief is best achieved by a coeliac plexus nerve block with alcohol, either at the time of operation or percutaneously under radiological control. Otherwise, reasonable analgesia can be achieved by the methods described in Chapter 6.

Exocrine and endocrine pancreatic insufficiency

The clinical features of this condition are malabsorption with weight loss and steatorrhoea. Pancreatic enzyme supplements are prescribed and the patient is advised to take as many with each meal as are necessary to control the loose motions.

Diabetes secondary to pancreatic cancer rarely requires insulin for control. Dietary carbohydrate restriction, occasionally supplemented by oral hypoglycaemic agents, is usually adequate.

Chemotherapy and radiotherapy

Chemotherapy

Regimens so far devised, either alone or in combination, are not curative. Chemotherapy regimens that have shown some palliative response (10–30%) are based on combination therapy using 5-flurouracil (5-FU), adriamycin, epirubicin and mitomycin or methotrexate. Newer, less toxic derivatives of platinum-based compounds and metalloproteinase inhibitors are also now being evaluated.

Radiotherapy

Radioactive iridium wires can be inserted into the malignant mass at operation. Alternatively, intraoperative beam radiotherapy to the exposed tumour has been used. These methods have shown little additional benefit.

External beam radiotherapy from a linear accelerator has been shown to prolong survival but is not curative.

Combinations of radiotherapy and chemotherapy are being evaluated in current clinical trials.

PROGNOSIS

Pancreatic cancer carries a poor prognosis and most patients are dead within 2 years of diagnosis – more than half within 6 months. Even for those patients fortunate to present with a surgically resectable lesion, the 5-year survival after successful removal is less than 20%.

Islet cell tumours

These tumours are discussed in detail in Chapter 31.

Acute abdominal conditions – surgical aspects

Acute abdomen

Urgent abdominal conditions form the bulk of the emergency activity of general surgeons. The range of causes is very wide and management often challenging. Many of the conditions are considered elsewhere in this text: intestinal obstruction (Ch. 23); trauma (Ch. 3); vascular emergencies (Ch. 28); acute urological disorders (Ch. 32); large bowel disorders and acute lower bowel haemorrhage (Ch. 24).

DEFINITION

The term 'acute abdomen' is a loose one encompassing all those conditions that present with clinical features of short duration (arbitrarily less than 10 days) which might indicate a progressive intra-abdominal condition that is threatening to life or capable of causing severe morbidity. Not all patients will turn out to have such a threatening condition but they need to be considered as being in danger until surgical evaluation has been completed. The majority of such patients have pain as their chief symptom. There are a very large number of possible causes but most patients are victims of a relatively small number of common conditions.

From the beginning of emergency abdominal surgery, at roughly the end of the 19th century, surgical practice has been largely dominated by a policy of management based on 'it is better to look and see rather than to wait and see', because of the often progressive nature of many causes of the acute abdomen. More recently, and with the development of new technologies (e.g. structured data sheets, computer assistance, laparoscopy and ultrasound – discussed below), the surgical objective has become to reach a management decision which separates those who must have an operation to prevent dangerous progression from those who do not. Often this decision involves making an accurate diagnosis of the cause, but this is not always immediately necessary. The important matter is to classify the patient correctly into one of three categories based on the evidence available:

1. operation necessary
2. operation not immediately necessary; further information should be sought but may be followed by the need for surgery
3. operation not necessary.

315

Acute abdominal conditions – surgical aspects

These categories span a spectrum of causes which can be graded in terms of their threat to life on a scale of 1 to 10 (1 = conditions which are never life-threatening; 10 = conditions which are associated with great risk of serious complications or death – Table 22.1). For example, a patient eventually labelled as having non-specific abdominal pain for which a cause is not identified and from which no physical adverse effect follows would be classed as 1, whereas a ruptured aortic aneurysm (Ch. 28) would be classed as 10. However, it is more difficult to allocate other conditions on the scale in such a precise way, because their severity is subject to variation between individuals (e.g. on the grounds of age and co-morbidity) and also depends upon the rapidity with which manage-ment is undertaken. Because of this, the causes of the acute abdomen shown in Table 22.1 are assigned a score of < 5, and > 5. All the standard features of history-taking and physical examination apply to the evaluation of a patient thought to have an acute abdomen. However, there are two features of clinical practice that have proved particularly useful:

- structured data sheets
- computer assistance.

Structured data sheets

These sheets were introduced to make sure that data entered into a computer were complete and uniform (Fig. 22.1); they force rigorous collection of information and have, in consequence, a power of their own to improve the analysis of the individual episode. Those who have made a special study of the acute abdomen strongly recommend them. They provide a useful reminder of the information required in any patient with a possible acute abdomen.

Computer assistance

One of the first applications of computers to clinical diagnostic problems was in the diagnosis of acute abdominal disorders characterised by pain. Although indubitably successful, the method has not found wide application, perhaps because it requires attitudes and equipment which are not uniformly available (this may change). Structured data sheets and sequential methods of analysis are almost equally effective in most common causes of the acute abdomen.

Table 22.1
Severity scale for causes of the acute abdomen

Condition	Grade		
	< 5	5	> 5
Non-specific abdominal pain	*		
Ruptured abdominal aortic aneurysm			*
Ovarian cyst rupture or torsion		*	
Perforated peptic ulcer		*	
Urinary tract infection	*		
Ectopic pregnancy rupture		*	
Mesenteric adenitis	*		
Diverticulitis		* ——	*
Renal colic	*		
Appendicitis		* ——	*
Pseudo-obstruction	*		
Small bowel obstruction		* ——	*
Fitz–Hugh Curtis syndrome	*		
Malignancy	*		
Salpingitis	*		
Cholecystitis	* ———————		*
Mesenteric adenitis	*		
Intestinal ischaemia		* ——	*
Terminal ileitis	*		
Intussusception		* ——	*
Gastritis/duodenitis	*		
Volvulus of the colon		*	*
Gastroenteritis	*		
Inflammatory bowel disease		* ——	*
Torsion of appendices		* ——	*
Meckel's diverticulum rupture			*
Testicular torsion			*
Sickle cell crisis	*		
Referred pain from chest (myocardial infarct, pneumonia)	*		
Abdominal tuberculosis		* ——	*
Porphyria		*	
Irritable bowel syndrome	*		
Diabetes mellitus	*		
Dysmenorrhoea	*		

GENERAL CLINICAL FEATURES

Pain

Abdominal pain has three origins:

- visceral
- parietal
- extra-abdominal.

Visceral pain is generated either because of muscular contraction (colic) in organs such as the gut or ureter or because of stretching of the wall of a hollow organ (gall bladder) or the capsule of a solid one (aching pain from an enlarged liver). Organs from which such pain arises do not have a precise surface representation so that the sensation is not accurately localised by the patient. However, pain which arises from the embryonic foregut (down to the second part of the duodenum) is usually located to the epigastrium; from the midgut (second part of the duodenum to the midtransverse colon) to the periumbilical region; and from the hindgut to the suprapubic area. Visceral pain is often severe and, in general, is central yet diffuse, as in bowel obstruction (Ch. 24) or biliary colic (Ch. 19); ureteric pain is ipsilateral (Ch. 32).

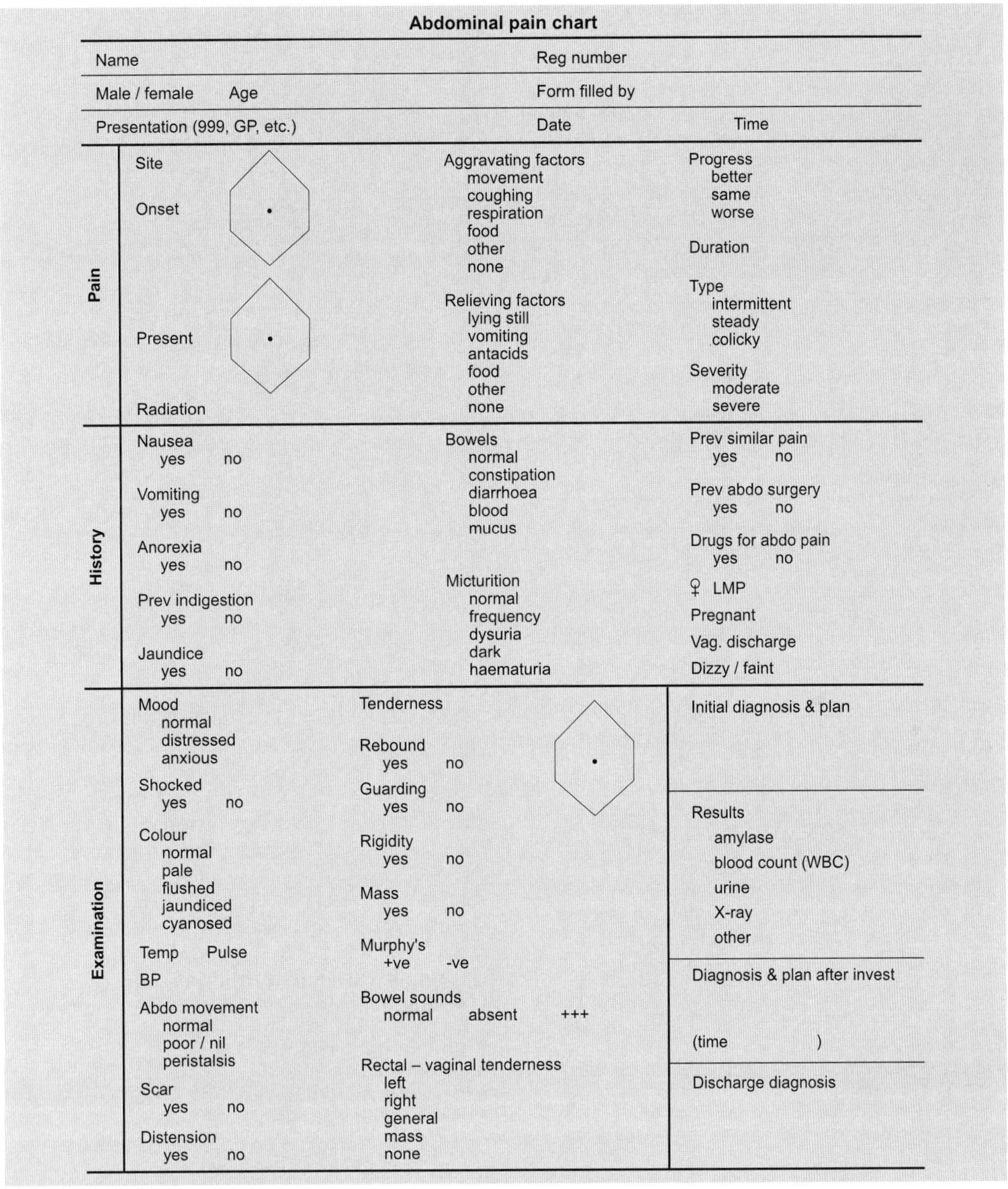

Abdominal pain chart

Name		Reg number	
Male / female	Age	Form filled by	
Presentation (999, GP, etc.)		Date	Time

Pain	Site Onset	Aggravating factors movement coughing respiration food other none	Progress better same worse Duration Type intermittent steady colicky
	Present Radiation	Relieving factors lying still vomiting antacids food other none	Severity moderate severe
History	Nausea yes　　no Vomiting yes　　no Anorexia yes　　no Prev indigestion yes　　no Jaundice yes　　no	Bowels normal constipation diarrhoea blood mucus Micturition normal frequency dysuria dark haematuria	Prev similar pain yes　　no Prev abdo surgery yes　　no Drugs for abdo pain yes　　no ♀ LMP Pregnant Vag. discharge Dizzy / faint
Examination	Mood normal distressed anxious Shocked yes　　no Colour normal pale flushed jaundiced cyanosed Temp　Pulse BP Abdo movement normal poor / nil peristalsis Scar yes　　no Distension yes　　no	Tenderness Rebound yes　　no Guarding yes　　no Rigidity yes　　no Mass yes　　no Murphy's +ve　　-ve Bowel sounds normal　absent　+++ Rectal – vaginal tenderness left right general mass none	Initial diagnosis & plan Results amylase blood count (WBC) urine X-ray other Diagnosis & plan after invest (time　　　) Discharge diagnosis

Fig 22.1 **Structured sheet for collection of data.**

In pain of visceral origin, a distinction should be made between colic, which truly comes and goes at (fairly) regular intervals, and distension, where the persistent tension on the wall or capsule of an organ produces pain of the same nature but which is more continuously present. In clinical practice the difference is often not appreciated but it help the clinician to think clearly about cause (see, for example, biliary colic, Ch. 19).

Parietal pain has its origin in the abdominal wall at any depth from the skin through to the peritoneum; the parietes have an accurate surface representation so that the patient can usually indicate where exactly is the pain: examples are peritonitis (see 'Appendicitis', Ch. 24) and abdominal wall bruising. Sudden onset of diffuse parietal pain, associated with physical findings of peritoneal irritation, usually means perforation of a hollow viscus, rupture of an abscess into the general peritoneal cavity or bleeding.

The combination of visceral pain and local irritation is characteristically seen in acute appendicitis (Ch. 24) or acute cholecystitis (Ch. 19), where the initial pain of obstruction to the lumen of the organ is manifest as central colic and then, when inflammation becomes manifest because of the obstruction and ischaemia, produces localised pain at the site where the organ is in contact with the parietal peritoneum of the anterior abdominal wall. As indicated below, there is a potential diagnostic trap when an area of peritoneal irritation is not in contact with the anterior abdominal wall and therefore does not produce pain.

Extra-abdominal pain may take two forms:

- pain that originates from sources that share innervation with the abdominal wall – approximately T9 to L1 – such as may occur in spinal cord conditions which involve the spinal nerves
- pain from a wide variety of disorders where the mechanism is not well understood.

Apparent pain. To the three origins – visceral, parietal and extra-abdominal – should be added two clinical occurrences of apparent abdominal pain:

- *Münchhausen's syndrome* (so-called because it recalls the tales of Baron Münchhausen who invented marvellous adventures). There are certain individuals of an unusual temperament who seem to need attention from the hospital service and present with dramatic symptoms which include (although are not always dependent upon) pain as a prominent feature. There is usually a convincing story of an acute abdomen but without a cause. It is easy to be taken in by such patients and they move from hospital to hospital undergoing needless investigation and surgery. There are attempts to set up registers in A&E departments in the UK to deal with this problem.
- *Drug-dependent patients* may feign pain to obtain analgesic drugs.

Pain patterns

The patterns of pain can often be helpful in diagnosis involving the acute abdomen. Radiation is when pain starts in one place and then spreads to another while the initial pain usually persists. Radiation of pain through to the back is characteristic of involvement of a retroperitoneal structure such as the pancreas (Ch. 21) or abdominal aorta (Ch. 28), while radiation of unilateral visceral pain to the testis in the male or groin in the female suggests a renal origin. Shoulder-tip pain may occur in irritation of the undersurface of the diaphragm – the phrenic nerve and the skin of the shoulder have a common segmental nerve supply (C3 and 4).

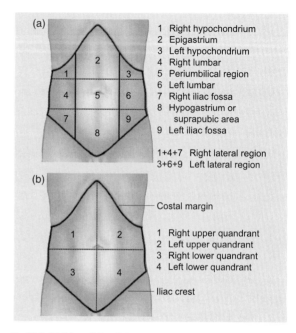

(a)
1 Right hypochondrium
2 Epigastrium
3 Left hypochondrium
4 Right lumbar
5 Periumbilical region
6 Left lumbar
7 Right iliac fossa
8 Hypogastrium or suprapubic area
9 Left iliac fossa

1+4+7 Right lateral region
3+6+9 Left lateral region

(b)
Costal margin
1 Right upper quandrant
2 Left upper quandrant
3 Right lower quandrant
4 Left lower quandrant
Iliac crest

Fig 22.2 **Division of the abdomen into sectors facilitates description and interpretation of findings**.

Pain localisation

Visceral pain is imprecisely localised. Parietal pain is more accurately localised and, when associated with the physical signs of inflammation in the same area, is frequently used to guide both further investigation and management. For example, a patient with pain in the right iliac fossa (possible acute appendicitis) is managed differently from one with the same features in the left iliac fossa (possible colonic diverticulitis) or right subcostal pain (possible cholecystitis) (Fig. 22.2).

Gastrointestinal disturbances

Vomiting indicates one of the following:

- gastrointestinal obstruction
- pyloric stenosis
- the reflex effect of an acute disturbance such as often occurs in the early stages of other causes of the acute abdomen, e.g. biliary or renal colic; it is rarely continuous.

Anorexia and nausea are present in many patients with an acute abdomen but are non-specific in relation to cause and can arise in many other circumstances.

PHYSICAL FINDINGS

Some common features are considered here.

Peritoneal irritation

When pressure is applied to the anterior abdominal wall over a site of irritation of the peritoneum, the clinical response is a spinal reflex which causes involuntary contraction of the overlying abdominal muscles – 'guarding' (see 'Murphy's sign'). Inflamed visceral peritoneum must be in contact with the abdominal wall for this to take place. A more advanced stage occurs in generalised peritonitis when the muscles are held rigid – the abdomen is 'board-like'. A consequence is that the abdomen is held still and breathing becomes increasingly thoracic (see 'Perforated peptic ulcer').

Rebound tenderness is elicited by gentle pressure with the hand followed by its rapid removal and is thought to indicate the parietal peritoneum parting company from an underlying inflamed viscus. It is not a very reliable indicator of peritoneal irritation, is uncomfortable for the patient and can more kindly be determined by asking the patient to cough or by percussion of the abdomen.

Auscultation

Bowel sounds are increased in intestinal obstruction and also in infective diarrhoea and are absent in paralytic ileus.

Pelvic examination

It has always been a surgical maxim that digital pelvic examination via the rectum is essential in the evaluation of the acute abdomen. Many clinicians put it more coarsely: 'If you do not put your finger in, you are liable to put your foot in.' Rectal examination is usually not needed in the assessment of children with suspected appendicitis. Per vaginal examination is also often helpful but can only be done when the hymen is no longer intact and even then should be used only when it is thought necessary to elucidate a problem. The value of both rectal and vaginal examination is that, in irritation of the pelvic peritoneum, the manoeuvre causes a complaint of pain which, although ill-localised, can often be identified as to the right or left side. There is a similar response to moving the cervix (cervical excitation). In addition, pelvic examination may give specific information about the presence of a pelvic mass and vaginal discharge, and a vaginal swab can be taken for culture.

INVESTIGATION

Circumstances, particularly the patient's general condition and the localisation of pain, determine the appropriate investigations. When the diagnosis remains in doubt there is a considerable variety of investigations that need to be considered and these are discussed under individual disorders. Provided that the condition is not judged to be life-threatening, a period of observation and review after a few hours (and by the same clinician) is useful.

Routine urine testing

The presence of red cells or white cells can focus attention on the urinary tract as a possible cause of the problem. Other findings, such as glucose and ketone bodies, may help in management. A pregnancy test may be helpful when a fertile woman complains of abdominal pain.

Blood

Routine blood examination for haematological and electrolyte components is traditional, but although it can be helpful in categorising diagnosis, it can also be misleading in that intra-abdominal inflammation in its early stages does not necessarily cause a raised white cell count (see 'Appendicitis' below). Screening for thalassaemia and sickle cell disease should be done in Afro-Caribbean patients. Electrolyte abnormalities (such as a low potassium concentration) occur with vomiting or diarrhoea and can cause management problems. Other blood investigations are considered under individual conditions. The serum amylase concentration must be measured in all patients with acute upper abdominal pain.

Imaging

Plain X-rays have a selective place. They may give positive information when a renal disorder is suspected and should confirm the diagnosis of intestinal obstruction. An erect chest X-ray may show separation of the liver from the undersurface of the diaphragm by free air if there is a gastrointestinal perforation, although this finding is positive only in 60%. It is often said that there are some patients who cannot tolerate being upright for a chest film; this is not so – the time required is small and help from others always makes this possible.

Contrast examinations. For the most part, these are unnecessary. However, water-soluble contrast enemas have an important place in intestinal obstruction and in paediatric surgery in relation to intussusception. Swallows have disadvantages in that they may provoke vomiting and aspiration; however, they can sometimes confirm that a leak from the gastrointestinal tract has sealed.

Intravenous urography. See Chapter 32.

Ultrasound. When this is available for the evaluation of patients with an acute abdomen, experienced operators contribute to an accurate diagnosis. In particular, visualisation of the appendix almost certainly indicates a swollen organ which is inflamed, while the presence of gallstones within a distended gall bladder indicates biliary colic or acute cholecystitis. An abdominal aortic aneurysm can be outlined (Ch. 28). Ultrasound also has a secondary place in management of the acute abdomen either for guided biopsy or in closed drainage of an effusion of abscess.

Peritoneal cytology. This technique has been validated but is not widely used. After the bladder has been emptied, either spontaneously or by catheter, a 14 gauge catheter is inserted under local anaesthesia into the peritoneal cavity midway between the umbilicus and the symphysis pubis. A fine catheter is inserted and suction applied. The aspirate is then expressed onto a slide, stained and the cell profile and percentage of neutrophils recorded. In females, a peritoneal neutrophil count of more than 50% indicates the presence of either appendicitis or pelvic inflammatory disease. In males, such a percentage means that laparoscopy or laparotomy is required as the next step.

Peritoneal cytology may also be useful in selected groups of patients who seem to have an acute abdomen. Those with abdominal tuberculosis may present with acute symptoms accompanied by clinical features suggestive of ascites. Fluid recovered by aspiration does not reveal bacilli in 50%, but a high activity of adenosine deaminase – an enzyme produced by lymphocytes and macrophages during the immune response – is a sensitive and specific marker.

Laparoscopy. Laparoscopy has a valued place in assessment and may also be used for therapy (e.g. appendicectomy, closure of perforated ulcers). Its chief role is when the diagnostic classification between operation necessary and operation not immediately necessary or not required remains uncertain. The common circumstance is of a female in whom the diagnosis may be either appendicitis or a number of other causes which do not require operation (including pelvic inflammatory disease) or in which the organ involved requires a different operative approach (Information Box 22.1). Laparoscopy can resolve the problem. The procedure is also useful when the clinical features in a suspected acute abdomen are atypical.

> ### *i* Information Box 22.1
>
> *Causes of non-traumatic right iliac fossa pain and tenderness in young women*
>
> - Appendicitis
> - Salpingitis
> - Ovarian cyst (rupture or torsion)
> - Mesenteric adenitis
> - Terminal ileitis (Crohn's diseasse, *Yersinia* infection, tuberculosis)
> - Right ureteric calculus
> - Urinary tract infection
> - Meckel's diverticulum (inflammation, perforation or torsion)
> - Cholecystitis
> - Perforated duodenal ulcer

Acute appendicitis

AETIOLOGY AND PATHOLOGICAL FEATURES

The cause of acute appendicitis is thought to be obstruction of the appendicular lumen by either a mass of inspissated faeces (faecolith) or oedema. Distal to this, bacterial multiplication takes place and tension rises. Blood supply is then compromised and progression to gangrene is common. The appendix then ruptures and a spreading peritonitis caused by enteric organisms (including Bacteroides) ensues. Alternatively, a severely inflamed appendix may be walled off by surrounding omentum and loops of bowel (an appendix mass) which will eventually contain pus (an appendix abscess). Appendicitis and many of the conditions that mimic it are commonest in the age range 2–40 years. Untreated, the condition threatens life and, although uncommon at the extremes of age, it is in the very young and the elderly that it has the highest mortality, mainly because the diagnosis is difficult.

The appendix may be in a number of different positions in relation to the caecum: medial; medial and below; extending over the pelvic brim into the pelvis; retrocaecal; or retroileal. The clinical features of inflammation are modified accordingly.

CLINICAL FEATURES

Symptoms

The history begins with central abdominal pain of a visceral type – ill-localised and usually around the umbilicus – accompanied by a variable amount of anorexia, nausea and one or more episodes of vomiting. As the organ becomes inflamed, local peritoneal irritation causes parietal pain felt in the right iliac fossa. Occasionally the progression to gangrene is so rapid that these symptoms are largely absent or unrecognised by the patient who presents with the generalised abdominal pain of peritonitis. Other variable features of the history are:

- previous similar attacks – not all surgeons accept the idea of recurrent appendicitis but there seems to be good evidence to support the concept
- more frequent vomiting if the appendix is retroileal
- variable urinary symptoms – frequency and dysuria – because of an inflamed appendix close to the right ureter
- mucous diarrhoea because of the formation of an appendix mass in the pelvis which irritates the wall of the rectosigmoid.

Physical findings

General. A coated tongue and foul breath accompanied by mild pyrexia are characteristic, but absence of all three does not exclude appendicitis.

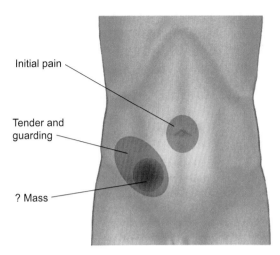

Initial pain

Tender and guarding

? Mass

Fig 22.3 **Area of maximal tenderness in most cases of acute appendicitis.**

Abdomen. Local tenderness and guarding at McBurney's point – the junction of the middle and outer thirds of a line which joins the umbilicus to the anterior superior iliac spine – is present when the appendix is in its most common position, medial to the caecum (Fig 22.3). However, these abdominal signs vary in position, are often much reduced in retroileal or particularly retrocaecal appendicitis, and may be absent if the organ is in the pelvis. It is often said that pressure applied in the left iliac fossa causes increased pain in the right lower quadrant (Rovsing's sign), but this is unreliable and not recommended as a diagnostic sign.

Pelvic examination is especially helpful when the inflamed appendix is in the pelvis. Rectal examination is usually sufficient but in young women, where pelvic inflammatory disease is a possibility, a vaginal examination is done to attempt to localise the side of maximum tenderness.

INVESTIGATION

When the clinical features are typical, the diagnosis is not difficult to make, but a wide variety of conditions can mimic appendicitis and, in the past, up to 25% of patients submitted to operation on a diagnosis of acute appendicitis did not have the condition and few had the need for an operation. Apart from the routine investigations indicated above, three techniques have been shown to be discriminatory and to help to reach a management decision:

- peritoneal cytology
- laparoscopy
- Ultrasound.

The first of these is not widely used. The second is most valuable in young (15–40) females, who may have either pelvic inflammatory disease or acute appen-

dicitis. Ultrasonography has a place in any patient where the diagnosis is in doubt and expert ultrasonographers are available immediately.

MANAGEMENT

Acute appendicitis with or without peritonitis

Once the diagnosis has been made, the likelihood of progression (or the presence already of spreading inflammation) demands the removal of the organ – appendicectomy (USA: appendectomy) – which may be done either through a small transverse incision in the right iliac fossa or via the laparoscope. Prophylactic antibiotic therapy (Ch. 9) reduces the incidence of wound or port-site infection.

Appendix mass

Some doubt surrounds the choice of management, and good clinical evidence is not available to resolve the issue. The choice is between:

- *Non-operative management*, with nothing by mouth, parenteral fluids, antibiotics and frequent reassessment of clinical state – the mass may resolve (the great majority), deterioration may ensue and require a change of plan, or an abscess may form.
- *Operative management*, in which case the mass is explored and the appendix removed, unless an abscess is found which it is judged better only to drain.

Appendix abscess

If it is clear either on clinical examination or by the use of ultrasound that an abscess has formed, this is drained by an incision over its most prominent point. If the appendix is easily accessible, it can be removed.

Elective appendicectomy

This procedure is carried out after successful non-operative management of an appendix mass. It is also done in some patients who will be out of reach of surgical facilities should they contract appendicitis (e.g. polar scientists and technicians, astronauts). Good evidence that either of these reasons is valid is absent.

Elective appendicectomy may also be recommended after undoubted recurrent attacks of appendicitis, but this is rare. Appendicectomy should not be done for vague right iliac fossa pain; the usual result is a patient who has had a surgical procedure and still has the pain.

Acute upper gastrointestinal bleeding

The usual presentation of upper gastrointestinal bleeding is haematemesis – the vomiting of blood – a dramatic symptom of life-threatening portent. It is an indication of bleeding into the gastrointestinal tract from the lower end of the oesophagus to the duodenojejunal flexure. Some blood usually passes downwards through the gut and is subject to digestion. As a result, haematemesis is usually accompanied or followed by melaena – the rectal discharge of altered dark blood. Occasionally upper gastrointestinal bleeding may be so rapid that bright unaltered blood is passed per rectum. Sometimes haematemesis may be absent in bleeding from the upper gastrointestinal tract and the only clinical feature is melaena.

EPIDEMIOLOGY AND AETIOLOGY

In the UK, upper gastrointestinal (UGI) bleeding leads to 50–100 hospital admissions per 100000 population each year. There are many possible causes but only a few are common. Peptic ulcers account for more than half, and oesophageal varices, caused by portal hypertension, accounts for about 5–10%. In many countries where liver disease is common, oesophageal varices are much more likely to be the cause of haematemesis than in the UK (up to 40%), although their incidence in Britain is on the increase. In severely ill patients with renal or hepatic failure, gastroduodenal erosions are a common source of bleeding.

Between a third and a half of patients who present with haematemesis are taking non-steroidal anti-inflammatory agents (NSAIDs), which can exacerbate peptic ulcer and also be associated with acute erosions. Table 22.2 gives the results of a world survey of 4431 patients who presented with upper GI bleeding. In 22%, multiple (or very rare) causes were found.

In the UK, the incidence of duodenal ulcer (DU) is much higher than that of ulcers in the stomach. However, more gastric than duodenal ulcers cause haematemesis (55% GU; 44% DU), and more deaths are attributable to bleeding from GU than from DU (55% GU; 45% DU). Unusual peptic ulcers which can also bleed are those in the lower end of the oesophagus and those associated with hypergastrinaemia (Zollinger–Ellison syndrome). Gastric cancer is a relatively rare cause of haematemesis, although blood oozes from the surface of the tumour to cause anaemia.

Table 22.2
Mortality for haematemesis – by diagnosis

Condition	Mortality (%)
Peptic ulcer	4.3
Varices	30.7
Erosions	7.1
Cancer	14.2
Mallory–Weiss syndrome	2.0

Table 22.3
Haematemesis from peptic ulcer in the United Kingdom (HIPE* figures 1964)

Cause	Number	Deaths	Percentage
GU	3705	521	14
DU	4684	432	9.8 (female: 15; male: 6)

Mortality

Upper gastrointestinal haemorrhage is a serious condition. Mortality rates for the common causes taken over all ages and from all the common causes are from 5 to 30% (Table 22.2) and have not changed much over the years. In a world survey, the mortality was highest for those with varices. The low mortality for bleeding peptic ulcer of 4.2% is, however, not typical; figures around 10% are common (Table 22.3). Death depends chiefly on three factors:

- age – e.g. in peptic ulcer it is very low in those under 50 years but very high in those over 80
- concomitant disease in the cardiorespiratory system
- cause of bleeding.

In some instances, bleeding is a terminal event in a patient already very ill or dying. In the UK there is evidence that bleeding increasingly occurs in the old and ill. In consequence, what are real advances in management for individual patients are not reflected in an overall fall in mortality.

CLINICAL FEATURES

Fresh blood may be present in the vomit. Alternatively, if it is retained for a short time in the stomach, it becomes darkened by the action of acid and when vomited has the appearance of coffee grounds. If acute bleeding is haemodynamically significant – in excess of a blood donation (500 mL) – the patient may feel faint and show pallor. The vomit may then contain large quantities of fresh blood or clot. The Valsalva effect of vomiting may further reduce venous return to the heart and cause a vasovagal syncope (faint). With larger losses, the classical signs of haemorrhage are usually present, with sweating, tachycardia and, depending on the volume lost, hypotension and air hunger. When the bleeding is severe, melaena may be an early feature: the passage of bright red blood in large quantities from the rectum indicates either a haemorrhage from below the duodenal flexure or massive, very rapid blood loss from the upper gastrointestinal tract.

IMMEDIATE DIAGNOSIS

Unless the bleeding is clearly minor, the initial history and physical examination should be brief and focused on the features essential to urgent management. There are three components to immediate diagnosis:

- Make sure that there has been acute loss of blood.
- Assess the amount and rate of bleeding – this, along with measures to restore circulating volume, is the first priority.
- Determine the cause, which often leads on to a decision as to how the episode should be treated.

Has bleeding occurred?

It is obviously important to establish that there has actually been a haematemesis. Measures which help are:

- Eliminate swallowed blood (e.g. from a nosebleed) as a cause.
- Examine what has been vomited – if it is not obviously fresh blood and clots are absent, test for haemoglobin; intestinal obstruction can produce what looks like coffee ground vomit.
- Do a rectal examination – fresh or altered blood gives confirmation of bleeding and can also be used in assessing the rate of loss.

Amount and rate of bleeding

- Make the usual observations of the circulation to assess the amount of blood lost.
- In haemodynamically significant bleeding, insert a central venous catheter for measurement of central venous pressure (CVP).

MANAGEMENT

It is increasingly recognised that a cooperative multi-disciplinary approach to management is essential because it makes key decision-making easy and rapid. A team who are specialised in the management of this emergency has been shown to be effective in reducing mortality.

Initial management

The methods of dealing with acute bleeding from any cause are followed. Frequent measurement of CVP is not only valuable in monitoring the success of volume replacement (particularly in the elderly), but also may give early warning of further bleeding before changes in pulse rate or blood pressure have occurred.

Requirement for blood

The objective should be to maintain a haemoglobin level greater than 10g/dL. The quantity of blood necessary to do this and to restore a normal level of CVP is an indicator of the volume lost in the acute phase, and in bleeding from peptic ulcer is also helpful in determining the type of treatment (see below). It has been shown that patients with peptic ulcer or erosive bleeding who vomit altered blood and do not have melaena and whose haemoglobin level remains above 12.10g/dL, are unlikely to re-bleed. Simple rules for the provision of blood are given in Table 22.4.

Table 22.4
Guidelines for cross-matching blood in haematemesis

Clinical state	Action
Without haemodynamic problems	None
With haemodynamic problems	4 units
Anaemic (haemoglobin less than 10 g/dL)	1 unit of blood for every 1 g deficit below 10 g/dL
Continued bleeding	Guided by clinical features but at least 4 units
Rebleed if under 60 years	No action unless there is haemodynamic instability
Rebleed if over 60 years	4 units

Diagnosis of cause

Given that the patient has a stable circulation, either because the loss is small or because it has been corrected, further details can be obtained for both history and physical findings.

History. The relevant features associated with different common causes are shown in Table 22.5

Physical findings. Signs of chronic liver disease should be sought, including neurological features suggestive of encephalopathy. Other findings vary with the cause, e.g. the presence of supraclavicular lymphadenopathy in bleeding from gastric carcinoma.

Upper gastrointestinal endoscopy is the key to achieving a diagnosis. If haemodynamic instability is present, it may be required as an emergency but can usually be deferred until the next scheduled endoscopy session. In the seriously ill, the procedure is not without some hazard, the main one being aspiration of regurgitated blood. Sedation should be kept to a minimum, particularly in the elderly.

To identify a lesion does not always imply that it is the cause of the haematemesis; for example, in patients with oesophageal varices because of alcoholic liver disease, up to 40% of episodes of bleeding are from peptic ulcer or acute gastric erosions. However, precise diagnosis can be achieved in nearly all instances and is the best basis of a management plan.

Definitive management

In any haematemesis from whatever cause, the management may be non-operative or operative. However, the distinction is now blurred by the increasing use of aggressive interventions undertaken endoscopically. The important decision to be made is whether or not the condition requires direct intervention by any method or whether it will resolve spontaneously; this is next considered under individual causes.

Peptic ulcer

MANAGEMENT

Many episodes of haematemesis from ulcers are self-limiting, and replacement of blood volume and with-

Table 22.5
Salient historical features in common cause of haematemesis

Cause	Mechanism	Historical features
Mucosal tear at cardia (Mallory–Weiss syndrome)	Forceful attempted vomiting	Acute inebriation Initial clear vomit Bright red haematemesis
Oesophageal varices	Rupture or erosion of mucosa over varix	Past liver disease Absence of peptic ulcer history Dark red haematemesis
NSAID-induced erosions	Breakdown of mucosal barrier to acid	Pain producing associated disorder (e.g. rheumatoid artiritis) Intake of NSAID
Peptic ulcer	Peptic digestion of vessel in base of ulcer; Fibrinoid necrosis of open vessel holding lumen open Exacerbation of ulceration by NSAIDs	Previous episodes of dyspepsia Diagnosed ulcer Recent worsening of symptoms Blood of variable colour with or without clots
Angiodysplasias	Rupture or mucosal digestion of a surface lesion	No history on initial occurrence
Other causes to consider	Varies with cause	Examples: History of anticoagulant intake Haematological disorders

drawal of precipitating factors (such as NSAIDs) are all that is required. Whether or not aggressive anti-ulcer therapy plays a part in urgent treatment is controversial, but it is good practice to continue it, usually with intravenous histamine H_2-receptor antagonists such as cimetidine and ranitidine or with proton pump blockers such as omeprazole.

However, continued bleeding or rebleeding within a few days can occur, especially in the elderly. Factors which help to predict the likely course of the patient are:

- age – those under 40 are unlikely to bleed continuously or to rebleed and, even if they do, are better able to respond satisfactorily to any haemodynamic disturbance
- ulcer size – those with a large (greater than 1.5 cm in diameter) lesion are more likely to rebleed
- endoscopic stigmas (see Box 22.1).

The presence of any of these adverse factors is an indication for local control of the bleeding ulcer at the

time of initial endoscopy. There are a number of methods:

- local injection of vasoconstrictor (adrenaline) or sclerosant
- thermal coagulation with a heater probe
- cold coagulation with a cryoprobe.

Any of these techniques can achieve control in the majority of episodes. Failure immediately to stop bleeding from a visible vessel is usually regarded as an indication for immediate operation.

Rebleeding after peptic ulcer haemorrhage is most likely within the first 3–4 days and is thought to be caused by peptic digestion of the clot, which seals the mouth of the vessel. The evidence for further loss is shown in Table 22.6. Repeated control by endoscopic methods can be attempted but, particularly in elderly patients with other problems such as cardiac or respiratory disease, operative intervention should be considered. The decision for or against operation is one that has to be made for each patient by the management team. A good dictum is: 'The elderly who are bleeding are usually not too old to be operated on; rather

---

Box 22.1

Endoscopic stigmas which suggest the likelihood of further bleeding from peptic ulcer

Actively bleeding vessel

Visible vessel in ulcer base

Adherent clot

Black spot in ulcer base

Table 22.6
Rebleeding in peptic ulcer

Class of evidence	Features
Haemodynamic evidence of continued blood loss after resuscitation	Persistent – low or falling CVP; tachycardia; hypotension
Clinical evidence of continued or repeated bleeding	Further fresh haematemesis (not old blood)
Re-endoscopy	Visible fresh bleeding
Haematological	Progressive haemodilution beyond 24 hours

Table 22.7
Indications for surgery for a bleeding duodenal ulcer

Timing	Age (years)	Basis of decision
Immediate	Any	Uncontrollable spurting vessel at endoscopy
		Clinical exsanguination
Delayed	Over 60	More than 4 units of blood required for haemodynamic stabilisation or more than 8 units over 48 hours
	Under 60	More than 8 units necessary for stabilisation or more than 12 units needed over 48 hours
On rebleeding	Over 60	One rebleed after initial successful control but while still in hospital
	Under 60	Two rebleeds after initial successful control but while still in hospital

they are too old not to be operated on.' The rules of thumb on which the decision is taken are given in Table 22.7.

Operations for bleeding peptic ulcer

Surgery is done first and foremost to save life. The aim is to stop the bleeding and to minimise the chance of it recurring.

Duodenal ulcer. The ulcer is exposed and the bleeding vessel underrun with a suture. Once control is achieved and blood volume restored, the operation is completed by a vagotomy (Ch. 18) and pyloroplasty. In a young fit patient, more conservative operations such as a proximal gastric vagotomy can be considered. Very large ulcers may require a Polya-type partial gastrectomy (Ch. 18).

Gastric ulcer. Attempts at limited surgery appear less effective than partial gastrectomy – usually of the Billroth I type (Ch. 18). A gastric cancer may be found at operation in a patient thought to have a bleeding gastric ulcer and is dealt with by a more radical resection.

Bleeding oesophageal varices

These are an increasingly common cause of upper GI bleeding and usually occur in patients with known liver disease or a history of alcoholism. Variceal bleeding in childhood or adolescence is the exception.

AETIOLOGY

The varices form at the junction of portal and systemic circulations at the lower end of the oesophagus or in the cardiac part of the stomach as a consequence of any interference with venous drainage from the portal into the systemic venous return.

EPIDEMIOLOGY

About 50% of those who have varices sustain a bleed, and 70% of those who bleed will do so again within a year. The mortality for each episode may be as high as 50% and is related to:

● the amount of blood lost
● ability to control the bleeding
● the severity of liver dysfunction.

MANAGEMENT

The treatment of bleeding varices is complicated and different regimens have proved both successful and unsuccessful in individual hands.

Lowering portal pressure

Lowering arterial input to the portal system, and therefore portal pressure, can be achieved by the intravenous infusion of vasopressin or one of its analogues and by a beta-blocker such as propranolol. This is the current mainstay of management. Alternatively, somatostatin may be used for the same purpose.

Tamponade

Balloon tubes (Sengstaken–Blakemore) will nearly always arrest bleeding but a rebleed is likely when the pressure is reduced – as it must be after 48 hours to avoid mucosal necrosis. There is a high incidence of respiratory complications.

Sclerosant injection

The basis of the method is similar to the obliteration of varicose veins elsewhere. The injection is made through the endoscope and can be repeated either to control further bleeding or to obliterate the varices and prevent recurrence. An alternative is to apply rubber bands to the varices, which is currently the most popular technique and probably the most effective.

Gastric transection

Dividing the oesophagogastric junction and re-anastomosis (usually with staples) interrupts the venous channels but requires an operation.

Relief of portal hypertension

None of the above methods does anything to relieve the portal hypertension and, in the past, definitive treatment for this was done by some surgeons in the treatment of bleeding. However, the operations involved are major and the mortality too high to justify their use in an emergency.

Gastric erosion (stress ulceration)

This cause of bleeding is associated with liver failure (multiple haematological factors affecting clotting), renal failure or other multi-organ failure particularly following trauma, especially burns where endoscopy in severe cases always shows gastric erosions although they do not always bleed. Bleeding from erosive gastritis may often be a terminal event in the seriously ill and does not necessarily justify treatment.

MANAGEMENT

Initially this is non-operative, with anti-ulcer agents such as cimetidine or ranitidine. Any possible cause should be corrected. Surgical intervention is rarely necessary, but occasionally gastric resection may save a seriously ill victim.

Incomplete lower oesophageal tear (Mallory–Weiss syndrome)

The mechanism is the same as that for a complete tear. The history is typically of an initial blood-free vomit followed by bright red haematemesis later. Most episodes of bleeding from this cause are usually minor and self-limiting but are occasionally severe and persistent. If this is the case, the stomach is exposed, opened and the tear oversewn, nearly always with good results.

Dieulafoy's lesion

A small punched-out mucosal hole erodes a vessel, usually high on the lesser curve of the stomach. The condition is uncommon and of unknown cause. Bleeding may be considerable and difficult to find either at endoscopy or at operation. Oversewing at operation is the correct treatment.

Rarer causes of haematemesis

- *Arteriovenous malformations* – these are rare but, in their various forms, may cause up to 4% of all haematemeses. Angiodysplasia is the commonest, although it is seen much more frequently in the colon. Vascular ectasias are more diffuse and give streaky appearances at endoscopy. Vascular lesions may also be part of a diffuse syndrome such as hereditary haemorrhagic telangiectasia. Management is complex and beyond the scope of this text.
- *Haemobilia*
- *Aortoenteric fistula.*

FURTHER READING

Brown A F T (1996) *Emergency Medicine: Diagnosis and Treatment.* Melbourne: Butterworth-Heineman

Brown N L (1997) *An Introduction to the Symptoms and Signs of Surgical Disease*, 3rd edn. London: Arnold

Ellis H (1997) *Clinical Anatomy* 9th edn. Oxford: Blackwell Science

23

Small bowel disease and intestinal obstruction

Diseases and disorders of the small bowel which may require surgical management are usually those associated with mechanical (such as obstruction), infective or bleeding problems. Clinical problems in the alimentary tract are now often dealt with by a gastroenterological team which includes physicians and surgeons working in consort with radiologists and others as occasion demands.

Vitellointestinal abnormalities

Persistence of the vitellointestinal duct takes a variety of forms:

- an open communication between the ileum and the umbilicus – vitellointestinal fistula
- a free diverticulum of the terminal ileum (Meckel's diverticulum), about 25–30 cm from the ileocaecal valve usually with a wide mouth; ectopic gastric mucosa may be present for reasons that are not known and may cause clinical problems
- a fibrous strand which is connected to the umbilicus and is attached either to the antimesenteric border of the ileum or to the apex of Meckel's diverticulum; acute intestinal obstruction may then occur often with strangulation.

ANATOMY

The length of the small bowel is an average of 6 m (22ft) in an adult. The duodenum is technically part of the small bowel but is usually considered separately. The small bowel proper begins at the duodenojejunal flexure to the left of the second lumbar vertebra in the root of the transverse mesocolon. Here there is a variable but usually well-developed fold of peritoneum known to surgeons as the ligament of Treitz. The mesenteric root extends obliquely downwards and to the right for 12–15 cm over the right sacroiliac joint. A conventional distinction is made between the proximal half (jejunum) and the distal half (ileum), but one merges smoothly into the other. The jejunum has a different pattern of vascular arcades and a wider diameter. Its wall is thicker because of the presence of prominent mucosal folds (valvulae conniventes) and, as its name implies, it usually seems to be empty. The valvulae are an important identifying feature on plain abdominal X-rays.

The turnover of intestinal mucosal cells is rapid and they have a life of only a few days before being discarded, their contents digested and recycled. The submucosa of the distal ileum contains well defined collections of lymphoid tissue – Peyer's patches. Their exact function is not well understood but they probably play a part in detection of intraluminal antigens derived from gut bacteria and elaborating antibodies to them. They may be the entry point of specialised organisms such as *M. tuberculosis* (see below). Inflammatory enlargement of an area of lymphoid tissue is almost certainly involved in the genesis of intussusception.

PHYSIOLOGY
Motility
There are two movements:

- *peristalsis* – a coordinated wave of contraction extending over some centimetres of the gut and propelling the contents forward
- *segmental movements* over a short distance which mix the bowel contents.

If there is an air/liquid interface, both actions produce bowel sounds. A peristaltic wave is characteristically associated with a gurgle (borborygmus) which lasts a second or more and may be quite audible to the unaided ear. Segmental movements produce fainter 'clicks' of shorter duration which are detected by auscultation anywhere on the abdominal wall (there is no need to move the bell of the stethoscope around but it is necessary to listen for 1 minute by the clock to be sure that bowel sounds are absent). Both types of sounds are louder and more frequent if small bowel activity is increased as in obstruction (see below) or diarrhoea.

Secretion and digestion
These processes, which begin in the mouth and stomach, continue and are completed in the small bowel, which secretes the succus entericus with an electrolyte concentration approximately the same as the extracellular fluid. The overall flux of liquid in 24 hours is large but the alimentary tract normally contains at any one moment only about 1 L of secretion. Diversion of intestinal content because of obstruction, the formation of a communication between the gut and the exterior (fistula) or diarrhoea rapidly causes extracellular fluid volume deficiency.

Absorption
Water and electrolyte are absorbed throughout the whole of the small bowel with high efficiency unless normal antegrade motility is interfered with.

Glucose, simple peptides and amino acids are almost completely absorbed in the jejunum (but see 'Adaptability' below).

Fat is emulsified by bile salts and broken down into fatty acids and monoglycerides which form micelles – small molecular aggregates of bile salts, monoglycerides, fatty acids and cholesterol which can then present their components to the mucosal surface for absorption. However, bile salts are not absorbed at this point (down to the mid-jejunum) but are recycled by the terminal

ileum from which they are transported by the portal blood to the hepatocytes for re-secretion into the bile. This *enterohepatic circulation* is a mechanism for preservation of molecules which require complex synthesis; removal or disease of the terminal ileum interrupts this. A further outcome is that the re-absorption of vitamin B_{12} intrinsic factor is also reduced, so that a macrocytic anaemia may develop.

Adaptability
Although, as described, absorption of different substances is to a degree localised, the small bowel is adaptable so that extensive resection can be done without obvious effects. Survival with a total length of 20 cm has been recorded, but it is a surgical principle to preserve as much healthy bowel as possible. Supplementary parenteral nutrition has been used in those with very short lengths of small bowel but transplantation is becoming increasingly feasible (see Ch. 13).

Fistula
An external communication between the bowel and the skin may be the result of disease (see, for example, Crohn's disease, below) or a complication of surgery where an anastomosis has failed to heal. The effects vary with the level in the bowel. A fistula high in the jejunum produces large losses of succus entericus and rapid extracellular fluid volume deficiency over a few days. In addition, the skin is digested by the high enzyme content of the escaping fluid. By contrast, a terminal ileostomy, say after resection of the large bowel (Ch. 24), may only result in an output of less than 1L and, although the skin is affected, should the content remain in contact with it, the digestive action is rarely as severe. A fistula in the large bowel is usually not associated with water and electrolyte disturbance.

Microbiology
Most organisms ingested by mouth are destroyed by the action of acid and pepsin in the stomach and the healthy small bowel is usually regarded as practically sterile. However, a large inoculum (as in gastroenteritis) or bacteria resistant to infection (e.g. *M. tuberculosis*) may survive. Any organisms in the small bowel are confined to the lumen by the protective action of the mucosal barrier. However, obstruction of the small bowel is associated with a variable breakdown of this protection. A similar loss is also seen with reduction in blood supply to the bowel either from local effects or as a result of general reduced perfusion from, for example, acute reduction in blood volume. Organisms, usually of faecal origin, increase in number and may penetrate the normally protective mucosal barrier and translocate into the interstitial space of the gut wall. It is thought possible that they may then migrate into the portal blood. The systemic effects of bacterial endotoxins which enter the circulation in this way are thought to be a factor in

the production of the systemic inflammatory response syndrome (SIRS) and multi-organ failure.

Intestinal obstruction

There are a bewildering number of different ways of defining and classifying obstruction of the alimentary tract distal to the stomach. A simple preliminary is to distinguish between mechanical and paralytic obstruction. In the first, there is a site (sometimes multiple) at which forward passage is prevented but above this the bowel is initially normal and active; in the second, the whole bowel is inactive. The word 'ileus' merely means obstruction, but in surgical practice it is usually reserved for the paralytic forms (see below), except that surgeons still speak of gallstone ileus which is an example of mechanical obstruction.

Mechanical obstruction

Further classification can be done in a variety of ways, all of which have their uses in individual circumstances. The clinical course may be acute, subacute or chronic. The condition may affect either the small or the large bowel. The cause may be specified – such as inflammatory adhesions or tumour – or described according to its position in relation to the bowel wall – i.e. luminal, mural or extramural (Box 23.1). The obstruction may be either 'open loop' – i.e. bowel content can escape proximally – or 'closed loop', in which a segment of gut is obstructed at both ends; large bowel obstruction is always potentially closed loop because the ileocaecal valve resists regurgitation from the caecum into the terminal ileum. Finally, the blood supply may also be obstructed – strangulation. The venous drainage is first interfered with and strangulating obstructions lead to haemorrhagic infarction.

PATHOPHYSIOLOGY

Proximal to an obstruction, intestinal contractions are increased in both magnitude and frequency. The bowel diameter increases and, because of this, contractions may eventually fail. The intestinal wall becomes oedematous and this, with reduced reabsorption of secretions, may cause extracellular volume deficiency. Strangulation causes blood loss into the affected loops and may produce hypovolaemia and, because of underperfusion of the affected segment, lactic acidosis. Eventually a strangulated loop will die (usually within 4–6 hours) and rupture, with the production of a severe bacterial peritonitis which is often fatal. Distension of the abdomen by the dilated loops may restrict diaphragmatic movement and so interfere with respiratory function. Vomiting may result in inhalation.

Box 23.1

Classification of mechanical obstruction

Luminal

Gallstone (gallstone ileus)

Food bolus

Meconium ileus

Mural

Stricture
    Congenital
    Inflammatory
    Ischaemic
    Neoplastic
Intussusception

Extramural

Adhesions
    Congenital
    Inflammatory
    Malignant
    Ischaemic

Hernia
    External
    Internal

Volvulus (twisting)
    Congenital
    Acquired

CLINICAL FEATURES

Symptoms

Abdominal pain is the first symptom and is central, ill-localised and characteristically of colic coming in waves with pain-free intervals of minutes. Large bowel obstruction causes lower abdominal colic and may eventually produce the more constant pain of distension. A strangulated loop in contact with the inner aspect of the abdominal wall causes well localised, often severe, pain.

Vomiting follows the pain, and the higher the level of obstruction, the earlier and more profuse it is. Initially, upper gastrointestinal contents are produced (food residue and dark greenish fluid) but, unless the obstruction is in the upper jejunum, dark brown, bitter, foul smelling (faeculent) material soon appears (vomiting of faeces is not a feature of intestinal obstruction but occurs in the relatively rare circumstance of an internal fistula between the large bowel and the stomach). In obstruction distal to the ileocaecal valve, vomiting may be absent because the small bowel can continue to propel its content into the distensible colon above the obstruction.

Distension is usually evident and is generally more marked the more distal the obstruction. Proximal jejunal obstruction (which is relatively uncommon) may be without distension.

Constipation. Most flatus passed per rectum is air that has been swallowed so that complete obstruction at any level is associated with absolute constipation for both stool and gas, which occurs early in large bowel obstruction and later in small bowel obstruction. Incomplete obstructions, as may occur in the large bowel from a progressively encircling tumour, cause reduction in the size and frequency of bowel motions with visible changes in the stool – mucus and blood (see Ch. 24).

Physical findings

General. Loss of water and electrolyte (and, in strangulating obstructions, blood) causes the circulatory changes that are discussed below. Temperature may be raised in a strangulating obstruction but in simple obstruction it is usually normal.

Abdomen. Distension is present which is approximately related to the level of obstruction – the lower the obstruction in the small bowel, the greater the distension. In large bowel obstruction, and because of the competence of the ileocaecal valve, the distension may outline the colon only with a visible caecum. An abdominal scar suggests but does not prove that the cause of a small bowel obstruction may be adhesions. Visible peristalsis may occasionally be seen in a thin patient and may coincide with an audible rush of peristalsis – see 'Auscultation' below.

Palpation may show:

- a mass anywhere in the abdomen – this suggests a specific cause for the obstruction
- an irreducible mass at a hernial orifice – strangulated hernia
- tenderness and guarding – this is highly suspicious of strangulation but can be difficult to assess in the first few days after an abdominal operation.

Percussion produces a tympanitic note because of the presence of gas-filled loops of bowel, although in a slowly developing low small bowel obstruction, fluid may predominate.

Auscultation reveals increased frequency of the segmenting sounds which are high pitched and tinkling and have been likened to the sound of water lapping against the side of a small boat. Loud peristaltic rushes may be heard and coincide with an attack of colic. When mechanical obstruction is indicated by other clinical findings but bowel sounds are absent, the condition is usually advanced or there is peritonitis which has resulted from perforation of an involved loop.

Rectal and (in females) pelvic examination is routine, and on occasion a mass may be detected. However, in small bowel obstruction, apart from the rectum being empty, the procedure is unhelpful.

INVESTIGATION

Imaging

Plain abdominal X-rays taken in the erect and supine positions are the standard and most reliable means of diagnosis. Some radiologists recommend supine films only because these usually provide all the information needed and reduce radiation exposure; certainly this is true if repeated observations for progress or resolution are required. Four questions are posed:

- Is this an obstruction?
- If so, is it in the small or large bowel?
- What is the level of obstruction in the small or large bowel?
- Can a specific cause be determined?

The characteristic appearance of small bowel obstruction is of a number of distended, gas- and fluid-filled loops of bowel with, in the erect posture, fluid levels. The levels are frequently arranged in a stepladder pattern (Fig. 23.1). Particularly in the jejunum, the valvulae conniventes may be visible. Adjacent loops may be separated by a variable distance which gives an indication of the amount of oedema fluid in the bowel wall. Gas is usually absent from the large bowel.

Large bowel obstruction causes accumulation of gas which outlines its wall proximally and which is maximal in the caecum. With a competent ileocaecal valve, the small bowel may be normal. The pattern of gas may give a nearly exact localisation of the cause with a cut-off point between distended proximal and collapsed distal colon.

Contrast X-rays are less commonly needed, but a water-soluble medium (Gastrografin) by mouth is sometimes needed when there is doubt about the diagnosis. Serial exposures can be made over some hours and the progress of the medium followed. Its entry into the

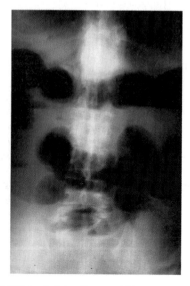

Fig 23.1 **Small bowel obstruction: erect X-ray.**

large bowel after 1–2 hours effectively excludes complete small bowel obstruction. When large bowel obstruction is clinically suspect, it is good surgical practice routinely to carry out a retrograde contrast study from the rectum, because experience has shown that the differential diagnosis of a truly mechanical obstruction from pseudo-obstruction – a disorder of motility which mimics it – is difficult (see 'Pseudo-obstruction', below).

Barium sulphate is never given by mouth in acute obstruction because it may make matters worse and is damaging if it is inhaled during an episode of vomiting. A clinical picture of chronic small bowel obstruction may be cautiously investigated by the use of barium.

Ultrasound is sometimes useful to elucidate the nature of a mass in the presence of intestinal obstruction.

Other special imaging techniques are considered under individual causes.

Haematological and biochemical

A raised white cell count suggests either an active inflammatory cause or strangulation, as does a metabolic acidosis. The disturbance of water and electrolyte metabolism which occurs in acute obstruction – particularly of the small bowel – requires routine tests both for diagnosis and to set up baselines for subsequent therapy. The concentration of amylase in the serum may be raised in acute obstruction so that, although it is useful in the differential diagnosis of acute pancreatitis (Ch. 21) in which there is often abdominal distension and other features that resemble obstruction, hyperamylassaemia is by no means a conclusive indication of pancreatic inflammation.

MANAGEMENT

Individual conditions are considered below but there are some general principles, the first being the choice between non-operative (conservative) and operative management.

Non-operative

The indications are:

- firm evidence that there is not a threat to the viability of the bowel – strangulation or perforation as suggested by signs of hypovolaemia, systemic inflammatory response and peritoneal irritation
- incomplete obstruction in either the small or large bowel with features which suggest non-progression, e.g. Crohn's disease in the small bowel and a left-sided carcinoma in the large bowel
- some instances of complete small bowel obstruction – the usual most suitable example is in adhesive obstruction (see below).

Conservative management involves:

- proximal decompression by a nasogastric tube with aspiration either continuously or on a regular intermittent basis

- water and electrolyte replacement
- repeated (4–6 hourly) evaluation of the clinical state – abdominal girth, development of tenderness, changes in bowel sounds and in cardiovascular status
- in individual circumstances, repeated straight X-rays or contrast studies and haematological and biochemical reassessment of the features of strangulation.

A limit of 5 days or less is usually placed on conservative management but special circumstances may alter this in either direction.

Operative

The indications are:

- established or suspected strangulation including those with irreducible external hernia
- complete large bowel obstruction with tenderness in the right iliac fossa – indicative of closed loop obstruction with possible perforation of the caecum
- failure of resolution after a period of non-operative management.

Operative management is preceded by a brief period of application of the measures outlined under non-operative management – gastric suction, water and electrolyte replacement. The only indication for urgent operation is when strangulation or other causes of non-viability of the bowel are likely. At operation, the obstruction is relieved and, if possible, the underlying cause removed. Dead or damaged intestine must be excised. Occasionally an irremovable obstruction (e.g. a fixed neoplasm) is bypassed.

Paralytic obstruction

This type of intestinal obstruction is caused by a failure of motility. The different forms are discussed in detail in the section on 'Common causes of ileus' (below).

Common causes of mechanical obstruction

Intraluminal

Gallstone 'ileus'

A sizeable stone in the gall bladder erodes through into adjacent duodenum or small bowel and is then carried distally until it impacts, usually in the relatively narrow ileum. The condition is now uncommon in the developed world because of the usual early treatment of gallstones.

CLINICAL FEATURES

Often there is a variable history which suggests bouts of intermittent obstruction. Eventually complete obstruction supervenes but the symptoms in a distal small bowel obstruction are sometimes difficult to interpret.

Physical findings are of considerable distension because of the long length of small bowel involved and with largely fluid-filled loops.

INVESTIGATION AND MANAGEMENT

The radiological findings are often diagnostic because, apart from the features of intestinal obstruction, air can often be seen in the biliary tree.

The gallstone is removed through an enterotomy slightly proximal to the point of impaction and the more proximal small bowel is examined for additional stones. A subsequent procedure may be done to deal with the disease in the biliary tree.

Food bolus

The common causes of food bolus are:

- poor chewing of food in an edentulous patient
- a previous gastric resection which has destroyed the pylorus
- high consumption of indigestible fibre (e.g. orange pith)
- occasionally, partial obstruction for some other reason with impaction of partially digested food at the site of narrowing.

The clinical features are similar to those of gallstone ileus – low small bowel obstruction.

MANAGEMENT

Operation is usually indicated even if a confident pre-operative diagnosis has been made, because there is always the risk of confusing the condition with another cause. The bolus can often be milked distally into the large intestine and it is rarely necessary to open the bowel and risk contamination of the peritoneal cavity.

Meconium 'ileus'

This is discussed in Chapter 35.

Mural

Neonatal obstructions and intussusception

These are discussed in Chapter 35.

Inflammatory

Crohn's disease, tuberculosis and, in the large bowel, diverticulitis may all produce obstruction by causing either inflammatory or fibrous strictures or by adherence of a loop of bowel to the inflammatory area. Diverticulosis of the large bowel rarely causes obstruction other than by:

- adhesions between the inflamed colon and the small bowel
- an inflammatory mass in the colon which leads to a clinical picture of large bowel obstruction.

In the small bowel, other causes of obstructive strictures are potassium chloride tablets (now rare because the current prescriptions are enteric-coated) and the ingestion of NSAIDs which may be associated not only with stricture but also with bleeding.

Extramural

Adhesions

Throughout the world, these are the commonest cause of small bowel obstruction after strangulated external hernia; in developed countries, where hernias are usually treated early, they are the leading cause.

AETIOLOGY

A small minority of adhesions are the result of developmental disturbances. The great majority are scars on the visceral peritoneum from inflammation.

The peritoneal mesothelial cells have a highly potent fibrinolytic mechanism based on the tissue conversion of plasminogen to plasmin. In consequence, any fibrin produced by inflammation in the peritoneal cavity does not usually consolidate and go on to be part of a scar. However, any persistent focus (Table 23.1) may overcome this fibrinolytic activity, particularly if there is local marginal ischaemia. Then the usual process of wound healing takes place and fibrous tissue is deposited. The small bowel, rather than moving freely within the peritoneal cavity, becomes attached to itself or to an adjacent fixed point and can therefore kink or twist (Fig. 23.1). Adhesions may be a simple isolated band or snare that can trap the bowel and narrow it from without, or may be complex and dense involving the whole peritoneal cavity.

The time course of adhesion formation is comparable to that of the inflammation/ischaemia which are the underlying causes. Acute processes can produce adhesions in a matter of days although this does not necessarily mean that obstruction follows and an adhesion can lie dormant for months or years. Thus post-surgical adhesive obstruction may be manifest either within a few days of an operation – when it may be

Table 23.1
Adhesions

Classification	Underlying cause	Examples
Congenital	Abnormality or arrest of development	Duodenal obstruction
	? Ischaemia	Persistent vitellointestinal duct with volvulus
Acquired		
Cell damage	Trauma	Post-surgical obstruction
	Irradiation	Peritoneal dialysis in renal failure
Intraperitoneal inflammation	Inhibition of fibrinolysis	Peritonitis, focal inflamed areas, e.g. diverticulitis of the colon
Ischaemia	Inhibition of fibrinolysis	Partially devascularised bowel, surgical procedures
Peritoneal loss	Lack of local fibrinolysis	Wide surgical excision
Intraperitoneal foreign materials	Foreign body inflammation	Surgical materials glove powder, sutures
Abnormality of fibrous tissue	Unknown	Colectomy for polyposis coli, stromal fibrous response to malignant disease

difficult to distinguish from a persistent paralytic ileus (see below) – or years or decades after the operation.

Apart from the causes shown in Table 23.1, it has often been postulated by exasperated surgeons, re-operating for the umpteenth time on a patient with adhesive obstruction, that there are patients who are 'adhesion formers'. The current evidence for this is unconvincing and usually some underlying cause can be found. Fortunately, the fibrinolytic properties of the peritoneum tend to resolution once individual episodes are dealt with.

CLINICAL FEATURES

There has long been controversy as to whether or not adhesions can cause symptoms other than intestinal obstruction. Chronic or recurrent pain is often ascribed to their presence. While this may be true, adhesions do not contain nerve tissue so that it is difficult to postulate mechanisms. For practical purposes it is best to assume that, with rare exceptions, adhesions present for treatment because they cause small bowel obstruction; large bowel obstruction of adhesive origin is extremely rare.

MANAGEMENT

This is on the lines outlined above. Strangulation is always a possibility which should be considered on the clinical evidence and which demands surgery.

External hernia

This is discussed in Chapter 26.

Internal hernia

This takes place into a recess of a peritoneal fold formed either during development (e.g. around the junction of the duodenum and jejunum at the ligament of Treitz)

or as a consequence of operation (e.g. lateral to a colostomy or ileostomy). They are rare.

CLINICAL FEATURES AND MANAGEMENT

Features are of intestinal obstruction without obvious cause. The clinical trap is that a loop of bowel may be strangulated but is not in contact with the anterior parietal peritoneum and therefore does not produce symptoms and signs of peritoneal irritation. In consequence, disastrous delay may occur.

Operation should be done on any patient who presents with acute small bowel obstruction with no obvious cause.

Volvulus

This is the general term for a twist of the bowel around its mesenteric axis. Both obstruction and ischaemia of the involved loop can occur. For neonatal volvulus see Chapter 35.

AETIOLOGY

Volvulus is less common in the small than in the large bowel.

Small bowel

The apex of the loop involved is tethered by an adhesion, often to the abdominal wall or other adjacent viscera at one point and rotation takes place around this. A rotation of more than 180° may result in strangulation.

Large bowel

Rotation may occur at two sites:

- *caecum* – when there is a persistent mesentery (uncommon)
- *sigmoid colon* – when the existing mesentery is usually more extensive than normal; this is the commoner cause of large bowel volvulus which,

although rare in the UK, is more frequently encountered in the developing world.

Caecal volvulus can occur in adults of 30 years of age or more, but sigmoid twists are more common in older people.

CLINICAL FEATURES AND MANAGEMENT

Small bowel

The clinical features are those of acute small bowel obstruction with localised abdominal pain if strangulation is added. Involvement of a considerable length of small bowel is, if strangulation occurs, associated with circulatory disturbance.

Operation is undertaken usually for small bowel obstruction of unknown cause. The volvulus is untwisted, the cause relieved and, if any bowel of doubtful viability is found, this is resected.

Large bowel

The features are those of large bowel obstruction occasionally with a background of repeated episodes. In caecal volvulus, although obvious intestinal obstruction is present, the clinical and radiological features may be confusing. An X-ray may show features that suggest gastric outflow obstruction.

Sigmoid volvulus is, in theory, more easy to diagnose. The patient is elderly. The features are those of large bowel obstruction, perhaps with previous episodes. The presentation is often acute with signs of circulatory insufficiency because of infarction. A grossly distended, drum-like abdomen is characteristic. The plain supine abdominal X-ray should be diagnostic with an Omega sign. As previously emphasised and for reasons that are discussed in more detail below (see 'Pseudo-obstruction', below), the clinical diagnosis of large bowel mechanical obstruction requires diagnostic confirmation by contrast retrograde enema using a water-soluble medium.

In caecal volvulus there is only a limited place for non-operative management because this is a closed loop obstruction. Particularly if signs of peritoneal irritation are present, operation is immediately undertaken, the ileum and right colon resected and the bowel reconstructed by ileotransverse anastomosis.

In sigmoid volvulus unlike caecal volvulus, non-operative treatment is the initial choice. A sigmoidoscope or colonoscope is introduced, a wide-bore flatus tube is passed along it and the sigmoid loop decompressed by careful negotiation of the obstructed loop. As one authority has remarked: 'protective clothing is recommended as the results of decompression are usually explosive'. Once decompression has been achieved, a decision on surgical excision of the mobile sigmoid colon can be taken at a later date, but this should usually be done because recurrence is common.

Failure to relieve the volvulus by these means or signs of peritoneal irritation that suggest strangulation require urgent operation. The colon is resected either with or without primary anastomosis.

Common causes of ileus

In cases of ileus, intestinal obstruction is present but the cause is failure of motility rather than a mechanical obstruction. Loss of forward propulsion must be recognised but the treatment is different from that of mechanical obstruction.

'Paralytic' (dysdynamic) ileus

AETIOLOGY

This condition predominantly affects the small bowel. The causes are either dysfunction of sympathetic outflow (the proximate cause of which is not well understood) or peripheral inhibition of peristalsis. A summary of causes is given in Table 23.2. There are two groups:

- *postoperative* – from handling of the bowel at surgical exploration; this is relatively transient (18–24 hours)
- *secondary causes* – either outwith or within the peritoneal cavity.

CLINICAL FEATURES

The features are those of intestinal obstruction but without pain and with the absence of evidence of intestinal activity, i.e. no bowel sounds. In the early postoperative period, it may be difficult to distinguish paralytic ileus from adhesive mechanical obstruction with a poorly functioning small bowel. The pain and the difficulty of examination produced by an incision may also confuse. Features that are helpful are:

- absence of colic
- abdominal silence on auscultation
- large and small bowel distension on plain X-ray with absence of a stepladder appearance of fluid levels.

MANAGEMENT

Ascertainment of the cause is basic to clinical management. If this can be eliminated or allowed to run its course, all that is needed is to keep the stomach empty by nasogastric suction or gastrostomy and to maintain water and electrolyte balance. Pharmacological methods of stimulating the gut have largely been abandoned. If the condition is prolonged in duration (more than 5 days), parenteral feeding may be required.

Table 23.2
Adynamic and dysdynamic ileus

Underlying cause	Mechanism	Examples
Sympathetic outflow dysfunction	Reflex inhibition	Temporary postoperative ileus
		Spinal injury
		Acute disorders, e.g. renal colic
	Pelvic and retroperitoneal bleeding or effusion	Trauma
		Anticoagulation
		Acute pancreatitis
	Malignant infiltration	Ogilvie's syndrome – ileus in association with malignant disease in the retroperitoneum
Local	Peritonitis	Bacterial infection
	Advanced mechanical obstruction	Overdistension
Biochemical	Interference with normal contractility of smooth muscle	Hypoxia
		Potassium deficiency
		Uraemia
		Diabetes mellitus
Pharmacological	As above	Anticholinergics
		Ganglion blockers
		Antidiarrhoretic agents

Pseudo-obstruction

This term is applied (somewhat inaccurately) to a dysdynamic ileus that affects the large bowel.

AETIOLOGY

The causes are similar to those given in Table 23.2 but the condition is more common in the elderly and in those confined to bed by another condition such as a hip fracture. Respiratory disease with hypoxia is a common accompaniment. The name *Ogilvie's syndrome* is sometimes used as a synonym for pseudo-obstruction but strictly should be limited to those instances which occur because of widespread retroperitoneal infiltration by malignant disease. Pseudo-obstruction is not the same as faecal impaction where there is a failure to defaecate usually with overflow incontinence of faeces but where the features of intestinal obstruction are absent.

CLINICAL FEATURES

The picture is of large bowel obstruction, but increased bowel sounds are not usually present. The caecum and transverse colon dilate (and caecal rupture can occur). Plain films do not show a typical cut-off point, which is often present in mechanical large bowel obstruction. As with paralytic ileus, the clinical problem is to distinguish between a patient with mechanical obstruction and dysdynamic pseudo-obstruction.

INVESTIGATION

To operate on a patient who turns out to have pseudo-obstruction, besides being unnecessary in most instances, carries a high mortality from accompanying or causatively associated illness. Because of this, a patient who is thought on clinical grounds to have large bowel obstruction, and in whom either there is no obvious cause or there are aetiological predisposing factors for pseudo-obstruction, should have a water-soluble contrast enema. Twenty per cent or more of such patients turn out to have pseudo-obstruction, but a smaller (though significant) number in whom a provisional diagnosis of pseudo-obstruction has been made prove to have a mechanical lesion. If the diagnosis is confirmed as pseudo-obstruction, the bowel is decompressed by passing a colonoscope, preferably leaving behind a long flatus tube to prevent re-dilatation. If identified, an underlying cause, such as hypoxia or hypokalaemia, is treated.

Neostigmine can also be used to relieve colonic pseudo-obstruction.

Vascular disturbances in the gut

The blood vessels of the gut have extensive anastomoses. In consequence, considerable vascular obstruction to input or drainage may exist without any clinical effects.

Table 23.3
Causes of acute vascular disturbances in the gut

Arterial	
Thrombosis on an atheromatous plaque	Usually at the ostium of a main vessel such as the superior mesenteric
Embolus	Atrial fibrillation
	Mural thrombus after myocardial infarction
	Detached atheromatous plaques
Reduced arterial flow	Low cardiac output – hypotension or heart failure
Desmoplastic obliteration	Carcinoid tumour
Venous	
Pharmacological	High-dose contraceptive pill – now rare
Stasis	Portal hypertension
Sepsis	
Coagulopathies	Sickle cell disease

Small bowel disease and intestinal obstruction

Acute presentation is the rule. Relatively rarely, chronic insufficiency occurs. The causes are summarised in Table 23.3.

Severe acute ischaemia; whether from arterial or venous causes, results in haemorrhagic infarction. Blood and extracellular fluid are lost into the affected loop, so producing hypovolaemia; the haemodynamic effects are potentiated by release of cytokines. Full-thickness ischaemia leads to gangrene with perforation and peritonitis.

A more gradual (subacute or chronic) reduction in arterial input may not have effects on the resting bowel, but with the increase in flow that accompanies digestion, the bowel contracts inappropriately and absorption is interfered with. The usual cause is an atheromatous plaque with narrowing at the ostium of the superior mesenteric artery.

Acute presentation

This is often an overwhelming and highly lethal event.

Clinical features

There is severe acute colicky abdominal pain, vomiting, rectal bleeding (usually darkened, altered blood) and symptoms of hypovolaemia. There may be a past history of an underlying disorder such as heart disease which could give rise to an embolus.

Clinical findings are hypovolaemia and signs of strangulation in the abdomen.

Investigation and management

Similar investigations are done as for intestinal obstruction. Special studies such as arteriography are occasionally indicated but the condition is usually so urgent that operation is required.

Management is by restoration of circulating blood volume and exploration of the abdomen. If possible, the gangrenous loop or loops are resected, but involvement of the whole small bowel (and often the right colon) carries a hopeless prognosis. Primary anastomosis may be done or the ends of the bowel are exteriorised until it is certain that further infarction has not taken place. If the cause is embolic, it is very occasionally possible to remove the clot and re-establish flow but this is the exception.

Subacute and chronic presentation

Clinical features

The history is often vague and the diagnosis is not made for some time. Features are:

- diffuse pain shortly after eating – so-called abdominal angina
- loss of weight – partly from malabsorption but also because the patient reduces intake to avoid pain
- occasionally diarrhoea.

The physical findings are non-specific. An abdominal bruit is sometimes detected on auscultation, but many abdominal bruits are not associated with vascular obstruction.

Investigation and management

If the condition is diagnosed on clinical grounds, selective angiography is done to outline the origins of the mesenteric vessels and plan treatment.

Untreated, the symptomatic patient often goes on to acute mesenteric infarction. A direct attack on the obstruction can be made either at operation or by balloon angioplasty. Alternatively, a bypass graft is sometimes feasible.

Crohn's disease (regional ileitis or enterocolitis)

AETIOLOGY

The cause of this condition is not known although various organisms have been associated with it and it is currently suggested that it is an inflammation produced by unusual strains of mycobacteria.

PATHOLOGICAL FEATURES

There is a transmural inflammation with oedema, fissures and non-caseating foci of epithelioid and giant cells leading on to fibrosis. Although the terminal ileum is most commonly involved, skip lesions can occur throughout the small bowel. Both oedema and fibrosis can cause intestinal obstruction but it is usually fibrous stricture that produces clinical manifestations. Internal fistulae may form between loops of bowel or into the retroperitoneal tissues or other structures. Healing is accompanied by fibrosis. The condition is often limited to the terminal ileum – where it is most common – either with or without a varying degree of involvement

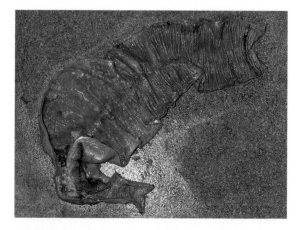

Fig 23.2 **Crohn's disease of the distal ileum — pathological specimen.**

of the large bowel (see Ch. 24), but it can occur anywhere in the gastrointestinal tract (Fig. 23.2). Associated perianal disease is common (Ch. 25).

CLINICAL FEATURES
Presentation may be acute or chronic, or a combination of both.

Acute
An episode of right iliac fossa pain and tenderness takes place which may mimic appendicitis (Ch. 24) or *Yersinia* ileitis and lead to surgical exploration. If a mass in the right iliac fossa is found, care should be taken not to explore – unless the matter is thought urgent – until investigation has established the nature and extent of the process.

Alternatively, the features may be those of low small bowel obstruction (see above).

Chronic
There are symptoms of general ill health with weight loss, colicky abdominal pain and diarrhoea. The physical findings are non-specific unless there is a mass present which is firm, irregular and often slightly tender.

INVESTIGATION

Imaging
Small bowel disease is best detected by barium meal (Fig. 23.3) and follow-through which shows:

- mucosal irregularities and ulceration
- strictures – especially the string sign of Kantor
- skip lesions with apparently normal bowel between them
- internal fistulae.

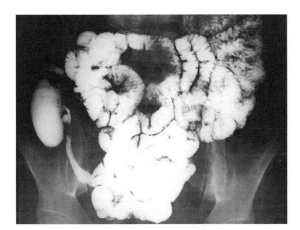

Fig 23.3 **Crohn's disease demonstrated with barium meal.**

Radiolabelled white blood cell imaging is a method of identifying active foci of disease which is particularly useful in patients suspected of having recurrent disease.

Biopsy
Even if symptoms of large bowel disease are absent, the rectal mucosa may be visibly abnormal or a biopsy may show typical appearances. Biopsies may also be obtained from the mucosa of the right side of the colon and terminal ileum at colonoscopy. If a patient is clinically diagnosed as having Crohn's disease at laparotomy – which may occur if the presentation mimics appendicitis – a biopsy of the bowel is avoided because there is a risk of fistula formation. However, a lymph node biopsy may be helpful, particularly in distinguishing the condition from tuberculosis.

MANAGEMENT
There is no specific treatment for Crohn's disease, although long-term antibiotics against enteric organisms are under trial. Many patients are managed symptomatically and with steroids by gastroenterologists. Immunosuppressive treatment with azathioprine has also been tried but is of doubtful value.

Surgical management is required when there is·

- intestinal obstruction
- abscess or fistula
- (sometimes) large bowel disease (see Ch. 24).

Surgery usually involves resection of a diseased segment of small bowel which may also be the cause of obstruction. Defining the margins of disease can be difficult and there is no guarantee against recurrence; half of all patients who have surgical treatment require further procedures within 10 years. Stricturoplasty can enlarge a narrow lumen provided the disease is no longer active and is less radical than excision. Bypass used to be done if resection was regarded as likely to be difficult but is not now used.

Tuberculosis

AETIOLOGY
The organism enters the gut via the lymphoid follicles found in the mucosa of the ileum. The source is either from without or from a focus of infection already present, such as an open pulmonary lesion with swallowed sputum. Both human and bovine strains of *M. tuberculosis* can be the cause but the latter is now very uncommon in the UK. In immunodeficiency states such as AIDS, unusual strains of mycobacteria, particularly *M. avium intracellulare*, may be found.

Tubercular infection in the small bowel is now uncommon in the developed world but remains a feature of communities with poor nutrition and continuing foci of tubercular infection elsewhere.

PATHOLOGICAL FEATURES

A typical tubercular inflammation takes place in the wall of the ileum with:

- ulceration
- lymph node enlargement and subsequent caseation and calcification
- healing with the formation of strictures.

In addition, tuberculosis may involve the peritoneum to produce tuberculous peritonitis characterised by the presence of military nodules and the development of ascites.

CLINICAL FEATURES

Weight loss, low-grade pyrexia, anaemia, diarrhoea and vague lower abdominal pain may be present. Ulceration causes blood loss and a frank rectal haemorrhage may occur. Either the inflammatory mass or the development of a stricture may cause acute intestinal obstruction.

A mass in the right iliac fossa has to be distinguished from one caused by Crohn's disease, which it resembles closely. Ascites may be present. There may be low-grade or frank intestinal obstruction.

INVESTIGATION

A barium follow-through can outline the terminal ileum and a contrast enema may show distortion of the caecum. Both appearances are difficult to distinguish from Crohn's disease, as are the findings on ultrasound examination of a mass. Half of patients with tuberculous ileitis also have a radiological pulmonary lesion.

MANAGEMENT

As with all other manifestations of tuberculosis, the primary treatment is with chemotherapy although this is becoming increasingly problematic with the development of resistant strains. The surgeon's tasks are:

- to establish the diagnosis by laparoscopy or laparotomy
- to manage complications such as bleeding and obstruction when it is usual to undertake resection of the affected area.

Radiotherapy effects

Rapidly dividing tissues which include the mucosa of the small and, to a lesser extent, the large bowel are sensitive to irradiation. Abdominal or pelvic radiotherapy to treat malignant disease can cause damage both to the mucosa and to the small blood vessels in the wall of the gut. Fortunately, with better radiotherapeutic techniques this is now less common.

CLINICAL PATHOLOGICAL FEATURES

The major pathological changes are mucosal atrophy and intramural fibrosis. Strictures with low-grade intestinal obstruction and ulceration with bleeding may follow. Presentation is with bleeding from the gut, intestinal obstruction, occasionally perforation and internal or external fistula formation.

MANAGEMENT

Surgical excision of the damaged loops may be required but reconstruction must use healthy unirradiated bowel or poor healing and anastomotic breakdown are common.

Diverticuli of the small bowel

Jejunal diverticuli

This uncommon problem is probably congenital but the cause is unknown. There are multiple herniated areas through the mesenteric aspect of the jejunum usually bulging to one side.

The clinical features are:

- vague dyspepsia
- perforation of one diverticulum
- macrocytic anaemia thought to be the consequence of infection
- enterolith formation with small bowel obstruction.

MANAGEMENT

Surgical intervention is required for emergencies, but otherwise the condition is managed without operation unless a local area of diverticulosis is definitely associated with remediable symptoms.

Meckel's diverticulum

ANATOMY AND EPIDEMIOLOGY

The embryological development and the forms the remnant may take have been considered previously. Occurrence follows a rough 'law of 2 s': 2% of the population; 2 ft (60 cm) from the ileocaecal valve; 2 inches (5 cm) in length; and twice as common in males as in females.

CLINICAL PRESENTATION

The diverticulum is notorious for the different ways in which it may present;

- persistent vitelloumbilical fistula (Fig. 23.4)
- acute diverticulitis which mimics appendicitis (see Ch. 24)
- perforation and peritonitis as a consequence of inflammation or from a retained foreign body such as a fishbone

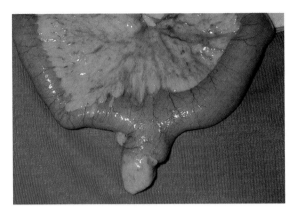

Fig 23.4 **Meckel's diverticulum.**

- intestinal obstruction when the diverticulum or an associated band is attached to the umbilicus and causes a small bowel volvulus or internal herniation
- ileo-ileal intussusception
- an ectopic peptic ulcer secondary to the presence of gastric mucosal cells.

The peptic ulcer occurs on the mesenteric border of the adjacent ileum and the presentation is of pain and lower small bowel bleeding (nearly always in children or young adults), which can be exsanguinating. Confirmation of its origin in a Meckel's diverticulum can sometimes be obtained by radionucleide scanning with $^{99}Tc^m$ sodium pertechnate.

MANAGEMENT
An *asymptomatic* diverticulum discovered at exploration for another reason is usually removed in a child, but in an adult over 30 years old it has already established that it is innocuous and may be left. *Symptomatic* diverticulae are dealt with according to the complications that they cause.

Small bowel neoplasms

EPIDEMIOLOGY AND AETIOLOGY
Primary tumours of the small bowel are relatively uncommon and account for only 5% of gastrointestinal neoplasms. Isolated benign smooth muscle tumours (leiomyomas) are of unknown cause but other factors are:

- gastroenterohepatic tumours
- developmental disorders
- immunocompromise – particularly Kaposi's sarcoma, adenocarcinoma and lymphoma
- Crohn's disease – this brings about a small increased risk of adenocarcinoma
- geographical location.

Developmental disorders
Small bowel tumours are associated with:

- Polyposis coli, although most of the neoplasms arise in the duodenum (see 'Familial polyposis coli')
- Peutz–Jegher syndrome – an ill-understood inherited relationship between intestinal polyps mainly in the jejunum and marginal pigmentation around the buccal and anal mucosa; the usual presentation is with intussusception
- Gardner's syndrome – this is a rare disorder in which small bowel adenomas and carcinomas are associated with skeletal abnormalities and desmoid tumours.

Immunocompromise
There are three circumstances:

- Coeliac disease in which there is gluten-sensitive enteropathy with a wide variety of other manifestations of atopy – there is a real although uncertain incidence of small bowel cancer
- Acquired immunodeficiency, as in AIDS, which makes the patient sporadically liable to Kaposi's sarcoma and lymphoma
- Immunosuppression, chiefly in transplant patients, is associated with small bowel lymphomas.

Geographical location
There is no doubt that lymphomas are more common in the Middle East than elsewhere. The cause is unknown but may reflect an infectious agent.

PATHOLOGICAL FEATURES
Benign tumours
Benign tumours – adenomas of various form – are, because of their hereditary association, commoner in the duodenum. Progression to carcinoma can occur. Other tumours are:

- *Leiomyomas* – these are intra- or extraluminal and give rise to bleeding and obstruction
- *Lipomas* – these are commoner in the large than in the small bowel and, because of their bulk, are liable to cause intussusception with abdominal colic and rectal bleeding
- *Neurofibromas* – can occur in isolation or as part of the general picture of neurofibromatosis; bleeding or obstruction may occur.

Malignant tumours
- *Lymphomas* – either primary or part of a more generalised disorder
- *Adenocarcinoma* – more common in the duodenum but also occurs elsewhere
- *Secondary tumours* – these are rare but occur in lung and breast cancer and also in malignant melanoma.

Management of obesity

DEFINITION AND EPIDEMIOLOGY

'Reference' or 'ideal' weights are obtained from population studies usually carried out for insurance purposes. It should be recognised that the figures obtained are what exists in the population and not what is necessarily physiologically ideal; for example, an increase of weight with age is very common in the western world but is not biologically advantageous. The definition of overweight is 10–20% above reference weight; and of obesity is more than 20%. An alternative and possibly more satisfactory method of expression is by the body mass index (BMI – weight [kg]/height [m²]) which should not exceed 20–23. The most recent studies assess the incidence of obesity in the UK as 8% of men and 12% of women.

CLINICAL SIGNIFICANCE

Mortality

Being fat increases mortality mainly from heart disease and diabetes mellitus.

Morbidity

Carrying excess weight puts strain on lower limb joints, and osteoarthritis of the hips and knees is common. Varicose veins and ulceration are frequent and more persistent in the obese.

Surgical procedures

If an operation is required for other disorders, there are:

- *management problems of associated diseases* – diabetes hypertension and gout
- *general perioperative complications* – myocardial ischaemia, pulmonary infections, deep vein thrombosis and pulmonary embolus
- *anaesthetic problems* – difficulty in intubation and altered metabolism of anaesthetic agents
- *surgical technical difficulties* of access and dissection
- *surgical complications* – wound infection and dehiscence.

Obesity contributes considerably to the risks of operation (Box 23.2).

AETIOLOGY

The great majority of the obese have a greater dietary intake over the years than they need to meet their energy requirements. This is a complex social matter which concerns physicians and others who are asked to advise management. A small minority have specific metabolic disorders (Box 23.3).

MANAGEMENT

All patients should be initially managed non-operatively

> **Box 23.2**
>
> *Surgical complications associated with obesity*
>
> Operative difficulties
>
> Cardiopulmonary complications
>
> Complications associated with general anaesthesia
>
> Wound complications
>
> Thromboembolism
>
> Associated medical complications

> **Box 23.3**
>
> *Causes of obesity*
>
> Excessive dietary intake
>
> Genetic syndromes associated with hypogonadism
>
> Hypothyroidism
>
> Cushing's syndrome
>
> Stein–Leventhal syndrome
>
> Drug-induced (e.g. corticosteroids)
>
> Hypothalamic damage

---

by treating any underlying disorder and by dietary control. However, it is well known that the obese have extreme difficulty in getting rid of their excess fat and, even if they do, frequently relapse. This has led to the involvement of surgeons in a variety of ways. All methods of treatment should be undertaken by a team and only after careful consideration of the motivation of the patient. The risks must be made clear and the possibility of failure explained.

Cosmetic procedures

Apronectomy. A sagging mass of fat and skin on the anterior abdominal wall can be removed by simple excision. The procedure is most useful in restoring self-image in a patient who has successfully lost weight.

Liposuction. Hypertonic saline and hyaluronidase are injected into the fat layer. The walls of adipocytes are broken down and the emulsion of fat which results is removed by suction. The procedure is potentially hazardous and may result in fat embolism, hypo-volaemia (from the osmotic effect of hypertonic saline) and postoperative anaemia.

Neither of these procedures attacks the root cause of the obesity, which is too high an intake.

Methods of reduce intake

Jaw wiring allows the intake of liquids only and often produces rapid weight loss provided access to high-energy drinks is prevented. Relapse is common and the method is now rarely used.

Jejuno-ileal bypass. The proximal jejunum is anastomosed to the distal ileum (10 cm proximal to the ileocaecal valve) so excluding the greater part of the absorptive surface of the small bowel. Weight loss is rapid but the morbidity is high (70%) from the consequences of malabsorption: hypoproteinaemia, hypocalcaemia, metabolic alkalosis and deficiency of trace elements. However, these problems usually improve after 6–12 months.

Gastric plication. A small (20 mL) proximal gastric pouch is constructed so that only a small meal is possible before the patient feels full. Stapling techniques can be used (vertical banded gastroplasty) and a laparoscopic approach is possible. A mean weight loss of 26 kg after a year has been reported and this procedure is currently the one of choice.

Laparoscopic banding. This is a relatively new and less invasive method of banding the stomach to create a small fundal gastric pouch.

24 Large bowel including appendix

The large bowel

STRUCTURE

Macroscopic

The large intestine is a muscular tube approximately 135 cm long extending from the ileocaecal valve to the junction of the rectum and anal canal. It has a greater diameter than the small intestine and is recognised by fatty appendages (appendices epiploicae) and by a sacculated appearance which is the consequence of the three longitudinal strips of smooth muscle (taeniae coli), which are shorter than the colon itself. The **caecum** is in the right iliac fossa and normally does not have a mesentery. The base of the appendix is attached to its posteromedial aspect below the ileocaecal valve. However, the position of the appendix in relation to the caecum is very variable, although the two commonest sites are:

- below and medial, overlying the pelvic brim
- behind the caecum in a recess of peritoneum – the retrocaecal space.

The caecum extends upwards to become the ascending colon, which turns to the left below the right lobe of the liver at the hepatic flexure to pass transversely across the abdomen as a long (~ 50 cm) dependent loop of transverse colon with a mesentery. Its course is in front of the right kidney and second part of the duodenum; the mesocolon is attached to the inferior border of the pancreas and the transverse colon ends at a relatively fixed splenic flexure. Here the bowel turns abruptly downwards as the descending colon in contact with the posterior abdominal wall to reach the brim of the pelvis. Below this point the bowel regains a mesentery and the loop (sigmoid colon) projects forwards into the pelvis before the colon retroperitoneal as the rectum.

Blood supply

Arterial supply is the consequence of the development of the first parts of the colon (caecum to splenic flexure) from the midgut and of the remainder from the hindgut (Fig. 24.1). The proximal arteries are branches of the superior mesenteric artery: the ileocolic, right and middle colic arteries. The descending colon and sigmoid are supplied by branches of the inferior mesenteric

343

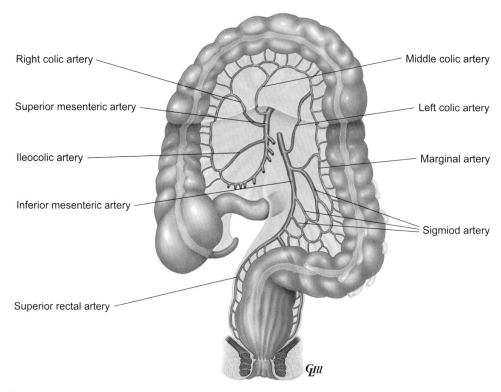

Right colic artery

Superior mesenteric artery

Ileocolic artery

Inferior mesenteric artery

Superior rectal artery

Middle colic artery

Left colic artery

Marginal artery

Sigmiod artery

Fig 24.1 **Blood supply to the colon and rectum.**

artery: left colic and sigmoid arteries. All of the colic vessels form anastomosing loops which extend from the distal ileum to the distal sigmoid and which create a continuous marginal artery about 1 cm from the bowel wall. The arrangement ensures a continued arterial input if local obstruction develops. However, the anastomosis is most tenuous in the region of splenic flexure (see 'Ischaemic colitis'). From the marginal artery, long and short vessels penetrate the bowel wall to supply muscle and mucosa, and their sites of penetration are points of potential weakness (see 'Diverticular disease', below).

Venous drainage corresponds to the arterial input. Blood from the proximal colon enters tributaries of the superior mesenteric vein, which is joined by the splenic vein to form the portal vein. The distal colon drains into tributaries of the inferior mesenteric vein which joins the splenic vein.

PHYSIOLOGY
Extensive or total colectomy is a frequently performed procedure (Box 24.1). Therefore, some understanding of the function of the colon (Box 24.2) is important.

Sodium and water absorption
Normally about 1.5 L of water, 200 mmol of sodium and 100 mmol of chloride pass through the ileocaecal valve every 24 hours. In transit through the colon, 95% of the sodium and water is reabsorbed across the mucosal colonocytes. In exceptional circumstances, water

---

Box 24.1

Indications for colectomy

Neoplasms of the colon

Diverticular disease

Ulcerative colitis

Crohn's disease

Volvulus

Slow-transit constipation

Ischaemia

Portasystemic encephalopathy

Box 24.2

Functions of the colon

Water absorption

Salt absorption

Bacterial metabolism and fermentation

Storage and evacuation of faeces

absorption can be increased three to four times and this ability can be used for rehydration when other routes, such as the intravenous one, are not available.

Sodium can diffuse down a chemical gradient; however, it is usually transported from the colon lumen across the colonocyte into the plasma by two energy-dependent mechanisms:

- sodium/potassium exchange in the cell membrane
- sodium/proton exchange at the luminal surface.

Chloride absorption is down an electrical gradient and by exchange for bicarbonate.

Water moves from the lumen into the cell because the latter is at a higher osmotic pressure, due to the active transport of solutes, principally sodium, chloride and short-chain fatty acids (see below).

Bacterial metabolism and fermentation

The colon contains 99% of the organisms in the gastrointestinal tract and more than 400 different types have been identified. Bacteria make up approximately 80% of the weight of normal faeces.

Bacteria in the colon are of surgical importance because:

- they cause fermentation (anaerobic release of energy) by breakdown of carbohydrates to produce short-chain fatty acids (SCFAs)
- they are the source of potentially lethal complications if the mucosal barrier is damaged.

Short-chain fatty acids are mainly the consequence of the action of bacteria on a substrate which is loosely called dietary fibre and which is composed mainly of complex polypeptides such as lecithin (a lipid), cellulose and hemicellulose. An increase in dietary fibre causes increased colonic motility and more rapid transit, partly because of the water-absorbing properties of fibre, but mostly because of increased bacterial activity and fermentation. SCFAs are reabsorbed and form part of the body's energy cycle. A by-product of these chemical reactions is gas (flatus), a mixture of carbon dioxide, hydrogen and methane with varying amounts of other gases, such as hydrogen sulphide, depending on the substrate.

Storage and evacuation of faeces

The content changes in consistency as it traverses the large bowel, from liquid in the right colon to a firm semi-solid stool on the left. The transit time between the caecum and evacuation via the rectum is very variable but is normally about 36 hours (slightly more in the female). Faeces are propelled by a combination of mass peristalsis and segmental contractions. Factors which influence colonic motility are:

- the fibre content of the diet
- amount of fluid in the colon
- contact laxatives such as bisacodyl

- hormones, e.g. cholecystokinin
- psychological factors such as stress
- food in the stomach, which can initiate a reflex colonic contraction (gastrocolic reflex).

Colonic motility is also subject to the circadian rhythm in that resting tone is considerably reduced at night.

Functional disorders

Constipation

This condition is defined as either excessive straining at stool or the passage of two or fewer stools in a week. It is a common complaint; prescriptions for laxatives in the UK cost the NHS about £15 million a year. The common causes are listed in Box 24.3. The commonest of these is inadequate dietary fibre, and the most important, which must be eliminated, is malignant disease of the left colon. When constipation occurs shortly after birth but with only minor or transient features of intestinal obstruction, Hirschsprung's disease should be considered. Very occasionally, the disease presents for the first time in adult life.

Slow transit constipation. A small number of patients, usually female, have chronic constipation which does not respond to increase of dietary fibre or laxatives; there is no structural abnormality but transit time is slow. The patient's complaint may be sufficiently severe to require treatment by total colectomy and anastomosis of the ileum to the rectum, but the results are not always satisfactory.

Box 24.3

Causes of constipation

Inadequate dietary fibre

Neoplasms of the colon, rectum and anus

Benign lesions of the anus

Endocrine disease, e.g. myxoedema

Drugs, e.g. codeine phosphate

Hirschsprung's disease

Slow-transit constipation

Psychological and behavioural abnormalities

Neurological causes
  Cerebral, e.g. stroke
  Spinal, e.g. multiple sclerosis, paraplegia, neoplasm

Inflammatory disease

Inflammation of the large bowel is known as colitis, and inflammation of the rectum and anus is known as proctitis. Boxes 24.4 and 24.5 list the non-bacterial and infective causes of colitis and proctitis, respectively.

Ulcerative colitis

EPIDEMIOLOGY AND AETIOLOGY
This condition is common in Scandinavia, the UK and North America. There is a higher incidence in rural dwellers and in those who smoke. Females are more commonly affected than males and the condition is prevalent in late adolescence and early adult life.

The cause is not known but the following may be involved.

Genetics
There is a higher familial incidence of ulcerative colitis than would be expected by chance. However, no clear genetic pattern of expression has been identified.

Transmissible agents
The histological and clinical features of the disease have some things in common with those that occur in acute bacterial infections of the colon, but in spite of intensive microbial investigation a specific organism has not been identified.

Diet
The prevalence of the disease in countries in which the diet is low in fibre and contains additives suggests that the use of highly milled flour and certain additives (e.g. carrageen) may be factors. A small number of patients with ulcerative colitis are made symptomatically worse by taking milk protein, which is the consequence of mucosal hypolactasia.

Psychodynamics
Introversion and depression are commonly seen and the symptoms are often made worse by psychological stress. However, it is probable that these matters are secondary rather than causative.

Immunology
The failure to find any infective agent has led to the suggestion that the destructive inflammation of the colonic mucosa is autoimmune, similar to that found in, for example, thyroiditis. However, markers of auto-immune disease such as antinuclear factor are no more common in these patients than in the normal population.

PATHOLOGICAL FEATURES
The major feature is inflammation of the mucosa with increased vascularity and haemorrhage. In spite of the name of the disease, macroscopic ulceration is not common except in very severe and advanced disease. The changes are usually most marked in the rectum (proctitis) and spread for a varying degree proximally into the colon. Rarely, the entire large bowel is involved but the disease does not extend proximal to the ileo-caecal valve. Box 24.6. lists the histological features; the most diagnostic of these is the crypt abscess (Fig. 24.2). Dysplastic change is thought to be a marker for the risk of malignant change (see below).

Box 24.4

Causes of colitis/proctitis

Ulcerative colitis

Crohn's disease

Ischaemic colitis

Infective colitis

Irradiation colitis

Box 24.5

Infective causes of colitis/proctitis

Bacterial
  Salmonella
  Shigella
  Mycobacterium tuberculosis
  Staphylococcus
  Gonococcus
  Campylobacter
  Clostridium difficile

Viral
  Enteroviruses
  Cytomegaloviruses
  Herpes

Spirochaetal
  Treponema pallidum

Chlamydial
  Lymphogranuloma pallidum

Protozoal
  Entamoeba histolytica

Metazoal
  Schistosoma mansoni

Mycotic
  Histoplasma capsulatum

- toxaemia
- anaemia from bleeding
- acute loss of water and electrolyte
- progressive abdominal distension.

The last of these may lead to perforation of the colon with general peritonitis, which carries a high mortality and gives the complication its sinister reputation.

Treatment is with blood transfusion, water and electrolyte replacement and parenteral steroid therapy. Intensive monitoring of both the systemic condition and the degree of colonic dilatation (by serial plain X-ray and measurement of the diameter of the caecum or ascending colon) is required to detect deterioration or the likelihood of perforation. In either event, urgent removal of the colon – usually leaving the rectum intact – and a diverting ileostomy may be required. Once the patient has recovered, further surgery may be considered as discussed below.

Massive haemorrhage
This is rare and usually responds to transfusion and intensive treatment of the disease.

Carcinoma
Adenocarcinoma develops as a result of dysplastic change in long-standing colitis. The risk is very small in those who have had the disease for less than 10 years. Thereafter, it increases in those who have *total colitis*, so that by 20 years it approaches 20%. The hazard is much less in patients with limited disease. The presence of a cancer is an absolute indication for surgery.

Complications other than in the gastrointestinal tract
Systemic complications (Box 24.7) are uncommon and are usually an indication of the severity of the colitis. If

---

Box 24.6

Histological features of ulcerative colitis

Lymphocyte and neutrophil infiltration of lamina propria

Crypt abscess formation

Goblet cell depletion

Destruction of surface epithelium (ulceration)

Mucosal oedema

Dysplasia

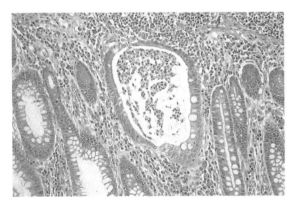

Fig 24.2 **Histological appearance of a crypt abscess in ulcerative colitis.**

CLINICAL FEATURES
Symptoms
The most characteristic symptom is bloody diarrhoea with associated social embarrassment and discomfort. There are periods of remission followed by acute relapse. Disease confined to the rectum is usually mild and without systemic effects. More extensive colonic involvement leads to ill health, weight loss, symptoms of anaemia and complaints of abdominal pain.

Physical findings
In mild disease, physical signs are few or absent. Those with a more severe or extensive condition look ill, show signs of weight loss, anaemia and dehydration. Abdominal examination may show colonic distension and tenderness.

COMPLICATIONS
Toxic megacolon (acute dilatation)
Severe inflammation may cause the colon (particularly the transverse part) to dilate. There is severe acute systemic disturbance with:

Box 24.7

Non-gastrointestinal complications of ulcerative colitis

Skin disorders, e.g. erythema nodosum, pyoderma gangrenosum

Eye disorders, e.g. iritis, episcleritis

Arthritis, e.g. ankylosing spondylitis, peripheral rheumatoid-type arthritis

Liver disorders, e.g. chronic active hepatitis, sclerosing cholangitis

Renal disorders, e.g. ureteric calculi following ileostomy, secondary amyloidosis, glomerulonephritis this is successfully treated, such conditions usually resolve. An exception is urinary calculus after removal of the colon and ileostomy. It is thought that this is partly the result of increased water loss via the ileostomy which leads to a more concentrated urine. However, disorders of oxalate metabolism may also be involved.

INVESTIGATION

All patients suspected of having ulcerative colitis should have a sigmoidoscopy and biopsy of the rectal mucosa. If there is the possibility of an infective cause for the symptoms, stool cultures are carried out. Except in the mildest cases, in which the proximal limit of the disease can be seen at sigmoidoscopy, a barium enema (Fig. 24.3) and a colonoscopy are necessary to determine the extent. The latter, accompanied by multiple biopsies, is the most precise method and may also reveal an unsuspected carcinoma.

MANAGEMENT

Medical

The majority of patients have minimal disease which can be adequately managed by a combination of prednisolone suppositories and oral salazopyrin. The first produces remission of symptoms and active disease, while the second reduces the risk of recurrence. Little steroid is absorbed from suppositories and the complications commonly associated with this class of

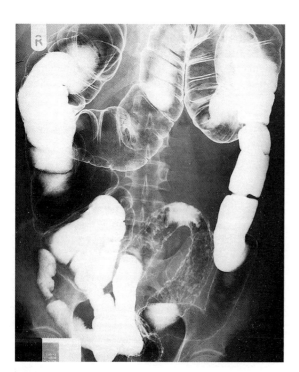

Fig 24.3 **Barium enema in a patient with ulcerative colitis.**

Box 24.8

Indications for surgery in ulcerative colitis

Severe exacerbations of colitis

Severe exacerbations of non-gastrointestinal manifestations

Toxic colon/acute dilatation

Chronic colitis refractory to medical treatment

Development of premalignant changes (dysplasia) in colon/rectum

Development of carcinoma of colon/rectum

---

agent are minimised. More extensive disease with incapacitating symptoms may require admission to hospital and systemic steroid therapy.

Surgical

Objective. Apart from special circumstances when a temporary diversion of the faecal stream by ileostomy alone is done, the objective of surgery is to remove all or nearly all diseased large bowel. The indications for surgery are given in Box 24.8.

Preoperative preparation. When there is time, electrolyte balance, toxaemia and anaemia are corrected. Mechanical preparation of the bowel is contraindicated because of the risk of perforation. Perioperative antibiotic prophylaxis is essential (Ch. 9). If either a temporary or a permanent stoma is contemplated (which is common – see below), a specialist in stoma care as well as the surgeon should discuss the matter with the patient.

OPERATIVE PROCEDURES

Proctocolectomy with permanent ileostomy

This is the standard procedure (Fig. 24.4): all diseased or potentially diseased bowel is removed and the patient is rapidly restored to full health. However, the permanent stoma requires an appliance to be worn and can have physical complications (Box 24.9), although these can usually be avoided.

Patients usually adapt well to the alteration of body image inevitably produced, but their occasional difficulty in doing so and a natural distaste for a stoma in both themselves and their surgeons has led to the development of other techniques.

Ileorectal anastomosis after colectomy

In some patients, the rectal disease may not be severe or may resolve after colectomy and temporary diverting ileostomy; ileorectal anastomosis (Fig. 24.5) may then

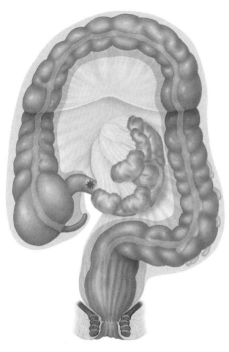

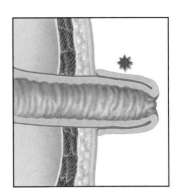

Fig 24.4 **Operation of proctocolectomy and ileostomy.**

produce a good functional result. However, there is risk of subsequent carcinoma in the rectum and inflammation may recur. Constant surveillance is necessary.

Continent ileostomy

The objective is to improve the cosmetic appearance of the stoma by avoiding a spout and to do away with the need for an appliance to be worn continuously.

The technique is to fold the distal ileum on itself to form a pouch with a valve at its end (Fig. 24.6). The pouch is emptied at the patient's convenience with a tube. The procedure is complex and has had a high incidence of complications and failure of continence.

Ileal pouch and ileo-anal anastomosis

The objective is the same as for continent ileostomy.

The technique is to form a similar pouch but to anastomose it to the anal verge after all large bowel mucosa has been removed (Fig. 24.7). Patients may either defaecate normally (although usually fairly frequently) or empty the pouch by per-anal tube. The operation is technically complex but is a major advance over proctocolectomy and permanent ileostomy.

Crohn's disease of the colon

The condition characteristically affects the small intestine (for more detailed treatment, see Ch. 23) but may involve the large bowel either in isolation or in combination with small intestinal disease.

CLINICAL FEATURES

Symptoms

The diarrhoea and other complaints are often indistinguishable from ulcerative colitis and the systemic upset is the same. There may be associated complaints of perianal problems such as fissure and fistula (Ch. 25).

Clinical findings

The abdominal findings are not specific. There is a high incidence of anal lesions such as

- fistula
- perianal abscess
- chronic fissure

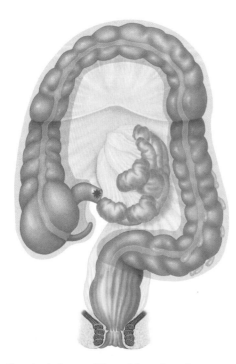

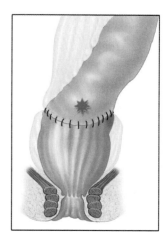

Fig 24.5 **Operation of colectomy and ileorectal anastomosis.**

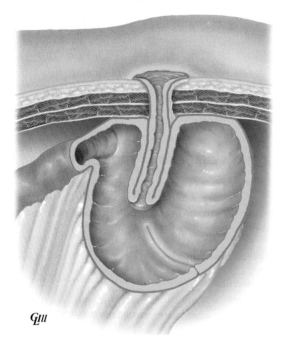

*GJ*II

Fig 24.6 **The continent ileostomy.**

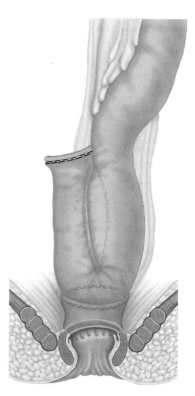

Fig 24.7 **Ileal pouch with ileo-anal anastomosis.**

- anal ulceration
- Oedematous skin tags.

INVESTIGATION

Sigmoidoscopy may not distinguish the disease from ulcerative colitis. Characteristic histopathological features may be found on biopsy. Barium enema (Fig. 24.8) shows segmental and discontinuous involvement of the large bowel and the presence of fissures

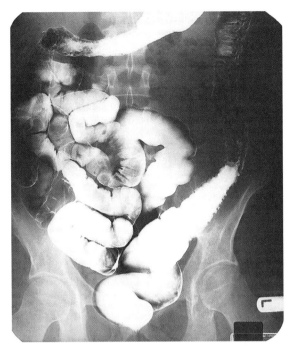

Fig 24.8 **Barium enema in a patient with Crohn's disease of the large bowel.** Note deep ulcers and sparing of rectum.

and fistulae in the bowel wall. Strictures are not uncommon.

MANAGEMENT

The medical treatment is similar to that for ulcerative colitis. Colectomy may be required for severe or intractable disease. The management of the disease in the small bowel, and particularly of obstruction, is given on in Chapter 23..

Ischaemic colitis

This condition is uncommon in those under the age of 50. The frequent occurrence at the splenic flexure, where the anastomotic loops are least well developed, suggests that the cause is reduced arterial input, perhaps from the development of degenerative arterial disease.

CLINICAL FEATURES

Symptoms are:

- acute left-sided abdominal pain
- dark red rectal bleeding.

  Clinical findings are:

- fever
- hypotension
- abdominal tenderness.

INVESTIGATION AND MANAGEMENT

A plain abdominal X-ray may show a distended splenic

flexure in which oedematous mucosa may be detected. This finding is confirmed by barium enema where the thumbprinting of the contrast medium by the mucosa is apparent.

Spontaneous resolution is the rule. Occasionally progression leads to gangrene for which emergency surgery is required. Intermediate between these is ischaemia that leads to late stricture for which surgery is needed.

Infective diseases

There are a wide variety of organisms capable of causing colitis (see Box 24.5) They are of surgical importance only because of the need to detect treatable infective agents in patients who may at first sight seem to have ulcerative colitis or Crohn's disease.

Diverticular disease

Diverticular disease is very rarely congenital in which case the walls of the diverticulae contain all layers of the normal colon. Much more commonly it is acquired and the diverticulae are serosa-covered outpouchings of mucosa alone through gaps in the muscularis which transmit the terminal blood vessels. The diverticulae are usually found in the left colon, especially the sigmoid, but quite frequently involve the entire colon.

EPIDEMIOLOGY AND AETIOLOGY

Acquired diverticular disease is very rare under the age of 35 after which there is a progressive increase in incidence, so that 50% of those in the eigth or ninth decade are affected though not necessarily symptomatic. The condition is common in Western countries but rare in China, India and Africa.

The most popular explanation of the cause is that a low-fibre diet is associated with increased intraluminal pressure which leads to pulsion herniation of mucosa alongside blood vessels. There is some physiological evidence to support this and the treatment of symptoms with a high-fibre diet is often successful. However, not all patients with diverticular disease consume a diet low in fibre and some Japanese have a particular form of the disorder exclusively in the right colon, a phenomenon which cannot be explained by the low-fibre theory.

PATHOLOGICAL FEATURES

The anatomical features are given above. Diverticulae have a narrow neck and inspissated faeces may accumulate within them. Inflammation may follow with a number of outcomes:

- persistent inflammation in a segment of bowel wall
- local inflammation of the affected diverticulum leading to perforation.

Perforation may in turn be:

- local into the pericolic tissues
- into the peritoneal cavity with generalised peritonitis
- into an adjacent organ such as the bladder with the formation of a fistula.

CLINICAL FEATURES

Symptoms

These are frequently absent and the diagnosis is made following a barium enema done for other reasons, chiefly to exclude a large bowel carcinoma.

There may be mild left lower abdominal pain which accompanies a long-standing irregularity of bowel habit with episodic slight diarrhoea or more usually constipation with the passage of small quantities of hard faecal pellets.

Signs

In uncomplicated disease, signs are absent or minimal. There is occasionally tenderness over the descending colon and this portion of the bowel may be palpable.

INVESTIGATION

Barium enema is the usual method of confirming the diagnosis (Fig. 24.9), but it should be deferred in patients with complications (see below). The diverticular openings may also be seen at colonoscopy. Diverticular disease is notorious for its ability, at barium enema examination, to conceal a coexistent carcinoma. It is possible to resolve doubt by a full colonoscopy.

MANAGEMENT

There is no evidence that increasing the amount of dietary fibre prevents the development of diverticulae. However, in the presence of mild symptoms (such as pain) attributed to their presence, the use of added fibre or other bulking agents (e.g. ispaghula) has been conclusively shown to be of benefit. If pain is severe or unresponsive, resection of the affected segment (usually the sigmoid) may be considered.

COMPLICATIONS

Inflammation

Involvement of a segment of the bowel wall may cause severe abdominal pain, pyrexia and tenderness over the affected segment. Progression to local perforation may take place, with a collection of inflammatory tissue and eventually pus around the sigmoid colon – a pericolic abscess. Its presence is indicated by a mass. Confirmation can be obtained by ultrasound examination or a CT scan. Although an early inflammatory process may settle with restricting oral intake and antibiotic therapy, a pericolic abscess must be drained.

It is thought that this is the result of a process similar to that of gangrenous appendicitis – a faecolith impacts in the mouth of the diverticulum and the blood supply is obstructed. The diverticulum becomes gangrenous and ruptures into an unprotected peritoneal cavity. The following features will be seen:

- generalised abdominal pain often accompanied by pain in the tip of the shoulder from the extensive pneumoperitoneum
- evidence of severe sepsis – fever and circulatory collapse
- abdominal tenderness and rigidity.

This complication is a surgical emergency, and laparotomy and surgical management of the site of perforation are essential.

Fistulation

The clinical features depend on the structures involved. A blind track into the pericolic tissues may only be found on barium enema. A bladder fistula is characterised by complaints of pneumaturia and recurrent bladder infection, and a fistula into the vagina is characterised by the passage of gas and faecal content per vaginam. Surgical treatment is required in both cases.

Haemorrhage

A degree of iron deficiency anaemia may be found in symptomatically mild diverticular disease but its cause is uncertain. Correction is by iron supplement. Much

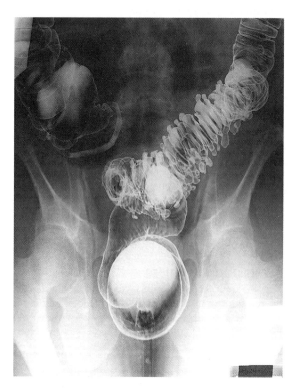

Fig 24.9 **Barium enema in a patient with diverticular disease.**

rarer is massive haemorrhage, which is thought to be the consequence of the erosion of a vessel in the neck of a diverticulum. Rapid exsanguination may be life-threatening in elderly patients. Diagnosis may be difficult not only because bleeding from vascular malformations (angiodysplasia) can occur in the elderly at any site in the large bowel, but also because haemorrhage from a diverticulum may be difficult to localise in patients with anatomically extensive disease. Selective angiography of the large bowel arteries is usually required, after which the treatment can be radiological or surgical.

Volvulus of the Large Bowel

See Chapter 23.

Neoplasia

Benign neoplasms

Adenomas

AETIOLOGY AND EPIDEMIOLOGY
Benign large bowel neoplasms are associated with a number of different conditions, many of which have a genetic component (see, for example, familial adenomatosis polyposis below). However, little is known about the proximate factors which cause the development of the lesions. Up to 10% of the Western world's population may have tumours, but elsewhere the condition is much more rare.

PATHOLOGICAL FEATURES
The most common and important neoplasm is an adenoma which arises from the glandular or epithelial cells. The tumour is most often a polyp with a stalk, but flat (sessile) lesions also occur. The histological appearance is a basis for classification into tubular, villous or tubulovillous (Fig. 24.10). Tubular polyps tend to be pedunculated and spherical; the other two types are more often multifronded and sessile. They may be single or multiple and in some hereditary syndromes many hundreds or thousands are present. The important clinicopathological correlate of an adenoma is that it is a premalignant lesion and exposure of its surface over the years to the faecal stream may initiate the development of an adenocarcinoma. This polyp–cancer sequence is most likely in lesions over 1 cm in diameter. Not all polyps are adenomas. The other causes of protrusions of mucosa that are anatomically polyps are given in Box 24.10.

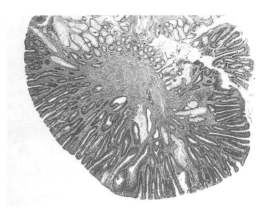

Fig 24.10 **Histological appearance of a tubular adenoma of the colon.**

Box 24.10

Classification of colorectal polyps

Neoplastic

Adenoma
   Tubular
   Tubulovillous
   Villous

Non-neoplastic

Hamartoma
   Juvenile
   Peutz–Jeghers

Inflammatory
   Lymphoid
   Inflammatory

Miscellaneous
   Metaplastic
   Connective tissue polyps

CLINICAL FEATURES AND DIAGNOSIS
Most adenomas are both asymptomatic and devoid of signs. Unless there is a family history or there are so many lesions that bleeding is obvious, the diagnosis is made either as the result of a screening programme or on incidental examination of the large bowel by colonoscopy or barium enema for unexplained iron deficiency anaemia or other symptoms.

A rare clinical syndrome is when a villous adenoma in the rectum is sufficiently large that large quantities of potassium-rich mucus are lost from it and the patient becomes hypokalaemic.

MANAGEMENT
The finding of an adenomatous polyp, particularly if it is larger than 1 cm, requires the following action:

1. Complete examination of the large bowel by colonoscopy to exclude or identify other similar neoplasms
2. Removal of all lesions, which can usually be achieved endoscopically
3. Regular lifelong surveillance for recurrence and/or the development of large bowel cancer.

Familial adenomatous polyposis

This is an autosomal dominant condition with a high degree of penetrance.

PATHOLOGICAL FEATURES
Multiple adenomatous polyps develop in the colon usually between the ages of 13 and 30 years, although sometimes this does not take place until the fourth decade. Progression through the polyp–cancer sequence is inevitable. Not infrequently, there are other manifestations outwith the colon.

CLINICAL FEATURES
The condition is initially asymptomatic, although a family history may be present. Blood from the rectum is the most common symptom and there may be other less specific complaints such as tenesmus and diarrhoea.

DIAGNOSIS AND MANAGEMENT
As in polyps, the diagnosis is made by endoscopy. Siblings should be examined.

Total colectomy is essential because of the universal progression to cancer. An ileoanal reconstruction is usually possible.

Malignant neoplasms

EPIDEMIOLOGY AND AETIOLOGY
Malignant tumours of the large bowel are common in the UK and second only to carcinoma of the bronchus as a cause of death. The highest incidence of adenocarcinoma, which accounts for 98% of the tumours, occurs in New Zealand, Australia, Western Europe and North America. The lowest is in Asia, Africa and South America, although Argentina is an exception. The disease can develop at any age from the second decade but the peak incidence is in the sixth and subsequent decades. The important aetiological factors are described below.

Dietary factors
Bile salt conversion. There is indirect evidence that a diet rich in animal fat is a major risk factor. It is suggested that such a diet, common in the Western world, produces an environment within the gut which favours bacteria that convert bile salts to carcino-

gens, and work on experimental animals supports this hypothesis.

Low intake of fibre has also been claimed to predispose to neoplasia because it slows transit and thus increases the time of exposure of the mucosa to carcinogens.

Adenomatous polyps
The polyp–cancer sequence is considered above. It probably accounts for the development of the great majority of large bowel cancers, a matter which emphasises the importance of screening.

Genetic factors
Familial adenomatous polyposis (FAP) as an inevitable cause of cancer is considered in Chapter 12. However, apart from this, there is a two to three times increased risk to a first-degree relative of a patient with adenocarcinoma and this hereditary non-polyposis colon cancer (HNPCC) probably accounts for about 10% of colon malignancies.

Inflammatory bowel disease
Long-standing and total ulcerative colitis as a cause is described above. Crohn's disease is also associated with a fourfold increase in the risk of colorectal carcinoma.

PATHOLOGICAL FEATURES

Distribution
The anatomical distribution is shown in Figure 24.11.

Synchronous lesions
Up to 3% of patients have one or more synchronous cancers and 75% have a benign adenoma.

Macroscopic classification
Tumours are classified as follows:

- polypoid
- ulcerative
- annular
- a combination of the above.

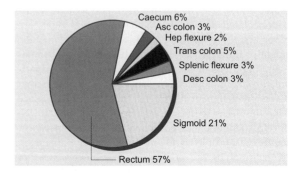

Fig 24.11 **Anatomical distribution of colonic carcinoma.**

Spread

Direct extension in the transverse axis of the bowel wall eventually causes complete encirclement. Tumour cells which arise in the mucosa penetrate the submucosa and muscle to reach the serosal surface of the bowel, or, where the bowel is extraperitoneal, as in the rectum, they spread into the fascia and the structures contained in it such as the sacral plexus (posteriorly), the ureters (laterally), and the bladder in the male or the uterus and cervix in the female (anteriorly).

Lymphatic permeation and embolisation carry tumour cells initially to local (paracolic) nodes and from there to nodes which lie on the course of the blood supply to the bowel. In consequence, spread is largely upwards towards the aorta and the portal vein.

Haematogenous. Malignant cells can often be seen within the lumen of capillaries and small veins in sections taken from colorectal tumours. They are probably the source of emboli which enter the tributaries of the portal vein and so reach the liver which may be involved at the time of treatment in up to 40% of cases. Spread beyond the liver to lung, kidney and bone is rare.

Transcoelomic implantation follows penetration to the serosal surface and causes ascites. Cells may also be implanted on the ovaries.

Direct implantation. Exfoliated cells remain viable within the lumen of the bowel and may be implanted if the mucosa is breached – as at the site of an ana-stomosis or in a haemorrhoidectomy wound if that procedure is carried out in a patient with an unsuspected proximal carcinoma.

Staging

The conventional method of staging is by Duke's classification (Fig. 24.12):

- *Stage A* – the neoplastic cells are confined to the mucosa. The 5-year survival is 90%.
- *Stage B* – the tumour has extended through all muscle layers and possibly reached the serosa; metastases to lymph nodes are absent. The 5-year survival is 60%.
- *Stage C* – as for stage B but with lymph node metastases. The 5-year survival is 30%. Stage C cases are often divided into C1 (local lymph node involvement only) and C2 (more proximal nodes involved). C2 carries a worse prognosis than C1.
- *Stage D* – this was not part of the original classification but is often used to describe a patient with disseminated metastatic disease.

SCREENING FOR COLORECTAL CANCER

The good results obtained in Duke's stage A cancer and the known polyp–cancer sequence have encouraged the idea that attempts should be made to detect asymptomatic polyps and early cancers. Two strategies are being explored:

- Surveillance of patients with known increased risk such as individuals with first-degree relatives who have had polyps or cancers. These high-risk subjects can be investigated by repeated routine colonoscopy.
- Faecal occult blood examination in patients over an agreed age – usually 50 years; those found positive are examined by colonoscopy.

These policies are still provisional but seem likely to result in the detection of a greater number of stage A tumours and the elimination of some polyps that would go on to malignant change.

CLINICAL FEATURES

Symptoms

The most important of these are listed in Box 24.11. A distinction can be drawn between the presentation

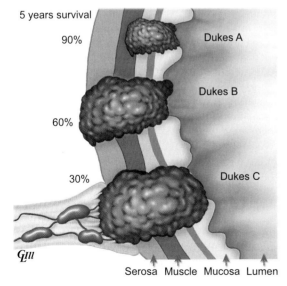

Fig 24.12 **Duke's staging of colonic carcinoma**

(5 years survival — 90% Dukes A, 60% Dukes B, 30% Dukes C — Serosa Muscle Mucosa Lumen)

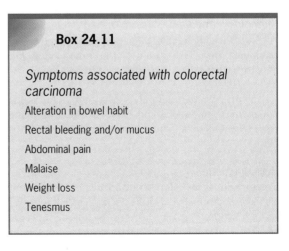

Box 24.11

Symptoms associated with colorectal carcinoma

Alteration in bowel habit

Rectal bleeding and/or mucus

Abdominal pain

Malaise

Weight loss

Tenesmus

of tumours in the right side, the left side and the rectum.

Right-sided tumours have non-specific complaints such as malaise, weight loss, vague abdominal pain and occasionally a self-detected mass in the abdomen. A frequent reason for the patient seeking medical advice is the development of symptoms of iron deficiency anaemia: any patient who does so and in whom the cause is not obvious should undergo full investigation of the large bowel at once. The liquid nature of the contents of the right side make presentation with intestinal obstruction rare.

Left-sided tumours are more likely to present with obstructive symptoms, because the stool is semi-solid or completely solid and the calibre of the bowel is less. There is colicky abdominal pain and a change in bowel habit which may include either constipation or diarrhoea, or alternation between the two. A distal tumour may lead to the passage of mucus which is confused with a loose motion. Visible blood in the stool is rare (10%). Acute intestinal obstruction may supervene.

Rectal tumours are more likely to be associated with rectal bleeding, usually on defaecation, and mucous discharge is common as is tenesmus.

A growth that has spread locally may cause:

- faecal incontinence from invasion of the anal sphincters
- back pain because of involvement of the sacral plexus
- urinary infection, a rectovesical fistula or renal failure through infiltration of the renal tract.

Physical findings

These are often absent. A mass may be palpable in the abdomen or on rectal examination. In advanced disease, weight loss may be obvious, there may be evidence of spread (ascites and hepatomegaly), and signs of bowel obstruction may be present.

INVESTIGATION

Sigmoidoscopy

All patients with symptoms that suggest a large bowel carcinoma must have a digital rectal examination and at least a sigmoidoscopy. Any mucosal abnormality is biopsied.

The investigation can only see, at best, as far as the mid-sigmoid colon (, 25 cm). Full visualisation of the large bowel requires barium enema or colonoscopy, or both.

Barium enema

Unless facilities for colonoscopy are available, a barium enema is done on all patients with suspected large bowel cancer (Fig. 24.13). Even if there is a clinically obvious rectal tumour, radiography and/or colonoscopy should

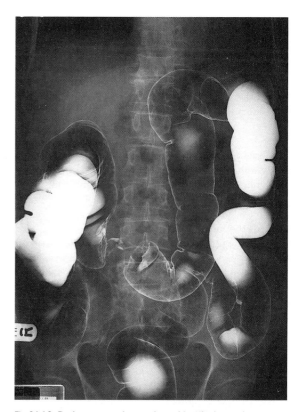

Fig 24.13 **Barium enema in a patient with colonic carcinoma.**

be considered to exclude a synchronous neoplasm and polyps.

Colonoscopy

Direct visualisation of the entire colon is the investigation of choice but the procedure is expensive in time and resources and can be technically difficult. It is gradually becoming more available although it may have to be reserved for special circumstances such as when radiology is unsuccessful.

Assessment of extent of disease and of spread

Carcinoembryonic antigen (CEA) does not play a part in selecting treatment but can be a useful marker of the elimination of disease and the emergence of recurrence. Therefore a pretreatment measurement is desirable. A preoperative CT Scan is desirable.

MANAGEMENT

Colon carcinoma

The treatment of Duke's A to C disease is primarily by surgical removal and this is accompanied in B and C tumours by adjuvant therapy. Right-sided tumours are removed by a right hemicolectomy and those on the left by a resection tailored to the segment of bowel involved (Fig. 24.14). The preoperative preparation and

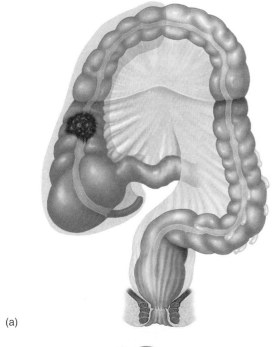

(a)

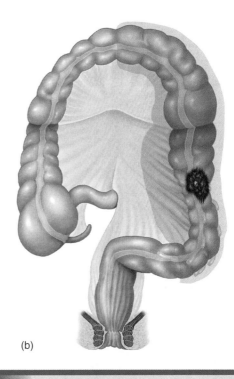

(b)

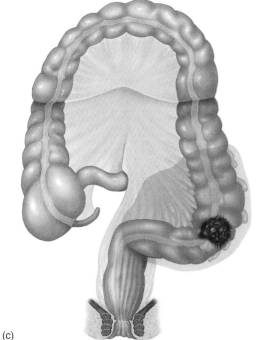

(c)

Fig 24.14 **Colectomy**. (Shaded areas resected).

the common complications of surgery are given in Boxes 24.12 and 24.13.

Rectal carcinoma

A tumour in the mid- or upper rectum is removed by resecting the distal colon and involved rectum and

---

> ## Box 24.12
>
> *Preoperative preparation for colectomy*
>
> Mechanical bowel preparation
>   Oral laxative
>   Whole gut irrigation
>   Enema/colonic irrigation
>
> Antibiotic chemoprophylaxis
>
> Thromboembolism prophylaxis
>
> Correct anaemia
>
> Correct electrolyte deficiencies

restoring continuity by joining the large bowel to the stump of rectum – anterior resection (Fig. 24.15a). The anastomosis may be done with either sutures or staples and the latter are particularly useful when the rectal stump is short and access difficult. A low rectal tumour requires the removal of the whole rectum and adjacent sphincters – abdominoperineal resection and end colostomy (Fig. 24.15b) – an operation usually carried out by two surgeons, one working within the abdomen and the other from the perineum.

Adjuvant therapy

Radiation

There is increasing evidence that patients with Duke's

Box 24.13

Complications of colectomy and rectal excision

Haemorrhage

Ureteric damage
    Urinary leakage
    Ureteric stricture

Damage to bladder function
    Acute retention
    Urinary incontinence

Damage to sexual function

Damage to duodenum (right hemicolectomy)

Damage to spleen (left hemicolectomy)

Anastomotic complications
    Stenosis
    Leakage

Complications of stoma
    Parastomal hernia
    Prolapse
    Electrolyte imbalance
    Ischaemia
    Stenosis

Diarrhoea/constipation

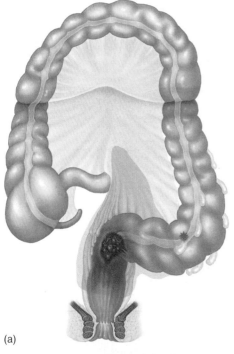

(a)

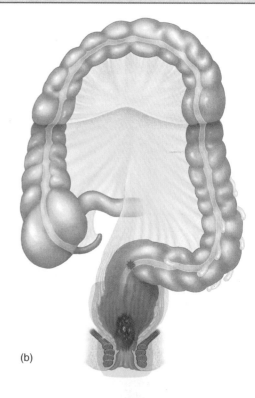

(b)

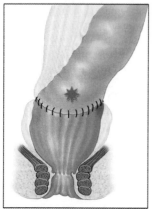

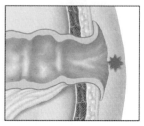

Fig 24.15 **Surgical management of rectal carcinoma.**
(**a**) Anterior resection of the rectum. (Shaded area resected).
(**b**) Abdominoperineal excision of the rectum and anus (shaded area resected).

B and C rectal carcinoma should receive local deep X-ray therapy.

Chemotherapy

Although solid tumours such as colorectal cancers are not very sensitive to chemotherapy there is evidence from clinical trials that results can be improved in Duke's stage B and C by the use of chemotherapy with 5-fluouracil either alone or in combination with other agents. Protocols are still being developed.

Advanced disease

Local disease and recurrence

When the local disease, particularly in the pelvis, cannot be removed and is causing substantial symptoms, radiotherapy and chemotherapy may be used, although the latter is more effective. Some recurrences (e.g. at a suture line) may be resectable, but this is uncommon.

Hepatic metastases

Some deposits in the liver are solitary and can be removed by surgery. A more radical approach is now used and has resulted in some improvement in survival. More diffuse hepatic secondaries are treated palliatively by chemotherapy.

Rectal bleeding

Rectal bleeding is a common symptom (Box 24.14). Usually the bleeding is of a minor nature and can be investigated on an elective basis. Rarely, bleeding is of a profuse nature requiring urgent investigation and treatment and occasionally urgent surgical intervention. In the younger patient, rectal bleeding is usually of benign origin (e.g. haemorrhoids) and can be effectively managed by non-surgical methods (see Ch. 25). In the older patient, malignancy must always be excluded. Where the patient presents with acute rectal bleeding, it may be appropriate to exclude upper gastrointestinal causes in the first instance (see Ch. 22). Once these have been excluded, the lower gastrointestinal tract needs to be investigated by urgent colonoscopy supplemented by arteriography. In the older patient, acute bleeding is likely to be the consequence of either diverticular disease or an aterio-venous malformation. Sometimes no cause can be identified for the haemorrhage and a 'blind' colectomy has to be performed by the surgeon.

Box 24.14

Causes of rectal bleeding

Haemorrhoids

Diverticular disease

Colorectal cancer

Colorectal polyps

Anteriovenous malformations

Ischaemia

Trauma

Colitis

Solitary rectal ulcer

Anal conditions
  Fissure
  Fistula
  Thrombosis
  Squamous carcinoma
  Warts

The Appendix

ANATOMY

The appendix is a blind ending tube varying from 2 to 20 cm in length (average approx. 9 cm) which arises from the posteromedial wall of the caecum and whose anatomical position in the pelvis may vary considerably:

- behind the caecum (retrocaecal) – 65%
- projects downwards into the pelvis (pelvic) – 31%
- immediately below the caecum (subcaecal) – 2%
- in front of the terminal ileum (pre-ileal) – 1%
- behind the ileum (post-ileal) – 0.4%.

The main artery is the appendicular artery which is a branch of the ileocolic that runs behind the terminal ileum to reach the base of the appendix and extend to its tip via the mesoappendix.

HISTOLOGY

The mucosa is similar to that of the colon in that it is of columnar type with crypts containing numerous mucus secreting glands. The distinguishing feature is the presence of extensive lymphoid tissue in the lamina propria which contains plasma cells, lymphocytes, eosinophils and macrophages embedded in a fibrocellular reticulum. In addition in this layer congregations of lymphocytes are seen so forming lymphoid follicles. The outer layers of the appendix are formed from the inner (circular) and outer (longitudinal) layers of smooth muscle which are continuous from the caecum and these in turn are covered by a complete serosal layer.

FUNCTION

In herbivores, the appendix and the caecum are highly

developed and are recognised to be of considerable importance in the digestion of cellulose by bacteria. In humans, the appendix is generally recognised to be vestigial, but the predominance of lymphocytes suggests that the organ may play a role in defence mechanisms against bacterial infections.

Appendix and disease

Appendicitis

The significance of the appendix to the surgeon lies in its importance as a common cause of the acute abdomen (see Ch. 22).

Mucocoele of the appendix

This is a rare condition which can be difficult to differentiate clinically from its malignant counterpart – cystadenocarcinoma (see below).

PATHOLOGY

A diffusely enlarged appendix develops as a result of a lumen filled with mucus. The latter in turn arises secondarily from obstruction of the lumen by mucosal hyperplasia, adenoma or cystadenocarcinoma. The diagnosis of carcinoma cannot usually be made on clinical grounds and can only be based on microscopic evidence of invasion of the appendix wall by mucin. Rupture of a mucocoele may result in pseudomyxoma peritonei. The latter syndrome is generally benign, although occasionally it may give rise to generalised inflammatory changes, ascites or intestinal obstruction.

CLINICAL FEATURES AND MANAGEMENT

Most mucocoeles are asymptomatic and are only discovered 'en passant' during laparotomy or at CT scanning.

Where symptoms occur appendicectomy is curative.

Tumours of the appendix

These are rare, accounting for less than 1% of all intestinal tumours, but because of their position, they can be extremely difficult to diagnose. The pathology of these tumours is as follows:

- Carcinoid – 85%
- Mucinous cystadenocarcinoma – 8%
- Colonic adenocarcinoma – 4%
- Miscellaneous – 2%

Carcinoid tumour

The incidence of carcinoid tumours is approximately 0.5% of appendicectomy specimens, and although the majority are benign, they have the potential to invade locally, metastasise and secrete biologically active substances.

PATHOLOGY AND CLINICAL FEATURES

These are small well circumscribed but non-encapsulated tumours usually located in the tip of the appendix and frequently only recognised microscopically (70% < 1.0 cm diameter). The tumour is composed of nests of uniform argyrophilic cells with occasional acinic development.

The majority are asymptomatic. Metastatic spread to the liver and carcinoid syndrome are extremely rare with appendix carcinoids.

TREATMENT

Most authorities agree that for small (microscopic) carcinoids, appendicectomy is sufficient treatment and such patients have a 99% 5-year survival. For more extensive local disease, more radical excisional surgery (e.g. right hemicolectomy) is advocated. Distant metastasis has only been recorded where the tumour exceeds 2 cm in diameter.

Mucinous Cystadenocarcinoma

These tumours are recognised by the presence of mucus-secreting epithelial mucosal cells. The mucin may penetrate the appendix wall and give rise to pseudomyxoma peritonei.

CLINICAL FEATURES

The tumour is usually asymptomatic but may, on occasions, give rise to appendicitis or present with an abdominal mass. At the time of presentation, approximately 50% of these tumours will have undergone intra-abdominal spread.

TREATMENT

These tumours are slow-growing; hence right hemicolectomy is usually adequate treatment and a 5-year survival of 70% can be expected. Simple appendicectomy is inadequate surgical treatment.

Colonic adenocarcinoma

Most of these tumours arise from the base of the appendix and thereby rapidly lead to occlusion of the appendix lumen and give rise to the pathological features of acute appendicitis.

CLINICAL FEATURES

Most tumours are symptomatic, giving rise to acute appendicitis.

TREATMENT

Since the operative findings are those of acute appendicitis, the danger is one of inadequate surgery, i.e. the surgeon performs appendicectomy alone. The presence of a firm mass at the base of the appendix should alert the surgeon to the possibility of malignancy and a radical right hemicolectomy is required. The prognosis is that of adenocarcinoma of the colon, i.e. it is dependent on histological grading and Duke's staging.

Anal and related disorders

The anal canal is a structure of considerable importance in that it controls two of humanity's most unsociable physiological needs – defaecation and the passage of flatus. Disturbances in its function or structure result in troublesome symptoms which need careful assessment if management is to be effective. At all times it must be remembered that disorders in the rectum and colon must be excluded before treatment is begun. The possibility of sexually transmitted diseases occurring in the anal region must also be kept in mind.

Introduction

ANATOMY AND PHYSIOLOGY

Embryology
The anal canal – the last 3–4 cm of the alimentary tract – is derived from a fusion of the embryological hind gut (entoderm) and the proctodeum (primitive skin – ectoderm – of the posterior perineum). Thus it is made up of both visceral and somatic structures and is also, because it is a junctional area, subject to developmental abnormalities.

Epithelial lining (Fig. 25.1)
Fusion between the hind gut and skin occurs at the transitional zone, which is proximal to a ring of the so-called mucosal anal valves. Distally there is the pecten where the canal is lined with stratified squamous epithelium and has the same sensitivity as that of the rest of the body. Hair-bearing skin follows.

Muscles (Fig. 25.2)
The internal sphincter is a condensation of the lower end of the circular smooth muscle of the rectum. The external sphincter is a complex plate of striated muscle which surrounds the anal canal and part of which is attached posteriorly to the coccyx. The function of both sphincters is related to defaecation and continence . The longitudinal smooth muscle of the rectum continues into the anal canal, within the intersphincteric space, traverses the internal sphincter and is attached to the epithelium and skin. It probably functions as a suspensory ligament for the epithelium of the canal.

In addition to the sphincters just described, the puborectalis sling is a specialised part of the levator ani in the floor of the pelvis. Its fibres, which run from the

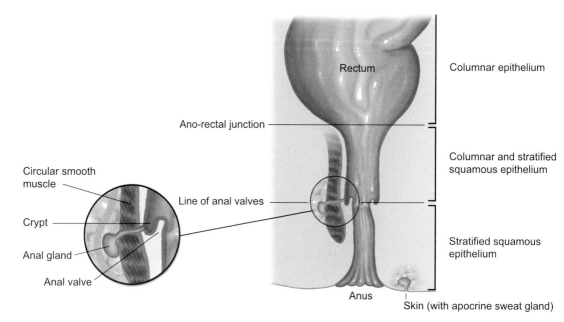

Fig 25.1 **The epithelium of the distal rectum and anal canal.**

Columnar epithelium

Columnar and stratified squamous epithelium

Stratified squamous epithelium

Skin (with apocrine sweat gland)

Rectum

Ano-rectal junction

Circular smooth muscle

Line of anal valves

Crypt

Anal gland

Anal valve

Anus

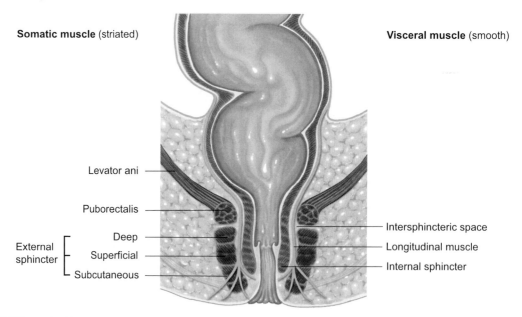

Fig 25.2 **The anal sphincters.**

Somatic muscle (striated)

Visceral muscle (smooth)

Levator ani

Puborectalis

External sphincter
- Deep
- Superficial
- Subcutaneous

Intersphincteric space

Longitudinal muscle

Internal sphincter

back of the pubis to the last two segments of the coccyx, also encircle the junction between the rectum and anus. Their contraction draws the junction anteriorly to create a 90°C angle between the anal canal and the rectum. The muscular contraction and angulation bring the anterior rectal wall into contact with the posterior proximal end of the anal canal so that a flap mechanism forms to counter a rise in intra-abdominal pressure. The arrangement is analogous to the ease with which flow from a garden hose is controlled by bending it to a right angle.

The intersphincteric space (outside the longitudinal muscle) represents a plane of fusion between the internal and external sphincters. It is an important surgical landmark, being utilised in a number of surgical procedures as well as being a pathway for the spread of perianal sepsis.

Nerve supply

Sensory

The sensation of rectal distension originates from sensory receptors within the muscles of the pelvic floor contiguous to and surrounding the rectum and is conveyed by the autonomic afferents (pelvic splanchnic nerves – S2 and S3). The central nervous system can, by mechanisms that are not fully understood, distinguish between the presence of faeces and flatus in the lower rectum and proximal anal canal – a property of considerable social utility. Information on pain travels with the parasympathetic and sympathetic nervous systems from the richly innervated anal papillae and surrounding tissues. The distal anal canal (because of its derivation from the proctoderm) is supplied by the pudendal nerve and shares the sensory characteristics of the rest of the skin of the body.

Motor

The levator ani muscles and the external sphincter are supplied by the pudendal nerve (S2 and S3) and the perineal branch of S4. The internal sphincter is innervated by both sympathetic and parasympathetic fibres, but it is the parasympathetic component which maintains constant contraction so keeping the anal canal normally closed with positive intra-anal resting pressure. The external sphincter also contributes to this but can contract voluntarily to meet challenges initiated by contraction of the rectum (see 'Defaecation' below).

Blood and lymphatic supply

Particular points to note are as follows:

- The anal canal is a watershed between the portal and systemic circulations, which is of special importance in relation to venous drainage.
- Venous plexuses lie in the subepithelial tissues both above and below the line of the anal valves.

In the left lateral, right posterior and right anterior positions, the venous plexuses, together with some arteriovenous anastomoses, are surrounded by smooth muscle, elastic and fibrous tissue to form three anal cushions. It is thought that their function is to complete the closure of the anal canal as sphincter tone brings them into contact with each other. An increase in the size of the cushions is the starting point of haemorrhoids.

Defaecation

This function is the result of the interplay of many factors not the least of which is activity within the colon and rectum.

Distension by flatus or faeces (which may be liquid or solid) causes a reflex small decrease in the contraction of the internal sphincter which allows a sample of rectal contents to enter the upper anal canal. Here they encounter sensory receptors at the dentate line which permits discrimination of their nature. At the same time muscular activity is also initiated in the rectum and pressure within it rises. If it is socially convenient for defaecation or the passage of flatus to take place, the internal sphincter and the puborectalis and external sphincter relax, the anorectal angle straightens and the bolus is passed. At the end of defaecation there is increased electrical activity in the external sphincter and puborectalis, the anal canal closes and the anorectal angle is restored. By contrast, if the moment is not convenient, the external sphincter and puborectalis continue to contract, returning the bolus to the rectum. Problems with this orderly sequence (incontinence) are discussed below.

SYMPTOMS OF ANAL DISORDER

Bleeding

Loss of blood from an anal lesion occurs characteristically at the time of defaecation and appears as a bright red streak or smear on the surface of the stool. Large quantities of blood in conjunction with or independent of the passage of a stool usually mean that the bleeding is higher in the gastrointestinal tract.

Pruritus

Itching can be either part of a generalised problem (jaundice or blood dyscrasia) or of local cause.

Pain

The embryological origin of the anal canal results in two types of pain. The mucosa of the proximal canal is insensitive to touch, gripping or cutting (hence it is possible to take a biopsy without anaesthetic). However, disorders deeper in the wall of the canal at this level may cause ill-localised pain felt in the perineum (see 'Anal sepsis'). The skin of the distal canal is sensitive and problems at this level are associated with well-localised pain. Pain is often brought on by defaecation.

Swelling or lump

The patient may report this either: because some normal component of the anal canal is appearing at the anal verge spontaneously or on straining; or because an abnormal structure has developed. Examples of the first are enlarged anal cushions (haemorrhoids) and prolapse of the rectal mucosa; of the second a new growth.

Discharge

There are three types of discharge:

- *faecal soiling* – usually the result of either distortion of the anal anatomy, say by a tumour, or of incontinence
- *mucoid* – a change in the mucosa of the rectum and/or proximal anal canal which is commonly inflammatory but may imply a mucus-secreting tumour
- *purulent* – almost always associated with sepsis.

Alteration in bowel function

A change in consistency and frequency of the stool (e.g. loose or hard motions) is generally the manifestation of an intestinal disorder. Loss of differentiation (flatus, liquid or solid stool) and faecal incontinence may be a manifestation of intestinal disorder, but is more usually the result of injury to the sphinctor complex.

CLINICAL EXAMINATION

Anal conditions cannot be diagnosed without clinical examination, which is an essential feature in the assessment of any patient with symptoms provisionally attributed to the anal canal and its surroundings. In addition, the rectum must always be examined to make certain that the underlying cause is not more proximal.

The position of the patient and adequate lighting are both important. In the UK, the left lateral position is found to be acceptable to most patients and is preferred. Should a vaginal examination be considered necessary, then the supine position is adopted.

Examination has three components – inspection, palpation and endoscopy – the last of which is by sigmoidoscopy and protoscopy. None of these is omitted.

Inspection

After initial inspection of the skin of the anorectal verge, the buttocks are separated, which usually brings the lower part of the anal canal into view. The patient should be asked to strain to see if mucosa emerges, especially if there is a history of prolapse. It is not always possible for the patient to do this and prolapse may be more satisfactorily confirmed with the patient in the squatting position. Some measure of the external sphincter's ability to contract can be obtained by eliciting the 'anal reflex' – touching the perianal skin with an orange stick or a pin which is followed by reflex contraction of the external sphincter. The response of the voluntary muscles to a request for contraction can also be assessed.

Palpation

The index finger is covered with a suitably soft thin rubber glove which is lubricated. First, the perianal skin is palpated to feel for induration which is an important sign of sepsis or malignancy. The finger is then passed into the anal canal superiorly and anteriorly to avoid the common sites of a painful lesion. Each quadrant is palpated to assess swelling or induration and also to get a feel for resting tone and voluntary contraction of the muscles. Finally the finger is inserted – preferably by extending the terminal digit of the examining finger – into the lower rectum. Here the contents (if any), the rectal wall and structures outside the rectum, such as those in the postrectal space, the prostate or, as far as they can be felt through the pouch of Douglas, the uterus and ovaries are all evaluated.

Endoscopic examination

There are two procedures for this: proctoscopy and sigmoidoscopy. The proctoscope is short – less than the index of most examiners – and therefore is only of value for examination of the anal canal. It is of no use to exclude rectal disease. However, it is relatively easy to do and can give some information about anorectal conditions such as haemorrhoids.

Sigmoidoscopy is done with either a rigid or a flexible instrument. The latter is able to traverse the

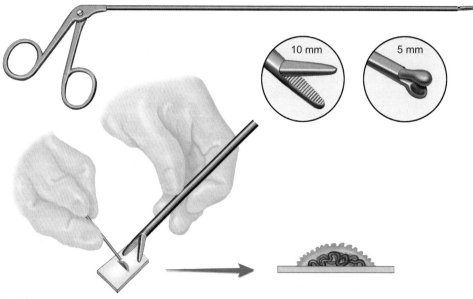

Fig 25.3 **Rectal biopsy.**

rectosigmoid angle more effectively but requires more skill to use. The rigid sigmoidoscope is used for initial examination and can nearly always inspect the rectum to at least 15 cm. Biopsies of the mucosa may be taken and should be correctly orientated on filter paper, before fixation in formalin to allow the best possible preparations for the histopathologist to examine (Fig. 25.3).

INVESTIGATION

Examination under anaesthesia (EUA)

Pain, discomfort and social resistance to being examined may mean that assessment of the lower bowel and anal canal can only be satisfactorily undertaken with the patient anaesthetised. Recourse to EUA should never be regarded as a sign of defeat and can often lead to a much more accurate assessment than in those who are able tolerate a rectal examination without anaesthesia. The procedure is the same as that outlined above.

Imaging

Contrast radiology by barium enema possibly supplemented by endoscopy with the flexible sigmoidoscope or colonoscope may be required in patients with anal disorders simply to establish normality in the colon and rectum.

Ultrasound. Intraluminal ultrasound provides very accurate information about the structure of the anal canal. Damage to the internal and/or external sphincters can be clearly identified by ultrasound and it can assist in localising perianal sepsis and fistulae. In addition, transrectal ultrasound can provide staging information on rectal neoplasms.

Magnetic resonance imaging (MRI) is currently the most accurate way of delineating perianal sepsis. It can very accurately identify primary and secondary fistula tracts as well as localised abscess. In addition, it can provide accurate data on extraluminal spread of rectal neoplasms as well as indicating with some accuracy lymphnode status.

Fistulography, rarely used, may assist the delineation of a fistula but is of little value in management. It is, however, useful to find the origin of discharge in the perineum when the primary disease is within the pelvis (e.g. diverticular disease).

Evacuation proctography – cinephotography of the expulsion of contrast medium from the rectum during actual or attempted defaecation – is used to assist in the diagnosis of obstructed defaecation.

Microbiological studies (Table 25.1)

Culture of pus in patients with acute abscesses may be helpful in determining whether or not a fistula is present – the presence of gut organisms usually means this is so – but is not usually crucial to management. By

Table 25.1
Bacteriological examination of anorectal material

Condition	Examination	Finding
Acute abscess	Standard cultures	Intestinal organisms – ? fistula
Gonorrhoea	Fresh swab and culture	*Neisseria gonorrhoea*
Syphillis	Dark ground examination	Spirochates
Fungal infection	Direct microscopy of scrapings of perianal skin Culture	Pathogenic organism
Tuberculosis	Histopathological examination	Caseating granulomas
	Culture for *Mycobacterium tuberculosis*	Organisms on Z-N stain Organism and sensitivity

contrast, it is essential for the diagnosis of certain sexually transmitted diseases and the uncommon fungal infections of the perianal skin.

Physiological studies

The following are widely used to evaluate patients with faecal incontinence:

- anal canal pressure – at rest, during voluntary contractions and in response to rectal distension
- electromyography of the external sphincter and its response to pudendal nerve stimulation.

Haemorrhoids

DEFINITION AND CLASSIFICATION

Most patients refer to any abnormality in the anorectal area as 'piles'. The word is, indeed, an alternative name for haemorrhoids, but to minimise confusion it is one best avoided in the description of clinical conditions.

Haemorrhoids are engorgement of the haemorrhoidal venous plexuses with redundancy of their coverings. The cushions may:

- remain in their usual position in the anal canal (internal)
- descend to involve the skin of the distal anal canal so that they prolapse on defaecation (interoexternal); but reduce spontaneously
- become of such a size that they are always partly outside the canal (external).

The alternative terms used are first-, second- and third-degree haemorrhoids.

Although they develop from the three cushions, and therefore have the positions of left lateral, right posterior and right anterior (the primary haemorrhoids), secondary haemorrhoids do occur in between these and in consequence the abnormality may become circumferential.

AETIOLOGY

Most patients with haemorrhoids do not have an obvious predisposing cause, although there may be a family history. In women, pregnancy may lead on to haemorrhoids as may pelvic tumours (ovarian and uterine). Constipation and straining at the time of defaecation may also be a factor. It has been suggested that patients with haemorrhoids have an increased resting anal canal pressure and the effort required to overcome this may be the underlying reason for straining at defaecation. The evidence to support this view is conflicting but it has provided the basis for one form of treatment.

It is sometimes suggested that carcinoma of the rectum may be an antecedent. This presumed relationship is probably coincidental because both conditions are relatively common and therefore may be present together.

CLINICAL FEATURES

Symptoms

- *Bleeding* – usually at defaecation but intermittent, bright red into the pan and/or on the toilet paper; spurting and dripping of blood may occur after defaecation and at other times of exertion
- *Discharge* – faecal soiling or a mucus leak because the haemorrhoids prevent complete anal closure
- *Pruritus* – if cleaning of the perianal skin becomes difficult or there is discharge
- *Discomfort* – when there is stretching of the sensitive external component
- *Swelling* – in intero-external or external haemorrhoids only
- *Prolapse* – often either not reported by the patient or called a swelling
- *Pain* – only when there are complications (see 'Thrombosis')
- *Bowel function* – many patients have a sluggish bowel function which leads to straining.

A traditional symptomatic classification of haemorrhoids based on only two of the above symptoms may give some guidance for management (Table 25.2).

Signs

The appearances of haemorrhoids vary from a slight increase in the size of the normal anal cushions, visible only at proctoscopy, to large intero-external haemorrhoids apparent on inspection of the anal verge. It is important to identify accurately what is seen. The external component of second- and third-degree haemorrhoids comprises the perianal skin and hair

Table 25.2
Symptomatic classification of haemorrhoids

Stage	Symptoms
Internal (first degree)	Bleeding
Intero-external (second degree)	Prolapse with spontaneous reduction; bleeding present or absent
External (third degree)	Prolapse which requires replacement; bleeding present or absent

Table 25.3
Conditions related to (and which may be confused with) haemorrhoids

Condition	Position
Anal skin tags	Anal margin
Fibrous anal polyps	Line of the anal valves
Prolapse of rectum	Similar to haemorrhoids but circumferental
Thrombosis in perianal skin (perianal haematoma)	Distal to mucocutaneous junction
Fissure	Primarily at the mucocutaneous junction but may have a distal skin tag
Benign tumours of the rectum	*Within* the rectum at sigmoidoscopy
Varices	Rare but almost impossible to distinguish
Haemangioma	Rare congenital abnormality

and, depending on the extent of prolapse, the pecten at the junction of the skin and mucosa. There is always a groove between the external and internal components which corresponds to the line of the anal valves. In patients with a prolonged history of prolapse, the normal intermingling of columnar and squamous epithelium at the transitional zone becomes all squamous and therefore opaque.

It may not always be possible to confirm the presence of prolapse at examination in the left lateral position. Straining assists the diagnosis, especially after the passage of a proctoscope.

Conditions that are related to haemorrhoids and which may cause diagnositic confusion are summarised in Table 25.3.

MANAGEMENT

Reassurance

Often all that is required is explanation of the symptoms to alleviate the fear of a more sinister diagnosis.

Bowel regulation

Because of the tendency to constipation, advice about ensuring a more regular bowel habit (increased intake of fluids, fruit and vegetables and the addition of bulk by the use of fibre) and the avoidance of prolonged straining is useful.

Proprietary suppositories

Most of these contain a variety of ingredients which include topical corticosteroids, local anaesthetics and antibiotics. There is no reason why such a cocktail should influence the symptoms of uncomplicated haemorrhoids and there is no objective evidence that they do. Their prescription is probably the outcome of ignorance about the cause of symptoms, an imprecise diagnosis and a poorly thought-out plan of management.

Treatments directed at the haemorrhoids

The various surgical treatments are considered in Table 25.4 in order of increasing severity and intervention from the patient's point of view. The various mechanisms of action are:

- *submucosal vascular occlusion* – produced in the main vessels to reduce bulk and fix redundant mucosa by fibrosis
- *excision of redundant tissue* – this is necessary for prolapse; lesser treatments may succeed unless there is symptomatic engorgement of the external venous plexus
- *reduction in anal canal pressure*.

Table 25.4 indicates that a given therapy may have more than one mode of action.

Injection sclerotherapy

This is usually the first treatment for those with bleeding or early prolapse. Phenol 5% in arachis oil is injected into the submucosa at the anorectal junction in amounts up to 5 mL at the three primary sites. The injection must be submucosal which can be observed by seeing the mucosa lifted from the muscle and assuming a pearly appearance (Fig. 25.4). A superficial intramucosal injection causes ulceration, and one that is too deep may result in an oleogranuloma – accumulation of the oil in the extrarectal tissues with low-grade inflammatory reaction. Too deep an anterior injection may also lead to prostatitis. Should the injection be

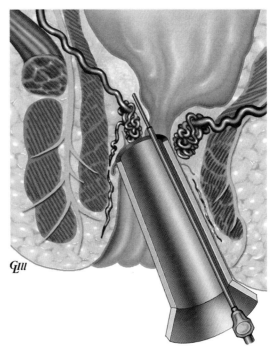

Fig 25.4 **Injection sclerotherapy.**

intravascular – avoided if the needle is kept on the move – severe pain may be felt in the right hypochondrium and injection must stop immediately.

The initial results are satisfactory for the control of bleeding – although it should be remembered that symptoms may be intermittent – but injection sclerotherapy may need to be repeated.

Infrared coagulation

A small burn is made in the mucosa and submucosa to a predetermined depth. This method, which is similar to injection sclerotherapy, is not widely practised and has secondary haemorrhage as a significant complication.

Table 25.4
Treatment of haemorrhoids

Method	Appropriate for	Occludes blood supply at anorectal junction	Fixes mucosa	Excises redundant tissue	Reduces anal canal pressure
Injection sclerotherapy[a]	First degree	*	*		
Infrared coaglation	First degree	*	*		
Band ligation[a]	Second degree	*	*	*	
Cryosurgery	Second degree	*	*	*	
Manual dilatation of the anus	Second degree				*
Lateral sphincterotomy	Second degree				*
Haemorrhoidectomy[a]	Second and third degree		*		

[a]Preferred methods

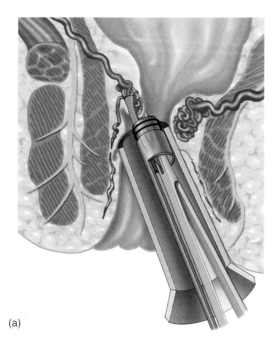

(a)

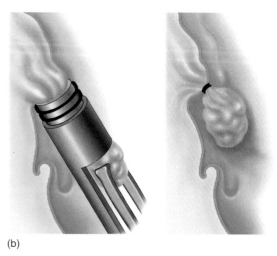

(b)

Fig 25.5 **Band ligation for haemorrhoids.**

Band ligation

This technique combines excision of redundant mucosal tissue with fixation of the mucosa to the underlying muscle (Fig. 25.5). There are two major problems: pain and haemorrhage after application of the bands. The first may occur immediately because of incorporation of sensitive epithelium from low in the anal canal or subsequently because of necrosis of the anal epithelium distal to the point of application. Bleeding may take place at any time up to 20 days after application and may be severe. However, band ligation is effective treatment for intero-external haemorrhoids.

Cryotherapy

This technique uses liquid nitrogen at −180°C to thrombose vessels and reduce the bulk of overlying tissue, but it has not gained popularity because of swelling and severe discharge after treatment which may last up to 6 weeks. There is a risk of incontinence if the internal sphincter is also frozen.

Manual dilatation of the anus

In addition to a reduction in anal canal pressure, which may be a contributory factor to the development of haemorrhoids, it is said that this procedure destroys tight fibromuscular fibres in the submucosa and the internal sphincter. The method has recently been popular but it is crude, does not help those with redundant tissue and may result in impaired control, especially if there is any pre-existing defect in external sphincter function. It is this risk, combined with a lack of precision, which suggests that it ought to be consigned to surgical history.

Lateral partial internal sphincterotomy

The distal half of the internal sphincter is divided, thus reducing resting anal canal pressure. The technique is not widely used nor is it recommended for the treatment of haemorrhoids, but it is effective in fissure.

Haemorrhoidectomy

This remains the most effective therapy for large prolapsing haemorrhoids. There are various techniques:

- *Ligature* – of the base of the haemorrhoid and excision of redundant tissue; the wounds heal by granulation and re-epithelialisation
- *Closed* – after ligation-excision, the mucocutaneous defect is closed by suture with the objective of primary union
- *Submucosal* – the enlarged cushions are dissected beneath their coverings and, as with the closed procedure, the defect closed.

All these procedures aim to excise as much redundant epithelium and vasculature as possible. The differences lie in how this is achieved and the manner in which the wounds are left at the end of the operation. In the UK, the technique of simple ligature and excision has always enjoyed much success and has been the routine. However, the other techniques are gaining in popularity because of reputed advantages in reduction of pain and speed of healing.

Haemorrhoidectomy has an unjustified reputation for severe postoperative pain and patients are often warned off the operation by the experience of others who have undergone it. With a better understanding of postoperative pain relief (Ch. 6), non-adherent dressings and the appropriate use of lubricant laxatives, the course after operation, although not without some discomfort, is coped with well by nearly all patients.

Stapled haemorrhoidectomy. Currently under trial, a modified circular stapling gun can be used to excise a circumferential strip of lower rectal mucosa pulling the redundant haemorrhoidal tissue back into its correct anatomical position. The remaining haemorrhoidal tissue is thus still of use for the maintenance of faecal continence.

COMPLICATIONS

Skin tags and anal polyps

These often coexist with haemorrhoids and require limited excision. Anal polyps should be transfixed before removal to avoid postoperative bleeding.

Thrombosis

Established haemorrhoids may develop thrombosis within their veins. A precipitating factor is the descent of intero-external haemorrhoids below the external sphincter and its subsequent contraction which cuts off venous drainage. The thrombosed haemorrhoid (or more usually haemorrhoids) is covered with both mucosa and squamous epithelium. The chief complaint is of pain and circumanal discomfort.

On examination there are obvious intero-external haemorrhoids with bluish discoloration, oedema and an ooze of blood.

The episode is best managed conservatively with local application of ice, the administration of non-constipating analgesics and lubricant laxatives and, if there are significant constitutional features, bed rest. Resolution always takes place and definitive treatment can be planned later. Occasionally the quickest relief of pain is by manual reduction of the thrombosed mass under general anaesthesia, but further prolapse may occur. Urgent haemorrhoidectomy, if carried out carefully and by an experienced operator, may well be advantageous particularly if there is concern over necrosis and sepsis in the thrombosed tissue. A very rare complication of thrombosis is infection and portal pyaemia.

Perianal haematoma

This condition is sometimes known as a 'thrombosed external pile' but it has nothing to do with haemorrhoids. The cause is obscure but what happens is thrombosis in a subcutaneous vein below the transitional zone and the precise term is a clotted venous saccule. The result is a discrete painful swelling said to look like a small blackcurrant. On examination there is a tender lump external to the anal canal which is blue or black depending on the duration of the episode.

Perianal haematoma may resolve with symptomatic management, although during this they may rupture and ulcerate (see below). If pain is severe, the haematoma is deroofed by a cruciate incision under local lignocaine anaesthesia with immediate relief, although it must be remembered that a vein has been opened and steps should be taken to ensure that bleeding does not occur.

Fissure in ano

Fissures are ulcers consequent upon tears of the mucosa at the anal margin which extend into the pecten.

AETIOLOGY

The cause is not always obvious, although constipation may initiate the problem both in children and in adults; however, constipation as a cause should not be confused with constipation as a result when patients become constipated because of the fear of painful defaecation. Trauma at childbirth and anal intercourse or other sexual manipulations may also be responsible in some instances. There seems little doubt that most patients have sustained hypertonicity of the internal anal sphincter – sphincter spasm. Whatever the precipitating event, a vicious cycle is set up of pain → sphincter spasm → constipation → greater difficulty on defaecation, which makes the local condition worse. Poor blood supply in the posterior midline may help to perpetuate a fissure.

ANATOMY AND PATHOLOGICAL FEATURES

The common site is posteriorly in the midline but it may be anterior or lateral. Depth may range from a simple superficial break in the epithelium to a chronic lesion with exposure of the fibres of the internal sphincter. Chronic lesions may have an associated skin tag (so-called 'sentinel pile'), an anal polyp of varying size and undermining of the edges. Sometimes sepsis may complicate a fissure with a resultant superficial fistula.

CLINICAL FEATURES

Symptoms

- *Pain* – usually occurs during defaecation and may be severe. It may continue for some time after defaecation but has usually eased before the passage of the next stool when the cycle is repeated. Pain is more common with an acute fissure, and some chronic, indolent lesions may be relatively pain-free.
- *Constipation* – may be the consequence of the patient's unwillingness to defaecate because of pain.

• *Bleeding* – this is not usually severe and may occur only on the toilet paper after defaecation.
• *Discharge of small quantities of pus* is uncommon but does occur.

Signs

In a patient with a painful acute lesion, separating the buttocks and gentle palpation of the anal verge reveal tenderness at the site of the fissure which is usually posteriorly in the midline. If a stable and satisfactory doctor–patient relationship is to be maintained, a digital examination should be avoided but it is often possible to see the lower end of the fissure by asking the patient to strain.

In more chronic lesions, a sentinel tag occasionally draws attention to the condition, as may discharge from a superficial fistula. A digital examination can usually be done and reveals thickening at the anorectal ring and a varying amount of tenderness, although this is not usually severe. Proctoscopy shows a lesion of varying depth in which the fibres of the external sphincter may be visible; there is granulation tissue and perhaps a small amount of bleeding.

Other causes of an ulcer at the anorectal verge include:

• Crohn's disease – perianal and intra-anal which can be extensive and associated with oedematous skin tags, sepsis and a bluish discoloration of the skin
• primary syphilitic chancre – more likely in homosexual patients
• herpes simplex – more likely in those who are HIV-positive
• lymphoma and leukaemia
• neoplasms – basal and squamous cell carcinoma
• excoriation (microulceration) associated with perianal skin disorders
• ruptured perianal haematoma.

MANAGEMENT

Acute fissure

This condition responds well to the application of a local anaesthetic gel (1% lignocaine) just before defaecation and the use of bulk laxatives. In those with considerable sphincter spasm, an anal dilator may also help. To be effective it should be well lubricated, preferably with a local anaesthetic gel, and passed into the anal canal twice or three times daily and held in place for up to 5 minutes.

There is some debate as to whether this instrument really helps and whether patients are happy to use it. In response to this, the dilator will do no harm and, if there is a chance that it might prevent the need for operative treatment, most patients are happy to give it a try.

Chronic fissure

Chronic fissure associated with a skin tag, anal polyp, undermining of the edges of the fissure and exposure of the fibres of the internal sphincter usually requires operative treatment.

Operation

The division of the fibres of the internal sphincter distal to the line of the anal valves (partial internal sphincterotomy) is most effective and is usually done laterally within the wall of the anal canal. It is an extremely effective procedure and relieves pain almost immediately. It does however carry a small but finite risk of passive incontinence, usually to flatus. Patients should be warned of this risk and care taken not to perform too extensive a sphincter division.

Nitric oxide donors

Chemical sphincterotomy is an attractive idea. It has the potential to relieve pain and heal a fissure but as it is temporary does not carry the risk of incontinence. Glyceryl trinitrate ointment (0.2%) has been evaluated and appears to have about a 60% success rate. It carries the down side of inducing headache in some patients and has a recurrence rate. However, it is currently favoured as first line therapy by many clinicians.

Anal sepsis

A variety of problems may present with suppuration – either an acute abscess or chronic purulent discharge. (Table 25.5).

Table 25.5
Conditions that are associated with perianal sepsis

Condition	Usual finding
Non-specific infection	Acute abscess
	Fistula in ano
Tuberculosis	Chronic infection
	Occasionally fistula
Crohn's disease	Chronic intractable infection
	Complex fistula
Hydradenitis suppurativa	Skin abscesses
	Anal canal rarely if ever involved
Skin sepsis	Usually *Staphylococcus aureus*
	Abscesses are often multiple
Trauma	External: sexual intercourse; accidental injury
	Internal: foreign body (ingested bone)
Intrapelvic sepsis	Diverticular disease; Crohn's disease
Sepsis in developmental cysts	Usually dermoid cysts
Malignant disease	Sepsis is an uncommon complication

Non-specific abscess and fistula

Infection of the anal intersphincteric glands with organisms found in the gastrointestinal tract – both aerobic (e.g. *E. coli*) and anaerobic (e.g. *Bacteroides* spp.) – is the cause of this common disorder. A variety of different anatomical abscesses and fistulae may present, an understanding of which is greatly simplified by knowledge of the routes taken by the spread of infection.

Spread of infection

Sepsis begins in the intersphincteric space and may spread in three ways:

- vertically (Fig. 25.6a)
- horizontally (Fig. 25.6b)
- circumferentially.

Anatomical sites of abscess

Five named abscesses are the consequence of spread in the above directions:

- intersphincteric
- perianal
- intermuscular
- supralevator
- ischiorectal

Formation of a fistula

When fistula follows acute non-specific inflammation, it is because pus from an abscess burrows in two directions: into and through the wall of the anorectal canal, perhaps along the track from where it may have originated; and superficially to emerge distal to the mucocutaneous junction. Two openings are formed – internal and external – and the track that now connects them is lined with granulation tissue. One or other opening may be, at any one time, closed, and if both seal, a further abscess develops. Repeated episodes of this kind may cause further and ever more complex tracks to form.

Classification of fistula

Classification is in relation to the anal musculature. There are two main types (Fig. 25.7):

- *Intersphincteric* – all the inflammatory tracks remain medial to the striated muscle
- *Transsphincteric* – there is a primary track across the external sphincter which may be at any level from just below the puborectalis to the lowest fibres of the external sphincter.

Other types of fistula include:

- *Superficial (cutaneous)* – confined to the superficial tissues with a bridge or bridges of skin between two or more openings; in effect this is a 'bridged fissure'.
- *suprasphincteric* – this is very rare and the primary track passes across the levator ani
- Extrasphincteric – this is usually the result of intrapelvic sepsis or inappropriate surgical treatment of another type of fistula and the track lies outside the whole sphincter complex.

CLINICAL FEATURES OF ABSCESS AND FISTULA

Symptoms

There may be a past history of similar episodes or one of intermittent or continuing discharge. The chief complaint in an abscess is of pain over a period of 3–4 days accompanied by swelling and difficulty on defaecation. In a fistula, discharge with or without occasional pain is usually less severe than that of an abscess.

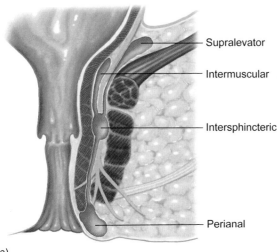

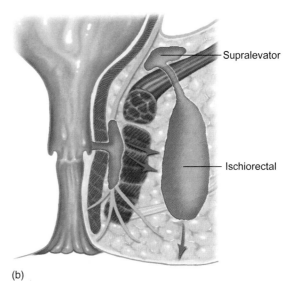

(a)　　　　　　　　　　　　　　(b)

Fig 25.6 **Spread of infection.** (a) Vertical spread. (b) Horizontal spread.

Anal and related disorders

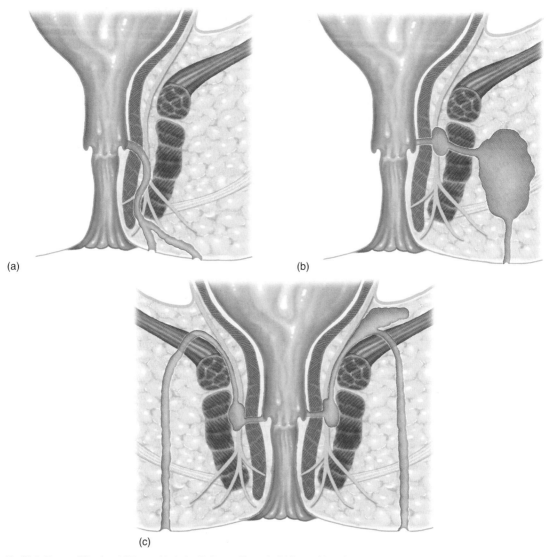

(a)

(b)

(c)

Fig 25.7 **Types of fistulae.** (a) Transsphincteric. (b) Suprasphincteric. (c) Extrasphincteric.

Signs

In an abscess, signs are the typical features of acute inflammation but it is unusual to find fluctuation even when the condition is of sufficient duration for pus to have formed. In a fistula there may be varying degrees of inflammation around the external opening; digital examination shows induration and it may be possible to express pus.

MANAGEMENT

Abscess

Antibiotics have little part to play – they cannot penetrate into the pus and there is often some necrosis of fatty tissue. An acute abscess requires surgical drainage. It is unwise to do anything more even though a fistula is suspected – swelling and hyperaemia mask the precise location of the sphincters. The pus should always be sent for microbiological examination because the presence of gut organisms indicates that a fistula is likely.

Fistula

A fistula is suspected if:

- discharge persists at the site of drainage of an abscess
- gut organisms are cultured
- abscess recurs
- induration is detected either clinically or under anaesthesia.

Treatment is based on eradication of the sepsis with the preservation of maximum anal function. A fistulous track must be laid open and allowed to heal from its base. The majority of superficial and intersphincteric fistulae (85%) are straightforward to deal with. The remainder (transsphincteric and suprasphincteric) are much more difficult and demand specialist care. Treatment is often prolonged and laying open can be extensive; it is carried out in stages so as to minimise damage to the sphincters. A fine thread of monofilament material (a seton) is often placed through the primary track around the external sphincter to act as a drain while the large wound exterior to the striated muscle of the external sphincter is allowed to heal.

Failure to heal satisfactorily may be the result of:

- inadequate initial treatment
- specific (but undiagnosed) cause e.g. Crohn's disease
- poor nutritional state
- poor wound care, e.g. epithelial bridging
- proliferation of granulation tissue which prevents epithelisation
- ingrowth of hair.

Given the first three causes are eliminated, the success of fistula surgery depends on good postoperative care of the wound. Dressings must be applied so as to ensure that wounds heal from their depths to the surface. Cleanliness is ensured by regular bathing, especially after defaecation, and by lavage with normal saline. Care is taken to ensure that bridging does not occur from the overgrowth of skin because this causes residual pockets of sepsis. Overgrowth of granulation tissue can usually be simply managed by cauterisation with silver nitrate but may require curettage. The wound edges are shaved to prevent ingrowth of hair.

Crohn's disease (see also Ch. 24)

The anal manifestations of Crohn's disease include:

- oedematous skin tags
- bluish hue
- ulceration
- sepsis.

The last of these is managed on similar lines to that of non-specific origin with great care not to divide muscle – any reduction in faecal control is a potential problem for patients with a major tendency to diarrhoea. However, this will only be a small, although important, part of overall management.

Tuberculosis

The possibility of tuberculous anal infection must always be remembered and chronic granulation tissue should be examined microscopically for caseating granulomas and cultured for *Mycobacterium tuberculosis*. The appropriate antimicrobial agent is required, followed by limited surgery.

Pilonidal disease

AETIOLOGY

The commonest site for pilonidal disease is the natal cleft. Other rarer sites include the umbilicus and the webs of the fingers in hairdressers. Hairs are found under the surface of the skin and may cause sepsis. In most instances, there is no clear explanation why this has happened, but one hypothesis is that shed hairs enter pits or crevices in the skin surface and then drill into the subcutaneous tissues. A contributory factor is puberty, with the changes in the skin that occur at this time.

CLINICAL FEATURES

Clinical presentation is because of sepsis sometimes precipitated by minor repeated trauma.

Symptoms

Pain, tenderness and discharge are the cause of the patient seeking attention. Recurrent episodes may have taken place over months or years.

Signs

There are one or more openings in the midline or to either side of it, perhaps with protruding tufts of hair (all the same length). The surrounding skin shows varying degrees of inflammation, and pus is either seen escaping or can be expressed from an opening. There may be confusion with anal fistula because of an opening some distance from the natal cleft, close to or even anterior to the anus.

MANAGEMENT

Management options are as follows:

- no specific treatment in those who are asymptomatic
- laying open of the septic area with curettage of the granulation tissue – it is necessary to make certain all side tracks are fully exposed
- Post-treatment shaving of the skin for 6 months – failure to do so is the commonest cause of recurrence.

More complicated methods of surgical management have been practised but, except in difficult recurrences, are no more successful than the above carefully undertaken.

Hydradenitis suppurativa

The apocrine sweat glands, which occur in the skin of the perineum, inguinal regions and the axilla, become the site of a mixed bacterial infection. Obesity, hormonal imbalance and poor hygiene are contributory factors. Varying degrees of sepsis occur, with pockets and tracks running widely in the subcutaneous tissue.

The condition may be confused with anal fistula, but the anal canal proximal to the skin is not involved. The treatment is to control the contributory factors and to lay open the septic areas. Healing is slow and plastic surgical procedures are sometimes necessary.

Pruritus ani

AETIOLOGY

Pruritus ani is a *symptom* not a diagnosis. The key to successful management is identification of the cause and possible causes include:

- *Post-defaecatory soiling* – soft sticky stools which cannot be cleaned away from the anal verge (soiling of the underwear is often associated); a funnel-shaped anus which is difficult to clean (10% after lateral sphincterotomy – see above); or lack of good hygienic practices. It is thought that metabolites (e.g. endopeptidases) from faecal bacteria produce the itching.
- *Anal disorders* – skin tags, haemorrhoids and fissures may make cleansing difficult and so contribute to poor perianal hygiene; purulent discharge also contaminates the skin with faecal organisms
- *Skin disorders* – dermatological diseases affecting the perianal skin include eczema, psoriasis, neurodermatitis, intertrigo, squamous cell carcinoma-in-situ (Bowen's disease) and extramammary Paget's disease (Ch. 27)
- *Infection* (rare) – bacterial (erythrasma) – infection with a Corynebacterium – and syphilis); viral (condylomata acuminata and molluscum contagiosum); fungal (diabetes and fungal vaginitis)
- *Infestation by parasites* (common) – lice (pediculosis) or threadworms (oxyuriasis)
- *Reactions to pharmaceuticals* – many properitary preparations, which contain a cocktail of ingredients (local anaesthetics and steroids), are used indiscriminately and can cause itching; prolonged application of local anaesthetics may lead to hypersensitivity reactions and steroids to skin atrophy
- *Systemic disorders* – generalised pruritus (obstructive jaundice, reticuloses) may also affect the perineal area
- *Sphincter dysfunction* – if a cause cannot be found, physiological assessment may reveal a sphincter defect which permits faecal leakage
- *Psychosocial problems* – These should always be borne in mind but only sought when all other possibilities have been excluded.

CLINICAL FEATURES

Symptoms
Itching in the perianal skin is the initial symptom, but if the causative factor persists, then soreness and even pain, especially on walking, may occur.

Signs
The skin may be normal but more commonly shows evidence of abrasion or of the presence of one of the specific causative factors described above.

INVESTIGATION

If at all possible, a precise diagnosis should be established by investigation appropriate to the expected cause. Threadworms may be seen on the perianal skin or the rectal mucosa at sigmoidoscopy. Biopsy may rarely be required to define the nature of visible perianal disease and in the patient with no obvious cause, sphincter dysfunction should be investigated.

MANAGEMENT

The key to successful management is the accurate determination and treatment of the cause, which can be achieved in 90% of instances:

- Medications which may be causative are withdrawn.
- Ointments for symptomatic management should only be used when a precise diagnosis has been made and normally for a defined period only.
- Severe inflammation or excoriation usually responds to a short course of a topical steroid (betamethazone 0.1%) sparingly applied twice daily for 2 weeks.
- Threadworms – oral piperazine (all family members require treatment).
- Faecal soiling (without sphincter dysfunction) – instruction in hygiene and the use of damp cotton wool rather than toilet paper; a thin piece of cotton wool on the end of the patient's index figure may be inserted up to three or four times a day to clean a funnel-shaped anus.
- Loose motions – if a cause is not found, a small dose of codeine phosphate or loperamide facilitates cleansing by making the stool firmer.

Faecal incontinence

Failure to have complete control of rectal contents causes considerable stress to the affected individual. A strong sense of social alienation develops so that imprisonment within the home is common from fear of embarrassment at work or in the presence of friends. It has long been recognised that incontinence is normal in infants and common in the very old, but the observation that there is a significant incidence in middle age is more recent. The increased awareness of the problem is the result of more concern by the caring professions such as doctors, nurses and social workers, less reluctance to discuss sensitive matters of body function and increasing attempts to manage the condition.

ANATOMY AND PATHOPHYSIOLOGY

The functional anatomy and physiology of the rectum and anal canal have been described above. Disturbances in these, either locally or because of neural disorders, are the basis of all incontinence.

DEFINITIONS

Urge incontinence

This is defined as an inability to defer defaecation for more than a few minutes. It is usually a sign of external sphincter injury or the result of the normal sphincter being overwhelmed, as in an acute diarrhoeal illness.

Passive incontinence

This is defined as loss of stool, or flatus without the patient being immediately aware that this has occurred. This is commonly a sign of internal sphincter injury.

AETIOLOGY

The causes of minor and major incontinence overlap and the distinction is chiefly one of the severity of the clinical features and the need for treatment.

Inadequate closure of the internal sphincter
The sphincter may be unable to close completely because of:

- large third-degree haemorrhoids
- rectal prolapse
- large faecal mass in the rectum – impacted faeces with liquid stool leaking past it and escaping through a lax sphincter
- anal canal tumour.

Damage to the sphincter complex
- Previous surgery, usually for perianal sepsis
- Overstretching – treatment of fissure; unusual sexual practices either voluntary or during sexual abuse
- Obstetric injury – third-degree perineal tear extending posteriorly from the vaginal wall into the anal sphincter.

Damage to the pelvic floor
- Obstetric injuries
- Pelvic fractures – shearing stresses on the pelvic floor with tearing of nerves.

Loss or absence of motor innervation to the internal sphincter
- Prolonged or complicated obstetric delivery – pressure on, or distraction of, the pudendal nerves
- Diabetic neuropathy
- Spina bifida or cauda equina tumour (both may interfere with the whole reflex arc of defaecation).

Loss of cerebrospinal regulation (upper motor neuron)
Disorder or disease in the CNS interferes with higher control of defaecation. Numerically these are relatively rare causes of incontinence with the exception of the central degenerative conditions of old age:

- trauma
- tumour in brain or spinal cord
- multiple sclerosis; motor neuron disease
- cerebral disease – Alzheimer's disease and other dementias; stroke.

Fistula between rectum and vagina
Developmental malformation of the anus may lead to an imperforate anus with termination of the rectum in the posterior wall of the vagina. A further cause of rectovesical fistula, very uncommon now in the developed world but still common in developing countries, is prolonged obstructed labour with pressure of the fetal head on the posterior vaginal wall and necrosis of this and the adjacent rectum. The bladder may also be involved.

From the above lists, it is clear that multifactorial obstetric events are amongst the commonest causes of faecal incontinence affecting younger women (Table 25.6).

CLINICAL FEATURES

Symptoms

There may be a relevant past history of one of the causes given above. In major incontinence, the patient recounts a life of misery and frequently brings to the clinic a map on which has been marked every known public facility they may need 'just in case'. Pads have to be worn and changed frequently and some patients, particularly those with neurological causes, have urinary incontinence as well.

A history of recent onset of the problem and its progressive development suggests a neurological lesion.

Table 25.6
Faecal incontinence caused by obstetric events

Event	Effect
Tear during delivery	Extension backwards to involve rectal wall and internal sphincter
Too large and episiotomy	As for tear
Difficult or prolonged delivery, perhaps with forceps assistance	Pressure and ischaemic damage to motor outflow in pudendal nerves – denervation of both sphincters and of muscles of pelvic floor
Obstructed labour	Necrosis of anterior wall of rectum and posterior wall of vagina leading rectovaginal fistula

Clinical examination

The local findings vary with the cause. There may be scarring of the perineum from surgery or obstetric intervention or other evidence of anal disease such as haemorrhoids or prolapse. On rectal examination, the anus may gape, and when a finger is inserted the resting anal pressure may be obviously reduced (weak internal sphincter). When asked to tighten the anus voluntarily, the response may be weak or absent (weak external sphincter).

The examination must include:

- full anorectal examination by sigmoidoscopy
- neurological examination beginning with testing the sensation of the perianal skin.

INVESTIGATION

Imaging

Ultrasound Anal ultrasound provides very accurate assessment of both internal and external sphincter. It can clearly identify damage to one or both of these structures.

Barium enema should always be considered if there is a history suggestive of either a neoplasm or inflammatory disease.

Anal manometry

Direct measure of the pressure in the anal canal at rest (internal sphincter) and on maximum voluntary contraction (external sphincter) may help to establish which muscle is at fault, although not necessarily the exact cause.

MANAGEMENT

Incontinence which is caused by inflammatory diarrhoea is usually manageable by treating the underlying condition. Faecal impaction is dealt with by manual removal of the faecal mass (enemas are useless) and regulation of the bowel with laxatives.

Minor incontinence from other causes (provided these are not an indication of progressive disease) may respond to a mild antimotility drug such as loperamide, an additional effect of which is to increase internal sphincter tone. Biofeedback uses the recording of the patient's own pressure trace to encourage increased tone and increase the ability of surviving muscle fibres to undergo hypertrophy; however, controlled trials have not been undertaken.

Surgical techniques

Intervention by surgery is indicated when:

- incapacitation has failed to respond to medical management
- there is a known cause which can be corrected by anatomical and physiological reconstruction
- A defect – such as neuropathy – can be compensated for by surgical means, e.g. reconstruction of the pelvic floor to restore the anorectal angle.

Based on these principles, anterior anal sphincter repair is successful in trauma from obstetric injury to the sphincter, while posterior anal repair can benefit those with neuropathic problems by restoring the anorectal angle and lengthening the anal canal. However, because denervation is long standing and usually irreversible, success in the latter is usually no more than 50%.

More controversial is the use of the gracilis muscle to create a neosphincter which encircles the anus. However, the gracilis does not have resting tone and the results are uncertain in spite of the usual confident reports from early applications. The procedure can be adapted to include the implantation of an electrical stimulator to provide tetanic stimulation; early results are (as is so often the case) encouraging and the financial costs are considerable.

When reconstructive surgery fails, a stoma to divert the faecal stream is a radical but appropriate alternative; an incontinent but manageable stoma on the anterior abdominal wall is greatly preferable to an incontinent but unmanageable opening in the perineum.

Tumours

Tumours of the anal canal are divided into those that arise in the anal canal above the line of the anal valves (the transitional zone) and those below at the anal margin. Anal canal tumours in the embryological junctional area tend to be more aggressive than those more distal which behave very much like other skin tumours.

AETIOLOGY AND PATHOLOGICAL FEATURES

Anal margin

Condylomata acuminata (Perianal warts)
These are the consequence of infection with the human papilloma virus (HPV) which is most often sexually transmitted in both sexes by anal intercourse. The condition is common in patients with HIV infection.

Keratoacanthoma
This benign squamous cell hyperplasia is occasionally found and without biopsy can cause diagnostic confusion.

Bowen's disease
This condition not uncommonly occurs at the anus.

Basal cell carcinoma and squamous carcinoma
Both of these are invasive lesions which, if unchecked, cause widespread local destruction and, in the latter, metastases in inguinal lymph nodes.

Anal canal

Squamous cell carcinoma, adenocarcinoma and *malignant melanoma* are all found in the transitional zone.

CLINICAL FEATURES

The clinical features have already been discussed under other headings above.

MANAGEMENT

A precise diagnosis is essential before treatment is planned. An incision biopsy may suffice, but for a small lesion a total excision biopsy is, in addition, effective treatment.

Anal margin

Condylomata acuminata are managed by excision with scissors, diathermy or laser. Keratoacanthoma and Bowen's disease are excised locally – the risk of invasive carcinoma is less than 20%. The latter may also respond to 5-fluorouracil ointment. Basal cell carcinoma and small cell squamous carcinomas may also respond to local excision. For larger lesions, radiotherapy with or without chemotherapy is currently the treatment of choice and avoids the need for an abdominoperineal excision of the rectum.

Anal canal

Tumours of squamous cell origin are best treated with radiotherapy with or without chemotherapy. Only if there is an incomplete response should radical surgery be required, as it is for adenocarcinoma. Malignant melanomas have a very poor prognosis despite radical treatment.

FURTHER READING

Keighley MRB, Williams NS (1993) *Surgery of the Anus, Rectum and Colon.* London: WB Saunders.

(1993) Surgery of colon, rectum and anus. In: Fielding LP, Goldberg SM (eds) *Rob and Smith's Operative Surgery,* 5th edn. Oxford: Butterworth-Heinemann.

Henry MM, Swash M (eds) (1992) *Coloproctology and the Pelvic Floor,* 2nd edn. Oxford: Butterworth-Heinemann.

Phillips RKS, Lunniss P (eds) (1995) *Fistula-in-ano.* London: Chapman Hall.

26

Hernia

No disease of the human body, belonging to the province of the surgeon, requires in its treatment a better combination of accurate, anatomical knowledge with surgical skill than hernia in all its variations.

Sir Astley Paton Cooper (1804)

General considerations

A hernia is a protrusion of a viscus or other structure beyond the normal coverings of the cavity in which it is contained or between two adjacent cavities such as the abdomen and thorax or into a subcompartment of a cavity. The first category is commonly called external and the second and third are internal. The most frequent hernias are external ones of the abdominal wall in the inguinal, femoral and umbilical regions and the account that follows concentrates chiefly on these.

EPIDEMIOLOGY
The first record of a hernia is in the Egyptian Papyrus Ebers (1550 BC) when it was regarded as a social stigma. Abdominal hernias are common. They occur at all ages and in both sexes and account for approximately 10% of the general surgical workload. Their relative frequencies are given in Table 26.1.

CLASSIFICATION
Hernias are best classified as congenital or acquired.

Congenital
In congenital hernias, there is a pre-formed sac which occurs as a consequence of the ordered or disordered process of intrauterine development – the patent processus vaginalis is a good example.

Table 26.1
Relative frequency of external abdominal hernias

Type of hernia	Incidence (%)
Epigastric	1
Umbilical	3
Incisional	10
Inguinal	78
Femoral	7
Other (rare)	1

Acquired

There are two types of acquired hernia:

Primary hernias occur at natural weak points, such as those where:

- structures penetrate the abdominal wall, e.g. the femoral vessels passing into the femoral canal
- muscles and aponeuroses fail to overlap normally, e.g. the lumbar region
- fibrous tissue normally develops to close a defect, e.g. at the umbilicus.

Secondary hernias develop at sites of surgical or other injury to the wall which normally constrains the contents of a body cavity (usually the abdomen), e.g. after laparotomy and penetrating injury.

AETIOLOGY

The two main factors predisposing to hernia are increased intracavity pressure and a weakened abdominal wall. In the abdomen, the former occurs as a result of:

- heavy lifting
- cough – chronic obstructive airways disease (but possibly lung cancer in a patient with a persistent cough of recent onset)
- straining to pass urine – benign prostatic hyperplasia, but recent rapid onset perhaps with backache might suggest carcinoma
- straining to pass faeces – more than 15% of men with large bowel cancer present with an inguinal hernia
- abdominal distension – which may indicate the presence of an intra-abdominal disorder
- change in abdominal contents – e.g. ascites, encysted fluid, benign or malignant tumour, pregnancy, fat.

A weakened (abdominal wall) occurs in:

- abnormal collagen metabolism
- advancing age
- malnutrition – either of macronutrients (protein, calorie) or micronutrients (e.g. vitamin C)
- damage to, or paralysis of, motor nerves.

Often, multiple factors are involved. For example, the presence of a patent, congenitally formed sac may not cause a hernia until an acquired abdominal wall weakness or raised intra-abdominal pressure allows abdominal contents to enter the sac.

ANATOMICAL FEATURES

A hernia consists of:

- a sac
- its coverings
- its contents

The sac comprises a mouth, neck, body and fundus (Fig. 26.1). The coverings of a hernia refer to the over-

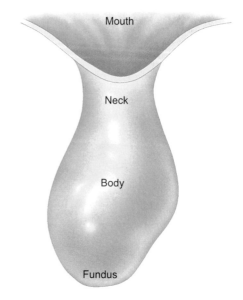

Fig 26.1 **Hernial sac.**

lying layers which are attenuated as the hernia emerges. Working from the outermost layer inwards, these are as follows:

- skin
- subcutaneous fat
- aponeurosis
- muscle
- endo-cavity fascia
- endothelial lining – peritoneum in the abdomen.

The contents of hernias vary, but most intracavity viscera have been reported. In the abdomen, the commonest contents are the small bowel and the greater omentum. Other possibilities include:

- the large bowel and appendix
- Meckel's diverticulum
- the bladder
- the ovary with or without the fallopian tube
- ascitic fluid.

NATURAL HISTORY AND COMPLICATIONS

The natural history of hernia development is progressive enlargement, not spontaneous regression, although there is the notable exception of congenital umbilical hernia in neonates, where the orifice may close over the years following birth. With the passage of time, the likelihood of a life-threatening complication increases.

Hernias may be reducible, irreducible, obstructed, strangulated or inflamed.

Reducible hernia

In this type of hernia, the contents can be returned from whence they came, but the sac persists. The contents do not necessarily reappear spontaneously, but do so when assisted by gravity or raised intra-abdominal pressure.

Irreducible hernia

The contents cannot be returned to the body cavity in this type of hernia. The causes of irreducibility are:

- narrow neck with rigid margins often in association with a capacious sac (e.g. femoral, umbilical)
- adhesion formation between the contents and the sac (usually long-standing hernias)

Irreducible hernias have a greater risk of obstruction and strangulation than do reducible ones.

Obstructed hernia

The obstructed hernia contains intestine in which the lumen has become occluded. Obstruction is usually at the neck of the sac but may be caused by adhesions within it. If the obstruction is at both ends of the loop, fluid accumulates within it and distension occurs (closed loop obstruction). Initially the blood supply to the obstructed loop of bowel is intact, but with time this becomes impeded and strangulation (see below) supervenes.

The term 'incarcerated' is sometimes used to describe a hernia that is irreducible but not strangulated. Thus, an irreducible, obstructed hernia can also be called an incarcerated one.

Strangulated hernia

Ten per cent of groin hernias present for the first time with strangulation. The blood supply to the contents of the hernia is cut off. The pathological sequence is venous and lymphatic occlusion; tissue fluid accumulation (oedema) causing further swelling; and a consequent increase in venous pressure. Venous haemorrhage develops and a vicious circle is set up, with swelling eventually impeding arterial inflow. The tissues undergo ischaemic necrosis. If the contents of the sac of an abdominal hernia are not bowel, e.g. omentum, the necrosis is sterile, but strangulation of bowel is by far the most common and leads to infected necrosis (gangrene). The mucosa sloughs and the bowel wall becomes permeable to bacteria, which translocate through it and into the sac and from there to the bloodstream. The infarcted, friable intestine perforates (usually at the neck of the sac) and the bacteria-laden luminal fluid spills into the peritoneal cavity to produce peritonitis. Septic shock ensues with circulatory failure and death.

Inflamed hernia

The contents are inflamed by any process that causes this in the tissue or organ that is not normally herniated, e.g.:

- acute appendicitis
- Meckel's diverticulitis
- acute salpingitis.

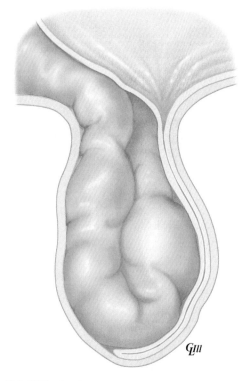

Fig 26.2 **Sliding hernia.**

It may be impossible to distinguish an inflamed hernia from one that is strangulated.

Special types of hernia

Sliding hernia (hernia en glissade)

This hernia is one in which an extraperitoneal structure forms part of the wall of the sac (Fig. 26.2). Five per cent of all hernias are sliding and indirect inguinal hernias account for the majority. On the right the caecum and ascending colon are involved, whereas on the left the sigmoid and descending colon are found in the sac. A portion of bladder may slide into a direct inguinal hernia. The incidence of sliding hernias increases with age and the duration of the hernia. Failure to recognise a sliding hernia at operation may result in damage to the structure involved.

Richter's hernia (Fig. 26.3)

In this type of hernia, only a portion of the circumference of the intestine (usually the small bowel) is trapped. The danger of this hernia is that the knuckle of bowel may become ischaemic without the development of obvious clinical features of obstruction (see 'Femoral hernia').

Hernia EN W – Maydl's hernia

This complicated disposition of intestine in an inguinal hernia is easier to illustrate (Fig. 26.4) than to describe.

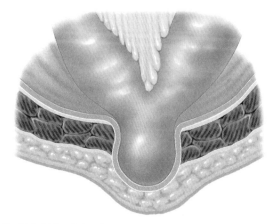

Fig 26.3 **Richter's hernia.**

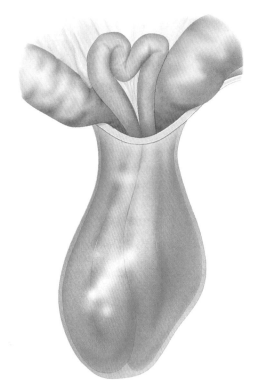

Fig 26.4 **Madyl's hernia.**

If strangulation occurs, the loop affected is within the abdominal cavity.

CLINICAL FEATURES

Symptoms

There may be a history of factors predisposing to increased' intracavity pressure (e.g. cough, heavy lifting – see 'Aetiology').

Local symptoms include:

- a lump which varies in size, may disappear when recumbent and reappears and enlarges on straining
- pain – local aching discomfort, but sometimes sharp.

Symptoms of complications may be:

- intestinal obstruction – colic, vomiting, distension and absolute constipation
- Strangulation – in addition to symptoms of intestinal obstruction, constant pain over the hernia, fever, tachycardia.

Signs

The patient should first be examined in the supine position and then, in all external abdominal hernias, standing. The area of the swelling is palpated to determine the exact position and then its physical characteristics. The lump's distinguishing features are reducibility and an expansile cough impulse – the lump gets bigger and more tense. On standing, bulges become more obvious and can be made additionally prominent by coughing.

When the patient lies down, it is possible to test for reducibility – if the swelling can be returned to the abdominal cavity it is said to be reducible. Control of the hernia is the ability to prevent its reappearance by digital pressure over the point at which reduction occurred. The patient is asked to cough: if the hernia does not reappear it has been controlled and the neck of the sac accurately located.

Other hernial sites should be examined, as bilateral and simultaneous hernias are common. Other causes of a lump that may be confused with abdominal wall hernias are shown in Table 26.2. A general physical examination is essential and includes a search for predisposing causes such as benign prostatic hyperplasia and colorectal cancer.

Signs associated with complications

Irreducibility. Locally there is a painless lump that does not reduce.

Obstruction. The hernia is tense, tender and irreducible. There may be distension of the abdomen and the other features of intestinal obstruction, although if the hernia does not contain bowel this is not necessarily the case.

Table 26.2
Other causes of lumps that must be differentiated from abdominal wall hernias

Tissue	Lump
Skin	Sebaceous or epidermoid cyst
Fat	Lipoma
Fascia	Fibroma
Muscle	Herniation through sheath; tumour
Artery	Aneurysm
Vein	Varicosity
Lymphatic	Enlarged lymph node
Gonad	Ectopic testis/ovary

Strangulation. Signs are as for an obstructed hernia but tenderness is more marked. The overlying skin may be warm, inflamed and indurated.

INVESTIGATION

Hernia is a clinical diagnosis. Investigations are rarely indicated or valuable.

Imaging

Herniography. This technique, which involves the injection of contrast medium into the peritoneal cavity and subsequent X-ray, is now rarely used in infants to identify a clinically undetectable contralateral hernia in the groin. It may occasionally be useful in confirming or refuting the presence of a hernia in a patient with chronic groin pain.

Ultrasound is being increasingly used to assess hernias that are difficult to define clinically, e.g. a Spigelian hernia.

CT and MRI have an occasional role in rare pelvic hernias (e.g. obturator hernia).

Laparoscopy

Unexpected hernias are sometimes discovered at the time of laparoscopy for undiagnosed abdominal pain.

Exploratory operation

In some infants with a convincing history from the mother, a hernia is not found on clinical examination. Exploratory operation can then be justified.

PRINCIPLES OF MANAGEMENT

The natural history of a hernia is one of progressive enlargement rather than of spontaneous resolution. The risks of irreducibility, obstruction and strangulation increase with time; that of strangulation is about 10%. For these reasons, surgical opinion now is that, with very few exceptions, hernias should be operatively repaired both to relieve the patient's symptoms and to eliminate the occurrence of complications, the most dangerous of which is strangulation. There is a particularly strong argument in favour of operation in those hernias that have a high incidence of this complication, i.e.:

- inguinal hernia with a narrow neck
- femoral hernia
- those that have become irreducible.

Advances in anaesthesia have made elective hernia surgery safe. A small number of patients may have associated disorders that make an operation inappropriate or may decline it; in these cases a truss (support belt) is used. For it to work the hernia must be reducible and the appliance must maintain the reduction when the patient stands and strains. It should be appreciated that a truss which does not control a hernia is a menace – by irritation and scar tissue formation it may actually increase the likelihood of incarceration and strangulation.

Presenting or predisposing conditions such as benign prostatic hyperplasia or obstructive airways disease may need treatment before the hernia is dealt with. In addition, in certain defined circumstances, preoperative preparation is necessary:

- Large hernias that warrant repair require particularly diligent preoperative preparation in order to minimise the risk of the operation and to ensure a favourable long-term outcome
- Weight reduction should be encouraged.
- Smoking is prohibited.
- Treatment of intercurrent disease (e.g. hypertension, diabetes) is essential.
- Therapeutic pneumoperitoneum is very occasionally necessary for giant hernias – when viscera are in a hernia sac for long periods of time, they lose the 'right of domicile' in the abdominal cavity; replacing them suddenly into the abdomen is associated with the dangers of respiratory embarrassment, compression of the inferior vena cava and paralytic ileus.

These complications can be averted by preparing the patient and the abdominal cavity by repeated intra-peritoneal injections of air over the 2 weeks before operation, up to a total of 2.5 L.

Elective operations are now largely done as either day or short stay procedures and patients are encouraged to resume normal activities as soon as possible. Groin hernias are often repaired by a laparoscopic approach, which has marginal benefits in reduction in pain and early return to work although long-term results are not yet available.

Strangulation is a surgical emergency which still carries a high mortality rate, particularly if, for any reason, operation is delayed.

Surgical techniques

Herniotomy is the removal of the sac and closure of its neck. It is the first step in nearly every hernia repair and in some instances (e.g. infant inguinal hernia – see below) may be all that is required.

Herniorrhaphy involves some sort of reconstruction to:

- restore the anatomy if this is disturbed
- increase the strength of the abdominal wall
- construct a barrier to recurrence.

The first of these is usually possible by suture. The second and third may be achieved with local tissue, but some form of darn or the insertion of prosthetic mesh is also widely used.

Obstruction and strangulation

The patient nearly always requires treatment of the associated obstruction of the gut.

Non-operative treatment can be considered in:

- infants
- obstructed hernia with a short history – less than 2 hours and previous evidence of reducibility. If the presentation is rapid (within 2 hours of onset) in a hernia that was previously reducible and there are no signs to suggest strangulation.

The patient is put in the head-down position and an ice pack may be applied; then an attempt is made to reduce the hernia by taxis, which consists of gentle manipulation of the swelling in the direction of the hernial orifice. Considerable experience is required. There is no place for vigorous manipulation, which carries the obvious danger of damage to the bowel or reduction en masse – reduction of the sac and its contents but with persistent trapping of the latter so that strangulation progresses.

Urgent operation is needed in the great majority of obstructed or strangulated hernias. The hernial sac and its contents are exposed and the constriction or other cause of obstruction relieved. Further surgery may be required to remove ischaemic bowel or omentum. For the reasons given above, strangulated bowel implies bacterial translocation and antibiotics are administered.

OUTCOME

Mortality

For elective repair the overall mortality is less than 0.5% but increases with age to approximately 0.5–1% for those over 60 years. For emergency operations it is 10 times greater. It is a sobering observation that the mortality for strangulated obstructing hernia has remained unchanged at around the 20% for the last 50 years. Death is dependent on:

- age – older patients have a higher incidence of intercurrent disease
- contents of the sac – gangrenous intestine (present in 10% of strangulated hernias) is associated with a 40% mortality rate.

Morbidity

The overall complication rate is around 7%. Any of the complications that beset surgery can occur during or after operations for hernia. Specific to the procedure are:

- persistent wound pain – often ascribed to a neuroma which forms after damage to or division of the ilio-inguinal or other nerve
- cutaneous anaesthesia – division of a nerve
- Recurrent hernia.

The rate of recurrence is between less than 1 to 10% for primary hernias (depending on the type) and 5–30% for recurrent hernias. Recurrence is associated with:

- age – the older the patient, the more likely is the hernia to recur
- presence or absence of predisposing factors
- site
- size – the larger the hernia, the more likely it is to have distorted the surrounding anatomy
- emergency or elective operation – the former being more likely to be associated with recurrence
- operation on a recurrent hernia – more difficult and more likely to fail
- experience of the surgeon.

See below for further consideration of recurrent hernias.

Specific hernias

Inguinal hernia

Inguinal hernias account for 80% of all external abdominal hernias. They occur at all ages, but are most common in infants and the elderly. Inguinal hernias are 20 times more common in men than in women, and more frequently occur on the right side.

ANATOMY

The inguinal canal (Fig. 26.5) runs in an antero-inferior direction from the internal to external inguinal rings

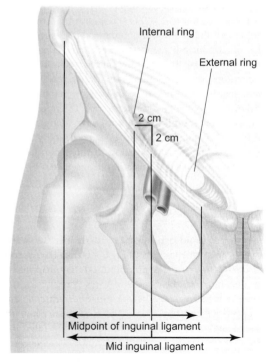

Fig 26.5 **The inguinal canal.**

and, in the male, is the path taken by the testis to reach the scrotum. In that sex, therefore, it contains the spermatic vessels and the vas deferens; in the female it only contains the round ligament. The internal ring lies 2 cm or slightly more above and 2 cm lateral to the mid-inguinal point – that point on the inguinal ligament midway between the anterior superior iliac spine and the symphysis pubis. To find it, the femoral artery is identified as it passes deep to the mid-inguinal point and the fingers are moved upwards and laterally. The medial aspect of the ring is bounded by the inferior epigastric branch of the femoral artery. The external ring is just above the pubic crest and tubercle to which the inguinal ligament is attached. In infants the internal and external rings are directly one behind the other but during growth they move apart.

The inguinal region and canal, particularly in the male, is a vulnerable area for the formation of hernia, but this is to some extent offset by contraction of the abdominal muscles, which compresses together the anterior and posterior walls of the canal and allows descent of the conjoint tendon to act as a partial shutter.

It is further thought that the cremaster muscle bunches the cord up into the canal so acting as a plug.

CLASSIFICATION

Indirect inguinal hernia
This passes through the internal ring lateral to the inferior epigastric artery and along the canal to emerge at the external ring above the pubic crest and tubercle. Its coverings are the attenuated layers of the cord.

Direct inguinal hernia
This hernia bulges through the posterior wall of the canal medial to the inferior epigastric artery and is therefore not covered by the layers of the cord.

Pantaloon hernia
This is a combination of both an indirect and a direct inguinal hernia.

AETIOLOGY

Indirect hernia
In an indirect hernia, there is a congenital sac or potential sac which is the remnant of the processus vaginalis. If the processus does not close, then an indirect hernia occurs in early life but other factors may lead to it reopening at any age. Indirect hernias are 20 times more common in men than in women. Sixty per cent occur on the right (possibly contributed to by damage to the motor nerves of the abdominal muscles at open appendicectomy), 40% on the left and 20% are bilateral.

Direct hernia
This is an acquired lesion. For reasons unknown

though contributed to by accessory factors such as the wear and tear of advancing age, repeated straining and raised intra-abdominal pressure, the posterior wall of the inguinal canal becomes attenuated. Direct hernia is therefore a condition of later life and is rarely seen under the age of 40.

CLINICAL FINDINGS
If it is impossible to get above a groin swelling it is most likely to be an inguinal hernia. In both indirect and direct hernias, the cough impulse that can be seen or palpated must be distinguished from normal diffuse bulging in the inguinal region, particularly in individuals of spare build. The principal differences between the two types of hernia on clinical examination are summarised in Table 26.3.

In addition to the features outlined in Table 26.3, an indirect hernia that extends beyond the external ring appears above and medial to the pubic tubercle, in contrast to a femoral hernia (see below) which is below and lateral to that bony point. The pubic tubercle can be found either by feeling laterally along the pubic crest from the upper border of the symphysis pubic or by following the adductor longus tendon from the medial side of the thigh to its origin from the body of the pubis. The tubercle is directly above.

One of the most useful methods of distinction between the two kinds of inguinal hernia is that a reducible indirect hernia can be completely controlled with a fingertip placed firmly over the internal ring.

For the clinical features and management of an infantile inguinal hernia, see Chapter 35.

Other causes of groin swelling
Although inguinal hernias are relatively easy to diagnose, there are a considerable number of other causes of

Table 26.3
Differences between an indirect and a direct inguinal hernia

	Indirect	Direct
Patient's age	Any age but usually young	Older
Cause	May be congenital	Acquired
Bilateral	20%	50%
Protrusion on coughing	Oblique	Straight
Appearance on standing	Does not reach full size immediately	Reaches full size immediately
Reduction on lying down	May not reduce immediately	Reduces immediately
Descent into scrotum	Common	Rare
Occlusion of internal ring	Controls	Does not control
Neck of sac	Narrow	Wide
Strangulation	Not uncommon	Unusual
Relation to inferior epigastric vessels	Lateral	Medial

swelling in this area that may require consideration when a lump is encountered. These include:

- femoral hernia
- hydrocele
- encysted hydrocele of the cord or of the peritoneovaginal canal
- undescended or ectopic testis
- lipoma of the cord
- epididymal cyst.

MANAGEMENT

The general principles of hernia management have been given above. Most adult inguinal hernias are repaired by open operation under local or general anaesthesia as a day case procedure. Elderly patients and those with serious medical problems require in-patient care. Open operation usually means a layered suture technique (Shouldice) or the insertion of a non-absorbable prosthetic mesh (Lichtenstein). Alternatively, mesh repair may be done through the endoscope – laparoscopy or pre-peritoneal endoscopy. These newer minimally invasive methods are currently being evaluated but, at least in the short term, appear to produce satisfactory results. They may find an additional role in the repair of recurrent and bilateral hernias (see below).

Specific complications

- *Urinary retention.* Because of the proximity of the inguinal region to urine excretion in the male, temporary problems may be encountered, but with modern techniques these are rare unless benign prostatic hyperplasia has been overlooked in the preoperative evaluation.
- *A scrotal haematoma* may follow extensive dissection.
- *Damage to the ilio-inguinal nerve* produces an area of anaesthesia over the pubic tubercle, scrotum or labia.

OUTCOME

Recurrence rates for inguinal hernia is one of the most hotly debated subjects in general surgery. With selection of patients only after adequate evaluation of contributing factors and with good technique, recurrence rates for groin hernias should be less than 1%. It is more widely quoted as 3% for primary hernias and up to 30% in the management of recurrence. However, such rates should be balanced against the population under study, the technique used and the quality of follow-up.

RECURRENT INGUINAL HERNIA

Even with what seems to be optimal operative technique, hernias recur. Factors involved in recurrence include:

- *Inadequate preoperative selection* – those with uncorrectable precipitating factors or on high-dose steroid therapy which interferes with healing

- *Type of hernia* – indirect hernias have a 1–7% recurrence rate but direct hernias reach 4–10%
- *Type of operation* – repairs under tension do not heal with adequate protection against recurrence
- *Postoperative wound infection.*

MANAGEMENT OF RECURRENCE

Recurrent inguinal hernias should be repaired in order to avoid the same complications that occur in primary hernias, which are even more likely when recurrence has taken place. Because of scarring, the dissection can be difficult and, in the male, orchidectomy is sometimes performed to allow closure of the deep ring. Recurrent hernias may be best managed by the endoscopic insertion of a mesh.

Femoral hernia

With femoral, the local pain the patient may not mention, while to the tiny lump in groin she does not call attention (On Strangulated Femoral Hernia – Zachary Cope, 1947).

Femoral hernias are acquired downward protrusions of peritoneum into the potential space of the femoral canal (Fig. 26.6). They account for 7% of all hernias but, in that they are four times more common in women than in men, 33% of groin hernias in females (5% in men). They are most common in late middle age and the

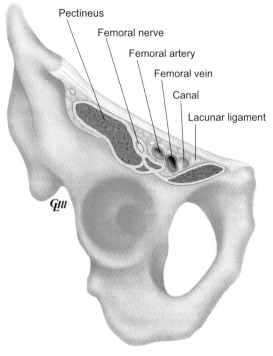

Fig 26.6 **Femoral hernia.**

multiparous and, unlike inguinal hernias, are rare in children. Bilateral hernias occur in 20%.

ANATOMY

The femoral canal is a 1.2 cm gap medial to the femoral sheath and femoral vein which contains a lymph node and fat. Its anterior (inguinal ligament), medial (lacunar part of the inguinal ligament) and posterior (pectineal part of the inguinal ligament) boundaries are rigid (Fig. 26.6): This narrow femoral ring produces a considerable risk of incarceration of any hernia that passes through it.

AETIOLOGY AND PATHOLOGICAL FEATURES

As mentioned above, the hernia is acquired. The wide pelvis of the female and the laxity of ligaments after repeated pregnancy are contributory factors, as is weight loss. As the sac develops, it passes forwards through the saphenous opening whose well-defined lower edge directs it upwards to lie over the inguinal ligament in the subcutaneous plane.

The narrow canal makes femoral hernia the one most likely to result in a Richter's hernia (30% of strangulated femoral hernias), although strangulation of an omental plug also takes place.

CLINICAL FEATURES

History

The patient is typically a middle-aged or elderly female, often of thin build, who complains of an intermittent lump low in the groin. However, a major problem is that she may not have noticed the lump and the first clinical presentation is with strangulation (see below), which occurs in 20%.

Signs

In a small hernia, a cough impulse is only rarely detected. A larger hernia may be seen to bulge on straining just below the medial part of the inguinal ligament. An irreducible hernia is a lump whose consistency varies according to its contents, which may for the reasons given above straddle the inguinal ligament. In consequence, it can be difficult to distinguish from an inguinal hernia but the upper medial border of a femoral hernia is always below and lateral to the pubic tubercle. The other conditions that should be taken into consideration when a femoral hernia is diagnosed are shown in Table 26.4.

Strangulation

In contrast to a strangulated inguinal hernia, in a strangulated femoral hernia there are often no localising symptoms and signs and the lump is often small, unimpressive and overlooked by the patient (and perhaps the clinician). The classic presentation is that of small bowel obstruction. However, the clinical features of this

Table 26.4
Inguinal swellings which may resemble a femoral hernia

Condition	Findings
Inguinal hernia	Swelling is above and medial to the public tubercle
Saphena varix	Compressible
	Palpable thrill on coughing
Enlarged lymph node	Usually multiple
	Not fixed on deep aspect and therefore more mobile
	Seek cause – infection, tumour, reticulosis
Lipoma	Soft but not reducible
Femoral artery aneurysm	Expanding pulsation
	Bruit
Psoas abscess	Fluctuant
	Lateral to femoral artery
	Associated swelling in the iliac fossa
Ectopic testis	Empty scrotum

may be modified by the presence of a Richter's hernia which only partly obstructs the lumen of the gut so that the symptoms and signs are more like gastroenteritis. This, combined with the difficulty in finding the hernia, makes for a late diagnosis, sometimes only after the gut has perforated and there is spreading peritonitis.

MANAGEMENT

All femoral hernias should be repaired without delay because of their great risk of strangulation. A truss has no place in management because it cannot control the hernia. The principles are given above. In elective operations, repair is usually by direct incision over the hernia, excision of the sac and sutured closure of the femoral canal. For operation on a patient with obstruction or strangulation, it may be necessary to open the abdomen to find the segment of gut that has been trapped should it reduce before it can be dealt with.

Umbilical hernia

Congenital (infantile) umbilical hernia

This condition is considered in Chapter 35.

Adult umbilical hernia

Only a small minority of adult umbilical hernias are the outcome of the persistence of a congenital defect.

AETIOLOGY AND ANATOMICAL AND PATHOLOGICAL FEATURES

Two types of hernia occur with overlapping but different aetiological factors of clinical importance.

True umbilical hernia (Fig. 26.7)

In this condition, the protrusion is through the umbilical scar, everting the umbilicus whose attenuated fibres are at the apex of the hernial sac. The cause is often secondary to an increase in the volume of contents of the abdominal cavity – e.g. due to obesity, ascites or large benign or malignant intra-abdominal tumours.

Para-umbilical hernia (Fig. 26.8)

The weakest area of the umbilical scar is at the superior aspect between the umbilical vein and the upper margin of the umbilical ring. It is at this point that a para-umbilical hernia develops. The emerging sac displaces the umbilical scar which lies below and slightly to one side.

These hernias are more common than true umbilical hernias and typically are found in the obese middle-aged patient. Women are affected five times more frequently than men. Generalised inadequacy of the musculofascial layers of the abdominal wall and repeated pregnancy are important contributory factors.

The neck of the hernia is often narrow. In consequence, tissues that enter have great difficulty leaving; adhesions form and the hernia becomes irreducible. The sac progressively acquires more contents and may become very large. The contents are usually omentum, often with small bowel or transverse colon. Frequently the sac becomes loculated when adhesions form between the omentum and the peritoneum. Not surprisingly, these hernias are at great risk of strangulation.

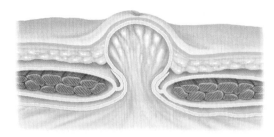

Fig 26.7 **Umbilical hernia.**

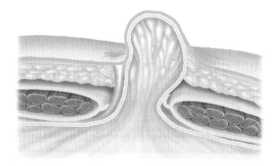

Fig 26.8 **Para-umbilical hernia.**

CLINICAL FEATURES

True umbilical hernia

Symptoms

These are often of an underlying cause of ascites or there may merely be gross obesity. Very rarely the patient will give a history which dates back to infancy or childhood.

Signs

Ascites may be obvious. The umbilicus is attenuated and sometimes paper-thin. Evidence of underlying malignancy should be sought both in the abdomen as a whole and at the umbilical opening where a nodule or nodules may be palpable.

Para-umbilical hernia

Symptoms

There is local pain and a swelling at the navel. Non-specific gastrointestinal symptoms are common and features of recurrent intestinal obstruction may have occurred.

Signs

The umbilicus assumes a crescent shape. Inspection and palpation reveal a swelling just above the umbilicus whose centre (in contrast to true umbilical hernia) is not attached to the apex of the protrusion. However, in grossly obese patients, the swelling may not be obvious to the naked eye and moreover is barely palpable. In others the hernia may be enormous. Usually it is reducible (at least in part) and there is a cough impulse. If reduction is possible, the palpable defect can be of any size, from one fingertip to admitting the fist.

Conditions that may be confused with a para-umbilical hernia include:

- cyst of the vitello-intestinal duct (rare)
- cyst of the urachus (also rare)
- metastatic tumour deposit.

MANAGEMENT

True umbilical hernia

Any underlying cause should be sought and dealt with. In the rare event that nothing is found and the hernia is causing symptoms, it is treated as a para-umbilical hernia.

Para-umbilical hernia

Symptomatic hernias require treatment. There is a high risk of strangulation and repair should be advised, even in the absence of symptoms. The usual procedure is to mobilise the sac and its contents, return the latter to the abdomen, close the neck and repair the abdominal wall by overlapping its layers (Fig. 26.9).

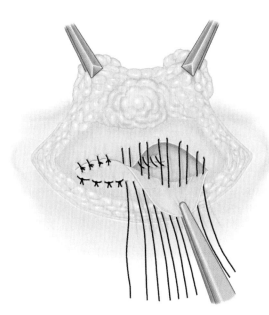

Fig 26.9 **Repair of a para-umbilical hernia.**

Strangulated umbilical hernia

The patient with severe abdominal pain and vomiting and a soft non-tender umbilical hernia is a diagnostic trap. The loculated nature of the hernia allows a strangulated portion of bowel (often of the Richter's type) to go unnoticed clinically. In other instances, the local features of strangulation may be obvious. The operative approach is as for an elective case, and the strangulating contents are dealt with according to their state.

Epigastric hernia

ANATOMY

The linea alba is the raphe formed by the junction of the rectus sheaths and the decussation of their fibres across the midline; it extends from the xiphoid process to the symphysis pubis. In its upper half, it is 1–3 cm wide and fibrous, but below the umbilicus it is a narrow cord.

PATHOLOGICAL FEATURES

The linea may be attenuated because of a congenital weakness in its lattice structure. Small neurovascular bundles that penetrate are also points of diminished resistance. Herniations of extraperitoneal fat through the linea usually occur in its upper half. They are found in 1% of the population from adolescence onwards. Males are three times more commonly affected than females and the protrusions are multiple in 20% of cases. The initial extraperitoneal fat protrusion may be followed by the formation of a peritoneal sac and omentum may enter this (visceral contents are rare).

Extraperitoneal fat or omentum is frequently incarcerated and may strangulate.

CLINICAL FEATURES

Symptoms

Three-quarters of epigastric hernias are asymptomatic and found incidentally on physical examination. When symptoms are present they are of two types:

- local pain – often exacerbated by physical exertion
- ill-defined pain – epigastric in site, often worse after meals (abdominal distension may strangulate the contents) and the clinical picture may mimic that of peptic ulceration.

Signs

The hernia may be visible if the patient is placed in an oblique light. The swelling is palpable in the midline and is usually tender and irreducible.

A patient who presents with vague upper abdominal symptoms and in whom an epigastric hernia is found should be fully investigated for the possibility of peptic ulcer, gall bladder or pancreatic disease before symptoms are attributed to the hernia.

MANAGEMENT

Patients with symptomatic hernias are offered repair. The herniated fat is excised. If a sac is present, the contents are reduced and the sac excised. The fascial defect is closed by suture. Any coincidental defects are similarly dealt with at the same time.

Incisional hernia

An incisional hernia is one that occurs through the wound of a previous operation. It has the same features as a hernia that is caused by non-surgical injury to the abdominal wall.

It is realistic to expect that 1% of transparietal abdominal incisions are followed by a hernia. Such hernias comprise 10% of the total number seen.

AETIOLOGY

Partial dehiscence of all or part of the deeper fascial layers occurs, but the skin remains intact or eventually heals. An incisional hernia is a postoperative complication and, like all such complications, its cause can be considered in terms of three factors:

- preoperative
- operative
- postoperative

Preoperative factors

- *Age* – the tissues of the elderly do not heal as well as those of the young

- *Malnutrition* – protein-calorie malnutrition, vitamin deficiency (vitamin C is essential for collagen maturation) and trace metal deficiency (zinc is required for epithelialisation).
- *Sepsis* – worsens malnutrition and delays anabolism
- *Uraemia* – inhibits fibroblast division
- *Jaundice* – impedes collagen maturation
- *Obesity* – predisposes to wound infection, seroma and haematoma
- *Diabetes mellitus* – predisposes to wound infection
- *Steroids* – have a generalised proteolytic effect
- *Peritoneal contamination (peritonitis)* – predisposes to wound infection.

Operative factors

- *Type of incision* – vertical incisions are more prone to hernia than are transverse ones
- *Technique and materials* – tension in the closure impedes blood supply to the wound; badly tied knots can work loose; closure with absorbable suture material fails to support the abdominal wall for a sufficient time to permit sound union
- *Type of operation* – operations involving the bowel or urinary tract are more likely to develop wound infection
- *Drains* – a drain passing through the wound often results in a hernia.

Postoperative factors

- *Wound infection* – equal in importance with the wrong choice of suture material: there is enzymic destruction of healing tissues; inflammatory swelling raises tissue tension and impedes blood supply; 5–20% of wound infections result in a hernia
- *Abdominal distension* – postoperative ileus increases the tension on a wound; stitches may cut out
- *Coughing* – generates wound tension.

Approximately 40% of incisional hernias occur with a documented episode of wound infection.

PATHOLOGICAL FEATURES

Most incisional hernias develop within 1 year of an operation, and it is unusual for a previously sound closure to become herniated after 3 years. Once a hernia has formed, mechanical forces ensure that it inexorably enlarges.

Incisional hernias are extremely variable. They may be wide or narrow-necked; often as contents accumulate, adhesions develop in the sac, and just deep to the neck, so that the hernia becomes both irreducible and loculated. Incarceration and strangulation then become real dangers. The sac can assume huge proportions, eventually housing much of the normal intraperitoneal contents.

CLINICAL FEATURES

Symptoms

There may have been a stormy convalescence from a surgical procedure. The complaint is of a bulge in the scar. As the hernia enlarges and loculates, symptoms of subacute intestinal obstruction are common. The hernia may give rise to local discomfort. The overlying skin may become thin and atrophic; eventually ulceration and even rupture can occur. Strangulation is a surgical emergency.

Signs

Examination reveals a readily apparent, usually reducible, hernia with a cough impulse at the site of an old scar. If the hernia is complex, many fibrous bands may be felt passing between the margins of the defect. When the patient is lying flat, these hernias are deceptively small but any manoeuvre that raises intra-abdominal pressure produces the hernia in all its glory.

MANAGEMENT

Even small symptomatic hernias should be repaired early. In asymptomatic hernias the risks of intestinal obstruction, strangulation and skin ulceration are such that repair, even in older patients, is also recommended. Protracted observation simply allows the hernia to increase in size and subsequent repair is rendered more difficult and hazardous. The surgical technique is the same as for paraumbilical hernias, but very large hernias may require prosthetic mesh reconstruction of the abdominal wall.

OUTCOME

The results of surgery are not as good as for primary hernias. Small incisional hernias have a recurrence rate of 2–5%, whereas in large ones it is 10–20%.

Rare but clinically important hernias

The following hernias comprise only 1% of the total but they are considered because their recognition is of clinical importance.

Interparietal hernia (Fig. 26.10)

The hernial sac lies between the layers of the abdominal wall. The cause may be congenital, when there is an associated abnormality of testicular descent, or acquired in an area of weakness in the lateral aspect of the deep inguinal ring and inguinal canal (when the sac usually communicates with a concomitant indirect inguinal hernia). The classification of such hernias is based on the anatomical location of the sac:

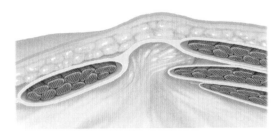

Fig 26.10 **Interparietal hernia.**

- properitoneal (20%)
- interstitial (60%)
- superficial (20%)

CLINICAL FEATURES

The *properitoneal* type of hernia is impalpable. The *interstitial* and *superficial* types often present with a small swelling above and lateral to the inguinal canal and deep ring. Such insignificant local features are ignored by patients, and 90% of these hernias present with intestinal obstruction that culminates in strangulation. The key to early diagnosis is to consider this type of hernia in any patient with the features of intestinal obstruction (simple or strangulating) with a palpable mass lateral to the deep ring and an abnormally placed testis.

MANAGEMENT

Operation (usually an emergency laparotomy for strangulating obstruction of unknown cause) reveals the hernial sac, which is excised and the fascial defect repaired.

Spigelian hernia

This is an interparietal hernia in the line of the linea semilunaris (the lateral margin of the rectus sheath, running from the tip of the ninth costal cartilage to the pubic crest). The hernia is usually at the level of the arcuate line, below which all aponeurotic layers are reflected anterior to the rectus muscle. The cause is related to the aponeurotic arrangement, which results in an area of weakness where fibres from the transversus aponeurosis fuse with those from the internal oblique. The hernial sac emerges and enlarges like a mushroom deep to the external oblique.

CLINICAL FEATURES

Symptoms

- Local pain that is worse on straining
- Lump
- Non-specific lower quadrant discomfort which needs to be investigated in its own right
- Features of obstruction or strangulation.

Signs

- Tenderness at the site of the hernial orifice
- Lump may be difficult or even impossible to feel.

INVESTIGATION AND MANAGEMENT

Recently, ultrasonography has proved useful in the demonstration of these hernias in patients with convincing histories but who lack clinical signs.

Repair is a simple matter of excising the sac and closing the defect.

Obturator hernia

In this condition, herniation occurs along the obturator canal which carries the obturator nerve and vessels out of the pelvis (Fig. 26.11). It is most commonly seen in frail old ladies. The hernia starts as a preperitoneal plug and gradually enlarges taking a sac of peritoneum with it. A loop of bowel may enter the sac and reduce spontaneously. Eventually a knuckle fails to reduce. Further loops can then be incorporated. A Richter's strangulation is common.

CLINICAL FEATURES

Symptoms

Lying deep to the pectineus, these hernias are largely asymptomatic until complicated by intestinal obstruction or strangulation. There is often a past history of intermittent symptoms of obstruction. In about 50% there may be the complaint of pain along the upper

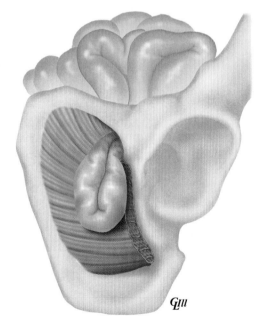

Fig 26.11 **Obturator hernia.**

medial side of the thigh which radiates down to the knee but, though present, this is not often elicited.

Signs

There are rarely any signs, except those of obstruction or strangulation. The diagnosis is made in most instances at the time of laparotomy for small bowel obstruction of unknown cause. With pressure on the obturator nerve, the patient holds the leg flexed to reduce the pain. In 20% of patients, the hernial sac protrudes medially around the pectineus and presents as a palpable swelling in the femoral triangle. Rectal and especially vaginal examination can reveal a swelling in the region of the obturator foramen.

MANAGEMENT

If discovered at laparotomy, the intestine is reduced, the sac withdrawn and the defect closed. If the diagnosis is made clinically, an elective procedure by the retropubic, pre-peritoneal approach can be done.

Lumbar hernia

Such hernias may be:

- congenital
- acquired primary
- acquired secondary – the result of surgical incision.

Acquired hernias through an incision for lumbar approach to the kidney are not uncommon, however, with the decline in open renal surgery they are becoming less common.

Acquired primary lumbar hernia

Hernias that occur through anatomical weak points in the lumbar region – the superior and inferior lumbar triangles (Fig. 26.12) – are uncommon.

CLINICAL FEATURES

Most present with a bulge or lump in the flank, associated with an aching discomfort. There is usually a cough impulse and the mass is reducible. The contents are most often small and large bowel – very rarely the kidney. Some 20% become incarcerated and 10% strangulate.

An irreducible lumbar hernia must be distinguished from;

- lipoma
- soft tissue tumour
- haematoma
- tuberculous cold abscess
- renal tumour.

MANAGEMENT

Primary hernias are managed by direct closure of the defect. Large incisional hernias require a mesh prosthesis.

Sciatic hernia

A sciatic hernia is the protrusion of a pelvic peritoneal sac through the greater or lesser sciatic foramen (Fig. 26.13).

CLINICAL FEATURES

Patients present with discomfort and a swelling in the buttock and there may be symptoms of sciatic nerve

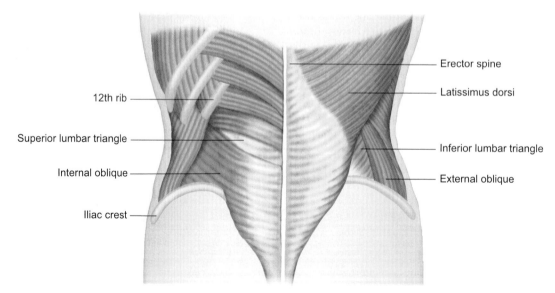

12th rib

Superior lumbar triangle

Internal oblique

Iliac crest

Erector spine

Latissimus dorsi

Inferior lumbar triangle

External oblique

Fig 26.12 **Lumbar hernia.**

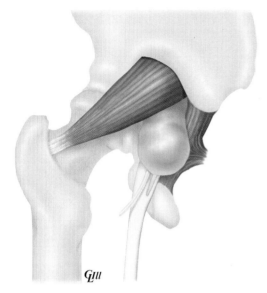

Fig 26.13 **Sciatic hernia.**

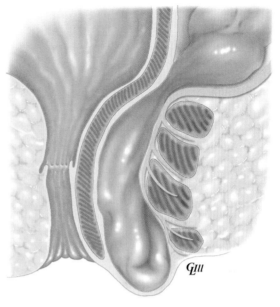

Fig 26.14 **Perineal hernia.**

compression. If the hernia is large, there is a reducible mass in the gluteal area, made larger on standing. Herniation of the ureters can cause urinary symptoms. There is an appreciable risk of strangulation.

MANAGEMENT
Treatment is by excision of the sac and closure of the defect by a transabdominal or transgluteal approach.

Perineal hernia

These may be:

- congenital
- primary acquired
- incisional.

Primary acquired perineal hernias occur in middle-aged, multiparous women. Their broad pelvis and the muscle-weakening effect of childbirth result in herniation

through the pelvic floor. Incisional perineal hernia follows 1% of combined abdominoperineal excisions of the rectum. Perineal hernia is classified on the basis of its relationship to the transverse perineal muscles (Fig. 26.14).

CLINICAL FEATURES
There is usually a perineal swelling and discomfort when sitting. A soft mass is found in the perineum, which is usually reducible. The wide neck has elastic margins. These hernias rarely have dangerous complications.

MANAGEMENT
Repair is by a combined abdominal and pelvic approach. The hernia is approached from below, the sac dissected free and reduced into the abdominal cavity. A laparotomy is performed and the pelvic floor repaired from above.

Breast disease

Breast symptoms are a common reason for patients to visit their doctor and many are concerned that they have breast cancer. In fact, only 1 in 10 patients referred to surgical clinics has a carcinoma – the remainder have a variety of conditions going under the general title of 'benign breast disease'. Many of the conditions that this term encompasses are not truly diseases but rather aberrations of normal development-involution of the breast that occur from puberty to old age. For this reason benign breast diseases are sometimes referred to under the ANDI classification (**Ab**Normal **D**evelopment and **I**nvolution) which highlights the relationship between normal stages of breast growth and the aberrations which represent a true disease.

Benign breast disease

Pubertal problems

Males
One of the earliest benign problems occurs in pubertal males rather than females when hormonal stimulation of male breast buds at the time of puberty results in often embarrassing rudimentary growth – *gynaecomastia*. The same condition occurs in old age when certain drugs (digoxin, diuretics, cimetidine) and conditions (cirrhosis of the liver) can, by interfering with sex hormone metabolism, induce growth of the breast buds. Very rarely the same problem can be induced by hormone-producing tumours.

Females
At puberty, excessive development is known as *juvenile hypertrophy* and is characterised by the growth of very large breasts which are both uncomfortable and embarrassing.

Common breast symptoms in benign disease

Patients present with one or more of the following symptoms or signs:

Breast disease

- pain – cyclical or non-cyclical
- lumpiness and lumps
- nipple discharge
- trauma
- infection.

The common conditions underlying these symptoms are summarised in Figure 27.1.

Pain

This is either cyclical or non-cyclical. The first follows the pattern of the menstrual cycle; the second is random in timing.

Cyclical pain

Onset is during the early phase of the cycle; intensity gradually worsens to reach a peak just before menstruation, easing with the start of the period. In its mildest form, the pain affects the upper outer quadrants of the breasts and causes only minor inconvenience. In more severe instances, the whole breast may feel engorged, tender and heavy; physical contact can be unbearable which often leads to psychological distress. Some postmenopausal women get breast pain which is often related to the use of hormone replacement therapy, in that this keeps the cells of the breast active.

Not every instance follows such a clear-cut clinical pattern. Pain may be in one breast only and some may experience pain nearly all the time, although this tends to get worse as menstruation approaches. There is no clear-cut explanation for these wide variations but they are probably related to subtle differences in hormone responsiveness and sensitivity within the breast which may vary throughout life. Such variable thresholds could also account for the fact that some patients go through very bad patches which disappear as abruptly as they start.

There are few clinical findings apart from tenderness and a firm nodular feel in the upper outer quadrants of the breast.

INVESTIGATION
In the presence of a typical history of bilateral cyclical pain, there is often little reason to embark on any investigations. Mammograms are of no diagnostic help and are difficult to interpret in women under 35, the group most frequently affected by this problem. The only value they may serve is to exclude an underlying cancer in patients whose pain is atypical or is coincidental with a lump. A pain chart in which patients record their pain and its intensity is sometimes useful in determining whether the problem is truly cyclical or non-cyclical.

MANAGEMENT
The most important aspect is reassurance that the condition is entirely benign and is not associated with either carcinoma or a tendency to its development in later life. Many are content to live with their discomfort if they can be reassured on both these counts.

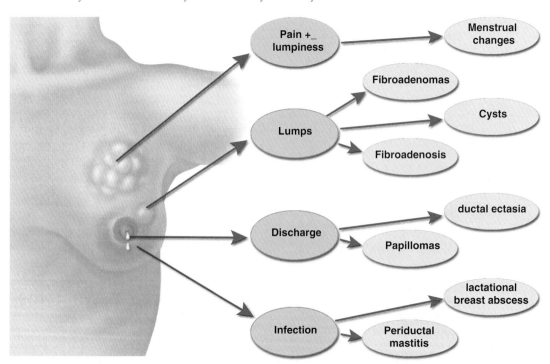

Fig 27.1 **Common causes of breast symptoms.**

For patients whose symptoms are severe enough for them to desire symptomatic treatment, three drugs are commonly used: gamma-linoleic acid, danazol and bromocriptine. Gamma-linoleic acid (most easily available in the form of evening primrose oil) is an essential fatty acid which is thought to work by rendering breast cells less sensitive to the effects of sex hormones; 60% of sufferers experience relief, but to be of therapeutic value it needs to be taken in full dose (320 mg daily) for 3–4 months before a benefit is really experienced.

Danazol interferes with the action of oestrogen on breast tissue and bromocriptine blocks the pituitary drive to produce follicle-stimulating hormone (FSH) and luteinising hormone (LH). Both danazol and bromocriptine are effective, but at the price of side-effects which are similar to those experienced in the menopause: danazol is usually given in doses of 200–300 mg daily and bromocriptine in gradually increasing doses of up to 5 mg daily.

These treatments are effective for typical cyclical pain but are less satisfactory when the pain is not quite so typical.

Non-cyclical pain

This may be intermittent or constant and confined to localised areas of one breast. It can be caused by conditions both within and without the breast, including:

- mammary duct ectasia
- periductal mastitis
- trauma
- Tietze's disorder – characterised by tenderness over the costochondral junctions.

It is often difficult to identify a specific cause of non-cyclical pain and a caring general physician may be the best person to look into the background of such patients.

INVESTIGATION

As with cyclical breast pain, investigation in those under the age of 35 is limited to clinical assessment. However, in older women, mammography is often a wise precaution, particularly if the pain is consistently localised to one spot or associated with a lump. A small number (10%) with such features have an underlying carcinoma.

MANAGEMENT

Non-cyclical pain is much more resistant to treatment than is cyclical breast pain. Hormonal manipulation is often ineffective but worth trying, as is firm support to the often large breasts. Simple NSAIDs, treatment of inflammatory conditions or an injection of lignocaine and steroid into the area may all be helpful. Quite a large number find all treatment of little benefit and end up having to live with their pain until it resolves by itself, which in the great majority it eventually does.

Breast lumpiness and lumps

The potential diagnoses in a patient who presents with a breast lump depend on whether it is a part of a diffuse lumpiness or a single discrete isolated lump. Other features which may influence the diagnosis are whether the lump is painful and the age of the patient.

Until recently, it was axiomatic that any palpable breast abnormality should undergo excision biopsy in case a cancer, however unlikely, might be overlooked. A recent major change in management has been a shift from this approach to the use of physical examination, radiological imaging (mammography) and fine needle biopsy to reach a definitive diagnosis – the 'triple approach'. In consequence, there are now fewer open biopsies which lead to a diagnosis of benign disease; the current ratio of benign to malignant biopsy is 0.6:1.

However, mammography is of little value in women under 35 years of age because the breasts are frequently too dense for small lesions to be seen. Some radiologists feel that this is also true for women up to the age of 40 and in consequence do not recommend mammography below this age. For women unsuitable for mammography, ultrasound offers a useful tool for evaluating palpable lesions but is a very poor method of general screening of the breast to exclude malignant disease.

Lumpiness. Lumpiness can present on its own but is frequently associated with cyclical breast pain. In common with pain, it is a manifestation of the cyclical changes that go on in the female breast during the menstrual years. A variety of descriptive terms have been applied to it:

- fibroadenosis
- cystic mastopathy
- fibrocystic disease
- cystic mastitis.

All are merely descriptive of the changes seen to a varying degree on histological examination and do not give any insight into cause. Their use carries the danger that the clinical condition becomes labelled as a disease when it is in fact part of the spectrum of normal behaviour of the breast which in some individuals is more pronounced.

Discrete single lump. The common causes of a lump are:

- fibroadenoma
- cyst
- very localised fibroadenosis.

The feature uniting them all is the well-defined nature of the lump.

Fibroadenosis

CLINICAL FEATURES

History

The encouragement of women to undertake regular self-examination may draw attention to the possible presence of a lump or of changes in consistency. Alternatively, cyclical or non-cyclical pain may lead to the discovery of what the patient regards as a lump. Usually, the upper outer quadrants are affected but, as with pain, one side alone may be involved. The majority of women who seek medical advice are young, often in the early years after the menarche.

Physical findings

There may be single or multiple lumps in one or both breasts, which may be acutely tender, particularly premenstrually.

INVESTIGATION

Imaging

Mammography is indicated in those over the age of 40 (see also 'Breast cancer', p. 000). In a lumpy breast, the appearances are those of dense fibrosis with micro- or macrocystic change.

Ultrasound is, as suggested above, indicated for those under 40 who may show cystic changes.

Fine needle aspiration cytology (FNAC)

Suspicious areas are aspirated under image control. Typical findings are of benign cells.

MANAGEMENT

Provided that imaging and FNAC have eliminated the diagnosis of malignancy, the essential treatment is reassurance based on the concept that the changes are part of the normal spectrum of the breast response to female sex hormones. If there is associated pain in a large breast, firm support may help.

Fibroadenoma

These tend to affect younger women and are infrequent after about 35–40 years of age.

PATHOLOGICAL FEATURES

Many remain static and a small proportion either regress or increase in size. In developing countries, they may reach a mass larger than the breast in which the growth occurs.

CLINICAL FEATURES

Generally, the patient discovers the lump. Pain and other symptoms are absent. A rare variant, usually in older women, is known as a phylloides tumour.

Physical findings are of a well defined lump, nearly always in an otherwise normal breast. The consistency is rubbery to firm or hard and there is such mobility that it may be difficult to find – hence the nickname 'breast mouse'.

INVESTIGATION AND MANAGEMENT

As with any discrete lump they should be subjected to triple assessment (clinical examination, imaging and FNAC). Provided all these support a diagnosis of fibroadenoma, small lesions can be left alone. However, larger lesions (> 4 cm) or those in older women may be better removed. Some authorities advocate repeating the assessment at 3 months if a conservative policy has been adopted.

Cysts

EPIDEMIOLOGY AND AETIOLOGY

Occurrence is usually at a slightly later stage of life than fibroadenoma – after 35 and through to the menopause. Cysts probably form under the same influences that cause the other cyclical breast changes. There has been some suggestion that multiple recurrent cysts are associated with an increased tendency to breast cancer.

CLINICAL FEATURES

The history is of a palpable and occasionally tender lump.

Physical findings are of a tense, discrete, mobile lump anywhere in the breast. Fluctuation can be difficult to elicit in a small cyst.

INVESTIGATION AND MANAGEMENT

Whenever a clinical diagnosis is made of a cyst, needle aspiration should be done at once; it yields straw-coloured fluid and causes collapse of the cyst. Equally important, it immediately reassures the patient although there have to be some exceptions:

- failure of the lump completely to disappear
- bloodstained aspirate.

Failure to disappear completely

Re-evaluation must take place within a few weeks. A persistent lump must be evaluated by mammography and either be subject to FNAC or excised for histological examination.

Bloodstained aspirate

The simple cause is a traumatic aspiration. However, this must be confirmed by cytological examination of the aspirate and mammography. Clinical reassessment, re-aspiration if a lump is present or excision biopsy is then the appropriate course.

In uncomplicated circumstances, follow-up is probably not necessary but it is reassuring to both patient and doctor for a single re-examination to take place about 6 weeks later. If there has not been recurrence, the patient is discharged with the caveat that any new lump must be subject to a repeat of the initial management.

Multiple cysts

Some patients have multiple cysts identified at mammography or which present clinically as a lumpy breast. Danazol (a dopamine receptor stimulant – see above) can be helpful in reducing the incidence of clinical recurrence. Given the possible risk of carcinoma, follow-up with mammography is necessary.

Nipple discharge

There are three common causes:

- mammary duct ectasia
- duct papilloma
- galactorrhoea.

An important point to establish is whether the discharge is from a single or from multiple ducts. That from a single duct, particularly if bloodstained, is more likely to be associated with a papilloma. Discharges are commoner in women over 35. In younger women they may be associated with the oral contraceptive.

Mammary duct ectasia

AETIOLOGY AND PATHOLOGICAL FEATURES

The cause, as with many breast disorders, is an exaggeration of the normal cyclical changes – a wear and tear process. The ducts adjacent to the nipple become dilated and engorged with breast secretions. Secondary infection and a retroareolar abscess may form, but even if this does not happen, fibrosis can cause nipple retraction.

CLINICAL FEATURES

History

The discharge can range from milky to dirty green and is often, but not always, bilateral. Occasionally it is associated with pain, usually cyclical. Acute infection causes pain and swelling.

Physical findings

The breast may have features of lumpiness (see above). The chronic inflammation often associated with the condition causes a characteristic retraction of the nipple which gives it a slit-like appearance that may be confused with carcinoma. In acute inflammation, an abscess forms which, if not treated at an early stage, discharges at the areolar margin. A small sinus (mammary fistula) then results which can be the focus of further attacks of inflammation.

INVESTIGATION AND MANAGEMENT

If qualified by age, patients should have a mammogram to establish the general state of the breast. Discharge is sent for cytological assessment.

Provided both the above investigations are normal, nothing further needs to be done other than to reassure the patient. If a discharge is very troublesome, excision of the duct system (Hadfield's operation) provides symptomatic relief.

Abscess

An abscess in this condition is followed, as described above, by a mammary fistula. In consequence, after drainage there is not only often a persistent discharge but also the risk of recurrence. The involved duct and its drainage area should be excised electively.

Duct papilloma

This is a relatively uncommon lesion.

CLINICAL FEATURES

There is a serous or bloodstained discharge from a single aspect of the nipple although the patient may not realise that the discharge is localised. Other symptoms are rarely present.

The breast is normal, but there is either the spontaneous appearance of discharge from one aspect of the nipple or 'milking', of a segment produces nipple discharge from the duct draining that segment.

INVESTIGATION

The main concern, particularly if the discharge is bloodstained, is that occasionally there is an underlying malignancy although duct papilloma is benign.

Investigations are the same as for mammary duct ectasia. However, in spite of negative cytological findings, it is nearly always necessary, in a bloodstained single duct discharge, to excise the involved system to establish that a papilloma is present.

Galactorrhoea

This is a rare cause of bilateral milky discharge. It follows lactation and is caused by a persistent elevation of prolactin.

MANAGEMENT

Bromocriptine is used until the discharge subsides. Prolactinomas should be considered in long persistent discharge but are rare.

Trauma

Trauma to the breast is relatively rare, although sexual

encounters and love bites may be responsible for local injury. A blunt impact can interfere with local blood supply and, together with a haematoma, cause fat necrosis. Another cause is the use of therapeutic anti-coagulants in patients with very large and pendulous breasts in which very minor trauma may precipitate extensive haemorrhage which may go on to necrosis.

CLINICAL FEATURES

Fat necrosis causes a hard painful lump usually following a story of minor local trauma.

A hard lump is often found, with some irregularity and occasionally tethering to the overlying skin. The appearances are suggestive of a carcinoma but the condition can usually be distinguished because of the history of trauma, associated bruising and resolution of the lump with observation.

INVESTIGATION AND MANAGEMENT

Investigation is the same as for any discrete lump. The condition resolves with time and specific treatment is not required.

Infection

There are two common causes of infection:

- lactational breast abscess
- periductal mastitis.

Lactational breast abscess

AETIOLOGY AND PATHOLOGICAL FEATURES

The condition is a complication of lactation and breast-feeding; the organism involved is nearly always *Staphylococcus aureus*. It is believed that bacteria get into the breast through cracks in the nipple during feeding. A segment of breast becomes inflamed so that there is initially cellulitis; however, the nature of staphylococcal infection means that there is a rapid build-up of tension, which is further contributed to by the lobular nature of the breast, and necrosis to produce an abscess occurs after a relatively short time. The abscess may break through into neighbouring segments and thus become multilocular.

CLINICAL FEATURES

History

The baby may be anything from a few days to some months old. The mother may have noticed an obvious crack in the nipple although this is unusual. Segmental pain in the affected breast rapidly becomes severe and sleep is often lost.

Physical findings

A tender red segment in the breast is seen, perhaps with evidence of nipple damage as a crack in its surface. Fluctuation is not a feature unless the abscess is advanced and beginning to point towards the skin which may ultimately show evidence of necrosis.

MANAGEMENT

If detected and treated early, acute mastitis can resolve. Anti-staphylococcal antibiotics are prescribed in full doses. If the nipple is obviously damaged, feeding on this side is stopped and the milk expressed from the healthy segments. Continued pain and loss of sleep suggest that there is an abscess which in its early stages can be aspirated with a wide-bore needle under local anaesthetic. Skin changes of thinning and necrosis require formal drainage and breakdown of all the loculi under general anaesthetic. Such an event usually puts an end to breast-feeding.

Ultrasound is a useful means of determining whether there is any pus to drain.

Periductal mastitis

AETIOLOGY AND PATHOLOGICAL FEATURES

This condition affects young women in their 30s and is associated with smoking. It is characterised histological by a low-grade inflammatory response around the ducts adjacent to the nipple. In consequence, an alternative name is 'plasma cell mastitis'. The bacteria involved are nearly always anaerobes.

CLINICAL FEATURES

Tenderness develops on one aspect of the areola. There is rarely any systemic disturbance. Recurrent bouts may occur before the patient seeks medical attention.

A tender swelling at the edge of the areolar is seen, which may progress to abscess formation with a peri-areolar sinus and discharge (see 'Mamillary duct fistula' above).

INVESTIGATION AND MANAGEMENT

Because there may be a discrete mass with only a few, if any, characteristics of inflammation, FNAC and mammography may be necessary to exclude an underlying carcinoma.

Inflammatory swellings may respond to antibiotics; however, when an abscess has formed it requires the same treatment as a lactational abscess which is usually drainage rather than aspiration. A complication of abscess is the formation of a mammary duct fistula, which discharges intermittently and may be associated with recurrent abscess formation. The duct segment must then be excised because, in the presence of a duct abnormality, attempts to eradicate sepsis with antibiotics are usually futile.

Malignant breast disease

The great majority of malignancies in the breast are adenocarcinomas.

Epidemiology

Breast cancer is the commonest form of cancer to affect women in the Western world. There are 24 000 new cases in the UK every year and it is directly responsible for 19% of all cancer-related deaths in women. England and Wales have the highest national age-adjusted mortality for breast cancer at 29.3 per 100 000 population, and Korea has the lowest at 2.6 per 100 000. The USA ranks 16th with 22.4 cases per 100 000 population.

The incidence also varies within population groups. Ethnic/cultural analysis shows, for example, that American Jews and nuns having a higher incidence than Mormons and American Indians. Such figures are hard to explain.

The incidence is on the increase in the Western world: the probabilities of developing the disease were estimated at 1:13 in 1970, 1:11 in 1980 and 1:9 in 1992. Although, in general, the less industralised nations tend to have lower rates of breast cancer, this difference is diminishing. Japan is an exception: a low incidence persists despite extensive industrialisation; however, in recent years, there has been a steady increase in Japanese incidence.

Aetiology

The risk factors for breast cancer are listed in Table 27.1. The most significant causes of an increase in relative risk are:

- age
- country of birth

Table 27.1
Factors affecting the risk of developing breast cancer

Factor	High risk	Low risk
Age	Greater than 50	Less than 35
Country of birth	Northern Europe North America	Asia or Africa
First-degree relative affected	Yes	
Age at first pregnancy	> 30 years	< 20 years
Nulliparity	Yes	
Previous breast cancer	Yes	
History of atypical hyperplasia	Yes	

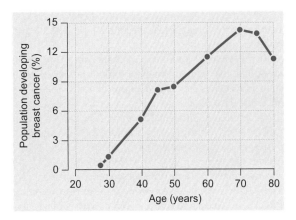

Fig 27.2 **Age and cancer of the breast.**

- genetic factors, particularly a history of breast cancer in a first-degree relative
- miscellaneous.

Age
Breast cancer is rare under the age of 35. Between the ages of 30 and 34 the incidence and mortality rates in the UK are 19.6 and 5.9 per 100 000 women, respectively; between 50 and 54 years these rise to 145.9 and 73.7 per 100 000 and they continue to increase further with age. (Fig. 27.2).

Genetic factors
Hereditary and familial breast cancer can be described using the Lynch system of classification, (see Box 27.1). If a satisfactory detailed family history is obtained, up to one-third will have some family history of breast cancer. Of these one-quarter will have true hereditary

---

Box 27.1

Lynch classification of inherited susceptibility to breast cancer

Hereditary breast cancer

A family history of breast cancer and, sometimes, related cancers – colonic, endometrial – forming part of the Lynch syndrome type II. This involves an autosomal dominant, highly penetrant cancer susceptibility factor. These patients tend to be younger than average, have multiple primaries and may also have other tumours.

Familial breast cancer

A family history of cancer of the breast including one or more first- or second-degree relatives with breast cancer that does not fit the hereditary breast cancer definition.

breast cancer: autosomal dominant gene expression pattern, early age of onset, excess bilateral disease and multiple other primary cancers.

Unfortunately definitive markers have not been identified that would facilitate early identification of such individuals and allow more intensive follow-up and earlier management.

Germline mutations in known and unknown breast cancer susceptibility genes account for an estimated 5–10% of cases of breast cancer. The two major breast cancer genes have now been identified: *BRCA1* on chromosome 17q and *BRCA2* on chromosome 13q. They both appear to be tumour suppressor genes: *BRCA1* is associated in particular with breast and ovarian cancer, and *BRCA2* with cancer of the breast and multiple other sites including the pancreas. Mutations in these genes are rare in the general population but it is now possible to offer predictive genetic testing, although the large number of associated mutations means that no reliable marker is available and testing can only be performed if DNA is available from an index case in the family tree. The risk of developing breast cancer associated with either gene is around 80–85% by the age of 70 years.

Miscellaneous factors

Menarche, menopause, child-bearing and fertility

Women who undergo early menarche and late menopause suffer from approximately twice the incidence of breast cancer as compared with their peers. A woman having a child before the age of 18 years has one-third the risk of developing breast cancer than a primiparous women over the age of 35. Infertility and nulliparity confer a higher probability of developing the disease and a first full-term pregnancy after the age of 30 increases the risk to greater than that for nulliparous women.

These effects are thought to be related to persistent exposure to endogenous oestrogen in the absence of appropriate progesterone concentrations.

Breast-feeding

Breast-feeding for a total time of greater than 36 months during a woman's reproductive years was thought to protect against the development of breast cancer. However, repeated observations have shown this to be untrue.

Diet

Dietary fat has been suggested as a risk factor although its exact role remains controversial. The different amounts of saturated and unsaturated fat available within specific diets may be important. Omega-3 unsaturated fatty acids are found in abundance in marine food sources and women such as Eskimos and the Japanese who have a high intake of them also have a relatively low incidence of breast cancer. Furthermore, in Japan, incidence has doubled with the adoption of a more Westernised diet. Studies on immigrants confirm this trend: third-generation Japanese immigrants to the United States have almost the same risk for breast cancer as the indigenous American population.

Obesity

The information available from the epidemiological studies on diet and breast cancer is further complicated by the fact that obesity is a definite risk factor in its own right. In postmenopausal women, obesity directly correlates with an increase in breast cancer risk of up to twofold. However, these women tend to come from the more affluent Western societies where saturated animal fats in the diet are common.

Exogenous hormones

There may be a slight risk of developing breast cancer if a high-dose oestrogen oral contraceptive has been taken for a prolonged time at an early age or before the first full-term pregnancy. This form of contraception is no longer in use and the risk from the low-dose oral contraceptive pill is considered negligible.

Oestrogen-containing hormone replacement therapy (HRT) may slightly increase the risk in postmenopausal women, especially those with pre-existing benign disease. The effect may, however, be related to the closer observation of women on HRT.

Previous cancer

The risk of a second primary breast cancer is reported to be up to five times the general risk and is inversely related to age at presentation of the first. An ipsilateral second primary is more common in women with a family history. In general, about 0.5% of women with a previous history of breast cancer will be expected to develop a second primary each year for the next 15 years.

Women with a previous history of primary ovarian or endometrial cancer are also at an increased risk, although probably less than twice that of the general population.

Irradiation

Exposure to radiation increases risk. The effect is accumulative and the incidence has been shown to be higher in survivors of nuclear weapon detonation and in women who have undergone multiple chest X-rays for monitoring of the progression of pulmonary tuberculosis (now uncommon).

Pregnancy

Pregnancy has been thought to be associated with a particularly aggressive form of breast cancer. Although more locally advanced cancers are diagnosed during pregnancy, there is not a higher incidence overall and the prognosis is similar stage for stage with the normal population. In theory, a subsequent pregnancy in a patient who has had a previous oestrogen receptor-positive tumour (see below) could shorten the disease-free interval. However, evidence for this is lacking, although it is rational for such women to avoid oestrogen-containing compounds.

Previous benign disease

The relative risk of developing breast cancer in the presence of proven benign disease is outlined in Box 27.2. Benign lesions may be either proliferative or non-proliferative, with subgroups within the various types of proliferative lesions conferring varying levels of risk.

Non-proliferative lesions such as fibrocystic disease and simple cysts with or without apocrine changes in the breast do not appear to be associated with an increased risk.

Proliferative lesions are distinguished by epithelial hyperplasia that implies an increased number of cells above the basement membrane. The degree of hyperplasia is related to the number of layers found, e.g. mild hyperplasia is associated with three or more cells above the basement membrane in a lobular unit or duct. The presence of atypical cells within the hyperplasia is significant in that it has a 4–5 times risk of progressing to a carcinoma. Atypical hyperplasia may be ductal or lobular in origin. It is thought that hyperplasia forms part of a spectrum of benign disorders that have the potential for malignant transformation. However, not all proliferative-type lesions are associated with increased risk; radial scars and so-called complex sclerosing lesions which are histologically similar to

---

Box 27.2

Relative risk of developing breast cancer in relation to previous benign disease

No risk

Apocrine change

Ductal ectasia

Mild hyperplasia (no atypia)

Slight risk

Moderate or florid hyperplasia (no atypia)

Sclerosing adenosis

Papilloma

Moderate risk

Atypical ductal or lobular hyperplasia

Box 27.3

Non-risk factors in breast cancer

Diazepam

Reserpine

Cholecystectomy

Thyroid disease

Hair dyes

Emotional stress

Cigarette smoking

Trauma to the breast with fat necrosis may *distort* the breast architecture but does not have malignant potential

---

sclerosing adenosis and also duct ectasia do not have malignant potential.

Fibroadenomas (see above) are benign tumours. For those women with a simple fibroadenoma there is no increase in the incidence of subsequent breast cancer.

Papillomas arise from the epithelium of the large ductal network of the breast. The centrally placed papilloma tends to be single and has no proven malignant potential. However, those that occur peripherally are often multiple and can contain areas of atypical hyperplasia and even ductal carcinoma in situ (see below).

Factors without proven risk

Many possible risks have been related to breast cancer but have subsequently been disproved although they remain a source of potential confusion (Box 27.3). Smoking is not a risk factor but because it is related to earlier menopause it has a popular but undeserved reputation as a protective factor. The balance of evidence supports neither a causative nor a protective role.

Natural history

Tumour doubling time is the time taken for the mass of cells which make up the malignancy to double in number or the tumour to double in size. Estimates of the doubling time for a breast cancer are about 100 days and, on this basis, a growth that originated from a single cell would take 8 years to become a 1 cm diameter, clinically detectable lump of 10⁹ cells. This theoretical calculation is modified by the fact that doubling time is governed in practice by more complex factors: in the first 30 doublings the growth rate is not constant, and thereafter the rate of growth is slowed by

Table 27.2
Survival in relation to axillary node status

Patient group	Survival (%)	
	5-year	10-year
All patients	64	46
Node-negative	78	65
Node-positive	47	25

the occurrence of cell death in the mass. A palpable breast tumour may therefore have been present for even longer than the simple calculation suggests. After 20 doublings the tumour acquires its own blood supply and from then on cancer cells can be shed into the blood. The possibility of early spread to distant parts of the body is therefore present from an early stage and is added to by the rich lymphatic network of the breast which can pick up cells from the intercellular spaces and transport them to the regional lymph nodes. However, successful implantation of the cells, either shed into the bloodstream or escaping from the primary tumour via lymphatics, seldom occurs before the 27th doubling (5 cm) because, before this, natural killer cells and other macrophages of the immune system are able to cope with the malignant cell load. Systemic dissemination is critical because more than 95% of patients who die of breast cancer do so from distant metastasis. That blood-borne implanted micrometastases take place relatively early is evident from the fact that 20–25% of patients who do not have tumour in their regional lymph nodes at the time of their removal still experience relapse because of distant disease. Once tumour has also spread via the lymphatics to regional nodes, the figure rises to between 50 and 75% (Table 27.2).

Staging

It was recognised even before the concept of early micrometastases was understood that some form of staging of the disease could be helpful in assessing the likelihood of survival, although it is realised that it is blurred by the possible presence of micrometastases which will develop subsequently into distant recurrences.

The international TNM classification (Ch. 12 and Table 27.3) allows grouping of the disease into clinical stages. Staging allows comparison between groups of patients and also defines those unsuitable for an attempt at surgical removal but who may be suitable for the other forms of adjuvant therapy.

Node status in the axilla may be established at operation by histological examination either of an en bloc removal (axillary clearance) or by sampling nodes closest to the tumour.

Table 27.3
TNM classification of breast cancer

TNM stage	Pathological description
Tis	Carcinoma in situ (pre-invasive)
	Paget's disease (no palpable tumour)
T0	No clinical evidence of primary tumour
T1	Tumour less than 2 cm
T2	Tumours 2–5 cm
T3	Tumour greater than 5 cm
T4	Tumour of any size but with direct extension to chest wall or skin:
	(a) Fixation to chest wall
	(b) Oedema, lymphocytic infiltration, ulceration of skin or satellite nodes
	(c) Both (a) and (b).
N0	No palpable ipsilateral axillary lymph nodes
N1	Palpable nodes not fixed
	(a) Inflammatory only
	(b) Containing tumour
N2	Fixed ipsilateral axillary nodes
N3	Ipsilateral supraclavicular or infraclavicular nodes or oedema of arm
M0	No evidence of distant metastasis
M1	Evidence of distant metastasis

The presence of distant metastasis is more difficult to establish with certainty because current techniques are not sensitive enough to detect microdeposits. The outcome of TNM classification is used to define a clinical stage which can be employed as a guide to treatment and prognosis (Table 27.4).

Other prognostic indicators

As well as stage and nodal status, there are many other factors that can be used for prediction (Table 27.5).

Histological
The following favourably affect prognosis:

- low tumour grade
- high degree of elastosis
- reactive changes in the regional lymph nodes
- positive oestrogen receptor status.

Table 27.4
Application of TNM classification to treatment and prognosis

UICC stage[a]	TNM	5-year survival treatment[b]
I	T1, N0, M0	84% Early cancer
II	T1, N1, M0; T2, N0–1, M0	71% Early cancer
III	Any T, N2–3 M0; T3, any N, M0	48% LABC[c]
IV	Any T, any N, M1	18% Metastatic

[a] UICC International Union Against Cancer.
[b] Details in text.
[c] LABC locally advanced breast cancer.

Table 27.5
Other prognostic variables in breast cancer

Size of tumour
Lymph node involvement
Distant metastasis

Biological factors	Favourable	Unfavourable
Histological type	Tubular, colloid, papillary	Scirrhous
Grade		
Necrosis	Absent	Present
Lymphocytic infiltration	Present	Absent
Oestrogen status	Positive	Negative
Reactive lymph nodes	Present	Absent
Proliferative rate	Low S phase	Aneuploid
Chromosomal defect		Deletion/ alteration 1, 3, 6, 7, 9 Shortening of allele on chromsome 11
Proto-oncogenes		c-erb-B/c-H-ras
Growth factors (GF)		Epidermal GF Transforming GF Platelet-derived GF Fibroblast GF Insulin-like GF

Other factors have an adverse effect:

● vascular and lymphocytic invasion by tumour
● extensive angiogenesis
● expression of the proto-oncogene C-erb B2 and loss of expression of the suppressor p53.

Screening

The relatively poor results in the past of conventional treatment have led to the view that the disease must be detected earlier at a presymptomatic stage (p. 000). Studies from New York and Scandinavia have shown that it is likely that finding hidden cancers by proactive measures improves long-term survival by allowing lesions to be removed before micrometastases have occurred. In the UK, women between the ages of 50 and 64 years who are registered with a general practitioner are called every 3 years for a screening mammogram. In the USA, screening is undertaken more frequently, with a baseline mammogram being performed between 35 and 39 years, then 1- to 2-yearly for 12–24 months and yearly from 50 years with no age limit. These intervals are aimed at reducing the chance that an interval cancer develops but remains undetected between mammogram episodes. In the UK this risk is thought to be low enough to warrant the 3-yearly interval.

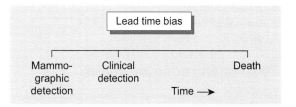

Fig 27.3 **Apparent reduction in mortality from cancer of the breast due to lead time bias.**

Controversial issues about the UK screening programme are:

● no screening for women under 50
● discontinuation of routine screening of women at 65 – after this age patients may present for screening but are not called as a routine; the reason given is that compliance falls off dramatically (but financial considerations are undoubtedly also of importance).

The 50–64 year group is the only one in which screening has so far been shown to reduce mortality. Mammographically detected cancers are smaller and axillary lymph node involvement is less common. A reduction of 30% in long-term mortality has been shown (Fig. 27.3) even if the 'lead time' is allowed for. Lead time is the difference in time between a tumour being sub-clinical and detectable only by screening methods, such as mammography, and when it would have become clinically apparent. If the patient still dies at the same point in time then an apparent survival advantage is gained due to the 'lead time bias'.

Several trials are currently in progress to evaluate screening for women under the age of 50 years. Current advice is that for high-risk women under the age of 50, a specialist clinic should coordinate a personal mammography programme. If the family history is of post-menopausal cancer, mammography may be delayed until 35 years. Where the family history is of premenopausal cancer, referral at any age 10 years younger than the first presentation of the parent is thought appropriate.

Pathological features

A feature of clinical interest is that most breast cancers are associated with fibrous tissue proliferation – they are *scirrhous*. The consequence is that the growth and surrounding tissue contracts so that dimpling of the skin and indrawing of the nipple may be seen. The growth is an adenocarcinoma arising from the epithelium lining the ducts and acini forming the lobules. It is therefore divided principally into ductal and lobular types.

The histological grade of tumour relates to the degree of differentiation:

- grade I – well differentiated
- grade II – moderately differentiated
- grade III – poorly differentiated.

Oestrogen receptor status

The majority of breast cancers are 'oestrogen dependent' tumours. As such they tend to express oestrogen receptors. The degree of expression can be measured with immunohistochemistry, and the breast cancers are labelled as either oestrogen receptor positive or negative. Oestrogen receptor positive breast cancer tends to respond to hormonal therapy and carries a better prognosis than oestrogen receptor negative tumours.

Carcinoma in situ (T[tumour]IS)

This term refers to the period during which normal epithelial cells undergo apparent malignant transformation but do not invade through the basement membrane. There are two forms:

- Lobular – LCIS
- Ductal – DCIS. DCIS represents all types of in situ carcinoma that are not identified as lobular. It can be further subdivided into:
  - comedo
  - solid
  - cribriform
  - micropapillary.

However, the distinction remains primarily between LCIS and DCIS, although comedo DCIS is a particularly menacing type of in situ carcinoma with reports of frequent association with microinvasive foci and lymph node metastasis. Necrosis and microcalcification are common and, because the second may be seen on mammography, the incidence may be increasing as earlier diagnosis becomes more widespread. By contrast, LCIS is not associated with any radiological markers and therefore may not be detected early.

The ratio of DCIS to LCIS is 3:1 with approximately 10–37% of those with LCIS and 30–50% of those with DCIS going on to develop invasive carcinoma.

With LCIS, future cancers may be in either breast regardless of the site of the in situ changes. A further confounding statistic is that approximately 50–65% of future malignancies are of ductal origin, which indicates that LCIS is a marker of increased risk of diffuse bilateral disease as opposed to a true anatomic precursor of lobular cancer.

However, with DCIS, the malignancies are ductal in origin, arise in the ipsilateral breast and usually are confined to the same quadrant from which the biopsy which yielded the diagnosis was taken.

Table 27.6
Relative frequency of histological types of breast cancer

Type	Frequency (%)
Ductal	80 (non-specific 50%)
Lobular/ductal combined	5
Medullary	6
Colloid	2
Other less common specific types (tubular, papillary)	2
Sarcoma and lymphoma	0.5

Invasive breast carcinoma

PATHOLOGICAL MANIFESTATIONS

The disease has protean pathological manifestations.

Ductal with productive fibrosis (infiltrating ductal)

This is the commonest form of cancer of the breast – approximately 80% (see Table 27.6). The most common form is of non-descript but highly variable histological type. Sheets, cords, nests and trabeculae of tumour cells may be present all in varying amounts. If the main bulk of tumour is of this type then the presence of more specific histological features in small amounts does not appear to alter the prognosis.

Medullary

This form comprises about 6% of the total. Histologically it has completely circumscribed borders with a syncytial sheet-like growth pattern, a diffuse infiltrate of lymphocytes and a variable number of plasma cells. Nearly 50% of these tumours are associated with intraductal carcinoma usually at the periphery of the main tumour.

Colloid (mucinous)

Largely confined to the elderly population, this tumour accounts for approximately 2% of breast cancers. Histologically, large pools of mucin are surrounded by variable groups of tumour cells. The classical signet ring appearance of mucinous tumours in other sites is not seen in breast colloid carcinoma.

Tubular

Clinically, tubular carcinoma is found in younger than average patients with the late 50s being the peak age, the diagnosis usually being made at mammography. In consequence, the lesion is still small (less than 1 cm) and up to a fifth of breast tumours identified at mammography may be of this type. Histologically they are well differentiated and have randomly arranged tubular elements in a loose stroma.

Papillary

This accounts for less than 2% of cases of breast carcinoma and usually present in the seventh decade.

Histologically, it is well circumscribed with marked papillary differentiation.

Other pathological types

Adenoid cystic carcinoma

This type accounts for less than 0.1% of breast cancers. Similar to the tumours of the same name found in the salivary glands, it also resembles cribriform intraductal carcinoma.

Lobular carcinoma

These lesions have a high propensity for bilaterality (up to 30%), multicentricity and multifocality. The age at presentation is similar to that of infiltrating ductal carcinoma and they constitute 5–10% of breast carcinomas. Histologically, lobular carcinoma has a characteristic appearance with homogeneous small cells with small nuclei, absent nucleoli and scanty cytoplasm. They characteristically permeate a desmoplastic stroma in single file, linear fashion (Indian filing) or surround terminal ductal lobular units in a circumferential targetoid way. When abundant mucin is produced by the tumour, the nuclei are displaced laterally and the cell comes to resemble the signet ring type of gastro-intestinal adenocarcinoma. Lobular carcinoma has a particular propensity for metastasising to membrane structures and forming diffusely involved metastasis. Structures that may be concerned include the peritoneum, the pleura and the meninges as meningeal carcinomatosis.

Clinical features

History

In nearly all women, presentation is with a solitary, non-tender breast lump of varying duration; often its presence has been denied by the patient for several months although 70% have discovered the lesion (the remaining are detected by the examining physician in 25% and by mammography in 5%). Pain is present in fewer than 5%. Table 27.7 outlines the frequency of presenting symptoms and signs. It is important to note the length of time the mass has been present. Much less common is the patient who has a small primary and only presents when symptoms of generalised malignant disease become manifest. Finally, denial may be carried to extreme when a patient realises that she has a lump and allows it to progress to ulceration (see also 'Paget's disease' below).

Physical findings

The mass is solitary, does not cause pain on palpation, is ill-defined and may show signs of tethering to the skin. In locally advanced disease, the lymphatic channels

Table 27.7
Methods of presentation of breast cancer

Symptom/sign	Frequency (%)
Lump	76
Pain	5
Nipple retraction	4
Nipple discharge	2
Skin retraction	1
Axillary mass	1

are obstructed and the skin becomes oedematous with thickening and the hair follicles more prominent although embedded in the rugose skin – so-called skin of the orange (peau d'orange).

In *medullary carcinoma*, the lump may be soft, haemorrhagic and bulky, deep in the breast but characteristically mobile.

Colloid carcinoma is usually a bulky mass in the sixth or seventh decade.

Tubular and papillary carcinoma do not have distinctive physical findings but tend to present in older women.

Other malignant tumours affecting the breast

Paget's disease

This condition presents clinically as a chronic, eczematoid eruption of the nipple. Indeed the diagnosis may be confused with eczema although there are distinct differences (Table 27.8). It constitutes approximately 2% of histological types and is almost always associated with an underlying intraductal or invasive carcinoma.

Inflammatory breast carcinoma

This tumour comprises 1% or slightly more of breast carcinomas. It is rapidly progressive and is characterised by erythema, peau d'orange and skin ridging with or without a palpable mass. Unlike other breast cancers, the commonest presenting feature is pain. The characteristic appearance of a diffusely enlarged breast is consequent upon the dissemination of tumour cells through the lymphatics of the dermis (Fig. 27.4). If the tumour cells remain within the superficial lymphatics and the blood vessels, then a condition known as telangiectatic carcinoma may arise with numerous

Table 27.8
Comparison of Paget's disease and eczema of the nipple

Paget's disease	Eczema
Unilateral	Bilateral
Progressive/continuous	Intermittent/variable
Moist or dry	Moist
Irregular/discrete	Indistinct
Nipple always involved	Nipple sparing
Pruritis absent	Pruritis present

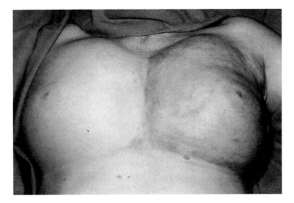

Fig 27.4 **'Peau d'orange' of cancer of the breast.**

purple papules and haemorrhagic, vesicle-like lesions covering the breast. Extensive involvement along tissue planes may produce a nodular pattern or, when associated with extensive fibrosis, a diffuse thickened lesion – a thoracic girdle (carcinoma en cuirasse).

Malignant phylloides tumour

This accounts for about 0.5% of all breast tumours. The name is derived from its fleshy leaf-like (phylloid) appearance. There are both stromal and epithelial components, although the stromal elements predominate. On histological examination, malignant phylloides tumours provide a spectrum of disease from frank sarcomatous malignancy to appearances almost indistinguishable from a fibroadenoma. Even with histological confirmation, its behaviour can be difficult to predict. The prognosis is generally good but unpredictable.

Clinical features. There is often a large, painless and nodular growth which is surprisingly mobile. With continuing enlargement of the tumour, the breast adopts a characteristic 'teardrop' appearance (Fig. 27.5). Treatment is by wide excision through normal tissues. However, as with other sarcomas, local recurrence can occur.

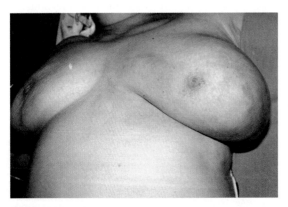

Fig 27.5 **'Teardrop' appearance of phylloides tumour of the breast.**

Lymphoma

Primary breast lymphoma is extremely rare, with only 207 cases having been reported in the literature to 1985. The malignancy does not differ structurally from the same growth in other sites. Treatment is by mastectomy with lymph node clearance, with radiotherapy for local recurrences and chemotherapy for disseminated disease. Prognosis is favourable.

Establishing a diagnosis of breast cancer

Any palpable breast abnormality should be assessed by the process of triple assessment:

- clinical evaluation
- radiological evaluation
- cytological/histological evaluation.

A thorough history should form part of any assessment because important information can be gained on the nature of the breast mass or condition that caused the individual to ask for medical advice and also the other risk factors mentioned above: family, menstrual and reproductive history, the use of hormones and a personal history of breast cancer or breast disease.

During the course of communication with patients with possible breast cancer, it is important to convey the fact that only 20% who consult do have the disease: 50% do not have breast disease as defined pathologically; 20% have benign (fibrocystic) disease; and most of the rest have a fibroadenoma.

Physical examination

The technique of examining the breast should involve inspection and palpation of the entire breast and lymph node-bearing areas (Fig. 27.6).

The patient must be undressed to the waist and sit facing the examiner. The breast is initially examined from the front with the arms first at the side, then raised above the head and finally placed on the hips – in this last case they should be both relaxed and pressed into the sides in order to tense the pectoralis muscle. The patient is asked to point out the supposed area of abnormality and this is examined first. However, in spite of any abnormality being discovered the following are also assessed:

- asymmetry
- visible lumps
- erythema
- cutaneous oedema (peau d'orange)
- contour flattening

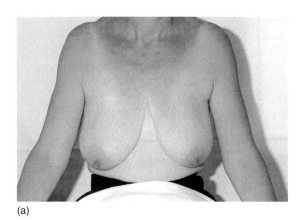

(a)

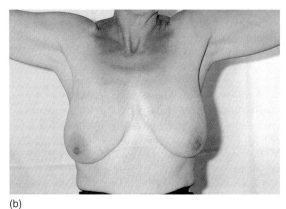

(b)

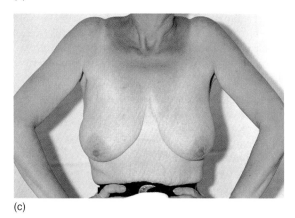

(c)

Fig 27.6 **Examination of the breast.** (a) From the front; (b) with arms raised; (c) with arms pushed into the side.

- skin tethering as identified by puckering, particularly when the arms are raised
- abnormal fixation
- retraction and altered axis of the nipples; in advanced cases there may be gross ulceration of the skin overlying the lesion (Fig. 27.7).

After this, with the arms extended forwards, the patient is asked to lean forward, once again looking for skin retraction (Fig. 27.8). The breasts are then re-examined, paying particular attention to the outer

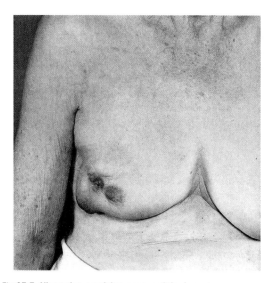

Fig 27.7 **Ulceration overlying cancer of the breast.**

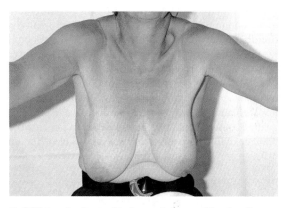

Fig 27.8 **Leaning forward to demonstrate any skin retraction.**

border of pectoralis major. Here lymph nodes may be felt. The supraclavicular, infraclavicular and axillary lymph nodes should be examined, the examiner taking the weight of the patient's arm either on the shoulder or on the opposite arm (Fig. 27.9).

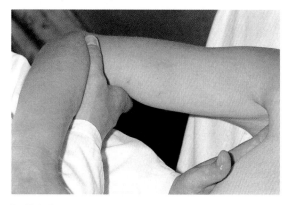

Fig 27.9 **Examination of the axillary nodes.**

Further palpation of the breast is best performed in the supine position. A pillow under the shoulder of the breast allows the breast tissue to flow along the chest wall. The breast is examined initially with the patient's hand behind the head and then to the side. Care must be taken to ensure the whole breast is examined, transversely from sternum to clavicle, posteriorly to latissimus dorsi and inferiorly to the rectus sheath. In order to achieve this, the breast is examined a quadrant at a time. The examination is carried out with a flat hand (Fig. 27.10), never grasping or pinching. The nipple/areola area should be carefully inspected for epithelial changes, retroareolar masses and nipple discharge. The significance of the different types of discharge are shown in Table 27.9.

Should a mass be felt, whether related to the breast substance or in the lymph node area that drains it, its position, size, consistency and any fixation to surrounding deep or superficial structures must be carefully assessed and recorded. Fixation to skin is evaluated by pinching up the overlying skin. Mobility in relation to muscle is evaluated by palpation with the pectoralis major both contracted and relaxed. Should the patient complain of discharge, then an attempt to reproduce this should be made. Methods include 'around the clock' palpation of the areola area, quadrant by quadrant, noting any dilated ducts or nodules and, if this fails to produce the discharge, gentle compression of the subareolar tissue. The number of ducts involved and the degree of dilatation

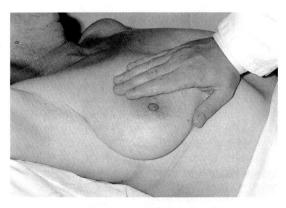

Fig 27.10 **Examination of the breast with a flat hand.**

Table 27.9
Discharge from the nipple

Type	Abnormality/cause	Cancer risk
Bloody	Hyperplasia/ectasia	Yes
	Papilloma	No
Serous	Hyperplasia/ectasia	Yes
Watery	Hyperplasia	Yes
Opalescent	Ectasia/cyst	No
Milk	Hormonal	No

should be assessed. Any discharge that is obtained should be tested for blood using a reagent stick and be sent for cytological examination.

Many surgeons use a prepared diagram and sheet for accurate recording of information following breast examination.

Investigation

Imaging

Mammography

Mammography was first used in 1913 by a German surgeon, Salomon. The change from xeromammography to film screening allowed a reduction in radiation dose so that the single-view mammogram gives an average dose of 2 mGy. The estimated risk of inducing a fatal breast cancer from one such examination is 1:100 000 for women aged between 50 and 65 years and twice this for women aged between 30 and 49 years.

A mediolateral oblique view taken from upper medial to lower lateral aspects is now standard and images the whole of the breast. It is usually combined with a craniocaudal view although, for screening asymptomatic women, a single view is considered adequate.

Generally, mammography in women under 35 years is often not helpful because they have particularly dense breasts at this age which can mask any underlying tumours and also make interpretation very difficult. However, it should be done if there is clinical suspicion of malignancy.

Mammographic abnormalities that warrant further investigation include:

- radiological masses undetected on clinical examination
- microcalcifications
- stellate densities
- architectural distortion
- change from a previous mammogram.

However, even with skilled interpreters, mammography has a false-negative rate of between 10 and 15%. Therefore it is only part of the spectrum of diagnosis and other tests must be integrated into a diagnosis.

Ultrasound

In use since the 1950s, ultrasound has been shown to be useful in discriminating solid from cystic masses and especially in the evaluation of the dense breast. Other uses include ultrasound-guided biopsy or needle localisation. In younger women, ultrasound may reveal more information than mammography and most surgeons would perform this test first in women less than 35. Masses smaller than 5–10 mm may not be visualised and masses in fatty breasts are also difficult to assess.

Blood flow assessment by Doppler ultrasound has been used in assessment because breast tumours have enhanced blood flow; however, this is currently only of research interest.

CT

This can be useful in staging the disease but does not have a role in diagnosis.

MRI

Initially, MRI mammography did not show any advantage over conventional techniques in the detection and evaluation of breast cancer. However, since the introduction of Gd-DTPA enhancement and true dynamic scanning, the results seem to indicate a use in evaluating the indeterminate breast mass or after treatment. Breast tumours are noted to enhance heterogeneously and rapidly in contrast to benign tumours, which have more homogeneous and uniform enhancement. Further research is being done to evaluate the sensitivity and specificity of this technique fully, but early results appear encouraging.

Aspiration cytology

Needle aspiration of a breast lump is done with a 21-gauge needle. The technique is outlined on page 000. The contents of the needle are expressed onto a slide, smeared and fixed (often in both air and alcohol) for cytological examination. In skilled hands, this method is very accurate with false-negative rates of less than 1 in 100. For impalpable lesions, stereotactic techniques can be used to localise the lesion for needle aspiration.

Wide bore core needle biopsy

The method provides a sample of tissue for histological rather than cytological examination. The pathological diagnosis which results should be more certain because cellular architecture can be assessed. Because of this, wide bore core needle biopsy is rapidly superseding the use of aspiration cytology in specialist breast clinics.

Open biopsy

Excision biopsy

This refers to the removal of all gross evidence of disease with a small rim of normal breast tissue. If the tumour is small enough, all macroscopic disease is removed. Incisions are made along Langer's lines (Fig. 27.11) for maximum cosmesis. The operation can usually be done as an outpatient procedure under local anaesthetic.

Incision biopsy

This is similar to excision biopsy except that only a part of the lump is removed. It is generally felt that this is not good surgical practice. The use of incision biopsy is therefore restricted to larger tumours, especially suspected sarcomatous lesions where the incision must be made in such a way as to facilitate later excision of the scar as part of removal of the whole lesion. The use of incision biopsy has largely been superseded by wide core bore needle biopsy.

Mammographic-guided needle biopsy

Screening mammography (above) demonstrates many clinically impalpable lesions. To localise these, a marking needle is placed under mammographic guidance before surgical excision. The tissue around the needle is then excised and further imaging done to ensure that the indicated lesion has in fact been removed (Figs 27.12 and 27.13). If it is not evident in the

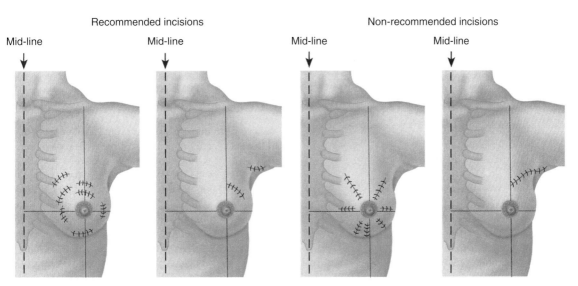

Fig 27.11 **Site of skin incision on the breast.**

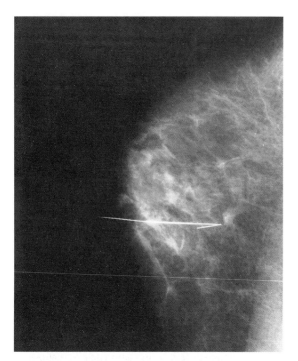

Fig 27.12 **Identification of tumour with a needle on mammogram.**

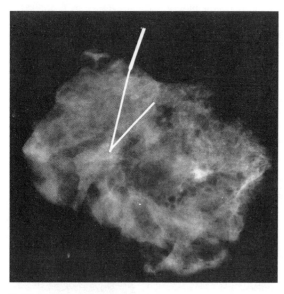

Fig 27.13 **X-ray of excised lump.**

sample, more tissue from around the site is taken until the lesion is identified.

Ultrasound-guided biopsy

Both the technique of needle-guided biopsy and real-time cyst aspiration can be used. Techniques of one or the other are dependent on the expertise available.

Nipple biopsy

Conditions affecting the nipple, especially an eczema-like appearance (see 'Paget's disease'), often warrant biopsy. A wedge of nipple–areolar complex can be excised under local anaesthetic with minimal cosmetic disruption to confirm or refute a diagnosis such as that of Paget's disease.

Management

Historical perspective

It would be inappropriate to describe the current therapeutic options available without providing an historical background.

The first documented reference to breast cancer occurs in the Edwin Smith Surgical papyrus (3000–2250 BC). The lesion was in a male but encompassed all the main features of breast cancer. Celsus later recognised the necessity and value of operation for early breast lesions and the difficulties encountered with advanced disease.

The Galenic system of medicine, laid down in the 2nd century AD, provided a classical description of the disease and ascribed it to an excess of black bile. The conclusion drawn from this was that excision could not cure the imbalance and this was the opinion held by the majority of established physicians until and including most of the Renaissance period.

In the 18th century, LeDran stated that cancer of the breast was a local disease that spread via the lymphatics to regional nodes. He removed these nodes in his cancer operations.

With the advent of deliberate surgery, which straddled the development of anaesthesia and anti-sepsis, surgeons in the late 19th century adapted LeDran's views and began to develop an operation designed to conform with the concept of progressive spread from the site of the primary. In 1877, at a presentation to the British Medical Association, Mitchell Banks of Liverpool supported Charles Moore of the Middlesex Hospital, London, in espousing wide removal of the breast with en bloc dissection of the axillary contents. He also advocated axillary dissection in the absence of clinically positive nodes, recognising the possibility of occult lymphatic spread.

In 1894, William S Halsted of the Johns Hopkins Medical School, Baltimore, and Willie Meyer of the New York Graduate School of Medicine simultaneously reported their results for local and regional recurrence following radical mastectomy. Halsted published the details of his operation and his results of 6% local recurrence with 45% 3-year survival improved greatly on those of his contemporaries. Therefore, Halsted's radical mastectomy with removal of the pectoralis muscle and radical lymph node dissection rapidly became accepted as the standard operation for breast cancer.

In the 1930s, D H Patey of the Middlesex Hospital, London, refined this to modified radical mastectomy with preservation of the pectoralis major muscle but resection of pectoralis minor to facilitate axillary node dissection.

It was not until the 1950s that surgeons began to realise that radical mastectomy was not the treatment of choice for all patients. Veronesi in Milan and Fisher in the USA postulated that breast cancer was not a regional curable disease but a systemic disease from the start. Lymph node involvement therefore represented a failure of the immune system to combat the disease rather than direct stepwise dissemination from a localised focus. Cure requires consideration of systemic anticancer treatment. With the advent of the current adjuvant regimens, the trend is now towards local excision with or without radiotherapy or chemotherapy. In 1971, 48% of patients with breast cancer in the USA underwent Halsted-type radical mastectomy; however, by 1981 this had dropped to 3%.

Current therapeutic options

The modern approach to breast cancer is multidisciplinary, with surgery, radiotherapy and chemotherapy all having important roles to play.

The treatment afforded to patients suffering from the disease depends on the stage of the cancer at the time of presentation.

Carcinoma in situ

DCIS and LCIS have different risks for the development of invasive cancer. As yet, their natural histories have not been fully elucidated.

DCIS presents an easier problem as it generally is unilateral and is thought to be a precursor of invasive disease. Trials of segmental excision with or without radiotherapy are currently underway but they must be judged against mastectomy which eliminates all the pre-invasive involved tissue. This is recommended when the disease has extensive foci and local excision margins are not clear of tumour and also for those patients who are at a high risk of developing local recurrence and reduced survival, defined as:

- size greater than 40 mm
- comedo appearances on histological examination
- high-grade tumour
- oestrogen receptor status negative.

Postoperative radiation is usually given to these patients. Breast-conserving therapy remains an option provided the patient understands the risks. The patient is followed up regularly with mammography and clinical examination, and if there is evidence of recurrent disease, a mastectomy is done.

The treatment for LCIS is confused by the fact that it is a marker for a disease that is often bilateral, multicentric and only sometimes goes on to invasive ductal cancer. Therefore the patient can elect to be observed closely or to undergo a curative bilateral mastectomy. Less than 1% of axillary nodes will be affected and clearance is not required.

Stages I and II

The results of prospective trials, based on the hypothesis that dissemination occurs early, show that long-term survival is not enhanced by radical surgical resection as opposed to breast conservation. In consequence, the pendulum has swung towards the principle of local control and, where possible, breast conservation. Local control is achieved by:

- complete removal of the tumour
- adjuvant local radiotherapy possibly supplemented by systemic cytotoxic therapy.

The following therapeutic approach is generally accepted for a tumour of less than 4 cm in diameter:

- unifocal disease
- breast volume of adequate size for a satisfactory cosmetic result
- wide local removal of tumour – either the lump alone (lumpectomy,) or removal of the involved breast quadrant (quadrantectomy) and local radiotherapy to reduce the risk of local recurrence from residual tumour cells
- excision margins shown to be clear on retrospective examination of the pathological specimen
- acceptability for the patient.

Breast-conserving surgery involves the removal of the tumour but leaving the majority of the breast intact so preserving, at least in part, an important feature of the female self-image with a better cosmetic result. Within the various techniques used for conservative therapy there is considerable variation in the amount of tissue removed. Wide local excision implies the removal of the tumour with a significant margin. Lumpectomy often refers to a less radical excision. Quadrantectomy involves the excision of the tumour and the associated breast quadrant and, although still classed as conservative breast surgery, a considerable amount of the surrounding breast tissue and skin is removed and the cosmetic and psychological results are not as good as for lumpectomy. Lumpectomy or wide local excision can be utilised for all tumours that fall into the above categories. The proponents of quadrantectomy claim a reduced local recurrence rate when compared with more local procedures.

Centrally placed lesions or diseases of the nipple are generally considered unsuitable for breast-conserving surgery although central incision including the nipple areolar complex can be considered if breast size allows.

In a tumour greater than 4 cm in diameter, mastectomy is more often recommended with or without local radiotherapy. Additional factors are:

● multifocal disease
● centrally placed tumours
● small breasts precluding good cosmesis from breast conservation
● excision margins not clear after wide local excision
● patient choice.

Local radiotherapy does not affect overall survival but local recurrence is slightly reduced at 10 years. Nevertheless many surgeons consider this advantage too small to recommend routine use of radiotherapy after mastectomy unless the patient has significant lymph node involvement or other risk factors for recurrence. However, after breast-conserving surgery, it is accepted that radiotherapy be given to the remaining breast in order to reduce the rate of local recurrence from as much as 30% down to approximately 10%.

It may be possible in the future to apply even more stringent selection criteria for radiotherapy after conservative breast surgery. For example, there is not any benefit for postmenopausal patients with tumours of less than 2 cm in diameter which are also:

● axillary node-negative
● low-grade
● oestrogen receptor status-positive
● non-comedo
● low intraductal component
● without local lymphatic or blood vessel involvement.

This could mean that currently 80% of women are receiving local radiotherapy unnecessarily. However, the role of local radiotherapy in the remaining 20% is confirmed and the selection criteria are so specific and the morbidity of modern radiotherapy so low that it would be difficult to justify attempting to select out these patients with the attendant risk of local recurrence. At the present time there is a large UK study investigating this issue.

The axilla in stage I and II disease

Assessment of the pathological status of axillary lymph nodes is judged essential for future management because it has been shown that it is one of the markers for prognosis. The presence of nodal metastasis implies systemic dissemination of the cancer and adjuvant cytotoxic or hormonal therapy should be considered. Clinical assessment is useless – 20–30% of involved nodes are impalpable clinically. The axillary nodes are

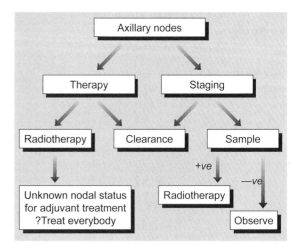

Fig 27.14 **Flow diagram showing management of axillary nodes.**

at three levels according to their relation to pectoralis minor:

● level I – inferior to the lower border of the muscle
● level II – immediately behind its belly
● level III – above and adjacent to the axillary vessels.

The nodal status can be assessed by removal of soft tissue (sampling) up to level II; at least four lymph nodes should be identified at histological examination. The alternative is axillary node clearance, which is both potentially therapeutic, in that it surgically clears the axilla of any tumour-bearing nodes, and also provides the nodes needed for staging.

The demonstration of lymph node involvement following axillary lymph node sampling requires that axillary radiotherapy be given to help control axillary nodal metastasis. However, if an axillary clearance is performed, radiotherapy for positive nodes is unnecessary – all the diseased nodes have been removed. In addition, after clearance, radiotherapy is associated with a high incidence of lymphoedema of the arm because of the combined surgical and X-ray damage to lymphatics (see 'Complications', below).

The overall concepts involved in the management of the axilla are represented in Figure 27.14.

Limitations of local resection (breast conservation)

There are additional limitations to those already mentioned. If the excision margins are not clear then many surgeons offer a further local excision. Histologically proven involvement of the excision margins of the second procedure results in the further offer of a mastectomy. Extensive local lymphatic and vascular invasion around the primary tumour is also an indicator of a high risk of local recurrence and a mastectomy is considered by some to be appropriate. Those with an extensive intraductal component

(EIC) are more likely to develop a recurrence. Women less than 35 years are also more likely to suffer local relapse.

Complications of local procedures

As with all surgical procedures, the complications can be divided into general and specific, immediate, early and late.

Specific immediate and early complications

The breast is a vascular organ with a rich blood supply. Haemorrhage during any operation on the breast can be considerable and it is usual to make preparations for possible blood transfusion before mastectomy.

Inadequate haemostasis at the time of operation leads to the formation of a postoperative haematoma which may require evacuation under general anaesthesia. Surgical interruption of the breast lymphatics increases the possibility of the accumulation of lymph to cause a postoperative seroma which requires repeated needle aspirations over several weeks but usually settles with time.

Infection of the skin flaps can lead to skin loss and, after mastectomy, grafting may be necessary to cover the defect. Infection is more likely to develop if the skin is fixed under tension, or is rendered ischaemic by a haematoma or seroma.

Complications associated with radiotherapy

Radiotherapy has specific complications, including cutaneous inflammatory reactions, photosensitisation and the development of fibrosis, and, in the long term, distortion of the breast. There have been reports of an increase in coronary artery disease in those women who have undergone irradiation to the left chest field and also of lung fibrosis. However, such complications were associated with older techniques, and modern treatment does not appear to have the same problems.

Late complications

Cosmetic

In addition to the distortion that may be caused by the fibrotic reaction initiated by the radiotherapy, surgical scarring after a breast conserving procedure can also lead to disfiguring distortion. Re-operation may be required to produce a better appearance.

Shoulder stiffness

Surgical dissection of the axilla and radiotherapy both carry this risk. Adequate analgesia and instruction by a physiotherapist should be utilised in order to facilitate an early return to as full a range of shoulder movement as can be achieved.

Brachial plexus damage

Persistent paraesthesia or numbness in the ipsilateral arm result. The symptoms may decrease with time. The possibility should be raised, although not exaggerated, in the pre-treatment interview.

Lymphoedema of the arm

This is the result usually of the combination of surgical axillary lymph node clearance and radiotherapy. A slight degree of temporary lymphoedema probably develops in most patients but it may progress to massive and disfiguring swelling with loss of function. The therapeutic combination is thus not acceptable. The treatment for established lymphoedema involves the use of sequential compression bandages and dynamic sequential compression if this is available. Very rarely, if the lymphoedema is massive or in the rare occurrence of malignant lymphangiosarcoma because of impairment of local immunity, an amputation may be the only method of achieving relief.

Management of more advanced disease and special problems

Stage III disease

A more extensive mastectomy may be necessary because of fixation of the tumour to surrounding tissues, particularly the pectoralis major. Radiotherapy must then follow. Survival generally approaches 45% at 5 years for stage III disease. Preoperative neoadjuvant combination chemotherapy over two to six drug cycles has been used to reduce tumour size (see below) – cyclophosphamide, doxorubicin and 5-fluorouracil (CAF). A response rate of 60–75% is expected. The effect on the tumour cells may not only cause shrinkage but also affect the tumour cells' kinetics such that the possibility of surgery exacerbating the progression of the disease is reduced.

Inflammatory carcinoma

The optimum treatment regimen for inflammatory breast cancer has yet to be developed. However, the best results to date confirm that a multimodality approach is required which utilises various combinations of surgery, radiotherapy and chemotherapy. After preoperative neoadjuvant radiotherapy and induction chemotherapy, a mastectomy with level III axillary lymph node removal is performed. Radiotherapy is administered to the wound site once this has healed and, if a favourable response to the chemotherapy has been noted, this may be continued, although the optimum duration of therapy has not been elucidated. Studies utilising combinations of chemotherapeutic agents have claimed up to 75% survival at 5 years; however, in general, survival remains at 30%.

Paget's disease

It is assumed that an underlying carcinoma is always present. A *palpable* growth is managed by mastectomy with either axillary clearance or sampling and, if lymph nodes are positive, local radiotherapy. The prognosis and further treatment are related to the menopausal state of the patient and the stage and grade of the primary tumour. Impalpable tumours are dealt with by mastectomy or central excision including the nipple areolar complex if breast size allows. The management of the axilla and other local treatments are guided by the final histology.

Adjuvant therapy

Both cytotoxic and hormonal therapies are used.

Cytotoxic therapy

The heterogeneous nature of breast cancer means that at any time during treatment the cancer cells contained within a metastasis may be at different stages of their cell cycle. Therefore, combination therapy that can affect the cell at different stages of its cycle is required to achieve the response rates in women with known axillary or distant metastasis.

The most effective agents are methotrexate and adriamycin given intravenously. They are often combined with cyclophosphamide and 5-fluorouracil as CMF and CAF, respectively. Response rates, as measured by objective shrinkage of metastatic deposits, vary between 20 and 70%. Complete response with eradication of tumour is very rare, less than 20%.

Chemotherapy is now considered beneficial for all women at high risk of relapse, including high-grade pre- and post-menopausal women regardless of nodal status. The maximum benefit however remains for pre-menopausal women with node-positive and oestrogen-receptor-negative disease.

Drug toxicity remains a problem and patients should be aware of this; side-effects include lassitude, temporary alopecia, blood dyscrasias (including profound leucopenia), immunosuppression and distressing gastro-intestinal symptoms including nausea, vomiting and diarrhoea. Alopecia can be managed by concealment with a wig. Upper gastrointestinal symptoms are much relieved by 5HT antagonists (ondansetron).

Hormonal manipulation

The rationale behind this method is that tumours which arise in tissue which is a target for hormones — such as the breast — may have their growth affected by either endocrine ablation or pharmacological blockade.

Hormone receptors in breast Cancer

The cytosol of breast cancer cells may contain both oestrogen (ER) and progesterone (PR) receptors. Approximately 60% possess some oestrogen receptor activity which is also a biochemical marker for the degree of differentiation and histological subtype. ER-positive tumours exhibit a 50–60% objective response rate to hormone therapies whereas only 10% of ER-negative tumours respond. The progesterone receptor is a marker of oestrogen action. Tumour which possess both ER and PR are more likely to respond to hormonal therapy than those with ER alone, but benefits are also seen in a substantial number of PR-negative tumours. Epidermal growth factor (EF) and the proto-oncogene erbB2 are transmembrane tyrosine kinase receptors that are over expressed in a proportion of breast cancers, these invariably being ER poor. However, when expressed in ER-positive patients there is evidence to suggest that they may predict a poor response to hormonal therapy. The situation as regards the ER receptor may even be more complex than currently understood as a second ER receptor (ER β) has recently been described that appears to be associated with a worse prognosis.

Pharmacological blockade

Tamoxifen is a triphenylamine anti-oestrogen that acts by binding to the oestrogen receptor and thus blocking the effect of endogenous oestrogen. Approximately 30% of all breast cancers respond to tamoxifen with this rising to 60% if they are receptor positive. It also reduces the subsequent incidence of contralateral breast cancer in postmenopausal patients by up to 40%. The maximal benefit appears to be gained by taking 20 mg of tamoxifen for 5 years with proportional mortality reductions of 12% for 1 year, 17% for 2 years and 26% for 5 years of treatment. The absolute improvement in 10-year survival rates with 5 years of tamoxifen is 10.9% for node positive patients and 5.6% for node negative patients. These benefits are present in both pre- and postmenopausal women, however the mortality reduction is not significant in ER nega-tive patients. Tamoxifen is associated with a 2-6 times increase in endometrial carcinoma but this type of malignancy is very rare and therefore a 6-times increase over the normal incidence makes little statistical impact when compared to the potential benefits. Recent interest has concentrated on the possible role of tamoxifen in prevention. Following the early publi-cation of the NSABP prevention study P-1 it is now recommended for high risk groups in the USA. However, the data is not fully mature and on-going trials in the UK are currently addressing these issues.

Some breast cancers are tamoxifen resistant or even respond unfavourably to tamoxifen. Primary resistance is usually associated with ER-negative status whilst there are various postulated mechanisms for the acquisition of secondary resistance. In addition, some

ER-positive tumours breast tumours occasionally respond unfavourably to tamoxifen and it appears that these tumours are erb B2 positive and for this group chemotherapy may be more appropriate. ERβ appears to stimulate breast cancer growth and may be associated with a positive erb B2 status. The implications for the use of tamoxifen, which is a partial agonist, in this group are clear.

Alternative methods of oestrogen modulation

Adipose tissue, breast cancer tissue and the adrenal cortex can all produce oestrogen. Tamoxifen is a selective oestrogen receptor modulator (SERM) but is only a partial antagonist and has pro-oestrogenic effects on the uterus, bone and vascular endothelium in addition to the concerns over tamoxifen resistance and possible worsening of prognosis in some patients. Alternative anti-oestrogens without intrinsic oestrogenic effect have therefore been developed. These SERMS include the pure antioestrogen ICI 182780 (faslodex). This has been shown to induce a response in tumours that have acquired or possessed inherent resistance to tamoxifen.

An alternative strategy is to utilise drugs that prevent the aromatisation of androgen to oestrogen. Two major types have been developed:

- **Type I inhibitors**. These inhibit the attachment of the androgen substrate to the enzymes catalytic site and include formestane and exemestane.
- **Type II inhibitors**. These interfere with the cytochrome p450 moiety of the enzyme and include anastrozole and letrozole.

These aromatase inhibitors have been shown to dramatically reduce the level of circulating oestrogen and to induce response in hormone-dependent breast cancer. Trials are currently underway to evaluate whether they are equivalent to tamoxifen and whether the addition of both an aromatase inhibitor with tamoxifen may be even more potent.

The majority of the new selective aromatase inhibitors are still under investigation and the progestogen-based drug megestrol remains the traditional second line hormonal therapy.

Aminoglutethimide is a non-selective aromatase inhibitor that produces an effective chemical adrenalectomy. Steroid replacement is required and side effects are common. Its use has therefore largely been abandoned in favour of the new aromatase inhibitors.

Castration

Castration can be achieved by surgical, medical or pharmacological means.

In premenopausal women, oophorectomy can be used either as a second line therapy for recurrent disease or as a primary therapy where it has been shown to be as effective as chemotherapy for all groups except oestrogen-receptor-negative, node-negative patients. By removing the ovaries or inactivating them with radiotherapy, the primary source of oestrogen is removed. Alternatively, a chemical oopherectomy can be performed utilising Gn-RH agonists. This effectively produces a medical castration and a resultant reduction in oestrogen release from the ovaries equivalent to surgical removal. Adrenalectomy and hypophysectomy have also been used in the past to suppress ovarian hormone production but have now been largely superseded by the above methods.

Psychological considerations in therapy

It must be stressed from the very beginning that the patient has an active role to play in the joint decision-making that necessarily accompanies successful treatment.

Mastectomy

One-third of women will suffer moderate or severe anxiety and depression after mastectomy. Concerns about body image, and effects on interpersonal relationships and family life can often lead to a dramatic withdrawal from society.

Even patients who have undergone breast-preserving procedures can have such symptoms because of persistent thoughts of recurrent or remaining disease. Counselling is required both pre- and postoperatively. It is not acceptable for a women to be anaesthetised for a breast operation without knowing exactly what is to happen to her body. A nurse specialised in such work is proving an increasingly useful ally.

Metastatic disease

Metastatic breast cancer is for the moment incurable. Despite this, the response to chemotherapy and actual survival rates are highly variable, which reflects the biological heterogeneity of the disease. There are a number of factors that are associated with the degree of aggressiveness of residual disease. Clinically, time interval between diagnosis and development of metastatic disease, organ sites involved and rate of tumour growth are indicators of aggressiveness. Biological characteristics include proliferative activity of the tumour, the hormone receptor status of the primary tumour and the amplification or overexpression of certain proto-oncogenes such as CerbB2. Host characteristics such as young age and Negro race may also be important adverse factors. Once the cancer has become disseminated systemically, surgery to the breast and subsequent radiotherapy are done only for local control. Combination chemotherapy can produce remission in up 70% with a median survival of 32 months if complete remission at initial treatment has been achieved. The most common combination in use for primary chemotherapy is the CMF regimen (cyclophosphamide, methotrexate, 5-fluorouracil), with second-line chemotherapy being a doxorubicin and vinblastine combination.

Follow-up

Review after treatment presents some particular problems. Patients who have undergone breast-conserving surgery have a lifelong risk of local recurrence which, although a source of anxiety for the patient, can be managed with a salvage mastectomy, or even further local excision, and does not mean impending death. Patients who have undergone mastectomy have a low rate of local recurrence, but its arrival generally heralds a significant progression of the disease. In the majority of instances, local recurrence is apparent within 3 years. If breast-conserving surgery has been done, then the remaining breast tissue will be distorted by postoperative scarring and associated fibrosis; clinical examination and mammography are both very difficult to interpret and local recurrence of the disease may be missed until it is well advanced. The detection of distant metastasis generally heralds the final phase of the disease and both further systemic and local therapy may be required to prolong life and reduce morbidity.

Follow-up is by annual mammograms and clinical examination for patients who have undergone breast conserving surgery and biannual or annual mammograms for patients with one remaining breast in order to detect a second primary – an assessment which continues for the rest of the patient's life. Other more specific investigations for metastases are only used if the patient complains of symptoms suggestive of secondary deposits.

Palliation of specific problems

Bone metastases

Seventy-three per cent of patients who die from the disease have skeletal metastases. However, less than half of these have symptoms and these lesions should be managed only when recognised as source of trouble. The exception is a lesion that threatens pathological fracture such as one in a weight-bearing bone which should be fixed internally and followed by radiotherapy. Palliative therapy should not be withheld because the median survival is as high as 48 months in patients with metastases confined to bone and 17 months for those with additional deposits at other sites. Pain from osseous metastasis can be controlled with radiotherapy, NSAIDs or opiates. Recently bisphosphonates have been shown to reduce the progression and morbidity associated with boney metastases even if they are not associated with hypercalcaemia.

Transient hypercalcaemia occurs in almost half of those with bone metastasis. Levels greater than 3 mmol/L are often associated with distressing gastro-intestinal and neurovascular symptoms.

Pleural and lung metastases

Pleural effusions and metastatic pleural disease are frequent problems. Up to 37% of all malignant pleural effusions are associated with metastatic breast cancer and are nearly always the result of haematogenous metastasis, but in some locally advanced tumours, spread may be directly through the chest wall. For this reason, bilateral effusions occur in 15%. The presence of pleural metastasis is an ominous feature because it is associated with metastasis in other sites in more than half of those who present with it.

Malignant pleural effusions are initially managed by removing the pleural liquid by either needle aspiration or intercostal drainage. However, reaccumulation is inevitable and pleurodesis is required. For this to succeed, the pleural surfaces must be in apposition, which is best achieved by intercostal drainage. An irritant such as tetracycline is successful in between 70 and 100%. Bleomycin may also be used either initially or after failed tetracycline therapy (85% success rate).

Individual lung metastases do not generally cause problems. However, diffuse infiltration of the pulmonary lymphatics produces a stiff lung often with bronchospasm and dyspnoea. Symptomatic relief can sometimes be obtained with bronchodilators and steroids.

Median survival is between 6 and 15 months. The median survival from diagnosis of the pleural effusion is 10 months, with half this group succumbing directly to their bronchopulmonary disease and half to distant metastasis to other sites.

CNS metastases

In autopsy series, about 30% of those who have died from breast cancer have been shown to have metastasis to the CNS. Of these, about 65% are asymptomatic and it is rare for a brain metastasis to be the cause of death. The dura is the most common site, with the cerebellum next. Solitary metastasis occurs in approximately 40%, with the incidence of cranial dural involvement increasing threefold if vertebral body metastases are present.

Symptoms may be either of raised intracranial pressure or focal neurological problems which depend on the site of the lesion.

Untreated survival is approximately 6 weeks. With aggressive combined therapy, which, in carefully selected patients, includes surgery, radiation therapy and chemotherapy, survival may be extended to approximately 50% at 1 year.

Spinal compression

After lung cancer, breast cancer is the second most common cause of symptomatic spinal cord compression. When it has occurred, approximately one-third develop irreversible hemiparalysis, so that an early diagnosis and urgent treatment are essential. Extramedullary disease accounts for more than 97%. The metastases reach the epidural space either by direct local extension from invasion of a vertebral body or by haematogenous spread. For diagnosis, a plain X-ray is more specific than a bone scan and can accurately predict the presence or absence of metastasis in over 80%. However, if, as is rarely the case, only the intervertebral disc is involved then plain X-ray is likely to be normal. Nevertheless, in a patient with breast cancer and back pain who has both a normal neurological examination and a normal plain film, spinal metastasis is very unlikely. CT and MRI scanning provide the diagnostic information necessary for planning treatment.

As mentioned above, treatment is a matter of urgency with the immediate introduction of dexamethasone to reduce oedema and subsequent radiotherapy. Approximately 50% respond to these measures. Indications for surgical decompression include:

- posteriorly placed lesions
- continued progression of disease in spite of radiotherapy
- recurrent compression after initial response to radiotherapy
- vertebral instability.

Radiotherapy is the best therapeutic option and should be given to all those treated surgically if they have not been previously irradiated at the site of compression.

Breast reconstruction following mastectomy

Reconstruction should not be considered a purely cosmetic procedure but rather a functional restoration of an important aspect of appearance and self-image.

There are five essential elements to any reconstructive procedure that also apply in breast cancer:

- coverage to allow survival of the procedure
- coverage to allow adequate tumour clearance
- repair of irradiated or scarred tissue by introduction of new blood supply as in flap reconstruction
- recreation of the form of the lost part
- replacement of function of the lost part.

The first three relate to soft tissue coverage and are dependent on the healing of the initial operation whatever that may have been. The last two relate to restoration of the form of the breast which is intricately interwoven with its perceived function.

Potential candidates are likely to have a set of goals that must be achieved in order to make reconstructive breast surgery worthwhile:

- symmetry
- adequate form, consistency and size
- lasting result
- no detrimental effects on treatment and outcome.

However, each may also have their own ideas about what reconstruction, if any, is desired and what quality of cosmetic result is sought. This must be thoroughly discussed before planning the exact nature of the operation.

In some instances, breast reconstruction may be carried out at the same time as the mastectomy, and for this the myocutaneous J-type latissimus dorsi flap is particularly suitable. Flaps of this kind with an independent blood supply allow radiotherapy and chemotherapy to begin after only 10 days, in contrast to other methods of skin coverage such as free flaps and skin grafts that require a longer healing period.

However, most patients are advised to wait for reconstruction until after their initial course of radiotherapy or chemotherapy has been completed. Reconstruction may be achieved using autogenous tissue or by a combination of implanted expanders and a prosthesis.

The basic shape of the breast can be achieved with a simple silicone implant provided the mastectomy flaps are not too tight (Fig. 27.15). These are now usually placed deep to the pectoralis major in order to reduce the formation of a deforming fibrous capsule – common in subcutaneous implants. Despite this advance, a prosthetic implant is often subject to deformity from scar encapsulation. Because of this, tissue expanders may be implanted at the time of mastectomy or later. Once sufficient skin is available, the expander is replaced with an implant. Scar encapsulation and subsequent deformity are much reduced. Recently combined prosthesis that act as expanders and also contain a permanent silicone component have been introduced. These do not have to be replaced once expansion is satisfactory and the final shape achieved.

Autogenous tissue transfer offers the only possibility of reconstructing a breast that will match the form, shape and consistency of the opposite side. Various myocutaneous flaps are available – including the standard latissimus dorsi flap – that can be used with an implant to increase its bulk. Flaps based on the rectus abdominis (transverse rectus abdominis myocutaneous – TRAM flap) (Fig. 27.16) have become the standard in breast reconstruction with autologous tissue and it is against this that all other methods must be considered. In certain circumstances, microvascular techniques can be employed in order to facilitate the transfer of free flaps from regions such as that supplied by the gluteal vessels. The general principles involved in breast reconstruction are illustrated in Fig. 27.17.

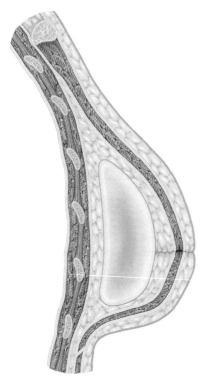

Fig 27.15 **Silicone implant.**

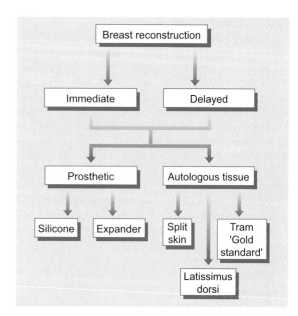

Fig 27.17 **General principles of breast reconstruction.**

Male breast cancer

Male breast cancer is rare – less than 1% of all cases. It is associated with high endogenous levels of oestrogen, and is preceded by gynaecomastia in 20%. Testicular feminisation, Klinefelter's syndrome (XXY), oestrogen therapy, irradiation and trauma are all risk factors. Stage for stage, the prognosis is the same as for female breast cancer although it tends to present late. The treatment options are also similar.

FURTHER READING

Benign breast disease

Dixon M, Sainsbury R (1998) *Handbook of diseases of the Breast.* 2nd ed. Edinburgh: Churchill Livingstone.

Hughes LE, Mansel RE, Webster DJT (2000) *Benign disorders and diseases of the breast.* 2nd ed. London: WB Saunders

Breast cancer

Dixon JM (1995) *The ABC of Breast Diseases.* London: BMJ Publishing Group.

Harris JR, Lippman ME, Morrow M, Hellman S, Henderson IC, Kinne DW (eds) (1996) *Diseases of the Breast.* Philadelphia: JB Lippincott.

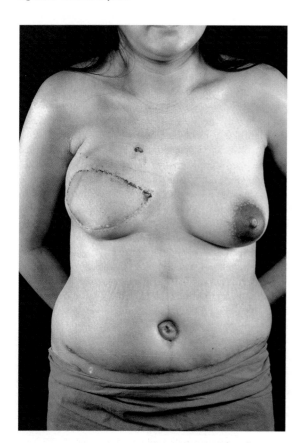

Fig 27.16 **Use of myocutaneous flap (TRAM).**

28

Arterial disease

Arterial physiology and anatomy

Arterial disease exerts major haemodynamic effects upon the circulation, which in turn cause the symptoms and signs of disease. In order to understand these processes, it is necessary to have a basic grasp of normal arterial physiology.

Normal arterial physiology

This subject can be understood in the context of blood flow, pressure and energy.

Blood flow is governed by the following parameters:

- blood pressure, velocity and blood viscosity
- the anatomy of the arterial tree
- the mechanical characteristics of the arterial wall
- the properties of the vascular endothelium.

Blood pressure

Conventionally, blood pressure (P) is measured in millimetres of mercury (mmHg). It is dependent upon:

- the force of cardiac contraction
- circulatory volume
- tone – the pressure exerted by the muscular effect of the arterioles.

Blood energy

Potential energy (E_p) is primarily determined by blood pressure. Kinetic energy (E_k) relates to the square of blood velocity (v). Blood flows through the circulation in response to changes in total blood energy (E), i.e. the sum of potential and kinetic energy.

Bernoulli's theorem states that when fluid flows from one point to another, provided flow is steady and there are no frictional losses, the total energy remains constant. As blood moves away from the heart, the total cross-sectional area of the arterial tree increases so that, if total flow is to remain constant, velocity must decrease. Kinetic energy is therefore converted to potential energy and, under idealised conditions where fluid energy is conserved, this is actually associated with a small increase in blood pressure. Although the arterial system is an extremely efficient conduit, it is not frictionless and contains bends and branches. In addition, arterial flow is pulsatile rather than steady. For these reasons the Bernoulli theorem, does not accurately describe events in vivo: fluid energy is dissipated, mainly as heat, through viscous and inertial losses.

Viscous energy losses

These are the consequence of frictional forces. Viscosity defines the resistance of a fluid to flow because of inter-molecular attractions and, in whole blood, is mainly determined by haematocrit and the concentration of plasma proteins. It is most conveniently expressed in relation to water (relative viscosity). The relative viscosity of whole blood is approximately 3–4 and plasma is about 1.8.

Inertial energy losses

These are changes in kinetic energy as a consequence of changes in blood velocity, the pattern of flow and its direction. In vivo inertial losses are more significant than viscous ones, especially in the presence of disease that leads to dilatation, tortuosity, narrowing or occlusion.

Resistance to flow

The diameter of peripheral vessels has the greatest effect on peripheral resistance and (given normal blood viscosity), at flow rates found within the human circulation, resistance increases markedly when vessel diameter falls below approximately 3 mm. Resistance in the human circulation is therefore from the:

- microcirculation – small arteries, arterioles and capillaries (70%)
- venous circulation (10%)
- large and medium-sized arteries (20%).

Thus, those arteries most commonly affected by athero-sclerosis in health offer little resistance to flow.

To summarise, as blood flows through the arterial tree, energy is lost through both viscous and inertial factors. Loss of kinetic energy is manifested by a reduction in blood velocity, and loss of potential energy by a reduction in blood pressure. In the presence of arterial disease, these losses may be excessive and may result in underperfusion of tissues and ischaemia.

Patterns of arterial flow

Three main forms are recognised:

- *Laminar* – when the motion of the blood can be described by a series of concentric rings parallel to the wall of the vessel; the flow velocity is greatest in the centre and least at the vessel wall (a so-called parabolic flow profile)
- *Turbulent* – a disorderly flow pattern where velocity varies randomly across the diameter of the vessel

- *Disturbed* – midway between laminar and turbulent where, at certain points in the circulation, there is transient disruption of laminar flow which is re-established further downstream.

In health, the only part of the human circulation in which there is turbulent flow is the ascending aorta, although disturbed flow may occur at the origin of branches. In the presence of atherosclerosis, turbulent flow is common.

Boundary effects

The boundary layer is the blood flowing adjacent to the vessel wall. At branch points and where the lumen suddenly changes size, the layer may slow down, change or even reverse its direction. Such boundary layer separation (BLS) leads to complex local flow patterns at arterial bifurcations, anastomoses and sites of arterial disease. Atherosclerotic plaques have been observed to occur particularly at points where BLS leads to reversed or stagnant flow, e.g. at the carotid bifurcation (Fig. 28.1). The reasons for this are unknown, but may relate to mechanical changes in frictional forces (shear stress) between the blood and the vessel wall or to prolonged contact between humoral factors in the blood and the endothelium at these points.

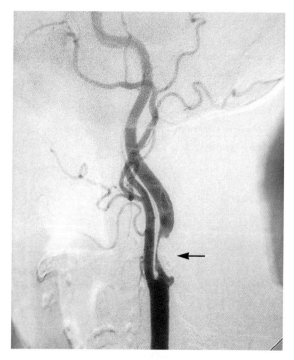

Fig 28.1 **Intra-arterial digital subtraction angiogram showing a 90% stenosis of the internal carotid artery (arrow).** Note how the vessels proximal and distal to the lesion appear almost normal. This is one of the few areas of the body where arterial disease is often localised and thus amenable to endarterectomy.

Pulsatile nature of flow

Blood flow in vivo is pulsatile. The haemodynamic principles outlined above are useful but depend upon steady laminar flow within a straight, frictionless tube. In consequence, they do not provide a precise description of the events which occur in the human circulation. Therefore, instead of using the term vascular resistance, 'vascular impedance' better describes the opposition of the circulation to pulsatile flow and includes the effects of viscosity, bends, branches, changes in diameter, arterial elasticity (compliance) and wave reflections. In order that blood should flow, mean arterial pressure (MAP) must fall although in health the gradient in MAP between the heart and the ankle is only of the order of 10 mmHg. Therefore, as the pressure wave moves distally, MAP and diastolic pressure fall. However, due to reflected waves from the distal circulation, systolic pressure actually increases and pulse pressure widens. It is for these reasons, in health the systolic ankle: brachial pressure index (ABPI) is normally greater than 1 and does not fall on exercise.

Phases of arterial flow

Arterial flow is normally triphasic, consisting of:

- an initial large forward flow caused by ventricular contraction
- a short period of reverse flow in early diastole
- a third phase of forward flow in late diastole.

The duration of the reverse flow phase depends upon peripheral resistance: when this increases (vasoconstriction on exposure to cold), the reverse flow period is extended; when it decreases (exercise, exposure to heat) the opposite is the case.

Structure of the arterial tree

Arterial wall compliance

In addition to arterial geometry, blood flow is determined by the physical characteristics of the arterial wall itself, which in turn depend upon the relative amounts of collagen, elastin and smooth muscle. The compliance (elasticity) of the artery allows blood energy to be stored during systole and to be returned to the blood in diastole. As the distance from the heart increases, the elastin:collagen ratio decreases so that the more distal arteries do not store as much energy in this way and act more as passive conduits.

Law of Laplace

For a thin-walled structure, this law describes the relationship between tangential tension (T), radius (r) and intraluminal pressure (P):

$$T = Pr$$

Thus, the greater the diameter, the greater the tension in its wall for a given blood pressure. This relationship also explains why blood pressure increases arterial wall stress and why hypertension is such a strong risk factor for aneurysmal dilatation, rupture and dissection (see below).

Abnormal arterial physiology

The above account of the normal physiology indicates the complexity of the principles that govern arterial flow. The forces at work in the presence of arterial disease are even more difficult to define.

Arterial narrowing (stenosis)

This is the commonest arterial lesion. Blood flow and blood pressure begin to be reduced at about the same magnitude of narrowing; further reductions in diameter or cross-sectional area affect flow and pressure at approximately the same rate. Because flow along the length of the artery at a localised stenosis must remain constant, velocity increases. Thus, potential energy (pressure) is converted into kinetic energy and back to potential energy. If the stenosis is short, smooth, tapering and low-grade, laminar flow is preserved and little energy is lost. By contrast if it is long, irregular, abrupt and high-grade, turbulence is produced and energy is dissipated.

Critical arterial stenosis

This is somewhat arbitrarily defined as a stenosis which produces a reduction in flow (and usually pressure) and is normally associated with a 50% reduction in diameter (~ 75% reduction in cross-sectional area). The greater the velocity of the blood which flows into the stenosis, the greater the inertial and viscous energy losses and so the greater the fall in pressure distal to the stenosis. Flow across a stenosis can be augmented by exercise or any other factor which results in peripheral vasodilatation and so reduces the vascular resistance of the distal circulation. Thus a stenosis may not be haemodynamically and symptomatically significant (critical) at rest but becomes so at high flow rates. This is the basis for exercise or 'stress' testing.

Atherosclerotic stenoses are frequently multiple. Because viscous energy losses are proportional to the length of the stenosis, one 4 cm stenosis is equivalent to two 2 cm stenoses of the same diameter. This is not true for inertial energy losses, because the two 2 cm stenoses cause more turbulence than a single 4 cm stenosis – a consequence of the doubling of entrance and exit effects on flow. Thus, a series of separately non-critical stenoses may act as one critical stenosis to reduce flow and pressure. When two lesions are of equal severity, both should be corrected; where they are not, the narrower one should be dealt with first. Arterial stenosis leads to loss of energy and loss of pressure. At first, only peak systolic pressure (PSP) is affected, MAP being preserved. Reduction in PSP is thus the most sensitive measure of stenosis. Stenosis also leads to changes in the normal triphasic waveform, with damping of the PSP, loss of the normal forward flow in late diastole (biphasic pattern) and then loss of normal reverse flow in early diastole (monophasic pattern). Such changes can be used to assess arterial disease by non-invasive means with ultrasound and plethysmographic techniques.

Collateral circulation

The increase in size of vessels that run parallel to a site of obstruction, and hence the creation of a bypass for flow (collateral circulation), is a vital compensatory mechanism that affects the clinical manifestations of arterial disease and the manner of treatment. Through mechanisms that are not well understood, but which almost certainly involve a response by the endothelium to shear stress, increased flow through an artery leads to hypertrophy and dilation. This enlargement of existing vessels provides an alternative pathway for blood flow. Effective collateral circulation is dependent upon the normal anatomy of the area involved. Disease of the superficial femoral artery with collateral flow through the profunda femoris system is perhaps the most common example of effective collateral flow and retinal artery obstruction of end-vessel occlusion.

Collateral dilatation takes time, so that *gradual* development of a stenosis has a better outcome than sudden narrowing or occlusion. The formation of a collateral circulation can be augmented through exercise because the reduction in peripheral resistance on walking increases flow through the alternative pathway. However, no matter how well a collateral circulation develops, the vessels are of less overall diameter than that which they replace, the peripheral resistance is greater and so the blood supply to the organ or limb is poorer.

Normal arterial anatomy

Arterial wall structure

Arteries are normally distensible, compliant and have three layers:

- *Intima* – a single-cell endothelial layer which rests on a basement membrane
- *Media* – separated from the intima by the internal elastic lamina, composed mostly of smooth muscle cells but also, in large vessels, containing numerous elastin fibres
- *Adventitia* – a meshwork of connective tissue which contains the vasa vasorum that provide blood to the media; between the media and adventitia is the external elastic lamina.

Box 28.1

Properties of the normal endothelium and arterial wall

Endothelium

Controls microvascular permeability

Non-thrombogenic, pro-fibrinolytic surface through production of prostacylin, heparins and activation of fibrinolytic cascade

Modulation of the inflammatory response through cytokine and adhesion molecule release or expression

Modulation and initiation of thrombus formation through platelet and coagulation cascade activation

Production of vasoactive substances such as nitric oxide, angiotensin-converting enzyme (ACE) and endothelin

Arterial wall

Storage of blood energy

Autoregulation – contraction and relaxation in response to myogenic and metabolic factors

Lipid metabolism

Production of connective tissue

Arterial repair through migration and proliferation of smooth muscle cells

---

Arterial endothelium

The endothelium is not merely an inert lining (Box 28.1). The biology of the endothelial cell is complex and still imperfectly understood. Any disease process that leads to endothelial dysfunction has major effects upon arterial autoregulation, blood coagulation and fibrinolysis.

Effects of ischaemia-reperfusion injury (IRI)

Ischaemic injury

All tissues rely on the circulation to deliver oxygen and nutrients and to remove the waste products of metabolism. Any pathological process that reduces the blood supply leads to the replacement of aerobic by anaerobic metabolism and the build-up of the potentially harmful products of metabolism, particularly carbon dioxide and lactic acid, with the accumulation of hydrogen ions. Through mechanisms which are poorly understood, tissues can adapt to a degree of ischaemia, especially if it develops gradually rather than acutely. However, after a certain point, cell membrane disruption and macromolecular denaturation occur, which lead to irreversible ischaemic injury and loss of function, even if normal arterial flow is eventually restored. Tissues differ widely in their tolerance of ischaemia; irreversible damage to neurons occurs after only a few minutes but skin may survive for up to 24 hours. This variability in tissue tolerance affects the clinical manifestations of arterial disease in different parts of the body as well as the urgency and success of surgical intervention.

Reperfusion injury (RI)

While it is easy to understand that tissues are damaged by ischaemia, it is more difficult to appreciate that as much, if not more, injury can be sustained when ischaemic tissue is reperfused. In vascular surgery, reperfusion is a common event. Every time a patient with claudication takes exercise and experiences pain, the leg muscles are ischaemic and on rest are reperfused; virtually every open operation upon an artery requires that the vessel which supplies a peripheral vascular bed is temporarily interrupted, which inevitably leads to a degree of distal ischaemia. After repair, when the circulation is restored, reperfusion occurs.

The mechanisms which underlie reperfusion injury are complex and imperfectly understood. Briefly, when tissues are rendered ischaemic, the endothelium lining that vascular bed is activated. Instead of providing a smooth, non-stick surface, activated endothelial cells release pro-coagulant substances, express adhesion molecules that attract and bind leucocytes and release cytokines that act upon the white cells to produce more cytokines and oxygen-derived free radicals. When the tissue is reperfused, leucocytes, platelets and thrombus adhere to the endothelium and imperil the microcirculation. An inflammatory response is initiated and tissues are damaged. In addition, some activated leucocytes and their products escape into the general circulation and can contribute to organ failure, such as renal failure and adult respiratory distress syndrome (ARDS, Ch. 16).

CLINICAL COMPLICATIONS

Compartment syndrome (see also Ch. 34)
When severely ischaemic tissues are reperfused, the microcirculation is very permeable and plasma leaks through the damaged capillary endothelium into the interstitial space. Ischaemic cells also swell because of membrane injury. The overall result is marked tissue swelling and oedema. Calf muscles are held within fascial compartments which do not allow expansion. Reperfusion is therefore associated with a marked increase in intracompartmental pressure such that,

despite normal arterial inflow, the microcirculation remains underperfused and cellular hypoxia persists. Fasciotomy is therefore necessary at the same time as revascularisation.

General metabolic effects
If a large embolus lodges at the aortic bifurcation (saddle embolus) to cause total ischaemia of the lower body, revascularisation by means of bilateral transfemoral embolectomy is usually achieved without difficulty. On reperfusion, however, deterioration rather than improvement often occurs because of the entry of metabolites, such as potassium and hydrogen ions, into the general circulation. Cardiac arrest several hours later is not uncommon.

Myoglobinuria
Irreversible damage to muscle cells causes release of myoglobin into the circulation on reperfusion. Renal tubular injury and renal failure may follow. Management comprises adequate hydration and a forced alkaline diuresis.

Surgeons and anaesthetists take all possible measures to reduce RI by minimising the duration of ischaemia through expeditious surgery and/or the use of shunts to maintain the blood supply to the distant organ while the operation is completed. In addition, attention to fluid balance, oxygenation and certain drugs such as mannitol, allopurinol and dopamine may help to attenuate the effects of RI and protect the kidneys and the lungs from these processes.

Pathological features of arterial disease

A distinction is drawn between macrovascular disorders which affect large vessels and microvascular ones which involve the distal parts of the arterial circulation – the smallest arteries and arterioles.

Atherosclerotic occlusive disease

This is the commonest cause of arterial disease in developed countries. It is also known as 'arteriosclerosis' or 'atheroma' and to lay people as 'hardening of the arteries'. Atherosclerosis is found in virtually 100% of adults from developed countries and is responsible for 50% of all deaths. The prevalence of atheroma increases with age but it is not regarded as an intrinsic part of the ageing process.

Definition

Atherosclerotic occlusive disease is a variable combination of changes in the intima which include focal accumulations of lipid, complex carbohydrates, blood and blood products, fibrous deposits and calcium deposits associated with secondary changes in the media (World Health Organization).

Development

It is still far from clear how atheroma develops. The first event is probably endothelial damage caused by:

- *Mechanical injury*. At certain points in the circulation the endothelium is exposed to particularly high shearing forces, especially in the presence of hypertension. In this context, the low pressure pulmonary circulation is very rarely affected.
- *Chemical injury*. One or more constituents of tobacco smoke almost certainly have a direct toxic affect on the endothelium. Certain lipids are also harmful.

Damaged endothelium ceases to be a functional barrier between the blood and the arterial wall, and lipoproteins, fibrinogen, leucocytes and platelets can transgress the intima. Through poorly understood mechanisms, smooth muscle cells are in turn stimulated to enter the intima from the media, take on the properties of fibroblasts and secrete collagen and matrix.

The end result is an atheromatous plaque which is elevated, pale yellow or grey, involves the intima and media, and consists of smooth muscle cells, fibroblasts, macrophages, collagen and intra- and extracellular lipid. The endothelium may be lost from the surface of the plaque to form an ulcer, with cholesterol and/or altered blood constituents (thrombus) at its base. Such a plaque is often described as 'complex'.

AETIOLOGY

Smoking

Tobacco smoking is the single largest risk factor for arterial disease and the risk is directly related to the number of 'pack-years' smoked. Tobacco smoke contains many hundreds of different chemicals and it is unclear which are directly toxic to vascular endothelium. In addition, smoking increases blood viscosity and activates leucocytes to make them less deformable and more likely to become involved in inflammatory processes. Raised blood levels of carbon monoxide may also be a factor. Cessation of smoking is associated with a rapid reversal of the adverse rheological changes and a reduction in the risk of future vascular clinical events. It is not known if atheroma regresses but certain studies suggest that it does.

Diabetes

Both insulin-dependent and non-insulin-dependent diabetes greatly increase the risk of atheroma. Lesions develop earlier in life and progress more rapidly. The distribution of atheroma may also differ from that found in non-diabetic patients (e.g. the tibial and foot vessels are more commonly affected). Both secondary increases in blood lipid levels and changes in endothelial cell metabolism may be involved.

Hyperlipidaemia

The normal plasma level of cholesterol varies between populations: in the UK, 5–6 mmol/L is usual. Many of those with arterial disease have much higher levels. Raised plasma levels result from:

- a high-fat diet
- a genetically determined reduction in the removal of lipid and lipoproteins from the circulation (primary hyperlipidaemia); hyperlipidaemia is one of the commonest inherited autosomal dominant conditions (approximately 1 in 500 of the UK population)
- secondary hyperlipidaemia caused by a variety of other conditions – diabetes, hypothyroidism, excessive alcohol intake and drugs (thiazide diuretics and corticosteroids).

There is increasing evidence that, in the presence of atheroma, reduction in cholesterol levels is associated with a decline in future vascular events, particularly myocardial infarction and stroke. Those with arterial disease should therefore have a measurement of lipid levels and, if there is an abnormality, efforts should be made to correct it.

ANATOMICAL DISTRIBUTION

Although atheroma can be found throughout the circulation, it does have a predilection for certain sites – the carotid bifurcation, the coronary arteries, the infrarenal aorta and the superficial femoral artery. In any one patient, not all may be affected equally or indeed at all.

COMPLICATIONS

An atheromatous plaque may cause:

- narrowing or occlusion, which can result in ischaemia and infarction
- thrombosis
- athero-embolism where fragments of plaque, cholesterol and thrombus break off and lodge in the distal circulation
- weakening of the arterial wall with aneurysmal dilation
- periarterial inflammation.

Aneurysmal disease

The term aneurysm denotes an abnormal localised dilatation of a blood vessel. Almost any artery may become aneurysmal, although the commonest large vessel is the infrarenal aorta, followed by the iliac and popliteal arteries.

CLASSIFICATION

- *Anatomical* – localised (saccular) and diffuse (fusiform)
- *Pathological* – true (lined by all three layers of the normal arterial wall) and false or pseudo (formed in the adventitia or completely outside the wall)
- *Aetiological* – see below.

AETIOLOGY

Atherosclerosis

There is continuing controversy over whether aneurysmal disease is just another manifestation of atherosclerosis. However, many believe it to be a separate condition – medial degenerative disease. Nevertheless, there is no doubt that aneurysmal disease shares the same risk factors as atheromatous occlusive disease (although hypertension appears a more important factor) and that aneurysmal and occlusive arterial disease often coexist. In addition, there is a strong familial element in aneurysmal but not in occlusive disease. Furthermore, there are patients, some of whom who have never smoked, who exhibit wide-spread aneurysmal dilatation (arterial ectasia or arteriomegaly) without any evidence of peripheral, cerebral or coronary occlusive disease. With the successful correction of life-threatening aneurysms, the long-term survival of such patients approximates to that of a population matched for age and sex but without aneurysmal disease. This is in sharp contrast to those with occlusive disease who have a poorer long-term prognosis because of cardiac and cerebrovascular events.

Inflammation

In some patients, atherosclerosis, whether associated with aneurysmal dilation or not, can lead to an intense periadventitial inflammatory and fibrotic response. The reasons are unclear but clinical problems can occur in consequence. Approximately 10% of abdominal aortic aneurysms (AAA) have an inflammatory element: the anterior wall is extremely thick and structures such as the ureters are often surrounded to cause obstruction and hydronephrosis or caval occlusion. There is no evidence that such aneurysms are any more or less likely to rupture, but operative repair can be technically very difficult. Patients frequently complain of abdominal or back pain and their erythrocyte sedimentation rate (ESR) is usually raised. On computed tomography the thickened aortic wall is seen to pervade surrounding tissues. Steroid treatment has been advocated to reduce inflammation and oedema in order to relieve pain, ureteric obstruction and to make aneurysm repair more

straightforward. However, there is no evidence that steroid treatment reduces, and it may even increase, the risk of rupture.

Dissection

Weakness of the aortic wall may result in an intimomedial tear and allow blood to track under pressure through and/or outwith the various layers of the wall. Such a dissecting aneurysm usually affects the thoraco-abdominal aorta. Rupture may occur outwards (usually fatal) or inwards into the aortic lumen with the subsequent formation of a large saccular aneurysm in the weakened section. Causes of the defect include:

- atherosclerosis usually with hypertension
- Marfan's syndrome (below) in which there is a structural defect in the biochemical nature of the media.

Infection

The arterial wall is normally highly resistant to bacterial and other infections. However, certain organisms (see 'Arteritis' below), notably *Salmonella* and *Treponema pallidum*, have a particular ability to infect, and thus to weaken, the aortic wall with the formation of a mycotic aneurysm and its rupture. In developed countries, mycotic aneurysms account for less than 1% of all aneurysms but they are still common elsewhere.

COMPLICATIONS

Surgeons operate on aneurysms to prevent or manage complications, the most notable of which is rupture. Other complications include thrombosis and distal embolism (e.g. popliteal and subclavian). Less frequently, aneurysms cause external compression or stretching of surrounding structures – the bronchus or recurrent laryngeal nerve (thoraco-abdominal) or the duodenum (infrarenal aorta).

Arteritis (vasculitis, angiitis)

Although the majority of such patients do not present to surgeons, arteritis can cause macrovascular complications such as ischaemia and aneurysm. Other patients may present with Raynaud's phenomenon.

AETIOLOGY

Vessels of any size may be infected by pyogenic bacteria, mycobacteria, fungi, viruses, protozoa, *Rickettsia*, and spirochetes such as *Treponema pallidum*. Infection may damage the vessel wall directly through effects on the endothelium and/or vasa vasorum or indirectly through immunological mechanisms.

A range of arteritides are attributed to immunologically mediated injury. They may or may not occur in association with arthritis, myositis and myocarditis as part of a defined autoimmune connective tissue disease such as systemic lupus erythematosus (SLE). In the majority, the inducing antigen is unknown. These hypersensitivity arteritides may be further classified on the basis of the histological changes in the arterial wall.

PATHOLOGICAL FEATURES

Inflammation may be acute or chronic and associated with necrosis, fibrosis or granuloma formation in the vessel wall. Neutrophils, macrophages and lymphocytes are involved, as is activation of the complement system and kinins. Systemic effects are associated with the release of acute-phase proteins and lead to fever and malaise. The clinical features depend largely upon the size, type and anatomical distribution of vessel(s) affected, together with the chronicity and severity of the inflammatory process. Acute forms may have a sudden and dramatic onset progressing to death with all the lesions at the same stage of development. Chronic forms may have an insidious onset, a waxing and waning course, with lesions in various stages of progression and remission. Early diagnosis is important because many patients respond quickly to medical treatment but, if left untreated, have a poor prognosis

(Table 28.1). Although there is no universally accepted classification of the arteritides, they may be grouped on the basis of aetiology, type of vessel affected and symptoms. There is an increasing tendency simply to use the term vasculitis.

The dominant feature may be:

- *Necrotising*. Inflammation is associated with segmental necrosis of the vessel wall which often contains a considerable amount of fibrin (fibrinoid necrosis).
- *Acute inflammatory*. There is a short history and usually an identifiable antigen, often a drug. Small veins, arteries and capillaries are affected by an acute inflammatory response. Lesions may progress rapidly (even to death), be self-limiting in response to withdrawal of antigen or may become chronic.
- *Chronic inflammatory*. Although these are characterised by a chronic inflammatory reaction, presumably in response to repeated exposure to an antigen, often the source is unknown.
- *Granulomatous*. Inflammation is associated with the development of granulomas, with or without the presence of giant cells.
- *Fibrosis*. Excessive fibrosis is found in the vessel wall.

Table 28.1
Investigation of vasculitis

Investigation	Results and comments
Acute phase proteins C-reactive protein (CRP) complement factors (C)	CRP, C3 and C4 usually elevated; useful for diagnosis and monitoring treatment
ESR	Usually elevated; less responsive than CRP
Autoantibodies Antinuclear antibody Anti-double-stranded DNA Anticentromere Extractable nuclear antigen Anticardiolipin Antineutrophil Rheumatoid factor	May be of primary pathogenic significance or may simply be secondary markers of tissue injury; most helpful in the diagnosis of defined connective tissue disorders such as SLE, scleroderma and CREST syndrome
Serum electrophoresis Cryoglobulins	Serum immunoglobulins (Ig) are usually non-specifically elevated; monoclonal Ig (paraproteins) may be present; some paraproteins (cryoglobulins) precipitate on cooling and damage skin vessels
Urinanalysis	High incidence of renal involvement in arteritis mandates examination of the urine for protein, blood, casts and red cells. Plasma creatinine as well as 24-hour urinary protein and creatinine clearance should be performed
Biopsy Renal Temporal artery	If positive may confirm arteritis and aid more precise diagnosis; negative biopsy does not exclude arteritis because lesions are focal and can be missed
Imaging CT MRI	May identify vasculitic lesions in deep organs
Echocardiography	Assesses myocardial and valvular function in patients with myocarditis, endocarditis, aortitis and coronary artery aneurysms (Kawasaki disease)
Angiography	Delineates the pattern of large vessel disease; allows planning of arterial reconstruction (Takayasu's disease)

Surgical arteritides
Giant cell arteritis

The temporal and retinal arteries are frequently involved in this condition. Arm vessels may also be affected.

CLINICAL FEATURES

Symptoms
In retinal artery disease, blindness is the leading symptom, which may cause presentation to a vascular surgeon with the mistaken diagnosis of a transient ischaemic episode from a lesion in the carotid artery.

Physical findings
Usual findings are:

- loss of vision
- evidence of hypertension
- a tender, thickened temporal artery.

INVESTIGATION
A markedly elevated ESR will be found. The diagnosis is confirmed by removal of a segment of temporal artery which shows the characteristic biopsy findings.

Takayasu's arteritis

This condition primarily affects the aortic arch (and its branches) in young women.

CLINICAL FEATURES

Symptoms
Most patients suffer a vague prodromal illness followed, after a variable period of time, by the symptoms and signs of vascular occlusion – most commonly arm claudication, syncopal attacks and visual disturbances.

Physical findings
These will depend on the arterial bed involved. Stenosis, occlusion, thrombosis, secondary atherosclerosis and aneurysmal dilation of affected vessels are all seen.

INVESTIGATION AND MANAGEMENT
Apart from an acute-phase response, there are no specific markers of the disease. Primary treatment is with steroids and immunosuppressants, but vascular reconstruction may be required.

Polyarteritis

This is a small vessel disease which may lead to ulceration and gangrene of the digits and abdominal pain from mesenteric ischaemia (Ch. 22).

Systemic sclerosis (scleroderma)

This condition commonly presents with Raynaud's syndrome (see below) many years before other features of the disease become apparent. It may progress to tissue loss with ulceration and gangrene of toes and fingers which may require amputation. The Calcinosis, Raynaud's, oEsophageal, Sclerodactyly, Telangiectasia (CREST) syndrome is a variant.

Systemic lupus erythematosus (SLE)

This may also present because of Raynaud's phenomenon.

Miscellaneous conditions

There are a number of other conditions which are associated with arterial disease.

Behçet's disease

This condition is characterised by orogenital ulceration and vasculitis. It is associated with venous thrombosis and thrombophlebitis as well as arterial aneurysm and occlusion.

Buerger's disease (thromboangiitis obliterans)

This may be a form of atherosclerosis or, perhaps more likely, a type of inflammatory arteritis. Small, rather than large and medium-sized arteries, are affected. Veins may also become involved and develop thrombophlebitis. Femoral and popliteal pulses are often normal, but pedal pulses are absent. Young male smokers are almost exclusively involved and there appears to be a genetic element in that the incidence is particularly high in certain ethnic groups. Symptoms of peripheral vascular insufficiency nearly always begin before the age of 30. Complete cessation of smoking allows collaterals to form and is associated with a good prognosis, but failure to refrain almost inevitably leads to major amputation.

Marfan's syndrome

This is a familial disorder in which the basic underlying defect is a mutation in the fibrillin gene on chromosome 15. The physical manifestations are:

- long fingers
- high arched palate

- lens dislocation
- focal medial necrosis of the aorta, which may lead to aortic valve root dilatation and incompetence, dissection of the ascending aorta and the development of thoracoabdominal aneurysm.

Ehlers–Danlos syndrome

This is a familial disorder of collagen. Patients are 'double-jointed', have wide scars and carry a high mortality from aneurysm rupture.

Fibromuscular hyperplasia

This is characterised by arterial stenoses and dilatations and results in a 'string of beads' appearance on angiography. It most often affects the renal and carotid arteries of young women and is amenable to angioplasty.

Patient assessment

Clinical

History

Enquire about the nature, severity, onset and duration of symptoms of the presenting complaint. Also ask about past medical history, with particular emphasis on cardiac disease (angina, myocardial infarction), hypertension (severity, duration, treatment and quality of control), cerebrovascular disease (transient ischaemic attacks [TIA], amaurosis fugax and stroke), renal disease (renal failure, requirement for dialysis) and diabetes.

Systematic enquiry

Ask the patient about the following:

- a history of allergy, particularly to iodine which may be considered as a contrast medium for arteriography
- drug therapy, past and present – particularly the use of beta-blockers, which may aggravate critical ischaemia; angiotensin-converting enzyme (ACE) inhibitors and non-steroidal anti-inflammatory agents (NSAIDs), which may precipitate renal failure in patients with renal artery stenosis and borderline renal function
- anticoagulant therapy, in case invasive investigations and/or surgery are being contemplated

- symptoms of arterial disease elsewhere (arterial disease is nearly always multisystem) – e.g. a patient with leg ischaemia frequently has significant coronary artery and cerebrovascular disease which predispose to myocardial infarction and stroke.

Information may not be volunteered because the presenting features may supersede or mask disease elsewhere (claudication in the leg may limit exercise tolerance so that angina is not manifest and, conversely, relief of leg pain may unmask cardiac pain).

Physical findings
General

The examination begins the moment the patient enters the consulting room. An impression of general health, vigour and mobility are important in the management of arterial disease, especially if major surgery to prolong life or to improve its quality comes to be considered. Tobacco on the breath and/or staining of the fingers suggest recent heavy cigarette smoking. Other relevant general findings are the presence of finger clubbing, anaemia, jaundice, lymphadenopathy, central cyanosis and degree of breathlessness, particularly the ability to lie flat on the examination couch (those with arterial disease often have a history of cardiorespiratory disease). Gouty tophi are infrequently found, but hyperuricaemia accelerates atheroma and is amenable to treatment. Xanthomata or xanthelasma may suggest treatable hyperlipidaemia.

Weight loss and cachexia are not usually caused by arterial disease except when the mesenteric vessels are involved. If they are a striking feature, the cause should usually be sought elsewhere.

Mental state and coherence are assessed. A past stroke may be evident from paralysis of a limb, hemiplegia or speech disturbance and can indicate carotid artery disease.

Walk with the patient and observe how he or she copes with a flight of stairs in order to determine the march tolerance and general level of fitness.

Cardiovascular examination

Pulse rate and rhythm, in particular the presence or absence of atrial fibrillation, are established. Blood pressure should be recorded in both arms because subclavian artery disease is relatively common. Although minor differences of 10–15 mmHg are not diagnostically significant, they may affect the accuracy and interpretation of future blood pressure monitoring. Subclavian artery disease may also preclude the use of an axillofemoral graft. Supra-aortic pulses (carotid, subclavian, axillary) should be gently palpated and the presence of bruits sought. A prominent carotid pulse usually signifies a tortuous vessel rather than an aneurysm.

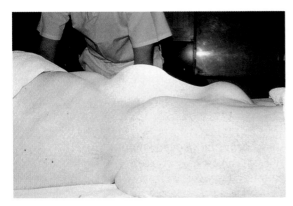

Fig 28.2 **A large abdominal aortic aneurysm is obvious on inspection of the abdomen in this thin patient.**

The heart and precordium are examined in the standard way. The presence of murmurs and evidence of left ventricular hypertrophy (displacement of the apex beat) should be sought.

The abdomen must be fully uncovered from xiphisternum to the groin. Look for abnormal pulsations (Fig. 28.2). Note any scars. Palpation is gentle because both normal, and aneurysmal aortas are often tender. The most important measurement in an aneurysm is width, not length, and allowance must be made for the thickness of the abdominal wall musculature and fat. It can be difficult to distinguish between the transmitted pulsation of an upper abdominal mass (including faeces in the transverse colon) which overlies the aorta and the expansile pulsation of an aneurysm. Positioning the patient so that the mass is no longer resting on the aorta may make the distinction obvious. Assessment of the possible presence of an aortic aneurysm, even by experts, is notoriously unreliable and physical findings should be confirmed by ultrasound. The normal aorta bifurcates at the level of the umbilicus (L3–4) and abnormal pulsations below this area are usually iliac in origin. Aortocaval fistula is associated with a machinery murmur on auscultation, and stenoses of the aortoiliac, mesenteric and renal arteries may produce a systolic bruit.

Lower limb pulses should be noted together with any accompanying bruits. If there is doubt whether it is the patient's pedal, or the examiner's own digital, pulse that is being felt, it is useful to simultaneously feel the patient's radial pulse. The femoral pulse is usually easy to feel at the mid-inguinal point (below the inguinal ligament midway between the anterior superior iliac spine and the pubic symphysis). The popliteal pulse is felt on deep palpation in the popliteal fossa with the knee flexed to relax the popliteal fascia. It is usually difficult to feel; if it is very obvious then the examiner should consider the possibility of a popliteal aneurysm. The posterior tibial pulse is felt between the medial malleolus and the Achilles tendon. The dorsalis pedis artery is a continuation of the anterior tibial and is felt on the dorsum of the foot just proximal to the groove between the first and second metatarsals, lateral to the tendon of extensor hallucis longus. In 10% of normal people it is congenitally absent, the dorsum of the foot being supplied by a perforating branch of the peroneal which may be felt 1 cm medial to the lateral malleolus at the ankle.

Neurogenic claudication

In a small proportion of patients with intermittent claudication, pedal pulses are palpable. It is then worth asking the patient to walk until the pain comes on and to reassess pulsation. If they have disappeared, it suggests that there is an arterial stenosis but that it only becomes haemodynamically significant when the demand for flow is increased (see p. 000). However, if pulses are still present, then arterial claudication is unlikely and the diagnosis of spinal or neurogenic claudication (p. 000), where pain is caused by nerve root compression, must be considered. In this condition, pain often affects the thigh and the calf equally, is present on standing not just walking, and is usually relieved only by sitting or lying down, not just by ceasing to walk. Straight leg raising may be impaired and there may be subjective and objective neurosensory loss. There may be muscle wasting or reduced reflexes and the femoral nerve stretch test may be positive.

Venous claudication

Venous claudication because of obstruction to venous outflow (Ch. 29) produces a bursting pain in the calf on walking. Unlike arterial and neurogenic claudication, the pain is usually only relieved by elevation, the leg is chronically swollen and there is usually a clear history of previous deep vein thrombosis.

Features of chronic ischaemia in the legs are loss of hair, pigmentation, ulceration, pallor or gangrene. Elevation of the severely ischaemic foot causes pallor and guttering of the veins. Dependency produces a reddish-blue appearance from the presence of desaturated blood within the skin – the sunset foot. Tissue loss is usually obvious although lesions of the heel and between the toes are easily missed if examination is cursory.

Investigations

An experienced vascular surgeon can often make the diagnosis of arterial disease and determine its severity and anatomical extent by a careful history and examination alone. The surgeon will also usually have at this point a fairly clear idea of the treatment options available.

Investigation must consider how to obtain the most information, in the safest and most pleasant way for the patient and for the least cost. There must also be a clear idea how the results of any particular test will affect the management. A significant proportion of patients do not require surgical intervention either because their symptoms are not vascular (or if vascular they are very mild) or because their general condition renders surgery too hazardous. In such patients, complex investigations are rarely indicated unless it is thought desirable to establish a baseline against which progression can be measured.

Although arteriography gives excellent anatomical information about the arterial circulation of the lower limb (the one which brings the majority of patients for investigation), it is expensive, not without hazard and should not be requested in every patient who presents with symptoms and signs of lower limb ischaemia. In addition, although intra-arterial pressures can be measured at angiography, the investigation provides little haemodynamic information. There is, therefore, a place for non-invasive studies that can be performed routinely and safely and which provide functional information through measurement of blood pressure, limb volume and flow velocity (see Ch. 4).

Risk factor assessment

Arterial disease has usually been present for many years before it becomes symptomatic. The concept that, by intervening early in its course, prevention of progression to symptoms can be achieved is termed primary prevention. Intervention to prevent progression and clinical deterioration once symptoms have developed is known as secondary prevention.

A major role of the vascular surgeon is to identify risk factors for arterial disease that influence primary and secondary prevention. For example, up to a fifth of patients with arterial occlusive disease are diabetic, although in up to half of these the diagnosis may not have been made before the onset of vascular symptoms. A third to a half of vascular patients may have hyperlipidaemia requiring control with diet and/or medication. Other risk factors include hypertension, smoking, lack of exercise and obesity.

Before investigations specific to the symptomatic part of the body are conducted, it is necessary to view the patient with arterial disease as a whole and to correct risks factors as far as is possible. Many large studies show that this is a highly worthwhile exercise. For example, reduction in blood cholesterol concentrations in patients with hyperlipidaemia and coronary artery disease can reduce death from myocardial infarction by up to a third. There is increasing evidence that careful glycaemic control in diabetics reduces the vascular complications of the disease, and treatment of even mild hypertension markedly reduces the risk of stroke. Cessation of smoking is associated with a reduction in vascular events and with increased long-term patency of arterial reconstruction.

Ultrasound

The principles of ultrasound investigation are discussed in Chapter 4.

Ankle brachial pressure index (ABPI)

Atherosclerotic stenoses cause a pressure drop between the arm and the foot. This can be measured by detection of pulsation at the elbow and ankle with a Doppler probe while the pressure is gradually reduced in cuffs on the upper arm and just above the ankle. Normal pedal pressure is usually 10–20 mmHg higher than brachial pressure and the normal ABPI around 1.1. An ABPI of less than 0.9 normally indicates a haemodynamically significant lesion (which may be asymptomatic); 0.5–0.8 is associated with claudication; 0.25–0.5 with rest pain; and less than 0.25 with tissue loss – ulceration or gangrene. There is considerable variation between patients, with proximal lesions and multilevel disease having a greater effect on the ABPI than isolated distal disease. For an individual, the trend in ABPI over time is more important than the absolute value. ABPI can also be used to assess the success or otherwise of intervention. After successful surgery or angioplasty, the ABPI should rise by at least 0.15; a subsequent similar fall suggests that re-occlusion has taken place.

Non-compressible vessels

Calcified crural vessels, most commonly but not exclusively found in diabetics, may not be compressible and the ABPI is then falsely elevated.

Post-exercise ABPI

Inertial energy losses across a stenosis are proportional to blood velocity. In low-flow states, lesser degrees of stenosis may not produce a pressure drop so that, at rest, the ABPI may approach normal. After exercise, increased cardiac output and reduced peripheral resistance raise flow velocity to the point where pressure across the stenosis begins to fall. A reduction in APBI after exercise may therefore unmask mild to moderate disease. Reactive hyperaemia may be used as an alternative to exercise when the general state precludes treadmill exercise. A cuff is placed on the thigh, inflated above systolic pressure for 5 minutes and then released. The temporary ischaemia distal to the cuff causes reactive vasodilatation which leads to a phase of hyperaemic flow when the cuff is removed. The fall in ABPI on reactive hyperaemia correlates well with that found after exercise, but treadmill testing has the advantage that it gives a better impression of the patient's overall disability and of cardiorespiratory function. For example, it is important to know whether walking is actually limited by angina or osteoarthritis rather than by claudication.

Segmental pressures

By placing cuffs around the upper thigh, lower thigh and calf, the level of lesions causing significant falls in pressure can be determined.

B-mode ultrasound

This procedure is principally used in vascular surgical practice to screen for, assess the size of and follow the time course of aneurysms, particularly in the abdominal aorta (Fig. 28.3).

Duplex ultrasound

This has revolutionised vascular surgery and yields simultaneous anatomical and physiological information on flow in a variety of arteries safely, non-invasively and, if necessary, repeatedly. Duplex is used in many areas affected by occlusive and aneurysmal arterial disease (Fig. 28.4). Disadvantages are that the equipment is expensive and the production and interpretation of the scans require considerable experience.

Assessment of stenosis

When blood flows through an arterial stenosis, velocity increases. The high-speed jet can be localised on B-mode ultrasound with the aid of colour flow mapping and the precise velocity of the jet measured. The increase in velocity is proportional to the degree of stenosis and so, by comparing the velocities proximal

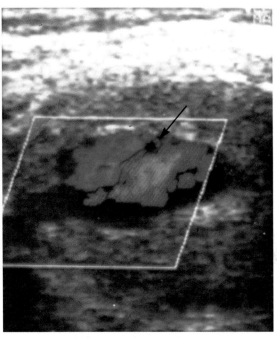

Fig 28.4 **A colour flow duplex scan of a longitudinal cross-sectional image of an aneurysm.** The B-mode facility demonstrates the aneurysmal wall (**arrow**), while the colour Doppler indicates flow within the lumen: red, flow towards the ultrasound probe; blue, flow away from the probe. The appearance of red and blue flow within the aneurysm is indicative of turbulence.

(V_1) and distal (V_2) to the stenosis (V_1/V_2 ratio), an estimate of the degree of stenosis can be made. For example, in the internal carotid artery, a V_1/V_2 ratio greater than 4 together with a peak systolic velocity greater than 120 cm/s and a peak diastolic velocity greater than 40 cm/s suggests a stenosis of greater than 70%. Similar assessments can be made at any other site where the artery lies superficially and can thus be insolated by the ultrasound beam. In thin patients, reliable information can even be obtained from the aortoiliac segments. Duplex can also be used to look for stenoses within arterial bypasses – graft surveillance.

Plaque morphology

Duplex ultrasound also provides useful information about the composition of a plaque. In the carotid artery this may relate to a plaque's propensity to cause a stroke. Thus, the more lipid-rich and the less fibrous a carotid plaque, the more likely it is to be a source of atheromatous emboli which lodge distally to cause a stroke, TIA or amaurosis fugax (transient unilateral loss of vision secondary to occlusion of the retinal artery or its branches).

Plethysmography

This is the measurement of volume change: during

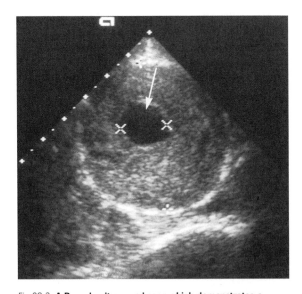

Fig 28.3 **A B-mode ultrasound scan which demonstrates a transverse cross-sectional image of a large abdominal aortic aneurysm.** The appearance has been likened to that of a fried egg. The bright circular band around the egg is the aneurysm wall; the white of the egg is the laminated thrombus within the aneurysm sac; and the yolk is the channel through the centre of the aneurysm where blood still flows (**arrow**).

systole the limb expands with arterial inflow and during diastole it contracts with venous outflow. Several types of instrument are available but the simplest to use is the air plethysmograph (APG), also known as the pulse volume recorder.

Pneumatic cuffs are placed around the thigh, calf and ankle, and the cuff at the site to be assessed is inflated with air to a pressure of 60 mmHg so that the cuff is brought in to light contact with the underlying leg. Any change in limb volume at that point produces changes in volume within the cuff such that the volume trace obtained closely resembles that of the arterial pressure wave. Air plethysmography is now more commonly used in the research assessment of the venous circulation.

Computed tomography (CT)

In vascular practice, CT is most commonly used to examine the brain in patients who present with carotid artery disease and the aorta in those with aneurysmal disease and/or dissection (Fig. 28.5). CT can be performed with and without intravascular contrast medium to highlight the arteries and veins. Modern computer software systems can also generate three-dimensional reconstructions of the vasculature. Such images are very pleasing to the eye but provide little additional clinical information.

Magnetic resonance imaging (MRI – see also Ch. 4)

By the use of different sequencing techniques, arteries and veins can be emphasised with or without the injection of contrast material. The use of MRI in cardiac imaging is relatively advanced and by gating pictures to the electrocardiogram, real-time cine-loop images of the moving chambers and valves can be obtained. Although peripheral MR angiography (MRA) is not yet so developed, it is a rapidly developing area. The main disadvantages of MRA are that it is still relatively expensive; the scanners and the software are not widely available; and interpretation of the pictures requires considerable expertise and understanding of the basic physical principles. It thus seems less 'user-friendly' to surgeons.

Angiography

Despite the advances in non-invasive assessment described above, most surgeons still rely primarily upon angiography when procedures are planned.

Digital subtraction angiography (DSA)

Nowadays, virtually all angiography is performed using digital subtraction (Ch. 4), which allows fine detail in images of small vessels, such as those in the foot, to be obtained with relatively small amounts of contrast and less radiation exposure (Fig. 28.6).

Route of contrast administration

Usually the contrast is injected directly into the artery to be examined – intra-arterial DSA (IA-DSA). This, of course, means that the arterial system has to be punctured, which has consequences: the potential for local wound complications; discomfort; and sometimes the need for the procedure to be done as an in-patient. Most often the common femoral artery is punctured in

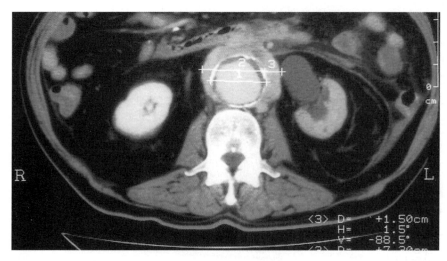

Fig 28.5 **Computed tomography (CT) scan to show a transverse cross-sectional image of a large abdominal aortic aneurysm.** The examination has been performed with contrast so that the blood in the aneurysm is white. The aneurysm is lined with a thin rim of thrombus. This particular aneurysm is an inflammatory one as indicated by the marked thickening of the aortic wall. On the left-hand side the ureter has become involved in the periaortic inflammatory processes and there is a hydronephrosis.

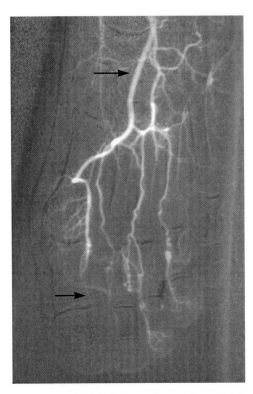

Fig 28.6 **Intra-arterial digital substraction arteriogram to show filling of the plantar arch of the foot from the dorsalis pedis artery (arrow, upper).** There is occlusion of the digital arteries to the great toe (**arrow, lower**) as a result of embolism from a proximal atheromatous plaque.

the groin. The brachial artery in the arm is also frequently used for coronary angiograms and when there is no femoral pulse. Some radiologists use the radial artery at the wrist to undertake IA-DSA as a day-case procedure.

Reasonable images may also be obtained when the contrast is injected peripherally into a vein – intravenous DSA (IV-DSA). The advantages of this approach for the patient are obvious. It also means that the procedure can be performed more quickly, less expensively and as an outpatient procedure. The disadvantages are that the images are not as clear, especially in the smaller peripheral arteries (as they are dependent upon a fast circulation time and a good cardiac output, which is often not the case in vascular patients) and more contrast is required.

Techniques

Vascular prostheses

Synthetic materials

Many of the techniques and prosthetic materials

available and very much taken for granted in modern day vascular surgical practice were not available as recently as 20 or 30 years ago. In particular, the development in the 1960s and 1970s of durable, non-thrombogenic, sterile, prosthetic materials for the construction of arterial bypasses was a major advance.

Prosthetic materials are used routinely in aortoiliac surgery where the long-term patency of a relatively short, large calibre, prosthetic replacement at a high-flow, high-pressure site is extremely good. The inner surface quickly becomes coated with protein and at each end there may be some limited endothelial ingrowth. However, in humans, as opposed to animals, a neo-endothelium never comes to line the entire length of any prosthetic conduit. Externally reinforced grafts are coated with rings or a spiral of polypropylene. Many surgeons now use them routinely in order to overcome fears of kinking or external compression, a particular hazard where a graft crosses a joint. In an axillofemoral graft, compression may be from a waist band or because the patient sleeps on the side of the graft.

Biological materials obtained from cadavers or animals (allografts or homografts) and chemically treated have been used since the late 1940s, but problems of availability, concern about cross-infection and late structural degeneration led to their abandonment after the advent of synthetic alternatives. New methods of preserving and sterilising these materials may allow their use in the future.

Vein

Autologous vein (usually the long saphenous [LSV] from the thigh) undoubtedly provides the best long-term results in medium to small calibre arterial reconstruction; specifically, the results of lower limb bypass with vein are better than with prosthetic materials. The longer the graft, the more distal the distal anastomosis, and the poorer the run-off vessels, the greater the advantage. However, in a proportion of patients, the ipsilateral LSV is either unusable because of disease or has been extirpated by varicose vein operations or for coronary bypass surgery. In such circumstances, vein can be harvested from other sites – the contralateral LSV, the short saphenous system or the arm. Another advantage of autologous material is resistance to infection. A potential disadvantage is the relatively small size of arm and leg veins, which makes them generally unsuitable for aortoiliac reconstruction. However, in exceptional circumstances such as a grossly contaminated field, lengths of veins can be spliced together in ingenious ways to form short lengths of large-calibre conduit.

Use of blood and blood products

Vascular operations are frequently associated with

Arterial disease

greater blood loss than are general surgical procedures, additionally contributed to by full anticoagulation. For these reasons, there is a particular requirement for effective and sometimes extremely rapid blood replacement. Interruption of the circulation to relieve occlusion or carry out bypass usually involves a temporary period of ischaemia for substantial areas of the body. The combination of loss of blood volume, ischaemia and reperfusion predisposes to coagulopathy, which may require correction with blood products such as fresh frozen plasma (FFP), cryoprecipitate and platelets.

Blood transfusion has its own shortcomings and complications. There is increasing enthusiasm for autotransfusion, which can be achieved in several different ways.

- *Predonation*. If the need for surgery can be predicted several weeks in advance, the patient can attend the blood bank and predonate their blood for their own later use. Although this overcomes problems with infection and incompatibility, the blood transfused still has the properties of that from the bank.
- *Isovolaemic haemodilution*. Blood is taken from the patient immediately before operation and replaced with crystalloid; it may then be transfused back during the procedure. The advantage is that the retransfusion is of fresh whole blood.
- *Autotransfusion (cell saving)*. Blood shed during operation can be collected by suction, washed and reinfused.

Anaesthetic considerations

(see also Ch. 6)

Patients who undergo vascular operations are usually older, have more cardiorespiratory and cerebrovascular comorbidity, are more likely to be diabetic, are on more medications, and suffer more postoperative morbidity

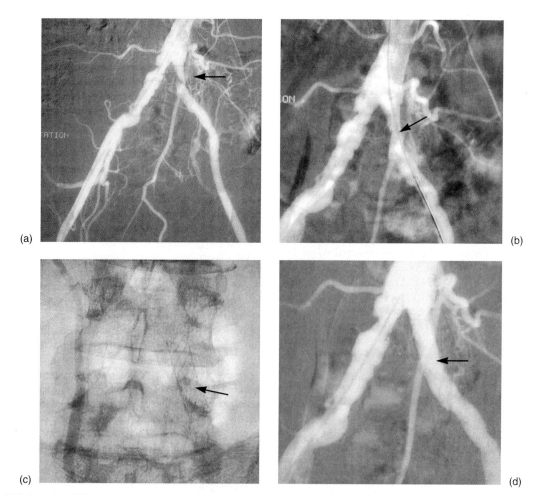

(a) (b) (c) (d)

Fig 28.7 **There is a 90% stenosis of the left common iliac artery (arrow, top left).** A guide wire (**arrow, top right**) has been passed across the stenosis from a left common femoral arterial puncture and the lesion has been stretched open by a 10 mm angioplasty balloon. A metal stent has been positioned across the lesion (**arrow, bottom left**) to prevent restenosis. A final angiogram shows a widely patent left common iliac artery without residual stenosis (**bottom right**).

and mortality than those who have general surgical procedures. Because of their widespread arterial disease and frequent lifelong heavy smoking, they are at especially high risk of cardiac, respiratory and cerebrovascular complications. The haemodynamic and metabolic stresses upon the heart consequent upon clamping major vessels, long periods of ischaemia followed by rapid reperfusion are noteworthy. The anaesthetist is therefore closely involved in pre-operative assessment and risk factor management, the operation itself and in postoperative care.

Percutaneous transluminal angioplasty (PTA)

A guide wire is passed through the site of stenosis or occlusion via a percutaneous puncture of an accessible adjacent artery. A catheter-mounted balloon is then inserted over the guide wire and the balloon is inflated within the lesion to open the artery by disruption of the plaque. A small metal mesh tube (stent) may then be placed over the guide wire and deployed within the recanalised artery to reduce the risk of re-stenosis (Fig. 28.7).

Since PTA was first described, there have been major technical advances in the available equipment, and interventional radiologists are becoming increasingly adventurous in the scope of the procedures done. Despite these trends, there appears to be no reduction in the number of open arterial reconstructions being carried out and PTA should be viewed as widening the scope of treatment rather than as a rival to surgery.

INDICATIONS AND RESULTS

Aortoiliac disease

The results of PTA are undoubtedly best in large, high-flow vessels and it is often the treatment of choice in stenoses and occlusions of the aortoiliac system. There is some evidence that, unless the lesion in question is a short stenosis, and the result of PTA alone is technically perfect, angioplasty should be followed by stent placement, although the initial cost is considerably increased.

Infra-inguinal disease

Except in a (uncommon) short, stenosis of the superficial femoral artery (Fig. 28.8), the results of infra-inguinal PTA (usually performed for claudication) are disappointing. Some interventional radiologists strongly disagree with that view and claim good long-term success even after recanalisation of long occlusions of arteries both above and below the knee.

Critical limb ischaemia

This is discussed in detail below.

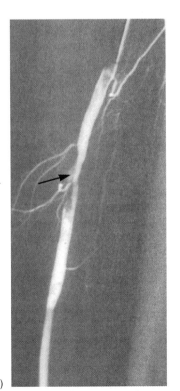
(a)

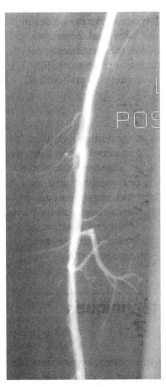
(b)

Fig 28.8 **Focal atheromatous plaque with attached thrombus in the right superficial femoral artery (arrow, left).** This plaque had been the source of emboli to the toes and was treated successfully by angioplasty (**right**) and 6 months of anticoagulation with warfarin.

Other sites

Although the bulk of PTA is performed for lower limb ischaemia, the technique has been used in the carotid, renal and mesenteric arteries. The long-term results of PTA and stenting in these areas remain to be defined. PTA is also used to dilate stenoses within bypass grafts (graft surveillance).

COMPLICATIONS

Although percutaneous techniques are associated with less morbidity and mortality than open surgery, they are not without complications and there is a significant early technical failure rate which depends on the clinical indications and the anatomical site. The main complications are related to the arterial puncture required to enter the arterial tree: haematoma, false aneurysm, occlusion and thrombosis. Although many of these can be treated non-operatively, a proportion require direct operative repair. Less commonly, angioplasty of a stenosed artery may lead to acute occlusion, worsening of ischaemia and the need for emergency surgical revascularisation.

Thrombolysis

Thrombolytic agents, such a streptokinase, urokinase and tissue plasminogen activator (TPA), are different from heparin and warfarin in that, rather than preventing clot formation, they actually lyse pre-formed thrombus. The technique involves infusing a drug into an artery in the hope that, after lysis, the diseased section that caused the thrombosis can be visualised and treated either by operation or PTA. The precise indications for thrombolysis are difficult to define.

COMPLICATIONS

Thrombolysis is not without morbidity and mortality especially in the elderly. Most complications are the consequence of haemorrhage. Therefore thrombolysis is contraindicated after recent surgery and in the presence of any other likely bleeding point such as a peptic ulcer or a recent haemorrhagic stroke. Dissolution of clot can lead to distal embolisation; particularly to be dreaded is embolus from the heart or carotid vessels to produce an ischaemic stroke.

Open surgical techniques

Endarterectomy

Before the advent of reliable prosthetic bypass materials, endarterectomy, (open removal – coring out – of atheroma from inside a diseased artery) was the standard operation for occlusive arterial disease,

especially that in large calibre vessels. However, the technique poses a number of problems:

- The operation is technically demanding and maximally invasive.
- Unlike bypass surgery (see below), endarterectomy requires a very wide dissection of all, or almost all, of the length of the artery to be cleared.
- Arterial disease is generalised and there are few instances where a diseased artery can be cleared to normal artery above and below the lesion: Thus there is always a point of transition between the endarterectomised surface and the diseased intima of the adjacent vessel which, especially downstream, can form a ridge or a flap which is a focus for thrombosis, vessel occlusion and distal embolisation.

Endarterectomy is now much less frequently done except in certain specific sites, notably the carotid bifurcation.

Bypass

This is now the commonest procedure for occlusive arterial disease.

TECHNIQUE

The operation proceeds as follows:

- Arteries above and below the occlusion are dissected out and controlled.
- A tunnel is made through the tissues to allow passage of the bypass.
- Systemic heparin is given.
- Arteries are clamped.
- Proximal and distal anastomoses are constructed.
- Native vessels and the graft are flushed to expel any air or clot.
- Anastomoses are completed.
- Clamps are removed.
- Flow is re-established.
- Adequacy of graft flow and distal perfusion are assessed.

Most bypasses done in the UK are for critical lower limb ischaemia, when failure to revascularise the leg often results in amputation.

Bypass grafts are usually described in terms of their inflow, outflow and conduit (e.g. femoral to popliteal with reversed vein). Bypasses can generally be grouped into those that are anatomical – the conduit follows more or less the same course as the native vessel (e.g. femoropopliteal) – and those that are extra-anatomical, where a different path is used (e.g. axillofemoral).

Embolectomy

There has been a steady decline in the proportion of

patients who develop acute ischaemia because of an embolus, as opposed to a thrombosis from chronic obliterative atherosclerosis. There are several reasons:

- a declining population of patients with atrial fibrillation and valve damage after rheumatic fever
- increased use of warfarin in the management of atrial fibrillation
- increased use of thrombolysis for myocardial infarction, which limits infarct size and the development of left ventricular mural thrombus.

Nevertheless, embolectomy is still frequently done especially in the arm where embolus has always been the commonest cause of acute ischaemia. Once the diagnosis of embolus has been reliably made on clinical assessment, perhaps supplemented by the use of angiography, the operation can be performed under local, regional or general anaesthesia.

TECHNIQUE

Briefly, the operation proceeds as follows:

- The relevant artery, usually the brachial in the arm or the common femoral in the leg, is dissected out and flow controlled proximally and distally with tapes or plastic slings.
- Heparin is given systemically.
- The artery is opened.
- Balloon catheters (Fogarty) are then passed into the artery with the balloon deflated and then removed with the balloon inflated to extract the clot.
- The adequacy of clot extraction is established clinically or by means of on-table angiography.
- The arteriotomy is closed (with a patch of vein if there is concern about the artery being narrowed at that point).
- Flow is re-established.

Postoperatively, anticoagulation is continued. A search for a definite source of the embolus is usually made, although its origin may prove elusive. In the absence of a proven source, a judgment must be made as to the appropriateness and duration of anticoagulation.

Although most emboli lodge in the arm or leg, any arterial bed may be involved, e.g. the carotid artery leading to stroke, or the superior mesenteric artery with bowel ischaemia (Ch. 23). Only a small minority of emboli are the result of infective endocarditis or of tumour. However, it is routine to send a portion of the extracted clot for bacteriological culture and histopathological examination.

Sympathectomy

Limb ischaemia

The sympathetic nervous system causes arteriolar constriction and in the past it was believed that by interrupting the sympathetic nerve supply to an ischaemic area, vasodilatation might improve the flow of blood. However, blood vessels in ischaemic tissues are already maximally dilated and, if sympathectomy does provide any benefit in severe distal ischaemia, it is likely that other mechanisms, such as alteration of pain perception, are responsible. With the increased use of arterial bypass for lower limb ischaemia, sympathectomy is used less and less.

Hyperhidrosis

The sympathetic nervous system also innervates sweat glands. Upper limb (cervical or thoracic) sympathectomy is most often used for severe axillary and palmar hyperhidrosis if medical treatment fails. The operation used to be performed through the root of the neck but is now done safely and expeditiously by thoracoscopy. Lumbar sympathectomy is also of value in patients with severe plantar hyperhidrosis. The effect on sweat gland function is usually permanent.

Raynaud's phenomenon

Cervical sympathectomy has been recommended for Raynaud's phenomenon (RP) but the long-term results in the hand are poor. For an unexplained reason, however, lumbar sympathectomy may provide long-lasting relief in RP which affects the toes.

Amputation

INDICATIONS

Ideally, no one with critical ischaemia should undergo major limb amputation for peripheral vascular disease without assessment by a vascular surgeon. Arterial reconstruction is by far the better option because of:

- Mortality – 10–20% for amputation
- Stump infection and ischaemia are both common and, in up to 10%, lead to further amputation at a higher level; deep venous thrombosis and pulmonary embolus are also well recognised complications
- Failed rehabilitation – 2 years later, less than two-thirds of below-knee and less than one-third of above-knee, unilateral amputees are independently mobile
- Financial cost – although a distal bypass operation for limb salvage may entail hospital expenditure in the region of £5000, a major limb amputation frequently costs 10 times as much once rehabilitation, artificial limbs and long-term care are considered.

It is a medical, humanitarian and economic disaster to do a reconstruction which fails early. However, in that 50–75% of patients with critical limb ischaemia are dead within 5 years (mostly from cardiac and cerebrovascular events), not all bypass procedures require to work for a prolonged period. Reconstruction should be attempted if there is at least a 75% chance of the bypass remaining functional for 2 years. Sometimes, however, amputation is the only option in those with unreconstructable arterial disease and advancing tissue loss or with symptoms that cannot be controlled by medical means.

LEVEL

Because rehabilitation is directly related to level of amputation, every effort should be made to preserve the knee, if it is mobile and there is a prospect of a prosthesis. Although numerous investigations have been proposed, there is not a single test which reliably predicts at which level an amputation will heal. Level remains, therefore, largely a matter of clinical judgement.

PERIOPERATIVE PAIN

Preoperative

Many patients who need amputation for ischaemia have considerable preoperative pain. Adequate analgesia around the time of operation is vital for both humane reasons and because it hastens recovery and rehabilitation. The anaesthetist is usually closely involved in this aspect of care (Ch. 6).

Postoperative

Phantom pain, a continuation or worsening of the pain experienced in the limb before amputation, often accompanied by a distressing sensation that the limb is still present, is common. Various treatments have been advocated such as electrical stimulation, the anticonvulsant carbamezepine and the tricyclic antidepressant amitriptyline. There is some evidence that, if the patient goes to the operating room completely pain-free, then the incidence of phantom pain is reduced. Epidural pain relief (Ch. 6) may achieve this end.

REHABILITATION

Although an amputation might be considered a technically straightforward procedure, there are important surgical principles which have to be observed if the chances of healing the amputation stump are to be maximised. In addition to the surgical team, the successful postoperative rehabilitation of an amputee depends upon the close cooperation of other disciplines – physiotherapists, occupational therapists and prosthetists.

Management of aneurysmal disease

Abdominal aortic aneurysm (AAA)

EPIDEMIOLOGY AND AETIOLOGY

This condition is present in 5% and responsible for the death of 1% of men over the age of 60. The principal cause of death is rupture, but distal embolism from thrombus in the aneurysm sac and, rarely, a thrombotic occlusion can also set the scene for death. The aetiology of aneurysmal disease is discussed above. The other complications of AAA are inflammation of the wall leading to abdominal or back pain and compression of surrounding structures.

PATHOLOGICAL FEATURES

In keeping with the law of Laplace, an aortic aneurysm inevitably slowly expands, a process made more likely by hypertension. The rate of expansion is highly variable both between patients and for an individual patient over time. Thus the lifetime threat posed by a 5 cm AAA is considerably greater for someone aged 50 years than it is for someone over 75. Eventually rupture takes place through all the attenuated layers, with either the initial formation of a retroperitoneal clot or immediate free bleeding into the peritoneal cavity sufficient to cause death. The risk of rupture is related to the size of the aneurysm: the normal aorta is 1.5–2.5 cm in diameter and is defined as aneurysmal when it attains twice that diameter – in excess of 4 cm. The reported annual risk of rupture varies quite widely but is probably in the region of:

- 4 cm: 1–2%
- 5 cm: 5–10%
- 6 cm: 10–15%
- 7 cm: more than 20%.

Only a third of patients with rupture live long enough to reach hospital, and of those that are operated upon, only half survive. Thus, the overall (community) mortality for rupture is as high as 80–90% and possibly many other deaths occur from rupture of an undiagnosed, asymptomatic aneurysm.

SCREENING

The mortality for elective AAA repair in asymptomatic or mildly symptomatic disease is, in the best centres, less than 5%. It thus makes clinical sense to detect and repair as many aneuryms as possible before rupture.

Ultrasound-based screening of a defined population has been used to find asymptomatic aneurysms with the inference that this will, in time, reduce the number who require operation for rupture and, in consequence, overall mortality. However, the resource implications of population screening remain to be defined, so that most vascular surgeons are forced to accept a more modest, opportunist, screening programme: those with arterial disease seen in the vascular clinic are actively examined clinically and by ultrasound for the presence of an aneurysm. The process may be extended to first-degree relatives of known patients with AAA and to other high-risk groups attending hypertension and cardiology outpatient clinics.

CLINICAL FEATURES

In thin patients, the aneurysm itself as well as its trans-mitted pulsation may be visible on inspection. On palpation there will be a pulsatile, expansile swelling in the midline of the abdomen, usually extending towards the left-hand side. However, it is important for the student to appreciate that clinical examination alone, even when performed by an experienced vascular surgeon, may be unreliable at confirming the presence or absence of aneurysmal disease and at estimating the size of the aorta. This is one reason why so many AAAs go unrecognised until there are life-threatening complications such as rupture. Any suspicion of AAA should therefore prompt an ultrasound examination, and indeed a number of experts have advocated ultrasound-based population screening for AAA. Although it is frequently taught that AAA tenderness indicates actual or impending rupture, or the presence of an inflammatory component, this too is unreliable. Healthy persons will often feel pain if their aorta is palpated firmly. There may be a bruit on auscultation in association with origin stenoses of the branches of the abdominal aorta (coeliac axis, superior mesenteric, renal arteries). There is an association between AAA and aneurysms elsewhere so the examiner should specifically exclude the presence of femoral and popliteal aneurysms. The surface marking of the aortic bifurcation is at the level of the umbilicus, so any pulsation felt below this level is likely to denote the presence of iliac aneurysmal disease.

MANAGEMENT

Although, as described above, most AAAs gradually increase in size, the unpredictable nature of this process means that vascular surgeons usually organise repeat ultrasound examination at 3- to 6-monthly intervals for those who do not require urgent management.

Indications for elective repair

The decision to operate involves weighing the known risk of leaving the AAA in place against that of operation. The first depends upon:

- size
- presence of symptoms
- age and physiological state.

The risk of operation depends primarily upon cardio-respiratory status. Anaesthetists (Ch. 6) and cardiologists can help the surgeon assess this, and also life expectancy, more precisely. There is no advantage to be gained in repairing a small aneurysm at low risk of rupture in an elderly person with severe myocardial disease whose cardiac prognosis is poor.

Technique
Briefly an elective AAA repair proceeds as follows:

- The abdomen is opened through a long vertical midline or transverse incision.
- The surgeon confirms the presence of an operable aneurysm and the absence of other disease which might affect prognosis, particularly colorectal cancer.
- The neck of the aneurysm is dissected free by mobilising the fourth part of the duodenum to the right with care to avoid injury to the left renal vein.
- The iliac arteries are also dissected free.
- A bolus dose of i.v. heparin, usually 3000–5000 units, is given and, after a delay of 1–2 minutes, first the iliac vessels to avoid distal embolism and then the aorta are clamped.
- The aneurysm is opened longitudinally and any back-bleeding from lumbar arteries or the inferior mesenteric artery is dealt with by suture ligation.
- Thrombus is evacuated – most aneurysms are full of organised blood clot with only a small central lumen to allow blood flow.
- An appropriately sized graft is then sutured end-to-end with non-absorbable sutures to the infrarenal neck of the aneurysm and then to the iliacs.
- Before the lower anastomosis is completed, the arteries and the graft are thoroughly flushed to expel any clot.
- Flow is then restored to the legs, one side at a time to minimise the stress on the heart of the fall in blood pressure upon reperfusion; haemostasis and lower limb perfusion are then evaluated.
- The sac of the aneurysm and the posterior peritoneum are closed over the graft to exclude it from the peritoneal cavity (inlay technique) and to separate the graft from the duodenum to minimise the risk of an aortoduodenal fistula.
- The abdomen is then closed in the standard manner.

Use of the high dependency or intensive therapy unit is routine (Ch. 10).

Operation for rupture proceeds in a similar manner except that systemic heparin is not given and the neck of the aneurysm is clamped before the iliacs to reduce the risk of exacerbation of the rupture.

Popliteal aneurysm

One in 10 patients with AAA also have a popliteal

artery aneurysm (PAA) and 50% of patients with PAA have an AAA.

PATHOLOGICAL FEATURES

This type of aneurysm develops in the same way as others. The main complication is thrombosis with or without distal embolisation. Because the aneurysm itself is nearly always asymptomatic, presentation is usually as an emergency with the symptoms of acute limb ischaemia, unless an incidental diagnosis has been made on vascular examination.

MANAGEMENT

Emergency

Acute thrombosis of a PAA is associated with a high rate of limb loss, because usually the distal calf vessels thrombose simultaneously. Small thrombi from within the PAA may have embolised to obliterate the vessels of the calf and foot which makes surgery technically difficult because there is no distal run-off for the surgeon to use for a bypass. Thrombosis in a PAA is an accepted indication for thrombolysis, which can be used to dissolve clot in the calf vessels either preoperatively by the radiologist through a femoral catheter or by the surgeon directly in the operating room. Despite these techniques, 50% of those who present with an acute thrombosis of a PAA lose the limb.

Elective

Many would operate when the diameter exceeds 2 cm or when a significant amount of thrombus has been seen on ultrasound. About 20% of patients have bilateral disease, so the other limb should be carefully examined and if a PAA is found it should be repaired.

Technique

A reversed vein bypass is constructed from the superficial femoral artery above to the popliteal artery below the aneurysm. The PAA is tied off and thus excluded from the circulation.

Thoraco-abdominal aneurysm (TAA)

EPIDEMIOLOGY

The general view has been that 90% of all AAAs affect the infrarenal aorta. However, with increased awareness and better imaging techniques, particularly CT, it has become apparent that a greater proportion of aortic aneurysms than was previously thought (perhaps 15–20%) involve the abdominal aorta above the level of the renal arteries and/or the thoracic aorta (Fig. 28.9).

The risk of rupture appears to the same as for infrarenal aneurysms. TAA may also lead to aortic dissection and compress surrounding structures such as the oesophagus to cause dysphagia or a main bronchus to produce lobar collapse and recurrent

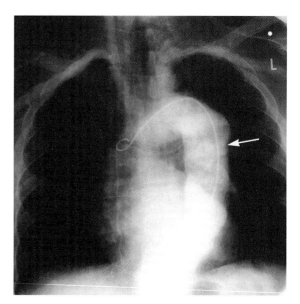

Fig 28.9 **Angiogram showing aneurysmal dilatation of the thoracic aorta**. The guide wire is lying within the lumen (**arrow**). Angiography may underestimate the size of an aneurysm because it only demonstrates the lumen and not the large amount of thrombus that also usually lies within the aneurysm sac.

pneumonia. TAA may also cause severe chest and back pain, especially if it is large and there is erosion into the vertebral column.

MANAGEMENT

Repair is attempted in only a few centres in the UK and the technique is highly specialised. The complexity, and thus the risks are considerably higher than for infrarenal AAA repair. As a result, many surgeons would defer TAA repair until the patient had severe symptoms or, in asymptomatic patients, the aneurysm had reached a size where the risk of rupture was thought to be particularly high.

False aneurysm

AETIOLOGY

In civilian practice, most false aneurysms are the consequence of arterial puncture of the common femoral artery. After the procedure, the hole in the artery fails to close and blood enters the perivascular space to form a haematoma which liquefies to create a fluid cavity into which arterial blood still circulates and which is walled off from surrounding tissues by a fibrous capsule.

MANAGEMENT

If a false aneurysm is small then it may close spontaneously provided that the patient is not on anticoagulants. It is also possible to induce thrombosis by compression under ultrasound guidance. However, if the aneurysm is large, too tender to compress and continuing to expand, then surgical repair is necessary. This is usually a straightforward procedure – closure of the hole in the artery and obliteration of the sac. More recently, false aneurysms have been treated successfully with thrombin injection.

Anastomotic false aneurysm

A false aneurysm can also develop at the site of an anastomosis between prosthetic material and native artery. In these circumstances, the surgeon should always consider the possibility of infection. Such anastomotic aneurysms may require operative repair to prevent rapid expansion and haemorrhage.

Chronic lower limb ischaemia

Intermittent claudication

Intermittent claudication (IC) is the mildest manifestation of lower limb ischaemia and affects approximately 5% of men over 60 years. In the majority it is the consequence of atherosclerotic narrowing or occlusion of the superficial femoral artery in the thigh.

CLINICAL FEATURES

Symptoms
Arterial insufficiency causes ischaemic muscle pain on walking which is relieved by rest. To begin walking again causes re-arrest after the same distance has been travelled. This depends on whether the patient is walking on the flat or uphill but otherwise is quite constant under the same conditions. At rest, the blood requirement is met by the collateral circulation through the profunda femoris system which joins the popliteal artery below the blockage usually just above the knee. However, exercise produces a demand which cannot be met and the calf muscles become ischaemic. Because the thigh muscles still have a normal blood supply, the pain is usually felt only in the calf. Cycling may be used as an alternative to walking because this activity depends primarily on the thigh rather than on the calf muscles. If stenosis is more proximal (aortoiliac), then pain is felt in the whole leg and even the buttock if the blood flow to the internal iliac artery is compromised. A penile erection may also be impossible or difficult to sustain (Leriche syndrome) consequent upon an aortoiliac obstruction.

Physical findings
On examination, the limb may be obviously ischaemic. Pulses are usually diminished or absent below the

femoral but, if they are present, exercise causes their disappearance.

DIAGNOSIS
There are many causes of pain in the leg, of which arterial disease is only one. Much of the time of a vascular service is spent excluding other disorders. Pain that radiates from the back, hip and knee joint, osteoarthritis and venous outflow obstruction (venous claudication, Ch. 29) may all be difficult to distinguish from true arterial claudication, especially if there is some coexistent but asymptomatic arterial disease.

MANAGEMENT
Arterial claudication is common, but progression to critical ischaemia is unlikely. Anxious patients should be reassured that amputation is unlikely. The risks for arterial surgery or amputation are less than 1–2% per year.

However, certain patients are at risk of disease progression, including those who:

- present with severe claudication of less than 50 m
- have low (less than 0.5) ABPI
- have multilevel or distal disease
- are diabetic
- continue to smoke.

Such patients need careful assessment, aggressive treatment of risk factors and the offer of reconstruction or endovascular therapy if and when critical limb ischaemia develops.

Medical therapy
For many years the standard treatment for the majority of patients has been *stop smoking and keep walking*. All should be:

- reassured that the legs are not in imminent danger
- warned about the hazards of continued smoking
- screened and treated for correctable risk factors (diabetes and hyperlipidaemia)
- told to exercise regularly to the point of pain in order to develop collateral circulation.

The majority accept the wisdom of this advice and attempt to alter lifestyle. However, a proportion will not comply and/or will not accept their level of disability and in these intervention may have to be considered.

Percutaneous transluminal angioplasty (PTA)
Experts disagree on the role of this procedure in claudication. There have been few direct comparisons between PTA and best medical therapy (BMT), but where patients have been randomly allocated to one or the other, PTA has not been shown to confer any additional long-term benefit. In the first 6 months, while BMT is taking effect, PTA of suitable

lesions might provide better short-term symptomatic improvement.

In the longer term, however, there are clear advantages to BMT because not only does it lessen symptoms bilaterally but it also increases longevity by reducing the risk of death from ischaemic heart disease, stroke and bronchial carcinoma – by far the most frequent causes in this group. Furthermore, PTA costs £500–1000 per procedure and, although arguably safer than open operation, is associated with a 1–2% major morbidity rate. To some extent, comparisons between BMT and PTA are clinically inappropriate and the two procedures should be viewed as complementary and not competitive. The fundamental question is not in which patients should PTA be considered instead of BMT, but rather in which patients will PTA augment the results of BMT.

There is no doubt that the results of PTA are better in the aorto-iliac than in the femoropopliteal segment. If clinical examination (reduced femoral pulse and/or the presence of a bruit) suggests that aortoiliac (inflow) disease is significantly contributing to symptoms, then angiography with a view to PTA should be considered. By contrast, if the femoral pulses are normal and the clinical diagnosis is one of femoropopliteal or infra-popliteal occlusion, routine investigation in greater detail is not indicated and is usually reserved for those with a threat to the limb or livelihood.

Operation

Contention also surrounds this option. As mentioned previously, the natural history is benign in terms of limb loss, and potential mortality or morbidity from intervention (both about 1%) must be set against this.

Aortoiliac (supra-inguinal) disease

There is a lower threshold for reconstruction in this arterial segment because:

- the ability to compensate for aortoiliac occlusion by formation of collaterals is not as good as it is in infra-inguinal disease
- the long-term result of aortoiliac reconstruction is considerably better than in infra-inguinal bypass; more than 80% of aortobifemoral grafts for claudication are patent at 10 years
- bilateral claudication can be corrected by a single operation
- those affected by aortoiliac disease are generally younger and more likely to have their livelihood threatened by their disability.

Infra-inguinal disease

By contrast, there is much less enthusiasm for infra-inguinal bypass because:

- compensation by collateral development is often good

- at 5 years, less than 70% of femoropopliteal grafts are still patent
- bilateral claudication is common, requires two operations and so doubles risk
- insertion of a bypass graft leads to involution of collateral pathways; if the graft blocks, the patient nearly always returns to a worse level of ischaemia than that present before operation
- rest pain may develop after a failed graft and force reoperation; the long-term results of such procedures are less impressive than those of primary reconstruction.

There can be few experienced vascular surgeons who have not seen a patient die or lose a limb as a result of vascular surgery done for claudication. In the UK, most adopt an extremely conservative approach and less than 10% of infra-inguinal grafts are for claudication.

Critical limb ischaemia (CLI)

Critical limb ischaemia is defined as rest pain which requires strong (opiate) analgesia for a period of 2 weeks or more, and tissue loss, in association with an ankle pressure of less than 50 mmHg (European Consensus Document). The inference is that, without intervention, a patient with CLI will come to major amputation within weeks or months.

CLINICAL FEATURES

Symptoms

Rest pain is indicative of severe ischaemia, usually felt in the forefoot and, typically, the pain is worst at night and disturbs sleep. The reasons for this are:

- Metabolic rate in the foot is increased under the warm bedclothes.
- Cardiac output and blood pressure fall during sleep.
- A beneficial affect of gravity on pedal blood pressure is lost.

For these reasons, relief at night is often sought by hanging the leg over the side of the bed or walking about on a cold floor.

Physical findings

In addition to findings of arterial insufficiency, there may be evidence of multilevel disease. Constant pain in the foot with single level arterial disease is uncommon and should lead to a search for other causes.

Ischaemic tissue is extremely sensitive to injury: even minor wounds fail to heal and ulceration follows.

Minor damage quickly leads to infection and bacterial toxins destroy yet more tissue. Frank gangrene then ensues and can spread extremely rapidly, especially in diabetics.

Relatively limited arterial occlusion may sometimes be present in CLI because the heart is inadequate – pump failure. For example, after myocardial infarction or another cardiac event, cardiac output and systolic blood pressure fall to a point where even a small increase in peripheral vascular resistance cannot be overcome. Management is difficult because of the hazards of major procedures and the outlook is poor.

MANAGEMENT
Medical
In contrast to a presentation with claudication, rest pain is a warning that tissue loss is imminent. In the great majority, CLI does not improve without surgical intervention but medical measures have important roles:

- assessment and treatment of heart failure, intercurrent infection and anaemia
- control of diabetes
- antibiotic therapy of local infection (although the poor blood supply limits the tissue concentration that can be achieved)
- pain relief
- use of anticoagulants and occasionally prostacyclin-based drugs when tissue loss is minimal.

All of these measures can ensure that an optimum condition is achieved before surgical intervention is performed.

Balloon angioplasty
The majority view is that, in patients with early rest pain and/or minimal tissue loss (subcritical ischaemia), PTA may tip the balance just enough to salvage the limb when surgical reconstruction is not feasible. However, some believe that all patients with CLI should in the first instance be managed with PTA and that operation should be reserved for those who do not respond.

Sympathectomy
This has little role to play in CLI, although those with early rest pain may achieve some relief.

Amputation
This is a last resort. Primary amputation can be the best option in the elderly frail patient with extensive tissue loss, but mortality is inevitably high.

Palliation
There are circumstances in which the patient and the family interests are best served by the provision of terminal care only.

Surgery
Bypass surgery and, to a far lesser extent, local endarterectomy are the mainstays of treatment, although the frequently present multisystem medical and vascular problems dictate a mortality for limb salvage surgery of up to 10%.

Aortoiliac disease
In CLI, this is usually associated with infra-inguinal disease. As already implied, the results of PTA and stenting are optimal at this site, as are the long-term results of open arterial reconstruction. In younger, fitter patients who are considered unsuitable for PTA, the standard operation is aortobifemoral bypass graft. In those not fit for aortic surgery, an extra-anatomical bypass may be suitable. For example, if there is an iliac occlusion on one side and a relatively disease-free vessel on the other, a femorofemoral crossover graft (Fig. 28.10) is possible. An alternative is an axillobi-femoral graft, where the inflow for the graft is taken from the axillary artery below the clavicle (Fig. 28.11).

Femorodistal bypass
This refers to an arterial reconstruction below the inguinal ligament in which common femoral or superficial femoral arteries are the site of proximal anastomosis and the popliteal or tibial vessels are the site of distal anastomosis. A popliteo-pedal bypass is a variant (Fig. 28.12).

Technical aspects of limb salvage surgery
Most femorodistal bypass grafts originate from the common femoral artery, but in certain patients, particularly diabetics, who have patent vessels to knee level and tibial vessel occlusion, there is no reason why the

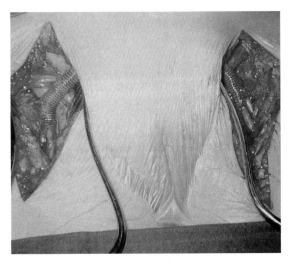

Fig 28.10 **An operative photography to show a Dacron graft carrying blood from the left to the right common femoral artery below a right iliac occlusion.**

447

Arterial disease

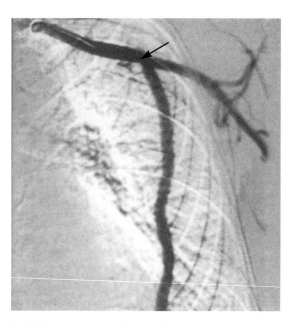

Fig 28.11 **Angiogram showing a graft using the left axillary artery as an inflow site (arrow) in order to revascularise both legs below an aortoiliac occlusion.** The patient was not considered fit enough to undergo aortic surgery.

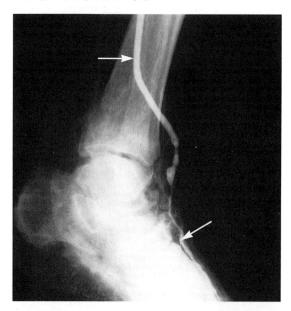

Fig 28.12 **An on-table angiogram to show flow of contrast from an in situ femorodistal vein graft (arrow, upper) in to the dorsalis pedis artery (arrow, lower) on the dorsum of the foot.** The operation was carried out for critical limb ischaemia in a diabetic patient.

graft should not come from the popliteal. In general, the shorter the graft, the easier it is to construct and the better the patency.

The requirements for a successful distal bypass are:

- good inflow
- a reliable conduit
- good outflow.

Inflow is usually provided by the ipsilateral iliac system and any iliac disease must be corrected by PTA with or without placement of a stent.

Conduit. There is no doubt that autogenous vein provides the best long-term results, especially if the distal anastomosis is below the knee. The patency of long prosthetic bypasses (PTFE or Dacron) can be improved by using a vein interposition cuff at the distal anastomosis. Vein grafts may be placed in a reverse manner or in situ (non-reversed). In the first, the vein is reversed to remove any obstruction to flow that may occur from intact valves. In the second, the vein is not reversed and the valves are cut. Although no significant difference in patency between the two techniques has ever been demonstrated, from a technical point of view there are advantages to the in situ technique when a long bypass to calf and foot vessels is to be constructed.

Outflow refers to the vessels into which the graft is to deliver blood. If the bypass is delivering blood to a dead end then thrombosis is inevitable.

Long-term patency

Femorodistal bypasses have a finite life expectancy which should be explained to the patient. Telephone contact should be available for those who feel that the graft may not be working. The chances of resurrecting a failed graft, particularly of vein, are often directly related to how quickly the problem can be tackled.

Most of those who have had a bypass are prescribed aspirin, because this both increases the rate of graft patency and reduces the risk of future coronary and cerebrovascular events. Anticoagulants are also sometimes used, although there is no definite evidence that these enhance patency, and anticoagulation in an elderly population is not without hazard.

Graft surveillance

It has been known for some time that certain grafts develop stenoses over time and that these predispose to occlusion. A graft with a tight stenosis that is presumed to be at risk of sudden occlusion is sometimes classified as a failing graft. There is some evidence that, if such a graft can be identified and corrective measures applied before thrombosis occurs, the long-term patency may be significantly improved.

Stenosis most frequently takes place either at the distal anastomosis or within the body of a vein graft. The cause is neointimal hyperplasia – in simple terms, scarring where the intima has been damaged and which then impinges on the lumen to create a stenosis. Detection is best achieved by colour-flow duplex ultrasound; the concept of duplex-based vein graft surveillance is now well established. The patient returns for a scan every 3 or 6 months. If a tight stenosis is detected, a confirmatory angiogram is done and the lesion is corrected by either PTA or open operation. Most stenoses develop within the first 18 months and, to save cost and effort, most graft surveillance does not routinely go beyond this point. Late failure is more often the result of disease progression in the native arteries proximal or distal to the bypass.

Management of thrombosis in a graft
The options are:

- If the leg is viable then it may be sensible to do nothing and wait for collaterals to develop. However, in that the majority of grafts are inserted for CLI, many (but not all) thromboses lead to redevelopment of a critical state.
- Thrombolysis – if successful, the underlying lesion which caused the graft to block can then be identified and corrected by either surgery or PTA.
- Thrombectomy – mechanical removal of thrombsis, followed by an operative angiogram to identify the underlying lesion and surgical correction
- Construction of a new graft – some believe that in virtually all circumstances, the graft must be replaced by a new bypass in order to optimise long-term patency.

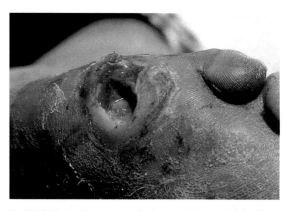

Fig 28.13 **Typical 'punched-out' ulcer over the head of the fifth metatarsal in a patient with diabetic peripheral vascular disease and neuropathy.**

The principles of management are best medical care for the diabetes, wide debridement of devitalised tissue, drainage of pus and, if ischaemia is present, revascularisation.

The diabetic foot

CLINICAL FEATURES

Diabetics have a tendency to develop, often quite suddenly, severe ischaemia and infection in the feet which progresses to rapid tissue necrosis and amputation. There are three reasons for this:

- *Vascular disease*, which, in diabetes, develops earlier in life and tends to be more extensive and distal. This makes intervention, by means of either angioplasty or surgery, more difficult and technically demanding. The clinical features are similar to non-diabetic vascular disease except that a palpable popliteal pulse is more frequently present, due to the more distal distribution of disease, particularly affecting the tibial vessels.
- *Sensory neuropathy* reduces or abolishes protective reactions to minor injury and to symptoms of infection or ischaemia
- *Autonomic neuropathy* causes a lack of sweating and the development of dry, fissured skin which permits entry of bacteria.
- *Motor neuropathy* results in wasting and weakness of the small muscles, loss of the longitudinal and transverse arches of the foot, and development of abnormal pressure areas such as over the metatarsal heads (Fig. 28.13).

MANAGEMENT

Tissue loss is neuropathic or ischaemic, or more commonly a combination of both (neuroischaemic).

Arterial disorders of the upper limb

The arm is affected by ischaemia eight times less commonly than the leg because:

- atherosclerosis affects the leg more frequently
- the arterial supply of the leg in relation to muscle bulk is much poorer than that of the arm
- the ability of the arm to derive collateral supply appears superior.

Unlike the leg, the commonest cause of ischaemia is embolism. Ischaemia can progress rapidly and loss of any part of the upper limb has a devastating functional result.

Thoracic outlet syndrome

AETIOLOGY
Thoracic outlet syndrome (TOS) occurs when the lower trunk of the brachial plexus and/or the subclavian vessels are compressed as they pass over the first rib or a cervical rib or cervical band which runs from the transverse process of the seventh vertebra towards the first rib. The majority of patients are female, and aged between 20 and 40 years.

CLINICAL FEATURES
Symptoms
The symptoms are predominantly neurological, typically pain, weakness, and/or paraesthesia over the ulnar

aspect of the hand and forearm, often extremely vague and difficult to assess. Compression of the subclavian vein at the thoracic outlet may cause axillary vein thrombosis (Ch. 29). Only 5% present primarily with arterial ischaemic symptoms, most commonly claudication or Raynaud's phenomenon (below). Turbulent flow caused by a subclavian stenosis may progress to post-stenotic dilatation of the subclavian artery, which in turn may develop into an aneurysm; thrombus within this may cause a distal embolism.

Physical findings

A cervical rib can be palpable. On external rotation and hyperabduction of the shoulder, the radial pulse may be lost and the hand may go pale and numb (these signs are not specific because a proportion of normal people will also lose the radial pulse). Wasting of the small muscles of the hand is always pathological but can occur in a wide variety of conditions. Obvious digital ischaemia may be present after embolisation (Fig. 28.14) but also occurs in Raynaud's phenomenon where it is, however, always bilateral.

INVESTIGATION

Plain radiography

A plain radiograph of the neck may show a cervical rib (Fig. 28.15) or a prominent transverse process which suggests but does not establish the presence of a fibrous band.

MRI

This is now the investigation of choice in that compression of the nerve roots and the artery can be demonstrated.

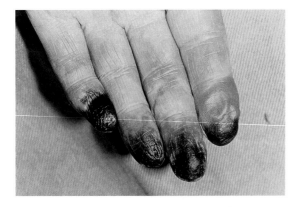

Fig 28.14 **Clinical photography showing extensive digital gangrene in a patient who had been treated medically for presumed Raynaud's phenomenon despite the fact that the symptoms had only ever affected one hand.** More recently, gangrene had developed over only a few weeks. In fact, this patient had a cervical rib associated with a subclavian aneurysm containing thrombus which had been embolising down into the digital arteries. The rib was excised, the subclavian aneurysm replaced with a PTEE graft and the tips of the affected fingers amputated.

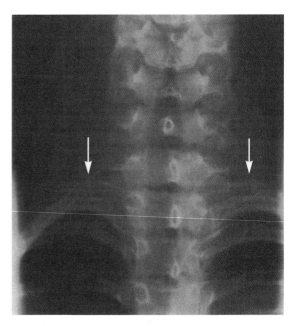

Fig 28.15 **Plain radiograph of the cervical spine showing the presence bilaterally of cervical ribs (arrows).**

Angiography

A fixed stenosis in the neutral position, especially when it is associated with post-stenotic dilatation or aneurysm, is always pathological and remains the clearest indication for arterial surgery. Stenosis present only on abduction is present in 10% of normals.

Duplex ultrasound

If present, a subclavian aneurysm together with any intraluminal thrombus can be identified, as can venous obstruction.

Venography

This investigation confirms venous obstruction and/or impingement.

Nerve conduction studies

These are useful in localising the problem to the thoracic outlet and should be considered before operation.

MANAGEMENT

Non-operative

In the absence of objective neurological damage or arterial ischaemia, treatment is symptomatic by physiotherapy in an attempt to improve posture and strengthen the muscles of the neck and shoulder girdle.

Surgery

Failure of conservative measures suggests the need for operative decompression. If a cervical rib or fibrous band is present, it can be excised via a supraclavicular approach. If not, many advocate excision of the first rib through a transaxillary approach; a few suggest this even if a cervical rib is present. A subclavian aneurysm is excised and replaced by a graft.

When the symptoms are clear-cut and the diagnosis certain, the results of surgery are good. In other circumstances, when the surgeon and the neurologist are uncertain and operation is done as a diagnostic test or as a last resort, they are poor.

Acute ischaemia of a limb

AETIOLOGY

The great majority of cases of acute limb ischaemia are caused either by embolism or by thrombosis at a site of previous atherosclerotic narrowing. Differentiation is of clinical importance because the management is quite different (Table 28.2). However, even the experienced may be unable to distinguish between the two with confidence and it is not uncommon for a patient with established peripheral vascular disease to have an embolus.

Embolism
Embolic material comes from:

- mural cardiac thrombus after a myocardial infarct
- left atrial appendix in atrial fibrillation
- vegetations from a heart valve in endocarditis or rheumatic disease
- thrombus from the aorta or other major vessel that is aneurysmal or atherosclerotic
- thrombus formed within a graft.

Embolic material tends to lodge at the site of major branches because of a match between it and the decreased vessel diameter.

Thrombosis
Surgical thrombectomy alone rarely succeeds because of early rethrombosis; some form of arterial bypass or thrombolysis is usually necessary.

CLINICAL FEATURES

Symptoms
Symptoms are often described as the six Ps:

- pulseless
- pain
- pallor
- perishing cold
- paralysis
- paraesthesia.

Physical findings
These reflect the symptoms. The limb is pulseless, pallid or cyanotic, cold and incapable of movement. In embolic occlusion, events occur rapidly with early loss of motor and sensory function. In these circumstances the diagnosis of ischaemia, as well as the need to act quickly, is usually obvious. In those with thrombosis the presentation is often acute on chronic.

MANAGEMENT
Faced with the acutely ischaemic limb, the following questions must be addressed:

- Is the limb salvageable?
- Is the limb threatened?

The non-viable limb
Features that indicate the limb is no longer salvageable include:

- fixed staining of tissues
- lack of blanching on pressure
- anaesthesia with rigid muscles – rigor mortis.

Acute-on-chronic limb ischaemia may be the manifestation of another terminal illness such as cardiac failure or malignancy. To subject such a patient to amputation just before death from the underlying disease is not good practice.

In all circumstances, the decision must be whether it is appropriate to offer amputation or palliation. The wishes of the patient must be respected. If informed consent cannot be obtained, then the next of kin or other relatives should be involved.

Table 28.2
Clinical features of acute embolism and thrombosis

Embolus	Thrombosis
Ischaemia is of sudden onset and very severe because of lack of preformed collaterals	Onset often insidious and less severe because of the pre-existence of collaterals
A source potential of embolus can usually be identified	No obvious source of embolus
Hospital records may indicate the presence of previous normal pulses	Previous records indicate long-standing peripheral pulse deficit
No history of arterial disease	History of arterial disease, e.g. myocardial infarction, stroke, peripheral vascular disease
Normal pulses in contralateral limb	Absent or reduced pulses in contralateral limb

The threatened limb

An ischaemic limb that is likely, in the absence of revascularisation, to become non-viable. Features include:

- loss of sensation
- loss of active movement
- pain on passive movement and when the calf muscles are squeezed.

When these features are present, there is a maximum of 6 hours in which to re-establish normal flow to avoid irreversible nerve and muscle injury. If embolism is obvious, embolectomy is performed, but if the diagnosis lacks certainty, an angiogram avoids a blind procedure; alternatively, operative angiography achieves the same purpose. The surgical revascularisation required depends on the images obtained. In those whose limb is threatened but whose general condition precludes long and complicated arterial surgery, amputation may be the only option.

The non-threatened limb

If sensation and movement are present and calf tenderness is absent, then the limb is not immediately threatened and it is safe to delay intervention. A period of medical optimisation and heparin therapy may lead to spontaneous improvement as a collateral circulation opens. Angiography and reconstruction can then be done on a semi-elective basis. An alternative is to start thrombolysis but this requires 12–24 hours to complete.

Vasospastic disorders (Raynaud's phenomenon)

Understanding of this area has been hampered by the use of inconsistent terms. Here, standard European definitions are used:

- *Raynaud's phenomenon* (RP) is the general term which describes the clinical features of episodic digital vasospasm in the absence of an identifiable associated disorder
- *Secondary Raynaud's syndrome* (RS) is when the phenomenon occurs secondary to one of the conditions listed in Box 28.2.

EPIDEMIOLOGY AND AETIOLOGY

Raynaud's phenomenon is 10 times commoner in women than in men and may, in a mild form, affect up to 25% of the young female population. An episode in the fingers typically occurs in response to cold and emotion, but other predisposing factors such as the oral contraceptive pill, certain migraine drugs and tobacco

---

Box 28.2

Conditions associated with Raynaud's syndrome

Connective tissue disorders
Systemic sclerosis (90%)
Systemic lupus erythematosus (30%)
Mixed connective tissue disease (80%)
Dermatomyositis/polymyositis (20%)
Sjögren's syndrome (30%)

Macrovascular disease
Thoracic outlet obstruction
Atherosclerosis
Buerger's disease
Radiation arteritis

Occupational trauma
Vibration white finger (VWF)
Chemical exposure, e.g. nitrates, polyvinyl chloride
Repeated exposure to extreme cold

Drugs
Cytotoxic drugs
Ergotamine
Beta-blockers
Cyclosporin

Miscellaneous
Malignancy
Reflex sympathetic dystrophy
Arteriovenous fistula

---

have been identified. The toes and other extremities may be involved and there is increasing evidence that RP may be a manifestation of a total body microvascular disorder.

CLINICAL FEATURES

There are three phases:

- *pallor* – because of digital artery spasm
- *cyanosis* – from the accumulation of deoxygenated blood
- *redness* (rubor) – reactive hyperaemia as blood flow returns.

Pain is unusual unless there are other complications, e.g. digital ulceration and gangrene.

DIAGNOSIS

In the majority, the diagnosis of RP can be made on symptoms and physical findings; additional investigations are not required unless secondary RS is suspected. The proportion of patients who have an underlying disorder is uncertain; experts who run specialist clinics tend to collect the more intractable and severe examples and, with adequate long-term follow-up, as many as 80% of all referred patients will eventually develop features of an underlying cause. Conversely, a GP who sees a small number of mildly affected patients may only occasionally identify one with a defined connective tissue disease (Box 28.2). Only a minority have clear evidence of connective tissue disease on presentation. However, those with current tissue loss or scars from its previous occurrence must be assumed to have secondary RS and a careful enquiry into the presence of isolated features of CTD should be made. Abnormal dilated nail-fold capillary loops, visible with an ophthalmoscope, are suggestive of, but not specific for, RS. Presentation for the first time in childhood or over the age of 30 increases the likelihood of RS. Eighty per cent of those who present at over 60 years of age have an underlying disorder, although it is most often atherosclerosis. An asymmetrical distribution should also alert the vascular surgeon to the possibility of microembolisation from a proximal lesion (TOS) and a full vascular examination should be done in all.

MANAGEMENT
Medical
Most often, reassurance about the usually benign nature of their condition, advice to stop smoking and to avoid exposure to cold are sufficient; chemical hand-warmers and electrically heated gloves are available. There is controversy over whether the oral contraceptive pill should be discontinued but hormone replacement therapy appears to be safe. Numerous drugs have been used, the best of which appears to be the calcium channel blocker nifedipine, although side-effects are relatively common. Vasodilators may also be useful. In those with severe attacks, admission to hospital for a 5-day infusion of prostacyclin may provide great symptomatic relief in the winter months and, for unknown reasons, the beneficial effects may last up to 6 weeks.

Surgical
Secondary Raynaud's syndrome caused by macro-vascular arterial disease (Fig. 28.14) is nearly always unilateral and may progress rapidly to tissue loss in the hand if the underlying lesion is not identified and treated expeditiously. In RS in the hand, sympathectomy is associated with poor long-term results but the procedure appears to be more useful in the feet. In the variant CREST syndrome, digits affected by severe ulceration or calcium deposits may require amputation, although every attempt should be made to preserve as much tissue as possible.

Cerebrovascular disease

Carotid artery disease
PATHOLOGICAL FEATURES
Approximately 80% of all strokes are ischaemic rather than haemorrhagic and, of these, as many as half are caused by atherosclerosis at the carotid artery bifurcation – leading to either distal embolisation or thrombotic occlusion.

CLINICAL FEATURES
Symptoms
Micro-embolisation to the eye leads to ipsilateral transient loss of vision (amaurosis fugax), often described by the patient as a black curtain coming across the eyes which usually lasts from a few seconds to a few minutes. A larger embolus may cause permanent blindness due to retinal infarct. Embolisation to the middle cerebral artery leads to hemispheric symptoms, usually a contralateral hemiparesis and, if the dominant hemisphere is affected, loss of speech. A cerebral event which lasts less than 24 hours and does not leave residual symptoms and signs is termed a transient ischaemic attack (TIA).

A completed stroke progresses to brain damage with a residuum of neurological features.

Physical findings
The neurological findings and their duration are consistent with the size of the area of brain affected.

DIAGNOSIS AND INVESTIGATION
Carotid artery stenosis may be visualised by angiography (Fig. 28.1) but this technique may be associated with a 1–2% stroke rate and is not suitable therefore as a first-line investigation. Colour flow duplex scanning can give accurate information on the presence and degree of stenosis, and an increasing number of centres use this investigation as a basis for operation. A CT brain scan before operation is commonly done to define the presence of pre-existing cerebral damage or to exclude other pathology.

MANAGEMENT
Indications for carotid endarterectomy (CEA)
Two large randomised controlled trials have indicated that in cases of amaurosis fugax, TIA or stroke with good recovery plus an internal carotid artery stenosis of 70% or greater, the risk of future stroke is significantly reduced by CEA carried out as a supplement to best medical therapy, as compared with best medical therapy alone. Most stenoses less than 70% should be treated medically. The risks of surgery in patients with

acute stroke and in those with completed stroke with poor recovery outweigh the benefits. There is also mounting evidence that patients with high-grade but asymptomatic stenosis may benefit from surgery, but in the UK the results of further trials are awaited.

Technique

The major complication of CEA is a stroke. The benefits of the operation depend crucially upon a low perioperative stroke rate, which should be less than:

- 7.5% after a previous stroke
- 5% in amaurosis fugax or TIA
- 3% in those who are asymptomatic.

Balloon angioplasty

Trials are underway to compare CEA with angioplasty and stenting. Early data indicate that the immediate complication rate from endovascular treatment is higher than that associated with CEA. However, in the future, with the development of new technology, at least a proportion may be treated non-operatively.

Carotid body tumour (CBT)

PATHOLOGICAL FEATURES

These rare lesions arise in the carotid body or less commonly in one of the adjacent nerves such as the vagus. They are paragangliomas, but it is not clear what proportion are malignant. Lymph node deposits may be found in up to 25% but distant metastases are extremely rare and local recurrence is uncommon.

CLINICAL FEATURES

The usual presentation is a painless lump in the neck. It is frequently mistaken for a lymph node or a parotid lesion and may have been explored previously.

The lump is not tender, is fleshy and, most importantly, can only be moved transversely in relation to the carotid sheath.

DIAGNOSIS

A typical lump in the neck is investigated by either angiography, duplex scanning, CT or MRI. Angiography reveals a tumour blush and typical splaying of the internal and external carotid arteries into a wine glass shape (Fig. 28.16). Other imaging gives more detailed information on the feasibility of resection. Few carotid body tumours secrete active substances and, in the absence of symptoms, there is no requirement to routinely check the levels of circulating catecholamines (see 'Phaeochromcytoma).

MANAGEMENT

Carotid body tumours should be excised because they grow locally and the larger the tumour the more diffi-

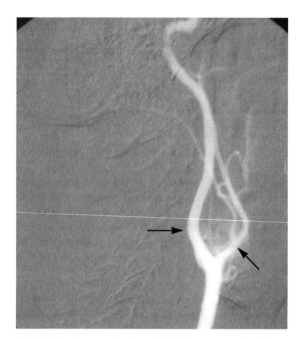

Fig 28.16 **Angiogram showing a 'blush' of contrast and splaying of the internal (arrow, left) and external (arrow, right) carotid arteries because of the presence of a carotid body tumour.**

cult the operation becomes. Radiotherapy is reserved for symptomatic treatment of an inoperable lesion.

Visceral ischaemia

Acute mesenteric ischaemia

This condition is discussed in detail in Chapter 23.

Chronic mesenteric ischaemia

The ability of the gastrointestinal circulation to develop collaterals ensures that the great majority of patients with arterial inflow obstruction are asymptomatic. It is generally believed that at least two of the three arteries which supply the gut (coeliac axis, superior and inferior mesenteric arteries) must be critically stenosed or occluded for symptoms to develop.

CLINICAL FEATURES

A typical complaint is of severe abdominal pain after eating – mesenteric angina. Fear of eating develops, so that mesenteric ischaemia is always associated with significant weight loss. This presentation mimics many other abdominal disorders and frequently the patient has had numerous inconclusive investigations before the diagnosis is finally made.

Apart from weight loss, which is universal, there are rarely any physical findings. Occasionally an epigastric bruit is present but this is often audible in those who are otherwise normal.

DIAGNOSIS AND MANAGEMENT

Although, in these slim patients, an experienced ultrasonographer can often identify mesenteric disease on duplex scanning, the diagnosis can only be made with certainty on angiography.

Surgical revascularisation is the mainstay of treatment, although balloon angioplasty is playing an increasing role. The commonest operation is to take a graft from the aorta to the superior mesenteric artery and the coeliac axis. This is a major surgical undertaking and is associated with significant risk, but the long-term results are good. The alternative is often a slow and painful death from progressive cachexia.

Renal artery disease

Renal artery stenosis

PATHOPHYSIOLOGICAL AND PATHOLOGICAL FEATURES

In most patients, renal artery stenosis (RAS) is asymptomatic and merely an incidental finding at postmortem or on angiography done for another indication (Fig. 28.17). RAS leads to decreased renal perfusion and the release of renin from the juxtaglomerular apparatus. Renin converts angiotensinogen

Table 28.3
Comparison of renal artery atherosclerosis and fibromuscular dysplasia

Atherosclerosis 60%	Fibromuscular dysplasia 40%
Males aged 60 years and over	Females usually aged 40–60 years; may affect children
Stenosis at or within 1–2 cm of ostium	Affects distal two-thirds of renal artery ± segmental branches
30% have aortic occlusive or aneurysmal disease	Often multifocal
Part of generalised atherosclerotic disease	'String of beads' on angiogram
10–20% may occlude in 3 years	Occlusion uncommon
30% have bilateral disease	Unknown aetiology

to angiotensin I, which is in turn converted to angiotensin II (ATII) in the lung. ATII causes vasoconstriction and the release of aldosterone from the adrenal cortex. The renal excretion of sodium is reduced and blood pressure rises, which may in the short term return renal perfusion to normal. However, a progressive stenosis leads to worsening ischaemia, hypertension, loss of nephrons, atrophy and irreversible renal failure. The two main causes of RAS are atheroma (60%) and fibromuscular dysplasia (up to 40%). These two disease processes are quite different (Table 28.3). Less common causes include renal artery aneurysm thrombosis and embolism arteritis and trauma.

CLINICAL FEATURES

Renovascular hypertension affects a large number of people. For example, in the UK, approximately 10% of the adult population is hypertensive and in these a renal cause is thought to be responsible for about 10%. Suggestive features are onset before the third and after the fifth decade and the presence of peripheral vascular disease. The hypertension is typically of abrupt onset, severe or malignant in nature and difficult to control with standard medical therapy.

Renal failure caused by RAS is much less common but it should always be considered in the differential diagnosis of renal failure, particularly when there is other evidence of peripheral vascular disease. Deterioration of renal function after administration of an angiotensin-converting enzyme (ACE) inhibitor may be the trigger for clinical detection because these drugs prevent the adaptive responses described above. Discontinuation of the ACE inhibitor usually returns renal function to pre-treatment levels.

DIAGNOSIS

Renovascular hypertension can be successfully corrected by surgical and/or radiological means and

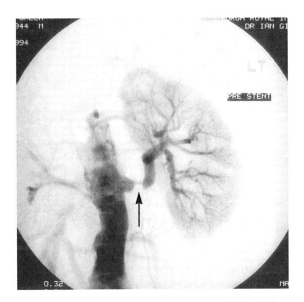

Fig 28.17 **Angiogram showing almost compete occlusion of the left renal artery from atherosclerosis (arrow).** This was successfully treated by percutaneous placement of a stent.

will reduce the long-term complications of hypertension (stroke and heart failure), the need to continue lifelong anti-hypertensive medication and the risk of renal failure. Therefore it is important to make a precise diagnosis, but this can be difficult. Clinically suspected RAS is usually confirmed by angiography. Although many other less invasive and expensive investigations have been advocated, none is sufficiently sensitive or specific to be a satisfactory screening test (Box 28.3). Occasionally the clinical significance of the diagnosis of RAS can only be confirmed by reduction in blood pressure and/or improvement in renal function after its correction.

Box 28.3

Investigations of patients with renal artery stenosis

Intravenous urography

Delayed appearance of poorly concentrated medium in the affected kidney which may be small

False-positive and negative results make it unsuitable as a screening test

Technetium (Tc)-labelled diethylenetriaminepentacetic acid (DTPA) or mercaptoacetyltriglycine (MAG3) scanning

Poor take-up radioisotope on affected side

Reveals RAS if greater than 60%, especially after administration of an ACE inhibitor which exacerbates renal hypoperfusion

Colour flow duplex ultrasound

Directly measures flow velocities in the renal arteries

Very operator-dependent

Probably not reliable at present

Renin levels

Can be measured in general circulation or in renal vein

High levels suggest renovascular hypertension but low sensitivity and specificity

Angiography

Expensive

Morbidity and mortality make it unsuitable as a screening test

Intravenous digital subtraction techniques often provide inadequate images

MRI

Provides images of the renal arteries without exposure to ionising radiation

At present there are still problems with expense, availability and software

---

MANAGEMENT

Medical

Drugs can control all but the most severe forms of hypertension and may limit hypertensive nephropathy in an unaffected contralateral kidney. However, medical treatment cannot arrest progression of stenosis, and information from non-randomised studies suggests that surgical correction is associated with an increased survival when compared with medical therapy. In particular, the risks of renal failure, stroke and myocardial infarction are reduced.

Surgical

Balloon angioplasty is now the first line treatment of most cases of RAS, particularly that associated with fibromuscular dysplasia. Although restenosis is relatively common, the procedure can be repeated and is associated with less risk than open surgery. The long-term results of angioplasty are considerably better in non-ostial than in ostial lesions. Placement of a stent may offer better long-term patency in ostial disease. Open operation provides better long-term results than PTA but requires considerable surgical skill and is associated with a significantly greater morbidity and mortality. Operation is usually reserved for instances in which medical therapy and PTA have failed. The commonest operation is aortorenal bypass with long saphenous vein. Extra-anatomic renal revascularisation can also be achieved through hepatorenal and splenorenal bypasses. These procedures can be expected to provide long-term blood pressure control in 85–90% of patients with a mortality of less than 5% and a major morbidity of less than 10%. If there is a small non-functioning kidney, nephrectomy may be the only option. Acute thrombosis of a chronically stenosed renal artery may not lead to renal infarction because of the development of collateral capsular supply, and surgical bypass or PTA with stenting can sometimes be successful.

Renal artery aneurysm

This is an uncommon disorder which may lead to renovascular hypertension and renal failure. Rupture also occurs and repair should be considered if the lesion exceeds 2 cm in diameter.

Vascular trauma

MECHANISMS

The commonest non-iatrogenic cause of injury to blood vessels in the UK is road traffic accidents (usually blunt injuries). Penetrating injuries – e.g. knife and gunshot wounds – are much less frequent. Iatrogenic injury to the brachial and common femoral arteries from angiography and angioplasty are by far the commonest examples. If the injury is caused by a sharp instrument such as a knife, the arterial or venous wound tends to be limited to the area of immediate injury and the remaining vessel is undamaged. In some, particularly high velocity, missile wounds (Ch. 3) or in blunt trauma, the extent of the injury is often more extensive, in terms of both the vascular injury and associated injuries in other systems.

CLINICAL FEATURES

The two principal consequences of arterial injury are:

● *Haemorrhage* – external and obvious or internal and thus clinically inapparent until hypovolaemia develops. Blood loss tends to be greater if there is only partial rather than complete transection, because in partial transection the laceration is held open by the continuity of part of the wall, whereas in complete transection vasospasm and intimal retraction with thrombosis occur, which limits loss.
● *Ischaemia* – this is often severe because the injury is acute and the vasculature has previously been normal; there has not been any opportunity for collaterals to become established.

History and symptoms

An obvious story of injury is common, but sometimes, in the context of multiple trauma, this may not be apparent. Otherwise the symptoms are those of acute vascular interruption.

Physical findings

In young people, provided that the systolic blood pressure is above 100 mmHg, peripheral pulses should be readily palpable. Absent or diminished pulsation should immediately alert the clinician to the likelihood of vascular injury. In closed injury, an expanding haematoma may be palpable.

Doppler examination. An audible Doppler signal may be present from a collateral circulation even if the artery is transected proximally. However, in the lower limb, if the ABPI does not equal that on the uninjured side, vascular injury should be suspected.

INVESTIGATION

Angiography should be considered in any instance where there is doubt about the diagnosis or where the site of injury is uncertain (Fig. 28.18).

MANAGEMENT

As in any acutely ill patient, management begins with resuscitation (Ch. 3). Immediate control of haemorrhage by direct pressure and then operation rapidly to restore normal flow are essential. The latter is achieved either by direct repair of the artery and accompanying large

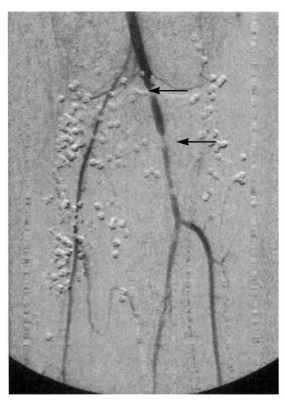

Fig 28.18 **This young man had a close-range shotgun wound of the knee.** Although peripheral pulses were still present, the angiogram indicates severe multilevel injury to the popliteal artery (**arrows**). The vessel was reconstructed successfully with a vein graft, but unfortunately, because of extensive nerve injury, above-knee amputation was eventually required. Numerous shotgun pellets are also seen in the soft tissues.

veins, if possible, or by means of a bypass graft. Because of the risk of infection, prosthetic materials should be avoided wherever possible.

All patients who sustain vascular trauma should received appropriate antibiotics and, when indicated, tetanus prophylaxis (Ch. 9). The use of thromboembolic prophylaxis has to be decided on an individual basis and must balance the risks of thrombosis against those of haemorrhage. The risk of reperfusion injury is greatest in vascular trauma and fasciotomy is frequently indicated for prevention (Fig. 28.19).

Traumatic arteriovenous fistula

If, as a result of trauma, there is damage to an adjacent artery and vein, a fistula between them may develop.

CLINICAL FEATURES

Symptoms include pain, swelling and sometimes other features of distal ischaemia. If the shunt is large, then, over some weeks and months, cardiac failure may develop.

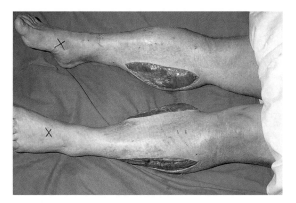

Fig 28.19 **Photograph showing bilateral fasciotomies done following revascularisation of bilateral severe leg ischaemia.** Note how the muscles are bulging through the skin incisions.

There is often a thrill on palpation and, on auscultation, a machinery bruit throughout the cardiac cycle. Distal venous engorgement may develop.

MANAGEMENT

Surgical repair is indicated, but various endovascular techniques such as embolisation and covering the fistulous opening in the artery with a stent may also be used.

False aneurysm

As discussed under 'Aneurysm', arterial injury may lead to false aneurysm. Treatment is by ultrasound guided compression, thrombin, surgical repair, or, in certain circumstances, embolisation with a coil or placement of a stent.

Arteriovenous malformation (AVM)

These types of malformation are congenital but not hereditary abnormalities, almost invariably present at birth, although they may not present for medical attention until much later in life. Haemangiomas, by contrast, present a few days or weeks after birth and are much more likely to regress spontaneously. The more proximal an AVM is in the circulation, the greater the transmitted flow. A proportion of malformations appear to be entirely venous.

CLINICAL FEATURES

Symptoms

Patients present at almost any age; onset of symptoms may be related to the appearance of the menarche, to

pregnancy or to an episode of minor trauma. There is swelling, discoloration and/or bleeding which is usually not life-threatening; pain, high-output cardiac failure, limb hypertrophy and ulceration are less common.

Physical findings

Lesions with an arterial component are usually pulsatile, a machinery-type murmur is heard on auscultation and, using a hand-held Doppler device, flow is easily detected in all phases of the cardiac cycle. Venous lesions engorge and empty with dependency and elevation, respectively.

DIAGNOSIS

Appearance in later life requires distinction from malignant lesions such as sarcoma and metastatic deposits. Apart from biopsy to exclude malignancy in cases of doubt, the diagnosis is usually clinical.

INVESTIGATION

In venous lesions, phleboliths may be seen on plain radiographs. A chest X-ray allows assessment of cardiac size. Ultrasound, with or without venography, can be used to assess venous lesions. CT and particularly MRI (now the investigation of choice) give valuable information about deep extent when excision is contemplated. Angiography is invasive, should not be done for diagnostic purposes and is reserved for those lesions in which therapeutic embolisation is under consideration.

MANAGEMENT

AVMs may not require treatment except for counselling and reassurance for both the patient and, in children, the parents. When necessary, the principles are control of symptoms and prevention of complications with minimal intervention. Radiologists, cardiologists and vascular, orthopaedic, plastic and maxillofacial surgeons may all be involved in therapy.

Occasionally operation may be required to exclude malignancy. Complete excision provides good long-term control but is rarely feasible. The technique of dissection and ligation of feeding arteries is always associated with recurrence, compromises arterial access for interventional radiologists and should not be performed. Amputation is sometimes required as a last resort. Therapeutic embolisation, in which the lesion is filled from within with thrombogenic coils or gel, is the mainstay of treatment but requires high skill and careful planning. This carries a risk of ischaemia in surrounding or distal vital tissues – inadvertent embolisation of neural tissues, fingers and toes is a particular concern. Venous lesions can be treated by direct injection of sclerosant and/or partial excision of prominent veins once the normality of the deep venous system (sometimes absent or hypoplastic) has been assured.

Future directions

Many of the techniques described in this chapter have only been developed over the last 20–30 years. This rapid pace of technological advance continues, particularly that of minimally invasive and endovascular techniques. For example, several centres in the UK now repair certain abdominal aortic aneurysms by a stent–graft combination placed percutaneously through the femoral artery without the need for an abdominal incision. Laparoscopic intra-abdominal arterial surgery, although still in its infancy, shows promise for the future.

Equally impressive have been the advances in non-invasive imaging. Within the next 10 years, conventional angiography and computed tomography may have been largely replaced by MRI in the assessment of the central and peripheral vascular systems. High-quality, real-time, colour flow duplex ultrasound imaging has already revolutionised the imaging of arteries and veins. New ultrasound contrast media may allow certain vessels such as the renal and mesenteric arteries, previously inaccessible to ultrasound diagnosis, to be imaged with increasing ease and accuracy.

It is likely that there will also be major advances in the development of prosthetic grafts to match the long-term performance of autologous vein. In addition, there is much basic science work directed towards allowing human cadaver and animal arteries to be used as arterial conduits in humans. With an ageing population and little evidence of a major decline in tobacco consumption or in the prevalence of diabetes, there is undoubtedly going to be a growing need for arterial surgery well in to the next millennium.

29 Venous and lymphatic disorders

Venous disorders

The venous system is affected by conditions that cause clotting within it and which may in turn have consequences for the return of blood from the tissues and input from the arterial side. In addition, anatomical abnormalities (usually in the valves of the veins) may interfere with the fluid dynamics of the venous circulation and impair tissue nutrition in the periphery.

ANATOMICAL AND PHYSIOLOGICAL CONSIDERATIONS

In surgical disorders, the important distinction is between the *superficial* and the *deep* systems (Fig. 29.1). Superficial veins in the limbs and head and neck drain the integument. They contain valves which permit central flow but oppose reflux. Each communication between the superficial and the deeper veins which takes place through the body's investing fascia is also provided with a valve so that blood passes only from

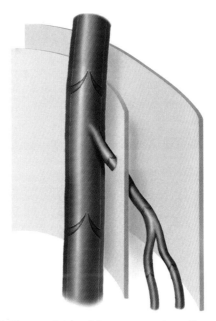

Fig 29.1 **The superficial and deep venous systems.** The superficial vein passes through deep fascia to the deep venous system. A valve exists between the superficial and deep vein, permitting one-way passage of venous blood from superficial to deep systems.

461

the superficial to the deep system. The definition of the deep system follows from this: it comprises all channels within the investing fascia. In the limbs, these contain valves similar to those in the superficial veins. However, in the trunk, the deep veins are without valves, so creating a central pool in which changes in pressure are uniformly distributed. Changes in central venous volume and pressure are one of the major methods by which cardiac output is maintained (see Ch. 17).

The detailed physiology of the veins of the lower limbs, whose function is much influenced by the upright posture of humans, is considered below.

PATHOLOGICAL FEATURES

Thrombosis

The fluidity of blood within veins is dependent on:

- free flow, although stagnation is probably only an accessory factor to other causes of thrombosis
- normality of composition
- an intact endothelial surface – all vessels, but veins in particular, contain plasminogen activators which can initiate the lysis of fibrin and so cause the dissolution of small accumulations of fibrin.

These three factors were first invoked as the underlying causes of venous thrombosis by the German pathologist Virchov. His 'triad' states venous thrombosis is likely to occur when there is (Table 29.1):

- stasis
- a change in the composition of the blood
- endothelial trauma.

Clotting of blood within a vein takes two clinicopathological forms (Fig. 29.2)

- *Thrombophlebitis* in which there is a strong element of endothelial trauma – either from physical causes or inflammation, or both
- *Venous thrombosis*, which may have a local (usually trauma) or general precipitating cause but in which acute inflammation is not initially present.

Table 29.1
Factors in the development of venous thrombosis (Virchov's triad)

Factor	Causes	Effects
Stasis	Obstruction	Encourages aggregation
	Varicosity	of platelets and margintion of leucocytes
Change in composition of blood	Increased platelets (thrombocytosis)	
	Cell surface factors (malignancy)	Affects factors?
	Surgery and trauma	Reduced fibrinolysis
Endothelial trauma	Direct injury	Provides point for adherence of platelets

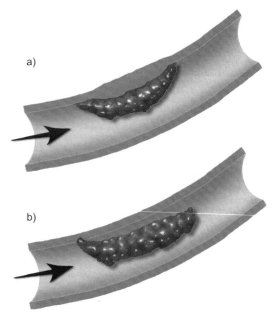

Fig 29.2 **Pathogenesis of venous clotting. (a)** Blood clotting in vein secondary to inflammation of endothelium of the vein: thrombophlebitis. **(b)** Blood clotting in vein due to stasis or factors other than inflammation: phlebothrombosis.

Although these are two distinct pathological entities, there may be an element of overlap in an individual case. The first is more common in superficial vessels and the second in the deep system.

The pathological distinction between the two types is of clinical importance. In thrombophlebitis, the clot is deposited on a damaged endothelium and is therefore attached to the vein wall throughout its length. Spread usually takes place proximally only to the point of the next venous confluence. In venous thrombosis, the clot is loosely attached to the vein wall at the point of origin and extension proximally is as a free-floating mass in the vein – propagated thrombus – which may be of considerable extent and can easily become detached to pass proximally into the heart and lungs. In both types of thrombosis (and in contrast to thrombosis in an artery – see Ch. 28), resolution takes place largely by fibrinolysis and the action of lysosomal enzymes secreted by leucocytes. The lumen is usually reestablished (recanalised) so that blood flow is restored. However, there may be a varying amount of damage to the wall of the vein so that it undergoes some fibrous replacement with loss of elasticity. In consequence:

- valves are destroyed or rendered incompetent
- there is dilatation and stagnation.

The effect on venous function in the lower limb is considered below.

The exception to the general rule of recanalisation is when the vein is kept empty during the thrombotic episode. Permanent obliteration then occurs – a process which is used in the management of varicose veins (see 'Sclerotherapy', below).

Varicose veins

A vein is said to be varicose when its normal anatomy is distorted by dilatation and tortuosity. Veins anywhere in the body can be affected, but for practical purposes this common condition affects the lower limbs. The following section considers the lower limb only.

ANATOMY

Venous drainage of the lower limb is by both the deep and superficial systems (Fig. 29.3)

- Superficial veins are in the subcutaneous tissue external to the deep fascia
- Deep veins are within the enveloping deep fascia and drain all structures within the fascial compartments, the most important of which are the muscles.

The two systems are connected by communicating veins, each of which contains a valve that permits flow only from the superficial to the deep. There are upwards of 100 in each leg, of which only a small number have clinical importance. The two major ones are:

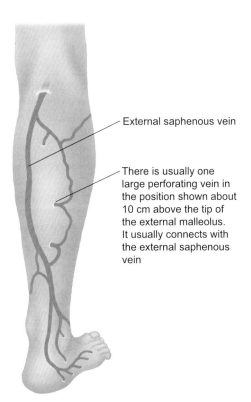

External saphenous vein

There is usually one large perforating vein in the position shown about 10 cm above the tip of the external malleolus. It usually connects with the external saphenous vein

Fig 29.3 **Venous drainage of the lower limb.**

- the entry of the long saphenous vein into the common femoral vein at the saphenous opening in the groin
- the junction of the short saphenous vein with the popliteal in the popliteal fossa.

Other communications are found along the line of the subsartorial canal and on the medial and lateral aspects of the leg below the knee.

The major deep veins follow the same paths as the arteries and, below the knee, are their vena comitans. Above the knee, the veins become a single companion trunk (femoral vein) which leaves the leg behind the inguinal ligament. In normal circumstances, the disposition of valves in the deep system prevents reflux.

VENOUS PHYSIOLOGY IN THE LOWER LIMB

The energy required to propel blood around the vascular system is generated by left ventricular contraction. In the erect position, the return of blood to the right side of the heart from the lower limbs is assisted by:

- inspiration, which lowers intrathoracic pressure
- the muscle pumps of the thigh, calf and feet – the second is by far the more important.

The pumps are driven by the contraction of muscles in the relatively rigid compartments deep to the investing fascia. Intracompartmental pressure rises, and the veins and sinuses in muscles are further compressed by the muscular contraction. Blood is expelled and can only flow proximally because of the valves in the communicating veins, which prevent its escape into the superficial system. This sequence can be illustrated by measurement of venous pressure in a superficial vein on the dorsum of the foot. With the patient horizontal and at rest, pressure is around 15 mmHg. On standing, but without muscle activity, blood continues to flow towards the heart but the pressure is increased to around 100 mmHg – an amount equivalent to the hydrostatic effect of a column of blood from the right atrium to the dorsum of the foot. Contraction of muscles in the calf and foot (e.g. by repeatedly rising on tiptoe) causes the pressure to fall to 40 mmHg as blood is expelled from the leg, the intracompartmental volume falls and flow takes place from the superficial to the deep system. Reflux of blood in the deep system – because of the effects of gravity – is largely prevented below the inguinal ligament by the valves in the large veins which break up the column of blood.

Just as with the cardiac pump, failure of either the muscle or the valves or the presence of obstruction affects performance and is reflected by a reduction in the degree of fall of superficial venous pressure on exercise and an accelerated return to resting standing pressure.

The common factor in the production of venous disease in the lower limbs is loss of venous valvular competence in the:

- superficial system – cosmetic tortuosities only without disturbance of pump function
- communicating veins – deep to superficial incompetence with reflux of blood and a sustained high pressure in the superficial systems on exercise
- deep valves – this raises pressure in the deep system and is associated with reflux of blood upon change of posture.

When the cause of malfunction is an episode of thrombosis in deep veins, deep to superficial incompetence and incompetence of valves in the deep veins are often both present (see 'Deep vein thrombosis', below). If pressure in the deep veins rises because of muscular contraction and there is deep to superficial incompetence, the action of the pump is associated with reflux from deep to superficial and consequential changes in subcutaneous venules and capillaries.

EPIDEMIOLOGY

The prevalence of varicose veins is around 2% with a female:male ratio of 3:1. Varices are less common in the young but as many as half of those between 65 and 75 years may have them.

The major complication of varices which occur either as a result of deep to superficial valvular incompetence or because of deep venous disease with valve destruction is the nutritional change in the skin which may eventually go on to ulceration.

CLASSIFICATION AND AETIOLOGY

It is customary to classify varicosities into:

- primary – there is deep to superficial incompetence only and the varicosities appear without an obvious underlying cause
- secondary – the varicosities occur because of some other cause: obstruction, or thrombo-inflammatory destruction of valves in both the communicating and deep veins.

Primary varicose veins

The exact mechanism by which valvular failure occurs is still disputed. It was originally assumed that a valve or valves in a communication between the deep and superficial systems became incompetent from above downwards, followed by progressive proximodistal destruction of the valves in the superficial system exposed to increased hydrostatic pressure – e.g. in the long saphenous system, saphenofemoral valve incompetence first, followed by dilatation of the vein itself and valve failure throughout its length. Studies with Doppler ultrasound, however, have suggested that branches of the long saphenous vein may become incompetent without or before incompetence at the saphenofemoral junction. In addition, use of the saphenous vein for cardiac and arterial surgery (see Chs. 9 and 19) suggests that its muscular wall makes it resistant to dilatation when pressure is raised.

There is little doubt that there is a familial component, but, this apart, there is not a convincing hypothesis of cause. Contributory factors are:

- obesity
- multiple pregnancy – possibly through hormonal effects on the muscle of the vein wall.

Secondary varicose veins

These are less common than the primary type but are still frequent in some groups of the population, such as women who have had multiple or complicated pregnancies. Causes are:

- deep or (less common) superficial venous thrombosis with recanalisation and consequent deep and/or deep to superficial valve destruction
- obstruction with venous hypertension – a proximal injury or obstruction from a tumour
- congenital or acquired arteriovenous fistulae with increased pressure and flow being transmitted from the arterial side of the circulation.

Secondary varicose veins are associated with the syndrome of chronic venous insufficiency, which is considered below.

SECONDARY EFFECTS

Perivenous tissue changes

The changes that occur in the skin and subcutaneous tissues of the lower limb are the consequence of venous hypertension. A rise in pressure at the venular end of the capillary loop causes:

- potential accumulation of interstitial oedema fluid which, at least initially, may be compensated for by increased lymph flow
- possible decreased oxygenation of cells with nutritional disturbance, which may make the skin liable to break down from minor trauma (so causing ulceration)
- ulceration.

Skin changes

The long-term changes in the skin and subcutaneous tissues from severe venous hypertension (usually but not exclusively in secondary varices associated with damage to the deep veins) have been attributed to a condition that is recognisable both clinically and microscopically: lipodermatosclerosis. This is characterised by:

- pigmentation – because of extrusion of red cells (diapedesis) and their subsequent dissolution

- thickening of the subcutaneous tissues – oedema and patchy fibrosis
- atrophy of the skin – often with depletion of normal pigment cells and white dermal patches.

Microscopic assessment of lipodermatosclerosis shows additional changes which stem from the venous hypertension and poor cellular nutrition:

- dilatation and tortuosity but a decrease in the number of capillaries
- trapping of white cells within capillary loops
- pericapillary deposition of a cuff of fibrin
- increased numbers of extravasated leucocytes.

All of these may have a role in the progression of the disorder. The dilated capillaries may be more permeable, so exacerbating the oedema. The fibrin cuff has been thought to reduce diffusion and so interfere with nutrition; however, this is currently regarded as unlikely and more probably a secondary phenomenon. Tissue oxygenation is certainly reduced, although this may be the consequence of lower oxygen extraction. White cell activation associated with the release of cytokines, proteolytic enzymes and free radicals that could result in further damage. Finally, tissue repair is inhibited by the physical presence of extravasated fibrinogen and by alpha-2-macroglobulin which binds growth factors so making them unavailable (trap hypothesis).

A further uncommon event is for squamous carcinoma to develop in a long-standing ulcer. Because of cell proliferation, the edge of a malignant ulcer becomes raised.

The pathological and other features of ulceration are considered in more detail below.

CLINICAL FEATURES

History and symptoms

A family history is obtained in more than a third of patients and is often coupled with onset at a relatively young age. In secondary varices, there may be a past history of deep vein thrombosis (see below) although absence of this does not exclude such an event having taken place.

A patient who is aware of the presence of varicose veins because of their visibility may, particularly if elderly, ascribe symptoms to them which have other causes. The common symptoms which it is reasonable to associate with varicose veins (some of which may have alternative causes) are listed in Table 29.2.

Discomfort. Aching is traditionally regarded by patients as a symptom they should have and may dominate the complaints even when the patient is in fact more concerned about the unsightliness. Relief of discomfort on elevation or through the use of an elastic stocking is common although non-specific. Patients who have incompetent or obstructed deep veins may complain of discomfort of a bursting type on exercise.

Table 29.2
Symptoms of varicose veins and alternative explanations

Symptom	Alternative causes
Ugly appearance	Obesity; vascular disorders
Aching	Simple fatigue; musculoskeletal disorders in limb or trunk (sciatica, arthritis of hip and knee)
Pain on exercise	Arterial claudication Spinal claudication
Ankle swelling	Oedema of other cause – cardiac, renal, lymphoedema
Restless legs	Neurological disorder
Pigmentation and depigmentation	Skin disorders
Eczema	Skin disorders
Attacks of superficial phlebitis	Systemic causes – neoplasia, thromboangiitis obliterans
Ulceration	See Table 29.11
Bleeding into the subcutaneous tissues	Blood disorders with reduced clotting ability or increased bleeding tendency

Pain may follow the development of a skin complication such as ulceration. Superficial thrombophlebitis is accompanied by acute pain along the line of the affected vein.

Bleeding may be one of the following:

- into the subcutaneous tissues where it is usually minor and causes only discomfort
- external from the rupture of a varix – precipitated by minor trauma; if the patient stays upright, there can be considerable blood loss because the haemorrhage is at high venous pressure. Deaths from such bleeding – which is in effect from the right side of the heart – have been recorded, although they are rare.

Eczema gives rise to itching which may lead the patient to scratch and further damage the skin.

Ulceration is usually painless, although episodes of inflammation may be associated with pain.

At the completion of the history in an individual patient, it is important to have developed some idea of the severity of the symptoms and the likelihood that they are related to the varicose veins or whether they are (as in more probable) the consequence of another disorder.

Signs in the lower limbs

Variceal pattern. The initial examination is in the upright position with the groin and foot fully exposed. The pattern of varices (Figs 29.4 and 29.5) is usually easily recognised as in the territory of either the long saphenous (most common) or the short saphenous (next most common), or both (unusual in primary varices). However, the patterns seen cannot be used on

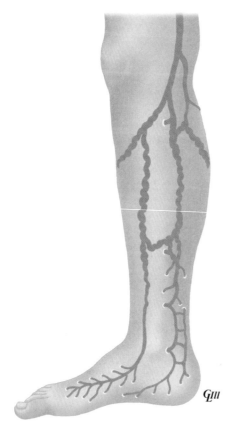

Fig 29.4 **Variceal pattern in long saphenous system in leg.**

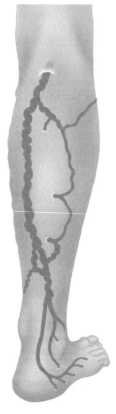

Fig 29.5 **Variceal pattern in short saphenous system in leg.**

their own to make an anatomical diagnosis because of intercommunication between the two systems. Unusual variations in the distribution of varices suggest a possible pelvic obstruction; if associated with an apparent enlargement of the limb and port wine stains of the skin, there is the possibility of an arteriovenous malformation or of the rare Klippel–Trenaunay–Weber syndrome (a complex developmental anomaly with multiple arteriovenous fistulae and overgrowth of the limb).

With the patient supine and on raising the leg, varices either disappear completely or reduce rapidly in size. The exception is when, in secondary varices, the cause is obstruction to venous outflow from the limb. The variceal pattern then includes the groin and adjacent abdominal wall.

Blow-outs – which are nothing more than localised dilatations – may be visible and palpable along the main course of either saphenous vein and are sometimes associated with a palpable defect in the deep fascia and the presence of an incompetent perforating vein. A pronounced dilatation is sometimes seen at the site of major incompetence between the deep and superficial systems: a saphena varix in the groin which must be distinguished from a femoral hernia (Ch. 26); and a mass of tortuous vessels in the popliteal fossa.

Oedema associated with primary varices is usually relatively mild, pits readily and is most often marked, particularly in men, at the site of the grip of an ankle sock. Gross oedema, except when associated with ulceration, is more likely to have a secondary cause: cardiac or renal disease, or lymphoedema.

Skin and subcutaneous tissues. In mild varices, the skin is usually normal. Where there has been long-standing superficial venous hypertension (whether caused by deep to superficial incompetence alone or associated with damage to the deep system), the characteristic changes of lipodermatosclerosis develop. The appearances are usually most obvious in the gaiter region (immediately above and usually on the medial side of the calf). The early stigmata are:

- visible tortuous veins
- thickening of the subcutaneous tissues – sometimes nodular in nature and a manifestation of the pathological change of lipodermatosclerosis
- an ankle flare – from capillary dilatation
- eczema – usually wet rather than dry and associated with scratch marks
- dark brown pigmentation from the deposition of haemosiderin
- atrophy with absence of normal pigment – white patches.

Acute active lipodermatosclerosis is easily recognised as painful, thickened and hard erythematous plaques in the subcutaneous tissue most often on the medial aspect of the lower calf.

GENERAL EXAMINATION

This may reveal underlying causes to explain symptoms and signs in patients who present with varices – particularly heart failure and musculoskeletal or pelvic disease in the elderly. Examination of the peripheral arterial system (skin temperature, nutritional changes and peripheral pulses) is essential to distinguish venous from arterial disorders or to assess the relative contribution of both to a complication such as ulceration.

Clinical tests of valve function

Percussion of the column of blood in a vein with the patient standing causes upward transmission of a palpable wave, especially when the vein is distended and thin-walled. In a varicose vein that has incompetent valves along its length, the wave is also transmitted downward. This procedure is most useful in the long saphenous system.

The Trendelenburg test (Fig. 29.6) is done by elevating the leg to 45∞ to empty the superficial veins by gravity which may be assisted by stroking them from distal to proximal. A tourniquet is then lightly applied to the leg (the degree can only be learnt by practice) just distal to the saphenofemoral junction and the patient asked to stand. If there is isolated saphenofemoral valve incompetence, the varicosities remain empty for at least 15–30 seconds and then gradually refill as blood continues to flow in from the arterial side

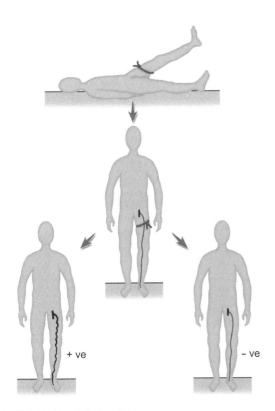

Fig 29.6 **The Trendelenburg test.**

of the circulation. The test is repeated with release of the tourniquet immediately on standing when momentary reflux from the deep system may be seen with the varicose veins filling at once. Finally, if the veins fill at once even with the tourniquet in place, the sequence is repeated, moving the tourniquet down the limb until the lowest point of deep to superficial incompetence is found. If there is still rapid filling when the compression is below the level of the termination of the popliteal vein, then it is likely that there are incompetent perforating veins in the calf. However, localisation of these is not usually successful by this simple clinical procedure.

The Trendelenburg test may be done with finger pressure alone rather than a tourniquet, but more experience is required; a precisely applied tourniquet is preferable.

INVESTIGATIONS

The investigations described below are for localisation of incompetent deep to superficial communications and for identification of valvular insufficiency in deep veins.

Continuous wave ultrasound

The simplest Doppler directional probe (see Ch. 3) generates continuous waves which, when the target is moving (as with blood), are altered in frequency on reflection; thus flow can be assessed. The principle is used to detect points of incompetence, e.g. at the saphenofemoral junction. With the probe just distal to this point, flow upwards in the saphenous vein is accelerated by compressing the calf. Release of compression in the presence of competent valve causes a sharp cut-off of the signal, but if there is incompetence, momentary reflux occurs and generates a new signal. The test can be repeated at other sites of suspected deep to superficial incompetence such as the popliteal fossa. However, the accuracy of this investigation, except at the saphenofemoral junction, is not very high and in complex instances other investigations, such as duplex Doppler scanning, are increasingly used.

Duplex doppler scanning

Duplex provides a combination of imaging the vessel with detection of the direction of flow (see Ch. 4). The underlying principles of assessment of flow are similar to those for the hand-held, continuous flow instrument. The advantages are:

- The anatomy, particularly at the saphenofemoral and saphenopopliteal junctions, can be clearly shown.
- Valves at these junctions and in the deep veins can be seen.
- Reflux is demonstrated by the reversal of the direction of flow using the same principle as with continuous flow Doppler.

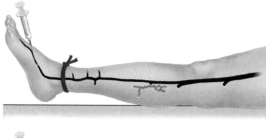

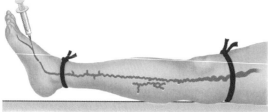

Fig 29.7 **Ascending venography.** The deep venous system is outlined in more detail by applying a tourniquet above the knee.

The recent instruments colour-code the direction of flow, which improves the precision with which reflux can be detected.

Venous pressure studies

The principle has been given above in the discussion of the venous muscular pump. They are not used in routine investigation but can be helpful in sorting out a complex problem of recurrence after surgery or of deep venous insufficiency.

Radiological imaging

Ascending venography is used to show the anatomical distribution of the deep veins. The contrast medium is injected into a dorsal vein on the foot and, by the application of a tourniquet at the ankle, fills the deep system. The latter is outlined in more detail by a venous tourniquet above the knee (Fig. 29.7). The technique can help to:

- identify sites of incompetent communicating veins (perforators) in the calf or thigh, although it does not necessarily reveal all of them.
- demonstrate evidence of present or previous damage to the deep veins from thrombosis – either persistent occlusion or valvular incompetence. Its use is reserved for difficult problems which are often associated with deep venous insufficiency.

Varicography. Injection of contrast medium directly into varices, particularly of the short saphenous vein, allows accurate determination of the anatomy – such as the confluence of the short saphenous with the popliteal – and therefore precise interruption by ligation. Unusually sited varices and recurrences after surgical treatment can also be studied by this technique.

MANAGEMENT OF PRIMARY VARICES

By definition, these are varices in the superficial system with:

- deep to superficial incompetence at one or more sites
- no evidence of disease in the deep veins.

Once it is certain that the symptoms and signs in the leg are associated with the varices, there are three options: compression hose, sclerotherapy or surgery.

Compression hose

The indications are:

- mild symptoms
- those without skin changes
- the elderly
- those who refuse other treatment
- most pregnant women.

The type of support and the choice are given in Table 29.3. It is important that any garments used should produce linear graduated compression, with the highest compression just above the malleoli and pressure decreasing towards the knee. Badly fitted supports or those which do not achieve graduated compression can produce more annoyance than relief and, on occasion, cause damage to the skin. Poor choice of stockings drastically increases the frequency of non-compliance. Patients should be instructed to apply compression hose before they get up in the morning and only to remove the support last thing at night.

Compression sclerotherapy

The principle is to produce sterile chemical inflammation in a vein kept empty by compression; thrombosis and obliteration of the lumen follow. The solutions most commonly used are 5% ethanolamine oleate or 3%

Table 29.3
Choice of support garment

Indication	Class	Pressure applied (at ankle mmHg)[a]	Garment
Young patients; mild symptoms	I	14–17	Compression tights
Severe varices; early skin changes	II	18–24	Graduated compression: elastic stockings
Advanced skin changes; ulcer	III	25–35	Heavy-duty elastic stockings or initially elastic bandaging

[a]The compression pressure quoted is obtained by measuring the elastic tension at different sites on the stocking and deriving pressure from Laplace's equation: pressure = tenxion × radius. Methods for measuring the pressure under the stocking when it is in use are also available.

Table 29.4
Complications of sclerotherapy

Cause	Reason	Outcome
Subcutaneous injection	Inexperience; failure to check reflux of blood into syringe	Pain, skin necrosis, ulceration
Intra-arterial injection	Failure to observe arterial pressure in syringe	Possible loss of limb from arterial thrombosis
Sclerosant entering deep veins	Inadequate compression	Deep vein thrombosis
Escape of sclerosant into general circulation	Inadequate compression	Anaphylaxis, haemolysis

sodium tetradecyl sulphate. The method is suitable only for isolated varices without a large site of deep to superficial incompetence, because, if this exists, recurrence rates are very high. Further uses are:

- obliteration of isolated incompetent perforating veins, especially after surgery
- vulval varices which persist after pregnancy.

Potential complications are given in Table 29.4. All are rare, but their possibility means that sclerotherapy should not be undertaken lightly.

Surgery

The indications and contraindications for surgery are given in Table 29.5. The aim is to interrupt by ligation the major points of incompetence between the superficial and deep venous systems and, if appropriate, to remove the varices for both functional and cosmetic reasons. The two most common operations are saphenofemoral and

Table 29.5
Indications for surgery in primary varicose veins

History or physical finding	Indication	Contraindication
Pain	Definite if established as not due to another cause	Doubt as to cause
Phlebitis	Varicose veins the only cause	Other conditions not excluded
Bleeding	Episode of considerable bleeding to exterior	Minor bleeding: systemic blood disorder not excluded
Skin and subcutaneous changes including eczema	To prevent ulceration	Deep venous disease must be excluded
Ulceration	Adjunct to healing	Surgery not able to correct venous hypertension

saphenopopliteal ligation (Fig. 29.8) both of which can be done using day-care facilities. In the first, great care has to be taken to demonstrate the anatomical arrangement of the tributary veins precisely, because failure to make a flush ligation of the junction of the saphenous with the femoral is the main cause of recurrence. The procedure is usually combined with removal of the saphenous trunk down to a variable level in the calf by stripping i.e. passing a flexible guide down the lumen of the vein, securing it to the divided vein and forcibly removing the vein subcutaneously. This not only improves the cosmetic result but seems also to be associated with fewer recurrences, perhaps because small incompetent perforating connections are avulsed.

If, in addition to saphenofemoral or saphenopopliteal incompetence, other sites have been identified, these are also ligated. Variceal channels are ligated and avulsed through minute stab incisions.

There are few complications after these procedures. Thrombosis in the remaining superficial channels may cause pain but is self-limiting. Very rarely a clot at the junction of the saphenous and femoral veins may give rise to a pulmonary embolus.

Recurrence after surgery on primary varices is low when adequate clinical assessment, supplemented if necessary by ancillary investigation, has been undertaken. The commonest causes are:

- poor operative technique
- failure to recognise concomitant short saphenous incompetence.

Recurrent primary varices require careful re-investigation by the methods already outlined.

Venous thrombosis

Thrombosis develops in superficial or deep veins anywhere in the body because of the events which constitute Virchov's triad (see Table 29.1), which occur in a wide variety of circumstances.

Superficial thrombophelebitis

AETIOLOGY

There are three main causes:

- stasis – varicose veins
- local trauma and inflammation – may be of any type but in surgical practice is frequently the result of i.v. therapy
- generalised hypercoaguability – malignancy and thromboangiitis obliterans.

Stasis is most often a contributory factor to the other two.

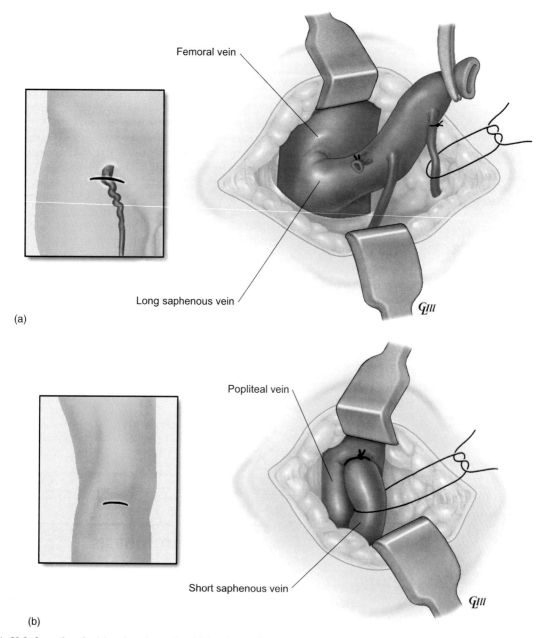

Femoral vein

Long saphenous vein

(a)

Popliteal vein

Short saphenous vein

(b)

Fig 29.8 **Operations for (a) saphenofemoral and (b) saphenopoliteal ligation.**

CLINICAL FEATURES

The affected vein becomes painful. There may be fever and, if the process is a pyogenic one, rigors as bacteria are shed into the general circulation.

An obvious cause, such as an intravenous infusion, may be present. There is a red line along the skin over the vein which is firm to hard and tender to touch. Systemic disturbance is variable.

MANAGEMENT

If there is a precipitating factor, this is removed. Thereafter the condition is usually self-limiting and is treated symptomatically with non-steroidal inflammatory agents. A spreading thrombophlebitis with systemic features may require blood culture and antibiotic therapy, and very occasionally there is suppuration for which drainage is necessary. In recurrent attacks of migratory phlebitis, a search should be instituted for either arterial disease or an underlying malignancy.

Deep vein thrombosis (DVT)

Although thrombosis in the deep veins of the lower

Table 29.6
Major antecedents of deep vein thrombosis

Factor	Circumstances
Immobilisation (venous stasis)	Bed rest during serious illness or injury Long distance air travel Unconsciousness
Changes in clotting	Contraceptive pill Injury and operation Childbirth Malignant disease Hyperviscosity (e.g. polycythaemia) Antithrombin III, protein S and protein C decificiency
Effects on vein wall	Trauma – accidental or from cannulation Extrinsic compression – inflammation, tumour bony abnormality

limb is allotted most attention because of its frequency and potentially serious consequences, the process is not limited to this part of the circulation and can occur anywhere in the deep system. The causes are summarised in Table 29.6 and follow the pattern of Virchov's triad (Table 29.1).

Axillary-subclavian vein thrombosis

AETIOLOGY

Only 2% of deep vein thromboses occur in these vessels. The condition is more frequent in men and is often associated with physical exercise which involves the shoulder girdle – butterfly swimming is a good example. Forcible abduction of the shoulder may cause intimal damage which is a starting point for thrombosis. Thrombophilia is another underlying cause – from use of the contraceptive pill and deficiencies in antithrombin 3, protein C or protein S. Finally, the common use of axillary-subclavian vein catheters for i.v. therapy may cause thrombosis from irritant solutions, local trauma or bacterial infection. It is said that deep vein thrombosis in the upper limb carries a 10% incidence of pulmonary embolus but this is rarely life-threatening.

CLINICAL FEATURES

History

There may or may not be an obvious precipitating cause. The onset is fairly rapid (2–3 days) with the development of swelling of the upper limb, dragging pain and heaviness.

Physical features

The limb is obviously swollen from its root to the fingers. The oedema initially pits readily but may become firm. Dilated veins coursing over the shoulder girdle are seen unless obscured by obesity or oedema.

INVESTIGATION

The diagnosis is usually obvious both from the circumstances and from the clinical examination. However, subsequent investigation for an underlying cause may be required once the acute condition has subsided.

MANAGEMENT

The limb is elevated to minimise the development of induration from prolonged oedema and to make the patient more comfortable. As the swelling subsides, an elastic support is substituted for elevation. Anticoagulant therapy, initially with heparin and thereafter with oral agents, is continued until the limb has returned to normal. Thrombolytic therapy with tissue plasminogen activator (t-PA) is increasingly used and, on occasion if there is an obvious local cause, surgical exploration or stenting is indicated. Provided an underlying cause is excluded, recurrence is rare.

Lower limb DVT

This is the condition that has attracted most attention because of its frequency and well established relation to surgical procedures, particularly in the elderly. However, because of the factors outlined in Table 29.6, it is not confined to the surgical patient, and those with serious illnesses that require or are traditionally associated with immobilisation, those with congestive heart failure and those with malignant disease are also at high risk.

ANATOMICAL CONSIDERATIONS

The deep venous system of the lower limb has been described above and comprises all the channels within the investing fascia. In clinical practice, lower limb thrombosis in the deep system commonly includes thrombus in the pelvic veins, in particular the external iliac and common iliac vein, either in isolation or in continuity with thrombus which originates in the leg. For both diagnosis and management, it is helpful to qualify a lower limb DVT by referring to the particular segment or segments of vessel involved, e.g. a popliteal vein thrombus or an iliofemoral vein thrombus.

AETIOLOGY AND EPIDEMIOLOGY

All the factors given in Table 29.2 apply to DVT in the legs. Of particular importance in the postoperative patient are:

- immobility during the operation and postoperatively
- techniques of anaesthesia that promote muscular flaccidity and low rates of blood flow – prolonged general anaesthesia with paralysis and assisted ventilation
- posture of the patient on the table – continuous pressure on the calves of the supine patient or the position used for hip replacement
- application of partial or full limb casts

- venous obstruction in the pelvis during a surgical procedure
- changes in clotting following surgical or other injury
- other changes in endothelial cell and leucocyte function after injury – this area in still under study.

The incidence has been best studied in the postoperative patient with which this account is chiefly concerned. Table 29.7 (compiled mainly from prospective studies which have employed highly sensitive detection techniques with radioisotope labelling of the thrombus) shows an average incidence of 30% in patients undergoing general surgical procedures. The incidence varies widely with age. Advancing age is associated with a rise, although this may partly reflect the type of surgery that is required, e.g. an incidence of more than 60% in hip replacement. The high figures do not necessarily reflect the need for therapy in that many small thrombi can undergo spontaneous lysis.

RISK FACTORS FOR DVT IN THE SURGICAL PATIENTS

The risk with various surgical procedures has been indicated in Table 29.7. Additional ones for individual patients are listed in Table 29.8. In practice it is important to remember that the following increase risk:

- age – particular over 40
- obesity
- operation for malignant disease
- a previous episode of DVT or pulmonary embolism

Table 29.7
Percentage risk of postoperative deep vein thrombosis without prophylaxis

Circumstance	Average risk (%)	Reported range (%)
General surgery		
Abdominal	30	3–50
Malignancy		40–70
Urology		10–50
Open prostatectomy	40	
Transurethral resection	10	
Vascular operations		
Femeropopliteal bypass	10	
Aortoiliac	5	
Traumatic operations in othropaedics		
Trauma	35	
Hip fracture		40–60
Tibial fracture		40–50
Elective orthopaedic procedures		
Hip replacement	50	40–60
Knee replacement	80	50–90

Table 29.8
Factors which increase the risk of deep vein thrombosis (DVT)

General conditions	Type of surgery	Medical
Age > 40 years	Duration of surgery greater than 30 minutes	Cardiac failure
Obesity	Prolonged operations	Stroke
Trauma	All surgery	
Oral contraception	Extensive dissection	Thrombocytosis
Pregnancy and puerperium	Surgery for malignancy	Poycythaemia
Immobilisation	All surgery but especially orthopaedics	Systemic lupus
Infection		
Previous DVT		

- continued consumption of the contraceptive pill – although this is less certain.

PATHOLOGICAL CONSIDERATIONS

Origin

Seventy-five per cent of thromboses originate in the calf, particularly the soleal sinusoids and in the valves of the calf veins; the remaining 25% are isolated to the proximal femoral or iliofemoral veins. Approximately 30% of thrombi in the calf spread in continuity to the popliteal and superficial femoral vein segments.

Natural history

As already indicated, many small calf vein thrombi undergo spontaneous lysis. When propagation occurs and occlusion of a main trunk such as the tibial or popliteal vein takes place, the thrombus is initially free-floating but after a relatively short time becomes adherent to the vessel wall and the process of organisation begins with either lysis or the replacement of fibrin by fibous tissue, or a combination of the two. The subsequent events are described in the section on the postphlebitic limb.

The possibility of a portion of clot becoming separated and a pulmonary embolus occurring is at its greatest while the clot remains free-floating and continues to acquire thrombus.

CLINICAL FEATURES

Symptoms

Particular in the postoperative patient, there are rarely, while the thrombus is confined to the small veins, any complaints. Extension into the main vessels may cause calf pain and swelling which is noticed by the patient.

Signs

Physical signs, particularly in the early stages, are also minimal and the accuracy of clinical diagnosis is no greater than 50% when compared to objective methods.

Calf tenderness. If possible, the knee should be flexed, the calf muscles relaxed and systematic bimanual palpation of each calf should take place up to the popliteal fossa. It is important to identify areas of tenderness, particularly in the soleal and gastrocnemius muscle masses. The consistency is compared in both limbs because the affected calf may feel more solid or less 'floppy' than the normal one.

Oedema. Ankle oedema in a limb that has not been the site of surgery and was not swollen before the operation should arouse suspicion. Spread onto the dorsum of the foot almost always means that, if venous thrombosis is responsible, the popliteal segment is involved.

Distension of superficial veins. Unilateral dilatation may be present but also occurs in association with hyperaemia or local infection.

Superficial thrombophlebitis can occur independent of DVT in the postoperative patient but may be associated with extension into the deep system. A tender cord-like thickening is easily palpable over the course of the normal or varicose superficial vein. The overlying skin is erythematous and the site itself is often extremely tender.

Limb discoloration. A diagnosis should have been made long before oedema has become so significant as to produce the pallor associated with obstruction to arterial inflow (see 'White leg').

Pain on dorsiflexion of the ankle (Homans' sign). This much quoted sign of pain in the calf on passive dorsiflexion of the ankle, is – as its originator always maintained – wholly unreliable and should be forgotten in the diagnosis of DVT.

DIAGNOSIS

All postoperative patients should be regarded as at risk of DVT and pulmonary embolus. This implies that, whatever procedure has been undertaken, the legs should be examined at least daily and that minor unexplained fluctuations in temperature should arouse suspicion. It is also important to ensure that the method of prophylaxis in use is being adhered to. Screening in high-risk groups is appropriate.

Many of the mechanical problems which can mimic DVT, such as a ruptured popliteal cyst or a tear of the fibres of the gastrocnemius, are rarely relevant in the postoperative patient. However, the diagnosis can be confounded by local trauma within the limb itself, such as surgery to varicose veins or hip replacement. Objective methods are then required to exclude thrombosis. Oedema from fluid overload, or cardiac or renal failure causes bilateral swelling. Haemorrhage into the limb may occur in a patient on anticoagulants, after an arterial puncture or direct arterial surgery. Superficial thrombophlebitis may be present in isolation but may coexist with DVT.

INVESTIGATION

The techniques used for the investigation of the peripheral veins have been described above.

Continuous wave ultrasound

In the presence of obstruction to major (axial) veins there is no change in flow rate on calf compression. The technique cannot, however, detect thrombi confined to the calf vessels. It can be a useful first-line approach when used regularly by an experienced operator, preferably a trained technician.

Duplex scanning

The vessel, the ability to compress it and the flow rate through it are both visible on the screen seen and, in skilled hands, the accuracy of diagnosis is more than 90%.

^{125}I fibrinogen uptake tests

Fibrinogen labelled with iodine-125 is taken up by an actively growing thrombus and can be detected as a hot spot by a scintillation counter. Its particular values are:

- investigation of the effectiveness of new methods of prophylaxis or treatment
- screening of patients who are at high risk following surgical procedures.

It is, however, not applicable in surgery that involves the limb below the inguinal ligament and is unhelpful in detecting thrombus above the mid-thigh and in the iliac segment. ^{125}I scanning is about 70–75% accurate but may take up to 5 days to establish a diagnosis if accretion to the thrombus is slow. It is now regarded as a research tool only, except in special circumstances.

Venography

Many of the above techniques were developed because of the invasive nature of venography. Until very recently, the contrast material used could itself cause thrombosis and, if extravasation occurred, tissue necrosis. With the development of low-osmolality contrast material, these risks have effectively disappeared. The only remaining disadvantages are the:

- discomfort of the needle insertion and the bursting sensation on injection of the contrast medium
- time and expense involved in any radiological technique.

Routine ascending phlebography is performed as described above. Because up to 50% of patients with DVT have involvement of both limbs, venography should be performed bilaterally. Thrombi show up as constant, lucent-filling defects (Fig. 29.9). The segment(s)

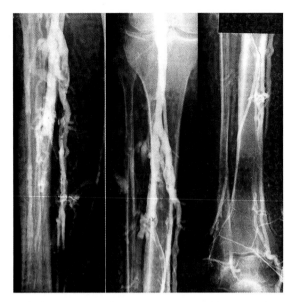

Fig 29.9 **Phlebogram of lower limb showing multiple thrombi in the tibial veins.**

involved can be defined and the upper limit outlined. It is difficult to recognise the age of a thrombus on venography but very fresh clot can be seen to float in the lumen. Although invasive, the method is more than 90% accurate and is the last court of appeal should the diagnosis remain in doubt after other investigations.

MANAGEMENT

It is a prerequisite of most clinical situations that an accurate diagnosis is obtained before treatment is begun, particularly where that treatment may have undesirable side-effects. This is true of the initial treatment of DVT with anticoagulants. Yet it is still unfortunately true to say that, in DVT, effective investigation may not precede diagnosis and treatment. This is perhaps more true of those who present *de novo* with a possible diagnosis of venous thrombosis than it is of post-surgical patients. Nevertheless, it should no longer be clinically acceptable to start and continue anticoagulant therapy without confirmed, objective non-invasive or phlebographic evidence of thrombus.

Once the diagnosis is established, treatment aims to:

- prevent extension
- reduce the chance of pulmonary embolisation
- limit the short- and long-term morbidity in the limb
- take measures to avoid late recurrence of thrombosis.

Anticoagulant therapy

Thrombus confined to the calf
Spontaneous lysis is common. Anticoagulant therapy can be avoided provided the patient is mobile. An

appropriately measured and fitted below-knee support and avoidance of sitting with the legs dependent are important supplementary measures.

About 20% of thrombi which begin in the calf extend proximally. If a decision is made to withhold anticoagulants, it is important to continue to monitor the limb.

Involvement of tibial, superficial femoral and popliteal veins and iliofemoral thrombosis
Immediate anticoagulation is essential provided there is not an absolute contraindication. Although heparin has been used for the treatment of DVT for more than 40 years, controversy still exists on the optimum dose and the duration of treatment. The clinical aim is the prompt resolution of pain and tenderness in the limb, and continuing pain at 24–48 hours suggests that anticoagulation is ineffective and thrombosis is continuing.

Heparin is administered by continuous i.v. infusion at a rate of 20–25 units/kg per hour. The patient's own pre-treatment accelerated partial thromboplastin time (APPT) should be at least doubled to ensure a therapeutic effect; comparison with a laboratory baseline normal is more likely to lead to inappropriate levels of anticoagulation. Plasma heparin levels should be maintained at more than 0.3 units/mL.

The duration of heparin therapy and the time when oral anticoagulation should be substituted remain debatable. Clinical experience suggests that in extensive DVT, it is correct to continue heparin therapy for up to 10 days, introducing oral anticoagulation with warfarin between days 5 and 7. This gives time for the international normalised ratio (INR) (Box 29.1) to reach the therapeutic range of 2–3.

Box 29.1

Calculation of the International Normalised Ratio (INR) for anticoagulant therapy with wafarin

Measurement – the time for fibrin clot to appear in citrated plasma after the addition of thromboplastin reagent and calcium – prothrombin time (PT)

Standardisation – all thromboplastin reagents are given an international sensitivity index (ISI) as recommended by the World Health Organization.

Calculations

$$\text{Prothrombin ratio} = \frac{\text{patient PT}}{\text{control PT}}$$

International normalised ratio (INR) = prothrombin ratio × ISI

To reduce discomfort and potential morbidity, the leg should be elevated during the early days of treatment and the patient should not be mobilised until the bulk of the swelling has subsided. Before mobilisation, the patient is fitted with a high-compression support, full-length or below-knee, depending on the extent of the thrombosis.

Complications of anticoagulant therapy

Bleeding may occur:

- subcutaneously or into joint spaces
- into the urine or gut
- from wounds or puncture sites.

Early warning signs are often the development of extensive areas of spontaneous bruising or ecchymoses in pressure areas which can only be detected by regular observation. Daily urine testing can reveal microscopic haematuria. In the postoperative patient, bleeding from surgical wounds and raw areas may take place, but the time course for the development of most thrombi is such that the risk is less than might be anticipated. Careful control of therapy is important but the risk of bleeding does not correlate well with the indirect tests used to monitor anticoagulation.

Heparin-induced thrombocytopenia is a well recognised but uncommon complication which also causes bleeding. When heparin is continued for more than 4 or 5 days, regular platelet counts should be done.

If there is bleeding, initial action is to stop the heparin (which has a relatively short half-life) and, if necessary, administer protamine sulphate by slow i.v. infusion: 1 mg neutralises 100 units of heparin and the dose is judged against the time since the infusion was stopped, in that heparin is rapidly excreted by the kidneys and has a half-life of less than 6 hours. Thrombocytopenia is an indication to discontinue the drug and substitute oral anticoagulants.

Continuing management

The risk of recurrent thrombosis is greatest in the first 3 months after an acute episode. When extensive DVT has occurred, a minimum of 6 months' oral anticoagulant therapy is prescribed. The role of subcutaneous low-molecular-weight heparin (see below) in the continuing management of established thrombosis is under assessment at present. It may well be that, when full anticoagulation is contraindicated, the antithrombotic effect of daily subcutaneous low-molecular-weight heparin will be an acceptable substitute.

Anticoagulant therapy does not alter the effect of established thrombus in causing damage to the deep veins. To endeavour to reduce the long-term local impact, patients should be discharged with instructions to wear high compression stockings. These should be worn continuously during oral anticoagulant therapy

and an assessment of venous function is carried out at the end of this period before a decision to discontinue support is made.

Alternative methods

Thrombolysis

In DVT after operation, thrombolytic therapy has little place because of the risk of hemorrhage. Its use is more appropriate in spontaneous extensive iliofemoral thrombosis where the limb itself is threatened (see 'White leg') and in pulmonary embolus.

Surgery

Removal of the thrombus by surgery (usually by the use of a balloon catheter passed through a small incision or percutaneously) is now seldom used. The remaining indication is threat to life or limb and failure to respond to non-operative management.

PROPHYLAXIS

Prophylaxis is much more effective in preventing morbidity from venous thrombosis and death from pulmonary embolus than is the treatment of the established condition. The development of methods of screening such as the 125I fibrinogen test has resulted in many studies over the last 20 years being done to establish the success or otherwise of prophylaxis, particularly in the postoperative patient. The methods studied and available (Table 29.9) are:

Table 29.9
Prophylaxis of deep vein thrombosis (especially postoperative)

Method	Efficacy	Disadvantages
Mechanical		
Physiotherapy by leg exercises	No proven effect	None
Early mobilisation	No proven effect although useful for other reasons	None
Graduated compressions stockings	Probably minor influence	Must be good quality and individually fitted
Intermittent calf compression	Known reduction	Cumbersome
Pharmacological		
Oral anticoagulants	Known reduction, especially orthopaedics	Takes time to be effective. Needs careful control. Increased bleeding risk
Low-dose unfractionated heparin	Successful in general surgery. Ineffective in orthopaedics	8- to 12-hourly injections
Low-molecular-weight heparin	Known reduction	Expense

- mechanical – preservation of calf muscle flow and emptying of veins in the leg
- pharmacological – alterations in the dynamics of the clotting mechanism designed to discourage venous thrombosis but not to lead to bleeding.

Mechanical

These techniques are less effective than pharmacological ones and are reserved for either low-risk patients or for specific surgical circumstances. Intermittent inflation of gaiters on the legs causes increased venous flow during (and sometimes after) operation. Low-compression graduated hose should also be used.

Pharmacological

These techniques interfere in different ways with normal blood coagulation. Their relative merits must be balanced against the possibility of causing excessive or uncontrollable bleeding, their time course of action and their ease of administration. In general surgery, the most commonly used form of prophylaxis is intermittent subcutaneous unfractionated heparin given at either 8- or 12-hour intervals. Such a regimen is most effective when the dose is calculated for each individual and based on a known response in preoperative APPT, or heparin levels. Calcium heparin is said by some to be more effective than sodium heparin when each is administered at a dose of 5000 units. The use of unfractionated heparin reduces the incidence of DVT by up to 60% in general surgery and up to 50% in most orthopaedic procedures. Prophylactic low-dose heparin also lowers the frequency of both fatal and non-fatal pulmonary emboli, and a list of suggested regimens dependent on the category of risk is given in Table 29.10. The ideal universal prophylactic has not yet been identified, but a substantial reduction in postoperative thrombosis can be obtained by employing the graded approach indicated. Prophylaxis should be routine in all surgical procedures which involve general anaesthesia and last more than 30 minutes and there must be compelling reasons to withhold it.

Recently, low-molecular-weight (LMW) heparins have been introduced because they cause a more specific antithrombotic effect through their ability to inhibit factor Xa and because, further, in experimental models they produce less bleeding for an equivalent antithrombotic effect. A similar or greater reduction in the incidence of venous thrombosis has been demonstrated in general surgical patients using a single daily dose begun the day before operation. In orthopaedic surgery (particularly hip replacement) the same may also be true, although a slightly higher dose is needed. The disadvantage of LMW heparins is their considerably greater cost compared with the unfractionated product.

Oral anticoagulants given in appropriate dosage clearly reduce the risk of thrombosis but they also carry

Table 29.10
Prophylaxis of DVT by risk category

Category of risk	Incidence	Suggested management
Low	Up to 10%	Early mobilisation Compression stockings
Medium (routine general surgery)	10–30%	Low-dose heparin Stockings where appropriate
High	Greater than 30%	
Major general surgery		Low-molecular-weight heparin
Surgery in malignant disease		Adjusted-dose heparin Oral anticoagulants Compression hose
Knee surgery compression		Intermittent
		Low-dose anticoagulants
Hip surgery		Low-molecular-weight heparin Oral anticoagulants Compression hose

a higher potential for bleeding complications unless their administration is very carefully controlled. The agent must be started several days before operation to prolong the prothrombin time so that the INR is approximately 2. A modification of this is to start the warfarin on the evening of surgery and to aim to bring the INR to a similar level by the fifth postoperative day.

Duration of prophylaxis

Subcutaneous heparin is continued for 7 days after operation or until the patient is fully mobile. In patients at high risk or with limited mobility, heparin may need to be prescribed for several weeks. Continuing self-administration at home of a single daily dose is a practical proposition.

Pulmonary embolism in DVT

The life-threatening complication of DVT is for the clot to become detached, be carried proximally and to lodge in the pulmonary artery or its branches so producing pulmonary embolism (PE).

AETIOLOGY

The great majority of PEs occur after surgical procedures complicated by the development of DVT. However, DVT and consequent PE can occur in immobilisation for any cause. The other causative factors have been listed in Table 29.8.

EPIDEMIOLOGY

In England and Wales (population c. 50 million) there are approximately 20 000 deaths a year from a pulmonary embolus. One in every 100 adult patients of all ages who undergo general surgical procedures, and 5 in every 100 who have a hip replacement, will die as a result of PE. The mortality of untreated symptomatic PE is 30%, and following massive PE, of those who die, 50–75% do so in the first hour.

PHYSIOLOGICAL AND PATHOLOGICAL CONSIDERATIONS

An embolus takes place when either the whole or the proximal propagated part of a free-floating clot becomes detached from the wall of a vein. The event may be spontaneous, or stripping of the attachment may occur as a result of an acute rise in venous pressure such as occurs during a Valsalva manoeuvre on defecation. The clot is swept proximally into the pulmonary artery and, if sufficiently large to be arrested in the main stem or across the bifurcation of the vessel, reduces cardiac output so much that death results instantly or within a very short time. Lodgement in branches produces a volume of lung tissue that is initially ventilated but underperfused. There is arteriolar spasm in the involved segment so reducing inflow and causing infarction. If the block to the pulmonary circulation is large, pressure in the right heart rises. Subsequently the segment becomes consolidated as a consequence of haemorrhage infarction. If the patient survives, the clot can lyse (50% within 2 weeks) and the circulation be restored. Alternatively, or even when there has been initial but incomplete lysis, organisation and fibrosis take place with a pulmonary scar detectable up to a year later on perfusion studies. Repeated emboli may, by this mechanism, cause the development of pulmonary artery hypertension and right heart failure.

CLINICAL FEATURES

Symptoms

There may be a sudden onset without warning. However, in retrospect, a swollen ankle or leg may have been present and it is a source of chagrin to notice this for the first time while trying to save the life of a patient with an acute circulatory collapse.

Size. Small emboli may not cause any symptoms. Those that involve up to half of the pulmonary circulation give rise to symptoms confined to the lung. Greater involvement causes additional cardiac and systemic effects. Pre-existing pulmonary disease increases the effects of a given amount of obstruction.

Chest pain. Infarction of the lung causes well localised pleuritic pain over the affected segment, worse on inspiration or coughing. A large embolus may be associated with crushing substernal rather than pleuritic pain and be rapidly followed by cardiac arrest.

Dyspnoea may be present but is not a striking feature except in very large emboli.

Haemoptysis may follow within minutes or hours in those that survive but is usually confined to blood streaking of the sputum.

Transient or prolonged loss of consciousness implies a large embolus with circulatory effects.

Signs

Circulatory. In a large embolus there is:

- arterial hypotension, usually with a pale, vasoconstricted skin, although sometimes with cyanosis
- raised jugular venous pressure
- tachycardia and, in large emboli, gallop rhythm
- variable arrhythmias.

Respiratory. Examination of the chest may show:

- pleural friction rub with associated crackles (*syn.* crepitations)
- later signs of consolidation
- pyrexia.

General. There may be evidence of DVT in the lower limbs, but detachment of the whole or the greater part of the clot from a relatively proximal vein may mean that the limb is normal.

INVESTIGATION

Chest X-ray

In small emboli there may be no abnormality. If infarction has occurred, a wedge of consolidation with its apex centrally located may be present or there may be evidence of areas of reduced vascularity – loss of vascular markings.

Pulmonary radio isotope scans

Technetium-99m-labelled albumin given intravenously may demonstrate areas of underperfusion of the lung. A normal scan excludes PE. Other causes of underperfusion (such as previous PE) may confuse, but in an abnormal scan there is approximately a 75% chance that a recent embolus is present. Specificity is greatly enhanced if ventilation is simultaneously assessed by the inhalation of xenon-133: there is a mismatch between perfusion (decreased) and ventilation (initially maintained).

Electrocardiography

In small to moderate-sized PE, the ECG is frequently normal. A large embolus, which produces dilatation of the right heart, causes tall and peaked P waves in lead II, and right axis deviation, right bundle branch block and T wave inversion in precordial leads. Large emboli can produce changes which are difficult to distinguish from inferior myocardial infarction.

Blood gas analysis

Reduction in Po_2 occurs if cardiac output is profoundly depressed and/or a very large volume of lung is underperfused. Dyspnoea increases the elimination of carbon dioxide and P_{CO_2} is therefore also reduced. This circumstance is uncommon except in collapse/consolidation of the lung (see Ch. 16) and, given the clinical circumstances, provides confirmatory evidence of PE.

Investigation of possible DVT
Provided the patient is in a stable circulatory state, if DVT has not been already looked for, the usual investigations are undertaken.

DIAGNOSIS
Other events may present the same clinical picture as a large embolus which produces circulatory effects:

- myocardial infarction – usually with the features of left rather than right ventricular failure
- massive fluid overload – generalised features are present in addition to right heart failure
- severe sepsis
- haemorrhage – the jugular venous pressure is low
- tension pneumothorax
- cardiac tamponade
- aortic dissection.

Pulmonary angiography
A catheter is passed from a peripheral vein into the pulmonary artery, contrast medium is introduced and serial X-rays or cine-angiography recorded. The diagnosis is confirmed by the demonstration of a filling defect in the pulmonary artery or arteries. Angiography is the definitive method of diagnosis and should precede any radical treatment. If the catheter is left in the artery, the circulatory course of the episode can be followed by pressure measurements.

MANAGEMENT

Resuscitation
When cardiac arrest is thought to have occurred, the standard techniques need to be instituted in an attempt to establish an adequate cardiac output and also to reach a diagnosis which is used to guide further treatment. An i.v. loading dose (10 000 units) of heparin should be given.

Continuing treatment
Resuscitation successful. An adequate cardiac output to sustain systemic perfusion is achieved. A continuous heparin infusion is begun at 25 units/kg per hour. Assuming progress is maintained, a similar regimen to that described for the management of venous thrombosis is followed and the patient is subsequently transferred to oral anticoagulation for a minimum of 6 months.

Resuscitation unsuccessful. Hypotension and an inadequate cardiac output persist. The options are (after establishing the diagnosis by angiography):

- establish cardiopulmonary bypass and remove the clot at open operation
- right heart catheterisation and regional administration of a thrombolytic agent such as streptokinase or altepase
- pulmonary artery catheterisation and suction removal of the clot – a method which can be combined with thrombolysis.

In the past, dramatic, occasionally successful, transthoracic embolectomies without cardiopulmonary bypass were described. However, without the availability of bypass, patients who survive to reach operation would also get to thrombolysis or direct suction.

Recurrent pulmonary emboli
Survival after a PE may not, if treatment of the DVT is rigorous, be followed by recurrence. However, further episodes of circulatory collapse, dyspnoea and chest pain are not infrequent. Extension of underperfusion or infraction in the lung can be confirmed by further isotope scanning or pulmonary angiography.

Management involves:

- Making sure that anticoagulation with heparin has been achieved and is at a therapeutic level
- Identifying the site of origin by venography
- Consideration of interruption of the venous pathway above the most proximal level of thrombosis.

The methods available for interruption are:

- surgical plication either by sutures or clips – now rarely used
- insertion of a filter into the vena cava below the renal veins.

Opinions vary about the need for such intervention if anticoagulation is adequate but they probably do have a small place.

White leg

Extensive venous thrombosis in the lower extremity can produce a clinical syndrome known as white leg or (the Latin term) *phlegmasia alba dolens* – an inflamed but white and painful leg – so called because it was originally thought that the condition had an inflammatory element.

AETIOLOGY
Rapid thrombosis along the whole length of the deep venous system and into the iliac segment so obstructs drainage that arterial input is reduced. The condition used to be common in the peurperium but is now more often seen in those with generalised hypercoaguability.

CLINICAL FEATURES

Symptoms

Pain and swelling in the whole limb are the dominant features. Systemic disturbance is often quite considerable.

Signs

The affected limb is:

- grossly swollen up to the inguinal ligament and oedema may spread onto the abdominal wall
- cool and white because of reduced arterial input
- often without arterial pulsation at the ankle from swelling, which makes it difficult to feel, but also because arterial pressure in the limb is reduced
- characterised by dusky cyanosis at the tips of the toes.

The last suggests that necrosis is about to supervene but in fact this is limited to the skin (see below).

MANAGEMENT

The initial treatment is that of any DVT with anticoagulants and limb elevation. Thrombolysis or clot extraction is reserved for those who do not improve in the first 24–36 hours or in whom there is extension of the distal cyanosis. Even then, it is doubtful if the results are improved over those of standard therapy, in that what appears to be a limb that requires major amputation (so-called venous gangrene) turns out, on continued non-intervention, to have only very limited loss of tissue in the skin and subcutaneous layers of the toes.

Once the acute episode is over, investigation of venous function follows the lines already outlined.

Other causes of deep vein thrombosis

Brief cross-references should be given here to sinus thrombosis in the head and venous thrombosis in the gut.

Postphlebitic limb – chronic venous insufficiency; calf pump failure syndrome

These and other terms are used to describe a limb in which there is damage to the deep veins, their valves and the valves in the communicating veins with the production of:

- raised static pressure in the deep veins
- transmission of this hypertension to the superficial system

- exacerbation of hypertension by the activity of the muscle pump which, in the presence of incompetent valves, allows deep to superficial reflux.

AETIOLOGY AND PATHOLOGICAL FEATURES

The most common cause is a previous deep vein thrombosis. It should be noted, however, that although destruction of deep veins is the rule, a number of patients with only severe long-standing deep to superficial incompetence can develop symptoms and signs which are clinically indistinguishable from those of chronic deep venous insufficiency. Furthermore, there may also be a group of patients who have deep venous incompetence without an underlying acquired cause.

Pathological features are of venous hypertension (described above) in the superficial tissues. Damage to the deep valves is usually secondary to a DVT with recannulation.

CLINICAL FEATURES

History

There may or may not be a history of a previous DVT, although its absence does not mean that a DVT did not take place without symptoms in the past. Over some years, the patient will have noticed the development of increased aching on exertion, ankle and calf oedema and the onset of nutritional lesions such as eczema and ulceration. A bursting feeling on walking is relatively common. Otherwise the symptoms are the same as for other causes of venous hypertension (see above).

Signs

The findings are of venous insufficiency as already described. Oedema is often quite marked and, although predominantly venous and compressible, may develop a lymphoedematous component which is firm.

INVESTIGATION

From the foregoing definition, it is clear that it is essential to establish whether or not there is deep vein involvement or whether the condition of the limb reflects only severe deep to superficial incompetence. The methods of achieving this have already been outlined.

MANAGEMENT

The potential for limb morbidity is poorly recognised by the physicians, geriatricians and dermatologists under whose management patients with advanced changes of venous hypertension such as ulceration are often placed. Surgery and the expertise of surgeons trained in the field of venous disease have much to offer, although they are not brought to bear as often as they should be.

Prophylaxis

Adequate prophylaxis and treatment of DVT and the subsequent use of effective well-tailored high-compression garments could be expected dramatically to reduce the development of the chronic changes of deep venous insufficiency such as intractable eczema and ulceration.

Treatment

Deep to superficial incompetence only. If clinical and other tests show that this is the cause, improvement up to complete cure can be produced by standard treatment with surgical ligation of points of incompetence, such as the saphenofemoral and saphenopopliteal junctions, and obliteration of varices. Long-term use of support hose is a valuable supplement.

Deep vein incompetence with deep to superficial incompetent communications but without ulceration. A full-length high-compression support is the least radical and the most acceptable method of treatment, coupled with sclerotherapy for obvious sites of perforating veins. A below-knee stocking may suffice in milder disorder: it must have a compression of 25–35 mm of mercury at the ankle and is measured up only after oedema has been reduced by elevation and ankle, calf and length measurements have been recorded to ensure an accurate fit. Techniques of venous bypass for obstruction and for valve reconstruction have been developed but follow-up is still short and they remain to be proven in the long term.

Leg ulceration

EPIDEMIOLOGY

Eighty to eighty-five per cent of leg ulcers are of venous origin, although, particularly in the elderly, an arterial element may be co-causative. Ten per cent are entirely the consequence of arterial disease. It is probable that approximately 1% of the population have, or have had, a leg ulcer and that, at any one time, between 30 and 40% of ulcers are active. Approximately 70% of those with active ulcers are over 70 years of age and there is a prevalence of 2% in the over-80s. Females exceed males by a factor of 3, perhaps reflecting the risks of pregnancy and childbirth.

It is estimated that management of leg ulceration caused by venous disease costs the NHS in the UK at least £55 000 000 a year.

AETIOLOGY

Oedema from venous hypertension and raised pressure at the venular end of the capillary loop, skin and subcutaneous hypoxia and an episode of minor trauma are the usual pathological antecedents of ulceration. They are

Table 29.11
Causes of ulceration of the leg

Underlying cause	Mechanism
Venous disease	Superficial venous hypertension: hypoxia, oedema, trauma
Arterial disease	Reduced inflow: hypoxia
Trauma	Skin loss, infection, persistent pressure in prolonged bed rest
Rheumatoid arthritis (often with an added arterial or venous component)	Autoimmune inflammation in subcutaneous tissues (vasculitis)
Pyoderma gangrenosum	
Systemic sclerosis	Inflammation of skin and subcutaneous tissues – cause unknown
Malignant disease	Squamous cell carcinoma (usually *de novo* but occasionally associated with long-standing varicose veins and ulceration) Malignant melanoma Basal cell carcinoma
Diabetes mellitus	Neuropathy; possibly an arterial component with skin infarction Lesions more frequent at pressure points – ball of foot and heel
Blood disorders	Microvascular thrombosis in sickle cell disease and spherocytosis

most likely to occur when there is damage to the valves of the deep veins, but long-standing superficial hypertension caused by deep to superficial incompetence alone is also a well recognised cause. Once an ulcer is established, healing of the poorly nourished skin is difficult, and granulation tissue and a fibrous base develops. The build-up of fibrosis with reduced input into the tissue from the arterial side of the circulation is a further impediment to healing. Ulcers may contain a small amount of slough in their base. Secondary infections by skin residents such as staphylococci are common and there is a varying amount of inflammatory change in the surrounding tissues. Spreading cellulitis does occur but is rare.

Other causes of leg ulceration may have to be taken into consideration in an individual patient; these are given in Table 29.11. Venous hypertension is, however, by far the commonest antecedent.

CLINICAL FEATURES

The lesion occurs almost exclusively just above or in relation to the medial malleolus. It is usually approximately oval, flat and without a raised edge, looks relatively healthy and has a granulating base. There is a thin layer of fibrin and weeping eczematous change in the surrounding skin which often arise from the use of inappropriate local applications. The tissues are indurated. There may be scarring in the adjacent paper-thin skin where healing has occurred in the past. Concomitant infection, with either surrounding erythema or extensive cellulitis, may be present.

A venous ulcer is recognised easily when it is situated in the typical position close to the medial malleolus, surrounded by pigmentation and oedema. However, venous ulcers also occur on the lateral side of the leg and on the foot, principally the dorsal surface. The circumferential size of the lesion does not indicate its cause and venous ulcers may be multiple.

DIAGNOSIS

An exact diagnosis must precede management. Apart from the obvious distinctions that have to be made from the conditions shown in Table 29.11, that between a venous and a predominantly or exclusively ischaemic ulcer is vital because the treatment is so different. The features that permit this are shown in Table 29.12.

Table 29.12
Distinctive characteristics of venous and arterial ulcers

	Venous	Arterial
History	Previous deep vein thrombosis; varicose veins	Intermittent claudication; ischaemic heart disease; hypertension; diabetes
Pain	Occurs only in severe oedema, secondary bacterial infection, thrombosis, varicose veins	Nearly always present; worse at night; relieved by dependency
Site	Usually near medial malleolus but do occur on lateral side of leg	Common on toes, heel, foot and lateral aspect
Size/ development	Variable but increases slowly if untreated	Variable but increases rapidly
Oedema	Common and worse at end of day	Uncommon unless the leg is dependent and patient immobile
Skin appearance	Pigmentation and atrophy; white patches; induration of subcutaneous tissues	Shiny, thin, atrophic nails
Skin temperature	Usually warm	Cool
Skin colour	Normal or slight cyanosis	Pallor made worse by elevation and slow to recover; cyanotic on dependency
Appearance of ulcer	Shallow flat margin; looks healthy; no deep invasion	Often involves deep fascia and fascia; tendon may be exposed
Foot pulses	Present, although can be difficult to feel because of oedema	Reduced or absent

Awareness of the association of ulceration with diabetes mellitus is well understood, but the relation with rheumatoid arthritis, systemic sclerosis (scleroderma) and other generalised diseases is less well recognised. The more elderly the patient, the more likely there are to be multiple aetiological factors.

It is rare in hospital practice to see an ulcer which has not been 'treated' for some considerable period of time elsewhere often without adequate determination of the cause – particularly the nature of the venous component.

MANAGEMENT

Most venous ulcers which are correctly diagnosed and treated early respond readily to conventional treatment, but even relatively small lesions can take up to 3 months to heal. More chronic lesions – the result of inappropriate or inadequate initial assessment and treatment – require a more precise regimen, as follows.

Step 1 is to establish if there is correctable superficial venous hypertension which is the consequence of deep to superficial incompetence only. If this is so, surgery as described above is indicated, although it is highly desirable to heal the ulcer first using the methods described below.

Step 2. If there are multiple points of incompetence or, what almost always amounts pathophysiologically to the same thing, deep venous damage, the starting point is non-operative management. The majority of venous leg ulcers fall into this category. The essential component is to apply effective compression to the limb and sustain it until the ulcer has healed. All venous ulcers heal if the patient is confined to bed with the foot elevated above the heart so that venous hypertension is abolished, the microenvironment improved and healing promoted. However, bed rest is a costly and therefore usually inappropriate method. Adequate local compression in a patient who is otherwise mobile is an effective alternative. The level physiologically appropriate is too high to be tolerable; however, compression of 25–30 mmHg at the ankle, falling to between 15 and 20 mmHg at the knee, is therapeutically adequate. It can be achieved by:

- Bandaging – usually multilayer and dependent on the skill of the nurse or doctor who applies it
- Shaped elasticated support (Tubigrip) – a single layer will produce compression of between 10 and 11 mmHg at the ankle and this can be doubled or tripled by applying either a second or third layer
- Fitted elastic hosiery with known compression – more expensive but does not require great expertise to apply.

Step 3, which runs concurrently with steps 1 and 2, is local management of the lesion. The inappropriate use of topical agents, including impregnated bandages, prescribed by either a physician or a nurse should be avoided. Dressings are kept simple, and pharmacologically active substances applied only for specific and logical reasons – which means hardly ever. If the underlying causes are treated, then bland dressings are all that is required (see also Ch. 3). In particular, antibiotics are not appropriate; all leg ulcers are contaminated with bacteria and most will yield a positive culture which frequently shows multiple organisms. Systemic therapy is indicated only if there is spreading cellulitis; topical applications are ineffective in controlling contamination unless the causes of the ulcer are dealt with.

Surgical measures in ulceration

On occasion, severely contaminated long-standing ulcers with infected granulation tissue at the base may benefit from surgical debridement (Ch. 3) before non-operative treatment is begun. Once other measures have been undertaken, but there is still an extensive area of skin loss, grafting may be considered to accelerate closure. Either split-skin or pinch grafts (Ch. 38) are used.

Surgery to varicosities

Once an ulcer is healed, surgical attention may need to turn to whether or not the venous hypertension can be corrected so as to prevent recurrence. The circumstance in which this may be possible has already been indicated – correctable deep to superficial valvular incompetence without incompetence in the valves of the deep veins. Whether or not surgery is undertaken, full support of the limb must be continued indefinitely.

Lymphatic disorders

ANATOMICAL AND PHYSIOLOGICAL CONSIDERATIONS

The lymphatic system is comprised of a network of capillaries and vessels lined by endothelial cells. The capillaries allow the absorption of protein-rich interstitial fluid across their walls and the vessels possess valves to prevent lymph reflux. Lymphatic vessels run alongside the venous system but drain directly to lymph nodes where the lymph fluid is filtered through lymphoid tissue. This permits phagocytosis of cellular and bacterial debris. In addition, lymph nodes provide the setting for the immunological response to foreign antigens. The efferent lymphatic vessels eventually drain into the central venous system.

PATHOLOGICAL CONDITIONS

These include lymphadenopathy (node enlargement), lymphangitis and lymphodema.

Lymphadenopathy may occur as the result of local infection or tissue injury, or as a feature of malignancy – either metastatic tumour (e.g. breast cancer, malignant

melanoma) or lymphoma. Node enlargement may be detected on examination or imaging such as ultrasound, CT or MR scanning (see Ch. 4). Open biopsy or fine needle aspiration cytology of an enlarged node should provide a pathological diagnosis when required and allow appropriate treatment, e.g. radiotherapy or cytotoxic chemotherapy for lymphoma. Excision of local and regional nodes with a primary cancer (e.g. breast, colon, stomach) is described as a radical operation, gives prognostic information by staging the tumour and may also improve local control and survival for some cancers (see Ch. 13).

Acute lymphangitis or inflammation of the lymphatic vessels occurs with streptococcal infections when tender red lines may be seen and palpated in the dermis. There is associated regional lymphadenopathy. Penicillin therapy combined with rest and elevation is usually effective.

Lymphoedema

Oedema is excess fluid between cells. *Lymphoedema* is the swelling which results from an increased quantity of fluid in the interstitial space of soft tissues in consequence of failure of function of the lymphatic drainage system.

CLASSIFICATION AND AETIOLOGY

The condition is classed as either primary (disorder of the lymphatic system itself) or secondary (some other condition outside the lymphatic system which interferes with drainage).

Primary lymphoedema

The subject is confused. The following factors are probably of importance:

- A very few patients are born with a hypoplastic lymphatic system, usually in the lower limb (*congenital hereditary lymphoedema.*)
- Obliteration by fibroids of unknown cause may develop at or after puberty.
- Obstruction of a group of lymph nodes (e.g. in the pelvis) may also occur for the same reason.
- Hyperplastic tortuous lymph channels can sometimes be shown at lymphangiography (see below) suggesting another type of congenital disease (often associated with capillary naevi); the defect may be in the valves of the lymphatics.

Primary lymphoedema is six times more common in women than men.

Secondary lymphoedema

In Western countries the causes are:

- Surgical removal of a group of lymph nodes – either in the axilla (mastectomy for breast cancer) or the groin (usually for malignant melanoma less commonly for other malignancies).

- Radiotherapy for malignancy. Usually both factors (surgical removal and radiotherapy) are involved in that it is not common for surgical excision alone to cause lymphoedema in the arm or the leg.
- Malignant invasion of lymphatics and nodes.
- Chronic venous disease may, particularly if infection occurs, cause secondary lymphoedema in addition to the hydrostatic oedema that is present because of raised venous pressure.

In developing and tropical countries intra-lymphatic infection is the commonest cause:

- *Filariasis* caused by the worm *Wucheria bancrofti* induces fibrosis in the lymphatics. The incubation period after the initial mosquito bite may be up to 18 months and, therefore, the condition should be borne in mind in those who have returned from tropical to temperate climates.
- Silica particles enter through the skin of those walking barefoot on silica rich soils; lymphatic drainage is interfered with and secondary infection of cuts further damages the partially obstructed lymphatics and nodes.

Functional classification

An alternative approach combines developmental lymphatic abnormalities with an acquired element (probably repeated infection). The lymphoedema that follows is either:

- obliterative from progressive intimal thickening
- obstructive from developmental abnormalities in proximal nodes and possible fibrotic replacement
- valvular from the presence of incompetence.

PATHOPHYSIOLOGICAL AND PATHOLOGICAL FEATURES

The interstitial space contains not only water and electrolytes but also proteins (mostly albumin), other large molecules, cellular debris and sometimes bacteria. Most of the water and electrolyte are reabsorbed at the venular end of the capillary loop. The rest enter the lymphatics and pass to the nodes and thence to the thoracic duct; in consequence, if lymph flow is obstructed, there is an increase in their concentration in the interstitial space. This stagnant fluid may:

- be invaded by granulations and become organised into fibrous tissue
- provide an ideal culture medium for pathogenic bacteria and so cause recurrent episodes of cellulitis which further aggravates interstitial fibrosis and destruction of lymph channels.

CLINICAL FEATURES

Although either primary or secondary lymphoedema may occur in any part of the body drained by lymphatics, the common clinical presentation is in the limbs — chiefly the lower — and the description that follows relates mainly to this. However, many of the principles apply elsewhere.

Primary lymphoedema

Symptoms

There is often a family history, particularly on the female side, though this may be confused with one of venous disease. The most typical presentation is a teenage girl with the insidious and apparently spontaneous onset of unilateral swelling of the dorsum of the foot and the ankle. At first the swelling is most obvious in warmer weather and tends to disappear with a night's rest but once it has been present for some time it fails completely to resolve. Pain is usually absent but discomfort is associated with heaviness as the swelling increases. Oedema gradually becomes more marked and frequently ascends into the calf and from the dorsum of the foot forward to the toes. Onset in older patients is often similar and may occur at a more proximal level in the limb, for example the thigh without foot and calf swelling. The skin remains healthy for many years and, in contrast to venous disease, complaints of pigmentation and ulceration are rare unless they develop because of recurrent cellulitis.

Signs

In half at initial presentation the oedema is unilateral but, if bilateral, one limb frequently shows more advanced changes. The early oedema principally accumulates on the dorsum of the foot and initially *pits* on pressure.

Even at a late stage there is frequently an element of removable fluid even though fibrosis may also have taken place. With more extensive oedema, this is uniformly distributed from the calf down into the toes. The skin is nearly always intact but may show visible and palpable thickening.

Secondary lymphoedema

Symptoms

There may be a history suggestive of the underlying cause and the onset of oedema may be closely related to this. Rapidity of onset may more closely mimic an acute venous thrombosis with which secondary lymphoedema may occasionally co-exist. Episodes of infection are more common in secondary disease.

Signs

The clinical appearances are similar to those of primary lymphoedema. When chronic venous disease is the cause, the features of venous hypertension may be apparent.

INVESTIGATION

The diagnosis is not usually in doubt but distinction of primary from secondary lymphoedema and, in both, detection of a cause may require further investigation.

Distinction between lymphoedema and venous disease

Ultrasonography excludes disease of the deep veins.

Distinction between obliterative and obstructive disease

A bolus injection of technetium-labelled rhenium/sulphur colloid into the web space of the foot produces slow clearance from the tissue and minimal uptake of isotope in the draining lymph nodes in obliterative disease. A CT scan may also indicate a lack or absence of nodes draining the area involved.

Cause of obstruction

When, on clinical grounds, the cause is thought to be obstructive and the condition is intractable to conservative management, *lymphangiography* is indicated. This combination of circumstances is rare — less than 10% of patients.

MANAGEMENT

Non-operative

- Reduction of oedema — elevation, distal-proximal massage, mechanical compression devices (Lymphopress™).
- Continuous support with compression garments such as elastic stockings.
- Prophylaxis of infection — control of fungal infection and good skin hygiene.

Constant encouragement and support is often required as patients consider that non-operative management implies that 'nothing can be done for me'.

Surgical

There is no current treatment that will reliably restore function to the lymphatic system.

Anastomotic and bridging procedures

- Improvement of lymphatic drainage in obstructive lymphoedema — microvascular anastomosis between lymphatics and veins.
- Provision of lymphatic *bridges* by anastomosis of an isolated loop of ileum without its mucosa to a lymph node just distal to an obstruction.

Debulking operations

- Removal of the skin and thickened subcutaneous tissue with free split-skin grafting of the raw area.
- Removal of much of the involved tissue with a dermal flap buried beneath the deep fascia which it

is hoped would provide new lymphatic pathways for drainage.
- Liposuction.

Symtomatic relief and cosmetic improvement may come from any of the above procedures. Selection is difficult and the operations are technically difficult. Liposuction is the least invasive.

....

Bacterial cellulitis as a complication of lymphoedema

The condition is both a complication of lymphoedema and a cause of secondary forms. It is common and frequently mis-diagnosed.

AETIOLOGY

Organisms, usually beta-haemolytic streptococci though occasionally a synergistic combination, gain entry either through an apparently inconsequential injury or an insect bite. More commonly, there is a history of chronic fungal infection in the web spaces of digits.

PATHOLOGICAL FEATURES

The condition is usually a self-limiting subcutaneous cellulitis but necrosis of skin or fascia can occur.

CLINICAL FEATURES

Symptoms

The onset is usually with an acute influenza-like illness, shivering and occasional rigors. Later, progressive swelling and erythema develop and spread with varying degrees of rapidity. If a limb is involved it is acutely painful.

Signs

The area involved is hot, red and tender. Swelling is increased. The regional lymph nodes — if they are present — are also tender.

MANAGEMENT

Early recognition and prompt antibiotic treatment in association with methods designed to reduce the oedema rapidly and enhance lymphatic drainage may reduce the immediate complication of skin necrosis and reduce the likelihood of further obliteration of lymphatics. The most effective initial antibiotic combination is high-dose penicillin 1.2 g four-hourly together with 500 mg of flucloxacillin 4 or 6 hourly. The initial site of entry should be dealt with, e.g. fungal infection in the web space.

Once the acute phase has subsided, oedema may be reduced by a high compression support. Six weeks of oral erythromycin is recommended for prophylaxis.

30

Neurosurgery

Neurosurgeons treat structural and, to a lesser extent, functional lesions of the brain, spinal cord and peripheral nerves. The common disorders treated are shown in Information box 30.1.

Basic clinical principles

Clinical findings

As with all branches of medicine, the fundamental approach in neurosurgery is to take a clear history, carry out a detailed examination and establish a differential diagnosis. Investigation then distinguishes between the diagnostic alternatives and allows a treatment plan to be drawn up. Taking a history from the patient may be impossible if the level of consciousness is impaired, but a history from relatives, friends and the emergency services may be helpful.

Special investigations

Lumbar puncture (LP)

Withdrawal of cerebrospinal fluid by tapping the subarachnoid space in the lumbar regions is used to diagnose subarachnoid haemorrhage (uniform blood

---

Information Box 30.1

Disorders treated by neurosurgeons
- Congenital abnormalities
- Trauma
- Tumours of the brain and spinal cord
- Cerebral haemorrhage
- Hydrocephalus
- Spinal degenerative disease
- Peripheral nerve entrapment
- Infections of the brain and spinal cord and their coverings
- Pain
- Movement disorders

485

staining and xanthochromia) and meningitis (pus cells and bacteria). LP must not be performed in the presence of any of the following:

- a history suggesting that intracranial pressure is raised
- impaired consciousness
- focal neurological signs
- papilloedema.

Computed tomography (CT)

This technique has revolutionised diagnostic neurology since its introduction in the mid-1970s (see Ch. 3). It allows imaging of brain, skull bones, soft tissues and spine and has become the first line of investigation for many conditions treated by neurosurgeons.

Magnetic resonance imaging (MRI)

The principles behind this technique are outlined in Chapter 3. The images are more detailed than CT but take a little longer to produce and patients need to remain very still thorughout the procedure. General anaesthesia may be needed in children and uncooperative adults.

Angiography

Contrast medium is injected into the cerebral or spinal arteries to see and delineate aneurysms and arteriovenous anomalies. The blood supply of a tumour can also be visualised.

Electrophysiology

The electroencephalogram (EEG) may be useful in the investigation of epilepsy. Nerve conduction studies are important in the diagnosis of peripheral nerve lesions.

Management of the unconscious patient

A patient in coma requires measures to save life and prevent deterioration before a precise diagnosis is made and definitive treatment undertaken. Whatever the cause of coma, management is along the following lines:

- establish and maintain a clear airway
- ensure adequate oxygenation, if necessary intubating the trachea and using artificial ventilation
- make sure the patient is fully resuscitated and has a normal blood pressure and good urine output which achieve adequate cerebral perfusion
- exclude metabolic causes of coma, especially hypo- or hyperglycaemia.

Once these objectives have been achieved, a diagnosis is made as soon as possible. Throughout it is necessary to pay attention to pressure areas, the state of

---

Box 30.1

The Glasgow Coma Scale

Event	Score
Eye opening occurs	
Spontaneously	4
In response to speech	3
On pain stimulation	2
Does not occur	1
Verbal response	
Alert and orientated	5
Confused	4
Inappropriate	3
Incomprehensible	2
Does not take place	1
Best motor response	
Commands are obeyed	6
Localises to pain	5
Withdraws to pain	4
Abnormal flexion to pain	3
Extension to pain	2
Not response to pain	1

---

the lungs, eyes, bladder and bowel function, general hygiene and nutrition.

Assessment of the level of consciousness

The Glasgow Coma Scale (see Box 30.1) is now universally used. It consists of three components which deteriorate as coma deepens.:

- the stimulus to produce eye opening.
- the patient's verbal response.
- the best motor response.

The score for each component is recorded and the total for the patient obtained. A fully conscious patient scores 15 points while one who is completely unresponsive scores 3. Coma is considered to be 8 points or less. Changes can be easily noted on a chart and the scale is simple enough to be reproduced accurately by all grades of nurses and doctors.

Congenital anomalies

With better intrauterine diagnosis, congenital anomalies of the central nervous system can be detected early in pregnancy. If the anomaly is untreatable and severe, a termination can be offered. Alternatively, if it is remediable, the need for early post-delivery or even pre-delivery treatment can be anticipated and arranged.

Spinal dysraphism

This is the general term for anomalies of fusion of the neural tube. It encompasses a range of conditions from asymptomatic spina bifida occulta to open myelo-meningoceles. In the latter, a baby may be paraplegic with no potential for sphincter control. If CSF is leaking through the defect, death from meningitis will usually occur; closure of the defect ensures survival but will not usually improve the neurological deficit, and the baby and its parents will have to deal with severe handicap for the rest of their lives. Difficult decisions about whether to treat these babies have to be taken in emotional circumstances bearing in mind the long-term consequences.

Milder forms of dysraphism occur with less or no neurological deficit. They include meningoceles, lipomas, sinuses and tethering of the cord. Some are able to be corrected surgically at an early age.

Encephaloceles

In this condition, fusion of the neural tube fails at the cranial end. Meninges and brain herniate through defects in the skull, most commonly in the occipital region and the frontonasal areas. They are surgically corrected at an early age.

Craniosynostosis

Premature fusion of one or more cranial sutures occurs. Single suture involvement is more common and causes excessive compensatory growth perpendicular to the fused suture. Thus children with sagittal suture fusion have elongated heads (scaphycephaly). More complex suture fusion can lead to craniofacial abnormalities which require a multidisciplinary approach to their correction. Brain growth is the main stimulus for the growth and shaping of the head and therefore any corrective surgery should be done within the first 2 years of life while the brain is still growing.

Trauma

Head injury is common, and spinal injury is about 1/10th as common as that to the head. Most head injury is trivial but there is a small group who develop potentially fatal complications which must be recognised and treated promptly. Many severe head injuries are hopeless from the moment they are sustained, but prompt and diligent care of some of these can lead to worthwhile recovery.

PATHOLOGICAL SEQUENCE AND PATHOPHYSIOLOGY

At impact, the brain is moved around within the skull, the movement being a combination of flexion, extension and rotation. This tears neurones and blood vessels within the brain substance, the degree of damage being proportional to the velocity of impact.

Thus low-velocity injuries such as a kick in the head will cause minor damage leading to a transient loss of consciousness or none at all and full recovery. The patient is said to be concussed. A higher velocity impact such as might occur in a road traffic accident causes more damage and can lead to prolonged coma, poor recovery and even death. In both cases, the mechanism of primary damage is the same, the only difference being the degree. Nothing can be done to reverse primary damage except to support the patient and hope for recovery.

A brain damaged by primary impact can be further damaged by secondary effects. These can be anticipated, prevented and sometimes reversed, but if unrecognised can turn a potential full recovery into a fatal result. The secondary effects are discussed below:

Respiration. Any interference with respiration leads to cerebral hypoxia, so causing further cerebral damage. The causes are airway obstruction, central respiratory depression and chest injury.

Perfusion. Failure of cerebral perfusion leads rapidly to cerebral hypoxia. A systolic blood pressure below 60 mmHg after head injury is rarely compatible with survival. Low blood pressure is rarely the outcome of the head injury and more often it is caused by some other injury such as a ruptured spleen which should be sought and corrected.

Blood clots (haematomas) within the brain substance, subdural space or extradural space cause cerebral compression. With intracerebral and subdural haematomas, there is usually associated primary damage, and cerebral compression is rapid with a poor prognosis. Extradural haematomas usually occur with minimal primary damage and slowly accumulate. Cerebral compression from an extradural haematoma (usually haemorrhage from the middle meningeal artery) leads to raised intracranial pressure with:

- progressive coma
- ipsilateral third nerve palsy
- contralateral hemiparesis.

Further compression leads to bilaterally fixed and dilated pupils, while the terminal stage of compression, coning (downward displacement of the brain stem into the foramen magnum), is associated with hypertension, bradycardia, respiratory arrest and finally cardiac arrest. Intervention at the stage of deteriorating conscious state can lead to a rapid full recovery but this is rare after coning has taken place.

Swelling. Primary and secondary damage cause brain swelling either by hyperaemia or an increase in extracellular fluid. Because the brain is enclosed in a rigid box, the increase in brain volume raises intracranial pressure. Cerebral perfusion pressure falls which leads to ischaemia, causing further brain swelling. A vicious circle develops, the degree of swelling usually reflecting the amount of primary damage.

Infection. The usual cause is a skull fracture with tearing of the meninges and a leak of CSF through an open wound or into an air sinus or the middle ear. There is meningitis or brain abscess, which can be disastrous. The presence of a leak is an indication for prophylactic antimicrobial chemotherapy.

Epilepsy. The brain uses glucose and oxygen abundantly when a fit is taking place and ischaemia develops rapidly if fits are not controlled.

CLINICAL TYPES OF HEAD INJURY

In the light of the pathological and pathophysiological features given above, there are only four fundamental types of head injury:

- *Trivial* – minimal or absent primary or secondary injury
- *Apparently trivial but potentially serious* – minimal or no primary injury but potentially serious secondary effects, e.g. extradural haematoma
- *Hopeless* – overwhelming primary injury
- *Apparently hopeless but potentially salvageable* – serious but survivable primary injury provided there is good care and secondary effects are minimalised.

When a patient speaks – even simple words – after head injury, the primary impact cannot have been severe and any deterioration is the consequence of secondary effects.

MANAGEMENT

Trivial injury

Aim

The aim is to identify and admit those who are at risk of developing secondary complications, especially haematomas. After taking a history and making an examination, the questions to be asked are:

- Should the patient have a skull X-ray?
- Should the patient be admitted?
- Should the patient be referred to a neurosurgeon?

Indications

For skull X-ray
- Loss of consciousness or amnesia
- Focal neurological signs
- Suspected CSF Leak or blood at the nostril or ear
- Suspected or obvious penetrating wound.
- Difficulty in assessing the patient, e.g. intoxication, after a fit and children.

For admission
- Focal neurological signs
- Skull fracture
- Depressed level of consciousness
- CSF leak, depressed fracture, penetrating wound
- Social circumstances.

For neurosurgical referral
- Deterioration
- Drowsiness in a patient with a skull fracture – this combination has a 1 in 4 chance of a significant clot being present and referral should be made before further deterioration takes place
- Depressed fracture/CSF leak
- Penetrating wound
- Failure to improve after 12–24 hours.

Patients who are admitted should be allowed to drink normally or an intravenous infusion should be started if they are vomiting or drowsy. They must not be allowed to become dehydrated. Regular observation is required and any fits controlled rapidly. Referral must be made at the earliest sign of a complication rather than waiting for deterioration to take place.

Most patients will be well enough to go home within 24–48 hours. They must be warned that even after mild head injury they may suffer headaches, dizziness and loss of concentration for a number of weeks. Reassurance is all that can be offered for this 'post-concussion syndrome'.

Severe injury

These patients will be brought to the accident and emergency department unconscious and often with other injuries. Management is along the following lines:

- Immediate intubation and ventilation. Fears of intubating a patient with an unstable spine and of masking physical signs by using sedatives/ paralysing agents are not valid. Unstable neck fractures are uncommon and patients will have a CT scan.
- Resuscitate.
- Examine thoroughly.
- X-ray – skull, spine, chest, pelvis and any obvious bony injuries.
- Plan treatment based on the injuries – the control of bleeding takes priority; if a laparotomy or thoracotomy is considered it should be done before the patient is transferred to a neurosurgical centre.

At the neurosurgical centre, treatment is along the following lines:

- In a stable patient, do a CT (Fig. 30.1).
- A haematoma is removed by craniotomy.
- Admit to the intensive care unit for a planned period of ventilation (e.g. 48 hours) to ensure

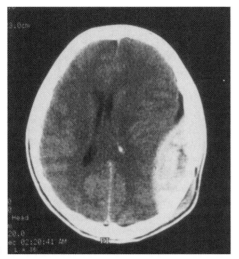
(a)

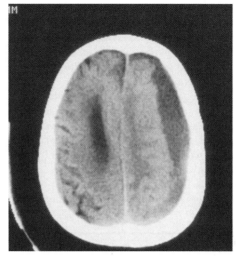
(b)

Fig 30.1 **CT scans (a)** Left extradural haematoma obliterating the ventricle and shifting the midline to the right. **(b)** Left chronic subdural haematoma.

oxygenation; hyperventilation may reduce intracranial pressure from brain swelling.

● Measure intracranial pressure using transducers in the ventricles, extradural or subdural spaces – if it is elevated, and there is not a haematoma, reduction is attempted by using ventilation, mannitol and sedation; steroids are of no value.

● Undertake intensive nursing care and physiotherapy.

OUTCOME AFTER HEAD INJURY

Other than the post-concussion syndrome, trivial injury rarely has any sequelae. Table 30.1 shows the outcome for those in coma on admission to hospital.

Moderately disabled patients usually have poor memory, personality changes, physical disability, epilepsy and depression either alone or in combination. Families may be wrecked by the difficulties of caring for these people and, other than self-help groups (e.g. Headway), there is often little assistance available.

Intensive rehabilitation with physiotherapy, speech therapy, occupational therapy and psychological help started soon after injury may reduce the difficulties and improve outcome but such resources are in short supply.

Table 30.1
Outcome in head injury with coma on admission

Status	Percentage of patients
Complete recovery	30%
Some disablement but able to look after themselves	20%
Severe disablement; vegetative state or unable to care for themselves	10%
Death	40%

Spinal injury

PATHOLOGICAL FEATURES AND PATHOPHYSIOLOGY

These are the same as those of head injury in that neurones suffer primary damage on impact and then are prone to the same secondary injuries from hypoxia, hypotension, haematoma and swelling. However, primary injury is the overwhelming problem and, when there is severe damage, spinal cord function at and below the level of the lesion is abolished. Thus a thoracic cord injury leads to paraplegia and cervical cord injury involves the upper limbs as well as the legs. Lesions above C5 cause complete tetraplegia, while lesions at C3 or above lead to respiratory paralysis and death unless early ventilation is undertaken.

As well as injury to the spinal cord, there may be damage to the vertebral column, usually fractures or fracture-dislocation. Spinal cord injury may occur without bony injury, and vice versa, but the two commonly coexist.

MANAGEMENT

The same principles of management as those for head injury apply: maintain oxygenation and perfusion pressure, remove compressing lesions (haematomas, bone fragments and acute disc prolapses) and reduce swelling. In addition, there are two fundamental questions which must be answered:

● Is the vertebral column stable?
● Is the spinal cord lesion complete or incomplete?

Until proven otherwise it must be assumed the vertebral column is unstable. Careful handling is required and the use of appliances such as spinal immobilising stretchers, cervical collars and traction should be considered. If spinal instability is present, it must be fixed using traction, bracing or internal fixation as appropriate.

Complete spinal cord injury is suspected when there is abolition of all spinal cord function below the level of the lesion. A flaccid paralysis with no sensation indicates a complete lesion with a poor prognosis for recovery, while preservation of any function, the sacral fibres being most resistant to damage, is a cause for cautious optimism.

Rehabilitation must begin early both to maximise recovery and to retrain the patient who will not recover. In contrast to head injury there are a large number of well established spinal injury units and, as a result of their work, fulfilling lives can be had despite severe handicap.

Tumours of the brain, meninges and spinal cord

The commonest brain tumour is metastatic cancer but they rarely present to neurosurgeons except when the diagnosis is unknown or a solitary slow growing metastasis is present.

Pathological types of primary brain tumour and their place of origin within the body are given in Table 30.2.

Gliomas

These tumours arise from the supporting tissues of the brain and their names reflects this: astrocytoma from the astrocyte; oligodendrocytoma from the oligodendrocyte; and ependymoma from ependyma. Their degree of malignancy is reflected in their cellular grading which considers features such as:

• cellularity
• mitoses
• pleomorphism
• necrosis.

Grade 1 tumours are slow-growing and may be benign in behaviour, while grade 4 tumours are aggressive and survival beyond 1 year is unlikely. Grades 2 and 3 are intermediate in prognosis.

Table 30.2
Tumours of the central nervous system

Tumour	Origin
Glioma	Supporting tissues
Meningiomas	Covering layers
Neuromas	Nervous tissues
Pituitary	Endocrine cells of anterior pituitary
Developmental	Abnormal islands of cells at points of closure of neural tube. Persistent primitive cells

Meningiomas

These tumours arise from the meninges and are usually benign although occasionally they may show malignant behaviour. Complete removal is rarely followed by recurrence.

Occasionally, multiple meningiomas occur and a meningioma may cause death because of its vital and inoperable position, e.g. a clivus meningioma which arises anterior to the brain stem between the foramen magnum and pituitary fossa.

Neuromas

The commonest of these is the acoustic neuroma which develops from the eighth nerve. They are usually benign.

Pituitary tumours

These tumours may be either endocrinologically active or inactive and present with hormonal dysfunction or by visual disturbance caused by upward growth of the tumour compressing the optic nerves in the region of the chiasma.

Developmental tumours

Craniopharyngioma, colloid cyst of the third ventricle, medulloblastoma and choroid plexus papilloma are the commonest of a large number of developmentally related tumours. The degree of malignancy varies.

In adults, these growths occur more commonly in the cerebral hemispheres; in children, posterior fossa tumours are commoner.

CLINICAL FEATURES

Except in very rare cases where tumours are found incidentally, e.g. on a CT scan done for head injury or stroke, they present in one of three ways:

• Raised intracranial pressure with headache that is worse in the morning and on straining. This is associated with papilloedema. Untreated raised ICP leads to coma and death.
• Fits. Late onset epilepsy needs investigation.
• Neurological deficit – this depends on the site of the tumour; rapid development of deficit often signifies malignancy whereas slow development usually means a benign tumour.

DIAGNOSIS

Once a tumour is suspected, the diagnosis is made by CT or MRI scanning.

MANAGEMENT

Benign tumours

If the tumour is obviously benign it is usually removed via a craniotomy. Should complete excision not be technically possible, as much of the tumour as can safely be removed is undertaken.

Malignant tumours

If the tumour appears to be malignant, there are a number of options:

- Craniotomy and removal of as much as possible; such treatment may be followed by no further action or by radiotherapy and/or chemotherapy
- Biopsy of the lesion unequivocally to establish the diagnosis and either do no more or use radiotherapy and/or chemotherapy of an incompletely removed lesion
- Undertake 'blind' radiotherapy/chemotherapy
- Do nothing.

For grade 4 tumours, the outlook is poor irrespective of the type of management. Depending on the site of the tumour, age and health of the patient and the surgeon's philosophy, any of the above options may be applied. It is the author's policy to always establish a tissue diagnosis, as cerebral abscess can occasionally mimic a tumour.

Cerebral haemorrhage

This is defined as spontaneous bleeding within the cranial cavity. Sites of haemorrhage are:

- within the brain substance (intracerebral haemorrhage)
- in the subarachnoid space (subarachnoid haemorrhage)
- in the subdural space (subdural haemorrhage).

Intracerebral haemorrhage

This occurs most often deep within the cerebral substance and is usually associated with hypertension or an underlying arterial anomaly such as an arteriovenous malformation or an aneurysm. Rarely, it may be the consequence of bleeding into a tumour or of a clotting defect.

CLINICAL FEATURES

The features are sudden onset of headache, neurological deficit and possibly coma.

MANAGEMENT

Removal of the haematoma is rarely of value; if the patient is in coma, taking out the clot rarely improves the clinical state. If the patient is alert with a deficit such as a hemiplegia, recovery is likely and will not usually be influenced by clot removal. Those patients

who are alert on presentation but who become gradually drowsier because of the size of the clot are most helped by clot removal. Cerebellar haematomas should be removed at an early stage as deterioration because of swelling within the closed posterior fossa is common.

Subarachnoid haemorrhage (SAH)

Bleeding into the subarachnoid space is caused by:

- ruptured aneurysm in 70%
- arteriovenous malformation (AVM) in 10%
- unknown cause in 20%.

CLINICAL FEATURES

There is sudden death in 40%. Headache and neck stiffness of sudden onset followed by drowsiness and coma are characteristic of the remainder.

PROGNOSIS

Thirty per cent of those who survive the initial episode die within the next 6 weeks from one of the following:

- failure to recover from the initial haemorrhage
- re-bleeding.
- cerebral ischaemia which is the result of arterial spasm 3–5 days after the haemorrhage.

However, ischaemia may be mild and without clinical effects, although if severe it is associated with hemiplegia and persistent coma.

MANAGEMENT

Establish the diagnosis by
- CT scan if this is available
- lumbar puncture if CT is not available or negative: the CSF is uniformly bloodstained and there is xanthochromia.

Bed rest. It is not necessary to nurse the patient flat as was once traditional.

Supportive care. Intravenous fluids, nimodipine (a calcium channel blocking agent) to reduce cerebral ischaemia and analgesia form the basis of supportive care.

Further investigation. If the patient is alert and has a minimal neurological deficit, cerebral angiography should be performed as soon as possible to establish the cause. Should an aneurysm be found, an operation may be done to exclude it from the circulation by placing a small metal clip across its neck without occluding the parent artery. Alternatively, the aneurysm may be occluded with platinum coils by endovascular techniques. An AVM, if superficial and in a suitable position, can be surgically excised. However, if deep or in an area of vital function, it can be treated by embolisation or stereotactically focused radiotherapy.

Subdural haematoma

PATHOGENESIS

Acute subdural bleeding is associated with trauma. Chronic subdural bleeding (SDH) is common in conditions of cerebral atrophy, notably old age and alcoholism. Minor trauma leads to a little insignificant bleeding in the subdural space. As this blood breaks down over the next few weeks or months, fluid is drawn into the subdural space because the breakdown products are hyperosmolal and a membrane forms. The collection gradually enlarges and compresses the brain, mimicking a tumour. Subdural haemorrhage in infants should always raise suspicion of non-accidental injury.

DIAGNOSIS AND TREATMENT

Diagnosis of a subdural haematoma is by CT scan.

Treatment is to let the fluid out of the subdural space via burr holes and to wash out the space.

Hydrocephalus

This condition is defined as enlargement of the normal cerebrospinal fluid (CSF) spaces.

PHYSIOLOGY

CSF is made by ultrafiltration through the choroid plexus mostly in the lateral ventricles. It passes via the foramen of Munro to the third ventricle and through the aqueduct to the fourth ventricle. It then leaves the ventricular system and passes into the subarachnoid space through the foramina of Luschka and Majendie and is reabsorbed into the bloodstream through the arachnoid granulations over the surface of the hemispheres (Fig. 30.2).

TYPES AND CAUSES

Communicating

In this type, CSF can reach the subarachnoid space but is not absorbed. Causes are anything that interferes with reabsorption by action on the arachnoid granulations, e.g.:

- subarachnoid haemorrhage
- head injury
- meningitis.

Non-communicating

Blockage prevents CSF reaching the subarachnoid space. Causes are:

- intraventricular haemorrhage
- congenital anomalies (Dandy–Walker cyst – aqueductal stenosis)
- tumours.

Overproduction of CSF

This is a rare condition that results from a papilloma of the choroid plexus.

CLINICAL FEATURES

Presentation depends on the age of the patient and the cause.

Infants
- Failure to thrive
- Enlarging head
- tense fontanelle
- Failure of upgaze (setting sun sign).

Adults
- Typical features of raised intracranial pressure
- Associated clinical signs of the cause – coma after head injury, subarachnoid haemorrhage or meningitis.

Elderly patients
A normal pressure hydrocephalus may occur in old age, which presents with:
- Confusion
- Ataxia
- Incontinence.

DIAGNOSIS AND MANAGEMENT

A CT or MRI will show the enlarged ventricles and may reveal a cause. In communicating hydrocephalus, lumbar puncture is safe, pressure can be measured and the effect of removing CSF can be assessed.

The principle of management is to drain off the excess CSF. Temporary drainage can be achieved by intermittent ventricular tap in infants or by continuous ventricular drainage. Permanent drainage is achieved by inserting a shunt, a silicon tube with a one way

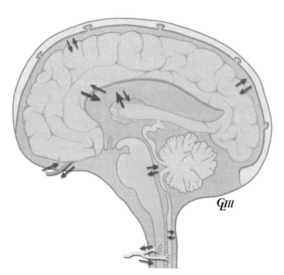

Fig 30.2 **The circulation of the CSF.**

valve of varying pressure ranges, between the ventricles and the peritoneum or the right atrium. Non-communicating hydrocephalus may be treated endoscopically.

Spinal degenerative disease

Degenerative disorders of the spinal skeleton are very common and make up a great deal of the workload of the neurosurgeon (both orthopaedic and neurosurgeons share this load). They affect the lumbar, cervical and thoracic regions in descending order of frequency.

Lumbar degenerative disease
Acute disc prolapse

This causes acute back pain of sudden onset radiating down the leg which is made worse by coughing or straining. Leg pain is often described as sciatica, but its distribution and other symptoms are dependent on the level of disc prolapse:

- Compression of the S1 root – pain down the back of the leg to the sole of the foot
- compression of the L4 root – pain on the inner aspect of the leg, weakness of ankle dorsiflexion and diminished ankle reflex
- compression of the L5 root – pain down the outside of the leg to the big toe and weakness of dorsiflexion of that digit.

INITIAL MANAGEMENT
Non-operative
Bed rest with adequate analgesia and muscle relaxants. Failure to improve or the development of a foot drop are indications for investigation by imaging with a view to surgery. MRI is the method of choice.

Surgery
Surgical options are to remove the prolapsed disc by open operation or to dissolve it by injecting the enzyme chymopapain. The latter is not widely popular.

Compression of the cauda equina

Occasionally a large central disc prolapse, usually at L5/S1, compresses the cauda equina and causes:

- back pain
- bilateral sciatica
- urinary retention.

Decompression must take place urgently to prevent permanent sphincter disturbance.

Lumbar canal stenosis

With increasing age and wear and tear on the spine, there is a general narrowing of the spinal canal by bony overgrowth and ligamentous hypertrophy. This gradually interferes with the blood supply to the cauda equina, leading to spinal claudication.

CLINICAL FEATURES
The patient develops numbness and weakness of the legs on walking, sometimes less than 100 metres. After a rest the symptoms resolve.

There are usually few physical findings unless the patient is walked beyond the distance where symptoms develop in which case some weakness may be evident.

INVESTIGATION AND MANAGEMENT
CT or MRI scanning will show a narrow spinal canal. Surgical treatment is by decompressive laminectomy.

Cervical degenerative disease

As with lumbar disease, presentation is either with acute disc prolapse or with the more chronic bony distortion (spondylitic type). Whatever the process, because the spinal canal is narrow, the spinal cord is likely to be involved (myelopathy). However, lateral compression of roots can lead to an isolated radiculopathy. Commonly the two coexist, with radiculopathy at the level of the lesion and myelopathy below it.

Myelopathy
CLINICAL FEATURES
An acute central disc prolapse or chronic cord compression from stenosis of the spinal canal can cause cord dysfunction which may be as severe as acute quadriplegia, although fortunately this is rare. Incomplete lesions are more common, usually of the central cord syndrome type with the arms more affected than the legs. The condition should be suspected whenever a patient complains of severe neck pain and has signs of an upper motor neurone lesion (hypertonia, brisk reflexes and an extensor planter response) in the legs, especially after minor trauma.

Chronic stenosis of the canal usually develops more slowly, often initially with numbness in the hands followed by difficulty in walking.

INVESTIGATION AND MANAGEMENT
In contrast to the lumbar spine, plain CT scanning is not of much value. If imaging is required, myelography or MRI scan is used.

MRI is the imaging of choice. When there are cord signs, immediate surgical decompression is indicated. In stenosis of the canal, surgical decompression by laminectomy is mainly to prevent progression, although occasionally reversals of the neurological deficit can occur.

Radiculopathy

CLINICAL FEATURES

An acute lateral disc prolapse or chronic osteophyte development can compress a nerve root in the lateral part of the spinal canal or the exit foramen. Pain occurs in the dermatome of the root (brachalgia) and, if severe, numbness and motor weakness develop. Appropriate reflexes are commonly lost, e.g. the biceps reflex with a C6 lesion, and triceps reflex with C7.

INVESTIGATION AND MANAGEMENT

Acute problems usually settle spontaneously with analgesia and cervical collar, but continuous pain or neurological signs need to be investigated by imaging (as for myelopathy). Surgery involves an anterior approach to the spine to remove the disc or osteophyte.

Thoracic degenerative disease

Thoracic degenerative disease is uncommon, probably because the thoracic spine is less mobile. Thoracic disc prolapses do occur and usually cause a chronic myelopathy. The treatment is surgical removal.

Rheumatoid arthritis

This disease affects the cervical spine as often as other joints, especially at the craniocervical junction. Occipital pain and spastic quadriparesis are typical features of rheumatic necks and may be helped by occipitocervical fusion or removal of the odontoid peg.

Spinal tumours

Spinal tumours are far less common than those in the brain. The anatomical site and the histological appearances are the two main methods of classification (Table 30.3).

CLINICAL PRESENTATION

Extradural
- Pain in the back which is usually non-specific but may be radicular
- Myelopathy.

Table 30.3
Tumours of the spinal cord

Site	Nature	Management
Extradural	Usually metastatic	Radiotherapy Surgery to prevent paralysis
Intradural extramedullary	Meningioma Neurofibroma	Surgical removal
Intradural intramedullary	Astrocytomas, ependymomas Cysts	Surgical decompression Radiotherapy

Intradural extramedullary
- Root pain
- myelopathy in late cases.

Intradural intramedullary
- Slow onset of central cord syndrome – clinical characteristics of lower motor neurone signs in the arms and upper motor neurone signs in the legs
- Detection by MRI.

MANAGEMENT

The management outlined in Table 30.3.

Peripheral nerve lesions

The common disorders are structural, e.g. trauma and entrapment.

Trauma

Injury may be by traction (e.g. a tear to the root of the brachial plexus when the arm is distracted in relation to the body) or by division in a penetrating wound.

Entrapment

Nerves that pass through bony or fibrous tunnels are affected (e.g. the median nerve in the carpal tunnel at the wrist and the ulnar nerve at the elbow).

CLINICAL FEATURES

Loss of function of lower motor type and anaesthesia follow trauma. Entrapment causes pain and tingling in the distribution of the nerve with muscle wasting if there is motor innervation.

INVESTIGATION AND MANAGEMENT

Further investigation is not required in obvious traumatic division, but a traction injury may require neurophysiological studies to confirm whether or not the injury is complete and therefore unlikely to recover. In entrapment, the symptoms and signs are often imprecise and nerve conduction studies are required for confirmation.

Repair of traumatic division can be primary in a clean wound but is better delayed if there is contamination. Results are variable but are improved by special techniques such as microsurgery. Entrapments are treated by surgical decompression.

Infections

PATHOLOGICAL FEATURES

Similar features occur in the brain and spinal cord. Acute infection is the result of:

- an opening which permits a CSF leak – a penetrating wound or a skull fracture which is compound into an air sinus
- contiguous infection
- metastasis from a source elsewhere in the body.

In most instances, a diffuse infection of the meninges results but an abscess may form within the brain. The latter is the result of:

- infection in the middle ear or air sinuses
- immunosuppression such as HIV infection (Ch. 9)
- an unknown source.

CLINICAL FEATURES

Meningitis
- Fever
- Headache
- Neck rigidity
- Decline in level of consciousness
- Fits.

Brain abscess
- Clinical manifestations as for a cerebral tumour
- Usually a swinging fever
- Spinal tenderness in an abscess within the spinal canal.

TREATMENT

Meningitis is managed with antibiotics, preferably after a bacteriological diagnosis has been made by lumbar puncture.

CSF leakage usually closes spontaneously but surgical management is occasionally required.

Abscess requires urgent drainage and several months of antibiotic therapy. The only exception is a tuberculous abscess which should be treated non-operatively with antibiotics.

Pain

With the development of more effective analgesics, surgery for pain is becoming less common. However, in intractable pain, neurosurgeons can be involved in implanting devices for delivery of analgesics directly to the CSF or epidural space, or in destroying pain tracts by cordotomy or producing lesions in the dorsal root entry zone. The work is specialised and best carried out within the framework of a dedicated pain clinic.

Movement disorders

Surgery can be carried out for movement disorders such as Parkinsonism, psychological disorders and epilepsy. Again these operations need to be carried out in super-specialist units with full support for investigation and treatment of the appropriate disorder.

Common to the treatment of the above conditions as well as to tumour biopsy and accurately aimed radiotherapy is the technique of stereotaxy. The principle is that if you wish to know where a submarine is, you need to know its longitude, latitude and depth. If you want to know where to find a point in the brain, you can fix a frame firmly on the head and undertake a CT or MRI scan. This gives three coordinates – x, y and z – relative to a fixed point on the frame, which are equivalent to longitude, latitude and depth. Needles and electrodes can therefore be placed very accurately into the brain allowing lesions to be made or biopsies to be taken.

FURTHER READING

Crockard A, Hayward R, Hoff J T (eds) (1999) *Neurosurgery: The Scientific Basis of Clinical Practice*. 3rd edn. Oxford: Blackwell Science
Fundamental facts for the career neurosurgeon

Jennett B, Linday K W (1994) *An Introduction to Neurosurgery* 5th edn. Oxford: Butterworth-Heinemann
A good basic overview for the student or house officer

Lindsay K W, Bone I (1997) *Neurology and Neurosurgery Illustrated* 3rd edn. Edinburgh
Slightly more detail than Jennette & Lindsay but also a good basic text for student and house officer

Perkin G D, Hochberg F H, Miller D C (1993) *Atlas of Clinical Neurology* Mosby: London
Clear detailed illustrations relevant to both neurology and neurosurgery

Surgery of the endocrine glands

Principles in endocrine surgery

Although surgeons have operated on the endocrine glands for more than a century, in the last 20–30 years, endocrine surgery has become a subspeciality. The reasons, apart from the technical demands, are that the biochemical and genetic understanding of the place of the endocrines in the body's function has greatly increased and that cooperation between surgeon and the specialist physician has become ever more necessary and productive. Nearly all endocrine disorders that have to be considered for surgical management fall into the following classes:

- neoplasia – either benign or malignant and, if the latter, either primary or secondary
- autoimmune
- genetic – and of varying inheritance.

In addition, disorders may or may not be associated with endocrine dysfunction, which is usually due to hypersecretion either of the hormone normally produced or of one or more of its analogues. Finally, hormones may be produced by tissues (usually neoplastic) which are not normally associated with an endocrine function (e.g. bronchial cancer, Ch. 16) to cause paraendocrine syndromes.

Before individual organs and their disorders are considered, some principles that underlie all surgery on the endocrine glands are outlined.

Diagnosis
A precise diagnosis is essential and has the following characteristics:

- The organ or organs involved; if an organ is paired (e.g. the adrenal) whether one or both are responsible
- Exclusion of a paraendocrine syndrome
- The exact nature of the disorder
  - neoplastic: whether benign or malignant (primary or secondary)
  - autoimmune: the process involved
  - genetic: the mode of inheritance and the influence of this on counselling of both the patient and relatives

- Consideration of the presence of endocrine disorders other than that which causes the patient to present (see 'Multiple endocrine neoplasia' (MEN))
- Secretory status – normal or abnormal and, if the latter, the qualitative and quantitative effects on other organs and systems.

Choice of management

Surgical treatment may not be the only option, and before it is undertaken other methods of management must be considered. Particularly in asymptomatic disorders (e.g. hypercalcaemia thought to be caused by a parathyroid adenoma or hyperplasia), the risks of operation must be balanced against those of progression of the disorder.

Localisation of a tumour

Accurate anatomical localisation is always of help, although in some special circumstances it can be omitted. Localising techniques are of three kinds:

- conventional imaging, including arteriography
- selective uptake of labelled precursors
- sampling of effluent blood from areas in the vicinity of the endocrine gland thought to be affected.

All of these techniques may also identify harmless, non-functioning adenomas which have been called (inelegantly) incidentalomas. The finding of such a lesion does not always confirm the clinical diagnosis of endocrine dysfunction. In addition, the presence of a tumour which has potential serious consequences must not be confused with one that is incidental.

Fitness for surgery

Even if the ultimate treatment is surgical, it is often necessary, by preoperative medical management, to correct any deleterious effects of hormonal dysfunction. An urgent operation for endocrine dysfunction is rarely required.

The thyroid

EMBRYOLOGY

The thyroid gland is derived from an epithelial proliferation in the floor of the pharynx at a point that is later indicated by the foramen caecum at the junction of the anterior two-thirds and the posterior third of the tongue in the midline. The gland migrates downwards in front of the foregut to come to lie anterior to the trachea but, during this movement, remains attached to the floor of the mouth by a narrow canal – the thyroglossal duct – which ultimately disappears. Its persistence results in:

- thyroglossal sinus
- thyroglossal cyst.

SURGICAL ANATOMY

The important matters are:

- Investment by a thick fibrous sheath (pretracheal fascia) which sends septa into the substance of the gland and also binds it to the larynx so that a normal gland rises on swallowing
- A rich blood supply from the paired superior and inferior thyroid arteries (Fig. 31.1) – increase in blood flow occurs in disease such as hyperthyroidism and may make surgical treatment more difficult
- Lymphatic drainage to the middle and lower deep jugular, pretracheal and mediastinal nodes – the first two groups are initially involved in some malignant disorders.
- Proximity of the recurrent laryngeal nerve to the inferior thyroid artery between whose branches it usually passes although this is variable (Fig. 31.1) – injury, with paralysis of the vocal cord on the same side, may occur during operation
- Application of the superior pole of the gland to the anterolateral aspect of the larynx across which passes the external laryngeal nerve to supply the cricopharyngeus (Fig. 31.1) – damage to the nerve interferes with reaching a high note in speech and singing
- The close, though variable, relationship of the parathyroid glands to the posterior aspect of the thyroid – extensive dissection and/or inadvertent removal during surgical operations on the thyroid may cause temporary or permanent hypoparathyroidism
- Pyramidal lobe – a vertical tongue of thyroid tissue of variable size which arises from the isthmus and extends towards the hyoid bone; it is a remnant of the embryological descent of the gland
- Aberrant thyroid tissue – found anywhere along embryological descent of the gland but always in the midline; common sites include the back of the tongue (lingual thyroid) and the anterior mediastinum (retrosternal extension).

Operations on the gland threaten adjacent vital structures and these and the effects of injury are summarised in Table 31.1.

HISTOLOGICAL FEATURES

The thyroid is composed of follicles (acini) which are roughly spherical with a diameter of $30\,\mu m$. Each is lined with epithelial cells which secrete the thyroid hormones that are stored in the colloid of the follicle. The cells are usually cuboidal but become columnar in response to the secretion of pituitary thyroid-stimulating hormone (TSH).

A second group of cells – C cells – between the follicles, manufacture and secrete calcitonin.

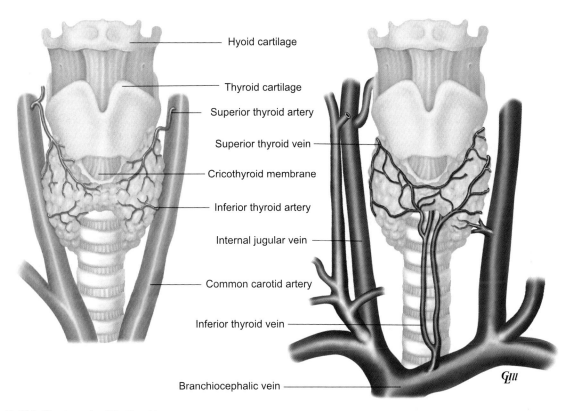

Fig 31.1 **Blood supply of the thyroid.**

Table 31.1
Important structures which must be safeguarded at thyroidectomy

Structure	Result of injury
Recurrent laryngeal nerve	Paresis or paralysis of vocal cord: Unilateral – hoarseness Bilateral – stridor; change in voice; risk of aspiration
Parathyroid glands	Hypocalcaemia – severity depends on amount of tissue that remains
External laryngeal nerve	Paresis or paralysis of cricothyroid muscle – inability to achieve high pitched notes

PHYSIOLOGICAL FEATURES

The gland produces two types of hormones:

- those that regulate metabolic rate – thyroxine and its analogues
- calcitonin, which is concerned with calcium homeostasis.

Thyroxine and its analogues

Iodine is trapped by follicular cells and bound to tyrosine residues on the glycoprotein thyroglobulin. The iodine-containing residues – mono-iodotyrosine (MIT) and di-iodotyrosine (DIT) – are cleaved and coupled to yield tri-iodotyrosine (T_3) and thyroxine (T_4). Both the iodination reaction and the cleavage of MIT and DIT are catalysed by the enzyme thyroid peroxidase, which is membrane-bound and located at the apex of the follicular cell. T_3 and T_4 are bound in the circulation to thyroxine-binding globulin, thyroxine-binding prealbumin and albumin. T_3 is believed to be the biologically active hormone formed predominantly from the peripheral de-iodination of circulating T_4.

The hypothalamic–thyroid axis regulates the production of T_3 and T_4. Thyrotrophin-releasing hormone (TRH) from the hypothalamus promotes the release of thyroid-stimulating hormone (TSH) from the anterior pituitary. TSH binds to its receptor on the follicular cell and stimulates synthesis and release of T_3 and T_4, whose presence in the blood decreases TRH and TSH output.

Thyroid hormones have wide-ranging metabolic and physiological effects, demonstrated by the variety of syndromes observed in both excess production (thyrotoxicosis) and deficiency (myxoedema).

Calcitonin

The hormone acts to decrease the concentration of calcium in the serum by inhibiting osteoclast-directed absorption of bone and by increased renal excretion of calcium.

GENERAL PATHOLOGICAL FEATURES

As described above, the thyroid is a target organ. It is influenced by:

- dietary intake of iodine – inadequate intake may cause hypertrophy (which may be followed by involution) because the gland seeks to extract as much of the element as possible so as to synthesise its hormones
- pituitary TSH
- other hormones – particularly oestrogens
- immune globulins which target the thyroid TSH receptor and may be important in causing thyrotoxicosis
- goitrogens – substances which block the normal pathways of synthesis of thyroid hormones.

In consequence, the gland undergoes cyclical hypertrophy and involution according to the internal environment to which it is exposed. Some pathological changes can follow. Repeated stimulation may result in areas of fibrosis – the gland becomes nodular, although only one nodule may be palpable. Most multinodular goitres are the consequence of this mechanism. Stimulation may be associated with clinical hyperactivity – thyrotoxicosis.

Evaluation of thyroid disease

The commonest symptom in thyroid disorder is goitre – an enlargement of the gland. Goitres vary considerably in size. The World Health Organization (WHO) has designed a simple and convenient system for grading goitres.

In clinical practice, goitres are often subdivided into:

- simple non-toxic
- toxic – associated with hyperthyroidism.

Simple goitre is any enlargement not associated with thyroid dysfunction and which does not result from inflammation or neoplasia. Hypothyroidism (myxoedema) may, however, develop as the end stage of a simple goitre.

CLINICAL FEATURES

History

Apart from presentation with a goitre, there may be other symptoms in the neck or of a change in thyroid hormonal status.

Associated neck symptoms are:

- dysphagia – compression of the oesophagus
- dyspnoea – compression or displacement of the trachea
- hoarse voice – infiltration of the recurrent laryngeal nerve usually by carcinoma
- other lumps – usually lymph nodes.

Table 31.2
Eye features in hyperthyroidism

Symptoms	Signs
Poor sight for both near and distant objects	Ophthalmoplegia
Double vision	
Grittiness in the eye	Conjunctival oedema (chemosis)
Exophthalmus – protrusion of the globes	Exophthalmus
	Lid retraction
	Lid *lag*

Functional state may be:

- euthyroid – a normal level of thyroid function
- hyperthyroid (thyrotoxic) – increased levels of circulating thyroid hormones
- hypothyroid – decreased levels of circulating hormones.

An individual with a goitre may be in any of these three states.

Symptoms related to thyroid hyperactivity are

- subjective – nervousness, irritability, behavioural change
- weight loss – in spite of a good appetite
- diarrhoea
- muscle weakness
- tremor
- intolerance of a hot environment, preference for cold
- loss of libido and, in addition, in women, oligomenorrhoea
- eye complaints (see Table 31.2).

Symptoms of hypothyroidism are:

- slowness, tiredness and malaise
- weight gain, despite poor appetite
- constipation
- depression, psychosis and (rarely) coma
- change in appearance – puffy eyes, dry skin and coarse hair
- poor libido and, in women, menorrhagia or oligomenorrhoea.

Features associated with cause are:

- place of long-term residence – an area of endemic goitre?
- family history – genetic causes
- drugs – antithyroid agents, iodide-containing medicines (asthma) and para-aminosalicylic acid (tuberculosis)
- age – puberty or the menopause
- pregnancy.

Physical findings

If a neck swelling is present and the thyroid is suspected as the cause, the matter can nearly always be decided by asking the patient to swallow: all thyroid swellings move upwards unless the neck is diffusely infiltrated with cancer.

Clinical features of thyrotoxicosis are:

- anxiety
- excessive purposeless movements
- diffuse fine tremor – best elicited in the outstretched fingers.
- signs of recent weight loss – loose skin, little subcutaneous fat
- warm and often moist peripheries with vasodilatation
- sinus tachycardia and systolic hypertension
- atrial fibrillation and cardiac failure, especially in the older patient
- eye signs (Table 31.2)
- pretibial myxoedema – infiltration of the shin present only in those with eye signs
- proximal myopathy – particularly in the upper limbs.

Signs of hypothyroidism are:

- hypersomnolence
- slow relaxing tendon reflexes
- nerve entrapments – carpal tunnel syndrome
- cool, dry and thickened skin
- peripheral and periorbital oedema
- hoarse voice
- bradycardia
- cardiomegaly.

Examination of the thyroid

In addition to determining the usual features of consistency and contour, this should include:

- Size according to the WHO grade
- Multiple nodules
- Mobility of the gland on swallowing
- Whether or not it is possible to get below any enlargement
- Movement on protrusion of the tongue – characteristic of thyroglossal cyst
- Palpation for a thrill and auscultation for a bruit – both features of an increased blood supply
- Detection of tracheal deviation.

DIAGNOSIS

After the history and clinical examination are complete, the clinical metabolic status (hyperthyroid, hypothyroid or euthyroid) and the nature of the goitre (diffuse, nodular or solitary nodule) will have been determined. This information allows the clinician to place the patient into a diagnostic category. However, some pitfalls of clinical assessment are as follows:

- Mild degrees of hyper- and hypothyroidism may not be clinically evident and may only be detected by tests of thyroid function.
- When a single nodule is thought to be present, there are often several others which are impalpable.

- Bruits may be transmitted from the precordium, notably in aortic stenosis.

Some common diagnostic categories of goitre are described below.

Euthyroid – smooth enlargement. This is a diffuse, smooth, often firm goitre – it is most commonly an endemic condition, the result of the thyroid attempting to extract more iodine from the blood in circumstances when there is iodine deficiency; this may be an early phase which progresses to multinodular goitre. Thyroid enlargement in pregnancy is a similar condition.

Euthyroid – multinodular goitre. The majority of patients present with this. The most common cause is endemic (iodine deficiency in the diet) or sporadic goitre (isolated occurrences affecting few people), but these features may be seen in long-standing goitres that are the consequence of cell hyperplasia, including autoimmune thyroiditis.

Euthyroid – single palpable nodule (clinical solitary nodule). In this case, the rest of the gland may be truly normal; alternatively there may be other impalpable nodules.

Hyperthyroid – diffuse goitre. The whole gland is enlarged and soft and its surface is smooth: typical of Graves' disease. Other features such as eye signs may be present.

Hyperthyroid – gland multinodular. This is the so-called secondary thyrotoxicosis seen commonly in the older patient who usually gives a history of long-standing goitre.

Hypothyroid – varying goitre, either smooth or multinodular. The typical clinical signs of Hashimoto's thyroiditis are seen.

INVESTIGATION

There are three general methods:

- tests of thyroid function
- imaging
- biopsy.

Thyroid function

Most laboratories measure blood levels of total thyroxine (T_4), free thyroxine, total tri-iodothyronine (T_3) and TSH. Many authorities recommend measurement of TSH as the initial investigation of patients with suspected hypo- or hyperthyroidism. If the outcome is abnormal, then measurement of output hormones is made.

Thyroid function tests may be unreliable in three circumstances:

- severe acute or chronic illness – total and free T_3 and T_4 tend to be low and basal TSH normal or low (sick euthyroid syndrome); values return to normal when the underlying illness has resolved

- pregnancy and in those taking oral contraceptives – levels of thyroid hormones are often greatly increased but do not cause clinical problems
- intake of drugs that affect thyroid hormone protein binding – these include antithyroid drugs, lithium and amiodarone.

Imaging

Techniques available are:

- X-ray of neck, thoracic inlet and chest
- ultrasound
- CT or MRI
- isotope scans – ^{131}I and ^{99m}Tc pertechnate.

These are used in three circumstances:

- hyperthyroidism – when the cause is thought to be a solitary nodule
- thyroid cancer
- ectopic thyroid.

Hyperthyroidism. ^{99m}Tc scan is the investigation of choice for patients assumed to be hyperthyroid. It is relatively cheap and exposes the patient to a lower dose of radiation than an iodine isotope scan. This imaging can reliably distinguish between the common causes of thyrotoxocosis.

Thyroid cancer. In primary tumour, ultrasound establishes whether the lesion is solid or cystic, and an isotope scan whether it is hot or cold (functioning or non-functioning). However, neither investigation can reliably determine if a lesion is benign or malignant.

When there is metastatic disease after the thyroid primary has been removed (usually by total thyroidectomy), total body scanning is very sensitive for the detection of deposits of differentiated thyroid cancer. Both CT and MRI are also important in assessing the extent of a proven malignant tumour.

In postoperative follow-up, iodine scanning is valuable to detect recurrent disease.

Ectopic thyroid tissue. Abnormal locations include the midline of the upper neck and the anterior mediastinum. A correct diagnosis must be made because of the risk of excising what is the only functional thyroid tissue. Scanning with ^{123}I is the best technique because it is more specific for thyroid tissues than ^{99m}Tc and avoids confusion with salivary glands which also take up technetium. The radiation dose for ^{123}I is much less than for ^{131}I and it is therefore safely used in the young.

Biopsy

There are two methods of biopsy:

- fine needle aspiration cytology (FNAC)
- core biopsy with a drill or wide-bore needle.

In both, a nodule is targeted either by palpation or with the help of ultrasound.

FNAC is a reliable method of providing a tissue diagnosis but is dependent on an experienced cytopathologist. The technique is useful in suspected malignancy, particularly a solitary nodule in which ultrasound imaging and isotope scanning lack specificity for the prediction of a histological diagnosis. Although FNAC has a low incidence of false-positive results, the false-negative rate may be as high as 20% and clinicians must be aware that a negative report does not exclude cancer. Liquid aspirates of cystic lesions are examined for malignant cells although these are rarely found.

Core biopsy using a Trucut or other wide-bore needle, is done under local anaesthesia and provides tissue that can be examined histologically. The risk of haemorrhage precludes its routine use other than in a hard, fixed mass such as a widely infiltrating carcinoma or lymphoma.

Non-toxic goitre

A simple hyperplastic goitre is caused by stimulation of the thyroid from a raised circulation level of TSH which is, in turn, the outcome of low levels of circulating thyroid hormones. The end stage of such hyperplasia is a multinodular goitre.

EPIDEMIOLOGY AND AETIOLOGY

The underlying factor is an absolute or relative deficiency in dietary iodine. Causes are:

- in endemic areas from iodine lack in the soil (geographically on high ground where, on a geological time scale, rain has washed out soluble elements such as iodine)
- change in physiological demand
- blockage of normal uptake or processing of iodine within the gland – usually goitrogens in the diet or in medications
- enzyme malfunction in the gland.

Endemic iodine deficiency causes the gland to enlarge and produce a goitre as it attempts to extract sufficient iodine from the diet where this is deficient.

Physiological variations such as puberty and pregnancy may alter demand for thyroid hormones and cause temporary enlargement of the gland. In pregnancy, increased renal iodine excretion, raised TRH concentration and direct stimulation of the thyroid by beta-HCG (human chorionic gonadotrophin) all induce hyperplasia.

Goitrogens are chemicals which interfere with thyroid hormone synthesis. They are found in foods such as cabbage and cassava, and goitres are common in areas where these are consumed in large quantities.

Enzyme malfunction is manifest clinically when, for example, peroxidase, responsible for organification of trapped iodine, is deficient. Syndromes of this type (e.g.

Pendred's syndrome, a combination of goitre and congenital deafness) are genetic.

Hyperplastic goitres can occur in childhood in endemic areas but those of physiological cause appear between 15 and 30 years. Goitres from goitrogens may be seen at any age. In almost all instances, females outnumber males by nearly 5:1.

CLINICAL FEATURES

History
The patient is euthyroid and complains of a painless, gradually progressive swelling in the neck. In later stages there may be discomfort or pain. Tracheal or oesophageal compression may develop with dyspnoea or dysphagia, particularly if there is retrosternal extension.

Physical findings
During the hyperplastic phase, the thyroid is often better seen than felt, its surface is smooth and the consistency soft. Later nodules develop and the gland often becomes large – sometimes enormous – and firm. Occasionally only one nodule is palpable, although there are microscopic changes throughout the gland. Such a single clinical nodule is often referred to as dominant. The trachea may be displaced and there may, in advanced enlargement, be signs of obstruction of the superior vena cava with distended veins coursing over the neck and chest. Regional lymphadenopathy or a hoarse voice suggests malignant change.

INVESTIGATION
The most important consideration is to establish whether or not there is a carcinoma. It used to be taught that multinodular goitres are almost never malignant, but recent studies indicate that the histological incidence of malignant change may be as high as 16%. However, in that the potential of such microscopic lesions to invade the thyroid capsule is not known, their clinical significance is questionable.

Thyroid function tests
Confirmation of the clinical status should be obtained. Most patients are euthyroid but some are hypothyroid. An older patient with a goitre and features of cardiac disease such as arrhythmia or heart failure may be thyrotoxic without any other clinical features of over-activity.

Imaging
Plain X-ray of the chest and thoracic inlet may show:

- tracheal compression and deviation
- retrosternal extension
- glandular calcification.

Ultrasound is the best way to demonstrate multiple nodules. High resolution can distinguish cysts from solid lesions.

Isotope scans show irregular uptake. Cold nodules may be areas of cystic degeneration, fibrosis or malignancy. The main indications for the use of an isotope scan are:

- possible retrosternal extension
- recurrent multinodular goitre in which the quantity of thyroid tissue is uncertain.

Biopsy
Fine needle aspiration cytology is indicated for nodules in which there is uncertainty on clinical or ultrasound assessment.

MANAGEMENT

Euthyroid goitre
This may well resolve spontaneously and requires reassurance only. Surgical intervention is necessary only if resolution does not occur and the goitre is cosmetically unacceptable, becomes nodular or produces complications.

Hypothyroid goitre
Thyroxine treatment is necessary to restore and maintain the euthyroid state. It provides an extraneous source of hormone and so suppresses the cellular hyperactivity that causes the goitre.

Multinodular goitre
Once nodules are associated with significant enlargement of the gland, return to normality with thyroid replacement is unlikely to succeed. Provided there is no suggestion of malignancy, it is acceptable to leave the gland alone and follow its progress by repeated clinical examination. Surgical excision is done if there is:

- suspicion of malignancy that has not been allayed by the investigations described above
- cosmetic problems
- pressure symptoms from tracheal or oesophageal compression.

In extensive disease, a near total excision may be necessary but must be done only by experienced surgeons because of the risk of damage to the parathyroids and recurrent laryngeal nerves.

Thyrotoxicosis and toxic goitre

Thyrotoxicosis or hyperthyroidism is the clinical syndrome which results from the peripheral actions of raised levels of circulating thyroid hormones.

CLINICAL CLASSIFICATION
Thyrotoxicosis is a relatively common problem affecting nearly 2% of females and 0.15% of males. It has several distinctive causes whose manifestations and treatment

are different. Ninety-five per cent of instances are the result of the three most common causes:

- diffuse toxic goitre – Graves' disease
- multinodular toxic goitre
- toxic solitary nodule or adenoma.

Rarely, manifestations of the disease are the consequence of self-administration of thyroxine (thyrotoxicosis factitia).

Graves' disease

This is the commonest cause of thyrotoxicosis and can occur at any age although the peak incidence is between 20 and 40 years. Women are affected five times more often than males.

AETIOLOGY

It is caused by an autoimmune process characterised by the presence of a spectrum of abnormal autoantibodies, whose actions are directed against the thyroid TSH receptor (long-acting thyroid stimulators, LATS). Why they are produced is unclear but there is evidence that genetic factors are concerned. The eyes may be involved (Graves' ophthalmopathy) possibly because of a cross-reaction between antibodies to eye muscles and thyroid antigens. There is a group of patients who have all the ocular features of Graves' disease but who are euthyroid – ophthalmic Graves' disease.

CLINICAL FEATURES

The natural history of Graves' disease is one of intermittent remission and relapse. Forty per cent of patients have a single episode only.

The symptoms of thyrotoxicosis have been summarised above. There may be a history of autoimmune disease. Eye involvement may produce double vision.

The thyroid is often uniformly enlarged, firm, smooth and moves on swallowing. There may be a bruit. When there are eye problems chemosis and periorbital oedema may be seen. The specific eye signs are summarised in Table 31.2.

INVESTIGATION

Thyroid function tests. These confirm thyrotoxicosis with an elevated T4 and reduced TSH.

Thyroid autoantibodies. Anti-thyroglobulin and anti-microsomal antibodies are present when the cause is autoimmune.

Multinodular toxic goitre (Plummer's syndrome)

This is sometimes referred to as secondary toxic goitre in that a goitre has been present for several years before the development of toxic features. The disease is more

Table 31.3
Comparison of multinodular toxic goitre and Grave's disease

Feature	Multinodular goitre	Grave's disease
Onset	Over 50	Puberty to early 20s
Symptoms related to nervous system	Uncommon	Common
Cardiac involvement	Common	Uncommon
Thyroid enlargement	Usually slight and irregular	Can be considerable – diffuse, smooth and soft
Tracheal displacement	Not uncommon	Rare

common in women and usually presents after the age of 50. Eye disease is unusual but cardiac arrhythmias and heart failure are common presenting features. The goitre is nodular and may be large, sometimes displacing the trachea. Features which distinguish multinodular toxic goitre from Graves' disease are summarised in Table 31.3

Toxic solitary adenoma/nodule

AETIOLOGY

This is a solitary autonomous adenoma. The cause of toxicity is not known but it is clear that LATS are not involved. The condition is responsible for nearly 5% of all hyperthyroidism. A single nodule in the gland becomes overactive and produces high levels of thyroxine, causing suppression of all surrounding thyroid tissue. This property permits diagnosis of a solitary toxic nodule on an isotope scan because the nodule takes up isotope but the surrounding gland does not. Eye disease is unusual in thyrotoxicosis caused by a solitary nodule.

Management of thyrotoxicosis

General principles

It is important to distinguish between the three types of thyrotoxic disease, as their specific treatments differ. However, a common principle is to make all patients euthyroid before any further action is contemplated. This is achieved either by:

- antithyroid agents
- therapeutic use of radioactive iodine.

The first is temporary but the second is permanent and therefore should not be used except as part of a long-term strategy of management.

In addition, other secondary problems should be brought under control although suppression of thyrotoxicosis may lead to their spontaneous resolution:

Table 31.4
Management of eye complications in Grave's disease

Problem	Treatment
Exposed cornea with drying	Methylcellulose eye drops for lubrication
Failure of lid closure in marked exophthalmos	Tarsorrhaphy
Inflammation	Systemic steroids
Deterioration in sight from compressive optic atrophy	Surgical decompression of both orbits
Severe diplopia	Corrective surgery to eye muscles

- eye complications (Table 31.4)
- cardiac complications – managed by medical means.

Antithyroid agents. Carbimazole and related drugs block thyroid peroxidase and therefore inhibit thyroxine synthesis. They are the agents of choice in the UK for the initial management of the thyrotoxic state. The dose is 30–60 mg daily and the major side-effect is agranulocytosis. However, the long half-life of T_4 means that the therapeutic response is slow – up to 8 weeks may be required to reduce the metabolic and other effects of excess levels.

Beta-adrenergic blocking agents are effective in reducing the effects of T_4 on the sympathetic system, which is the way in which thyrotoxicosis is manifest both physiologically and clinically. Propranolol is most commonly used. It may be administered parenterally in a severely toxic patient.

Thyroxine is added to the above therapies in some instances to enable a larger dose of antithyroid drug to be given to suppress the gland as much as possible without producing hypothyroidism (block and replace regimen).

MANAGEMENT OF SPECIFIC CAUSES OF THYROTOXICOSIS

Graves' disease

Non-operative
The nature of the disease and the possibility that only one episode will occur makes non-operative management preferable. Antithyroid agents are continued for 6–18 months. Half of those treated become permanently euthyroid. The majority of those who relapse do so in the first 2 years after treatment is stopped.

Operation
Thyroidectomy is indicated for:

- patients unwilling to undergo prolonged drug treatment
- relapse after drug therapy
- intractable side-effects of therapy
- failure of compliance
- large goitre after effective drug treatment.

Subtotal thyroidectomy is the standard operation, leaving a small remnant of about 5 g of tissue on each side.

Specific complications of thyroidectomy for Graves' disease are:

- recurrence of hyperthyroidism (3%) – managed by antithyroid agents or therapeutic radioiodine
- hypothyroidism (10% of patients within 1 year of operation) – it is particularly likely if microsomal antibodies were present before the operation because they continue to destroy the thyroid remnant; the proportion rises with time.

Treatment of eye problems
Eye disease may improve or regress completely when the patient has reached a euthyroid state, but not always. The management is given in Table 31.4.

Multinodular toxic goitre
Antithyroid drugs very uncommonly induce remission. Radioactive iodine is the definitive treatment for those with:

- small goitres
- absence of pressure symptoms
- disorders which preclude surgery – usually severe heart disease
- refusal of an operation.

Subtotal thyroidectomy
In large goitres, pressure symptoms may persist after medical treatment for thyrotoxicosis unless the bulk of the thyroid tissue is removed. In such instances, subtotal thyroidectomy is the preferred treatment provided that the risk is low for the individual patient. Subsequent thyroid replacement therapy may be required and management of pre-existing heart disease may have to be continued indefinitely.

Solitary toxic nodule
Radioactive iodine ablation is probably the best option. The remainder of the thyroid does not concentrate the ^{131}I because it has been suppressed secondary to the undetectable level of TSH. An alternative strategy is to surgically excise the nodule together with the lobe in which it is contained.

Clinical solitary thyroid nodule

AETIOLOGY AND PATHOLOGICAL FEATURES
Between 1 and 3% of the population have an isolated thyroid nodule and the proper approach to its presence must be understood. The causes are summarised in Box 31.1. The chance of malignancy being present is about 10%. Risk factors include:

Causes of a clinical solitary nodule

- Cyst
- Focal subacute thyroiditis
- Localised Hashimoto's disease
- Non-functioning adenoma
- Functioning adenoma
- Malignant disease
- Metastatic deposit

- previous neck irradiation
- iodine deficiency
- family history of thyroid carcinoma.

CLINICAL FEATURES

The history and physical findings are the same as in multinodular goitre, but only a single nodule is found in an otherwise apparently normal gland.

INVESTIGATION

Thyroid function tests

These are done to exclude toxicity, but in the majority the state is euthyroid.

Imaging

Ultrasound determines whether the nodule is truly solitary or multiple – a dominant nodule in a multinodular goitre is the commonest cause of a clinical solitary nodule. A cystic lump can also be distinguished from a solid one; this is of some importance in that cysts are less likely to be malignant.

Isotope imaging. Malignancy is extremely rare in nodules that are hot and the incidence of malignancy for a cold nodule is about 15%.

FNAC

Is the preferred method of diagnosis and often makes a pre-operative diagnosis available. However, as indicated above, in certain circumstances it may be unreliable.

MANAGEMENT

If a definite diagnosis of malignancy has not been achieved preoperatively, the operation is a total thyroid lobectomy. The resected tissue is examined histologically at once by frozen section while the patient is still in the operation room – a procedure that takes about 20 minutes at the most. If the result is unequivocally malignant, a total thyroidectomy is done. If the diagnosis is benign or inconclusive, the wound is closed and the result of more formal histological examination awaited.

Management of patients who are to undergo thyroid operations

It is now almost unknown for a patient to be operated upon without having been rendered euthyroid and without the other toxicity effects, such as cardiac arrythmias, having been treated.

Investigation

Investigations specific to operations on the thyroid (and the parathyroids) are:

- indirect laryngoscopy to assess vocal cord function
- measurement of baseline plasma calcium concentration
- white cell count in patients who have received antithyroid agents.

Information

A full explanation of possible complications – bleeding, nerve injury, transient hypocalcaemia and long-term hypoparathyroidism – must be given as part of obtaining informed consent.

Medication

Antithyroid agents and beta-adrenergic blockers are continued up to the day of operation.

Operation

Dissection must be precise and structures at risk of injury should be formally identified. Because of the serious nature of bleeding into the neck, haemostasis must be rigorous and drains are usually positioned to the site of dissection.

Complications

Bleeding into the neck causes dyspnoea and stridor (respiratory obstruction) usually within 24 hours of operation. This is an emergency and may require the wound to be opened without return to the operating room. Alternatively reintubation and formal drainage may be necessary.

Hypocalcaemia. The condition is unusual if only one lobe has been operated upon. After an operation which has involved resection of portions of both lobes, the calcium level is routinely measured on the day after the operation and, if it is low, prophylactic administration of oral calcium carbonate may be indicated. The first clinical features are paraesthesia around the mouth and in the digits; later there is muscle spasm and finally tetany. The two typical clinical signs are:

- Trousseau's – occlusion of the circulation to the hand causes small muscle spasm
- Chvostek–Weiss – tapping the facial nerve in front of and just below the ear induces spasm of the facial muscles.

Although not life-threatening, the condition is disturbing and is managed by the intravenous administration of calcium gluconate.

Nerve injury. The nerves at risk are the recurrent and superior laryngeal. Identification of injury to the recurrent laryngeal nerve at the time of surgery is followed by immediate repair. If recurrent nerve injury is diagnosed after operation (more commonly the case) the patient should be promptly referred to a specialist ear, nose and throat surgeon. Invasive treatment is withheld for about nine months as nerves that have been stretched or bruised can recover, and patients are prescribed speech therapy. If severe disability persists beyond this time, techniques including injection of polytetrafluoroethylene (PTFE) into the vocal cord and surgical lateral fixation may be considered.

Thyrotoxic storm (syn. crisis). Adequate preoperative treatment to restore a euthyroid state has now almost abolished this major complication, which had a mortality of 10%. The cause is the release of large amounts of thyroxine into the circulation. Ancillary factors which may be involved in the thyrotoxic subject are:

- stress or infection
- operations, other than those on the thyroid
- therapeutic doses of radioactive iodine with consequent cell destruction.

The condition was most common in the early postoperative period after manipulation and resection of the thyroid. Its clinical features include restlessness, confusion, tachycardia and hyperpyrexia. In severe cases, the patient may become hypotensive and may suffer cardiac arrest.

Prevention is to ensure the euthyroid state before operation which, if there are urgent indications, can be done within a week by the use of a combination of carbimazole, iodine and, most importantly, a beta-adrenergic blocking agent.

Treatment is urgent and is with full doses of propranolol, potassium iodide and antithyroid drugs; propylthiouracil is preferred.

Thyroiditis

Hashimoto's thyroiditis

This is an autoimmune disease of unknown cause. The thyroid is diffusely infiltrated by lymphoid and plasma cells with the formation of germinal centres and destruction of thyroid follicles.

CLINICAL FEATURES

History
In the early stages of the disorder, there may be thyrotoxicosis, but with progression, symptoms of hypothyroidism are typical. A goitre may occasionally be the presenting feature and produce pressure symptoms.

Physical findings
A diffuse goitre is characteristic and is firm with an irregular (bosselated) surface. Less commonly the disease is focal and there is a solitary nodule.

INVESTIGATION AND MANAGEMENT
Titres of autoantibodies directed against thyroglobulin and thyroid microsomes are markedly elevated. The biochemical pattern of hypothyroidism (raised TSH and low T_4) is present. There is no need for isotope scanning. In focal thyroiditis, FNAC is used to confirm the diagnosis.

Management is by life-long thyroxine suppression. Most goitres shrink to a minimal size but those that persist may require subtotal thyroidectomy.

De Quervain's thyroiditis

This is an uncommon condition caused by viral infection. There is an acute inflammatory reaction in the gland with histiocytes, multinucleate giant cells and granuloma formation.

CLINICAL FEATURES
The history is of an acute pain in the neck, accompanied by malaise and pyrexia. A tender enlarged thyroid will be seen.

INVESTIGATION AND MANAGEMENT
The ESR is raised and, in the early stages, there may be an elevated T_4 and a low TSH consistent with hyperthyroidism. Thyroid antibodies are absent.

The condition is self-limiting and analgesics and NSAIDs are all that is required.

Reidel's thyroiditis

This is an exceptionally rare condition of unknown cause. There is dense fibrosis, not confined to the gland but extending into the surrounding soft tissues of the neck. It may occur in isolation or with other analogous disorders such as retroperitoneal fibrosis, sclerosing cholangitis and mediastinal fibrosis.

CLINICAL FEATURES
A rapidly increasing goitre is noticed by the patient, often with features of tracheal or oesophageal compression.

A hard, woody goitre which is palpable will be found an examination.

INVESTIGATION AND MANAGEMENT

Diagnostic criteria do not exist. The priority is to exclude malignant disease. FNAC demonstrates scanty fibroblasts, but open biopsy may be required for diagnostic certainty.

Decompression of neck structures may be required and occasionally tracheostomy is necessary.

Cancer of the thyroid

This condition is relatively uncommon, causing less than 0.5% of all deaths from malignant disease, but, perhaps because of interesting biological features, has attracted considerable clinical and research interest.

AETIOLOGY

The cause of most thyroid cancers is not known. However, certain predisposing factors are:

- Genetic – medullary carcinoma of the thyroid is a familial condition and is associated with neoplasms in other endocrine organs
- Radiation – either from external beam radiotherapy, previously frequently given for a variety of benign and malignant conditions of the head and neck, or from the environment (^{131}I), where exposure occurs because of high natural levels or from nuclear explosions (Hiroshima and Nagasaki) or accidents (Chernobyl)
- Goitre – carcinoma is more common in regions where goitre is endemic; the reason is not entirely clear, but increased stimulation by TSH with repeated hyperplasia and involution may be responsible.

PATHOLOGICAL CLASSIFICATION

There are four common types of thyroid cancers:

- papillary
- follicular
- medullary
- anaplastic.

The first two are usually grouped together as differentiated carcinoma. The pathological features and behaviour are so different that they are considered in relation to each type of growth.

MODES OF PRESENTATION

Incidental finding
Occult thyroid tumours may be encountered either within a resection specimen or at the time of surgery for benign disease.

Primary tumour
The patient notices a painless lump in the neck and examination reveals a solitary thyroid nodule. Physical signs of local invasion are:

- hoarseness – typical of invasion of the recurrent laryngeal nerve
- stridor
- fixity of the lump.

Metastatic disease
An enlarged lymph node in the neck may first call attention to the disease, as may distant spread to lung, bone or brain.

Differentiated cancer

Papillary carcinoma

Pathological features
Papillary carcinoma accounts for two-thirds of all thyroid malignancies and is generally a slow-growing tumour with a good prognosis. Many tumours are found only at postmortem examination (13–28%). Histologically, finger-like tumour papillae are present and the growth is often multifocal. Psammoma bodies are typical. The tumour invades lymphatics and over 50% of patients have cervical lymph node involvement at presentation.

Investigation
Euthyroidism is the rule. The diagnostic investigation is FNAC. Ultrasound shows a solid lesion and may reveal enlarged lymph nodes.

Follicular carcinoma

Pathological features
Follicular carcinoma is a well encapsulated solitary tumour which comprises 20% of all thyroid malignancies and has a favourable prognosis. There is a uniform follicular structure and the diagnosis of cancer as distinct from a follicular adenoma is dependent on the presence of extracapsular or venous invasion. Other strongly suggestive features of malignancy are:

- nuclear polymorphism
- increased nuclear to cytoplasmic ratio.

The tumour spreads by the bloodstream and cervical node involvement is found in only 5%.

Investigation
Euthyroidism is always the case. FNAC is unreliable in distinguishing between follicular adenoma and carcinoma. Aspiration cytology that yields follicular cells should be followed by removal of the involved lobe and histological examination for the features of cancer.

MANAGEMENT OF DIFFERENTIATED CARCINOMA

Primary tumour

The minimal procedure is total thyroid lobectomy with resection of the isthmus. Thereafter, clinical opinion (rather than prospective studies) supports either thyroxine suppression of TSH production or total thyroid ablation by surgical removal or therapeutic doses of ^{131}I for the same process. The thinking underlying the use of ablation is as follows:

- Papillary tumours are multifocal.
- Follow-up by repeated measurements of thyroglobulin and ^{131}I diagnostic scanning is more sensitive.
- The incidence of local recurrence is reduced.

However, total thyroid lobectomy with thyroid suppression is adequate treatment for most slow growing tumours and avoids the greater morbidity of total thyroidectomy, including hypoparathyroidism and damage to the recurrent laryngeal nerves. Opinion is therefore divided. Adverse prognostic indicators that influence surgeons to undertake total ablation are:

- age over 50 years
- tumour diameter greater than 4 cm
- presence of local invasion or distant metastases
- pronounced angio-invasion in follicular carcinoma.

Metastases

Cervical lymph nodes. Involvement of these by tumour is not an indicator of survival. Involved nodes are best resected because this reduces the incidence of local recurrence.

Distant metastases. The majority of differentiated tumours are functional, i.e. they concentrate iodine. This property not only facilitates their detection by a radioisotope scan but also their treatment with ^{131}I. However, metastases are only detected once the whole thyroid has been ablated and thyroxine replacement has to be withheld for 6 weeks before scanning or radioiodine therapy. For the uncommon tumours that do not concentrate iodine, external beam radiotherapy is used.

FOLLOW-UP

Total body iodine scanning

In addition to regular clinical examination, patients who have undergone total thyroid ablation have a total body radioiodine scan, although, as already stated, this necessitates stopping replacement therapy with thyroxine for 6 weeks.

Thyroglobulin

Most differentiated tumours produce this substance; it is therefore a useful postoperative tumour marker. Most clinicians measure the thyroglobulin on an annual basis and resort to total body scanning when a rise is detected.

Medullary carcinoma

AETIOLOGY AND PATHOLOGICAL FEATURES

These tumours account for 5–10% of thyroid malignancies and are derived from C cells, which means that they produce calcitonin that can be detected in the blood. Three-quarters occur sporadically but there is a genetic basis for the other quarter. Such familial medullary carcinoma:

- is inherited in an autosomal dominant manner with an age-related penetrance
- frequently has a pre-invasive phase – C-cell hyperplasia – which is diffusely distributed throughout the gland
- is often multifocal
- can be associated with other endocrine disorders such as phaeochromocytoma and parathyroid hyperplasia (see 'MEN II syndrome').

SCREENING OF RELATIVES

The relatives of those with medullary carcinoma (including all patients with MEN syndrome) must be screened at the time of diagnosis. Until recently, this has relied on biochemical tests of the blood and urine (plasma calcium concentration and 24-hour urinary excretion of VMA), but negative results do not exclude involvement because the disorder may only become apparent in relatives several years after screening. The development of genetic tests for the presence of the specific mutations associated with MEN syndromes can remove the requirement for repeated screening when an individual is shown to be unaffected and may also lead to prophylactic action such as a thyroidectomy.

CLINICAL FEATURES

History

For those with a family history, the diagnosis may be established by screening at a stage when symptoms are absent. Otherwise, the history is of a lump in the neck or of distant metastases. Rarely there is diarrhoea because of high plasma concentrations of calcitonin.

Physical findings

These vary with the stage of the disease:

- thyroid nodule or nodules
- mass in the neck either from lymph node metastases or advanced local disease
- features of distant metastases
- marfinoid phenotype (see MEN II).

INVESTIGATION

Familial tumours

Selective screening of relatives is dealt with above.

Children of affected patients are screened by measurement of plasma concentrations of calcitonin, annually from the age of 3. The sensitivity of this is increased by stimulating production of calcitonin by the administration of gastrin intravenously. The recently discovered association of a defect in the *ret* proto-oncogene in those with medullary cancer is likely to transform screening and permit the use of a single blood test. Prophylactic thyroidectomy may then follow.

Sporadic tumours

Blood examination. Plasma calcitonin is elevated.

FNAC is done on a thyroid mass or lymph node enlargement.

Imaging. ^{99}Tc-dimercaptosuccinic acid (DMSA) body scan is useful to detect both the primary tumour and secondary deposits.

MANAGEMENT

Total thyroidectomy and thyroid replacement therapy comprise the initial treatment. In the postoperative period, patients are studied by measurements of plasma calcitonin. Surgical resection is favoured for local recurrence and radiotherapy for distant metastases.

Prognosis is favourable given early diagnosis.

Anaplastic carcinoma

These are aggressive tumours and are believed to arise from previously unrecognised differentiated tumours. They are more common in areas where endemic goitre is prevalent but the incidence is decreasing. Usually the presentation is at or above 60 years.

CLINICAL FEATURES

A long-standing goitre may have been present which has recently increased in size and perhaps caused pressure symptoms.

Physical findings are of a hard woody mass with fixation to surrounding structures. Clinically the condition can be confused with Reidel's thyroiditis or lymphoma.

INVESTIGATION AND MANAGEMENT

FNAC or, if this is equivocal, open biopsy will confirm the diagnosis. Lung metastases are frequently found on a chest X-ray.

As much of the tumour as possible is excised and the patient is treated by external beam radiotherapy, both to endeavour to eliminate local residual growth and to prevent fungation through the operation wound. These tumours do not respond to radioiodine.

Anaplastic carcinoma has a uniformly poor prognosis and few patients survive beyond 12 months.

Lymphoma

This is a rare growth (1% of thyroid malignancies) typically affecting elderly females. Long-standing Hashimoto's thyroiditis is the only known risk factor. The condition is part of the non-Hodgkin's B-cell lymphoma group.

The presentation is similar to anaplastic carcinoma.

INVESTIGATION AND MANAGEMENT

The diagnosis is made on histology rather than cytology which requires an incisional biopsy. The tumour can also be imaged by a gallium-67 isotope scan.

Treatment is specialised and determined by the stage and grade of the tumour. At an early stage, removal of all visible tumour (debulking) is done combined with radiotherapy. Advanced disease is generally managed by a combination of chemo- and radiotherapy. The prognosis is much better than that for anaplastic carcinoma and to make the distinction is therefore important.

Parathyroid

EMBRYOLOGY

The superior parathyroid glands (IV) are derived from the fourth pharyngeal pouch, whereas the inferior glands (III) are from the more cephalad third pharyngeal pouch. The explanation for this apparent paradox is that of the common origin of the inferior glands and the thymus. From the fifth week of gestation, the thymus gland (also derived from the third pouch) descends into the superior mediastinum, taking the inferior parathyroids with it. In consequence, some surgeons refer to the inferior parathyroids as 'parathymic'.

ANATOMY

Because of their complicated embryological derivation, the precise location of individual glands is variable, although it tends to be symmetrical. The superior glands are usually found adjacent to the thyroid, typically within a 1 cm radius, above the junction of the inferior thyroid artery and the recurrent laryngeal nerve. The inferior glands are usually located in a condensation of fascia between the lower pole of the thyroid and the thymus (the parathymic ligament). However, they may lie in the superior mediastinum or within the carotid sheath. The typical parathyroid gland is only 1 mm × 3 mm × 5 mm and weighs approximately 30 mg: the total weight of parathyroid tissue is thus about 120 mg. The blood supply for both pairs of glands is usually from the inferior thyroid artery. Less than 5% of individuals have five or more glands, with the supernumerary ones usually located within the thymus.

The cellular structure of the parathyroid gland is:

- abundant chief cells which manufacture and secrete parathyroid hormone
- sparse oxophil cells whose function is poorly understood.

PHYSIOLOGY OF THE CONTROL OF THE LEVEL OF SERUM CALCIUM

The concentration of plasma calcium is tightly controlled between 2.2 and 2.6 mmol/L by parathyroid hormone (PTH) and vitamin D, possibly supplemented by the effects of calcitonin from the thyroid.

Parathyroid hormone (PTH)

The main product of the parathyroid glands has three principal actions:

- Stimulation of the activity of osteoclasts in bone and thus mobilisation of calcium from bone into the bloodstream
- Enhancement of the absorption of calcium from the gut into the bloodstream, an action facilitated by vitamin D
- Increase of the reabsorption of calcium by the renal tubules, thereby reducing urinary calcium excretion.

All of these tend to increase serum calcium concentration, which then has negative feedback on the secretion of PTH.

Vitamin D

Vitamin D_3 is generally regarded as being produced in the skin from the action of ultraviolet light upon 7-dehydrocholesterol; it is also ingested in the diet. This inactive form undergoes a two-stage hydroxylation process in the liver and kidney (Fig. 31.2) to produce the active vitamin D: 1,25-dihydroxycholecalciferol. The second hydroxylation is stimulated by PTH. Active vitamin D_3 enhances intestinal calcium absorption by PTH and facilitates bone mineralisation and stimulates bone resorption.

Calcitonin

Calcitonin is secreted by the parafollicular or C cells of the thyroid. Its actions are the direct opposite of those of PTH and, in particular, it decreases osteoclastic activity. However, its biological importance in calcium homeostasis is uncertain. Serum calcium concentration is normal both in patients who have undergone total thyroidectomy (and who therefore have negligible serum levels of calcitonin) and in those with medullary thyroid carcinoma (high levels of calcitonin).

Hyperparathyroidism

In this condition, there is overactivity of one or more

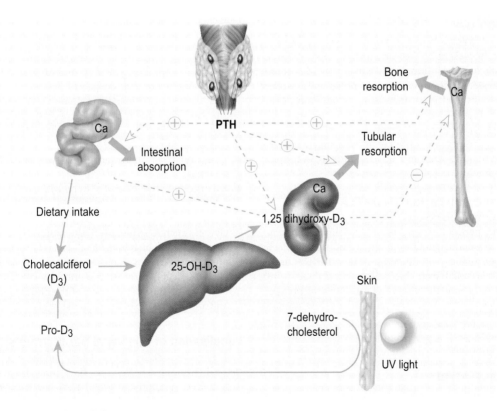

Fig 31.2 **Metabolism of vitamin D.**

parathyroid glands with secretion of excessive amounts of PTH. Three subtypes are recognised:

- *Primary hyperparathyroidism.* Without any demonstrable stimulation, the parathyroid gland(s) secrete inappropriately raised amounts of PTH. Serum calcium concentration is raised and negative feedback is abolished, so the level of PTH is inappropriately high for the level of calcium. The cause is most commonly adenomatous change in one parathyroid, but less frequently there may be hyperplasia of all four or a carcinoma of one.
- *Secondary hyperparathyroidism.* This occurs in chronic renal failure (failure of tubular reabsorption) and intestinal malabsorption. There is a reduction in the plasma concentration of calcium which causes hyperplasia of all four glands. Increased production of PTH is therefore appropriate and, if the cause of hypocalcaemia can be corrected, in most instances the parathyroids return to normal.
- *Tertiary hyperparathyroidism.* If the stimulus in secondary hyperparathyroidism continues unchecked, parathyroid overactivity may become autonomous. Following renal transplantation the new kidney retains the ability to activate vitamin D which, in the presence of continuing parathyroid overactivity, leads to hypercalcaemia.

Primary hyperparathyroidism

EPIDEMIOLOGY

Primary hyperparathyroidism is the commonest subtype to present to the surgeon. The availability of the multichannel autoanalyser, which provides serum calcium concentrations on blood samples sent for other tests, has resulted in an increasing recognition of this disorder. It can occur at any age but is uncommon in the first decade. The peak incidence is between 20 and 50 years. Women are more commonly affected. It has been reported to occur in 1 in 1000 patients in hospital but community prevalence is much less.

AETIOLOGY AND PATHOLOGICAL FEATURES

The cause remains obscure.

Eighty per cent of patients have a solitary adenoma. The adenomatous gland is enlarged and the chief cells are hypertrophied and numerous. The other glands are suppressed, small, their chief cells few and their stroma contains an abundant amount of fat. In 5% of patients, adenomas are multiple. The remainder (15–20%) have multiple gland hyperplasia. Patients with hyperplasia may suffer from the multiple endocrine adenoma (MEN) syndrome.

CLINICAL FEATURES

History

The symptoms are those of complications of the

disorder, often summarised as 'stones, bones, abdominal groans and psychic moans' but more formally listed as:

- urinary tract stones – mainly renal colic (Ch. 32)
- bone decalcification, which may cause bone pain or a pathological fracture
- abdominal pain – often of obscure cause but occasionally consequent on the presence of a peptic ulcer or recurrent pancreatitis (Ch. 21)
- psychological disturbances of altered mood – mainly depression which may remain unrecognised by the patient or the doctor until successful treatment alters the mental state for the better.

Acute disturbances. Occasionally a rise of serum calcium concentration above 3.5 mmol/L produces a syndrome of vomiting, dehydration, renal failure and coma. The event may be potentially lethal.

Asymptomatic. Increasingly (up to 80%) patients are without symptoms and the possibility of the condition is signalled by an abnormal result on the autoanalyser profile.

Physical findings

Examination rarely reveals any abnormality. It is most unusual to find a lump in the neck. Features of the complications outlined above may be present.

INVESTIGATION

Diagnostic criteria are as follows:

- Unequivocal hypercalcaemia – blood is taken without applying a tourniquet to the arm because this may raise serum calcium concentration by provoking regional acidosis. At least three measurements are made on different occasions; since most calcium in serum is bound to albumin, results are adjusted to a standard albumin concentration of 40 g/L.
- Detection of simultaneous raised levels of PTH in the blood.
- Exclusion of other causes of hypercalcaemia (see Table 31.5).
- X-ray of the hands. Even in the absence of gross changes such as generalised osteoporosis or bone cysts, both of which occur in advanced disease but are rarely seen now that detection tends to be early, subperiosteal bone erosion is often revealed; it is best seen on the lateral aspect of the middle phalanx and around the top of the terminal phalanx (Fig. 31.3).

Localisation of abnormal parathyroid(s)

This is not necessary for a patient undergoing parathyroid exploration for the first time because an experienced surgeon can identify no less than 95% of glands during neck exploration. However, if the first operation fails to discover and remove the abnormal

Table 31.5
Other causes of hypercalcaemia to be excluded in the diagnosis of primary hyperparathyroidism

Cause	Method of exclusion
Secondary carcinoma of bone (common sites: breast, bronchus, thyroid, kidney and prostate)	History Typical bone X-rays Bone scan
Multiple myeloma	Typical bone X-rays Plasma electrophoresis Bence–Jones proteinuria
Vitamin D intoxication	History of intake
Sarcoidosis	
Thyrotoxicosis	
Rare tumours (usually carcinoma of bronchus) which secrete PTH-related peptide	
Familial hypercalcaemic hypocalciuria – diminished renal calcium excretion	Family history Low renal calcium output

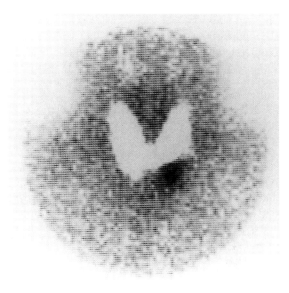

Fig 31.4 **Isotope scan highlights an adenoma of the left inferior parathyroid gland.** (By courtesy of Dr K Meeran, Hammersmith Hospital)

- *Invasive*
  - digital subtraction arteriography demonstrates the arterial anatomy and may reveal a blush from a hyperplastic or adenomatous gland
  - selective venous sampling from veins draining the neck structures directs the surgeon to the area in which the abnormality lies.

MANAGEMENT

Non-operative

Immediate treatment of serum calcium concentrations above 3.5 mmol/L and with the general symptoms given under 'Acute disturbances' consists of rehydration and the administration of bisphosphonates, which inhibit osteoclastic bone resorption. Calcium concentrations are measured at least daily and often need to be followed more frequently. Moderate hypercalcaemia (3.0–3.5 mmol/L) is usually controlled by intravenous rehydration.

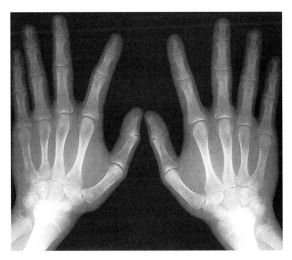

Fig 31.3 **X-ray of the hands in primary hyperparathyroidism.** There is subperiosteal bone erosion on the radial aspect of the middle phalanges and tufting of terminal phalanges. (By courtesy of Dr. C Cousins, Hammersmith Hospital)

gland(s), accurate localisation must be attempted before a repeat operation. There are two reasons:

- There is a greater chance that the disorder is in a gland (or glands) at an unusual site.
- Re-exploration of the neck carries a sixfold greater risk to the recurrent laryngeal nerves and successful lateralisation of the parathyroid reduces this.

Methods of localisation are:

- *Minimally invasive*
  - neck ultrasound: unreliable
  - CT and MRI: more reliable than ultrasound
  - isotope scanning: technetium-sestamibi subtraction scanning correctly lateralise glands with up to 90% success in special centres (Fig. 31.4) and more recently sestamibi-only scanning.

Surgical

Surgical removal offers the only cure for primary hyperparathyroidism and should be offered to all symptomatic patients and those asymptomatic patients whose calcium concentration exceeds 3.0 mmol/L. The high success rate and low morbidity of exploration of the neck have led towards an aggressive surgical policy for asymptomatic patients with a plasma calcium between 2.75 and 2.95 mmol/L.

The preoperative preparation is as for thyroidectomy. Facilities must be available for perioperative frozen section examination and weighing of all material excised at operation.

Operation

The approach and exposure are the same as for thyroidectomy. All four parathyroid glands must be clearly identified. If an adenoma is found, it is removed carefully and a small biopsy taken of another gland to confirm that suppression is present.

The surgical treatment of multi-gland hyperplasia is more difficult. The conventional management is subtotal parathyroidectomy (removal of three and a half glands), leaving half a gland in the neck. However, there is a chance of recurrence, and neck re-exploration is then more difficult and dangerous. Some surgeons now autograft the remaining half gland into the forearm. The graft survival rate is high (more than 90%) and further surgery in the neck is avoided. A third option is to cryopreserve some parathyroid tissue and delay its transplantation until hypocalcaemia is documented; however, graft survival is much lower. The fourth option is to excise all parathyroid tissue and place the patient on lifelong calcium and vitamin D supplements.

Postoperative care

Serum calcium concentration is measured as soon as the patient returns from the operating room and twice daily thereafter. After a successful procedure, the calcium level often falls below normal before it rises to the normal range. If the calcium level does not fall, or returns to its original level after a transient decrease, the surgeon has failed to remove the disordered tissue.

The patient is questioned for early signs of hypocalcaemia such as paraesthesiae of the hands and lips. Trousseau's and Chvostek's signs may be elicited. It may be necessary to give oral calcium and vitamin D until the suppressed parathyroids recover.

Complications

Recurrent hypercalcaemia is the consequence of failure to remove an adenoma or enough hyperplastic tissue.

Re-exploration must be carried out, but only by an experienced surgeon because the complication rate is much higher than for a first operation.

Hypoparathyroidism. Transient hypocalcaemia is common even after successful removal of a diseased gland but recovery occurs within a week. Permanent hypocalcaemia follows removal of too much parathyroid tissue. If cryopreserved tissue is available, some of it is implanted as already described; otherwise, the patient is treated with calcium and vitamin D for life.

Parathyroid carcinoma

This condition is very rare. Usually there is invasion of local tissues and recurrence after excision. Metastases are uncommon. Death is often caused by hypercalcaemia.

CLINICAL FEATURES

There may be symptoms of metastatic disease in addition to the progressive effects of hyperparathyroidism.

Physical findings are of a mass in the neck which may be palpable; this should alert the surgeon to the possibility of carcinoma.

INVESTIGATION AND MANAGEMENT

The plasma calcium concentration is typically very high and is accompanied by a high level of PTH. CT of the neck demonstrates the local anatomy and a chest X-ray should be taken to look for secondary spread.

The surgical strategy is en-bloc resection of the tumour. Adjuvant oncotherapy should be considered and bisphosphonates may be required to control the hypercalcaemia.

Adrenals

EMBRYOLOGY

The glands are derived from two components: The cortex and the medulla. The cortex is formed during the fifth week of life from proliferation of mesodermal cells. This is then invaded by ectodermal cells which have migrated from the neural crest (ectoderm) to form the adrenal medulla; these cells either differentiate into chromaffin cells containing granules of catecholamines (phaeochromocytes) or non-chromaffin sympathetic ganglion cells.

Neural crest cells are widely dispersed throughout the embryo but are usually replaced by lymphatic tissue shortly after birth. Ectopic rests of cells have been described in diverse sites including the urinary bladder, gonads and gastrointestinal tract. Persistence of these cells may give rise to extra adrenal medullary neoplasms.

ANATOMY

The adrenal glands are paired and similarly placed, bilaterally, above the kidneys; however, they are far from symmetrical. Each normal gland weighs approximately 5 g and is 5 cm long, 3 cm wide and approximately 1 cm thick. The right gland is pyramidal while the left is semilunar. The blood supply arises from three arteries: branches from the aorta, renal and phrenic arteries.

PHYSIOLOGY

The cortex secretes steroid hormones from three distinct zones. The outer zona glomerulosa secretes the mineralocorticoid aldosterone whose major actions are in the control of renal sodium and potassium excretion in conjunction with renin and angiotensin. The middle zona fasciculata secretes the glucocorticoid cortisol whose many physiological effects include hepatic gluconeogenesis, protein catabolism, some mineralo-corticoid effects and regulation of the response to inflammation. Secretion of cortisol is regulated by adrenocorticotrophic hormone (ACTH) from the anterior pituitary. The inner zona reticularis secretes adrenal androgens and accounts for 15–20% of total androgen activity. The cells of the adrenal medulla are part of the amine precursor uptake and decarboxylation (APUD) system and secrete catecholamines noradrenaline and adrenaline.

PATHOLOGICAL FEATURES

The variety of disorders which arise from adrenal hyperplasia and tumours are summarised in Box 31.2.

The adrenal cortex

CLASSIFICATION OF DISORDERS

Hyperplasia or neoplasia of the adrenal cortex produces characteristic syndromes which are dependent on the zone of origin:

- zona glomerulosa – primary hyperaldosteronism
- zona fasciculata – Cushing's syndrome
- zona reticularis – virilism.

These entities can occur on their own or there may be a mixed picture which is suggestive of an adrenal carcinoma.

Primary hyperaldosteronism

EPIDEMIOLOGY AND PATHOLOGICAL FEATURES

This condition is relatively rare, occurring in less than 2% of patients with hypertension. It presents most commonly between the ages of 20 and 50 years and is more common in men. There are two subtypes:

- idiopathic hyperaldosteronism – bilateral adrenal hyperplasia
- Conn's syndrome – a single, usually small, canary-yellow tumour of the adrenal cortex, which is nearly always benign (98%).

Idiopathic hyperaldosteronism is three times less common than Conn's syndrome as a cause of primary hyperaldosteronism. It is important to distinguish between a single tumour, which is best treated surgically, and bilateral adrenal hyperplasia which can be managed medically.

Inappropriate autonomous oversecretion of aldosterone leads to sodium retention and potassium loss, causing hypertension and muscle weakness. High levels of aldosterone suppress the renin–angiotensin–aldosterone axis and, in consequence, the plasma renin concentration is low.

CLINICAL FEATURES

Symptoms are either vague or absent. Patients may complain of lethargy, muscle weakness and thirst. Clinical examination is normal but there is hypertension.

INVESTIGATION

There are two stages of investigation: initially to confirm the diagnosis and then to localise a tumour if one is thought to be present.

Initial
- Confirm primary hyperaldosteronism
- Differentiate between Conn's syndrome and adrenal hyperplasia.

Localisation
CT scan may show a small (1 cm) tumour (Fig. 31.5) but it must be remembered that there is a significant incidence of adrenal incidentalomas.

Scanning with radioactive-labelled cholesterol can distinguish a solitary functional adrenal tumour from bilateral increased uptake. If there is still doubt, it may be necessary to perform adrenal venous sampling to measure aldosterone concentrations. However, this technique carries a risk of infarction to one or both adrenals.

MANAGEMENT

Non-operative
If a tumour has been diagnosed, it is essential that

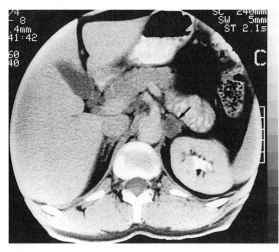

Fig 31.5 **Abdominal CT scan demonstrating a left adrenal tumour (arrow) in a patient with Conn's syndrome.** Note the typical appearance of the normal right adrenal with its very dark medulla. (By courtesy of Dr A. L. Hine, Central Middlesex Hospital)

serum potassium concentration is returned to normal before surgical treatment is considered; this can be achieved by the use of spironolactone which blocks aldosterone receptors and reduces aldosterone secretion; 200–400 mg/day is used for 3–6 weeks before operation. Hyperplasia is not an indication for exploration and bilateral adrenalectomy because this renders the patient permanently dependent on steroids and restores the blood pressure to normal in only one-third of all patients. Spironolactone in doses of 200–400 mg/day controls the hypokalaemia but other agents may be necessary to reduce blood pressure.

Operative

Adenomas are treated by unilateral adrenalectomy. This can be achieved either through a posterior approach or at laparoscopy. There is a high cure rate and virtually no morbidity or mortality. The hypokalaemia of primary aldosteronism is almost universally cured, but hypertension persists in 30% of patients and may recur in a further 20%, with, therefore, a long-term cure of hypertension of only 50%.

Cushing's syndrome

This condition is characterised by glucocorticoid excess. The underlying causes are shown in Box. 31.3.

EPIDEMIOLOGY

Cushing's syndrome affects patients between 20 and 40 years old and has a predilection for women; however, ectopic ACTH secretion has an equal sex incidence which reflects the chief cause which is bronchogenic carcinoma. Adrenocortical carcinoma as a cause is very rare.

> **Box 31.3**
>
> *Causes of cushing's syndrome*
>
> *ACTH-dependent*
> - Ectopic ACTH secretion (see also p. 000) – 15%
> - Cushing's 'disease' – 65%
>
> *ACTH-independent*
> - Adrenocortical adenoma – 10%
> - Adrenocortical carcinoma – 10%
> - Iatrogenic steroid therapy – variable but should never be forgotten

PATHOPHYSIOLOGY

Primary ACTH-secreting tumours of the pituitary are described later in this chapter. Ectopic ACTH production stimulates both adrenal glands to produce excess cortisol. Adrenocortical adenomas and carcinomas secrete excess levels of cortisol with suppression of ACTH, and each accounts for about 10% of patients with Cushing's syndrome.

CLINICAL FEATURES

History

The effects of excess cortisol on the body are wide-ranging and produce characteristic clinical features. Typical symptoms are:

- facial and truncal obesity
- menstrual irregularity
- hirsuitism
- muscles weakness
- osteoporosis.

Clinical findings

The typical physical signs are (Fig. 31.6):

- moon face
- buffalo hump
- central obesity ('lemon-on-sticks' appearance)
- muscle wasting and weakness
- striae
- hirsuitism
- ecchymoses
- hypertension.

Adrenal carcinomas tend to be large and a mass may be palpated. Patients with ectopic ACTH production are usually pigmented and may have clinical signs of a primary bronchial neoplasm.

INVESTIGATION

Biochemical and endocrinological

The following are used to confirm the presence of the disorder:

secretion are best treated by resecting the primary source, but all too often this is either not technically feasible or the patients have advanced secondary disease and a poor prognosis. In such circumstances, drugs which block steroid synthesis, such as metyrapone and aminoglutethimide, are used.

Surgical

Adenomas are treated by unilateral adrenalectomy. Adrenal carcinomas are usually advanced and metastases are common. Despite their poor prognosis (less than 50% survival at 2 years), surgery is the treatment of choice in an attempt to reduce the bulk of the tumour and palliate the symptoms of steroid excess. This can be aided in part by the use of Mitotane (o,p′-.DDD), a mitochondrial poison which, in the majority of patients, reduces the secretion of both cortisol and adrenal androgens.

Virilising tumours

Overproduction of sex steroid hormones can lead to either virilisation (excess androgen) or feminisation (excess oestrogen). The cause is usually a congenital enzyme defect or an adrenal tumour.

Congenital adrenal hyperplasia

Pathophysiology

The underlying cause in 90% is an enzyme deficiency – absence of 21-hydroxylase, an enzyme essential for cortisol synthesis. The consequent reduction in plasma cortisol levels leads to an excess of ACTH, which in turn results in an increase of intermediate metabolites which become channelled into testosterone production.

Clinical features

The usual presentation is at birth with pseudo-hermaphrodite external genitalia in female children and precocious sexual maturation in affected males.

Investigation

The diagnosis is confirmed by finding high concentrations of the steroid precursors in blood and urine. The karyotype must be checked in affected females.

Management

Medical. Cortisol deficiency is corrected so as to suppress the ACTH secretion. Hydrocortisone $25\ \text{mg}/\text{m}^2$ is given daily in two or three divided doses.

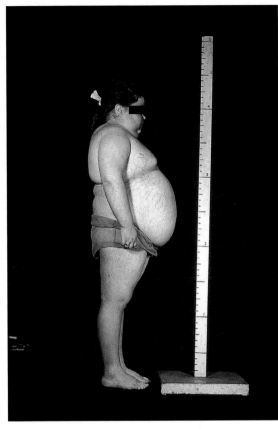

Fig 31.6 **Cushingoid ('lemon-on-sticks') appearance of a female adolescent.** (By courtesy of Professor S. R. Bloom, Hammersmith Hospital)

- The 24-hour urinary free cortisol is elevated and a low-dose dexamethasone suppression test depresses the hypothalamic–pituitary axis in normals but not in Cushing's syndrome.
- ACTH-dependent and -independent disorders are distinguished by the methods given in Table 31.6.

Localisation of a tumour

Methods used are CT and selective venous sampling.

MANAGEMENT

Medical

If an operation is indicated, steroid cover with hydrocortisone must be given both preoperatively and perioperatively and reduced to a maintenance dose of 20–30 mg/day of hydrocortisone usually within 10 days after operation. Patients with ectopic ACTH

Table 31.6
Methods to distinguish between ACTH-dependent and ACTH-independent disorders

Test	Cushing's disease	Adrenal tumour	Ectopic ACTH
Plasma ACTH	Normal to elevated	Undetectable	Elevated ++
High-dose dexamethasone suppression test	Suppression	No suppression	No suppression

Surgical. On occasions, surgical correction of the abnormal genitalia may be necessary.

Adrenocortical adenoma and carcinoma

Acquired syndromes of sex steroid excess are rare and usually secondary to an underlying adrenocortical tumour. Androgen-secreting tumours are much more common than are the feminising tumours.

Investigation and management

The diagnosis is made by a combination of selective venous sampling, CT and radionucleotide Scanning (seleno-cholesterol is the most favoured viewing agent).

When there is a benign tumour of the adrenal, surgical removal is curative. By contrast, adrenal carcinoma carries a poor prognosis.

The adrenal medulla

Tumours are the only conditions of surgical importance and are derived either from chromaffin cells (phaeochromocytoma) or non-chromaffin cells (neuroblastoma, ganglioneuroma and ganglioneuroblastoma).

Phaeochromocytoma

This is a catecholamine-secreting tumour of chromaffin cells in the adrenal medulla or in the paraganglionic tissues adjacent to the sympathetic chain at any level.

It is a rare tumour with an incidence of 1 in 2 million and which therefore accounts for less than 1% of cases of hypertension.

PATHOLOGICAL FEATURES

It has been called the '10% tumour' because 10% are bilateral, 10% are malignant and 10% are extra-adrenal. Extra-adrenal tumours are more likely to be malignant and can be found anywhere from the pelvis to the base of the skull. The most common extra-adrenal site is the organ of Zuckerkandl, which lies at the aortic bifurcation, but instances in the urinary bladder, the mediastinum and the neck have all been described.

Malignancy is usually characterised by the presence of established metastases in liver, lymph nodes, bones and lungs.

Phaeochromocytoma occurs in half of patients with MEN-II and is also associated with other uncommon disorders such as von Hippel–Lindau disease (phaeochromocytoma, angioma, renal carcinoma), neurofibromatosis and tuberose sclerosis.

CLINICAL FEATURES

History

The typical symptoms are secondary to the effects of excessive α-adrenoreceptor stimulation. Sweating is very common in phaeochromocytoma and occurs in almost 90% of patients. Attacks are usually spontaneous, but sometimes they are precipitated by exercise, overeating, defaecation or sexual intercourse. Patients describe them as consisting of:

- paroxysmal headache
- palpitations
- profuse perspiration
- sometimes precordial pain
- a fearful feeling of impending death (angor animi).

These rarely last more than 15 minutes but tend to become more frequent over time.

Death from cardiovascular episodes and myocardial infarction has occurred during an attack. It must be remembered that invasive investigative procedures may precipitate an acute episode – an important consideration in efforts to localise the tumour.

Physical findings

Hypertension is the most common finding: over 50% of patients have persistent and sustained hypertension, but in the other 50% it is intermittent. Examination is otherwise normal but an abdominal tumour is occasionally found.

INVESTIGATION

Blood examination

The circulating plasma volume may be reduced by a combination of intense vasoconstriction and hypertension. A secondary rise in haematocrit is then evident.

Cardiac

There may be evidence of left ventricular hypertrophy on the ECG.

Hormonal

Twenty-four hour measurement of the urinary metabolites of adrenaline and noradrenaline – vanillylmandelic acid (VMA) and metanephrines – is an effective screening test and is rarely normal in patients with symptomatic disease. If VMA levels are high then plasma catecholamines are measured. Once an endocrine diagnosis has been made, a CT scan of the abdomen will usually localise the tumour.

MANAGEMENT

Medical

Phaeochromocytomas are potentially lethal and the major advance in their management has been the preoperative use of α- and β-adrenergic blocking agents which have reduced operative mortality to 1%. Alpha-receptor blockade is mandatory before removal of the tumour and, when cardiac function is compromised, must be introduced gradually; phenoxybenzamine, a non-selective α-blocker, is the agent of choice. Phenoxybenzamine decreases the vasoconstriction so that mild to severe postural hypotension develops and the blood volume may need to be restored by increased oral fluid intake. The subjective symptoms are relieved and the patient may appear to be drowsy as though sedated. Tachycardia may increase so that β-blockade becomes necessary but only after α-blockade is well established and the circulating blood volume has been restored.

Surgical

After the above preparation and precise localisation of the tumour, exploration and removal comprise the treatment of choice.

Neuroblastoma

Neuroblastoma is the third most common malignancy of childhood (after leukaemia and cerebral malignancy) and, in the UK, affects approximately 1 in 10 000 children alive at birth.

PATHOLOGICAL FEATURES

Neuroblastomas arise from the most primitive cells of the adrenal medulla. Local invasion of surrounding structures is frequent. Blood-borne metastases are common, particularly to the skull and orbit from left-sided primaries (Hutchinson type) and liver from right-sided primaries (Pepper type).

CLINICAL FEATURES

The child typically presents with malaise and weight loss. An abdominal mass will be felt. Hypertension is not usually a feature.

INVESTIGATION AND MANAGEMENT

Urinary levels of VMA are usually elevated.

Referral to a specialised centre is essential to ensure the highest rate of survival. A triad of chemotherapy, radiotherapy and de-bulking surgery occasionally produces excellent results. The overall prognosis, however, is poor although dependent upon how advanced the disease is at the time of diagnosis.

Acute adrenal insufficiency

This is essentially a medical condition but surgeons may encounter adrenal insufficiency as a post-traumatic (including postoperative) complication. It may be either acute or chronic and the common causes are shown in Box 31.4.

CLINICAL FEATURES

In acute adrenal failure, patients present with hypotension, vomiting, abdominal pain and mental confusion.

Box 31.4

Causes of adrenal insufficiency

Acute
- Primary – Addison's disease
- Secondary – adrenal apoplexy in the newborn
- Sepsis – especially meningococcal (Waterhouse–Friderichsen syndrome)
- Bilateral adrenalectomy
- Postoperative haemorrhage

Chronic
- Idiopathic atrophy
- Adrenal destruction
  — tuberculosis
  — histoplasmosis
  — metastatic disease
  — lymphoma
  — amyloidosis
  — haemochromatosis
- Hypothalamic–pituitary axis disease
  — tumour
  — irradiation
  — infarction

There is typically a history of recent surgery or associated sepsis, coagulation defect or cancer. Hypotension and circulatory collapse inevitably develop.

INVESTIGATION AND MANAGEMENT

The classical picture of hyponatraemia and hyperkalaemia may take several days to become apparent and can be confused by concomitant intravenous fluid regimens. A low plasma cortisol is diagnostic but the fundamental necessity is to be aware of the diagnosis.

Management is by urgent steroid replacement with the cooperation of an endocrinologist.

Gastroenteropancreatic tumours

These are slow-growing tumours and tend to cause symptoms by their secreted peptides rather than by any bulk effect, although pressure and other mechanical events may occur in the late stages. With the exception of insulinoma, most gastroenteropancreatic tumours are malignant. However, despite extensive hepatic and other metastases, which are often present at the time of the original diagnosis, many patients may survive for years.

Insulinoma

EPIDEMIOLOGY

Insulinomas constitute about 70% of all pancreatic endocrine tumours and occur in approximately 1 in 1 million of the population. Although they are rare in children, in infants there may be an associated entity of nesidioblastosis – a very rare condition of β-cell hyperplasia which is diffuse throughout the pancreas and causes symptomatic hyperinsulinaemia and usually necessitates either a distal subtotal or a total pancreatectomy.

PATHOLOGICAL AND PATHOPHYSIOLOGICAL FEATURES

The tumour arises from the beta islet cells and 70–90% are benign, usually small (less than 2 cm in diameter) and equally distributed throughout the pancreas. Less than 10% are multiple and about 10% are associated with MEN-1. They intermittently secrete insulin with consequent hypoglycaemic attacks.

CLINICAL FEATURES

History

Pre-coma – light-headedness, disorientation and sometimes disturbances of mood such as bad temper and rage – may go on to frank unconsciousness usually with spontaneous recovery although brain damage may occasionally occur. Many patients have previously been investigated for mental illness, epilepsy or suspected drug abuse before the diagnosis is finally established.

Physical findings

Clinical signs are usually absent although patients tend to be obese because they eat to avoid hypoglycaemia. The diagnosis is suspected when three criteria are met (Whipple's triad):

- attacks are precipitated by fasting
- hypoglycaemia (less than 2.0 mmol/L) is documented at the time of an attack
- symptoms are relieved by the administration of glucose.

INVESTIGATION

Biochemical and endocrine

Patients are fasted and the plasma glucose is monitored. When the plasma glucose falls to 2.0 mmol/L or less, further samples are taken for insulin, C-peptide and sulphonylurea. C-peptide is cleaved from the pro-insulin molecule and should therefore be elevated in the presence of a raised endogenous insulin, which is not the case if self-injection of insulin is taking place. Patients may need to be rescued from a fast with intravenous 50% dextrose.

Sulphonylurea assay will not be detectable unless the patient is in a self-induced hypoglycaemic attack.

Localisation

Once hypoglycaemia in the presence of hyper-insulinaemia has been verified, attempts are made to localise the tumour. This can be achieved with a combination of CT scans, visceral angiography, portal venous sampling and intraoperative ultrasound scanning.

MANAGEMENT

Medical

Before surgical exploration is contemplated, diazoxide, which inhibits the release of insulin, is administered to return the blood sugar concentration to normal. In the perioperative period, patients receive an intravenous infusion of 10% dextrose and potassium 40 meq/L.

Surgical

The only curative treatment for insulinoma is removal. Tumours can usually be enucleated, but for large ones (10%) it may be necessary to resect part of the pancreas.

Glucagonoma

This is a very rare malignant tumour with an estimated annual incidence of 1 in 20 million. It is an α-cell tumour of the pancreas which secretes glucagon. Most glucagonomas are solitary and, in the majority, liver and lung metastases have already occurred at the time of presentation.

CLINICAL FEATURES

There is a characteristic syndrome of migratory, necrolytic erythema, diabetes mellitus and weight loss. The rash is so typical that a pancreatic endocrine tumour may be diagnosed from this alone. Its cause is uncertain but it may be consequent upon a deficiency of zinc in the skin.

INVESTIGATION

Confirmation of the diagnosis is achieved by demonstrating an elevated plasma level of glucagon in the absence of other causes of hyperglucagonaemia (e.g. renal or hepatic failure). Most tumours are large and readily detected on CT.

MANAGEMENT

Medical

Before attempted removal by operation, patients may require nasogastric or parenteral feeding. Zinc deficiency is corrected. Octreotide, a somatostatin analogue, often improves the rash but does not confer any survival benefit.

Surgical

Surgical resection for cure is the treatment of choice but is open to only a minority of patients. For those with extensive and metastatic disease, debulking of the tumour and selective hepatic artery embolisation of liver secondaries achieve reasonable palliation.

Gastrinoma

EPIDEMIOLOGY

This is the second commonest islet cell tumour, although it frequently occurs in extrapancreatic sites, particularly the duodenum. Approximately one-third of patients with gastrinomas have the MEN I syndrome.

PATHOPHYSIOLOGY

Thirty per cent of gastrinomas are malignant and over 70% of these present with metastases. Their secretion of gastrin stimulates an excess production of gastric acid and leads to the development of the Zollinger–Ellison syndrome – severe peptic ulceration, often multiple, with a progressive and complicated course and sometimes found in the distal rather than the proximal duodenum.

CLINICAL FEATURES

Symptoms

Patients typically complain of epigastric pain secondary to peptic ulceration. Other symptoms include:

- diarrhoea
- weight loss
- dysphagia secondary to oesophagitis.

Physical findings

Physical examination is usually normal. Clinicians are alerted to the diagnosis by the atypical nature and severity of peptic ulcers seen on upper intestinal endoscopy and which are refractory to conventional anti-ulcer medication.

INVESTIGATION

Biochemical and hormonal

In the absence of anti-ulcer medication, the biochemical criteria for a diagnosis of gastrinoma are:

- elevated fasting levels of serum gastrin
- Increased gastric acid secretion.

Gastrin in the serum can also be elevated in achlorhydria, pernicious anaemia, atrophic gastritis, renal failure and hyperparathyroidism. In doubtful instances, the level of gastrin rises in response to provocation with secretin.

Imaging

The role of preoperative imaging for localisation is controversial and many tumours are not found until the patient is explored.

MANAGEMENT

Treatment is directed at both the tumour and the complications it produces.

Medical

Historically, the management of a gastrinoma syndrome was by total gastrectomy, which removed the target organ rather than the tumour so preventing the complication of peptic ulcer. The advent of omeprazole, a proton-pump inhibitor, has provided a very effective means of palliating the symptoms/complications of excess gastric acid and rendered gastric surgery virtually obsolete.

Surgical

A well localised tumour should be removed to endeavour to achieve a cure. However, half of those who undergo resection develop recurrence; nevertheless the tumours are usually slow-growing and up to 30% will survive many years on long-term omeprazole, even in the presence of a large tumour load.

VIPoma

The estimated annual incidence of VIPoma is 1 in 10 million. These islet cell tumours are always malignant and oversecrete vasointestinal peptide (VIP). They produce the Verner–Morrison syndrome of watery diarrhoea, hypokalaemic acidosis and achlorhydria.

CLINICAL FEATURES

In addition to the increased stool volume, patients may complain of lethargy and flushing.

Clinical examination is typically normal, although occasionally an abdominal mass and hepatomegaly are found.

INVESTIGATION

The diagnosis is made by detecting an elevated concentration of VIP in the serum in patients with hypokalaemic alkalosis. A combination of CT, ultrasound and visceral angiography localises the tumour.

MANAGEMENT

Medical

The electrolyte disturbances are corrected with intravenous fluids. Octreotide dramatically improves the secretory diarrhoea by inhibiting the release of VIP. In the presence of extensive metastases, the mainstay of treatment is cytotoxic chemotherapy rather than surgery.

Surgical
Resection of tumours is reserved for patients without metastases (approximately 50%).

Carcinoid tumours

Carcinoid tumours are clinically uncommon, although pathologically they are the commonest neuroendocrine tumour of the gastrointestinal tract (1% of those submitted to postmortem).

PATHOPHYSIOLOGY
Carcinoid tumours arise from the enterochromaffin (Kulchitsky) cells located throughout the body but principally within the intestinal submucosa (85%) and the main bronchi (10%). These cells are part of the amine precursor and uptake system (APUD). Carcinoid tumours secrete vasoactive substances (serotonin, bradykinin, prostaglandin, substance P), which are rapidly metabolised by the liver. A characteristic desmoplastic reaction is found in the mesentery with fibrosis and contraction and this may compound bowel obstruction or cause mesenteric angina.

CLINICAL FEATURES
Carcinoid tumours may present in a number of ways:

- incidental finding at laparotomy
- local physical complications – bowel obstruction, perforation, haemorrhage
- features of metastatic disease
- carcinoid syndrome (see below).

  Clinical examination is often normal.

INVESTIGATION
In the absence of secondary disease, these tumours may be difficult to localise. They are predominantly submucosal and are not seen on contrast examination of the gastrointestinal tract. Visceral angiography may detect the tumour from the corkscrew appearance of the mesenteric vessels produced by the desmoplastic reaction. The tumour expresses somatostatin receptors on its cell surface. Radiolabelled agents which bind to these receptors (e.g. octeotride) can be used to make a diagnosis by scintigraphic scanning.

MANAGEMENT
Gastrointestinal carcinoid tumours are classified according to their embryological site of origin.

Foregut. Gastric carcinoids are often (60%) associated with hypergastrinaemia, occasionally as part of the Zollinger–Ellison syndrome. In these instances the clinical course is typically indolent and the tumours can be adequately resected and progress kept under observation with the endoscope. The sporadic tumours (not associated with hypergastrinaemia) display a more aggressive tendency and necessitate surgical resection. Duodenal carcinoids are rare and usually adequately managed by local resection.

Midgut. Small bowel carcinoids present in a non-specific way, usually with abdominal pain. Two-thirds of patients develop metastases and one-third carcinoid syndrome. Tumours are sometimes multiple and associated with other malignancies, in particular adenocarcinoma of the small intestine.

Appendicular carcinoids are found in approximately 1:200 appendices, usually incidental findings during surgery for appendicitis. They most commonly occur at the tip of the appendix (90%) and appendicectomy is curative. If a tumour is at the base or larger than 2 cm in diameter, a right hemicolectomy is recommended.

Hindgut. Colorectal carcinoid tumours have a predilection for the right colon and typically present with abdominal pain and haemorrhage. Treatment consists of regional hemicolectomy with removal of lymph node metastases.

Metastatic disease. Even in the presence of metastases, resection of the primary is recommended to avoid bowel complications. In selected patients, it may be feasible to resect an hepatic metastasis.

PROGNOSIS
The prognosis of patients with a carcinoid tumour is relatively good. The most important factors are the site and stage of the primary disease. Favourable sites are the appendix and the bronchus where 5-year survival rates of over 94% can be achieved in small tumours. Liver metastases reduce 5-year survival to about 30%.

Carcinoid syndrome
PATHOPHYSIOLOGY
Carcinoid syndrome occurs when vasoactive substances (mainly 5-hydroxytryptamine – serotonin) are secreted and reach the systemic circulation in sufficient concentration to have a pharmacological effect. There are two circumstances:

- Large amounts of serotonin produced from a gut tumour saturate hepatic metabolic pathways.
- Hepatic or other metastases secrete directly into the systemic circulation.

  In more than 90%, the underlying cause is a primary tumour of midgut origin.

CLINICAL FEATURES
The characteristic symptoms of the syndrome are:

- cutaneous flushing
- diarrhoea
- valvular disease on the right side of the heart – tricuspid and pulmonary valve stenosis
- Bronchospasm.

In addition to hepatomegaly, the patient may be flushed and a heart murmur may be heard. Bowel sounds are often hyperactive.

INVESTIGATION
The syndrome is diagnosed by detecting elevated levels of 24-hour urinary 5-hydroxy-indolacetic acid (5-HIAA), the breakdown product of serotonin. CT and ultrasound demonstrate the presence of hepatic metastases.

MANAGEMENT
The liver is usually diffusely involved and less than 5% of affected patients have liver tumours amenable to surgical excision. The mainstay of treatment is octreotide, which suppresses hormone release. In addition, hepatic metastases may be embolised at selective hepatic angiography and this procedure can be repeated. Any patient undergoing operation must have preoperative preparation with octreotide in order to avoid a carcinoid crisis, a potentially fatal event caused by a surge in the release of secretory products at the time of operation.

Pituitary

EMBRYOLOGY
The pituitary gland develops from two distinct elements:

- An ectodermal outpocketing of the stomodeum known as Rathke's pouch produces the anterior lobe
- A downward extension of the diencephalon forms the posterior lobe.

ANATOMY AND PHYSIOLOGY
The normal pituitary is bean-shaped with a concave upper surface bearing the pituitary stalk of the posterior lobe which is attached to the hypothalamus. The gland lies in the pituitary fossa and is surrounded by a capsule which is continuous with the dura mater and is perforated on its upper surface for the pituitary stalk.

The pituitary gland produces many hormones whose secretion is regulated by the adjacent hypothalamus.

Tumours of the anterior pituitary

EPIDEMIOLOGY AND PATHOLOGICAL FEATURES
Tumours of the pituitary account for approximately 10% of intracranial neoplasms. Carcinoma of the pituitary is very rare. In general, pituitary tumours are benign, epithelial neoplasms three-quarters of which secrete inappropriate amounts of pituitary hormones.

Most secrete only one hormone. Those that produce either prolactin, growth hormone or ACTH account for 90–95% of secreting tumours. Rarely, these form part of the multiple endocrine neoplasia type 1 (MEN-1) syndrome.

CLINICAL FEATURES
History
The mode of presentation depends upon:

- local pressure effects
- the endocrine consequences of hypersecretion of a specific hormone.

Non-secreting tumours cause symptoms of raised intracranial pressure and visual field defects because of the proximity of the optic chiasm.

Physical findings
In addition to the features of the individual endocrine syndrome, there may be visual field defects, signs of raised intracranial pressure and other cranial nerve lesions.

INVESTIGATION
Lateral skull X-rays may show enlargement of the pituitary fossa or erosion of its floor. MRI reveals in great detail the surrounding soft tissue structures such as the pituitary stalk and optic chiasm. To show small tumours, it is possible to enhance the pictures using gadolinium-DTPA (diethylene-triamine-penta-acetic acid). The sensitivity of detection of tumours with MRI is over 90%, compared with about 50% with CT (Fig. 31.7), and, if available, it is the investigation of choice. When doubt

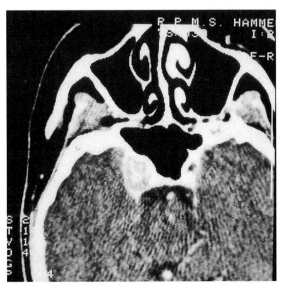

Fig 31.7 **CT of a pituitary tumour adjacent to right spenoidal sinus.** (By courtesy of Professor S. R. Bloom, Hammersmith Hospital)

exists after MRI, angiography and selective venous sampling of the petrosal sinuses may localise a tumour.

Prolactinoma

PATHOLOGICAL FEATURES

Prolactin-secreting tumours less than 1 cm in diameter (microprolactinomas) may be present in up to 10% of postmortems; most are clinically without significance. Tumours larger than 1 cm (macroprolactinomas) have specific effects in women and in men.

PATHOPHYSIOLOGY AND CLINICAL FEATURES

In women
- Delay in the onset of menstruation
- The menstrual periods may range from amenorrhoea to
- oligonemorrhoea although they are occasionally normal
- Sterility is present even if the periods are normal
- Galactorrhoea can vary from large quantities of milk production to a minor discharge
- Reduction in libido is common.

In men
- Galactorrhoea
- Decreased libido with associated impotence
- Change in secondary sexual characteristics such as reduced growth of facial and body hair and small soft testicles associated with apathy and weight gain.

MANAGEMENT

Medical
Bromocriptine, an agent derived from ergot, is a dopamine agonist and inhibits the release of prolactin. In the majority of patients, it returns the prolactin concentration to normal. Menstruation is quite rapidly restored and galactorrhoea is reduced. The drug is not always well tolerated because of side-effects, including nausea and vomiting, which can sometimes be limited by careful adjustment of the dose or by taking tablets intravaginally. If intolerance is severe, other ergot derivatives may be tried.

Surgical
Long-term treatment with bromocriptine for micro-prolactinomas is popular because their prolactin secretion is very modest. Some expert centres do, however, consider microsurgery (transsphenoidal microadenom-ectomy) which has the advantage that it can potentially cure the patient. For most macroprolactinomas, surgery is not curative and, when attempted, causes hypo-pituitism. Bromocriptine often induces tumour shrink-age. Radiotherapy may be added in an attempt to induce a cure.

Syndromes of growth hormone excess

Giantism

Growth hormone-secreting pituitary adenomas are manifest as gigantism in the prepubertal population before fusion of the bony epiphyses arrests growth. Affected individuals can reach an abnormal height, although what is truly abnormal must be judged against the standards of the local population. However, this end-point is rarely seen nowadays because of early recognition and prompt surgical excision of the tumour.

Acromegaly

Growth hormone excess after fusion of the epiphyses is a more insidious disorder often not diagnosed until many years after its onset. It is a rare condition with a prevalence of only 40 cases per million.

CLINICAL FEATURES
The main appearances are of overgrowth of the hands and feet and coarse facial features (Fig 31.8). In addition, there are physiological disturbances:

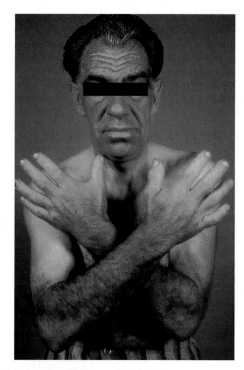

Fig 31.8 **Acromegaly.** Note coarse facial features due to increased growth of connective tissue and cartilage together with the typical broadening and enlargement of the fingers. (By courtesy of Professor S. R. Bloom, Hammersmith Hospital)

- glucose intolerance – diabetes mellitus
- osteoporsis
- hypertension.

INVESTIGATION

The diagnosis is confirmed by finding elevated plasma growth hormone levels which are not suppressed by a glucose tolerance test and by identifying a tumour as described above.

MANAGEMENT

General

It is important to make a distinction between cure and control. Cure is achieved when growth hormone levels are undetectable on random blood samples or in response to a glucose tolerance test; control is obtained when levels of growth hormone are significantly reduced. Most centres attempt to control rather than eradicate the excess of growth hormone. The treatment of acromegaly in part depends on the expertise of the local centre.

Operation or radiotherapy

Transsphenoidal operation or the use of radiotherapy often shrinks rather than completely removes the tumour and both are equally effective. The disadvantages of radiotherapy are that it takes several years for the growth hormone level to fall to an acceptable value but continued decline may eventually result in hypopituitarism.

Medical

Octreotide (a somatostatin analogue) administered as an adjunct to surgery or radiotherapy is effective in further reducing growth hormone levels.

Cushing's disease

AETIOLOGY

Cushing's disease is pituitary-dependent bilateral adrenocortico-hyperplasia secondary to ACTH secretion by a pituitary adenoma. The majority of affected patients are female, and they present with cushingoid features. The clinical description and diagnostic tests are detailed above. The differential diagnoses are adrenocortical adenoma/carcinoma, ectopic ACTH secretion and steroid therapy.

MANAGEMENT

Surgical

Transsphenoidal removal of the pituitary is considered the first-line treatment and gives an 80% chance of cure. For the remaining 20% of patients, it may be necessary to irradiate the pituitary. Used in isolation, radiotherapy can cure approximately 50% of adults but has a remark-

able 80% success rate in children. Bilateral adrenalectomy remains an option, particularly in patients not cured by either surgery or radiotherapy, but it is considered a salvage technique in the presence of failure of other treatments.

Medical

There is little role for long-term drug treatment unless there has been a failure of radiotherapy or surgery. Metyrapone, which blocks steroid synthesis by the adrenal gland, is used preoperatively.

Complications of management of pituitary disorders

Nelson's syndrome

This is a combination of skin hyperpigmentation and a rapidly expanding pituitary tumour which may arise as a consequence of adrenalectomy for Cushing's disease. The lessening of feedback inhibition by cortisol results in markedly elevated levels of ACTH, associated with a transformation of a microadenoma into a fast-growing and aggressive pituitary tumour. Pigmentation occurs as a direct effect of the high concentration of plasma ACTH, whose molecular structure closely resembles melanocyte-stimulating hormone (MSH). This hyperpigmentation is also observed in ectopic ACTH syndrome. To prevent Nelson's syndrome after bilateral adrenalectomy, the pituitary must be irradiated.

Diabetes insipidus

A deficiency of vasopressin (antidiuretic hormone, ADH) which is normally secreted from the posterior lobe. Its commonest cause is as a complication of operations on the pituitary. There is polyuria and compensatory polydipsia. Dehydration (pure water lack) may result. The diagnosis is confirmed by a high plasma osmolality in the presence of a low urine osmolality. Treatment is with synthetic vasopressin (DDAVP) administerd as a nasal spray.

Mixed tumours of the pituitary

It is sometimes possible to demonstrate production of more than one hormone by the cells of a pituitary tumour. Adenomas that produce both growth hormone and prolactin may cause acromegaly and mild features of hyperprolactinaemia. When surgical tumour samples are maintained in cell culture, it may be possible to demonstrate the secretion of multiple hormones in vitro which are not paralleled by multiple endocrine manifestations in vivo.

Thyrotrophic adenomas (TSH-producing adenomas)

These tumours are rare, very aggressive and account

for approximately 1% of pituitary neoplasms. They present with mild thyrotoxicosis and are best treated by radical surgery.

Gonadotrophin-producing tumours

These tumours are exceptionally rare and large, often with compression of the pituitary stalk. Patients therefore present with the unusual combination of panhypopituitarism with retained libido and potency because of the effects of luteinising hormone on testosterone secretion. Treatment is by transsphenoidal hypophysectomy.

Craniopharyngioma

It is believed that this tumour arises from nests of misplaced tissue of the hypophyseal recess (Rathke's pouch). Although most are suprasellar, some develop within the pituitary fossa. They account for approximately 3% of all pituitary tumours and have been reported at birth. Increase in tumour size is slow and presentation is with headaches, visual defects and failure of normal growth. Local pressure on the surrounding hypothalamic tissue by the tumour produces an intense gliosis, making total excision by the neurosurgeon not only difficult but also extremely dangerous.

Null-cell adenomas

So-called functionless tumours of the pituitary were in the past thought to be quite common. Many such adenomas are now shown by immunocytochemistry or tissue culture techniques to secrete a variety of hormones although these are produced at an insufficient level to cause endocrine syndromes. Their major presentation is with severe headaches associated with destruction of the pituitary, consequent hypopituitarism and associated severe visual defects. Small tumours are often found incidentally at postmortem.

Carcinoma of the pituitary and secondary deposits

Carcinoma of the pituitary is exceptionally rare and, when it occurs, rarely metastasises outside the brain. Secondary deposits in the pituitary are quite common. They are blood-borne and associated with carcinomatosis, particularly from primary growths in the bronchus or breast. It is rare for these tumours to produce specific clinical entities.

Multiple endocrine neoplasia

During embryonic life, the cells destined to form the endocrine organs arise from a single group in the neuroectoderm of the fetus. These cells, despite their widespread location in the body, have common histochemical features summarised by the acronym APUD (amine precursor uptake and decarboxylation). When such a tumour arises from one endocrine gland, it is likely that it is associated with tumour in other endocrine organs. The distribution of these tumours is not haphazard; certain associations are more common. Multiple endocrine neoplasia types I and II (MEN I, MEN II) are such autosomal dominant familial cancer syndromes.

MEN I

This is the more common type and involves the MEN 1 tumour suppressor gene on chromosome 11. The syndrome comprises neoplasia or hyperplasia of the parathyroids, the pancreatic islet cells, the pituitary and the thyroid, and rarely adrenal cortical tumours, carcinoids and lipomas. The pattern of neoplasia most commonly present is shown in Table 31.7. Not all tumours are present in any one patient. The likelihood of a particular tumour being found in a patient with MEN I and the effects of these disorders is also shown.

MANAGEMENT
Parathyroid hyperplasia

There is a very high recurrence rate following subtotal parathyroidectomy and some surgeons advocate total parathyroidectomy and lifelong maintenance with calcium and vitamin D supplementation.

Pancreatic islet cell hyperplasia

Pancreatic adenomas tend to be multiple and recur after partial pancreatectomy. A conservative approach is therefore adopted for gastrinomas with reliance on medical treatment. Insulinomas are treated by either distal pancreatectomy or enucleation of tumours that are in the pancreatic head.

Table 31.7
The pattern of neoplasia in MEN I.

Gland(s)	Abnormality	Frequency	Effect
Parathyroids	Hyperplasia	90%	Hyperparathyroidism
Pancreatic islets	Multiple adenomas	60–80%	Zollinger Ellison syndrome or insulinoma or glucagonoma or VIPoma
Pituitary chromophobes	Adenoma	50–70%	Prolactinoma or acromegaly
Thyroid	Adenoma	20%	Non-functional

Pituitary adenomas

These can be treated medically (see above) or by excision if medical treatment is unsuccessful.

Thyroid adenoma

The main consideration is to exclude malignancy and for this reason the adenoma is best excised.

MEN II

This is an inherited cancer syndrome characterised by medullary thyroid cancer (MTC) and its precursor C-cell hyperplasia. There are three distinct subtypes:

- familial – MTC is the sole feature
- MEN IIa – MTC, phaeochromocytoma and parathyroid hyperplasia
- MEN IIB – as with MEN IIA (although parathyroid involvement is rare) but with the additional developmental abnormalities of marfanoid features, mucosal neuromas and intestinal ganglioneuromas.

GENETICS

The MEN II gene has been identified as the *ret* proto-oncogene on chromosome 10 which encodes the transcellular tyrosine kinase receptor. Mutations of the *ret* proto-oncogene have also been identified in patients with Hirschprung's disease.

MANAGEMENT

Thyroid medullary carcinomas

See above for a discussion.

Adrenal tumours

These must be removed. Recurrence is likely and patients must be carefully followed up.

Parathyroid hyperplasia

The disease is usually mild and surgical resection is limited to the enlarged gland(s).

Screening relatives

See 'Medullary thyroid carcinoma' (above).

Urology deals with diseases and disorders of the male genitourinary and female urinary tracts. Urologists have been responsible for the introduction of many new techniques. These include the development and widespread use of endoscopes, lithotripsy and prosthetic inserts for hollow organs (stents).

Kidneys and ureters

SYMPTOMS ARISING FROM THE KIDNEY AND URETER

Systemic

Fever
Acute pyelonephritis is usually associated with a high fever (40°C). In infants and children there may not be any associated urinary symptoms. Chronic pyelonephritis is not associated with fever. Swinging pyrexia is often a feature of renal carcinoma.

General malaise and weight loss
These are often seen – as in diseases of other systems – with cancer or chronic infection. They may also be features of chronic renal failure.

Pain
Pain may be perceived at the surface directly over the area of involvement: local renal pain is felt in the flank and costovertebral angle. It is typically a dull, constant ache and related to distension of the renal capsule. However, many renal diseases progress slowly and may not be associated with such pain until some secondary event occurs to cause acute capsular distention. Examples are cancer, tuberculosis, polycystic disease, staghorn calculi and hydronephrosis secondary to congenital pelviureteric junction obstruction (Fig. 32.1).

Pain may also be experienced at the surface further away from the site of origin. Such pain is often called 'referred', but it is being felt at the surface representation of the segment in which it originates. Thus the severe pain of ureteric colic which occurs in waves and is often associated with vomiting may be felt in the testicle (T11 to T12). A stone in the lower ureter may cause pain in the scrotal wall (L1) and in the bladder.

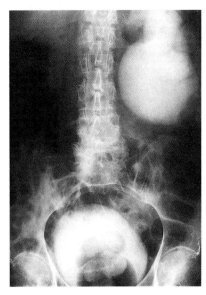

Fig 32.1 **An intravenous urogram of a congenital obstruction of the left pelviureteric junction.**

Table 32.1
Common causes of haematuria

Systemic	Nephrological	Urological
Anticoagulants	Mesangial IgA disease	Carcinoma of kidney
Sickle cell disease	Glomerulonephritis	Urothelial tumours
Bacterial endocarditis (emboli)	Renal infarcts	Stones
Henoch–Schönlein purpura	Urinary infection Tuberculosis	Schistosomiasis Benign prostatic hypertrophy
	Polycystic disease	Trauma Infection
Cyclophosphamide Non-steroidal anti-inflammatory agents		

Oliguria and anuria

A reduced or absent urine output may be caused by underperfusion of the kidney as a result of shock from blood, water and electrolyte loss or in sepsis. Bilateral ureteric obstruction or injury to a solitary kidney are other causes.

Anaemia and its symptoms

These are invariable in chronic renal failure but also occur as a result of renal tumours, chronic infection and blood loss.

Local

Haematuria

Haematuria always requires full investigation. The additional presence of proteinuria and abnormal red cell morphology on microscopy are more suggestive of a renal cause. Common causes of haematuria are shown in Table 32.1.

CLINICAL EXAMINATION OF THE UPPER URINARY TRACT

Tongue

In that water and electrolyte disturbance are common in urological disease, the tongue should be examined for dryness and at the same time the breath smelt for the characteristic fishy smell of uraemia.

Abdominal inspection

In children, inspection is the most reliable method of identifying a renal mass, which may be seen in the upper abdomen or inferred from fullness or oedema in this area, the latter implying perinephric infection.

Palpation

The patient should lie supine on a firm surface. The kidney is lifted by one hand placed in the costovertebral angle. On deep inspiration, the kidney moves downwards. When it is at its lowest, the other (anterior) hand is pressed firmly backwards beneath the costal margin in an effort to trap the kidney below that point. The anterior hand can then palpate the size, shape and consistency of the kidney as it slips back into its normal position. The left kidney should be examined from the left side. The right kidney lies lower than the left and it is sometimes possible to feel the lower pole even if it is normal. The left cannot usually be felt unless it is enlarged or displaced.

Enlargement of the kidney suggests polycystic disease, a renal cyst, tumour or hydronephrosis.

Percussion

Renal masses are frequently soft and difficult to feel. They can often be more easily outlined by percussion.

Auscultation

A bruit may be heard over the upper abdomen. Possible causes are renal artery stenosis, aneurysm of the renal artery and an arteriovenous fistula.

INVESTIGATION

A combination of haematological, biochemical, bacteriological, radiological, isotopic and endoscopic examination is needed to achieve an accurate, rapid, cost-effective determination of the probable diagnosis and requirements for treatment.

Examination of the urine

Technique. A timed urine collection may be required for assessment of renal function (see 'Creatinine clearance' below), proteinuria or the excretion of substances associated with stone formation.

It is best to examine a freshly voided specimen taken midway through the act of micturition. Many of the details in the collection of this midstream (MSU) sample are shrouded in rituals which are mostly a waste of time and money. Specimens collected from women who have not undergone any special preparation and who void into disposable plastic cups show a 95% concordance with a catheter specimen. In addition, genital cleaning makes little difference to the bacterial count. The most important factor is rapid transport of specimens to the laboratory.

They are usually collected into a clean polystyrene cup and then transferred without spillage to a sterile universal container. In younger children, a plastic bag is attached around the urethral meatus. In girls, catheterisation with a fine catheter is appropriate, although, in either sex, suprapubic needle aspiration is easy to perform, particularly if hydration is adequate and the bladder full. The suprapubic area is cleansed, local anaesthetic injected to raise an intradermal wheal 1–2 cm above the pubic symphysis. A 10 mL syringe with a 22 gauge needle is inserted perpendicularly through the abdominal wall into the bladder, maintaining gentle suction with the syringe so that the urine is aspirated as soon as the bladder is entered.

Colour and appearance. Overtly, bloody urine is usually unmistakable. However, red urine can result from:

- betacyanin excretion after beetroot ingestion
- myoglobinuria, the result of muscle trauma
- haemoglobinuria after haemolysis.

Chemical tests. Chemically impregnated reagent strips permit the simultaneous rapid performance of a number of tests, including the presence of blood, protein, ketones, glucose, nitrites and leucocyte esterase. These tests can be useful for screening and show excellent correlation with more extensive laboratory examination.

Microscopy. Examination of the centrifuged urinary sediment allows identification of red blood cells (which always requires further investigation), white blood cells, bacteria and casts. Cytological examination for malignant cells is also possible.

The presence of five to eight white blood cells per high-powered field is abnormal (pyuria) and, if associated with bacteria, indicates a urinary infection. Sterile pyuria – white blood cells but without bacteria – occurs in:

- tuberculosis of the urinary tract
- urinary stones
- recovery from urinary infection.

Culture enables the organism present to be identified and a prediction made of which antibiotics may be effective in treatment.

Serum creatinine concentration and creatinine clearance

Creatinine in serum is the end-product of the metabolism of creatine in skeletal muscle which takes place at a

---

Box 32.1

Creatinine clearance

Requirements

Timed urine sample (usually 24 hour)

Blood sample for creatinine concentration taken during the 24-hour urine collection period

Measurements

Urine volume (mL/min or per 24 hours) = V

Urine creatinine concentration (mmol/L) = U

Plasma creatinine concentration (mmol/L) = P

Calculation

$$\text{Clearance} = \frac{U \times V}{P} \text{ mL/min}$$

Interpretation

The creatinine clearance is the amount of blood completely cleared of the substance per minute and, because creatinine is completely filtered through the glomerulus, clearance approximates glomerular filtration rate (GFR).

---

fairly steady rate. The molecule is filtered through the glomerulus and its clearance is approximately equal to the glomerular filtration rate (GFR). The serum creatinine concentration remains within the normal range until approximately 50% of renal function has been lost. The determination of creatinine clearance is shown in Box 32.1.

Blood urea concentration

The amount of urea in the blood is also related to the GFR. However, it is more influenced by factors external to the kidney, e.g.:

- dietary protein intake
- endogenous sources of nitrogen in the gut such as a gastrointestinal haemorrhage
- rate of urine production, which is the outcome of a number of factors including the state of hydration.

Approximately two-thirds of renal function must be lost before a significant rise in the blood urea concentration takes place. The measurement is less specific as an index of renal function than is creatinine clearance.

Serum calcium concentration

The level of serum calcium should be routinely measured in patients with renal stones to identify hyperparathyroidism and alterations in vitamin D metabolism in those with renal failure. Calcium concentration may also be elevated in patients with renal cell carcinoma either as part of a paraneoplastic syndrome caused by the secretion of parathyroid hormone-like substance or from bone destruction by secondary deposits.

Serum alkaline phosphatase

The concentration may be elevated as part of a paraneoplastic syndrome in renal cell carcinoma or from bone deposits in patients with genitourinary or other cancer.

Radiography

Abdominal plain film is frequently called a KUB (kidneys, ureter, bladder) and is the preliminary exposure taken in any radiological study of the urinary tract. It is always the first film to be examined before reporting on any contrast study and can avoid pitfalls (Fig. 32.2) and yield a great deal of information (Fig. 32.3).

X-ray contrast studies. Some water-soluble preparations that contain iodine can be administered by several routes, including directly into blood vessels. All procedures which use intravascular contrast media carry a small but definite (~ 5%) risk of an adverse reaction. Most are minor and include nausea, vomiting, itching, rash or flushing. Cardiopulmonary adverse reactions can occur but are rare (1:40 000), although they may be life-threatening or fatal. The contraindications to the use of intravascular contrast to image the urinary tract are shown in Box 32.2.

Patients with relative allergic contraindications can be given corticosteroids. However, there is little evidence to indicate conclusively that their prophylactic use is efficacious.

Intravenous urogram (IVU) is the most frequently used contrast investigation. Many of the items listed in

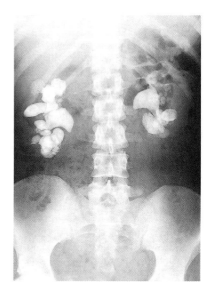

Fig 32.2 **Plain film of the abdomen.** Bilateral renal calculi which could be mistaken for an intravenous urogram are shown.

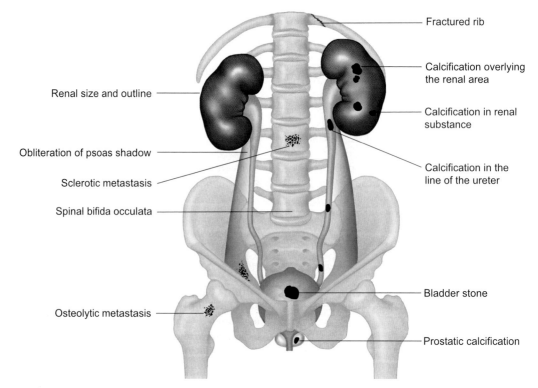

Fractured rib

Calcification overlying the renal area

Calcification in renal substance

Calcification in the line of the ureter

Renal size and outline

Obliteration of psoas shadow

Sclerotic metastasis

Spinal bifida occulata

Bladder stone

Prostatic calcification

Osteolytic metastasis

Fig 32.3 **A guide to the interpretation of a plain abdominal X-ray.**

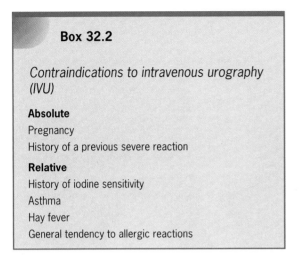

Box 32.2

Contraindications to intravenous urography (IVU)

Absolute
Pregnancy
History of a previous severe reaction

Relative
History of iodine sensitivity
Asthma
Hay fever
General tendency to allergic reactions

Figure 32.4 may also be elicited or confirmed by urography and additional information also obtained (Fig. 32.5).

Those with moderate renal failure are unable to excrete the usual dose of contrast media at a concentration sufficient to provide an image, and a larger than usual dose is required. It is usual to restrict fluids before an IVU so as to concentrate the urine, but this should not be done in diabetics.

Retrograde ureterography may be necessary if the IVU is unsatisfactory. A cystoscopy and the placement

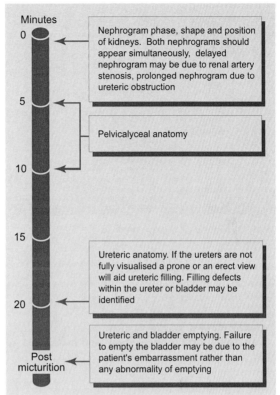

Minutes

0 — Nephrogram phase, shape and position of kidneys. Both nephrograms should appear simultaneously, delayed nephrogram may be due to renal artery stenosis, prolonged nephrogram due to ureteric obstruction

5 — Pelvicalyceal anatomy

10

15 — Ureteric anatomy. If the ureters are not fully visualised a prone or an erect view will aid ureteric filling. Filling defects within the ureter or bladder may be identified

20

Post micturition — Ureteric and bladder emptying. Failure to empty the bladder may be due to the patient's embarrassment rather than any abnormality of emptying

Fig 32.5 **Additional information from an IVU.**

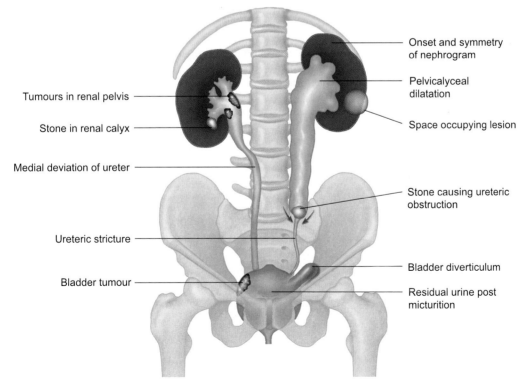

Onset and symmetry of nephrogram

Pelvicalyceal dilatation

Space occupying lesion

Tumours in renal pelvis

Stone in renal calyx

Medial deviation of ureter

Stone causing ureteric obstruction

Ureteric stricture

Bladder diverticulum

Bladder tumour

Residual urine post micturition

Fig 32.4 **A guide to the interpretation of an intravenous urogram.**

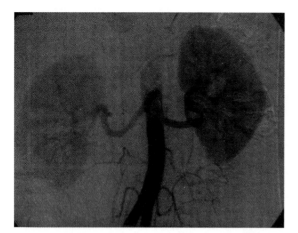

Fig 32.6 **A normal renal arteriogram showing single arteries to both kidneys.**

of a catheter in the ureter are required. Radio-opaque contrast medium is then introduced directly into the renal pelvis or ureter.

Antegrade pyelography Contrast media is introduced either through a nephrostomy tube (nephrostogram) or by direct injection into the renal pelvis via a percutaneous needle puncture.

Arteriography (Fig. 32.6) is most frequently done to evaluate:

- possible causes of renovascular hypertension
- anatomical suitability of potential live related kidney donors
- vascular anatomy before surgery.

Arteriographic techniques can also be used for therapy. Arteriovenous fistulae and bleeding vascular renal tumours can be embolised and renal artery stenoses dilated.

Micturating cystourethrography is done to determine the presence of vesicoureteric reflux. Contrast medium is introduced into the bladder via a urethral catheter which is then removed. Dynamic X-ray studies are made during voiding and contrast may be seen to reflux up the ureter(s) (Fig. 32.7). The urethra is also delineated and an assessment of residual urine can be made.

Ultrasonography

Ultrasound is used in the upper urinary tract to:

- determine the size of the kidneys and the presence of pelvicalyceal dilatation, which may be due to obstruction in patients with renal failure when intravenous urography is unlikely to be effective
- distinguish between solid and cystic renal masses
- identify non-opaque renal stones.

Ultrasonography cannot provide detailed visualisation of the calyces and pelvis, nor does it outline an

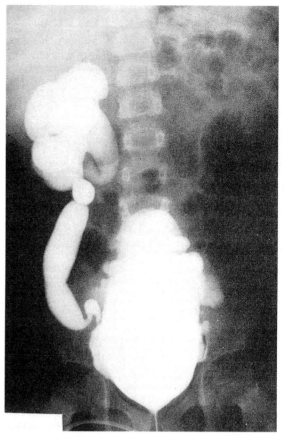

Fig 32.7 **A micturating cystogram which shows reflux and renal scarring.**

undilated ureter or provide functional information about the upper urinary tract.

Computed tomography (CT)

The principal uses of CT are:

- diagnosis and staging of tumours (Fig. 32.8)
- delineation and diagnosis of retroperitoneal masses
- identification and classification of renal trauma.

Magnetic resonance imaging (MRI)

The main advantages of MRI are as follows:

- it does not involve the use of ionising radiation
- it permits multiplanar imaging
- it is non-invasive
- it allows greater tissue contrast than do other modalities.

Patients who should not undergo MRI include:

- those with cardiac pacemakers
- those with ferromagnetic metallic foreign bodies, including ones that have been placed surgically.

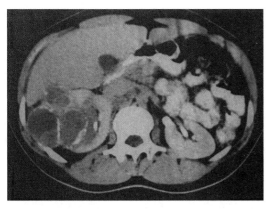

Fig 32.8 **A CT scan showing a right renal tumour with extension into the vena cava.**

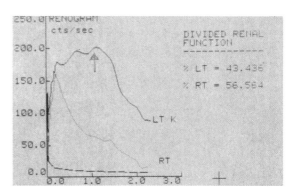

Fig 32.10 **A DTPA renogram following frusemide (arrow) showing clearance of the isotope which refutes a diagnosis of obstruction.**

Radioisotope studies

There are two types of radioisotope study:

- *dynamic*, in which the function of the kidney is examined over a period of time
- *static*, which involve imaging of a radiopharmaceutical taken up and retained by the renal tubules.

Dynamic. Diethylene-triamine-penta-acetic acid (DTPA) is actively secreted by the renal tubules. It is labelled with technetium-99m and administered intravenously. There is a progressive accumulation of the isotope followed by excretion which is recorded over each kidney by a gamma camera (Fig. 32.9) to give quantitative data on excretory function. The information can be used to demonstrate the degree of obstruction in one kidney. Progressive uptake of isotope may also occur in a dilated but unobstructed system, but this can be distinguished from obstruction by the rapid clearance of the isotope after the intravenous injection of frusemide (Fig. 32.10). Technetium-99m mercaptoacetyltriglycine (MAG3) is rapidly cleared by tubular secretion and is not retained in the parenchyma of normal kidneys. Due to a much smaller volume of distribution and faster clearance, MAG3 is replacing DTPA in diuretic renography.

Static Dimercaptosuccinic acid (DMSA) is taken up by tubular cells in proportion to their function. The same technique is used as for DTPA scanning: labelling with ^{99m}Tm, intravenous injection and counting with a gamma camera. The relative function of each kidney can then be determined. The investigation is of value in identifying ectopic kidneys, renal scarring and pseudo-tumours in which normally functioning renal tissue is abnormally placed within the substance of the kidney.

Disorders of the kidney

Congenital anatomical abnormalities

The developing kidney is lobulated and becomes kidney-shaped at around 34 weeks of intrauterine life. Persistence of such lobulation into adult life is not of significance. *Renal agenesis* (the absence of a kidney, ureter and half the trigone of the bladder) has an incidence of 1:450 and is important in the context of trauma. A solitary kidney undergoes compensatory hypertrophy. *Renal aplasia* is associated with a small

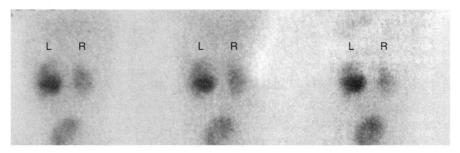

Fig 32.9 **A DTPA renogram which is suggestive of an obstructed left kidney.**

number of nephrons and undeveloped pelvis and ureter. A *hypoplastic kidney* is a miniature adult organ commonly associated with the development of hypertension and infection for either of which nephrectomy may be indicated. An *ectopic kidney* may cause confusion by presenting as an abdominal or, more usually, a pelvic swelling.

Renal cysts

True cysts occur in three circumstances:

- a solitary cyst
- multicystic kidney
- polycystic kidney

Solitary cysts

The aetiology is unknown. Symptoms are usually absent and the cyst is found during investigation of the urinary tract for other reasons. Very occasionally there may be pain or obstruction of urine drainage and only then is treatment required by percutaneous aspiration under ultrasound guidance.

Multicystic kidney

Multiple cysts may be found in either dysplastic or otherwise normal organs. In a poorly functioning dysplastic kidney, a nephrectomy is indicated if pain, infection or hypertension is a feature. Multiple cysts in an adult kidney with normal function do not usually warrant treatment. However, if there is pain, aspiration under ultrasound guidance is done.

Polycystic kidney disease

There are two types: infantile and adult.

Autorecessive polycystic renal disease

Infantile disease is inherited as an autosomal recessive and presents within the first 9 months of life with gross abdominal distension because of renal masses. The child is pale, has easily palpable kidneys and renal failure. Most infantile polycystic disease has a hopeless prognosis and, without dialysis or transplantation (see Ch. 13), death takes place before the age of 18 months.

Autodominant polycystic renal disease

This is ten times more common than autorecessive disease. The relatively common occurrence of this condition makes it important, especially as 10% of patients who require renal replacement therapy have this condition.

Aetiology and pathological features
A single gene defect linked to the alpha-haemoglobin gene on the short arm of chromosome 16 is inherited as an autosomal dominant. The precise mechanism of cyst formation is unknown. They are present in infancy and, with advancing age, enlarge to cause progressive loss of intervening renal tissue and the development of renal failure. The following can be associated:

- berry aneurysms of the cerebral vessels
- malignant renal neoplasms
- polycythaemia
- cysts in other organs – liver, thyroid, breast and pancreas
- hypertension.

Clinical features
The common presenting age is between 25 and 50 years. Symptoms include:

- loin pain from increase in size of the kidneys
- acute loin pain with haematuria because of haemorrhage into the cysts
- hypertension and its associated sequelae.

General examination commonly reveals hypertension. There may be features of chronic renal failure. The kidneys are large and irregular (Fig. 32.11). Occasionally there is hepatomegaly from cystic involvement of that organ.

Diagnosis
A definitive diagnosis can be made by intravenous urography, which shows the pelvis of each kidney elongated and attenuated by the smooth surface of adjacent cysts. However, ultrasonography is less invasive and more directly confirms the presence of multiple cysts in the kidneys and other organs. The investigation should be used to screen children who are the offspring of parents known to have the condition.

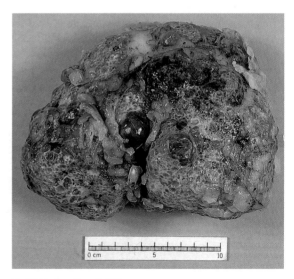

Fig 32.11 **A polycystic kidney.**

MANAGEMENT

In the majority, the disease is progressive and ultimately necessitates renal replacement by dialysis and/or transplantation (Ch. 13). Failure to control hypertension accelerates the loss of kidney function.

Urinary infection

Urinary tract infection is the most common bacterial infection in humans of all ages. The incidence and sequelae of urinary infections, their diagnosis and treatment all vary with age. By the time adolescence is reached, 1–2% of boys and 5% of girls will have had a urinary infection.

Infection in children

AETIOLOGY AND PATHOLOGICAL FEATURES

Organisms that ascend from the urethral meatus are usually Gram-negative faecal flora. *E. coli* and *Proteus* spp. are the commonest. Vesicoureteric reflux or other anatomical abnormalities may be associated. If infection ascends to the growing kidneys (up to the age of 5 years) and is repeated, renal damage occurs with progressive scarring (the outcome of healing of a cortical abscess) and the development of renal failure and hypertension. Infection is one of the few preventable forms of renal failure.

CLINICAL FEATURES

The younger the child, the more non-specific the symptoms (see Box 32.3). Older children may complain of:

- loin pain
- increased frequency
- burning on micturition
- haematuria
- enuresis

Box 32.3

Non-specific symptoms associated with urinary tract infection in children

Vomiting and diarrhoea
Jaundice
Weight loss
High fever
Unexplained screaming attacks

Specific signs are absent but there may be some tenderness in one or both renal angles.

INVESTIGATION

Bacterial culture

Urine should be obtained for culture and antibiotic sensitivities before antibiotic therapy is begun.

Imaging

Any child with an infection must be thoroughly investigated to find out if there is an anatomical abnormality.

Ultrasound identifies congenital abnormalities, dilatation of the renal pelvis and ureter, urinary stones and renal scarring.

Micturating cystourethrography is done, after the urine has been made sterile, to identify and quantitate vesicoureteral reflux, scarring and the adequacy of bladder emptying (Fig. 32.7).

DMSA renography is the best way of identifying renal scarring.

MANAGEMENT

Infants and children with a normal IVU and micturating cystogram

A single course of an appropriate broad-spectrum antibiotic (amoxycillin, trimethoprin, augmentin and cephalosporins are among the most effective) should be given for 5–7 days. Thereafter, follow-up for a year with monthly urine specimens for bacterial analysis. Because of the risk of renal scarring in infants, prophylactic low-dose antibiotics are given until the age of 2 years. In older children, prophylaxis is limited to 6 months. Clinical recurrence requires further antibiotic therapy and full investigation.

Children with vesicoureteric reflux and/or renal scarring

The treatment of the acute episode is as above. Thereafter, prophylaxis up to the age of 5 years is essential. Ultrasound examination of the kidneys is done at yearly intervals. A direct cystogram is done up to the age of 2 years, if the reflux has not resolved. An indirect cystogram using MAG3 renography is performed annually up to the age of 5 years. The reflux resolves spontaneously in 80% and, in consequence, there has been a move away from its surgical correction. Indications for surgery are not clearly defined but include:

- recurrent infection in the presence of antibiotic prophylaxis
- persistent loin pain or fever
- poor compliance with prophylaxis
- progressive scarring.

Acute pyelonephritis

AETIOLOGY

Aerobic Gram-negative bacteria which ascend from the urethra and genital tract are the principal cause; haematogenous infection is infrequent. Once infection is established in the bladder, its ascent to the kidney is the consequence of:

- microbial virulence
- presence of vesicoureteric reflux
- quality of ureteric peristalsis.

CLINICAL FEATURES

Symptoms are:

- high fever, sweating and often vomiting
- dull ache in the loin
- increased frequency
- dysuria
- haematuria.

The only specific sign is loin tenderness.

INVESTIGATION

Urine

This is turbid and contains protein and blood. Organisms, red cells, white blood cells and debris may be seen on direct microscopy. Culture is essential.

Blood

Apart from routine investigations, a blood culture may identify the pathogen responsible.

Imaging

KUB may show renal enlargement or obliteration of the renal outline by perirenal oedema or the presence of a radio-opaque stone. An IVU in the acute phase of the disease is of little value because renal excretion is reduced.

Ultrasonography may identify a radiolucent stone but, more importantly, may show dilatation of the renal pelvis which suggests an obstruction that needs urgent relief (Fig. 32.12).

MANAGEMENT

There is no need to wait for the results of bacterial culture and sensitivity tests. Antibiotic therapy should begin at once. The majority of infections are caused by organisms that are sensitive to trimethoprim, amoxycillin or cephalosporins. The urine is re-cultured a week after treatment is complete to ensure that the infection has been eradicated. In women, a high vaginal swab should also be taken to exclude the development of candidiasis which is a common sequel of treatment with broad-spectrum antibiotics and can cause recurrent infection of the lower urinary tract.

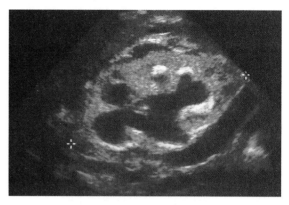

Fig 32.12 **Ultrasound examination showing dilatation of the renal pelvis, a result of ureteric obstruction.**

Once the acute episode has settled, any correctable precipitating cause is dealt with.

Chronic pyelonephritis

This is a confusing term. It is largely a radiological diagnosis based on the finding of shrunken kidneys with an irregular outline because of cortical scarring – the end result of cortical abscesses. The calcyes are clubbed (Fig. 32.13).

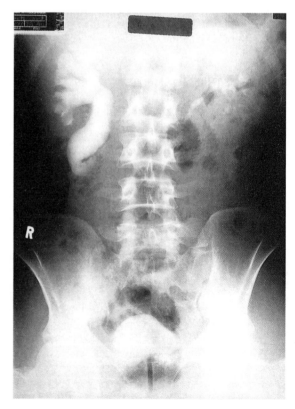

Fig 32.13 **An IVU showing chronic pyelonephritis, a shrunken scarred right kidney with calyceal clubbing.**

CLINICAL FEATURES

The symptoms are those of:

- urinary tract infection
- renal failure
- hypertension.

There are no specific signs. Most patients are hypertensive, while some are normotensive due to the development of a salt (Na^+) losing nephropathy.

MANAGEMENT

Existing infection must be eradicated and recurrence prevented by long-term continuous antimicrobial prophylaxis. If hypertension is associated with unilateral disease, a nephrectomy may be indicated.

Renal abscess

AETIOLOGY AND PATHOLOGICAL FEATURES

There are two causes:

- *Haematogenous spread* – usually of *Staphylococcus aureus* – from a distant site. The condition is common in drug abusers and diabetics. Abscesses are usually multiple and in the cortex.
- *Acute pyelonephritis*, often with obstruction, causes medullary abscesses which are more common.

CLINICAL FEATURES

Symptoms

There may be a history of recurrent urinary tract infection or parenteral administration of therapeutic (insulin) or other non-therapeutic substances. The patient is often acutely ill with high fever and loin pain.

Signs

In *cortical abscess*, signs are of:

- flank tenderness
- palpable mass
- erythema of the skin of the loin
- clear urine.

In *medullary abscess*, signs are of:

- flank tenderness
- obvious pyuria.

INVESTIGATION

This is as for acute pyelonephritis. Ultrasonography can identify a renal abscess but it is difficult to distinguish this from a cystic-necrotic renal carcinoma. However, percutaneous needle aspiration, under ultrasound guidance, confirms the presence of pus.

MANAGEMENT

Management is with systemic antibiotic therapy. Percutaneous drainage of any collections seen on ultrasound is carried out. In medullary abscess, there is subsequent correction of any precipitating factor.

Perinephric abscess

AETIOLOGY AND PATHOLOGICAL FEATURES

The majority of perinephric abscesses result from rupture of a cortical abscess into the perinephric tissue. They therefore lie between the renal capsule and perirenal fascia. A large collection may point posterolaterally over the iliac crest (Fig. 32.14). The organisms are the same as those found in renal abscesses. There may be an underlying infected hydronephrosis (pyonephrosis).

CLINICAL FEATURES

The onset tends to be slower than in renal abscess. The patient has a fever and complains of loin pain.

Signs are of:

- tenderness over the affected kidney
- large mass
- pleural effusion on chest examination.

INVESTIGATION

Blood

There will be a marked leucocytosis.

Imaging

Plain X-ray of the abdomen shows a soft tissue mass in the flank with obliteration of the renal and

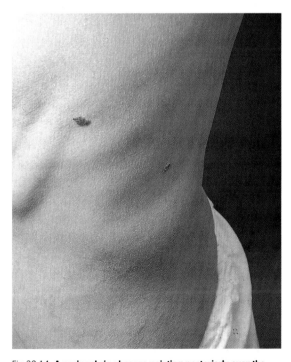

Fig 32.14 **A perinephric abscess pointing posteriorly over the iliac crest.**

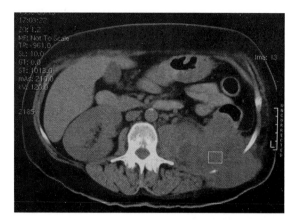

Fig 32.15 **A CT scan of a patient with a perinephric abscess and pyonephrosis.**

psoas shadows. A stone in the renal pelvis may be seen. Because of spasm of the lumbar muscles, there is often a scoliosis with the concavity towards the affected kidney. Gas – produced by coliform or other organisms – may be seen in the renal collecting system or around the kidney. An IVU may show delayed excretion or non-function.

Ultrasonography may demonstrate a hydronephrosis as well as delineating the extent of the abscess.

CT scan may also outline the mass (Fig. 32.15).

MANAGEMENT

Percutaneous drainage under ultrasound guidance may be adequate but an open operation is sometimes required. Nephrectomy is often needed because of underlying kidney disease.

COMPLICATIONS

Ureteric stenosis because of periureteric fibrosis is a common sequel. If the kidney has not been removed, the patency of the ureter should be assessed after 1 month.

Renal tuberculosis

EPIDEMIOLOGY

The condition is on the increase in the UK. There are three known reasons:

- influx of migrants from developing countries where the disease is endemic
- tuberculosis in patients with the acquired immune deficiency syndrome (AIDS)
- tuberculosis in drug users.

However, in addition, renal tuberculosis is reappearing in those that do not meet the above criteria.

AETIOLOGY AND PATHOLOGICAL FEATURES

The organism reaches the genitourinary tract by haematogenous spread from a focus in the lung which is often asymptomatic. The kidney is usually the primary site and other organs become involved by shedding of bacteria into the urine. The progress of the disease is slow and, in a patient who is otherwise in good condition, it may take many years to destroy the kidney. Involvement of the renal pelvis and ureter may lead to stricture and hydronephrosis. Infection of the bladder wall causes progressive fibrosis and ultimately a shrunken bladder.

CLINICAL FEATURES

The slow evolution of the disease means that, in a patient with an involved kidney, years may elapse before symptoms occur, although occasionally there may be a dull ache in the flank and haematuria. Spread to the bladder may cause increased frequency and pain on moderate bladder distension and at micturition. Rarely, the first presentation is when the patient discovers a painless epididymal swelling.

There are no specific signs.

INVESTIGATION

Urine

The finding of persistent pyuria without pyogenic organisms on ordinary culture is an indication to collect a first morning specimen on at least three separate occasions for culture for tubercle bacilli. Although a negative result does not exclude the disease, a positive one – which is obtained in a high percentage of samples – is confirmatory. If there is strong presumptive evidence for the presence of tuberculosis, but a negative result, cultures should be repeated, because not only is it necessary to be certain that genitourinary tuberculosis is present, but also the antimicrobial sensitivity must be determined before treatment is begun.

Imaging

Chest X-ray may show evidence of tuberculosis.

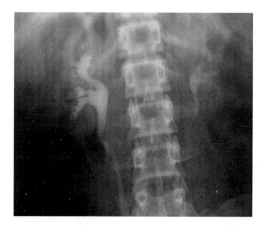

Fig 32.16 **A tuberculous abscess cavity in the upper pole of the right kidney in a patient who presented with an epididymal swelling.**

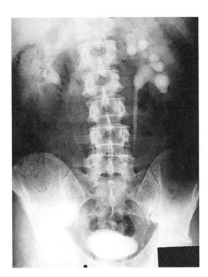

Fig 32.17 **An IVU which demonstrates a left ureteric stricture after treatment for renal tuberculosis.**

IVU may demonstrate calcification in the kidney, an abscess cavity or dilated calcyes (Fig. 32.16). Absence of function is a consequence of complete destruction – auto-nephrectomy.

MANAGEMENT

Management is by chemotherapy. Treatment does not usually need to exceed 9 months and consists of a combination of rifampicin, isoniazid and pyrazinamide. During this treatment, repeated examination by ultrasound or IVU is required to make sure that a ureteric stricture does not develop as the tuberculous lesions heal (Fig. 32.17).

Renal trauma

Injury to the kidney is not uncommon, but it rarely results in an urgent life-threatening problem.

AETIOLOGY AND PATHOLOGICAL FEATURES

Closed trauma follows road traffic accidents and sporting injuries and may be accompanied by fracture of the 11th and 12th ribs and injuries to the liver and spleen.

Penetrating injuries by knives, bullets and a diagnostic biopsy may, in the first two instances, be associated with other abdominal and thoracic damage. A classification of renal injuries is in Box 32.4.

CLINICAL FEATURES

No symptoms may be attributable to the kidney especially in multiple trauma (p. 000). An otherwise well patient may complain of loin pain and haematuria.

Signs of renal trauma are:

Box 32.4

Classification of renal injuries

1. **Minor renal trauma** (85% of cases) – renal contusion, subcapsular haematoma, superficial cortical laceration. These injuries rarely require surgical exploration.

2. **Major renal trauma** (15% of cases) – deep corticomedullary lacerations which may extend into the collecting system. Extravasation of urine into the perirenal space may occur along with large retroperitoneal and perinephric haematomas.

3. **Vascular injury** (1% of blunt trauma) – there may be total avulsion of the artery or vein or partial avulsion of the segmental branches of these vessels

- haematuria
- bruising over the ribs posteriorly
- evidence of penetrating injury
- tenderness and guarding in the loin
- hypotension
- expanding mass
- localised bruit in arteriovenous fistula.

INVESTIGATION

Imaging

Plain X-ray may show fractures of the 10th, 11th or 12th ribs.

CT scan with contrast is now the investigation of choice. It will accurately assess:

- absence of function on the affected side but a normal contralateral kidney
- absence of function and no contralateral kidney
- the extent of injury
- lacerations
- extravasation
- surrounding haemorrhage
- vessel injury
- non-renal injuries.

Renal angiography is required in the following circumstances:

- non-function on CT
- persistent severe haematuria which might require embolisation
- presence or development of a bruit
- late development of hypertension in a patient who has recovered from an injury.

MANAGEMENT

Any patient with a renal injury should be at rest in bed and have the usual observations All urine passed is examined for blood.

Penetrating injury

Because there is a high risk of injuries to other organs, surgical exploration is usual. Other injuries take priority and the kidney is explored only if there is evidence on preoperative evaluation or at operation of major damage. Nephrectomy may be inevitable.

Closed injury

Treatment is initially non-operative with careful continued assessment. Prophylactic antibiotics are administered. Unless one of the more severe injuries listed in Box 32.4 is present, most injuries resolve, although a relatively prolonged period of stay in hospital may be required. The incidence of later surgical intervention to manage complications is also increased but, in contrast to early exploration, nephrectomy is less commonly needed.

Persistent haematuria or arteriovenous fistula

Selective arterial embolisation of the site is the management of choice.

Renal tumours

Tumours of the kidney account for approximately 2% of all malignancies. Benign tumours are extremely rare.

There are four types of malignant tumour, apart from the very rare fibro- and liposarcomas:

- nephroblastoma (Wilm's tumour)
- adenocarcinoma (hypernephroma)
- transitional cell carcinoma of the renal pelvis
- squamous carcinoma of the renal pelvis.

Nephroblastoma

This is also known as a Wilm's tumour. This is the commonest genitourinary neoplasm in infants and second only to brain tumours as a cause of death in this age group. Sex distribution is equal, there is a peak incidence at 2 years and the tumour is bilateral in 5%.

PATHOLOGICAL FEATURES

It is an undifferentiated embryonic tumour which contains primitive glomeruli and tubules as well as irregular areas of collagen, cartilage, bone and adipose tissue. Spread is by direct infiltration of the kidney and surrounding structures, by lymphatics and by the bloodstream to the liver, lungs, long bones and brain.

CLINICAL FEATURES

There is often failure to thrive, and a thin, ill infant or child presents with a visible abdominal mass. One-third have haematuria.

INVESTIGATION

Imaging

IVU. The preliminary film may show areas of speckled calcification. There is usually renal cortical and calyceal distortion. Evidence either of normality or of involvement of the other kidney is also obtained.

Ultrasonography demonstrates a solid renal mass.

MANAGEMENT

Surgery

In all patients, a radical nephrectomy (a procedure in which, through an abdominal approach, the kidney, perirenal soft tissue and adjacent lymph nodes are removed as a block and the renal vessels divided as close to their origin as possible) is done. The renal vessels are ligated early in the operation to reduce the risk of escape of malignant cells during manipulation.

Additional treatment with radiotherapy and/or chemotherapy depends on the stage of the disease.

PROGNOSIS

For localised tumours, there is a 5-year survival of 80%, but this falls to 30% in the presence of lymph node metastases. Survival is zero for those with metastases to solid organs.

Adenocarcinoma

EPIDEMIOLOGY AND PATHOLOGICAL FEATURES

The peak incidence is in the fifth generation and the condition is commoner in men. The tumour arises from the renal tubules, is usually well-encapsulated and contains areas of haemorrhage and necrosis. On histological examination, it consists of columnar or cuboidal cells with clear cytoplasm and dark nuclei. Spread is by local infiltration and chiefly by the blood to distant organs. Direct growth may take place into the renal vein and vena cava. Paraneoplastic syndromes may occur (Table 32.2).

Table 32.2
Paraneoplastic syndromes in renal cell carcinoma

Event	Cause
Raised ESR	Changes in plasma proteins
Anaemia	Depressed erythropoiesis and haemolysis
Polycythaemia	Erythropoietin secretion
Hypercalcaemia	Tumour secretion of parathormone-like substance
Raised alkaline phosphatase concentration	Secretion from the tumour
Pyrexia	Circulating pyrogens
Hypertension	Secretion of renin
Amyloid deposition	Unknown
Peripheral neuropathy and myopathy	Unknown

Table 32.3
T component of TNM staging of carcinoma of the kidney

Stage	Findings
T1	Tumour < 2.5 cm limited to kidney
T2	Tumour > 2.5 cm limited to kidney
T3	Tumour extends into major veins or invades adrenal or perinephric tissue but not beyond Gerota's fascia
T4	Tumour invades beyond Gerota's fascia

Table 32.4
N and M component of TNM staging of carcinoma of the kidney

Stage	Findings
N	
NX	Regional lymph nodes cannot be assessed
N0	No regional lymph node metastases
N1	Metastases in a single lymph node < 2.0 cm in diameter
N2	Metastases in single lymph node > 2–5 cm in greatest diameter or multiple lymph nodes, none > 5 cm in greatest diameter
N3	Metastases in the lymph node > 5 cm in greatest diameter
M	
M0	No metastases
M1	Distant metastases

STAGING

TNM staging is used, based on the preoperative investigations, operative findings and the histological examination of the excised tissues. T stages are shown in Table 32.3 and N and M stages in Table 32.4.

CLINICAL FEATURES

Twenty per cent of tumours are detected on ultrasound examination during the course of investigations for non-specific symptoms or for features that suggest a paraneoplastic syndrome.

Symptoms

Specific symptoms are not common but there are some which are semi-specific:

- aching loin pain
- episodes of acute pain – caused by haemorrhage into the tumour and sometimes of sufficient severity for the patient to present as an emergency
- haematuria (60%)
- symptoms of paraneoplastic syndromes (Table 32.2)
- pathological fracture.

Signs

A loin mass is the only finding unless there is clinical evidence of distant metastases. By the time that the triad of loin pain, loin mass and haematuria is present, the tumour is usually advanced.

INVESTIGATION

Urine

Haematuria should be sought. Significant proteinuria may indicate involvement of the renal vein.

Blood

Analysis should be done for any of the paraneoplastic syndromes. Hypercalcaemia or a raised alkaline phosphatase does not necessarily imply metastatic disease.

Imaging

Chest X-ray may show typical cannon ball metastases.

IVU demonstrates a space-occupying lesion best seen in the nephrogram phase and also calcyeal distortion.

Ultrasonography can distinguish between a cyst and a solid tumour and is an effective way of identifying involvement of the renal vein and the vena cava.

CT Scan is the most precise way of staging the tumour (Tables 32.3 and 32.4; Fig. 32.8).

Renal angiography is less commonly used but is essential in bilateral tumours or a tumour in a solitary kidney.

MANAGEMENT

Surgery

Radical nephrectomy is the primary treatment in the absence of metastatic disease.

Non-operative treatment

In symptomatic patients who are unsuitable for surgical treatment, embolisation of the renal artery is effective in controlling pain and haematuria.

Radiotherapy to the primary tumour is ineffective but may help in reducing the pain of a bony metastasis. Endocrine and chemotherapy are both ineffective. Other treatments that have been used include alpha-interferon and interleukin-2 for patients with metastatic disease. Some partial responses have been recorded.

PROGNOSIS

Seventy per cent of those with T1 tumours survive for 5 years and prolonged survival has been reported after removal of secondary deposits. However, there may be long intervals between the presentation of the primary and of metastases. Very rarely, secondary deposits may regress after removal of the primary. Nevertheless, very few patients who present with evidence of metastatic disease survive for more than 2 years.

Carcinoma of the renal pelvis

Carcinoma of the renal pelvis accounts for 10% of all renal tumours, and may be bilateral in up to 25% of cases.

AETIOLOGY AND PATHOLOGICAL FEATURES

Ninety per cent are derived from the transitional epithelium (urothelium) and are likely to be associated with similar tumours elsewhere in the urinary tract. However, urothelial tumours of the bladder are 60 times more common than those of the renal pelvis. The remaining 10% in the renal pelvis are squamous carcinomas – a consequence of metaplastic change – and are almost invariably associated with stones. The aetiological factors for transitional cell cancer are similar to those for the same lesion in the bladder.

CLINICAL FEATURES

These are loin pain and haematuria.

INVESTIGATION

Cytology

Malignant urothelial cells may be present in the urine.

Imaging

An IVU shows a filling defect in the calyces or renal pelvis which must be distinguished from a non-opaque renal calculus by ultrasound.

MANAGEMENT

Management is by removal of the kidney and ureter together with a cuff of bladder mucosa around the ureteric orifice. The reason for such radical surgery is the possibility of the occurrence of a further tumour; in the bladder it is simple to diagnose by cystoscopy, but the ureteric stump cannot easily be examined.

More conservative management has been attempted by endoscopic resection through a percutaneous nephrostomy tube direct instrumentation of the ureter or instillation of chemotherapeutic agents directly into the renal pelvis.

PROGNOSIS

In localised transitional cell tumours of the renal pelvis, the outlook is good but squamous cell carcinoma of the renal pelvis has a poor prognosis.

Stone disease

EPIDEMIOLOGY

The incidence and site of occurrence of urinary stones vary in different parts of the world and in different parts of the UK. Renal stones are more common in affluent communities while bladder stones remain the common site in developing countries. In the UK, the incidence of upper urinary tract stones varies from 15 per 100 000 in the north of England (Burnley) to 47 per 100 000 in the south-east (Canterbury). There are similar differences in the type of stone between countries: uric acid stones make up only 5% of the total in the UK, but this rises to 40% in Israel.

Box 32.5

Metabolic causes of urinary tract stones

Hypercalcaemia and hypercalciuria
Hyperparathyroidism
Idiopathic hypercalcuria
Hypervitaminosis D
Disseminated malignant disease
Myeloma
Prolonged immobilisation
Sarcoidosis
Milk alkali syndrome
Cushing's disease
Hyperthyroidism

Increase in other substances
Cystinuria (tubular transport defect for cystine, lysine, ornithine and arginine)
Xanthinuria
Primary hyperoxaluria
Secondary hyperoxaluria (ileostomy)
Hyperuricuria (gout; chemotherapy for leukaemia)
Indinavir therapy

AETIOLOGY

In the majority of instances this is unknown.

Metabolic disorders

Conditions that alter the composition of the urine, chiefly (but not exclusively) to increase its calcium content, are shown in Box 32.5.

Other causes

The commonest of these is infection with the urea-splitting organism Proteus sp. The result is the production of ammonia, an alkaline urine and triple phosphate stones (Staghorn calculi) (Fig. 32.2), which are a mixture of calcium, magnesium and ammonium phosphate. Others factors are dehydration and immobilisation.

CHARACTERISTICS OF STONES

These are given in Table 32.5.

CLINICAL FEATURES

Symptoms

These depend on the size and position of the stone and the presence or absence of infection. The patient may be asymptomatic or give a history of occasional haematuria or dysuria. In cystine stone, there may be a family history, and in all stones there may have been previous

Table 32.5
Characteristics of stones

Stone	Incidence	Colour	Appearance	Radio-opacity
Calcium oxalate (mulberry stone)	80%	Pale yellow-brown	Sharp projections	Opaque
Triple phosphate[a] (staghorn calculus)	10%	Chalky white	Soft	Opaque
Uric acid	5%	Light brown	Facetted	Lucent
Cystine[b]	2%	Yellow brown	Smooth	Moderately opaque
Xanthine	Rare	Yellow brown	Lucent	

[a] Often associated with infection with urea-splitting organisms, e.g. *Proteus* sp.
[b] Often a family history and/or episodes of repeated stone formation.

episodes. A stone lodged at the neck of a calyx or at the pelviureteric junction causes renal colic, in which there are waves of increasing pain in the loin often superimposed on a background of continuous nagging pain at the same site. Radiation downwards into the groin or scrotum is not common, in contrast to the symptoms of a stone in the ureter. The pain from a stone in the renal pelvis is continuous in the loin and often aggravated by movement.

Physical findings
Tenderness may be found in the loin and is increased in severity if there is infection or obstruction when pyrexia is common.

Differential diagnosis
Pain in stone disease is notorious for causing diagnostic confusion with other acute abdominal conditions, some of which require urgent surgical management. They include:

- appendicitis
- cholecystitis
- diverticulitis
- pyelonephritis
- leaking aortic aneurysm.

There are two reasons for making as precise a diagnosis as possible: first, to undertake relief of pain when one of the alternative conditions is present may mask the clinical features and compound the misdiagnosis; second, many substance abusers have learned the symptoms of renal colic in order to obtain analgesics or narcotics.

INVESTIGATION
Any patient who has formed a renal stone stands a greater than 20% chance of producing another. It is important to identify metabolic or structural abnormalities because appropriate management may reduce the risk of recurrence.

Urine
- Culture and sensitivity, measurement of pH and screening for cystine

- Two 24-hour collections with the patient on a normal diet for measurement of calcium, uric acid and citrate concentrations.

Blood
Concentrations of the following are measured:

- urea
- creatinine
- electrolytes
- total protein
- calcium
- alkaline phosphatase
- uric acid
- phosphate.

In a patient with a stone causing complete obstruction, the bladder urine may be sterile. Urine should then be obtained by the insertion of a percutaneous nephrostomy, which is almost certainly required for relief of obstruction.

Imaging
A patient who presents with acute symptoms and signs and a suspected stone must have an urgent IVU. The diagnosis can be firmly established, the size of the stone determined, together with the degree of obstruction, the likelihood of the stone passing spontaneously, and the need for hospital admission.

NON-OPERATIVE MANAGEMENT
Asymptomatic stone
A small asymptomatic non-obstructing stone in an elderly, unfit patient can be left alone.

Acute episode
The pain of renal colic is severe and is treated with narcotic analgesics, antispasmodics such as Buscopan and non-steroidal anti-inflammatory agents such as Voltarol. Stones less than 0.5 cm in diameter will usually pass spontaneously and, if they are opaque, their progress can be assessed by repeated plain abdominal X-ray.

Urology

Oxalate stones

The commonest abnormality detected is idiopathic hypercalciuria. A low calcium diet and a high fluid intake to dilute urine calcium concentration is often recommended. However, it is usually unsuccessful in that tap water in many areas contains significant amounts of calcium and a reduction in dietary calcium intake leads to an increased intestinal absorption of oxalate.

Attempts to reduce urine calcium excretion with bendrofluazide have only been shown to reduce calcium stone formation after prolonged periods of therapy. Sodium cellulose phosphate decreases calcium excretion but is often unacceptable because of the foul diarrhoea it may cause.

Cystine stones

Cystinuria is an inherited defect of amino acid transport involving cystine, ornithine, lysine and arginine. Cystine is relatively insoluble, particularly in acid urine, and this can lead to stone formation. Because its excretion is relatively constant, the stones can be both dissolved and prevented by maintaining a high fluid intake throughout the 24 hours and alkalinising the urine. The latter can be achieved with either sodium bicarbonate or potassium citrate, or a combination of both. If this fails, treatment with penicillamine, which produces a more soluble cystine–penicillamine complex, is sometimes successful. However, it may be associated with the development of skin rashes and the nephrotic syndrome.

Uric acid stones

Uric acid is less soluble in acid urine and, as a result, patients with chronic diarrhoea or an ileostomy are more likely to produce uric acid stones. They can be dissolved or prevented by increasing the fluid intake and alkalinisation of the urine. In addition, allopurinol (100mg thee times a day) should be given to those with an elevated serum level.

Triple phosphate stones

The prevention of recurrent phosphate stones associated with infection is dependent on three factors:

- complete removal of the initial stone(s)
- correction of any anatomical abnormalities of urine drainage
- maintenance of sterile urine.

The last can be achieved with long-term low-dose antibiotic therapy. If this proves difficult, treatment with a urease inhibitor (acetohydroxamic acid) should be considered.

Surgical management

Indications for intervention

Urgent percutaneous nephrostomy drainage is required when:

- fever does not resolve after 24 hours of appropriate antibiotic therapy in a patient with an obstructed kidney
- severe pain persists inspite of the medical management outlined above.

The nephrostomy track can be used at a later stage for endoscopic stone destruction or removal. An indwelling stent can be inserted to establish drainage down the ureter before treatment by lithotripsy (see below).

Intervention in persistent stone

Major advances have been made in the management of stones over the past decade by techniques other than open operation.

Destruction of the stone in situ can be done with:

- extracorporeal transcutaneous techniques (extracorporeal shock wave lithotripsy, ESWL)
- direct application of shock waves or laser to the stone by a probe inserted endoscopically or percutaneously.

Removal can be achieved either endoscopically or percutaneously.

Disorders of the ureter

Congenital anatomical abnormalities

Ureteric duplication

Incomplete duplication is much more common than complete ureteric duplication and occurs in approximately 1% of individuals. Complete duplication is present in about 1 in every 500–600 individuals. The extent of incomplete ureteral duplication may vary from a bifid renal pelvis (which could be considered as a normal variant) to two separate ureters joining with each other at some point during their course. A complete duplication results in two separate ureters with two separate ureteric openings in the bladder. The orifice of the upper segment ureter always enters the bladder more medial and caudal to the lower segment orifice. The ureter from the lower part of the kidney is more likely to be associated with vesicoureteric reflux, as the orifice of this ureter is more lateral and cephalic. As the orifice of the ureter from the upper pole is more caudal, it can be located in an ectopic position which may open at the level of the bladder neck, urethra, vestibule or vagina and may result in either obstruction or incontinence.

CLINICAL FEATURES

Duplication of the ureters is commonly asymptomatic. Vesicoureteral reflux into the lower moeity can result in infection, haematuria or flank pain.

MANAGEMENT

Asymptomatic duplications do not require any treatment. If one of the moieties of the kidney is non-functioning, a heminephroureterectomy is the procedure of choice. In cases of complete duplication, vesicoureteral reflux is managed in the usual way. An ectopic ureter can either be reimplanted or a heminephroureterectomy can be performed depending on the function of that portion of the kidney.

Congenital obstruction at the pelviureteric junction (PUJ)

The PUJ is the most common site of obstruction in the upper urinary tract.

AETIOLOGY

In the *congenital type*, intrinsic abnormalities of the PUJ are the most common cause of obstruction. They result from an aperistaltic segment at the level of the PUJ, resulting in a functional obstruction to the passage of urine. In some cases, valve-like processes and polyps have been found.

Extrinsic abnormalities are seen in about one-third of patients with PUJ obstruction. Abberant vessels may cause obstruction, especially when they cross in front of the PUJ or when the ureter appears to be trapped between two such vessels. PUJ obstruction occurs in approximately 1:1500 births. It is more common in males and is bilateral in 5% of cases. Obstruction is acquired as a result of stricture formation following surgery for stones, trauma or tuberculosis.

CLINICAL FEATURES

Symptoms

The typical clinical presentation has changed since the advent of widespread antenatal sonographic screening. A significant number of babies with antenatal hydronephrosis are subsequently found to have a PUJ obstruction.

In infants and children
- Abdominal mass
- Urinary tract infection
- Haematuria
- Failure to thrive.

In adults
- Intermittent loin pain sometimes associated with alcohol consumption

- Urinary infection
- Haematuria following mild trauma
- Symptoms of stones.

Signs

In infants and children
- Abdominal mass

In adults
- Loin tenderness
- Rarely, abdominal mass
- An incidental finding during the course of investigation for another condition.

INVESTIGATION

To diagnose PUJ obstruction, both anatomical and functional studies of the kidney are required. Anatomical information of the kidney can be obtained by ultrasound examination. Ultrasound examination reveals dilatation of the pelvicalyceal system and also demonstrates the state of the renal cortex.

Intravenous urography (IVU) with diuretic enhancement of urine flow

IVU gives an indication of the anatomical as well as the functional state of the kidney (Fig. 32.5) IVU can also be combined with diuretic enhancement of urine flow by giving 40 mg frusemide intravenously. Following contrast and frusemide injection, if there is no increase of dilatation of the pelvicalyceal system and good washout of contrast, this indicates a non-obstructed system.

Nuclear isotope scan

A prolonged excretory third phase occurs when there is pelvicalyceal dilatation. If frusemide is given, the counts may rise (obstructed) or fall (non-obstructed).

MANAGEMENT

Broad options of management include:

- observation
- surgical reconstruction
- percutaneous balloon dilatation
- retrograde balloon dilatation
- percutaneous incision (endopyelotomy).

Most PUJ obstructions are now discovered antenatally and hence are asymptomatic. Management is decided on the basis of anatomical and functional information provided by different scans. After birth, the kidneys are observed by repeated scanning with ultrasound and/or isotope renography.

Indications for surgery

These are:

- deterioration of renal function
- worsening of renal dilatation

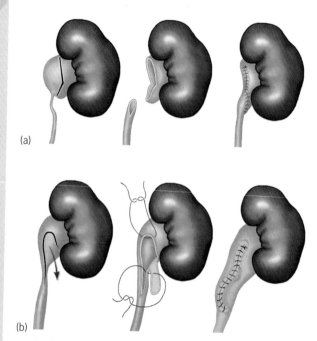

(a)

(b)

Fig 32.18 **Pyeloplasty operations. (a)** Anderson Hynes. **(b)** Culp.

- thining of renal cortex
- the presence of symptoms, pain, haematuria or infection.

For primary PUJ obstruction, if operative intervention is required, surgical reconstruction is the method of choice. The percutaneous or retrograde dilatation/incision techniques are usually reserved for secondary PUJ obstruction. The most common surgical technique is the Anderson–Hynes pyeloplasty which disconnects the pelvis from the ureter, reduces the size of the pelvis but requires re-anastomosis of the ureter to the pelvis. A Culp pyeloplasty is useful for those with a small extrarenal pelvis. Re-anastomosis of the ureter is not required (Fig. 32.18).

Ureteric disorders that may be either congenital or acquired

Megaureter

AETIOLOGY
The underlying cause of the congenital variety is the same as that of PUJ obstruction, but the muscular imbalance in megaureter is at the ureterovesical junction. The ureter proximal to this becomes dilated and hypertrophied. The condition may be bilateral and a secondary hydronephrosis may develop with the formation of stones.

Secondary megaureter, schistosomiasis or bladder outflow obstruction.

Box 32.6

Pathophysiological classification of megaureter

Congenital	or	Secondary
Non-refluxing or refluxing		Non-refluxing or refluxing
Non-obstructed or obstructed		Non-obstructed or obstructed

PATHOPHYSIOLOGY
Classification on the basis of reflux and the presence of obstruction to flow is shown in Box 32.6 and is used to guide management. Very rarely, reflux and obstruction may coexist. A combination of IVU, micturating cystograms and renography permits appropriate categorisation.

CLINICAL FEATURES
Symptoms of megaureter are:

- incidental finding during investigation for another condition
- loin pain
- urinary infection.

MANAGEMENT
Non-obstructed, non-refluxing megaureters do not require treatment.

Congenitally obstructed megaureters should be reimplantated after the narrowing at the distal end has been removed. Those with reflux are treated along the lines of management of vesicoureteric reflux. A *secondarily obstructed* megaureter requires treatment of its cause.

Vesicoureteric reflux

AETIOLOGY AND PATHOLOGICAL FEATURES
Primary reflux is the result of a defective valvular mechanism at the ureterovesical junction; when compared with a normal ureter, the intramural course is short and more horizontally directed. The condition is bilateral in 50%, and 90% of affected patients are female. There is a familial incidence. As the ureterovesical junction matures, reflux may cease spontaneously.

Secondary reflux may occur because of bladder outlet or urethral obstruction or in neurogenic bladders. Inflammatory conditions of the bladder wall (schistosomiasis tuberculosis) can hold the ureteric orifice open.

CLINICAL FEATURES
In primary reflux, the onset is in the first decade. Symptoms may include fever, lethargy, anorexia, nausea and vomiting. There is often mild haematuria but the

main symptoms are those of recurrent urinary infections. Older children may complain of pain in the loin or on micturition. In secondary disease, the onset is later and again symptoms of infection predominate.

There are no specific signs.

INVESTIGATION

IVU. This is often normal but may show ureteric dilatation or renal scarring.

Micturating cystogram. Cystoureteric reflux is best demonstrated at the time of micturition (Fig. 32.7).

Isotope scanning. A DMSA scan can be used to identify current renal damage.

MANAGEMENT

The majority of patients can be satisfactorily managed by antibiotic therapy. Long-term therapy to suppress infection is necessary up to the age of 6 years. The incidence of renal scarring after this age is very low. Surgical reimplantation of the ureter is indicated when medical management fails to suppress the development of new urinary infections or there is non-compliance with antibiotic treatment. The injection of inert, nonabsorbable substances around the ureteric orifice to prevent reflux offers a non-surgical option to treat this condition.

Ureterocele

Ureterocele is a cystic dilatation of the terminal portion of the ureter and may occur in either a normally placed ureter or rarely in an ectopic one. This usually involves the upper segment ureter of a duplex system. They may become very large and occupy most of the available space in the bladder. A stone impacted in the lower end of the ureter is one cause.

CLINICAL FEATURES

Some patients are asymptomatic. When symptoms do occur, they are usually secondary to complications, such as:

- obstruction of the bladder outlet
- infection
- loin pain.

Signs are minimal. An ectopic ureterocele in a female may present as a vaginal tumour at birth or in childhood. Occasionally they may present at the urethral meatus.

DIAGNOSIS

The diagnosis is made on an IVU which shows a rounded swelling in the bladder associated with a dilatation of the ureter – hydroureter.

MANAGEMENT

Asymptomatic ureteroceles do not need treatment. If the ureter is dilated or there is a stone, the ureterocele

can be transected endoscopically. The cut is made on the inferior surface because this makes reflux less likely. Ectopic ureteroceles require a heminephroureterectomy.

Acquired conditions

Ureteric injuries

AETIOLOGY

Open injuries occur from gunshot or stabbing. A closed avulsion of the ureter from the renal pelvis may follow rapid deceleration. However, surgical injuries during abdominal or pelvic operations are the commonest cause. The ureter is at particular risk if it is displaced from its usual anatomical position by the condition under treatment The operations most frequently associated with ureteric injury include:

- Gynaecological
  - hysterectomy
  - ovarian cystectomy
  - repair of vesicovaginal fistula
  - anterior colporrhaphy
- General surgery
  - sigmoid colectomy
  - abdominoperineal resection of the rectum
  - repair of aortic aneurysm
- Urology
  - excision of bladder diverticulae
  - ureterolithotomy
  - ureteroscopy.

PATHOLOGICAL FEATURES

One or both ureters may be ligated. The kidney stops secreting once the intraureteric pressure has risen to the filtration pressure. In consequence, dilatation of the renal pelvis is mild and, if the condition goes untreated, atrophy of the kidney takes place. Less commonly the lumen is incompletely obstructed by inclusion in a stitch in which case the kidney continues to secrete and hydronephrosis develops often with accompanying infection. Alternatively, the ureter is divided or suffers a crushing injury. The latter may be ischaemic. Urine then leaks to the exterior or into the retroperitoneal tissues and, less commonly, the peritoneal cavity.

CLINICAL FEATURES

The injury may be recognised at the time of surgery. If not, bilateral ligation will be recognised very soon. Leak usually presents around the fifth postoperative day but may be delayed for 10–14 days if it results from ureteric ischaemia. The features are:

- bilateral ligation – immediate postoperative anuria
- unilateral ligation – either absence of clinical features or, if there is proximal infection, fever and persistent loin pain

- division – urine appears from the drain, the wound or the vagina
- retroperitoneal leakage of sterile urine leads to abdominal distension secondary to ileus and intraperitoneal leakage to signs of free fluid in the peritoneal cavity
- retro- or intraperitoneal leakage of infected urine is associated with the features of peritonitis and generalised sepsis.

INVESTIGATION

In the early stages of complete obstruction, an IVU shows a nephrographic effect – contrast medium outlines the whole kidney but little change in radiodensity is seen in the renal pelvis or ureter. In incomplete obstruction or transesction, there is some delay in excretion, and ureteric dilatation on the side of the injury down to the site of damage is usually seen. If, however, this is not identified, retrograde ureterography may help.

MANAGEMENT

Prevention

An IVU should be done before any operation in which the ureters are at risk, particularly if there is the possibility of ureteric displacement.

Treatment

The insertion of a ureteric stent may allow a small fistula to close. In critically ill patients, a temporary percutaneous nephrostomy is the procedure of choice to allow drainage of the obstructed and usually infected kidney. In all other instances, surgical repair is necessary, and complicated procedures may be required.

If the injury is recognised at the time of surgery, ligatures should be removed, the crushed area resected, the cut ends should be spatulated and a primary anastomosis performed over a ureteric stent. Other techniques include (Fig. 32.19):

- reimplantation of the damaged ureter into the bladder
- anastomosis of one ureter to the other
- replacement of the ureter by small intestine
- use of the bladder flap (Boari) to replace the damaged segment

Retroperitoneal fibrosis

AETIOLOGY

There are two forms: idiopathic and secondary. In the first, as its name implies, the cause is not known. Secondary retroperitoneal fibrosis may follow:

(a)　　　　　　　　　　　　(b)

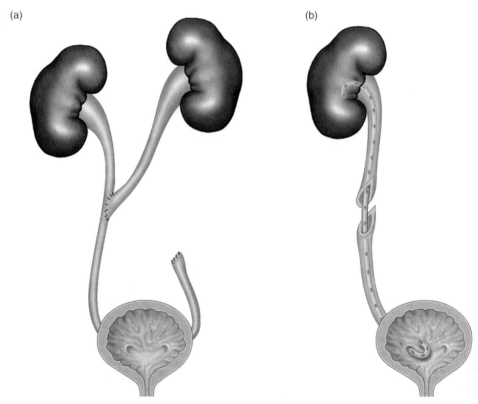

Fig 32.19 **Techniques which may be used for repair of an injured ureter.**

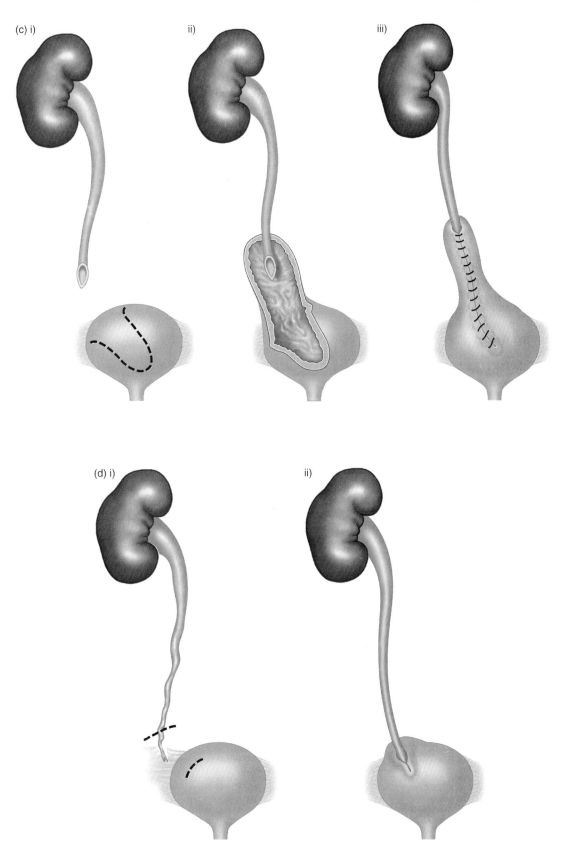

Fig 32.19 **(c, d)**

- treatment with methysergide
- extravasation of urine
- retroperitoneal sepsis
- aortic or iliac aneurysms
- radiotherapy
- most commonly, retroperitoneal spread of malignant disease – cervix, ovary, testis, prostate and lymphomas.

PATHOLOGICAL FEATURES

In the primary idiopathic form, one or both ureters become encased in and obstructed by a retroperitoneal plaque of fibrous tissue between the pelviureteric junction and the pelvic brim, although involvement may be more extensive.

CLINICAL FEATURES

Symptoms are non-specific but include backache, low-grade fever and malaise, as well as those of hypertension, renal failure or anuria.

The physical findings are also non-specific and related to the renal failure or hypertension.

INVESTIGATION

ESR is invariably raised.

Ultrasound may show upper urinary tract dilatation.

IVU shows upper urinary tract dilatation, with medial deviation of one or both ureters. However, if renal function is poor and the IVU inadequate to define the ureters, percutaneous nephrostomy tubes are inserted to improve renal function and allow subsequent identification of the site of obstruction.

Bilateral retrograde ureterography often results in complete anuria from ureteric oedema and should be avoided.

CT scan is useful to define the extent of the retroperitoneal mass.

MANAGEMENT

Treatment is surgical. A definitive diagnosis of possible underlying causes can only be made by histological examination of tissue from the retroperitoneum, and ureterolysis can be done at the same time. To prevent recurrence of obstruction, both ureters are either wrapped in omentum or brought laterally and intraperitoneally to distance them from the fibrotic mass. Idiopathic retroperitoneal fibrosis does respond to treatment with steroids, but long-term therapy is required. A histological diagnosis to exclude retroperitoneal malignancy is not made unless therapy is preceded by surgical exploration.

Ureteric stone

AETIOLOGY AND SITE OF LODGEMENT

These stones originate in the kidney and migrate downwards. Arrest is likely at the three sites of relative narrowing: the pelviureteric junction, the pelvic brim where the ureter crosses the iliac vessels, and the intravesical termination.

CLINICAL FEATURES

Ureteric stones almost always cause renal colic and account for one of the most frequent urological presentations in the accident and emergency department.

Symptoms

The patient is in severe pain which is intermittent and radiates from the loin to the groin and sometimes into the testicle, scrotum or labia. Vomiting frequently occurs and the patient is unable to find any comfortable position or to lie still. The urine is often bloodstained.

Signs

Fever suggests the presence of a pyonephrosis. The abdomen is tender with slight guarding. An impacted stone may be complicated by paralytic ileus which produces a silent distended abdomen.

INVESTIGATION

Urine

Examination of the urine is carried out for red blood cells and bacterial culture.

Imaging

A plain abdominal X-ray may show a calcified opacity lying in the course of the ureter. An IVU should always be done urgently to confirm the diagnosis and to assess the degree of obstruction and the likelihood of the stone passing spontaneously; 90% of stones less than 0.5 cm in diameter will do so (Fig. 32.20).

MANAGEMENT

Most patients are admitted to hospital for relief of pain, although the majority require only one parenteral injection of opiate. Anti-spasmodics and non-steroidal anti-inflammatory agents are effective thereafter.

Indications for intervention

- Evidence of infection
- Recurrent or persistent pain
- Failure of the stone to progress downwards
- Deterioration of renal function determined by isotope scanning.

Methods of intervention

In an emergency, intervention is by either percutaneous nephrostomy or the passage of a ureteric stent to bypass the obstruction (Fig. 32.21).

Definitive treatment is as follows:

- extraction – snaring small stones in the lower 5 cm of ureter in a basket passed up the ureter; or very rarely by open ureterolithotomy

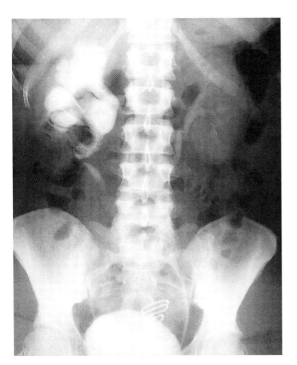

Fig 32.20 **An intravenous urogram showing clubbed calyces secondary to ureteric obstruction.**

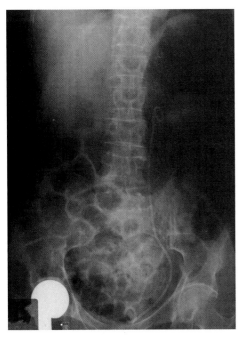

Fig 32.21 **Double pigtail catheter providing drainage of the renal pelvis and stenting of the left ureter.**

- extracorporeal destruction by shock wave lithotripsy
- in situ destruction with lithotripsy or laser via a ureteroscope.

Urinary diversion

Decompression or drainage of the urinary tract is frequently employed in urological practice. It is now usually done under radiological control rather than at open operation.

Nephrostomy and pyelostomy

In nephrostomy, a drainage tube is passed through the kidney substance into its pelvis; in pyelostomy the pelvis is intubated direct. Either procedure is most frequently employed to decompress and drain a kidney obstructed at the pelviureteric outflow. Decompression may also be needed after operations such as reconstruction of the pelviureteric junction. An external drainage bag can be avoided if it is possible to intubate an obstruction or suture line by placing a ureteric stent across it so that one end lies in the renal pelvis and the other in the bladder (Fig. 32.21). The technique is frequently used before lithotripsy, to prevent fragments of stone causing ureteric obstruction.

Other forms of urinary diversion

Surgical diversion of urine to the exterior is required if the bladder is removed or is so congenitally deformed (exstrophy) or diseased that adequate function is impossible. Diversion is most frequently achieved by using an isolated segment of ileum into which the ureters are implanted. The segment acts as a conduit to bring the urine to the abdominal wall (Fig. 32.22). Intestine can also be used to make a new bladder with a continent external opening on the abdominal wall which the patient catheterises intermittently (cf. continent ileostomy). Rarely, the ureters may be implanted into the intact sigmoid colon. However, that technique often leads to ascending urinary infection and chronic pyelonephritis; and, because of reabsorption of urinary constituents from the intestine, hyperchloraemic acidosis develops. Yet a further complication is the development of adeno-carcinoma at the site of ureteric implantation. This procedure has now been superseded by the creation of a pouch in the sigmoid colon (Mainz II). This has a much lower incidence of complications.

The lower urinary tract

SYMPTOMS IN THE LOWER GENITOURINARY TRACT
Bladder pain
This may be sharp or dull and is located in the midline

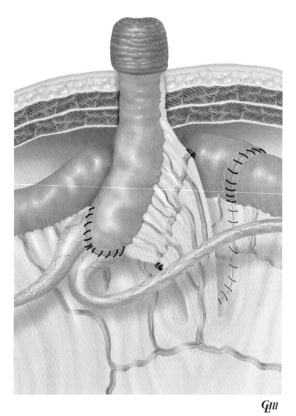

Fig 32.22 **An ileal conduit.**

of the lower abdomen. Rapid overdistension of a previously normal bladder causes severe pain, but if the distension is gradual over weeks or months, pain is absent.

Prostatic pain
This is a dull ache which may be felt in the lower abdomen, the rectum, perineum and anterior thighs.

Urethral pain
This is usually felt at the tip of the penis and ranges from a mere tickling discomfort to severe and sharp pain exacerbated by passing urine.

Scrotal pain
Pain may be referred to the scrotum as in renal colic. Similarly, pain arising from the scrotal contents may be referred to the groin or abdomen. Most scrotal pain is the result of stretching of the tunica albuginea: if this happens acutely, pain is severe, but slow distension, as in a tumour, causes a dragging sensation or a dull ache.

Disorders of micturition
Increased frequency may occur during the day and the night (nocturia) and may be a response to an excess fluid intake or failure of the kidneys to concentrate the

urine, as occurs in diabetes insipidus, hypercalcaemia, chronic renal failure and diseases which produce a high solute load such as diabetes mellitus.

Urological causes of increased frequency are:

- urinary infection
- incomplete bladder emptying
- detrusor irritability
- small bladder volume
- bladder cancer.

Dysuria. The term describes a burning sensation during the passage of urine. It may occur throughout micturition or just at its end (terminal dysuria). Infection with inflammation of the urethra is the commonest cause.

Strangury is a repeated desire to pass urine but with little to show for it other than pain related to the urethra or the penile tip. Infection is likely.

Intermittency. The urine stream is interrupted during micturition. The symptom is associated with bladder stones, ureteroceles and benign prostatic obstruction.

Hesitancy is the need to wait before the urine stream begins. Prostatic obstruction to urine flow and stricture are causes.

Incomplete emptying is, as the phrase implies, a feeling that the bladder is not emptied at the end of micturition. Prostatic disease and detrusor dysfunction are possible causes.

Terminal dribbling is a progressive reduction in the rate of urine flow at the end of the urine stream and is associated with prostatic obstruction.

Postmicturition dribbling is leakage after the patient believes that micturition is complete and is associated with detrusor irritability, urethral diverticulae or the failure to empty the urethra manually after micturition.

Incontinence is of five types:

- True – a fistula between the urinary tract and the exterior
- Giggle – in young girls provoked by bouts of unrestrained mirth
- Stress – leakage during a transient increase in abdominal pressure such as coughing or laughing
- Urge – a desire to pass urine of such severity that the patient is unable to reach the toilet; it may be associated with urinary infection, bladder stones, detrusor instability or bladder cancer
- Dribbling or overflow – there is a continual loss of urine from a chronically distended bladder.

Abnormal urine stream. The stream may be:

- slow – prostatic obstruction or detrusor insufficiency
- forked – often associated with a urethral stricture.

EXAMINATION
A distended bladder is visible and palpable in most

patients examined in the supine position. Dullness to percussion in the midline of the abdomen above the pubic symphysis nearly always means bladder distension in a male.

The external genitalia are often not examined because of embarrassment. The foreskin, glans penis and urethral meatus must be examined for meatal stenosis, phimosis, anatomical abnormalities such as hypospadias, penile tumours and warts. The scrotal contents are examined with the patient both supine and standing to aid identification of a varicocele.

Rectal examination

In the UK, it is traditional to examine the male in the left lateral position. The purpose is to identify abnormalities within the anal canal and rectum and to determine the size, contour and consistency of the prostate. A similar position is used in the female but is usually preceded by a vaginal examination with the patient supine and the knees flexed. In the latter, oestrogenisation of the perineum, urethral prolapse, urethral diverticulae and gynaecological abnormalities of the vagina, cervix, uterus and its adnexae can be detected.

INVESTIGATION

General

Bacteriological and biochemical investigation for the upper urinary tract are also relevant to the lower tract.

Imaging

Urethrography. Water-soluble contrast medium is introduced into the urethra via a catheter to outline urethral strictures, urethral diverticulae and urethral injuries.

Ultrasonography. Transabdominal, transurethral and transrectal routes are available. The techniques provide precise information on:

- residual urine
- bladder tumours
- prostatic size
- nature of prostatic enlargement – benign or possibly malignant
- staging prostatic cancer.

Transrectal ultrasound (TRUS) guidance also improves the accuracy with which a prostatic biopsy is obtained when confirmation of malignant disease is required.

CT and MRI are the most accurate way of assessing the depth of invasion of bladder and prostate cancer.

Bladder function

Urinary flow rate. The patient voids into a device which records the rate of accumulation of the expelled urine (flow meter). The total voided, which should be greater than 150 mL, and the peak and mean flows are recorded (Fig. 32.23). A peak flow of less than 15 mL/s may indicate bladder outflow obstruction or detrusor failure.

Urodynamics. The investigations are more invasive to the extent that urethral catheterisation with a filling catheter and a pressure transducer is required. A further pressure transducer is placed in the rectum to measure intra-abdominal pressure. Subtraction of pressures recorded by the two catheters is done automatically and gives a true intravesical pressure which is measured both during bladder filling and on micturition (Fig. 32.24). After micturition, residual volume is measured by emptying the bladder through the filling catheter.

Endoscopy. A flexible cystoscope passed under local anaesthetic or a small rigid cystoscope using sedation or general anaesthesia is used. The whole of the urethra and bladder can be examined and ureteric catheters passed.

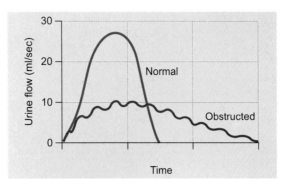

Fig 32.23 **Measurement of urinary flow rate using a flow meter.**

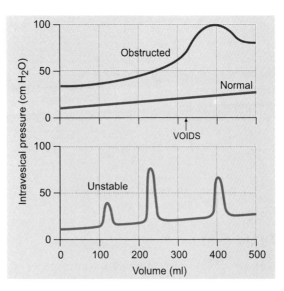

Fig 32.24 **Urodynamic pressure studies showing obstructed and unstable responses.**

Disorders and disease of the bladder

Congenital abnormalities

Urachus

Failure of the urachus to close results in a urachal fistula with leakage of urine from the umbilicus at birth. Persistence of the mid-part of the urachus produces an urachal cyst palpable in the midline below the umbilicus which may undergo malignant change.

Exstrophy of the bladder (ectopia vesicae)

EPIDEMIOLOGY AND AETIOLOGY

The incidence is approximately 1:50 000 live births with 50% being male and 50% female. The cause is unknown but the bladder does not infold so that its mucosa is exposed as a flat plate on the surface of the abdomen.

PATHOLOGICAL FINDINGS

There is failure of development of the anterior wall of the urogenital sinus and of the lower abdominal wall. The abnormality is associated with:

- wide separation of the symphysis pubis
- epispadias – failure of dorsal closure of the urethra
- inguinal hernia
- imperforate anus.

A secondary problem is the development of adenocarcinoma if the exposed bladder mucosa remains untreated.

MANAGEMENT

The bladder and penis are reconstructed in stages after a pelvic osteotomy to allow approximation of the symphysis pubis. The insertion of an artificial sphincter is usually necessary to maintain continence. Urinary diversion and excision of the deformed bladder may be required. Continence can be achieved in 80% of cases.

Infections of the lower urinary tract

Acute cystitis

In men, this is invariably bacterial and often associated with other bladder abnormalities such as outflow obstruction, foreign bodies, stones and tumours. In women, it is most commonly bacterial but may also be allergic or chemical. The agent responsible can easily ascend the short female urethra.

CLINICAL FEATURES

Frequency, dysuria, lower abdominal pain, strangury, haematuria and pyrexia all occur to a varying degree.

Mild suprapubic tenderness may be present and the urethral meatus may be inflamed. Apart from these, specific signs are absent unless there is evidence of underlying disease.

INVESTIGATION

Urine

It is essential to send a urine specimen for culture and sensitivity before antibiotic therapy is begun. In females, a high vaginal swab should be sent for analysis to exclude *Candida*, *Trichomonas* and other vaginal pathogens, because such infections may precipitate an attack of cystitis.

Imaging

Patients who present with haematuria must have both an IVV and a cystoscopy, which are also indicated when the MSU shows no bacterial growth. Carcinoma in situ of the bladder may present with cystitis-like symptoms.

MANAGEMENT

An episode requires bed rest, a high fluid intake and antibiotic administration based on the results of urine culture. Seven days after the course of antibiotics, a further MSU and high vaginal swab should be obtained to ensure that bacteria have been eradicated. In women, it is essential to identify those who have developed *Candida*, because this needs to be treated to stop the development of a vicious cycle of cystitis → antibiotic administration → persistent *Candida* infection → further symptoms.

Chronic cystitis

The cause is usually inadequate treatment and investigation of an acute attack. Postmenopausal women are prone to recurrent episodes of cystitis and can benefit from topical or systemic oestrogen replacement therapy. Ten per cent of patients who receive pelvic irradiation suffer from haemorrhagic cystitis without bacterial infection. Most cases subside spontaneously during the 12–18 months after completion of therapy, although it may lead to bladder fibrosis with a small contracted bladder.

Interstitial cystitis

This occurs most frequently in women who have irritative voiding symptoms and negative urine cultures. Many develop severe bladder pain, frequency, urgency and incontinence.

Tuberculosis of the bladder

In those who present with intractable symptoms that resemble cystitis and have a sterile pyuria, repeated examinations of early morning urine should be carried out to identify the tubercle bacillus.

MANAGEMENT

The treatment of contracted bladder is considered below.

Schistosomiasis (*Bilharzia*)

EPIDEMIOLOGY AND AETIOLOGY

The blood fluke *Schistosoma haematobium* is endemic in the Middle East and the Nile valley and other rivers and lakes of eastern and southern Africa. Human infestation is acquired by contact with infected water. Adult worms produce ova in the pelvic and vesical veins. The ova migrate through the bladder wall into the urine which is passed into the irrigation ditches where miracidia penetrate the water snail. These develop into cercaria which can pass through human skin and are carried to the pelvic venous plexuses where they develop into the adult fluke (Fig. 32.25).

PATHOLOGICAL FEATURES

The eggs in the bladder wall cause an inflammatory reaction which goes on to fibrosis, calcification and secondary infection. Stone formation and squamous carcinoma are secondary consequences. The ureters may be involved directly or may become secondarily dilated because of the small, thick-walled and fibrotic bladder.

CLINICAL FEATURES

Symptoms

In acute presentations, pyrexia, itching, dysuria,

frequency and haematuria are seen. In those who are in a chronic state, frequency, haematuria and episodes of infection resistant to treatment are usual.

INVESTIGATION

Urine examination and bladder biopsy

Eggs can be identified in either the urine or on bladder biopsy.

Imaging

IVU may show dilated ureters, stone formation or a small contracted bladder.

Cystoscopy. There is a small bladder and there may be small sandy patches around the ureteric orifices because of calcified granulomas. Areas of squamous malignancy may be obvious.

MANAGEMENT

Medical treatment is with praziquantel. Surgery may be required to reconstruct the ureters and the small contracted bladder.

Bladder trauma

Because of its anatomy, the bladder may rupture into either the peritoneal cavity or the extra-peritoneal plane. The differences in cause between the two forms of rupture are summarised in Box 32.7.

Intraperitoneal rupture

CLINICAL FEATURES

Symptoms

Usually there is a history of injury. Patients with a very full bladder have often consumed large quantities of

---

Box 32.7

Causes of bladder rupture

Intraperitoneal
Blunt abdominal trauma with a full bladder
Penetrating injury (rare)
Gross overdistension at endoscopy
During endoscopic surgery on the bladder vault

Extraperitoneal
Fracture of the pelvis
Resection of prostate
Difficult lower abdominal surgery
During repair of a direct hernia with bladder in the medial aspect of the sac.

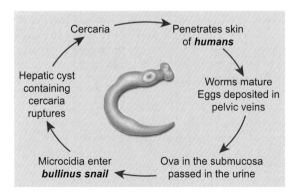

Fig 32.25 **Life cycle of *Schistosoma haematobium*.**

alcohol and a clear history may be difficult to obtain. There is usually also severe lower abdominal pain – modified by the patient's clinical state – and anuria.

Signs

These are as follows:

- If the urine is sterile, increasing abdominal distention and discomfort
- If the urine is infected, features of peritonitis
- Attempted micturition results in the passage of a few millilitres of bloodstained urine
- Urethral catheterisation is easy but urine is not forthcoming, although there may be a little blood.

MANAGEMENT

The abdomen is explored, the bladder laceration repaired and the bladder drained.

Extraperitoneal rupture

Trauma is the only cause – a fracture of the pelvis, or during transurethral resection of the prostate or bladder tumours.

CLINICAL FEATURES

There is a history of injury, either accidental or surgical. Symptoms are:

- lower abdominal pain, although this may be masked by the effects of pelvic fracture
- inability to micturate or, at most, a few drops of bloodstained urine.

Urine and blood extravasated into the perivesical space cause the following:

- tender suprapubic thickening
- palpable mass (occasionally).

MANAGEMENT

Extravasation of urine after transurethral resection of the prostate or of a bladder tumour usually responds to a period of urethral catheterisation. For severe injuries which are a consequence of pelvic fracture, suprapubic drainage of the bladder and drainage of the retropubic space are required.

Bladder tumours

The bladder, like the rest of the urinary tract, is lined with transitional cell epithelium and, because it acts as a store for urine and any carcinogens that may be present, it is the commonest site for the development of malignant urinary tract tumours. Benign tumours of the urothelium are exceedingly rare, as are benign tumours of the bladder muscle. Rhabdomyosarcomas

of the latter occur in childhood. However, the great majority of bladder tumours arise from the urothelium, 95% of which are transitional cell lesions. Carcinoma in situ (CIS) refers to flat areas of epithelium composed of cells with anaplastic features and disorderly pattern of growth without extension into the bladder lumen. They are multicentric and commonly occur in association with obvious transitional cell tumours. Squamous cell tumours occur in schistosomiasis, and adeno-carcinomas are the consequence of untreated bladder exstrophy or an urachal remnant.

EPIDEMIOLOGY

For urothelial cancer there is a 5:1 male predominance, although the incidence in females is increasing and may be related to cigarette smoking. The highest incidence of bladder cancer is in the sixth and seventh decades.

AETIOLOGY

Chronic irritation and carcinogenic chemicals are associated with the development of the disease:

Chronic irritation
- Schistosomiasis
- Exstrophy with persistent infection and physical trauma.

Carcinogens
- Cigarette smoking
- Chemical industry – aniline dyes, printing, rubber processing, pesticides.

Because of the known association with the above industries, there are now regular surveillance pro-grammes which use cytological examination of the urine. If a worker in an industry that is known to have a high risk develops bladder cancer, both the victim and dependents may be entitled to compensation.

CLINICAL FEATURES

Symptoms

The great majority of patients present with painless haematuria. A small proportion have urinary infections. A few tumours are found coincidentally in patients who undergo a cystoscopy for other reasons. Advanced cases have lower abdominal pain, severe dysuria, strangury and incontinence of bloodstained urine. Similar irritative findings are found in patients with carcinoma in situ and must be distinguished from bacterial cystitis.

Signs

Unless the disease is advanced, abnormalities are usually absent. A careful bimanual examination may reveal a mass in the bladder wall, but if the diagnosis is established by other means (usually endoscopically) then bimanual examination is better done under anaesthesia to stage the lesion.

INVESTIGATION

Urothelial tumours are often multicentric. Any patient who presents with symptoms suggestive of a urothelial tumour requires full investigation of the urinary tract, which includes:

- urine microscopy and culture for evidence of haematuria and infection
- cytological examination of the urine – most likely to be positive in those with carcinoma in situ or well differentiated tumours
- assessment of renal function
- IVU to search for other tumours in the renal pelvis, ureter or bladder (Fig. 32.26), although small tumours may be difficult to detect
- endoscopic examination of the urethra and bladder; endoscopy identifies the number, position and macroscopic type of urethral or bladder tumours and obtains a biopsy for histological examination of both the tumours and apparently normal mucosa
- bimanual examination (rectum and abdomen in the male; vagina and abdomen in the female) to assess spread of tumour beyond the bladder wall
- chest X-ray and bone scan to seek distant metastases.

In tumours which show histological evidence of invasion into bladder muscle, a CT or MRI scan is essential to determine the stage of the disease (see below) and the need for more radical treatment.

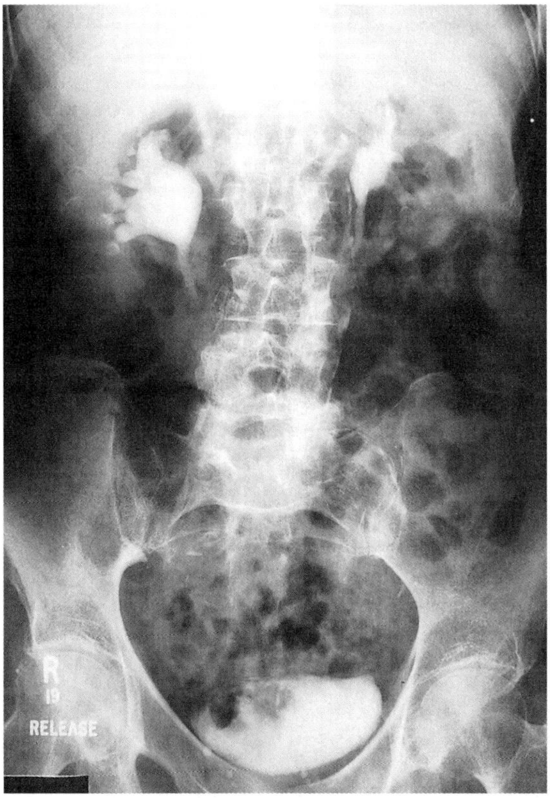

Histological grading

The grades used are:

- carcinoma in situ – this is a high-grade lesion
- well differentiated
- moderately differentiated
- Undifferentiated.

Most tumours contain a mixture of cell types. Grade is assigned on the worst pattern of differentiation.

Tumour staging

The TNM classification is used.

Tumour category is best assessed by histological examination of the resected specimen (pT category). The depth of penetration into or through the bladder wall is used as the criterion for the T component. A tumour is nominally regarded as superficial (pT1A–pT1B) if it has penetrated no further than the basement membrane (Table 32.6). Tumours that have transgressed the bladder wall to a greater degree are pT2–pT4 and their classification is based on a combination of histological and bimanual examination (Table 32.7).

Node category. The lymphatic spread is to nodes on the surface of the bladder, the internal iliac and para-aortic nodes and then more proximally. The classification is shown in Table 32.8.

Fig 32.26 **Intravenous urogram showing a large filling defect in the right side of the bladder as a result of a tumour.**

Table 32.6
Local staging of superficial bladder cancer from histological examination of the resected specimen

Stage	Histological findings
pTiS	Carcinoma in situ
pT1A	Papillary carcinoma with basement membrane intact
pT1B	Tumour has penetrated the basement membrane

Table 32.7
Local staging of bladder cancer that is no longer superficial

Stage	Findings
T2	Superficial muscle is involved
T3A	Deep bladder muscles is involved
T3B	Extending beyond muscle but bladder still mobile
T4A	Adjacent structures involved
T4B	Fixed to pelvic wall

Table 32.8
Nodal staging in bladder cancer

Stage	Findings
N0	No nodes involved
N1	Single regional node
N2	Multiple regional nodes
N3	Fixed regional nodes
N4	Distant lymph nodes

MANAGEMENT

Treatment depends on the site, size and histological grading of the tumour. At the initial endoscopic examination, the tumour is resected as far as possible, with deeper areas of resection being sent separately for histological examination to assess spread into the bladder muscle. Random biopsies of apparently normal bladder mucosa should also be obtained, as these may show changes of dysplasia or carcinoma in situ and provide useful prognostic information on the likelihood of recurrence. The treatment of superficial cancer (pT1S– pT1B) is summarised in Table 32.9. pT2 and pT4 tumours, unless they have advanced nodal involvement (N3–N4) or distant metastases, are managed by radical resection, radical radiotherapy or systemic chemotherapy, or a combination of these.

SURVEILLANCE

Once a diagnosis of urothelial carcinoma has been made, regular lifelong follow up is required; 50% of patients will develop further tumours.

PROGNOSIS

Five-year survivals are summarised in Table 32.10; 95% of those with pT1A tumours survive 5 years.

Bladder diverticulae

A diverticulum is a protrusion of mucosa through the bladder muscle (Fig. 32.27).

Table 32.9
Management of superficial bladder cancer

Stage	Treatment
pTIS	Endoscopic removal of local areas and intravesical BCG
pT1A	Transurethral resection (TUR)
pT1B	TUR
	For recurrence – repeated resection and intravesical BCG, adriamycin or mitomycin
pT1B with poorly differentiated tumour	Radiotherapy or radical cystectomy

Table 32.10
Survival in bladder cancer

Stage	Grade	5-year survival (%)
pT1S		75
pT1A	1	95
pT1B	1	72
pT1	3	39
pT2		45
pT3		39
pT4		5

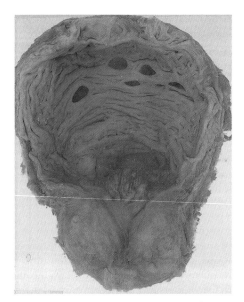

Fig 32.27 **Bladder showing the openings of multiple diverticulae.**

AETIOLOGY AND PATHOLOGICAL FEATURES

The majority are acquired and associated with bladder outflow obstruction.

Diverticulae are often multiple, not surrounded by muscle fibres and therefore unable to empty when the detrusor contracts. Stagnation of urine in a diverticulum or the urinary tract leads to infection, stone formation and squamous metaplasia with the possibility of tumour. A tumour in a diverticulum has a worse prognosis than one in the intact bladder because invasion into surrounding tissues occurs earlier.

CLINICAL FEATURES

Uncomplicated single or multiple diverticula are usually asymptomatic and found coincidentally during the course of investigation of a patient with bladder outflow obstruction. Complications lead to haematuria, dysuria and frequency.

There are no signs which are specific to the condition but infection may cause local tenderness.

INVESTIGATION AND MANAGEMENT

Diverticulae are frequently seen on ultrasound, intravenous urography and at cystoscopy.

Bladder outflow obstruction should be relieved. If diverticulae do not cause problems thereafter, treatment is not required. Persistent infection is an indication for removal.

Bladder fistulae

A fistula is an epithelial-lined track between one hollow viscus and another or between a viscus and the exterior. Bladder fistulae are classified in Table 32.11.

Table 32.11
Classification of bladder fistulae

Type	Origin	Condition
Bladder to exterior	Congenital	Extrophy of bladder Urachal fistula
Bladder to vagina	Acquired	Injury (prolonged obstructed labour) Hysterectomy Cancer Radiotherapy
Bladder to colon	Acquired	Diverticular disease Cancer Radiotherapy
Bladder to small intestine	Acquired	Crohn's disease Radiotherapy
Bladder to rectum	Acquired	Post-prostatectomy Carcinoma of rectum Radiotherapy for prostatic cancer Laser therapy to the prostate
Bladder to uterus	Acquired	Malignancy of either organ Caesarian section Radiotherapy

Vesicovaginal fistula

AETIOLOGY AND PATHOLOGICAL FEATURES
The commonest cause of vesicovaginal fistula in developing countries is prolonged obstructed labour and ischaemic necrosis by the descending fetal head of the anterior vaginal wall. In developed countries, they occur as a result of gynaecological surgery, pelvic malignancy and irradiation damage to the vagina and bladder during treatment for cervical cancer.

CLINICAL FEATURES
There is a constant leak of urine through the vagina.

There may be features of the underlying cause apparent. Examination of the vagina shows urine trickling down from the vault and the fistula may be thickened and palpable.

INVESTIGATION
IVU
An intravenous urogram is mandatory to exclude a ureterovaginal fistula.

Dye test
If there is doubt about the source of leakage, a swab is placed into the vagina and methylene blue inserted into the bladder via a urethral catheter. Blue staining of the swab in the vagina confirms the presence of vesicovaginal fistula. A swab soaked in clear urine suggests a ureterovaginal fistula. Patients with a vesicovaginal fistula often have multiple fistulae. The dye test should be repeated without the swab and the vagina examined directly using a Sim's speculum.

MANAGEMENT
Very few fistulae close spontaneously, however prolonged is bladder drainage.

Fistulae caused by irradiation or malignancy
Urinary diversion via an ileal conduit is most appropriate because the tissues are unsuitable for repair and life expectancy is short. In women with a long life expectancy, a continent urine diversion or Mainz II pouch may be appropriate.

Obstetric and post-traumatic fistulae
Repair should not be attempted within 3 months of confinement to allow control of infection and revascularisation of the ischaemic tissues. For postoperative fistulae, an immediate repair is done.

Fistulae from bladder to gut (enteric fistulae)

These are usually between the large bowel and the bladder.

CLINICAL FEATURES
The patient complains of:

- recurrent urinary infections
- bubbles in the urine (pneumaturia)
- faecal material in the urine (uncommon).

Signs are non-specific but include those of cystitis.

INVESTIGATION AND MANAGEMENT
The diagnosis is not usually in much doubt but a barium enema often identifies the site and extent of underlying disease. This is usually diverticular disease or, more rarely, carcinoma of the large bowel.

Management is by resection of the abnormal bowel and closure of the bladder.

Neuropathic bladder

This term is used to describe bladder dysfunction of neural origin. The neurophysiology of bladder function is incompletely understood and therefore clinical classifications are the most useful in therapy and widely used. Three types are recognised:

- acute atonic bladder
- chronic atonic bladder
- hyperreflexic bladder

AETIOLOGY
The causes may be divided into congenital and acquired.

Urology

The latter are further divisible into trauma, cord compression, primary central nervous system disease, and spinal cord disease secondary to that elsewhere.

PATHOLOGICAL FEATURES

Whatever the type of neuropathy, the secondary effects are:

- urinary stasis with dilatation of the upper urinary tract
- recurrent ascending infection
- progressive loss of renal function
- secondary stone formation.

CLINICAL FEATURES

Symptoms

These range from painless retention of urine to uncontrolled incontinence, frequency, urgency and poor urine stream. In long-standing neuropathy, there may be systemic symptoms of renal failure.

Signs

There is commonly evidence of other neurological involvement from the underlying cause. A full neurological examination is essential. Depending on the clinical nature of the neuropathy, the bladder may be distended with a trickle of overflow or empty with urine constantly emerging from the urethral meatus.

INVESTIGATION

Urine

Because of the likelihood of infection, bacterial culture is carried out repeatedly.

Renal function

Standard techniques are used.

Ultrasonography

Upper urinary tract dilatation and bladder emptying can be assessed.

Urinary flow studies

These are an essential part of the diagnosis and management of the neuropathic bladder. The patient with a full bladder voids into a machine which measures both the volume voided and the maximum flow (Q_{max} in mL/s). The pattern of voiding can also be observed. Voided volumes of < 150 mL may lead to erroneous results. A patient who has a normal bladder outlet and normally functioning detrusor will void with a flow rate of > 15 mL/s.

Pressure flow studies
Bladder and intra-abdominal pressure (usually rectal) are measured simultaneously. The abdominal pressure is automatically subtracted from the bladder pressure to give detrusor pressure. The bladder is filled at a standard rate and the detrusor pressure measured. Rises in pressure during filling are recorded, as is the detrusor pressure at maximal urine flow. After completion of voiding, the residual urine can be measured. Bladder emptying can be recorded using a video system.

MANAGEMENT OF CLINICAL TYPES OF NEUROPATHY

The general aims of treatment are to restore continence and preserve renal function.

Acute atony

This condition typically occurs after spinal cord injury in the stage of spinal shock (see Ch. 30) and may last up to 3 months. The internal involuntary sphincter remains closed and the detrusor inactive so that the bladder is distended and empties by overflow. However, this situation should not be allowed to occur because it results in delay of return of function to the bladder spinal reflex centres (sacral 2, 3 and 4). Intermittent urethral catheterisation performed by either the patient or the carer four to five times a day, best carried out in a specialised centre, prevents distension. The eventual result is an automatic bladder which empties involuntarily every 2 or 3 hours or a bladder from which the urine can be expelled by manual compression.

Chronic atony

The cause is either a peripheral neuropathy or long-standing outflow obstruction. The former is usually irreversible and either intermittent self-catheterisation or urinary diversion should be considered. It may be possible to correct the latter without producing incontinence (see 'Prostatic hyperplasia'). Urodynamic studies are essential in assessing residual detrusor function and the likelihood of the bladder being able to empty once the obstruction is relieved.

Hyperreflexia

Uninhibited high-pressure detrusor contractions are found on urodynamic studies but are not diagnostic of systemic neuropathy. Other features which may be found are:

- detrusor sphincter incoordination
- high voiding pressure
- significant residual volume
- poor and intermittent flow rate.

The bladder assumes a fir tree appearance on IVU or cystography (Fig. 32.28)

MANAGEMENT

This includes:

- *Bladder conditioning*. The patient is asked to delay voiding for longer and longer periods.

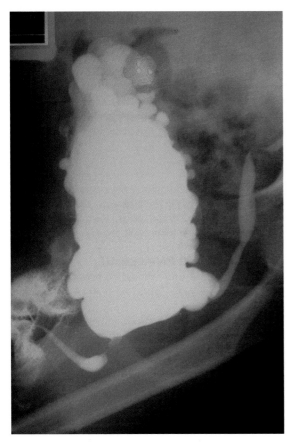

Fig 32.28 **Fir tree appearance of a neuropathic bladder.**

- *Anticholinergics.* These are usually used in combination with bladder conditioning and are effective in mild to moderate cases.
- *Clam cystoplasty.* An opened segment of small bowel is sutured into the opened bladder. This decreases the bladder pressure and increases the bladder volume. The reduction in bladder pressure results in poor bladder emptying, and intermittent self-catheterisation is usually necessary.
- *Urine diversion* may be indicated.

Incontinence

Incontinence is the involuntary passage of urine from the urethra and occurs as a result of either sphincter weakness or bladder instability.

The most common cause of stress incontinence in women is due to descent of the bladder neck so that any sudden increase in abdominal pressure acts only on the bladder and not the sphincter mechanism. In men it results from a prostatecyomy.

CLINICAL FEATURES

Symptoms
Stress incontinence results in involuntary loss of urine whenever intra-abdominal pressure is raised – coughing, sneezing or exercise. Symptoms of detrusor instability include frequency, urgency, urge incontinence, nocturia and bed-wetting. Not all of these symptoms may be present.

Signs
Patients with detrusor instability may have evidence of a neuropathy. Stress incontinence may be demonstrable when the patient coughs or strains.

INVESTIGATION

Urine examination
Bacterial culture is essential. Cytology should be obtained because the clinical features of detrusor instability can be mimicked by carcinoma in situ of the bladder. The two conditions can coexist.

Urodynamic studies
Patients with symptoms of detrusor instability may have normal urodynamic findings.

MANAGEMENT

Sphincter weakness
Conservative treatment includes:

- weight loss
- pelvic floor exercises
- pelvic floor stimulation
- local or systemic oestrogen therapy
- ephedrine 15–30 mg t.d.s. (at least 3 months' treatment is usually required).

In men pelvic floor exercises and ephedrine are worth a trial. Failure to respond requires surgical therapy with the insertion of an artificial sphincter or injection of inert substances into the sphincter area.

In women who have failed to respond to a conservative regimen, surgical treatment aims to elevate the bladder neck and can be achieved via either a transvaginal or a suprapubic approach. Long-term results of injections of collagen or other inert substances into the sphincter area are still being assessed.

Detrusor instability
Whether or not detrusor instability has been identified by urodynamic studies, the majority of patients respond to bladder training. After a full explanation of the condition, the patient is asked not to pass urine for increasingly lengthy periods. An accurate fluid chart of input and output and of the timing of micturition is also kept. In the few patients who fail to respond, anticholinergic agents are of value (e.g. oxybutinine

hydrochloride 5 mg t.d.s.), but they must not be used in patients with a history of glaucoma.

The prostate

The gland is subject to humoral influences throughout life. In utero, it is stimulated by maternal oestrogen and an alteration in the androgen oestrogen balance may be responsible for the enlargement of the prostate which occurs in later life. During the active sexual period, androgenic stimulation predominates. Testosterone produced by the testes, adrenals and the peripheral conversion of other steroids is converted in the prostate by the enzyme 5-alpha-reductase to dihydrotestosterone, the most active androgen within the prostate.

Clinical assessment

Rectal examination allows direct assessment of the size, shape, consistency and other features of the gland by digital palpation through the anterior wall of the rectum. The normal gland has the following characteristics:

- it is soft to firm
- it has a well defined median sulcus
- it is not tender.

  Abnormalities are as follows:

- Increased size causes the prostate to bulge backwards into the rectum so that the finger inserted through the anus passes a posterior overhang. The median sulcus becomes less obvious
- Changes in consistency are either diffuse or localised. A very hard and irregular gland is characteristic of prostatic cancer but can occur in other conditions.
- Tenderness is present in inflammation.

  It is notoriously difficult to judge accurately absolute prostatic size.

Diseases of the prostate

The prostate is subject to three major disorders:

- infection
- benign hyperplasia (BPH)
- carcinoma.

Infections

There are three clinical entities:

- acute bacterial prostatitis
- non-bacterial chronic prostatitis
- prostatodynia

Acute bacterial prostatitis

AETIOLOGY

This condition is more common in patients with diabetes mellitus. *E . coli*, *Staphylococcus aureus* and *Neisseria gonorrhoea* are the common organisms. *Chlamydia* may also be found. The route by which these organisms reach the prostate is unknown, but some instances may be by retrograde spread from the urethra.

CLINICAL FEATURES

There is general malaise with fever, rigors, dysuria and, frequency. Pain is felt in the perineum, the rectum, and the suprapubic and sacral areas. Rectal examination reveals an acutely tender but soft prostate.

INVESTIGATION AND MANAGEMENT

Bacterial culture of urine should be performed and, if possible, fluid obtained from the urethra after gentle prostatic massage.

Management is with bed rest and appropriate antibiotic therapy. If *Chlamydia* is identified, tetracycline or erythromycin are the agents of choice. The patient's partner will also need to be treated.

Non-bacterial (chronic) prostatitis

AETIOLOGY

This condition may arise as a result of a blood-borne infection or failure adequately to treat an episode of acute prostatitis. The prostate becomes the site of chronic inflammation with fibrous tissue formation.

CLINICAL FEATURES

There are symptoms of generalised ill health, frequency, dysuria, haematuria, haemospermia and perineal discomfort.

Rectal examination reveals a tender, hard and sometimes slightly irregular prostate. The prostate may also be normal.

INVESTIGATION AND MANAGEMENT

Culture of expressed prostatic secretion usually does not result in a growth of bacteria, but white blood cells are present.

The condition is difficult to eradicate. Long-term antibiotic therapy with a quinolone antibiotic, trimethoprim or tetracycline may be of value with alpha-adrenergic blocking agents to relax the smooth muscle of the prostate.

Prostatodynia

These patients do not have prostatic infection but suffer from chronic pelvic pain and require symptomatic relief.

Benign prostatic hyperplasia (BPH)

This condition is present in all men over the age of 40. The only method of prevention – unlikely to receive much support from the male population – is castration before puberty. Benign prostatic hypertrophy occurs in 75% of men in the eighth decade, and 20% of men over the age of 40 will require treatment during their lifetime for bladder outflow obstruction.

AETIOLOGY AND PATHOLOGICAL FEATURES

The cause of BPH is unknown but it is generally regarded as a consequence of fluctuating levels of both androgen and oestrogen (and consequently the ratio between them) at different times of life. The effect is to produce hyperplasia of the glandular cells of the central zone with associated myoepithelial and fibrous tissue development. The cells involved vary in their proportionate contribution in any one patient. Perhaps because of this, the condition is variably referred to as benign prostatic hyperplasia and benign prostatic hypertrophy, but both are subsumed under the shorthand BPH. The hyperplastic central zone cells displace the peripheral zone so that a pseudo-capsule is formed. Hyperplasia also variably compresses the urethral lumen but this has little relationship to the overall size – glands of less than 40 g can cause as much trouble as those in excess of 100 g. The only relevance of the size of the prostate is that it may affect the type of treatment given.

CLINICAL FEATURES

The patient may present in one of three ways:

- benign prostatic obstruction
- acute retention of urine
- chronic retention of urine.

Prostatic obstruction

Symptoms are:
- hesitancy
- poor stream
- intermittency
- terminal dribbling
- increased frequency, particularly at night
- urinary infection.

The last two, in part, are due to incomplete bladder emptying. In addition, patients with prostatic outflow obstruction frequently have detrusor instability and may therefore also complain of urgency and urge incontinence and postmicturition dribbling.

Signs are usually absent. Rectal examination shows that the prostate is enlarged with a regular contour.

Acute urinary retention

Forty per cent of patients who present in this way do not have a preceding history of prostatic outflow obstruction. The episode may be precipitated by anticholinergic drugs, diuretics (including alcohol), prolonged voluntary suppression of micturition and surgery for conditions outwith the urinary tract.

Symptoms are a sudden inability to pass urine and, after a very short period, acute severe suprapubic pain because of distension of what is usually a previously normal bladder.

Signs. The patient is in severe pain and frequently unable to stay still. The bladder is palpable and tender in the midline above the pubis and below the umbilicus. Rectal examination shows an enlarged prostate but the gland is pushed down by the overfull bladder so that the size may be exaggerated.

Chronic retention

Symptoms. Chronic retention is painless. The patient may be ill from the metabolic effects of back pressure on the kidneys. There is characteristically the passage at frequent intervals of small quantities of urine and of rising on a number of occasions at night.

Signs. The patient's clothes and underwear may be wet and smell of urine. Apart from the systemic features of renal failure, there is a visible suprapubic swelling, dull to percussion. A search is made for any neurological abnormality because a painless bladder enlargement from such a cause may be confused with BPH and chronic retention.

Rectal examination shows the same general features as those of acute retention.

INVESTIGATION

Bladder outflow obstruction

Urine is taken for culture.

Renal function is assessed as described previously.

Plain X-ray is done to exclude stones. There is no role for an IVU in the assessment of a patient with prostatic outflow obstruction because of BPH.

Ultrasonography is done to assess dilatation of the upper urinary tract and to estimate residual urine and prostatic size.

Micturition flow rate is measured. Ninety per cent of men with a flow rate of less than 12 m L/s have bladder outflow obstruction.

MANAGEMENT

Prostatic outflow obstruction

Not all men require treatment and a period of watchful waiting to see whether they become more symptomatic is justifiable.

Conservative treatment

This includes:

- alpha-adrenergic blocking agents
- 5-alpha-reductase inhibitors (finasteride) for men with glands greater than 40 g
- thermotherapy
- temporary prostatic stents.

Surgical treatment

The treatment of choice for a prostate estimated to weigh less than 100 g is a transurethral resection (TUR). If the gland is estimated to be larger than this, an open operation may be indicated. The use of lasers and prostatic vaporisation is still being assessed.

Acute retention of urine

The patient is in severe pain and catheterisation is required. It is best achieved by the suprapubic route. The advantages of a suprapubic catheter include:

- lack of damage to the urethra
- urethral stricture from an indwelling catheter does not occur
- false passages are avoided
- ease of introduction in a patient with a large prostate
- trial of voiding is simple
- the operative field is left clear for a subsequent TUR.

Because 40% of patients with acute retention have no previous history of outflow obstruction, it is reasonable to allow them to attempt to void after clamping the suprapubic catheter. Those who are able to void usually had a residual urine of less than 700 mL when initially catheterised and avoid a prostatectomy in the short term. Patients who revert back into retention require a prostatectomy.

Chronic retention

The treatment is by prostatectomy. The only indication for preoperative catheter drainage is in patients with impaired renal function secondary to back pressure on the kidneys. Catheterisation eventually leads to the development of a urinary infection, which increases the morbidity and mortality of a subsequent operation and is difficult to eradicate in a large floppy bladder. If a catheter is required, attempts should be made to decompress the bladder slowly, as this reduces but does not completely do away with the development of severe bleeding from distended submucosal veins. The renal concentrating mechanism is usually impaired and bladder catheterisation may result in diuresis leading to dehydration, hypotension and further impairment of renal function. Close monitoring of the patient's weight, blood pressure, pulse, fluid input and urine output is required. Once renal function has improved and stabilised, definitive surgery can be undertaken.

Prostatectomy

The operation of choice for glands less than 100 g is a transurethral resection in which the greater part of the adenomatous hyperplasia inside the pseudo-capsule of compressed peripheral zone is removed piecemeal by diathermy. For larger glands, a retropubic prostatectomy which incises the pseudo-capsule and enucleates the adenoma is preferred.

The advantages of transurethral prostatectomy are:

- absence of wound infection
- significant reduction in pain
- less frequent urinary infection
- postoperative incontinence reduced
- lower incidence of general complications such as chest infection, deep vein thrombosis and pulmonary embolus
- hospital stay and early mortality are reduced.

Disadvantages include:

- long period of training is required to learn the technique
- high incidence of re-operation for recurrent disease
- possible increased incidence of later postoperative mortality.

Complications

- Bleeding – primary, reactionary or secondary haemorrhage
- Absorption of irrigation fluid into the systemic circulation which can cause hyponatraemia with epileptiform fits and cardiovascular collapse (the TUR syndrome)
- Failure to void
- Urinary infection
- Epididymo-orchitis
- Incontinence
- Erectile dysfunction.

Retrograde ejaculation is an invariable sequel of prostatectomy about which patients must be warned.

Prognosis

Only 70% of patients are satisfied with the result of a prostatectomy. The main reasons for this are that either the operation was performed for detrusor instability rather than bladder outflow obstruction or, where both conditions existed, detrusor instability did not resolve after prostatectomy.

Carcinoma of the prostate

EPIDEMIOLOGY

This tumour is rapidly becoming the most common malignancy to affect men. The disease is one of ageing, rarely discovered under the age of 50 and with a peak incidence in the 70s. Examination of serial sections of the prostate of men who have died from other causes has demonstrated that 29% of those aged between 50 and 60, 49% of men in the age group 70–79 and 67% of those aged 80–89 had unsuspected prostate cancer. Not all are clinically apparent and, even when identified, they do not express the same malignant potential. At one extreme are those tumours which are found only at death, while at the other there are rapidly progressive tumours with invasive and metastatic potential. In between there are tumours with intermediate degrees of aggression and long periods of local growth only. However, current techniques are unable to identify which are which. In consequence, there is much confusion and controversy about whether or not to screen for the condition. To do so would lead to a significant over-treatment of the many men discovered. The same dilemma exists about treatment: diagnosis does not necessarily imply progression or a need to treat.

AETIOLOGY

Apart from the relationship to ageing, the cause is unknown, although there is probably some relationship with the hormonal environment. Some men have a strong family history.

PATHOLOGICAL FEATURES

The tumour is an adenocarcinoma usually arising in the periphery of the prostate and confined within the prostatic capsule. Its spread is:

- local in the periprostatic and perirectal soft tissues and upwards into the pelvis
- lymphatic to the iliac and para-aortic nodes
- blood-borne, principally to bone.

CLINICAL FEATURES

Symptoms
These include:
- bladder outflow obstruction (see above)
- metastatic disease – bone pain, leg swelling from lymphatic obstruction
- renal failure from bilateral ureteric obstruction.

Signs
- A nodule in a palpably benign gland
- Hard irregular prostate on rectal examination sometimes with perirectal and periprostatic thickening
- Ankle and leg oedema
- Other signs of metastases.

The disease may only be discovered at an incidental rectal examination or on histological examination of prostatic tissue removed during a prostatectomy for clinically benign disease.

INVESTIGATION

A histological or cytological diagnosis must be made and can be achieved by:
- transrectal or transperineal biopsy, preferably guided by ultrasound
- aspiration cytology
- transurethral resection.

Other investigations
These include:

- routine evaluation of renal function
- serum alkaline phosphatase concentration – elevated in patients with bone metastases.

Serum prostate-specific antigen (PSA) concentration

Prostate-specific antigen is secreted into the serum by both benign and malignant prostatic tissue. Its level relates to the volume of prostatic tissue and there is considerable overlap in the serum levels of patients with benign and malignant prostatic disease, particularly in the range associated with confined and hence potentially curable prostate cancer. Many men with mildly elevated PSA levels will not have prostate cancer and 20% of those with cancer will have a 'normal' PSA. In consequence, its use as a screening test for prostatic cancer is severely limited. However, it has value in monitoring the progression of the disease and response to treatment.

Ultrasonography
Abdominal ultrasound may identify unilateral or bilateral hydronephrosis because of ureteric involvement. Transrectal ultrasound is used both as an aid to diagnosis and for staging prostate cancer, but unfortunately it is not particularly accurate in either. It is unable to detect microscopic spread beyond the prostate.

Bone scanning
Radioisotope bone scan can detect areas of increased bone activity irrespective of their cause (Fig. 32.29). Confirmatory X-rays need to be taken of areas of increased isotope uptake.

Staging
Prostate cancer is staged by the TNM classification. The T stage is most accurately assessed with the patient anaesthetised; a description is given in Table 32.12.

MANAGEMENT
As yet there have been no useful randomised clinical trials in the treatment of prostate cancer. As a result, no hard and fast rules can be given on optimal treatment. Decisions should be based on the patient's age and general state. Options include:

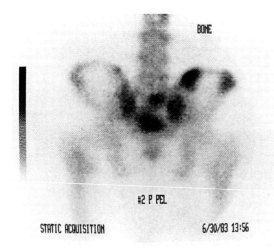

Fig 32.29 **A bone scan showing multiple hot spots caused by metastatic carcinoma of the prostate.**

Table 32.12
Staging of prostate cancer

Stage	Findings
T1a	An incidental finding of tumour with low biological potential for aggressive behaviour in a prostate removed for clinically benign disease
T1b	An incidental finding of a tumour with potentially biological aggressive behaviour found in a prostate removed for clinically benign disease (high-grade or diffuse)
T1c	Tumour identified because of an elevated serum prostate-specific antigen
T2a	Tumour involving half a lobe or less
T2b	More than half a lobe but not both
T2c	Both lobes
T3	Tumour extends through capsule and may involve seminal vesicle
T4	Tumour fixed invasive adjacent structures other than seminal vesicle

- no treatment with assessment of progress
- endocrine therapy
- radiotherapy
- surgery.

No treatment

Men with asymptomatic low-stage, low-grade disease and those with significant comorbidity can be offered follow-up with regular observation. Those who show signs of disease progression can then be treated with one of the therapies outlined below.

Early treatment by hormone therapy provides a slight survival advantage and reduction in morbidity from disease progression in men who have asymptomatic advanced localised or metastatic prostate cancer.

Endocrine therapy

Most of the cells of the prostate are dependent for their multiplication on the male hormone testosterone. Ninety per cent of circulating testosterone is produced by the testes under the influence of luteinising hormone (LH) which is in turn controlled by the hypothalamic secretion of luteinising hormone-releasing hormone (LHRH, Fig. 32.30). The remaining 10% of testosterone is produced by the adrenals and by peripheral conversion of other steroids. Eighty per cent of patients with symptomatic prostate cancer respond subjectively and 60% respond objectively to androgen suppression or ablation. The mean duration of response is 2 years. Once the tumour is no longer hormone-responsive, the mean survival is 6 months.

Androgen suppression. This is only used in men with locally advanced or metastatic disease. LHRH analogues initially stimulate the pituitary, but after approximately 7 days the pituitary receptors become blocked and down regulation occurs. Serum testosterone falls to castrate levels. These substances are long-acting and are administered subcutaneously every

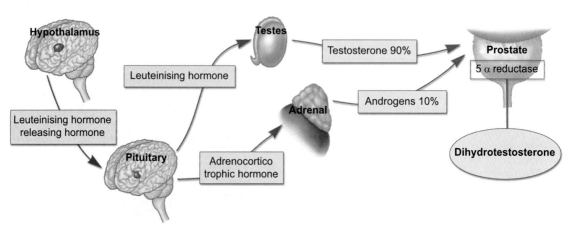

Fig 32.30 **Hormonal control of the prostate.**

1 or 3 months. Because of the initial stimulation of the pituitary, an anti-androgen should be given for 10–14 days before the analogue is given to prevent disease progression.

Androgen ablation is by bilateral subcapsular orchidectomy, which can be done under local anaesthesia as an outpatient and removes the testosterone-producing part of the testicle. There is no difference in response between orchidectomy and LHRH analogue therapy and the choice of treatment should lie with the patient.

Radiotherapy

Radiotherapy is effective in controlling the pain of bony metastases. It is also used for the treatment of the primary if it is thought that the tumour is confined to the prostate. There have been no useful randomised controlled trials to assess its benefit compared with radical surgery.

Surgical treatment

Transurethral resection is used in patients who present with symptoms of outflow obstruction or acute retention.

Radical prostatectomy is one of the most controversial aspects of the treatment of carcinoma of the prostate. Its use for disease that is believed to be localised to the prostate is widespread in the USA and Europe and is increasing in the UK. The reasons why its use in the UK has been slow to increase are:

- The purpose of the operation is to remove the whole of the prostate with its confined cancer, but current staging techniques cannot accurately identify patients in this class.
- Radical prostatectomy fails in its objective of removing the whole of the prostate in 50% of those submitted to it.
- Bilateral lymphadenectomy is required.
- A high proportion of prostatic cancers have low malignant potential and radical prostatectomy is over-treatment.
- There is a mortality of at least 1%
- Morbidity is considerable and includes incontinence, erectile dysfunction and anastomotic strictures.

Against this, it is probably indicated in men with poorly differentiated tumours which are thought to be localised to the prostate and who would otherwise have a 10-year life expectancy. A radical prostatectomy correctly performed will eradicate the disease if it is confined to the prostate. Until it is possible to accurately identify confined disease preoperatively, a substantial proportion of men 'suitable' for radical prostatectomy will not be cured.

PROGNOSIS

In men with prostate cancer confined within the capsule who undergo radical prostatectomy, approximately 55% survive 10 years, in comparison with those who have metastatic disease at presentation, of whom only 25% can be expected to survive 5 years with current therapy.

The male urethra

Congenital abnormalities

These are:

- urethral valves
- hypospadias
- epispadias.

Urethral valves

PATHOLOGICAL FEATURES

Folds of urothelium develop in the posterior urethra in utero to form a valve-like obstruction to the passage of urine. Gross dilatation of the prostatic urethra (Fig. 32.31), distention of the bladder and ureters and hydronephrosis result. Severe renal impairment follows. With increasing use of antenatal ultrasound, many boys with urethral valves are diagnosed in utero by antenatal screening.

CLINICAL FEATURES

The bladder may be palpable and the infant constantly

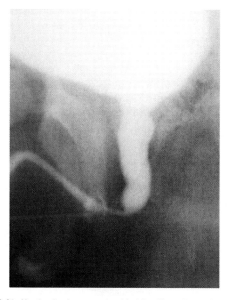

Fig 32.31 **Urethral valves causing bladder distention and dilatation of the prostatic urethra.**

dribbles urine. The development of a urinary infection may draw attention to the problem before end-stage renal failure develops.

MANAGEMENT

When diagnosed in utero, a stent can be inserted to drain the baby's bladder into the amniotic cavity, so preserving renal function. Endoscopic division of the valves is required, sometimes with urinary diversion to improve renal function.

Hypospadias

AETIOLOGY

The two genital folds on the ventral aspect of the phallus fail to fuse and form the anterior urethra of the male. The meatus is therefore displaced posteriorly for a variable distance. Hypospadias is classified according to where the opening lies (Fig. 32.32). Other genital abnormalities, such as failure of testicular descent, are often present and there may be a family history.

CLINICAL FEATURES

Apart from the abnormal opening of the urethra, the foreskin is hooded and the penis is bent (chordee) ventrally because of secondary fibrosis in the area of the absent urethra.

MANAGEMENT

Surgical repair, usually utilising the foreskin, is carried

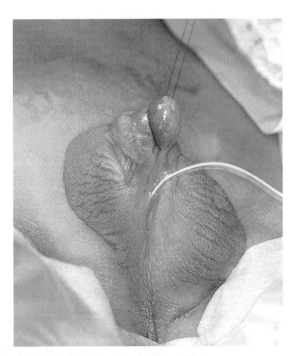

Fig 32.32 **An example of a penile hypospadias.**

out at around the age of 3 years before the child goes to school and has to face his 'normal' contemporaries.

Epispadias

This is extremely rare. The urethra opens on the dorsum of the penis and there may be exstrophy of the bladder. No clear embryological mechanism has been formulated. Complex repair is required.

Urethral injury

AETIOLOGY

The male urethra is more frequently injured than that of the female. The most common cause is instrumentation of the urethra by a catheter or cystoscope. Up to 30% of pelvic fractures are associated with urethral damage and 10% of urethral trauma, beyond the pelvic floor, is caused by a fall-astride injury.

CLINICAL FEATURES

History

A urethral injury should always be suspected in a patient who has been injured and who presents with any of the following:

- blood at the urethral meatus
- haematuria
- anuria.

Signs

Physical examination may reveal a palpable bladder. Lower abdominal tenderness is always present in a patient with a pelvic fracture and does not necessarily imply bladder or urethral damage. In fall-astride injuries there may be bruising and swelling in the perineum. In rupture of the membranous urethra, the prostatic area is said to be boggy and the prostate high-riding. However, anyone who has attempted to perform a rectal examination in a man with a fractured pelvis realises how difficult this physical sign is to elicit.

INVESTIGATION

It is unwise to make repeated attempts to pass a urethral catheter. If the diagnosis is in doubt, urethrography using water-soluble contrast media is done.

MANAGEMENT

The urethral injury takes low priority in the overall management of patients subjected to severe multiple trauma.

Anterior urethral injuries

If the rupture is *complete*, the perineal haematoma is evacuated and a primary repair done. If *incomplete*, either a well lubricated soft, small urethral catheter should be passed by an experienced urologist and left in situ for 10 days or a suprapubic catheter inserted.

Posterior urethral injuries

Either a suprapubic catheter should be inserted or a urethral catheter should be railroaded into the bladder (Fig. 32.33). This allows alignment of the divided ends, and if a stricture develops, subsequent management may be easier.

COMPLICATIONS

These are as follows:

- urethral stricture
- incontinence
- erectile dysfunction (neurogenic and vascular).

Urethral stricture

AETIOLOGY

Strictures may be congenital, traumatic or inflammatory (Box 32.8).

CLINICAL FEATURES

There may be a history related to the underlying cause. The patient complains of difficult and incomplete micturition with a poor stream.

There is a thin, divergent urine stream with terminal dribbling. The bladder may be palpable.

INVESTIGATION AND MANAGEMENT

Urine flow rate is reduced and prolonged with intermittent peaks due to temporarily improved flow due to abdominal strain. Urethrography demonstrates the site, length and number of strictures.

Urethral dilatation used to be the only treatment but invariably had to be continued indefinitely to prevent

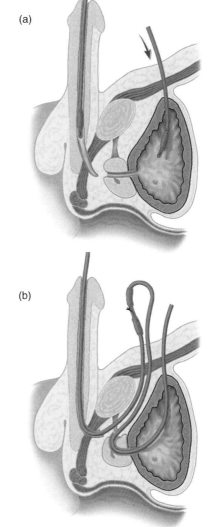
(a)

(b)

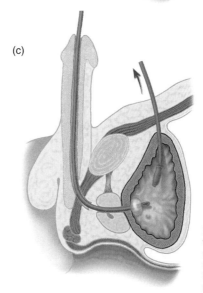
(c)

Fig 32.33 **A technique for railroading a urethral catheter in a patient with a ruptured urethra.**

Box 32.8

Causes of urethral stricture

Congenital
Meatal stenosis

Traumatic
Urethral catheterisation
Cystoscopy
Transurethral resection
After rupture of urethra

Inflammatory
Gonorrhoea
Non-specific urethritis

recurrence. Today the treatment of choice is direct endoscopic incision or a urethroplasty.

Penis

Phimosis

DEFINITION AND AETIOLOGY
This is inability to retract the foreskin.

Congenital
It is not usually possible to retract the foreskin without the application of undue force until the age of 2–3 years, because the inner surface of the foreskin adheres to the glans. No active measures are required for uncomplicated, unretractile foreskin even when the foreskin is reported as ballooning when the child passes urine.

Acquired
This is the result of:

- recurrent infections (balanitis) of which diabetes mellitus is an associate
- underlying tumour of the glans penis.

CLINICAL FEATURES
The preputial orifice is white and scarred and indurated, presenting symptoms including secondary untractability of the foreskin, irritation at or bleeding from the preputial orifice, dysuria and occasionally acute urinary retention.

MANAGEMENT
Treatment is by circumcision. The operation should not be carried out until infection is under control.

Paraphimosis

AETIOLOGY AND PATHOLOGICAL FEATURES
The foreskin contains fibrous tissue because of previous attacks of inflammation usually as a result of forceful retraction of the prepuce. It normally cannot be retracted, but if this occurs either by manipulation or during sexual intercourse, the fibrous band encircles the penis in the subcoronal area to cause congestion of the glans.

CLINICAL FEATURES
There may be a suggestive history. Pain in the glans is usually moderate to severe and there may be difficulty on micturition.

It is not possible to reduce the retracted foreskin. The glans is oedematous. A tight band may be palpable in the subcoronal area.

MANAGEMENT
An injection of hyaluronidase with lignocaine into the constricted area, followed by gentle pressure and traction, will usually result in reduction. Failure necessitates incision of the constricting band. Patients should subsequently be circumcised if it is a recurrent problem.

Circumcision

INDICATIONS
- Religious ritual circumcision – Muslims, Arabs and Jews
- Phimosis
- Paraphimosis
- Recurrent balanitis
- Preputial injuries.

COMPLICATIONS
The operation should not be undertaken lightly. There is an anaesthetic mortality. In addition there may be:

- primary or secondary haemorrhage
- secondary infection
- meatal ulceration and stenosis because of the absence of protection by the foreskin
- injury to the glans
- over-radical excision with scarring.

Peyronie's disease

AETIOLOGY AND PATHOLOGICAL FEATURES
The cause of this condition is unknown. There is fibrous thickening in the corpora cavernosae which results in bending or angulation of the penis when erect. Circumferential fibrosis may result in distal flaccidity during an erection.

CLINICAL FEATURES
The penis is angulated during erection which may make intercourse impossible or painful (Fig. 32.34). The

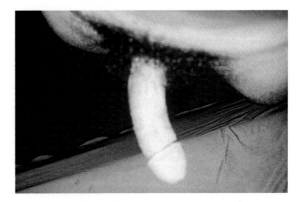

Fig 32.34 **Peyronie's disease with penile bending.**

degree of angulation can be assessed by inducing an artificial erection with an injection of intracavernosal prostaglandin E_1.

MANAGEMENT

The penis can be straightened but made shorter by excising a wedge from the corpora opposite to the maximum angulation. Resuturing the excised edges straightens the penis.

Priapism

This is a persistent and painful erection of the penis.

AETIOLOGY AND PATHOLOGICAL FEATURES

The great majority (80%) have no underlying cause. Those known are summarised in Box 32.9 and some relate to episodes of blood sludging. If detumescence does not take place within 8 hours, venous and arterial thrombosis ensues with fibrosis in the corpora and permanent erectile failure.

MANAGEMENT

Because of the risk of irreversible damage to the erectile apparatus, this is a urological emergency. Aspiration of the thick viscid blood from the corpora may be sufficient. If that fails, a shunt is created between the corpora cavernosa and the glans penis, the corpora cavernosa and the corpora spongiosa or the corpora cavernosa and the saphenous vein.

Carcinoma of the penis

AETIOLOGY

The occurrence of the disease mainly in the uncircumcised and elderly suggests that poor standards of subpreputial hygiene allow the accumulation of carcinogens but there is no direct evidence for this. The tumour is a squamous carcinoma. It is now rare in developed countries.

CLINICAL FEATURES

There is an offensive bloody discharge issuing from

Box 32.9

Causes of priapism

Idiopathic (80%)
Intracavernosal injections of vasoactive drugs for the treatment of erectile dysfunction
Sickle cell anaemia
Leukaemia
Malignancy

---

beneath a non-retractile foreskin. Inguinal lymphadenopathy is invariably present as a result of either infection or secondary spread.

MANAGEMENT

This depends on the extent of the disease. Treatment options include:

- partial amputation
- radical amputation with block dissection of inguinal lymph nodes
- radiotherapy
- chemotherapy.

Testis, epididymis and cord

Undescended testis

EPIDEMIOLOGY

Both testes are undescended in 30% of premature infants: at term this has fallen to 3%; and at one year 1%. Spontaneous descent after 1 year is exceedingly rare.

AETIOLOGY

The cause is failure of migration along the normal line of descent. In an ectopic testis the testicle deviates away from the line and may lie in front of the penis in the superficial inguinal pouch, in the perineum or in the thigh. The cause is not known.

CLINICAL FEATURES

An empty scrotal sac or hemiscrotum at 1 year indicates that the testicle is:

- proximal to the external inguinal ring (undescended)
- truly absent
- retractile – the cremaster muscle reflexly pulls the organ up towards the inguinal canal
- ectopic.

A retractile testis can usually be coaxed into the scrotal sac, or will enter spontaneously if the child is asked to crouch. An ectopic testicle may be palpable in the areas described above but cannot be brought into the scrotum. An incompletely descended testis may be palpable at the external ring or in the neck of the scrotum. A testicle in the inguinal canal is impalpable.

COMPLICATIONS

- Infertility – inevitable in bilateral and common in unilateral undescent, and frequent in those who have had undescent treated
- Torsion
- Trauma

- Inguinal hernia
- Malignant disease.

INVESTIGATION

If the testicle is not palpable, ultrasonography, CT and laparoscopy are useful investigations to determine whether the testicle is truly absent and, if not, where it is situated.

MANAGEMENT

The aim is to bring the testicle with its blood supply into the scrotum as early as possible, usually between 1 and 2 years. Boys who present with a well developed undescended testis before puberty should undergo an orchidopexy and operation to bring the testicle and its blood supply into the scrotum. However, if the testis is poorly developed an orchidectomy is advised. Beyond puberty, orchidectomy should be done. A testicular prosthesis can be placed in the scrotum.

Torsion

AETIOLOGY AND PATHOLOGICAL FEATURES

Torsion is a recognised complication of testicular maldescent. The episode occurs any time between birth and early adolescence but is uncommon thereafter. A horizontally lying testicle with a long mesorchium and cord within the vaginal sac, so that the testis hangs like the clapper of a bell, is most prone to torsion. This anatomical arrangement is usually bilateral so that both testes are at risk. The twist deprives the organ of its blood supply and, if untwisting does not take place within 6 hours, ischaemia is irreversible, gangrene develops and the testis either suppurates or atrophies.

CLINICAL FEATURES

There may be a history of previous episodes of testicular pain. The pain may be initially felt in the iliac fossa or over the cord and is often associated with vomiting.

The testicle is extremely tender, swollen and drawn up in the scrotum. The unaffected testicle may have a horizontal lie.

Other conditions which must be considered

- Torsion of an appendix of the testis
- Acute epididymo-orchitis
- Idiopathic scrotal oedema.

MANAGEMENT

Treatment of testicular torsion is, for the reasons given above, a surgical emergency.

Non-operative

It may be possible to de-rotate the testis. Standing at the foot of the bed, the testis is rotated towards the thigh and this may have to be rotated through two or three turns. If this manoeuvre is successful, the testicle and that on the other side should be surgically fixed on the next operating list.

Surgical

Failure of non-operative reduction requires immediate operation. The testis is de-rotated and fixed. The unaffected testis is dealt with at the same operation. A gangrenous testis is removed.

Orchitis and epididymo-orchitis

AETIOLOGY AND PATHOLOGICAL FEATURES

Primary orchitis is rare except in association with mumps. The testis is often secondarily infected from epididymitis which originates by retrograde spread from the prostate and seminal vesicle; a blood-borne infection is the alternative source. A surgical procedure on the lower urinary tract such as a TUR may also be a precipitating factor. The organisms are *Neisseria gonorrhoea*, *Escherichia coli* and *Chlamydia*. Chronic infection or a discharging sinus may be the consequence of tuberculosis.

CLINICAL FEATURES

There may be a preceding history of an operation or of dysuria, frequency and haematuria. Pain in the scrotum is acute and the patient is conscious of swelling. Fever and rigors are not uncommon.

The epididymis is acutely tender and enlarged, although it may be difficult to distinguish it from the equally tender testis. Overlying redness and oedema may be present.

INVESTIGATION

Blood count. Leucocytosis is present.

Blood culture. A positive culture is useful to direct antibiotic treatment, although this should be started on an empirical basis before the result is available.

Urinalysis. This will reveal a pyuria and the organism may be revealed by culture.

Aspiration of the epididymis. *Chlamydia* is best grown from this source.

Ultrasonography. Increased blood flow may be demonstrated.

MANAGEMENT

In a young man the commonest infecting organism is *Chlamydia*. Bed rest, scrotal elevation and tetracycline or erythromycin are appropriate. Other antibiotics may be needed according to the bacteriological analysis. The partner should also be investigated and treated.

Scrotal swellings

A non-inflammatory swelling of the scrotal contents may be a:

- testicular tumour
- epididymal cyst (spermatocele)
- varicocele
- hydrocele
- hernia.

CLINICAL EXAMINATION
The following points enable distinctions to be made:

- If it is possible to get above the swelling and palpate a normal cord, the swelling is not a hernia.
- If there is a cough impulse in the groin or, with the patient lying flat, the scrotal mass disappears or is reducible, the swelling is a hernia.
- If the testicle lies anteriorly and the epididymis posteriorly, gentle palpation establishes where the swelling lies and therefore its origin.
- Hydroceles transilluminate.
- Varicoceles are more apparent with the patient standing and feel like a bag of worms.

Hydrocele

AETIOLOGY
These may be congenital or acquired. *Congenital* hydroceles follow failure of obliteration of the processus vaginalis. Peritoneal fluid can then enter the scrotum. The great majority of *acquired* hydroceles are of unknown origin, but 10% are associated with tumour or infection of the testicle.

CLINICAL FEATURES
An infant presents with a large scrotal sac and the hydrocele is easily demonstrated by transillumination.

In adult life, there is a firm painless transilluminable swelling which it is possible to get above.

MANAGEMENT
The majority of congenital hydroceles resolve spontaneously by the age of 3, but persistence beyond this time requires operative treatment by division and ligation of the processus. In acquired hydrocele, aspiration is first done to allow examination of the testicle for any underlying cause. Sometimes this is therapeutic and the hydrocele does not recur. If it does, surgical excision of the outer wall of the hydrocele is required.

Epididymal cysts and spermatoceles

These may be single or multiple and are usually related to the head of the epididymis. They lie posterior or superior to the testicle and may transilluminate.

MANAGEMENT
Asymptomatic cysts do not require treatment. If they cause discomfort, simple aspiration is often satisfactory: spermatoceles yield a turbid milky fluid and epididymal cysts a fluid the colour of lemon barley water. Should recurrence occur after aspiration, surgical excision is required.

Varicocele

AETIOLOGY AND PATHOLOGICAL FEATURES
The venous valve at the junction of the left spermatic vein with the renal vein is incompetent or becomes so. It is most uncommon for the same to take place on the right. Very occasionally, a tumour in the kidney with extension along the renal vein may be present. Varicocele is a common finding in men presenting with subfertility but is equally common in men requesting vasectomy for contraception. The veins of the pampiniform plexus become enlarged and tortuous.

CLINICAL FEATURES
There is a dragging sensation in the scrotum which is worse in hot weather and on prolonged standing. Subfertility may be mentioned.

Physical examination reveals the 'bag of worms', which becomes more obvious if the patient stands. A cough impulse is present in the same position. The left testicle may be smaller than the right.

MANAGEMENT
Treatment is required for those with symptoms and for those with subfertility. The procedure of choice is embolisation of the testicular vein under radiological control.

Testicular tumours

Benign, interstitial cell and Leydig cell tumours of the testis are exceedingly rare. Malignant tumours are uncommon (1–2% of all neoplasms in males) but do occur in young adults with an otherwise long expectation of life. In the age range 20–35 years, testes tumours are the most common malignancy excluding leukaemia. The psychological effects of a diagnosis of malignancy are, in consequence, considerable.

AETIOLOGY AND EPIDEMIOLOGY
Maldescended testes – particularly those retained within the abdomen – have a 40% greater chance of malignant change than does a normal testis. Otherwise

Box 32.10

Teratomatous tumours of the testis

Differentiated (TD) – teratoma differentiated

Intermediate (MTI) – malignant teratoma intermediate

Undifferentiated (embryonal) carcinoma (MTU) – malignant teratoma undifferentiated

Trophoblastic (chorionic) carcinoma (MTT) – malignant teratoma trophoblastic

the cause is unknown. The overall incidence is 2–3 per 100000 of the population per year. They are rare before puberty. Teratomas (see below), which account for 60% of germ cell tumours, have a peak incidence at 20–30 years. Seminomas (see below), which account for the remaining 35%, have a peak incidence at 30–40 years. Lymphomas, which are often bilateral, occur in the 60–70 year age range.

PATHOLOGICAL FEATURES

Classification of germ cell tumours is as follows:

- seminoma
- teratoma
- mixed – these consist of both seminomatous and teratomatous elements but should be treated as teratomas.

The further subdivision of teratomas is shown in Box 32.10.

CLINICAL FEATURES

Symptoms

Ten per cent of patients give a history of previous orchidopexy, and in 5% the tumour is bilateral. There is often a recent history of trauma although this is not a cause but merely draws the patient's attention to the presence of a lump. The most frequent complaint is of a painless swelling which causes a dragging sensation in the scrotum. In one-third, the swelling is painful. Patients with a choriocarcinoma may develop gynaecomastia. Others present with symptoms from secondary deposits such as backache, haemoptysis or neurological complaints.

Signs

These include:

- a hard lump in the body of the testis
- diffuse testicular enlargement
- absence of tenderness on gently squeezing the testicle
- hydrocele.

INVESTIGATION

Tumour markers

Testicular teratomas secrete alpha-fetoprotein (AFP) and beta-human chorionic gonadotrophin (beta-HCG). Both teratomas and seminomas may secrete lactic dehydrogenase, and seminomas may secrete placental alkaline phosphatase. These should be measured preoperatively and at regular intervals postoperatively. They are good indictors of the likelihood of complete excision of the tumour or, alternatively, the presence of residual disease which requires further treatment.

Imaging

Ultrasound. If it is not possible to determine the nature of the mass in the testicle clinically, ultrasound is particularly helpful. The normal testis has a homogeneous appearance. Malignant tumours are inhomogeneous, may be cystic and are often associated with speckled calcification.

CT scan of the chest and abdomen is done to identify pulmonary deposits and lymphadenopathy. Regular repeated examination is required postoperatively.

STAGING

The stage of an individual tumour and its pathological type have considerable influence on management (see below). The clinical stages are summarised in Table 32.13.

MANAGEMENT

Patients with testicular tumours should be dealt with in specialist centres. There is no doubt that the earlier the diagnosis, the better the results. Improvements in therapy mean that the majority of testicular tumours should be regarded as curable.

Surgery

Orchidectomy is done through a groin incision – operations through the scrotum have a high incidence of tumour implantation. In order to reduce the risk of disseminating malignant cells by manipulation of the testis, the cord is mobilised and occluded with a non-crushing intestinal clamp before the testis is delivered from the scrotum. In men with a small or atrophic contralateral testis, or a history of subfertility, a biopsy from the contralateral testis should be taken. Up to 5% of men will have carcinoma in situ involving the other testis.

Table 32.13
Clinical staging of testicular tumours

Stage	Findings
I	Tumour limited to testis
II	Tumour of testis and retro-peritoneal lymph nodes
III	Involvement of infra- and supra-diaphragmatic lymph nodes
IV	Extra-lymphatic metastases

Table 32.14
Supplementary management of seminoma and teratoma after orchidectomy

Stage	Seminoma	Teratoma
I	Pelvic and para-aortic irradiation for relapse	Surveillance Platinum-based chemotherapy for relapse
IIa & b	Irradiation	Platinum-based chemotherapy Radical retroperitoneal lymphadenectomy for residual disease
IIc	Platinum-based combination chemotherapy	Platinum-based chemotherapy Radical retroperitoneal lymphadenectomy for residual disease

Supplementary management

The management options of seminoma and teratoma are given in Table 32.14. If chemotherapy is to be used, the patient should be advised to store semen prior to the chemotherapy. Patients with testicular tumours are often subfertile and chemotherapy may result in irreversible germ cell damage.

PROGNOSIS

In stage 1, 100% of patients survive. In stage 2–3, 5-year survival is between 80 and 90%

Seminoma. For a tumour localised to the testis, over 95% of patients should survive 5 years. For those who present with metastatic disease, the 5-year survival is approximately 75%.

Non-seminomatous germ cell tumours. For those with a tumour confined to the testis and low tumour markers, 90% survive 5 years. If the tumour markers are grossly elevated and metastases are confined only to the lungs, 80% survive 5 years, but if there are visceral metastases and grossly elevated tumour markers, the 5-year survival falls to 45%.

Andrology

Infertility

Ten per cent of couples have difficulty in conception. In approximately one-third, the problem lies with the male and in a further one-third there are contributory factors from both. Unless the male is found to be azoospermic (a complete absence of sperm) investigations of both partners should proceed simultaneously. The purpose of investigation is to give the couple a prognosis on the likelihood of conception. Couples who have been trying for more than 5 years with regular unprotected intercourse are unlikely to conceive without assisted conception.

CLINICAL FEATURES

History
Relevant questions include:

- age of both partners
- length of time trying to conceive

- previous children of both
- frequency of intercourse
- whether intercourse is taking place in the vagina.

A previous medical history of orchitis, venereal disease, inguinal or scrotal surgery, testicular injury or fallopian tube injury or disease should be sought. The occupation of both may be of significance, as may their general health and social habits (drug and alcohol intake).

Physical examination
In the male, testicular and epididymal size should be assessed, the presence of a vas on both sides confirmed and gynaecomastia excluded.

In the female, further examination is the province of a gynaecologist and is not further considered here.

INVESTIGATION

Semen analysis
This is the most useful investigation. The patient should abstain from intercourse for at least 4 days, and the specimen should be produced by masturbation into a sterile container and examined within 1 hour of production. The measurements provided by the laboratory and their normal values are shown in Table 32.15.

If white blood cells are found, a further semen specimen should be cultured for bacteria. The mixed agglutination reaction (MAR) test screens for antisperm antibodies and should be negative.

Endocrine analysis
Measurements of testosterone and prolactin are only required if a patient complains of lack of libido. In those with small testes, the FSH concentration in the

Table 32.15
Semen analysis

Measurement	Normal value
Volume	2–6 mL
Sperm concentration	More than 50 million/mL
Sperm motility	More than 60%
Abnormal sperms	Not more than 30%
White blood cells	None
Mixed agglutination reaction (MAR)	Negative

blood should be measured. If it is elevated and the patient has azoospermia, no further action is required as no treatment is available.

MANAGEMENT

In patients with oligospermia, it may be possible to separate out the most actively motile sperm and use these for artificial insemination. Azoospermia and a normal FSH suggest a diagnosis of testicular obstruction, which may be amenable to surgical correction.

Treatment of varicocele may improve both the sperm count and motility but not necessarily conception. Infected semen is an indication for treatment with antibiotics as for prostatitis. In the presence of antisperm antibodies, there is some evidence that treatment with prednisolone improves pregnancy rates, but using high-dose steroids has significant risks and side-effects. It is now possible to directly aspirate sperm from the epididymis or extract viable sperm from a testicular biopsy. These sperm can be directly implanted into an ovum. These techniques are used in cases of severe oligospermia.

Impotence

A better term is erectile dysfunction. The definition is the inability to achieve and maintain an erection for completion of satisfactory intercourse. Approximately 80% of men have a predominantly organic cause, but the fact that they cannot make love introduces an additional psychological element.

AETIOLOGY

Organic

- Generalised atheroslcerosis
- Diabetes mellitus
- Multiple sclerosis
- Pelvic fracture with urethral injury
- Arterial disease at the aortic bifurcation
- Endocrine dysfunction
- Anti-hypertensive therapy
- Corporeal venous dysfunction
- Other drugs.

Psychogenic

The psychodyamics are poorly understood and probably multifactorial.

CLINICAL FEATURES

Organic

The findings are those of the underlying cause.

Psychogenic

In this form, the following are more likely to be present:

- age less than 50
- non-smoker

- absence of neurological or endocrine disorder
- no anti-hypertensive therapy
- nocturnal and early morning erections
- erections with different partners
- erection is present up to the time of attempted penetration.

INVESTIGATION

These are required only in the following situations:

- The patient presents with lack of libido when measurements of serum testosterone and prolactin concentrations are required
- Young patients with impotence as a result of pelvic trauma to ensure that there is not a correctable arterial problem
- Failure to respond to an artificial erection test with vasoactive drugs – corporeal venous incompetence may be present and requires specialist investigation.

MANAGEMENT

Those with obvious psychogenic causes may benefit from psychosexual counselling. Correctable organic disease should be treated.

Therapies are as outlined below:

- *Sildenafil* is a type 5 phosphodiesterase inhibitor which prevents the breakdown of cyclic GMP, a second messenger for smooth muscle relaxation. It improves erectile ability sufficient to allow intercourse to take place in approximately 60% of men with organic disease.
- *Intraurethral prostaglandin E_1.* A small pellet of prostaglandin is inserted into the anterior urethra in men with organic erectile dysfunction – 66% achieve an erection satisfactory for intercourse.
- *Intracavernosal prostaglandin E_1.* The patient administers an injection of prostaglandin E_1 directly into the corpora cavernosum – 80% of men with organic erectile dysfunction achieve an erection.
- *Vacuum erection devices.* These consist of a plastic cylinder placed around the penis. By creating a vacuum within the cylinder, the penis becomes erect. The erection is maintained by placing a rubber constriction device around the base of the penis prior to removal of the cylinder.
- *Penile prostheses.* These are of two types: a semi-malleable and an inflatable. They are inserted at operation into both corpora cavernosae. They should only be used when other treatments have failed.

COMPLICATIONS.

- Sildenafil – facial flushing, headache, visual disturbances
- Intraurethral prostaglandins – penile pain and discomfort

- Intracavernosal prostaglandin – penile discomfort, penile fibrosis, prolonged erection
- Penile prostheses – pain, infection, extrusion
- Vacuum devices – penile oedema and bruising.

FURTHER READING

Whitfield HN (ed) (1993) Rob & Smith's Operative Surgery, Genitourinary Surgery, Vols 1–3, 5th edn. Oxford: Butterworth-Heinemann.

Whitfield HN, Hendry WF, Kirby RS, Duckett JW (1998) *Textbook of Genitourinary Surgery*, 2nd edn. Oxford: Blackwell Science.

Principles of orthopaedics

Orthopaedics is concerned with the surgical treatment of bone and joint conditions. The word is derived from the Greek for 'straight child' and the symbol that has been adopted by most orthopaedic associations is the twisted sapling (the bent child) lashed to a straight supporting stick.

Orthopaedic terms. A number of terms with particular definitions are used in orthopaedic practice and these are summarised in Information Box 33.1.

Special features of orthopaedic history and examination

History

Pain

This is usually the presenting symptom. Onset and duration are important. Was it sudden or was it slow over a few months? Is the pain constant or exacerbated by standing? The site is obviously important. There are some characteristic patterns: hip pain is classically felt in the groin but may also be apparent in the knee, particularly in children; if there is a nerve root trapped at the spine, pain may radiate down the arm or leg. Factors that may bring about relief include rest, load reduction with a walking stick, or drugs. Exacerbation from causes other than weight-bearing include particular movements such as a twist of the knee with a meniscal tear or lifting in low back pain. Night pain is an important symptom: it is common with arthritic joints when muscular tone relaxes. When sleep is lost, this may be an indication for joint replacement. Pain at night is also classical in benign osteoid osteoma.

Trauma

Is there a history of injury? Secondary osteoarthritis may follow:

- direct disruption of a joint
- malunion which places undue loads on a joint.

Need to use an 'aid'

The need for a walking stick or special cutlery may give an indication of the severity of the problem or of the

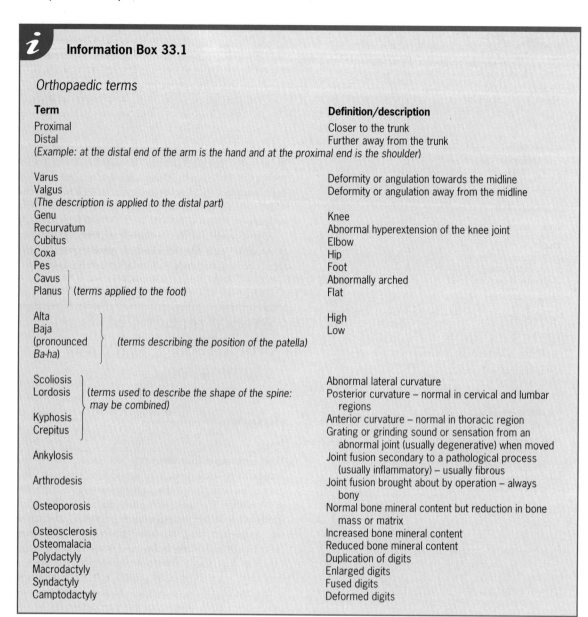

Information Box 33.1

Orthopaedic terms

Term	Definition/description
Proximal	Closer to the trunk
Distal	Further away from the trunk
(*Example: at the distal end of the arm is the hand and at the proximal end is the shoulder*)	
Varus	Deformity or angulation towards the midline
Valgus	Deformity or angulation away from the midline
(*The description is applied to the distal part*)	
Genu	Knee
Recurvatum	Abnormal hyperextension of the knee joint
Cubitus	Elbow
Coxa	Hip
Pes	Foot
Cavus	Abnormally arched
Planus } (*terms applied to the foot*)	Flat
Alta	High
Baja	Low
(pronounced *Ba-ha*) } (*terms describing the position of the patella*)	
Scoliosis	Abnormal lateral curvature
Lordosis } (*terms used to describe the shape of the spine: may be combined*)	Posterior curvature – normal in cervical and lumbar regions
Kyphosis	Anterior curvature – normal in thoracic region
Crepitus	Grating or grinding sound or sensation from an abnormal joint (usually degenerative) when moved
Ankylosis	Joint fusion secondary to a pathological process (usually inflammatory) – usually fibrous
Arthrodesis	Joint fusion brought about by operation – always bony
Osteoporosis	Normal bone mineral content but reduction in bone mass or matrix
Osteosclerosis	Increased bone mineral content
Osteomalacia	Reduced bone mineral content
Polydactyly	Duplication of digits
Macrodactyly	Enlarged digits
Syndactyly	Fused digits
Camptodactyly	Deformed digits

use of past conservative management by the patient or doctors.

Occupation

Certain occupations predispose to repetitive strain injury (RSI) such as tenosynovitis or carpal tunnel syndrome in typists, chicken pluckers or keyboard operators. Osteoarthritis of the spine is seen in miners and farm workers. Osteonecrosis of the femoral heads occurs in divers.

If surgery is proposed for the condition identified, will resumption of the previous occupation be possible or will it be necessary to consider retraining?

Dominant hand

The dominant hand may be affected more commonly, as in carpal tunnel syndrome.

Past medical history

This includes:

- similar problem on the contralateral side
- recent infections – urethritis, gastroenteritis or a streptococcal sore throat, all of which predispose to reactive arthritis
- pregnancy – which often precipitates low back pain or carpal tunnel syndrome.

Family history

Dupuytren's contracture, gout, rheumatoid arthritis and bone dysplasias may all run in families.

Medication

Current and past medication should be identified. The use of steroids predisposes to osteonecrosis of the femoral head. Patients on steroids often have problems with wound healing. Dupuytren's contracture is observed in association with phenytoin.

Examination

General assessment

Two classes of information result:

- specific indications of the cause of the problem
- suitability and fitness for surgery to correct the condition.

Joints

The examination of any joint has four components:

- Look
- Feel
- Measure (not always applicable)
- Move.

Look at:

- gait – assessment is made when the patient walks into the clinic or takes a few steps on the ward; normal gait has four phases (Table 33.1) which flow smoothly one into the other but there are many abnormalities (Information Box 33.2)
- skin – for scars and colour
- shape of the joint in general, the presence of swelling and lumps, and the position of the limb.

Feel for:

- temperature
- crepitus
- abnormal movement
- loose bodies

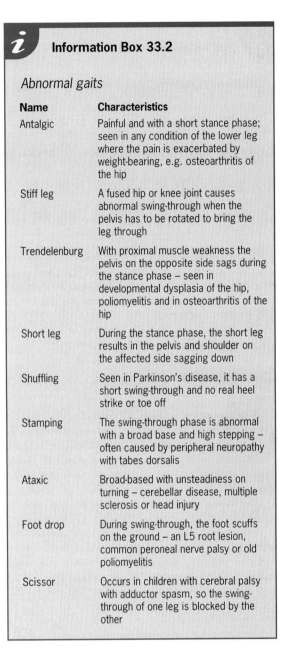

Information Box 33.2

Abnormal gaits

Name	Characteristics
Antalgic	Painful and with a short stance phase; seen in any condition of the lower leg where the pain is exacerbated by weight-bearing, e.g. osteoarthritis of the hip
Stiff leg	A fused hip or knee joint causes abnormal swing-through when the pelvis has to be rotated to bring the leg through
Trendelenburg	With proximal muscle weakness the pelvis on the opposite side sags during the stance phase – seen in developmental dysplasia of the hip, poliomyelitis and in osteoarthritis of the hip
Short leg	During the stance phase, the short leg results in the pelvis and shoulder on the affected side sagging down
Shuffling	Seen in Parkinson's disease, it has a short swing-through and no real heel strike or toe off
Stamping	The swing-through phase is abnormal with a broad base and high stepping – often caused by peripheral neuropathy with tabes dorsalis
Ataxic	Broad-based with unsteadiness on turning – cerebellar disease, multiple sclerosis or head injury
Foot drop	During swing-through, the foot scuffs on the ground – an L5 root lesion, common peroneal nerve palsy or old poliomyelitis
Scissor	Occurs in children with cerebral palsy with adductor spasm, so the swing-through of one leg is blocked by the other

- swelling – is it fluctuant and therefore fluid, or soft tissue or bone?

Measure the length of the limb to determine inequality in the two sides by using the distance between fixed bony points. Is it possible to determine if the whole limb or only a part of it is short?

Move. Joint movement may be painful and care should be taken not to cause pain. First, the patient is asked to actively move the joint in question. This gives the examiner an indication of the degree of pain and disability within an affected joint. Next the limb is passively moved. Often there is no significant difference between the active and passive ranges. Local

Table 33.1
Phases of normal gait

Phase	Movement
Heel strike	The heel makes contact with the ground
Stance	Weight is being transferred from the heel to the toes
Toe off	A final push is given to the foot as it leaves the ground
Swing through	The leg is brought forward with the knee slightly flexed to allow the foot to clear the ground

---

Information Box 33.3

Normal degrees of large joint movement

Joint	Flexion	Extension	Abduction	Adduction	External rotation	Internal rotation
Shoulder	180	50	180	30	80	100
Elbow	150	5	–	–	–	–
Wrist	Dorsi- 90	Palmar 90	Ulnar 30	Radial 15	Supination 90	Pronation 90
Hip	130	10	45	30	80	45
Knee	140	10				
Ankle	Dorsi- 15	Plantar 70	Eversion 10	Inversion 25		

---

weakness due to muscular or neurological dysfunction may result in limited active movement but a full range of passive movement; in the shoulder, rotator cuff lesions may limit active abduction but passive abduction is often unaffected.

The range of movement is recorded in the notes to allow for later comparisons (see Information Box 33.3).

Investigation

Imaging

Plain X-rays can allow differentiation between a disorder in bone and one in soft tissue and will nearly always confirm its nature. Old trauma may be evident. If arthritis is present, the type may be apparent (Table 33.2). Calcification within the joint may suggest an abnormality (Fig. 33.1).

Arthrography. Injection of a radio-opaque contrast medium into a joint delineates its anatomical boundaries and shows abnormal communications such as those that occur in rotator cuff tears of the shoulder. Intra-articular structures become apparent, e.g. loose bodies or the meniscii in the knee (Fig. 33.2). Arthrography can be combined with CT to give further information. The most frequent use of arthrography has been in the shoulder and the knee but, with the advent of magnetic resonance imaging (MRI), its use is declining.

Tomography. This technique is outlined in Chapter 4. Figure 33.3 shows an example of its use in the foot. It is increasingly being replaced by MRI.

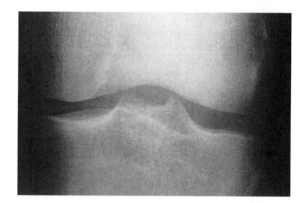

Fig 33.1 **Radiological calcification in a meniscus in the knee joint.**

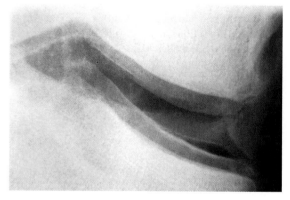

Fig 33.2 **Arthrogram of the knee.**

Computed tomography (CT). In orthopaedics, this technique is used for imaging the spine and bone tumours.

Magnetic resonance imaging (MRI). This technique (Ch. 4) provides excellent images in both coronal and sagittal planes, and with appropriate computer software, three-dimensional reconstruction is possible. MRI of the brain and spinal cord now provides

Table 33.2
Radiological appearances in arthritis

Feature	Osteoarthritis	Rheumatoid arthritis
Loss of joint space	Yes	Yes
Sclerosis	Yes	No
Osteophytes	Yes	No
Subchondral cysts	Yes	No
Erosions	No	Yes
Osteoporosis	No	Yes

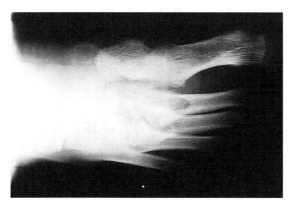

Fig 33.3 **Tomogram of a metatarsal.**

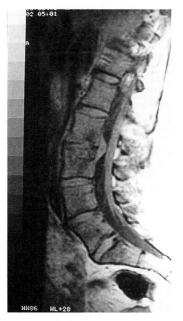

Fig 33.4 **MRI of a disc abscess in the spine.**

unparalleled detail (Fig. 33.4). MRI scans are also useful in the staging of bone tumours: intra-osseous spread can be identified and local oedema defined.

Isotope scanning (see Ch.4) is frequently used in orthopaedics. Technetium-99m di-phosphonate is concentrated in areas of increased osteoblastic activity usually associated with increased blood supply. These areas occur in such conditions as arthritis or bone secondaries. Scans also reveal zones of relative underactivity when the blood supply is reduced in osteonecrosis. Labelled white blood cells are used to localise infection within a painful joint replacement or a nidus of osteomyelitis (see below).

Blood investigations

ESR and C-reactive protein are non-specific markers of inflammation which can be used to follow the course of an orthopaedic disease and its treatment. They are raised in such conditions as an infected joint replacement, osteomyelitis, active rheumatoid arthritis and malignant disease.

Rheumatoid factor is an IgM autoantibody present in the serum of patients with a number of conditions, including rheumatoid arthritis (80%), Sjögren's syndrome (90%) and systemic lupus erythematosus (50%).

Uric acid. Raised levels in the serum are often confirmatory of the presence of gout.

Antistreptolysin (ASO) titres are increased in recent streptococcal infection which may be helpful in confirming an occult infection in a joint replacement.

Protein electrophoresis for a specific monoclonal antibody is of help in myeloma.

Alkaline phosphatase is raised in Paget's disease, secondary malignancy in bone and osteomalacia.

Synovial fluid examination

Joint aspiration is an outpatient procedure which may reveal:

- the presence of crystals in both gout and pseudogout
- organisms and a very high white cell count $(50 \times 10^9/L)$ in septic arthritis and lower levels in any inflammatory arthritis $(1–3 \times 10^9/L)$.

Arthroscopy

Endoscopic principles are considered in Chapter 4. The interior of the knee joint was first examined in 1918, using a cystoscope. The techniques were refined over subsequent years until 1957 when the first purpose-built instrument was introduced. An arthroscope is a rigid instrument with an outer sheath and an inner lens system. Different lenses are available to provide different viewing angles at the tip. Common viewing angles include 0°, 30° and 70°.

Almost any joint can be arthroscoped although some require specialised instrumentation. The commonest ones are the knee (most frequent), shoulder, elbow, wrist, hip and ankle. Arthroscopy of the phalangeal joints has been described, as well as that of the facet joints of the lumbar spine.

The technique consists of the introduction of the sheath into the joint by a small puncture wound (portal) followed by distension with saline. The lens system can be slid down within the sheath and the joint inspected.

Procedures can be done by introducing instruments through other portals. A large variety is available. They range from simple hooked probes to scissors, grasping forceps, knives, specialised meniscal sutures and powered tools to shave or cut. The Holmium–YAG laser is being used to trim intra-articular structures such as the menisci.

Arthritis

Osteoarthritis

EPIDEMIOLOGY AND AETIOLOGY

Osteoarthritis (OA) is the most frequent type of arthritis and is more common in women than in men. The incidence increases with age, and by 80 years, 80–90% of hips show radiographic evidence of osteoarthritis. The condition is usually primary but can be secondary to another condition (Box 33.1). Primary OA is of unknown cause although repeated minor trauma and a genetic predisposition are probable factors. It affects the main weight-bearing joints – the spine, hips and knees. The distal interphalangeal joints of the hand and, in the thumb, the carpometacarpal joints can also be sites of the disorder. Secondary osteoarthritis can affect any joint.

CLINICAL FEATURES

History

Joint pain and stiffness are usual and tend to be progressive over time but they may be variable from day to day. Pain initially occurs on weight-bearing, then at rest and subsequently wakes the patient at night. As well as pain during movement, joint crepitus may be felt and heard by the patient.

Deformity of the affected joint from local swelling and destruction may be noted and, on weight-bearing, these may increase.

Physical findings

- *Look* for:
  - local swelling
  - deformity – weight-bearing may make this worse
  - scars or sinuses that suggests a secondary cause.
- *Feel* to detect if:
  - the swelling is bone, soft tissue or fluid
  - crepitus is present.
- *Move* the joint to test:
  - active and then passive range of movement
  - stability of ligaments.

INVESTIGATION

Few investigations are required. Plain X-rays are needed to assess the extent of the disease but the radiological appearances (Table 33.2) may not correlate well with clinical symptoms.

Rheumatoid arthritis

EPIDEMIOLOGY AND AETIOLOGY

This is a systemic inflammatory disease which affects 3% of the female and 1% of the male UK population.

Box 33.1

The causes of osteoarthritis

Primary (or idiopathic)

Unknown

Secondary
Abnormal joint contour
Trauma (dislocation in particular)
Developmental dysplasia of the hip
Slipped upper femoral epiphysis
Osteonecrosis
Keinbock's disease of the lunate
Panner's disease of the capitellum
Scheuermann's disease of the vertebral end plates
Perthe's disease of the hip
Osgood–Schlatter's disease of the tibial tuberosity
Sever's disease of the calcaneum
Kohler's disease of the navicular
Freiburg's disease of the metatarsal heads
Drugs
    Systemic steroids and cytotoxics
    Intra-articular steroids
Local radiotherapy
Sickle cell disease
Alcoholism
Neoplasia – leukaemia and lymphoma
Occupational – Caisson's disease
Cartilage destruction
    Infection
    Recurrent haemarthrosis – haemophilia
    Gout and pseudogout
    Rheumatoid arthritis

Metabolic and endocrine disorders
Alkaptonuria
Wilson's disease
Acromegaly

Neuropathic disorders
Diabetes mellitus
Tabes dorsalis

Small joints in the hands and wrists, elbows, shoulders, cervical spine and feet are particularly involved, but any joints may be affected except the lumbar spine and the distal interphalangeal joints. The cause remains unknown although various organisms and an exaggerated immune response to them have frequently been invoked.

CLINICAL FEATURES

History

There is usually a long history of systemic illness with multiple joint involvement and extra-articular problems including weight loss, low grade fever, subcutaneous nodules, arteritis and tendon sheath involvement.

Joint symptoms are pain, morning stiffness and progressive deformity with loss of function.

Physical findings

- *Look*:
  - at the hands, which have the characteristic deformity of ulnar deviation of the fingers and subluxation at the metacarpophalangeal joints
  - for nodules on the subcutaneous border of the ulna.
- *Feel* for:
  - subcutaneous nodules
  - local warmth in the affected joint
  - soft tissue swelling around joints and tendon sheaths
  - joint crepitus.
- *Move* to detect:
  - active rather than the passive range of movement
  - abnormal joint mobility secondary to subluxation.

INVESTIGATION

The diagnosis of rheumatoid arthritis has usually been made by the time the patient is seen in the orthopaedic clinic.

Imaging

Plain X-ray may help to confirm the diagnosis (Table 33.2). However, there may be radiological features of superimposed osteoarthritis.

Blood examination

Anaemia is common and is either a leuco-erythroblastic type or reflects iron deficiency (secondary to chronic gastrointestinal bleeding after NSAID ingestion).

ESR is usually raised.

Rheumatoid factor is detectable in 80%

MANAGEMENT

Rheumatoid arthritis is predominantly managed by medical means. Patients are referred to the orthopaedic clinic or to one conducted jointly with rheumatologists when correction of deformity and restoration of function may be beneficial.

Other arthritides

Systemic lupus erythematosus (SLE)

This systemic inflammatory condition affects young women. Ninety per cent of patients develop joint symptoms that include polyarthritis of the hands.

Polymyalgia rheumatica

This affects the elderly and is more common in women. It presents with aching and stiffness in the shoulders and pelvis. Locally, there is muscle tenderness and a reduced range of active movement but normal passive movement. There may be associated temporal arteritis. The ESR is markedly raised. Management is directed at symptomatic relief, often with steroid therapy.

Gout

Arthropathy with urate crystal deposition affects mostly men at the metacarpophalangeal joint of the big toe, although the knee is also a common additional site. Acute attacks may occur spontaneously or be precipitated by local trauma. Gout may also be secondary to myeloproliferative disorders with increased purine production or renal disease with reduced urate excretion. Urate crystals may also be deposited as tophi in soft tissues: the Achilles tendon, around joints, in bursae and on the external ear. The diagnosis is made by demonstrating the presence of urate crystals within the joint or soft tissues. Management includes treatment of the acute attack with NSAIDs and long-term prophylaxis with allopurinol.

Management of arthritis

Arthritis is rarely reversible and treatment is directed at symptomatic relief and the preservation or restoration of function.

Non-operative

Conservative management

Conservative measures should always be tried initially. Pain relief with simple analgesics or NSAIDs will be helpful.

Intra-articular steroid injection

The role of this is controversial. Whilst an intra-articular injection will provide some pain relief, because the inflammatory reaction within the joint is reduced, repeated steroid injections are likely to increase joint degeneration by the inhibition of the normal processes of repair. In general, two or three injections is the maximum for any one joint.

Weight reduction

Weight loss is encouraged. Not only is the load transmitted through the damaged joint reduced, but also obesity is associated with an increase in the complications of operation should this ultimately be required.

Aids to daily living (ADL)

These should be considered; they include walking sticks and crutches. The rheumatoid patient with limited hand function may require special large-handled cutlery and easy-open containers for their medication.

Operative

When conservative measures have failed, surgical options need to be considered.

Arthroscopy

A joint that is swollen and inflamed will usually benefit from an arthroscopic washout which removes inflammatory mediators and fragments of cartilage.

Synovectomy

Surgical excision of the synovium or tendon sheath in rheumatoid arthritis can be beneficial. In the past it was done as an open procedure with consequent considerable joint morbidity, but this has been replaced by arthroscopic synovectomy with special powered instruments.

Joint surgery

Long-term or permanent relief of the symptoms of arthritis requires surgery on the bones of the affected joint. A variety of options are available (Table 33.3) and the choice depends on a number of factors, including:

- age
- expectations of the patient
- occupation
- the joint affected.

In the younger patient with osteoarthritis, prosthetic replacement (Table 33.4) is avoided, if possible, because of the limited lifespan of the prosthesis. The results of further replacements after initial failure (revision surgery) are not as good as the primary procedure and with each subsequent attempt, the surgery becomes more challenging.

Almost any joint in the arm or leg can be replaced. Usually the replacement consists of a metal component bearing on a high-density polyethylene surface. The prosthesis may be cemented into place with methyl-methacrylate bone cement or be uncemented, with the surface textured to encourage bone ingrowth. New surfaces include the use of hydroxyapatite (HA) which is the basic mineral of bone. With HA chemically bonded to the surface of the prosthesis, the patient's bone can directly bind the implant.

The first modern replacement was the hip joint developed by Charnley in 1961, although previous attempts had been made to replace the hip with wood or ivory. The modern hip joint can be expected to last for 15–20 years but this depends upon:

- surgical experience
- state of the recipient bone

Table 33.3
Surgical options for an arthritic joint

Procedure	Effects	Example
Arthrodesis	Stiff but pain-free joint	Fusion of the lumbar spine or ankle
Excision	Removal of one aspect of the joint may relieve pain; shortening of the limb beyond the resection	Keller's operation on the big toe for hallux valgus
Osteotomy	Alteration of the line of load transmission to an unaffected part of the joint	High tibial osteotomy for unicompartmental osteoarthritis of the knee
Prosthetic replacement	Excision of diseased joint surfaces and replacement of surfaces with metal and high-density polyethylene	Hip, knee and shoulder

Table 33.4
Joint replacement[a]

Type	Nature	Comments	Examples
Constrained	Simple hinge	Loosening because of inevitable rotational movement	Elbow Wrist
Semi-constrained	Simple hinge, but some rotation possible	Still subject to loosening	Elbow Wrist
Unconstrained	Two independent parts so that stability depends on sound anchorage in bone and the soft tissues	Most common type in use; highly satisfactory	Hip Knee Ankle Shoulder Elbow

[a] In the knee, the replacement can be unicompartmental if one side only is affected; more usually, all three compartments are replaced.

- prosthesis design
- stresses placed upon the implant.

About 50 000 hips and 40 000 knees are implanted each year in the UK.

Complications of joint replacement surgery include:

- general complications of any major operation
- specific complications of the procedure, including intraoperative fractures, postoperative dislocations and fractures, infection of the implant and loosening.

Loosening may be secondary to infection or an aseptic mechanical process. If the prosthesis is mechanically loose, it can be removed and replaced, but when infection is present, the safest option is to remove all the foreign material, identify the infective agent and treat this vigorously. At a second procedure, it may then be possible to insert another prosthesis.

Joint replacement surgery in rheumatoid arthritis carries particular risks. The immune response is altered and infection rates are higher. At operation, the bones are often osteoporotic with an increased risk of intra-operative fractures. When multiple joints are involved, the surgeon may be embarking on an extended programme of replacement.

Infections

Acute osteomyelitis

Before the introduction of antibiotics, acute osteomyelitis was a common infection with a 50% mortality. In the Western world the condition has now become much less common – although the reason for this is not entirely clear – and fatalities are rare.

AETIOLOGY

Haematogenous

Organisms transported by the bloodstream from a distant site lodge in the capillaries of bone (usually, but not always, the metaphysis of a long bone) and set up a focus. Their origin is usually not clear but occasionally there may be a distant infected focus, such as a boil or the unhealed stump of the umbilical cord. Localisation of the infection may be determined by a minor injury to the bone, although this is not well established in patho-logical terms. Individuals of any age may be infected but the condition is more common in children.

Exogenous

Direct inoculation of bone from the outside takes place as a result of some surgical procedure or after an open fracture.

PATHOLOGICAL FEATURES

Organisms

In haematogenous osteomyelitis, the agent is most commonly *Staphylococcus aureus* (85%), now usually penicillin-resistant. *Streptococcus pyogenes* and *Pseudomonas aeruginosa.* are other pus-producing organ-isms sometimes involved. Occasionally, *Salmonella typhimurium* is found either with or without an intestinal infection and is commoner in patients with sickle cell disease. *E. coli* may infect the bones of neonates.

Infection from without can be with any organism and is often mixed.

Pathological course

In haematogenous osteomyelitis, a short period of intense inflammation is speedily followed by pus formation within the medulla. Because bone is not expandable, pressure rises rapidly with two effects:

- pus is forced through the Haversian canals to reach the periosteum and lift this, so forming a subperiosteal abscess
- blood vessels thrombose and the bone dies; stripping of periosteum contributes to this infarction.

Eventually, if treatment does not take place, pus breaks through the periosteum, tracks up to the skin surface and discharges to produce an infected sinus. There is dead bone in its depths which gradually separates to form a sequestrum.

Exogenous infection does not usually pursue such an acute course and damage to bone is less. However, it is often persistent and chronic.

CLINICAL FEATURES

History

There is often a history of minor trauma. The patient, usually a child, is unwell with a high pyrexia and – if old enough to voice this – a complaint of severe localised bone pain. The affected limb is held still (pseudoparalysis).

Physical findings
- *Look*:
  - redness and oedema may be seen over the affected metaphysis
  - the limb is held still.
- *Feel*:
  - warmth at the affected site
  - focal bony tenderness – an important sign
  - fluctuant swelling overlying the bone
- *Move*:
  - pain on movement.

INVESTIGATION

Imaging

Plain X-ray is initially normal. Changes occur after 10–14 days, when the periosteum is lifted and there is local rarefaction. Later, dead bone and sequestra show up as sclerosis.

Ultrasound may identify a subperiosteal abscess.

Radioisotope bone scan shows increased activity in the early stages, well before anything is seen on X-ray.

MRI is extremely sensitive in identifying intra-osseous oedema and pus.

Blood examination

- Raised white cell count, ESR and CRP
- Blood culture (before the administration of antibiotics) is positive in half of those with haematogenous osteomyelitis.

MANAGEMENT

Non-operative

High-dose intravenous antibiotics are begun imme-diately after a blood culture has been taken. The affected limb is elevated and splinted because this helps to relieve pain. Antibiotic therapy is continued until the ESR has returned to normal, which may take 6 weeks.

Surgical

If the patient fails to respond by speedy return of temperature to normal and relief of pain, or if there is a fluctuant abscess on presentation, then the site is explored. The periosteum is incised and the underlying bone drilled to drain and decompress the medullary cavity.

COMPLICATIONS

- Acute septic arthritis secondary to direct spread from adjacent bone
- Pathological fracture through bone that is rarefied because of infection
- Growth impairment from epiphyseal involvement
- Chronicity because of dead bone
- Chronic osteomyelitis.

Chronic osteomyelitis

This condition occurs because of inadequate treatment of acute osteomyelitis or it may complicate the manage-ment of an open fracture or the surgical treatment of a closed one. It is now rare in the UK.

CLINICAL FEATURES

History

There has usually been an episode of acute haemato-genous osteomyelitis often followed by a discharging sinus. Evidence of infection is dormant for months or years with an occasional flare-up in which there is local pain and swelling with discharge of pus.

Physical findings

There are often scars from old sinuses, one or more of which may still be open with a purulent discharge.

INVESTIGATION

Imaging

Plain X-rays show grossly abnormal bone with areas of rarefaction and sclerosis. A sequestrum appears as a separate piece of dense bone lying within a cavity.

Isotope bone scan may show increased activity although, if there is a sequestrum, reduced uptake is present in relation to it.

CT may give useful information on the exact size and position of a sequestrum.

Examination of the blood

This is usually unhelpful, but the ESR may be raised. Blood culture is negative except during a flare-up.

MANAGEMENT

Non-operative

Antibiotics do not usually help because they are unable to penetrate the dense soft tissue fibrosis and the relatively ischaemic bone. The occasional flare-up can be managed with dry dressings until the sinus stops discharging.

Surgical

The aim of surgery is to remove all dead bone and infected material. A chain of antibiotic impregnated beads can then be implanted in the cavity to give a very high but localised concentration of antibiotic.

COMPLICATIONS

- Pathological fracture
- Amyloidosis
- Squamous cell carcinoma in the sinus tract.

Septic arthritis

In that it often follows osteomyelitis, this condition is now rare in the UK. Any joint may be affected but the common site is the knee.

AETIOLOGY

- Haematogenous spread from a distant focus of infection
- Secondary to acute osteomyelitis
- Direct inoculation after trauma or surgery – the incidence after arthroscopy is less than 0.2%.

PATHOLOGICAL FEATURES

Organisms
- *Staphylococcus aureus*
- *Streptococcus pyogenes*
- *Neisseria gonorrhoea*.

Course
The hyaline cartilage is destroyed by a combination of ischaemia and toxic enzymes released by white blood cells and bacteria. As with osteomyelitis, unchecked development of pus eventually ruptures the joint capsule and discharge occurs through the skin. Such a damaged joint heals with either a fibrous or a bony ankylosis.

CLINICAL FEATURES

History
The patient complains of increasingly severe pain in the joint and is unwell with a high swinging pyrexia.

Physical findings
- *Look* for:
  - a red and swollen joint
  - evidence of a local wound
  - immobility because of pain.
- *Feel* for:
  - local warmth
  - local tenderness.
- *Move:*
  - marked pain on movement.

INVESTIGATION

Imaging
Plain X-Rays are normal in the early stages. After 2–3 weeks, there is local rarefaction of the adjacent bone and loss of joint space. Still later, the necrosis of cartilage reduces the joint space still further. Finally, bony ankylosis can be seen.

Blood examination
The white cell count and ESR are raised and blood culture may be positive.

Joint aspiration
This should always be done and is both diagnostic and therapeutic. The aspirate is sent for culture. At the same time, the toxic content of the effusion can be reduced by washing out the joint cavity. The reduction of intra-articular pressure provides relief from pain.

MANAGEMENT

Non-operative
High-dose intravenous antibiotics are begun, adjusted on the results of culture and continued until the ESR has returned to normal, which may take 6 weeks. The joint is rested.

Surgical
The knee, ankle, shoulder and elbow can easily be reached through the arthroscope and the joint washed out. This is simply, because of the larger bore of the instrument, a more efficient form of aspiration.

COMPLICATIONS
- Dislocation – in particular, the hip in children
- Joint stiffness
- Secondary osteoarthritis.

Bone tumours

These are either primary or secondary. Primary tumours may be either benign or malignant but some are in an intermediate group which, although showing locally invasive features, do not metastasise. A detailed classification is given in Table 33.5.

CLINICAL FEATURES

History
When the tumour is secondary, there may be symptoms from the primary malignancy, although sometimes the first presentation is with bone pain or a pathological fracture. Pain is common and is localised

Table 33.5
Bone tumours

Cell of origin	Benign	Intermediate	Malignant
Osteoblast	Osteoid osteoma	Osteoblastoma	Osteosarcoma
Osteoclast		Giant cell tumour (osteoclastoma)	
Chondroblast	Chondroma		Chondrosarcoma
	Osteochondroma		
Fibroblast	Non-ossifying fibroma (unicameral bone cyst)		Fibrosarcoma
Vascular	Haemangioma	Aneurysmal bone cyst	Haemangiosarcoma
Marrow		Plasmacytoma	Ewing's sarcoma
			Lymphoma
			Myeloma
			Leukaemia

Table 33.6
Common sites of primary in secondary bone tumour

Site	Incidence (%)
Breast	35
Prostate	30
Bronchus	10
Kidney	5
Thyroid	2

at the site of the tumour. It is usually constant with no relieving factors and often worse at night. A lump may be noticed.

Physical findings

A thorough general examination is required. Most bone tumours are secondary deposits and so the common sites of a possible primary (breast, lung and prostate) must be examined (Table 33.6):

- *Look* for a lump.
- *Feel* for:
  - a lump
  - local bony tenderness
  - crepitus under the fingers when there is a history of possible pathological fracture.
- *Move* – possible abnormal movement in the presence of a pathological fracture.

INVESTIGATION

Imaging

Plain X-ray is always needed. Benign tumours have a sharp margin and the cortex is intact. By contrast, malignant growths are expansive with indistinct margins and destruction of the cortex. In osteosarcoma, new bone formation is seen – so-called 'sun-ray spicules'.

Isotope scan differentiates secondary deposits – which produce multiple areas of increased activity – from a primary tumour in which there is usually a solitary active area.

CT is required to assess the local spread of malignant tumours and so to aid in the planning of surgery. The lungs are scanned for evidence of metastases.

MRI is also useful for the assessment of local spread within the bone and adjacent soft tissues.

Benign tumours

These occur in young adults. They may be found in any bone; however, chondromas favour metacarpals, metatarsals and the phalanges.

CLINICAL FEATURES

History

Benign tumours are often without symptoms unless a pathological fracture occurs Constant local pain often worse at night may be the presenting feature. In osteoid

osteoma, relief is obtained from aspirin but not opioid analgesics.

Physical finding

- *Look* for any evidence of a fracture – chiefly deformity.
- *Feel* for:
  - a hard lump
  - localised bony tenderness
  - crepitus.
- *Test* for unusual movement – indicative of a pathological fracture.

MANAGEMENT

If there are symptoms, curettage and bone grafting may be required. A pathological fracture through the tumour can lead to spontaneous cure.

Intermediate tumours

These tumours are not truly malignant in that metastatic spread is very rare. There is, however, local destruction and, after surgery, there may be local recurrence.

Aneurysmal bone cysts

These are blood-filled cavities that usually occur in the spine and at the ends of long bones. On plain X-ray, the cyst is seen as an expansive lesion with thinning of the cortex. The management is curettage and bone grafting which is usually curative. Radiotherapy may be required for recurrent lesions.

Giant cell tumour (osteoclastoma)

This occurs at the end of long bones in young adults – the knee is a common site. There is local pain and possibly a pathological fracture. The X-ray appearance is that of a multiloculated or 'soap bubble' lesion; the tumour extends up to the joint surface. Metastases are rare but can occur especially after local recurrence.

Curettage with bone grafting is often followed by recurrence. The cavity should be filled with bone cement which sets by an exothermic reaction that is cytotoxic to residual tumour cells. Local recurrence necessitates wide excision and then either bone grafting or a prosthesis.

Malignant tumours

These are rare – only 150 new osteosarcomas and 40 new chondrosarcomas a year in the UK. They spread via the bloodstream to the lungs and other sites.

Osteosarcoma

This tumour occurs mainly in the young between the ages of 10 and 30 years. There is a second peak in the elderly in association with Paget's disease of bone. The tumour occurs in the metaphyseal region of long bones, the knee being the most common site. Its management used to be by amputation, but now, with more effective chemotherapeutic agents and consequently a better prognosis, surgical resection is less radical. Excision of the affected bone and replacement with a custom-made or modular prosthesis now form the standard approach. Radiotherapy is usually reserved for inaccessible sites or for recurrence. With radical surgery and chemotherapy, there is a 90% survival at 1 year and over 50% at 3 years. Survival for more than 3 years means a probable cure.

Chrondrosarcoma

This occurs in an older age group than that of osteosarcoma: 30–50 years. Tumours commonly involve the flat bones: scapula, ribs and pelvis. They vary widely in their degree of differentiation, from high-grade anaplastic to low-grade with only slow growth. Their management is by wide local excision with bone grafting or reconstruction with a custom-made prosthesis. Radiotherapy is ineffective. The 5-year survival ranges from 20 to 80%, depending on size, location and histological grade.

Fibrosarcoma

This is a rare growth in the age range of 40–60 and occurs at any site. Management is surgical, with wide excision or amputation. The outlook is poor with a 5-year survival rate of about 30%.

Ewing's sarcoma

This is a highly malignant tumour that affects children and adolescents of 5–20 years. Males are slightly more frequently affected. The common site is the diaphyseal region of long bones. The clinical features, in addition to local pain and a lump, may include general ill health and fever. The lump may be red and warm. Ewing's sarcoma is often intially misdiagnosed as acute osteomyelitis. On the plain X-ray, a characteristic 'onion peel' appearance is typically seen. Management is by chemotherapy followed by surgical excision and radiotherapy. The outlook has been poor. However, with radical and aggressive treatment, survival rates are now approaching 50% or more at 5 years.

Plasmacytoma

This condition is rare and consists of a mass of plasma cells in bone or soft tissue which may prove to be a focal manifestation of multiple myeloma. Isolated lesions are excised followed by a course of radiotherapy.

Secondary tumours

Secondary bone tumours are common: about 30% of patients who die of a malignancy have bone secondaries. Common sources of the primary growth are given in Table 33.6.

The patients are often over 60, because of the nature of the primary. Any bone may be affected, but the skull, vertebrae, ribs and pelvis are common sites. On plain X-ray, most secondary tumours are osteolytic but bone deposits from carcinoma of the prostate and about 10% of breast cancers are osteosclerotic. Treatment which is appropriate for the primary – such as hormone manipulation in breast and prostate cancer and chemotherapy – may alleviate the symptoms of secondary deposits. The pain may respond to anti-inflammatory drugs and local radiotherapy. Pathological fractures do not unite spontaneously and should therefore be internally fixed, in that quality of life is improved and nursing made easier, although life expectancy remains unchanged. Prophylactic internal fixation should be considered when there is:

- rapid increase in local pain
- destruction of 50% or more of shaft diameter in a long bone
- a femoral lesion greater than 3 cm in diameter.

Shoulder

The shoulder is the most mobile of all joints and, with the elbow, has the prime function of manoeuvring the hand to the best position required for function, particularly to the mouth.

GENERAL CLINICAL FEATURES

History

Pain is felt over the deltoid insertion in impingement syndromes (see below); at the front in arthritis; and at the top in acromioclavicular disorders. Radiation down the arm is common. Pain around the shoulder may also be the result of reference from other sites such as the heart, lung, diaphragm or cervical spine.

Stiffness is a common symptom in shoulder disease and loss of function such as inability to brush the hair can be socially embarrassing.

Trauma frequently figures in the history and may cause fractures, dislocations or soft tissue injury to the joint capsule, particularly the rotator cuff.

Mechanical derangement may be a presenting symptom as in recurrent dislocation.

Physical findings
- *Look* for:
  — muscle wasting of the deltoid, biceps, supraspinatus and infraspinatus
  — scars – indications of previous injury or surgery
  — the contour of the shoulder – in dislocation, the normal rounded appearance is lost and the

shoulder looks squared off because of the prominence of the acromion
— winging of the scapula because of weakness of the serratus anterior muscle.
- *Feel* for the belly of biceps during resisted elbow flexion – rupture of the long head of biceps tendon results in an abnormal contour of the muscle.
- *Move*:
— through the active and passive ranges (Information Box 33.3)
— note any painful arcs of movement during elevation of the arm – pain during mid-elevation is caused by subacromial impingement, but pain at full elevation is from an acromioclavicular disorder.

INVESTIGATION

Imaging

Plain X-rays are required, both anteroposterior and an axillary view. They can show degenerative arthritis, loose bodies and abnormal calcification – usually in tendons. In recurrent dislocation, a defect (Broca's defect or the Hill–Sachs lesion) may be seen on the humeral head and is caused by repeated impingement of the rim of the glenoid on the humerus.

Arthrograms have been commonly performed. Rotator cuff tears are demonstrated by leakage of contrast medium into the subacromial bursa.

CT and MRI are of increasing value. The tear may be visualised, loose bodies seen and bicipital tendinitis can be diagnedsed.

Arthroscopy

The procedure is both a diagnostic tool and of therapeutic value. It is possible to repair tears in the labrum of the glenoid, to decompress the subacromial space, to stabilise the shoulder in recurrent dislocation and remove loose bodies.

Acromioclavicular disorders
Acromioclavicular osteoarthritis

AETIOLOGY

This condition is often secondary to trauma with dislocation of the joint.

CLINICAL FEATURES

History

Pain is the usual feature often felt on the top of the shoulder in relation to the joint and aggravated by lifting the arm above the head or across the body.

Physical findings
- *Look* for:
— prominence of the acromioclavicular joint
— muscle wasting, in particular in the supraspinatus.
- *Feel* for:
— ·localised tenderness at the joint
— crepitus on movement.
- *Test* movement – pain is found when passive movement above shoulder level is attempted.

MANAGEMENT

Surgical excision of the outer end of the clavicle provides relief; however, after surgery there is some weakness.

Rheumatoid arthritis

The shoulder and acromioclavicular joint are often affected by rheumatoid arthritis. In addition to pain, there is often prominent swelling.

MANAGEMENT

Non-operative

Medical management of the disease is important and provides pain relief.

Surgical

Excision of the outer end of the clavicle is performed.

Subacromial disorders

The subacromial bursa, the rotator cuff and the tendon of biceps lie between the acromion and the head of the humerus. Any one of these structures may become trapped between the two bones and causes pain.

Impingement

This often affects the rotator cuff tendons of subscapularis and supraspinatus.

CLINICAL FEATURES

A painful arc occurs on abduction of the humerus. On examination, the arc is confirmed and can be precisely defined.

MANAGEMENT

Non-operative

Analgesics such as non-steroidal anti-inflammatory agents may help the local swelling to settle. Local steroid injection into the subacromial space is also helpful.

Surgical

If symptoms fail to improve with conservative measures then surgery is advisable. The subacromial space is decompressed by excising the undersurface of the acromion as a wedge.

Rotator cuff tears

There are two causes:

- acute injury as a result of trauma
- chronic lesions from degeneration within the cuff; there may have been a preceding associated dislocation of the shoulder.

PATHOLOGICAL FEATURES

There is a spectrum of disorders that are interconnected and which ranges from superficial abrasions of the rotator cuff from impingement through incomplete (partial thickness) tears to complete full-thickness ones. However, there is not inevitable progression from one to another. Other factors such as ischaemic degeneration within the cuff coupled with trauma may determine the extent of tear.

CLINICAL FEATURES

History

There may be a history of significant shoulder injury, but more usually there is chronic shoulder pain felt over the deltoid muscle, especially at one point of abduction. Adduction may also be difficult.

Physical findings

- *Look* for muscle wasting – especially in the supraspinatus.
- *Feel* for localised tenderness along the lateral border of the acromion.
- *Test* for shoulder movement – active movement, particularly abduction, is reduced but there is a full range of passive movement.

MANAGEMENT

Non-operative

Partial tears of the cuff heal and the symptoms settle after resting the shoulder. Once acute symptoms have settled, a graduated programme of rehabilitation is begun. Tears in the elderly should be managed conservatively; surgical repair in this age group is difficult and severe stiffness after surgery is likely.

Surgical

When symptoms fail to settle, then it is likely that the tear is complete. In the young, it should be repaired. The rotator cuff is exposed and repaired with interrupted sutures. Very large tears may require grafts of fascia lata to close the defect.

Calcific tendinitis

Deposition of calcium hydroxyapatite within the tendon of supraspinatus may occur for unknown reasons. There is a local inflammatory reaction.

CLINICAL FEATURES

History

The inflammation that takes place causes pain that is dull initially but over a few hours becomes increasingly severe. There is considerable muscle spasm and a septic arthritis may be suspected but the joint itself is not inflamed.

Physical findings

- *Look* for:
  - a pale, sweaty patient in severe pain
  - the arm held still by the side.
- *Feel* for diffuse tenderness of the whole shoulder region.
- *Test* for movement which will be resisted because of pain.

MANAGEMENT

Non-operative

Rest, anti-inflammatory drugs and local anaesthetic injections may help.

Surgical

Incising the tendon releases the calcific deposit. It squeezes out under pressure like toothpaste from a tube and pain relief is immediate.

Adhesive capsulitis (frozen shoulder)

This condition is characterised by increasing pain and relative immobility of the joint. The aetiology is unknown but there may be a history of minor trauma and the disorder may also complicate other illnesses such as a myocardial infarct or pneumonia.

CLINICAL FEATURES

Pain and stiffness are the only complaints. Joint movement is limited and attempts to increase the range of passive movement cause pain. Over a period of about a year, the symptoms gradually improve, and within 2 years the shoulder may have returned to normal.

MANAGEMENT

Non-operative

The mainstay of treatment is that resolution eventually takes place. Cautious physiotherapy is helpful and steroid injections into the shoulder joint may also help.

Surgical

When recovery is slow, a manipulation under anaesthesia is often beneficial.

Glenohumeral disorders

Osteoarthritis

This condition is uncommon and usually secondary to trauma. Pain is felt at the front of the joint and may radiate through to the posterior aspect. Conservative measures such as anti-inflammatory agents and steroid injections into the joint help in the early stages. Persistent disability requires:

- arthroscopy – the joint is washed out and any loose bodies are removed, which gives some relief for most patients
- arthroplasty – replacement with a prosthesis; many designs are available but most consist of a metal humeral head and a high-density polyethylene glenoid
- arthrodesis – fusion of the shoulder is less commonly done except as a salvage procedure after failed joint replacement.

Rheumatoid arthritis

The shoulder is commonly affected by this disease. Management is usually non-operative by treating the underlying condition and using intra-articular steroid injections. Surgical options are the same as for osteoarthritis.

Avascular necrosis of the humeral head

This is much less common than the same condition in the femoral head. The causes and mechanisms are the same. Management is by treating any underlying cause and by the use of anti-inflammatory agents and physiotherapy. Surgical core decompression is indicated in early disease to arrest progress. In the late stages, when there has been collapse of the humeral head and secondary osteoarthritis has developed, an arthroplasty may be required.

Elbow

The elbow joint is a hinge that works in consort with the shoulder in positioning the hand.

GENERAL CLINICAL FEATURES

History

Stiffness is noticed early by patients because of difficulty in getting the hand to the mouth.

Pain is common and often aggravated by movement.

Locking is an occasional feature particularly in degenerative disease.

Past trauma to the joint is not uncommon.

Physical findings

- *Look* at:
  - the shape of the joint – compare with the other side
  - contour for swellings – a bursa, rheumatoid nodule or effusion
  - carrying angle of the arm in extension – normal is 8–10° of valgus.
- *Feel* for:
  - crepitus
  - bony landmarks – two epicondyles and the olecranon: do they form an equilateral triangle (Fig. 33.5)?
  - effusion – best felt between the lateral epicondyle and the olecranon; the normal hollow is filled out by a soft swelling
  - radial head during pronation and supination – does it dislocate as the forearm moves?
- *Test* for:
  - ulnar nerve function in the hand

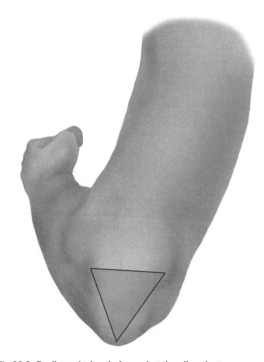

Fig 33.5 **Equilateral triangle formed at the elbow by two epicondyles and the olecranon.**

movements – ask the patient to demonstrate the active range of movement; measure the passive range of movement (Information Box 33).

INVESTIGATION

Imaging
Plain X-ray is usually the only investigation required and can show old injuries, the presence of arthritis, loose bodies and subluxation of the radial head.

Nerve function
If an ulnar nerve lesion is suspected, electromyography is required.

Osteoarthritis

CLINICAL FEATURES
The condition is almost always secondary to trauma. Pain and stiffness are the common symptoms. Locking can sometimes occur.

MANAGEMENT

Non-operative
The usual initial – and often the only – treatment required consists of analgesia, local strapping and physiotherapy.

Surgical
The indications for surgery are:

- symptomatic loose bodies which can be removed arthroscopically
- ulnar neuritis – usually the consequence of a valgus deformity, this is treated by transposition of the nerve in front of the medial epicondyle.

Fusion is indicated when there is failure of conservative treatment with severe pain. The joint is fixed in a position of function that allows the hand to reach the mouth – about 100° of flexion.

Total elbow replacement is possible but the technique is relatively new and the long-term results are less satisfactory in the joint with degenerative disease as compared with rheumatoid arthritis.

Rheumatoid arthritis

The elbow is often involved in rheumatoid arthritis and chemical features are of pain, swelling and stiffness.

MANAGEMENT

Non-operative
Most patients can be managed by control of the systemic disease and local measures including splints.

Operative
If conservative measures are not sufficient, then there are a number of surgical options.

Synovectomy can produce good relief of pain and is usually done through the arthroscope.

Excision of the radial head can reduce symptoms if this structure is particularly involved.

Fusion and replacement can both be considered.

Hand and wrist

Loss of hand function is very disabling in that nearly all daily activities require the hands to a greater or lesser extent. The wrist, in conjunction with the elbow and shoulder, positions the hand in space while the fingers and thumb hold and manipulate.

GENERAL CLINICAL FEATURES

History
Pain is often felt in the wrist but less commonly in the hand. Pain which originates in the hand may be felt across the wrist joint or be localised to a styloid process. In the fingers, it is usually related to pathological change in a joint. Pain at night which affects the hand and is associated with numbness is characteristic of compression of nerves in the carpal tunnel.

Stiffness in the wrist may not cause significant problems, but in the fingers it is an early complaint because it is so disabling.

Swelling in the hand or fingers is noticed early. Rings may become tight and so draw attention to the fingers.

Paraesthesia is usually in the distribution of a peripheral nerve.

Weakness is a common symptom in median or ulnar nerve lesions. Patients often complain of difficulty in fine finger movements such as knitting or writing.

Physical findings
- *Look* for:
  - the position of the hand at rest – are the fingers in fixed flexion because of fascial contractures in the palm (Dupuytren's contracture)?
  - finger deviation with ulnar drift as seen in the rheumatoid hand
  - muscle function in the hand – the thenar eminence may be atrophied in median nerve compression; and the hypothenar eminence and interossei in ulnar nerve compression
  - the pattern of any swelling at the joints of the fingers; Heberden's nodes are seen at the distal interphalangeal joints in osteoarthritis.

- *Feel*:
  - the palmar aponeurosis – thickened areas may indicate aponeurotic fibrosis
  - the skin – warmth and dryness are present if there is a peripheral nerve lesion.
- *Test*:
  - sensation to light touch and pinprick and establish the distribution of any loss found
  - for crepitus at the wrist on movement
  - ulnar and median nerves for Tinel's sign; this is often positive in fascial compression at the wrist or other causes of nerve excitability
  - active and passive ranges of movement (Information Box 33.3).

INVESTIGATION

Imaging

Plain X-ray is often needed and can confirm if a lump arises from bone. Arthritic change and its underlying cause can be demonstrated (Table 33.2). Old trauma may be evident. Unusual conditions such as Kienbock's disease (osteochondrosis of the lunate – often post-traumatic) or Madelung's deformity (subluxation of the distal radioulnar joint, see p. 000) can be confirmed.

Electromyography (EMG)

If a peripheral nerve lesion is suspected, EMG is essential. It confirms the diagnosis and site of the lesion and may help to avoid unnecessary surgery.

Arthritis at the wrist

At the wrist, osteoarthritis is often secondary to trauma. Rheumatoid arthritis also affects the wrist.

CLINICAL FEATURES

The symptoms are pain, stiffness and swelling. The swelling is often accompanied by deformity from a previous fracture. Crepitus may be felt.

MANAGEMENT

Non-operative

Measures such as a removable wrist splint can relieve symptoms, as do mild analgesics.

Surgical

The indications for surgery are pain and incapacity which have failed to respond to non-operative measures, such as in the young adult with post-traumatic arthritis. Of the options available (Table 33.3), fusion is the procedure of choice. The joint is removed and a bone graft inserted. A plate is normally required for stabilisation until the bone unites.

Wrist joint replacement is technically feasible but remains controversial.

Arthritis of the hand

The distribution in the hand follows a pattern characteristic of the cause.

CLINICAL FEATURES

Stiffness and deformity of the fingers are common symptoms. In rheumatoid arthritis, the hand deforms in a characteristic way. Progressive destruction of the metacarpophalangeal joints causes the fingers to drift to the ulnar side, and later there is subluxation at these joints. In addition, inflammatory tenosynovitis may lead to tendon rupture with one or more dropped (semi-immobile and flexed) fingers.

MANAGEMENT

Because arthritis, in particular rheumatoid, is a continuing process, management varies with the stage of the disease. A series of procedures may be required as deformities develop and progress.

Non-operative

Physiotherapy to conserve and improve hand function is essential. The occupational therapist can provide crucial aids to assist in the activities of daily living: modified cutlery with curved or flattened handles, special fasteners for clothes, and other devices may all preserve independence. Hand splints are often used. They rarely prevent deformity but do allow rheumatoid joints to be rested during an acute exacerbation of the disease.

Surgical

Various operative procedures are appropriate at different stages of the disease, but the potential problems of undertaking surgery should always be carefully discussed. Many badly deformed hands are still able to function usefully. Ruptured tendons should be repaired and, in rheumatoid arthritis, early synovectomy may delay destruction. In later stages, or in osteoarthritis, damaged joints may be replaced by silastic implants. These correct deformities and relieve pain but rarely increase grip strength and some residual stiffness persists.

Dupuytren's contracture

This is a condition of the hand in which there is thickening and contraction of the palmar aponeurosis, possibly from a local change in collagen metabolism.

AETIOLOGY AND PATHOLOGICAL FEATURES

The precise cause is not known but there are nevertheless a number of well recognised associated factors, including:

- a family history
- male sex

- regular high consumption of alcohol
- diabetes mellitus
- phenytoin therapy
- trauma.

Contracture is bilateral in 45%; similar lesions in the plantar aponeurosis occur in 5%; and the penile fascia is affected in 3%.

CLINICAL FEATURES

The usual first development is at the base of the ring and little fingers. As the lesion progresses, the fingers gradually develop fixed flexion deformities and the thumb web may also be involved.

MANAGEMENT

Non-operative

Although many measures have been tried, none is effective. The condition may be self-limiting but is usually progressive.

Surgical

Five operations may be considered and these are outlined in Table 33.7. The choice depends on the extent of the disease, the degree of disability and whether or not previous operations have been done.

Nerve entrapment syndromes

These commonly affect the hand. Usually it is compression of the median nerve that gives rise to symptoms, but ulnar nerve entrapment at the elbow or occasionally the wrist can also occur.

AETIOLOGY

Median nerve compression in the carpal tunnel is usually without an identifiable cause, but any abnormal structure within the tunnel can produce the condition. Examples are:

- wrist fracture – early from local haematoma and oedema or late because of a malunion and bony encroachment
- ganglion within the carpal tunnel
- tenosynovitis from rheumatoid arthritis or repetitive strain injury
- changes in the interstitial space – obesity, diabetes mellitus, hypothyroidism, pregnancy, acromegaly and amyloidosis.

Ulnar nerve compression is usually at the elbow adjacent to the medial epicondyle of the humerus. There may not be an obvious cause, but a fracture which causes a valgus deformity of the elbow may attenuate the nerve. Compression at the wrist in the ulnar canal between the pisiform and the hook of the hamate is less common.

CLINICAL FEATURES

History

In *median nerve compression* – the characteristic carpal tunnel syndrome – there is often pain in the distribution of the median nerve and this is frequently worse at night. Loss of grip and clumsiness in handling objects are other complaints.

In *ulnar nerve compression* at the elbow there may be a past history of trauma in the region of the joint. Weakness and clumsiness of the hand are the chief complaints.

Physical findings

Median nerve. Wasting of the thenar eminence and the first dorsal interosseus is seen. There is loss of sensation in the median nerve territory.

Ulnar nerve. If the compression is at the elbow, evidence of elbow deformity may be apparent with an abnormal carrying angle. An elbow lesion also causes weakness of the ulnar half of flexor digitorum profundus, but flexor carpi ulnaris is weak only when the lesion is above the elbow. Wasting of the

Table 33.7
Operations for Dupuytren's contracture of the palmar fascia

Procedure	Technique	Outcome
Percutaneous fasciotomy	Simple division of fibrous bands though percutaneous stab wounds	Recurrence rates high and damage may occur to nerves and blood vessels
Selective fasciectomy	Thickened areas are excised	Most common operation; successful in limited disease
Complete fasciectomy	Whole aponeurosis excised even if not obviously involved	Potentially curative but high incidence of skin necrosis
Complete fasciectomy and skin graft	Aponeurosis excised together with the skin of the palm followed by split-skin grafting	Curative but requires high skills
Amputation	Removal of a single digit (usually little finger), severely contracted into the palm and interfering with hand function	Can be procedure of choice in special circumstances

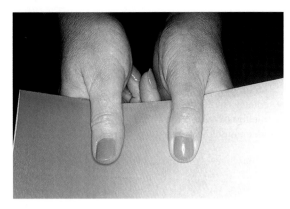

Fig 33.6 **Froment's sign.**

hypothenar and interosseus muscles is present (most noticeable in the first web space). The hand may appear flattened with the ring and metacarpophalangeal joints hyperextended because of lumbrical paralysis. Attempts to grip a sheet of paper between the thumb and index finger cause the trick movement of flexion of the distal phalanx of the thumb to compensate for the weak interossei (Froment's sign – Fig. 33.6).

MANAGEMENT

Non-operative
Underlying causes at the wrist are treated. In pregnancy, the symptoms often resolve rapidly after delivery. Injections of steroid into the carpal tunnel may help in mild cases but should not be repeated more than twice or irreversible fibrosis may take place in the median nerve. Non-operative treatment of ulnar nerve problems usually fails.

Surgical
Median nerve. Decompression of the median nerve by dividing the carpal ligament is a highly effective and simple procedure that can be carried out under local or general anaesthesia. Relief of symptoms is often immediate and any thenar wasting recovers with time. The procedure can now be performed endoscopically.

Ulnar nerve. For lesions with their cause at the elbow, the nerve is transposed to lie in front of the medial epicondyle after dividing the medial inter-muscular septum which, if left intact, can chafe the nerve and cause persistent problems. At the wrist, the ulnar canal is explored and decompressed. Recovery is slow compared with the median nerve but symptoms do generally improve.

Ganglion

Ganglions are tense cysts containing viscous, jelly-like material. They often occur on the dorsum of the wrist and are associated with joints or tendon sheaths. They may also be found in the hand and in the foot. Less commonly, subperiosteal ganglia are formed on long bones after trauma. The periosteum is raised by the contents of the lesions with resorption of underlying bone.

AETIOLOGY AND PATHOLOGICAL FEATURES
Many explanations have been advanced but none has been conclusively established. It is possible that they are derived from small extra-articular fragments of synovium and this would certainly explain both their inspissated contents and their tendency to recur if incompletely removed.

CLINICAL FEATURES
Symptoms are cosmetic only unless previous in-adequate surgery has caused secondary problems.

Signs are of a tense, fluctuant usually globular swelling deep to skin and incompletely mobile on the deep aspect because of attachment to a neighbouring joint or tendon sheath.

MANAGEMENT

Non-operative
An asymptomatic lesion which does not cause cosmetic embarrassment is best left alone. Traditional treatment has also included subcutaneous rupture – the family bible was often used as the weapon. More modern therapy consists of aspiration followed by steroid injection, but 15% or more recur.

Surgical
Excision of the ganglion is effective provided the technique is meticulous and undertaken in a bloodless field.

Trigger finger

The cause is unknown. There is localised thickening of a flexor tendon with associated narrowing of the sheath. The thickened part is then unable to pass smoothly under the entrance to the synovial sheath at the base of the finger.

CLINICAL FEATURES
The patient recognises that the affected finger catches in flexion and straightens suddenly with assistance and a snap. The features can usually be produced to order.

MANAGEMENT
Surgical treatment is the only option. The sheath is incised to allow the tendon to move freely.

de Quervain's syndrome

Tenosynovitis of the tendon sheaths of extensor pollicis brevis and abductor pollicis longus may be the result of local trauma but usually no cause is found. It is most frequent in middle-aged women.

CLINICAL FEATURES

The symptoms are pain and weakness of the thumb.

The sheath is palpably thickened and tender. Adducting and flexing the thumb and wrist (Finkelstein's test) are painful.

MANAGEMENT

Non-operative

Injection of steroid into the tendon sheath is often effective but it is important that only the sheath (and not the tendon) is injected because the tendon may otherwise be weakened and rupture.

Surgical

The tendon sheath is slit, so freeing up movement. The procedure is curative and that of choice if the condition is chronic.

Kienbock's disease

This condition is avascular necrosis of the lunate. In most instances the cause is unknown, but it may occasionally follow dislocation of the bone.

The patient – a young adult – complains of local ache and stiffness at the wrist. There are no clinical findings except slight tenderness over the dorsum of the wrist.

INVESTIGATION AND MANAGEMENT

Plain X-ray shows sclerosis of the lunate. As the condition progresses, there is fragmentation and secondary osteoarthritis develops in the wrist joint.

In the early stages a splint may help. Attempts have been made to revascularise the bone with part of the pronator quadratus muscle but these have met with limited success. Other surgical options include:

- removal of the bone and insertion of a Silastic prosthesis
- shortening of the radius to decompress the lunate
- fusion if osteoarthritis is present.

Madelung's deformity

This is a growth disorder of the distal radial epiphysis. It becomes apparent after the age of 10 years and is more common in girls.

The patient complains of a prominent lump alongside the ulnar styloid with stiffness at the wrist. Examination of the mother's wrist often reveals the same deformity. There is some limitation of the range of movement.

INVESTIGATION AND MANAGEMENT

Plain X-rays show the distal radius to be shortened slightly and curved, with the lunate tending to sublux between the radius and ulna. The ulna is of normal length and therefore appears more prominent.

Operations should be avoided. Excision of the distal ulna leaves an unsightly scar and a weak wrist. In gross deformity, elongation of the abnormal radius may improve the appearance and function of the wrist.

The hip

GENERAL CLINICAL FEATURES AND EXAMINATION

History

Pain originating from the hip tends to be felt in the groin or thigh. It may be referred to the knee, particularly in children. Pain is worse at the end of the day and on weight-bearing. Nocturnal pain may cause much loss of sleep.

Past trauma. In chronic disorders there may be a past history of trauma, e.g. fracture of the pelvis and dislocation or fracture-dislocation of the femur.

Limp and gait. Limp may be noticed by others or by the patient and there may be increasing difficulty in walking. Causes may be:

- pain as the patient tries to protect the joint
- short leg
- muscle weakness.

For abnormal gaits associated with hip disorders, see Information Box 33.2.

Physical findings

- *Look* at:
  - skin for scars
  - the position of the hip – in established osteoarthritis of the hip is in fixed flexion, internal rotation and adduction
  - gait; this can be protective (antalgic), Trendelenburg, short- or stiff-legged.
- *Feel:*
  - for crepitus on movement
  - to measure leg length – from the anterior superior iliac spine to the medial malleolus.
- *Move* to:
  - establish active range of movement
  - measure the passive range of movement.

The normal range is shown in Information Box 33.3.

It is important to ensure that movement is taking place at the hip alone and not the pelvis as well. On flexion, a hand under the lumbar spine can feel when the pelvis starts to tilt. During abduction and adduction, a forearm across the pelvis prevents pelvic tilt. Fully flexing the other hip to abolish the normal lumbar lordosis demonstrates a fixed flexion deformity as the affected leg rises up off the examination couch.

INVESTIGATION

Imaging

Plain X-ray is usually sufficient to confirm a clinical diagnosis.

Isotope scan. In lytic lesions, there is increased uptake; avascular necrosis appears as a relatively dense area.

CT and MRI can help to determine the site or extent of bony and other damage in more detail.

Blood examination

In osteoarthritis, the erythrocyte sedimentation rate is normal and rheumatoid factor is absent. The reverse is true in rheumatoid arthritis.

Osteoarthritis

This condition is extremely common. Its treatment to relieve pain and restore mobility has been revolutionised by the development of prosthetic hip joints.

EPIDEMIOLOGY AND AETIOLOGY

The factors that can contribute to the development of the condition have been discussed above. By far the commonest is wear and tear on the joint in a population with an increased life expectancy – by the age of 80 years, 80–90% of hips show radiographic evidence of the condition. Women are more commonly affected than men (3:1). The condition can be unilateral or bilateral. More than 10% of unilateral instances become bilateral over 5–8 years.

MANAGEMENT

Decisions on management depend on:

- what the patient wants
- age – although with modern techniques of surgery and anaesthesia, chronological age is rarely a bar to operation
- general physical condition
- degree of disability and its interaction with lifestyle.

Non-operative

Those with only minor symptoms can be managed by losing weight, physiotherapy, foam heel wedges, a walking stick and NSAIDs. Loss of 1 kg of body weight reduces the forces acting across the hip by roughly 3 kg.

Surgical

Surgery for osteoarthritis of the hip is now essentially joint replacement, although in the past there were other options (Table 33.3). Arthrodesis may still be considered in a young adult with a demanding physical occupation. An osteotomy can provide short-term relief of pain but a subsequent joint replacement may be difficult because of the altered anatomy. Excision is reserved for the infected hip replacement. The modern total hip replacement was introduced in 1961 and can be expected to last for at least 15–20 years. However, this depends on a number of factors, as described above.

The chief causes of failure are:

- infection, which should be less than 1%
- loosening without infection and recrudescence of pain.

Infection means that the prosthesis must be removed, although it may be possible to insert a replacement after the organism has been eliminated. Loosening without infection is treated by a revision procedure.

Rheumatoid arthritis (RA)

This is a systemic condition which is initially managed medically. The hip and knee are involved but, in particular, it affects the the upper limbs and the feet. There are a number of problems encountered with hip joint replacement in the patient with RA. When, as is often the case, multiple joints are involved, rehabilitation may be difficult. Bone quality is often poor so that intraoperative fractures occur. Infection rates are higher than for replacement in OA.

Nevertheless, hip replacement for RA has a definite place provided that the joint is the principal site of the problem and there is a good chance of restoring mobility.

Osteonecrosis of the femoral head

In this condition, the femoral head becomes ischaemic and infarcts. As a result, there is structural weakness and collapse of the bone.

AETIOLOGY

The underlying process is not fully understood. The following have been postulated:

- arterial insufficiency following a fracture or dislocation
- venous occlusion – a feature of Perthe's disease
- raised intraosseous pressure – possibly the cause in sickle cell disease, alcoholism, systemic steroids and decompression from high atmospheric pressure with the formation of gas bubbles.

MANAGEMENT

Non-operative

Treatment of any correctable underlying cause is instituted. Anti-inflammatory drugs are symptomatically helpful.

Surgical

Surgery is often required to provide pain relief:

- core decompression – drilling a core of bone out of the femoral head and neck is thought to be effective by reducing the intraosseous pressure and improving venous drainage but is less helpful in later stages III or IV
- arthroplasty is reserved for the late stages when there is collapse and secondary osteoarthritis.

Tuberculosis

AETIOLOGY AND PATHOLOGICAL MANIFESTATIONS

The disease is now less common although the incidence has recently increased in the poor and groups with immunosuppression from such causes as AIDS. The route of infection is haematogenous and the pathological features are the same as for tuberculosis in other organs – tissue destruction, abscess formation and fibrosis. Untreated, the joint progresses to bony ankylosis.

CLINICAL FEATURES

As well as systemic symptoms of malaise and fever, local ones include a mild ache and limp.

Initially, there is little to be found – only the features of an irritable hip. Later, there is marked wasting, joint stiffness, pain and shortening. This chronic picture is in contrast to the acute, severe pattern of septic arthritis.

INVESTIGATION AND MANAGEMENT

X-ray changes are of osteoporosis and, later, joint destruction.

As in septic arthritis, pus is drained, the organism is cultured to establish sensitivity to chemotherapy and appropriate anti-tuberculosis therapy begun. With these measures, damage can be limited. A hip that heals with bony ankylosis may require a raised shoe when walking is resumed. A painful joint may need to be arthrodesed. Arthroplasty is considered with caution because reactivation of the infection can occur.

The knee

GENERAL CLINICAL FEATURES

History

Age. Young adults commonly suffer injury in sport; their first presentation is often to general practitioners and casualty departments. In older individuals, the joint is more frequently affected by osteoarthritis, although injury may be a precipitating factor. In an acute event, the patient may be able to pinpoint the exact moment of injury.

Pain. Generalised or localised pain is a frequent symptom. The location is important because it may indicate the diagnosis. Generalised pain over the whole knee is a feature of arthritis and acute injury. In meniscal tears, pain is localised to the joint line, including posteriorly in the popliteal fossa. Collateral sprains cause pain above or below the joint line. Anterior pain is a symptom of disorders of the patella such as chondromalacia. Such anterior pain is frequently worse when the knee is loaded in flexion – characteristically when going up stairs. Deficiency of the anterior cruciate ligament is often associated with pain at the anterior joint line; after the knee gives way, the pain is diffuse.

Mechanism in injuries. Commonly, there is a twisting injury, with an associated tearing or popping noise from the joint which is accompanied by pain. The patient may well fall to the ground. Alternatively there is a long history of heavy load-bearing.

Swelling may be immediate and implies an acute haemarthrosis (the usual causes are given in Table 33.8). Delay for up to a day suggests a meniscal injury. Arthritic knees are chronically swollen from either an effusion or thickened synovium.

Locking and giving way occur when the knee is unstable. Locking may fix the knee, usually in flexion, or it may unlock with a pop or a click. The arthritic knee may also give way because of instability and may lock because of loose bodies trapped within it.

Physical findings

- *Look* for:
  - swelling – by assessing contour
  - wasting of the quadriceps
  - position at rest – is the joint in fixed flexion or is there a varus or valgus deformity?
  - scars – previous arthroscopy portals can be missed unless examination is meticulous
  - abnormal skin colour.

Table 33.8
Causes of acute haemarthrosis of the knee

Lesion[a]	Percentage
Anterior cruciate ligament rupture	39
Peripheral meniscal tear	26
Collateral ligament injury	13
Capsular tear	9
Osteochondral fracture	7
Posterior cruciate ligament rupture	6

[a] Seventy per cent have more than one lesion, 29% have only one lesion, and in 1% no cause is found.

- *Feel* for:
  - swelling – if present, is it bone, boggy synovial thickening or fluid?
  - the presence of an effusion (see below)
  - altered temperature
  - the joint line – medially, laterally and in the popliteal fossa
  - local tenderness, which suggests a meniscal tear
  - tenderness over the femoral condyles when the knee is flexed; they may be tender when damaged, as occurs in arthritis
  - the patella – is it very mobile; when pushed laterally, does the patient flinch (such positive apprehension is seen with recurrent dislocation of the patella); is there tenderness on the retropatellar surface?
  - loose bodies which may shoot from under the fingers
  - crepitus when the joint is moved.

Effusion is diagnosed by two methods. The first, cross-fluctuation, is the more sensitive of the two. The second, patellar tap, confirms a large effusion but may not be elicited with a small collection.

Cross-fluctuation. The suprapatellar pouch is emptied by placing one hand proximal to the patella, so pushing any fluid down into the main cavity of the joint. The hand stays in position and the medial and lateral sides are examined. In the normal knee, a soft hollow is seen but this is absent with a large effusion. With a stroking motion of the other hand to the medial and lateral sides, fluid can be pushed across the joint. In the presence of an effusion, a soft swelling appears on the opposite side of the knee to the hand.

Patella tap. The suprapatellar pouch is emptied as before and kept empty by leaving the hand above the patella. The other hand gently presses the patella down onto the underlying femoral condyles. There is a distinct feeling of the patella sinking down and coming to a sudden stop when it hits the condyles with a 'tap'.

Collateral ligament stability is assessed with the knee in 20° of flexion. A varus strain is applied to test the lateral collateral ligament; a valgus strain for the medial collateral

Cruciate ligaments. The integrity of the anterior cruciate is assessed performing the Lachman test (Fig. 33.7); and the posterior cruciate by looking for 'posterior sag' (Fig. 33.8).

Quadriceps wasting. The circumference of the leg is measured on both sides at a fixed distance (usually 10 cm) above the upper border of the patella.

Movement. The patient is asked to walk. On bearing weight, does the knee go into a valgus or varus deformity? There may be an antalgic, short leg or stiff leg gait (Information Box 33.2).

The range of active movement is then assessed and compared with the passive range. Is it possible to get

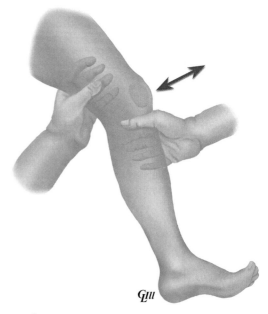

Fig 33.7 **Lachman's test for integrity of the anterior cruciate.**

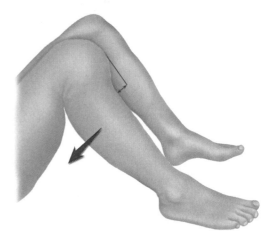

Fig 33.8 **Posterior sag in a lesion of the posterior cruciate.**

the knee to full extension, or is there a block? Finally, in a normal knee, the patella tracks evenly on the trochlear surface of the femur. Maltracking occurs when it is seen to sublux or dislocate laterally as the knee moves.

INVESTIGATION

Imaging

Plain X-rays reveal any arthritis. Loose bodies may be seen, often in the intercondylar notch. On the lateral film, the patella height should be about equal to the distance from the inferior pole of the patella to the tibial tuberosity. If it is less than this, then the patella is riding high (patella alta) and is liable to dislocate.

Skyline views show the patellofemoral joint and are taken with the knee flexed. The patella should be horizontal and centrally positioned within its trochlear groove.

Tunnel views are taken with the knee flexed to 45° and provide a view of the intercondylar notch. They are useful if loose bodies are suspected. If an avulsion of the anterior cruciate is possible, then a small flake of bone torn off the tibial plateau may be seen.

Weight-bearing films accentuate any loss of joint space and also show up varus/valgus deformities.

Arthrography can show meniscal and capsular tears. With the advent of MRI and diagnostic arthroscopy, its use is declining.

CT is not often used in the knee but can show arthritis, loose bodies and patella malalignment.

MRI can demonstrate meniscal and cruciate injuries. It is non-invasive and in many centres has replaced arthrography.

Radioisotope scan shows increased activity in degenerative conditions which may be localised to one compartment.

Meniscal injuries

A meniscus trapped between the joint surfaces may tear. There are five main types of tear (Fig. 33.9). The distribution is:

- medial meniscus – 70%
- lateral meniscus – 25%
- both – 5%.

The frequent involvement of the medial meniscus is because it is firmly adherent to the medial capsule and therefore less mobile than the lateral one.

CLINICAL FEATURES

History

There has usually been a painful twisting injury, often during sport. There may be an associated 'pop', 'crack' or tearing sensation within the joint and swelling quickly appears. Subsequently there is persistent swelling and a feeling of something catching. Occasionally the knee locks for some hours as the torn meniscus becomes lodged between the joint.

Physical findings

- *Look* for:
  - effusion
  - wasted quadriceps by comparison with the other side.
- *Feel* for:
  - effusion
  - tenderness at the joint line.
- *Test movement* for:
  - springy feel in a locked knee

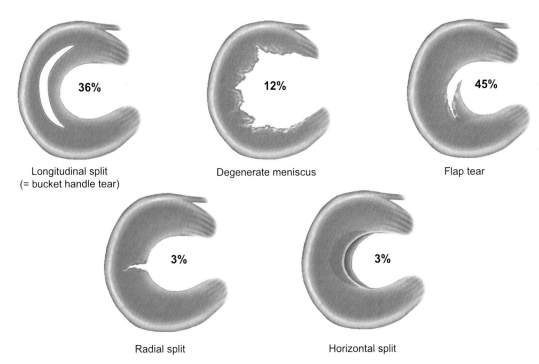

Longitudinal split (= bucket handle tear) — 36%

Degenerate meniscus — 12%

Flap tear — 45%

Radial split — 3%

Horizontal split — 3%

Fig 33.9 **Types of meniscal tear in the knee.**

— McMurray's test – with the knee at 90° of flexion, the tibia is rotated on the femur to try to trap the meniscal tear between the two bones; internal rotation of the tibia catches a lateral meniscus and external rotation the medial; in either event pain is felt at the joint line.

MANAGEMENT

Non-operative

When there is doubt about the diagnosis, then it is reasonable to treat the symptoms with a review in 2–3 weeks. In those with improvement, a graduated programme of knee rehabilitation is continued. When symptoms and signs persist, surgery should be considered.

Surgical

When the clinical features are typical, then the management is surgical. Arthroscopy (see below) is both diagnostic and therapeutic – the tear can be seen and then excised. After operation, it is vital that formal rehabilitation is undertaken to avoid further injury to the joint. This starts immediately with quadriceps exercises, and once the portals have healed, swimming, cycling and weight training of the muscles can begin. Only when all these activities are managed with ease is return to exercise which involves weight-bearing on the knee surface allowed (such as jogging, low-impact aerobics and finally contact or high-impact sporting activities).

Anterior cruciate ligament (ACL) injuries

MECHANISM AND PATHOLOGICAL FEATURES

These injuries are sustained after twisting and valgus strain are applied to the knee. Typically they are seen in the footballer who twists on the knee during a tackle on an opposing player. The medial collateral ligament and medial meniscus are often damaged at the same time. Hyperextension on its own can also produce an isolated ACL rupture. Occasionally, any of these mechanisms may avulse a fragment of bone at the insertion of the ACL onto the tibial plateau.

CLINICAL FEATURES

Physical examination demonstrates only about 70% of ruptures of the ACL. The diagnosis is often made at arthroscopy.

MANAGEMENT

Non-operative

The knee with a ruptured ACL can often be managed without resort to surgery. Intensive rehabilitation is used to strengthen the hamstring and quadricep muscles and improve proprioception at the knee. Swimming, cycling and weight training followed by gentle jogging can then be attempted. Change in lifestyle with withdrawal from some sports or other activities may be necessary. A brace can help to stabilise the knee. A large variety are available but all rely on firm strapping above and below the knee with metal or carbon fibre supports for tennis or skiing.

Surgical

With effective non-operative management, surgery may often be avoided. If it is, urgent operation has no advantage over delayed repair. The only unequivocal indication for early repair is when a fragment of bone has been avulsed from the tibial plateau which should be reattached with a screw.

Delayed reconstruction may be required if the ACL has failed to unite with nonoperative management. There are two types of operation:

- *extra-articular* – strengthening the lateral side of the knee with a strip of fascia lata reduces the tendency for the knee to rotate internally as it gives way
- *intra-articular* – the remnants of the ACL are replaced; a large variety of materials have been used including bovine collagen, cadaveric transplants, the patient's patellar ligament or hamstring tendons and synthetic substitutes of PTFE, carbon fibre or Dacron.

Most ACL reconstructions utilise the patients own patellar tendon or hamstring tendons.

Posterior cruciate ligament (PCL) injuries

Rupture of the posterior cruciate is much less common than that of the ACL and is often not recognised. The tibia is forced posteriorly on the femoral condyles – as in a head-on car crash when the lower leg hits the dashboard.

CLINICAL FEATURES

The functional instability after PCL rupture may be minimal, with the symptoms of pain, stiffness and an effusion only developing after degenerative changes in the knee have occurred.

In an acute injury there is a tense haemarthrosis with perhaps soft tissue abrasions on the front of the tibia.

INVESTIGATION AND MANAGEMENT

Plain X-ray shows an effusion and perhaps a piece of bone that has been avulsed off the tibia.

A change in lifestyle, including the form of sporting activity, may allow the patient to lead a near-normal life.

An avulsed fragment should be exposed through the popliteal fossa and reattached. In a rupture with chronic problems, the indications for surgical treatment are the same as for repair of the ACL and the methods are also similar.

Recurrent dislocation of the patella

The patella is a mobile sesamoid within the quadriceps tendon and is in a vulnerable position in front of the knee. True dislocation must be differentiated from maltracking in which there is painful subluxation.

CLINICAL FEATURES

History

Full dislocation. The patella always dislocates laterally and there is usually a history of direct trauma to the medial side, often during sport. The patient sees and feels the bone displaced and the knee is locked in 30°–40° of flexion. Anterior pain and rapid swelling develop.

Subluxation. The patella is felt to 'pop' out of place, often during a turning movement. Pain is momentary and sharp over the front of the knee, which may feel unstable or give way. Minor swelling is noted over 24 hours.

Physical findings
- *Look* for:
  - the patella on the lateral side of the knee
  - knee locked in flexion
  - effusion.
- *Feel* for:
  - position of the bone to the lateral side
  - tenderness on the medial side of the patella after reduction
  - effusion.
- *Test* for reducibility by applying firm pressure on the lateral side and simultaneously extending the knee; the bone may reduce with a 'snap'.

INVESTIGATION

Plain X-rays show the displacement. After reduction, patella alta (see below) may be seen. Skyline views are helpful and may reveal an osteochrondral fracture that occurs as the patella dislocates over the lateral femoral condyle.

In subluxation, X-rays may be normal or show patella alta.

Arthritis

Arthritis of the knee is very common and the usual form is osteoarthritis. Rheumatoid arthritis also occurs but less frequently. As in the hip; the management of this painful, disabling condition has been transformed by the development of prosthetic replacement.

CLINICAL FEATURES

History

Pain is the main complaint. Initially this is felt only after walking but later also at rest. Accompanying stiffness and swelling, initially intermittent but eventually permanent, occur. Locking because of loose bodies and acute painful giving way are both common.

Physical findings
- *Look* for:
  - varus or valgus deformity with the patient standing
  - swelling.
- *Feel* for:
  - effusion
  - tenderness at the joint lines and over the femoral condyles
  - crepitus.
- *Test* for:
  - movement – fixed flexion deformity is common
  - collateral ligament laxity when there is varus or valgus deformity.

MANAGEMENT

Non-operative
Weight loss, analgesics, physiotherapy, a walking stick and foam heel wedges all help in those with mild symptoms.

Surgical
There are several surgical options. The choice depends on:

- wishes of the patient
- age
- degree of disability.

Arthroscopy is a useful first step and allows the surgeon to assess the extent of the disorder. Debris in the joint is washed out and can provide pain relief for a year or more. Loose bodies can be removed and degenerative meniscal tears trimmed. In rheumatoid arthritis, an arthroscopic synovectomy is symptomatically useful in that synovial hypertrophy contributes to the inflammatory process.

Osteotomy. Often the medial compartment of the knee is affected by the arthritis but the lateral side is relatively spared. An osteotomy can be performed to realign the knee and forces are transferred to the relatively healthy side. This procedure is of use in the younger patient and may provide 8–10 years of pain relief. Once the lateral side starts to wear, a knee replacement can be done.

Total knee replacement. Knee replacements with a hinge were inserted in the early 1950s and later in that decade metal discs were interposed but with poor results. However, it was not until the early 1970s, with the development of unconstrained prostheses, that the results improved. 'Unconstrained' means that stability relies on the surrounding tissue tension to hold the two parts in correct alignment. A large variety of knee replacements is now available which fall into the three main groups as shown in Table 33.4.

Arthrodesis. This operation has largely been superseded by joint replacement. It can be a salvage procedure after joint replacement has failed. The knee is fused in a functional position of about 20° of flexion which allows the limb to be swung through during the relevant phase of the gait cycle.

The ankle and foot

....

The ankle

GENERAL CLINICAL FEATURES

History

Pain from the ankle joint is often felt as a band across its front. When there is a problem at the malleolus, the symptoms may be to one side or the other. Pain from the subtalar joint tends to be felt below the ankle and may radiate forward into the foot.

Instability is a sensation of unusual movement usually from side to side and is common because of the frequent exposure of the ankle to twisting strains.

Swelling around the ankle may be the consequence of local disease such as arthritis or of more general problems – cardiac or renal. In chronic instability, it is often localised at one or other malleolus.

Trauma is often an important factor. In addition to predisposing to chronic instability, it can also cause secondary osteoarthritis – the result of joint surface irregularity or of avascular necrosis in a fragment of a fractured talus.

Physical findings
- Look for:
  - swelling
  - scars.
- *Feel* for:
  - localised tenderness in the malleoli
  - crepitus (gently) in the area as a whole
  - swelling – boggy synovial thickening, pitting oedema or an effusion within the joint
  - local warmth.
- *Move* the ankle for:
  - walking – the gait (Information box 33.2) may attempt to avoid pain or there may be foot drop, which causes the toes to contact the ground when normally the heel should strike first; this gait is seen after injury to the sciatic nerve at the

buttock, or the common peroneal nerve at the knee
  - active and passive range – the ankle joint is capable of both plantarflexion and dorsiflexion from a neutral position; inversion and eversion occur at the subtalar joint; the test is done by holding the lower leg with one hand and grasping the heel with the other so that the subtalar joint can then be moved separately
  - excessive movement – laxity of the collateral ligaments is detected on inversion and eversion; drawing the foot forwards and backwards on the lower leg may reveal subluxation.

INVESTIGATION

Imaging

Plain X-ray may show arthritis or evidence of old trauma. When the history is one of instability, there may be localised arthritic changes at the malleolus with perhaps a loose body at the tip of the malleolus from an old avulsion fracture. Avascular necrosis of the talus results in sclerosis and collapse of the bone. If the history and examination suggest that the site of the problem is in the subtalar joint, it may be necessary to request plain films of this joint.

Stress X-ray is done by applying a valgus or varus strain to the joint while films are taken – when this is painful, general anaesthesia may be required. If there is significant instability, the talus may be shown to tilt within the mortice of the ankle joint.

Isotope bone scan may show an increase in activity in the ankle or subtalar joint or at a malleolus. In avascular necrosis of the talus, there is an area of reduced uptake.

CT confirms the presence of arthritis and is also helpful when avascular necrosis is suspected as its extent can be clearly seen.

Chronic instability

This condition is better prevented than cured. The cause is an inversion or eversion injury that tears the collateral ligament which is put under stress.

CLINICAL FEATURES

There is usually a history of the relevant injury. There is tenderness over the ligament just distal to the malleolus. Evidence of bruising is only present in the early stages.

INVESTIGATION AND MANAGEMENT

Stress X-rays will demonstrate talar tilt, although these may be difficult in the acute phase because of pain.

In a patient with an acute injury in whom a diagnosis of a collateral tear has been made, the traditional treatment has been 6 weeks in a below-knee plaster cast to allow the ligament to heal. More recently, early intensive physiotherapy with proprioceptive training on a 'wobble board' (a board balanced on a ball) has been advocated and the results are possibly better.

In spite of adequate treatment, chronic instability may become established and is treated:

- *Non-operatively* – which may be sufficient if the patient alters lifestyle, changes to a different sport or wears boots that support the ankle
- *Surgically* – a number of operations have been described; as well as reconstituting the affected ligament, further support is provided by using a local structure such as the tendon of peroneus brevis or augmenting the repair with carbon fibre.

Arthritis

As a weight-bearing joint, the ankle is prone to osteo-arthritis but much less commonly than the hip or the knee. The reason is unclear but may be in part because the ankle is essentially a hinge joint whereas at the hip and knee there is also rotation and therefore extra shear forces on the cartilage. Nevertheless, post-traumatic secondary osteoarthritis of the ankle is common in young adults involved in athletics.

Involvement by rheumatoid arthritis is to a similar extent as the hip and knee.

MANAGEMENT

Non-operative
This is the most common method: a walking stick, firm boots to limit movement at the joint and anti-inflammatory drugs.

Surgical
Operation is less satisfactory in the ankle than in the hip or knee; the options are fusion, which is disabling, or arthroplasty.

Prosthetic replacements are available but the long-term results are not as good, at the moment, as at the hip or knee. Their use is confined to the patient with rheumatoid disease and they are certainly not indicated in a young adult.

The foot

Painful feet are common and their owners come to all general and orthopaedic outpatient clinics. The hazard of attempts at surgical management of an individual lesion is that it may merely transfer the problem from one part of the foot to another and so never achieve a cure.

CLINICAL FEATURES

History
Pain is the usual presentation, most commonly localised to one point, but it may radiate, be worse on weight-bearing and be relieved by rest. There is often difficulty in finding shoes that can be worn without pain.

Physical findings
The appearance of the foot can be the presenting feature.
- *Look* for:
  - shape, including any callosities and their site
  - the shoes and in what areas they show signs of wear – an indication of how load is being transferred
  - evidence of vascular insufficiency – the presence of peripheral vascular disease may contra-indicate surgery on the foot.
- *Feel* for:
  - local tenderness
  - pulses in the foot.
- *Move:*
  - the midtarsal joint by holding the heel with one hand and the forefoot with the other
  - the toes – are any deformities correctable?

INVESTIGATION

Imaging
Plain X-ray of the foot may be required so as to plan an operation. The presence of radiological evidence of arthritis may influence what procedure, if any, is performed.

Films taken during weight-bearing may be useful: a small metal marker can be placed on a callosity and a film taken which will identify the structure at the pressure point.

Other investigations
Pedobarography produces a pressure profile of the foot. However, the device is not widely available. It can confirm the areas of high pressure and can be used to assess the effect of surgical procedures.

Most other investigations are usually not helpful. A painful and swollen first metatarsophalangeal joint may raise the suspicion of gout which can be confirmed if the serum level of uric acid is raised.

Hallux valgus

This is a progressive valgus deformity of the big toe. Once the toe starts to angulate, progression is inevitable because the pull of the tendons increases the deformity.

AETIOLOGY
A number of factors can be identified in the development of hallux valgus:

- family history
- sex – more common in females
- age – tends to occur in the middle-aged; with the passage of time the foot tends to splay, so making any deforming forces worse
- metatarsus primus varus – if the first metatarsal is in varus, there is a greater tendency for the big toe to go into valgus because of the pull of the extensor tendon
- shoes – modern shoes tend to be very tight at the toes, so forcing the big toe into valgus; hallux valgus is uncommon in barefoot communities.

CLINICAL FEATURES

History

There is cosmetic deformity and discomfort over the prominent bunion at the metatarsophalangeal joint. Inflammation occurs as this rubs on the shoes. Crossing of the first toe over the second and third increases discomfort.

Physical findings

- *Look* for the deformity and the bunion.
- *Feel* for localised tenderness.
- *Test* for movement, which is often reduced, and to find out if the valgus deformity is reducible.

MANAGEMENT

Non-operative

In the elderly with poor peripheral blood flow, conservative management is best. Surgical shoes can be made to fit the foot, as opposed to the normal practice of squashing the deformed toe and foot into the shoe. Regular chiropody is important to care for the skin and nails.

Surgical

Over 40 operations have been described for hallux valgus. A simple bunionectomy is usually not enough because the deformity will reoccur. When there is osteoarthritis at the joint, surgery is either an excisional arthroplasty (Keller's) or joint replacement with a Silastic implant. These relieve the pain and correct the deformity but the joint is often stiffer than normal and, after a Keller's procedure, the big toe is short. In the younger age group, surgery is directed at correcting the underlying deformity – the varus displacement of the first metatarsal. Various operations have been described to lateralise the big toe and therefore correct the deformity.

Hallux rigidus

This condition of a stiff, painful big toe is caused by degenerative arthritis at the first metatarsophalangeal joint. During walking, the big toe is unable to extend as the foot rolls forwards to toe-off (see gait cycle, Table 33.1). This is painful.

MANAGEMENT

Non-operative

A rocker-bottom sole on the shoe allows the foot to roll forward more easily during walking. This is often cosmetically unacceptable and so is of use only in those unable to undergo an operation.

Surgical

A dorsal cheilectomy is performed. This operation involves excision of the dorsal osteophytes and so allows a greater range of extension. A Keller's excisional arthroplasty or a Silastic joint replacement or a formal joint fusion can also be done.

Metatarsalgia

In this condition, the distal foot is painful. The source of the pain is high pressure on the metatarsal heads as the patient walks. It is often associated with claw toes (see below), and as a result, instead of the toes sharing in weight-bearing, all the weight is taken on the metatarsal heads. It can also occur when the foot has a high longitudinal arch (pes cavus) for either unknown reasons or in neuromuscular conditions such as cerebral palsy, spina bifida or Friedreich's ataxia.

Morton's metatarsalgia is a specific condition in which there is an interdigital neuroma between the metatarsal heads. This is then irritated by the adjacent bones, so resulting in pain and sensory disturbance at the corresponding cleft.

MANAGEMENT

Non-operative

A padded metatarsal bar fitted into the shoes helps to spread the load across the foot. Surgical shoes may also be required to accommodate the foot comfortably.

Surgical

An oblique osteotomy of the metatarsal necks allows the heads of the metatarsals to ride up. It is important to divide the second, third and fourth metatarsals because operating on one alone is not sufficient. In Morton's metatarsalgia, the affected space is explored and the neuroma excised. After operation, sensation is absent in the cleft.

Claw toes

Toes hyperextended at the metatarsophalangeal joints and flexed at the interphalangeal joints are clawed and do not touch the ground. As a result, they rub on the shoes and callosities develop over the proximal interphalangeal joints. There is also a tendency to develop an associated metatarsalgia. The cause is usually unknown but claw toes are seen in neuromuscular disorders such as spina bifida.

MANAGEMENT

Non-operative
Local measures such as felt pads and attention to footwear may be sufficient.

Surgical
Fusion of the proximal interphalangeal joint allows the toe to straighten. This is usually done by excising the joint and then using a small wire to hold the toe straight for 6 weeks until the bone ends unite. A single, grossly deformed toe should be amputated.

Plantar fasciitis

This is a painful condition of the heel caused by a localised area of inflammation of the plantar fascia at its origin from the os calcis. It is sometimes precipitated by local trauma or excessive weight-bearing.

CLINICAL FEATURES
A relevant history of focal trauma may be obtained. Otherwise, the only complaint is of well-localised pain in the heel on weight-bearing.

There is tenderness over the most prominent point of the calcaneus in the sole of the foot.

INVESTIGATION AND MANAGEMENT
Plain X-ray may show a spur on the plantar aspect of the os calcis.

Non-operative management measures are best – a foam heel wedge or local steroid injection. Surgery to release the plantar fascia is occasionally required.

Achilles tendinitis

This is a similar condition to plantar fasciitis in which there is an area of local inflammation at the insertion of the Achilles tendon. It may be precipitated by local trauma or a new pair of shoes that rub on the heel. Treatment consists of a heel wedge to reduce the tension in the tendon and a local steroid injection to the tendon sheath. Surgery is occasionally required to incise the inflamed tendon sheath.

Freiberg's disease

This condition is of an unknown cause in which there is fragmentation and collapse of the second metatarsal head. It occurs in young adults and there may be a history of local trauma. The enlarged metatarsal head produces local pressure symptoms and metatarsalgia. Treatment is conservative with felt pads to relieve pressure. Surgery is occasionally done to reduce the size of the metatarsal head.

Gout

This is a medical condition which does not usually concern the orthopaedic surgeon, but patients may present initially to the A&E department or the orthopaedic clinic. The metatarsophalangeal joint is red, hot, swollen and extremely painful. There may be a precipitating history of minor trauma to the big toe, dietary excess, recent surgery or the use of drugs such as a thiazide diuretic. In the acute stage, the treatment is with NSAIDs. Prophylaxis with allopurinol may prevent recurrent attacks and should be undertaken if these are frequent.

Paediatric orthopaedics

The hip

Problems with the hip are common. Patients present with a limp and pain which may be felt in the knee alone and any child with knee pain must have his or her hip examined. Whilst trauma and infection can occur at any age, other conditions tend to occur within particular age brackets (Table 33.9).

Developmental dysplasia of the hip

The hip is unstable at birth either because of ligamentous laxity or because of dislocation out of an undeveloped (dysplastic) acetabular socket.

EPIDEMIOLOGY
The incidence is 15/1000 at birth but falls to 1.5/1000 at 6 weeks. The left side is affected in 60%, the right in 20% and the condition is bilateral in 20%.

Table 33.9
Age ranges for paediatric orthopaedic conditions

Age	Condition
0–5 years	Congenital dislocation of the hip
5–10 years	Perthe's disease
10–15 years	Slipped upper femoral epiphysis

AETIOLOGY

Genetic

There may be a family history:

- affected sibling – 6% chance
- affected mother – 12% chance
- affected sibling and mother – 35% chance.

Sex

It is more common in girls than in boys in a ratio of 9:1. This is probably because the girl fetus is more sensitive to the maternal hormone relaxin secreted during pregnancy.

Perinatal

Associated factors are:

- first birth
- an extended breech presentation
- coexistent talipes (see below)
- any other congenital anomaly
- oligohydramnios.

Postnatal

Wrapping the infant in extension and adduction can cause hip dislocation.

CLINICAL FEATURES

History

Often the condition is diagnosed at birth, as part of the routine postnatal check. Occasionally, the parents may notice asymmetry of the skin creases. In older children there is a history of abnormal gait (Information Box 33.2).

Physical findings

- *Look*:
  - at the skin creases – there may be asymmetry of the gluteal creases but not if the condition is bilateral

---

Box 33.2

Special tests for developmental dysplasia of the hip

Barlow's test

With the hips adducted and flexed to 90°, gentle pressure is applied along the femoral shaft to dislocate the head posteriorly.

Ortolani's test

The femoral head is dislocated as for Barlow's test. The hips are then abducted and the head is felt to relocate with a 'clunk'.

  - for limited abduction in flexion
  - at the gait of an older child – it is a characteristic Trendelenburg gait.
- *Feel and move* – the head may dislocate and relocate when Ortolani's or Barlow's tests are performed (Box 33.2); they must be done gently and not repeated, because avascular necrosis of the femoral head may result.

INVESTIGATION

Plain X-ray. Up to 15 signs can be identified on a plain X-ray of the pelvis. The common ones are shown in Figure 33.10. The ossification centre of the femoral head does not appear until the age of five months. For the acetabulum to develop normally, the femoral head must be within it. If not, it remains shallow with a large acetabular angle.

Ultrasound. In experienced hands as well as being diagnostic, it is a useful screening technique.

Arthrography is required only for planning surgical correction in the older child.

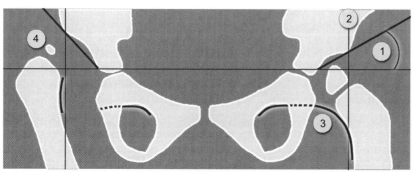

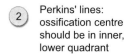

1. Acetabular angle: should be <30°
2. Perkins' lines: ossification centre should be in inner, lower quadrant
3. Shentons line: broken on dislocated side
4. Ossification centre: smaller on dislocated side

DDH   Normal

Fig 33.10 **Common radiological features of the dislocated hip.**

MANAGEMENT

The final result depends to a great extent on the age at which the diagnosis is made and treatment begun. If this is at birth, the developed hip is normal. The aim of treatment is to achieve a complete and stable reduction. Patients who are missed at birth may present late – up to the age of 3 or 4 years – and in these circumstances the outlook for good function is poor and treatment difficult.

Birth to 6 months

A splint is used to hold the hip joint in about 60° of abduction and 90° of flexion. A variety are available but the common types used are the Pavlik harness and the von Rosen splint. They are worn all the time until the acetabulum is seen to be developing normally.

Six months to walking

At this age, the hip is dislocated. Gentle traction is applied over a few weeks with progressive abduction (an adductor tenotomy may be required). The hip is then assessed under a general anaesthetic. If it is stable, a plaster of Paris hip spica is applied. If unstable or still dislocated, then an arthrogram is done which may show an inverted, thickened and folded acetabular labrum (limbus). This requires surgical removal to permit reduction.

The older child

An open operation is required to remove the limbus which is in the way of reduction of the femoral head into its socket. At a later stage, femoral osteotomy may also be required. Over 7 years of age, there is a case for non-operative management and, when secondary osteoarthritis develops in adult life, a total hip replacement.

Perthe's disease

There is, in this condition, a variable degree of avascular necrosis of the femoral head.

AETIOLOGY AND PATHOLOGICAL FEATURES

The cause is essentially unknown. An effusion forms, perhaps as a result of minor trauma or a viral infection. Pressure within the joint rises and impairs venous return from the femoral head which then undergoes avascular necrosis. The incidence is 1:9000 and the condition occurs four times more frequently in boys than in girls. It is bilateral in 10%.

The degree of collapse of the femoral head and the subsequent secondary arthritis is such that, by the age of 45, nearly half require a hip replacement, and by 65, secondary osteoarthritis is evident in 86%.

CLINICAL FEATURES

The age of onset is between 5 and 10 years with a limp and a complaint of a dull ache. There are few signs, but abduction in flexion is reduced.

INVESTIGATION

Imaging

Plain X-ray. An effusion may be seen. As the condition progresses, the femoral head becomes increasingly sclerotic and fragmented. Collapse of the head is associated with lateral subluxation.

Bone scan is rarely required but, if undertaken, shows an area of reduced uptake that corresponds to the femoral head.

Blood examination

Standard tests are normal, but very rarely an acute lymphoblastic leukaemia may present with features which resemble the irritable hip of Perthe's disease.

MANAGEMENT

Non-operative

Weight-bearing should be avoided while there is pain. The child should rest the hip whilst it is painful. A conservative approach can be employed if the progression of the disease is slow with limited involvement of the femoral head.

Surgical

If the femoral head subluxes laterally, surgery is aimed at containing it within the acetabulum. This can be achieved by wide abduction of the hip in a hip spica, or a femoral osteotomy to bring the head back into the acetabulum.

Slipped upper femoral epiphysis

The upper femoral epiphysis can sometimes slip on the adjacent cartilaginous growth plate (physis). The epiphysis then slides off posteriorly.

EPIDEMIOLOGY

The incidence varies with race. In Caucasians it is 2 in 100 000, but in Afro-Caribbeans it is 7 in 100 000. Boys are affected twice as often as girls. The age of onset is between 10 and 15 years and is younger in girls (12 years) than in boys (14 years). The condition is slightly more common on the left side and is bilateral at presentation in 10%. If one side slips, there is a 25% chance that the other side will follow.

AETIOLOGY

Trauma

There may be an acute slip after injury to the hip.

Hormonal

A relative deficiency of sex hormones which play a part

in the ossification of cartilage is thought to be a factor in the development of a chronic slip. As growth progresses, the cartilaginous plate is then unable to resist the increasing load placed upon it.

CLINICAL FEATURES

History

In 70%, the history is of chronic pain and a limp. In 30%, there is an acute slip with a correspondingly short history.

Physical findings

- *Look*:
  - the child is often fat and sexually underdeveloped
  - the hip is held in extension, external rotation and adduction.
- *Measure* – the leg is short by 1–2 cm.
- *Move*:
  - abduction in flexion is reduced – there may be fixed external rotation
  - possibly a Trendelenburg gait (Information Box 33.2).

INVESTIGATION

On an anteroposterior X-ray, the presence of a mild slip may be missed: look at Trethowan's line (Fig. 33.11). On a lateral film, however, the slip is easily seen. The amount is usually expressed as the percentage of the head uncovered on the lateral film.

MANAGEMENT

There is no place for conservative management. When there is a mild slip of up to 30%, the epiphysis should be pinned where it is without attempting reduction, because forcible manipulation may precipitate avascular necrosis. Greater than 30% displacement is managed by either of the following:

- open reduction and pinning – there is a 14% risk of avascular necrosis of the femoral head
- pinning without reduction and later femoral osteotomy to bring the epiphysis back into the correct position.

Late secondary osteoarthritis frequently occurs when there has been a slip of 50% or more.

It is generally accepted that if there is unreliable parental care or follow-up, consideration should be given to pinning the contralateral hip. However, a consensus on this is lacking.

Talipes

This term is applied to a congenital deformity of the foot. A more detailed classification follows below.

EPIDEMIOLOGY AND AETIOLOGY

The incidence is 2 in 1000 of live births in the UK. It is twice as common in boys as in girls and is bilateral in one-third.

In most instances, the condition is present at birth and it used to be thought that the intrauterine position might be causative. However, deformities from this cause rapidly recover after birth. Other causes are neuromuscular, e.g. spina bifida, polio and arthrogryposis – the last is a joint malformation of unknown but possible neurogenic cause.

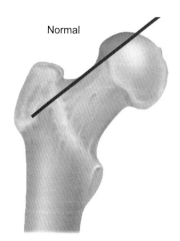
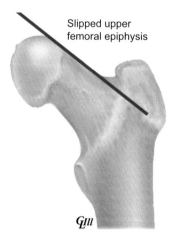

Fig 33.11 **Trethowan's line in slipped femoral epiphysis compared with normal.**

TYPES

The disorder is classified by the direction in which the heel points and the deviation of the forefoot. A foot that points down is said to be in equinus and one that points up in calcaneus. The forefoot may be in either varus or valgus.

The types in order of frequency are then:

- equinovarus – most common
- calcaneovalgus – second most common; may be associated with congenital dislocation of the hip
- equinovalgus – rare
- Calcaneovarus – rare.

CLINICAL FEATURES

The deformity is usually noticed at routine postnatal examination or by the parents within a few days or weeks of birth.

Physical findings are of uncorrectable deformity in one of the directions described above

MANAGEMENT

Non-operative

The initial treatment is to stretch the foot and strap it daily in a neutral or in a slightly more opposite position to the deformity present. This is continued for 6 weeks. At this time, if the deformity has been corrected, then strapping and, later, special shoes are continued until growth is complete.

Surgical

If at 6 weeks the deformity has not been corrected, then in the common equinovarus forms the Achilles tendon is lengthened, combined with a release of the soft tissue on the medial side. Any later relapses are managed by further soft tissue releases. After the age of 5, continued deformity requires surgery to the bone and is a specialised subject.

Minor leg deformities

Knock-knees, bow-legs and an in-toeing gait are all common and a source of much parental anxiety.

Knock-knee and bow-leg

In babies and toddlers, there is physiological bowing that corrects at 2–3 years of age. Later, at 4 or 5, there may be knock-knee of unknown cause. All but 2% of these correct spontaneously.

In a few children there is an underlying cause. Rickets is rare in the UK (but not unknown in some dark-skinned ethnic groups accustomed to more sunlight than they get in Britain). However, worldwide it is a common cause. Osteochondrosis deformans is a rare epiphyseal dysplasia which is associated with knock-knee.

In-toeing

This is the consequence of torsional deformity of either the tibia or the femur. Children then have a tendency to trip over their own feet. Treatment is not required until at least 6 or 7 years because almost all will correct spontaneously. If correction is required, then the affected long bone is derotated by an osteotomy.

Principles of management of fractures, joint injuries and peripheral nerve injuries

Surgeons tend to forget that they are not masters but only servants. They can assist the natural powers within all living flesh but cannot replace them.

(John Hunter)

Fractures

A fracture is a break in the continuity of a bone, ranging from an incomplete hairline crack to a complete break with many fragments. The majority of fractures are the result of violence, but if the bone is weakened by disease it may appear to break spontaneously, although this is usually as a result of minor injury (pathological fracture, see below).

CLASSIFICATION

The shape of the surfaces that result from fracture are the outcome of the extent and direction of the damaging forces applied. Their careful study allows these forces to be reversed at the time of reduction and also indicates the extent of soft tissue damage. In consequence, it is necessary to have some idea of the types of surfaces produced (Fig. 34.1).

Transverse

These are caused by direct (local) violence and are accompanied by local tissue damage.

Oblique and spiral

A twisting force (torque) applied at a distance is responsible for this type of fracture. Soft tissue damage at a site away from the fracture may be evident.

Greenstick

The bones of children are more yielding because they contain more connective tissue matrix and less mineral than do those of adults. The resulting greenstick fracture is an incomplete break.

Crush

Direct compression of cancellous bone may cause its trabeculae to collapse so that there is a crush fracture. Common sites include the os calcis and the vertebral bodies.

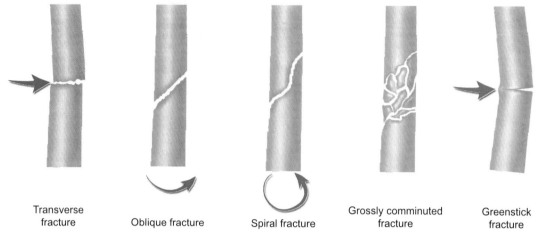

Transverse fracture

Oblique fracture

Spiral fracture

Grossly comminuted fracture

Greenstick fracture

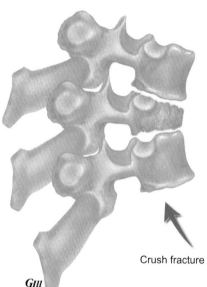

Crush fracture

G^{III}

Fig 34.1 **Types of fracture and surfaces produced.**

by disease. Often, it gives way after a trivial application of force such as might be encountered in normal

Table 34.1
Classification of open (compound) fractures. (After Gustilo & Anderson)

Type	Surface wound	Associations	Risk of infection (%)
I	1 cm or less	Low velocity Minimal soft tissue damage	0–2%
II	Greater than 1 cm	Low velocity Minimal soft tissue damage	0–10%
III*	Any size	High velocity or severe soft tissue injury Gross contamination as in military or agricultural injuries	Greater than 10%

* Type III injuries are further subdivided for treatment into:

IIIA – adequate cover of exposed bone still possible
IIIB – wide periosteal stripping with possible devascularisation of bone
IIIC – vascular (usually arterial) injury which requires repair.

Table 34.2
Causes of pathological fracture

Class	Example
Congenital	Osteogenesis imperfecta
Infection	Chronic osteomyelitis
Metabolic	Osteomalacia Hyperparathyroidism Osteoporosis
Benign neoplasms	Bone cyst Enchondroma
Malignant neoplasms	Primary bone tumours (rare) Metastatic carcinoma (common are breast, kidney, prostate, thyroid, lung)
Other	Paget's disease of bone

Comminuted

In this type of fracture, there are more than two fragments. Gross comminution occurs as a result of severe violence; significant soft tissue injury is usual.

Closed and open

A closed (syn. simple) fracture is not in contact with the exterior. By contrast, in an open (syn. compound) fracture, there is a communication between the site of fracture and the surface of the body. Most often this is through a wound of the skin and subcutaneous tissues but it can also take place (e.g. in the skull) through a mucous membrane.

Open fractures are classified as shown in Table 34.1.

Pathological

In a pathological fracture, the bone is weakened

activity. The common underlying causes are given in Table 34.2.

FRACTURE HEALING

Nearly all fractures can and will heal without surgical intervention at the site of the break. However, the surgeon harnesses the ability of the body for repair and this requires a thorough knowledge of the mechanisms and course of fracture union. As with healing of a soft tissue wound (Ch. 2), different stages in healing can be identified, but these form a continuum and blend into one another to varying degrees in different bones and in different circumstances. They are summarised in Figure 34.2.

Haematoma formation

A fracture tears blood vessels in the surrounding soft tissue, periosteum and medulla. A haematoma forms around and between the ends of the bone. Osteocytes in the fractured ends are deprived of nutrition and local cell death occurs. If a fragment of bone becomes completely detached from its blood supply, it undergoes avascular necrosis.

Cellular proliferation and organisation (inflammatory phase)

The next stage is similar to that in healing soft tissues (see Ch. 2) – an acute inflammatory reaction with vasodilatation, plasma exudation and inward migration of acute inflammatory cells. The haematoma is organised by granulation tissue with slender capillary loops in a loose connective tissue.

Formation of callus

Specialised cells from three sources invade the granulation tissue:

- capillary endothelium
- damaged endosteum and periosteum
- the systemic circulation, which supplies cells of unknown origin capable of differentiating into bone-forming cells.

The cells are stimulated to produce a randomly organised mass of fibrous tissue, cartilage and immature (woven) bone which provides an enveloping scaffolding of callus, usually visible radiologically from about 2 weeks in a child and 3 weeks in an adult. This initial phase of reformation of bone requires a small amount of movement: completely rigid fixation of the fracture eliminates it.

Randomly organised callus is at first weak and flexible so that stressing the fracture at this stage is associated with some movement and pain. Callus is progressively replaced – from 3 weeks onwards in a

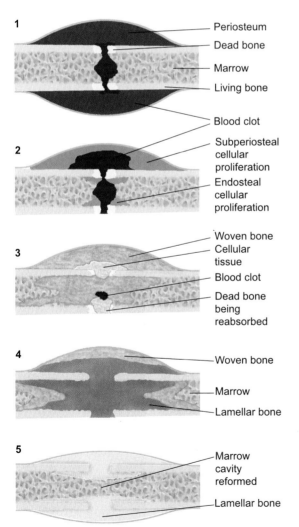

1
— Periosteum
— Dead bone
— Marrow
— Living bone
— Blood clot

2
— Subperiosteal cellular proliferation
— Endosteal cellular proliferation

3
— Woven bone
— Cellular tissue
— Blood clot
— Dead bone being reabsorbed

4
— Woven bone
— Marrow
— Lamellar bone

5
— Marrow cavity reformed
— Lamellar bone

Fig 34.2 **Stages of fracture healing.**

Box 34.1

Assessment of union of a fracture

Clinical

Absence of tenderness on direct pressure over the fracture site

Little or no pain when the fracture site is stressed by angulation or rotation

Absence of movement at the fracture site

Radiological

No evidence of a gap at the fracture side and continuity of bone trabeculae across it

*Radiological evidence usually occurs a few weeks after clinical evidence.

child and 4 weeks onwards in an adult long bone – by mature (lamellar) bone with a Haversian structure strong enough to immobilise the fracture site and produce union. The practical assessment of union is summarised in Box 34.1.

When the fracture is regarded as having united, immobilisation – usually by external splints – should be discarded. As a general rule, external splintage needs to be maintained for 4–8 weeks for fractures in cancellous bones and 6–12 weeks for fractures in long bones in adults. Fractures in children heal in approximately half these times.

Consolidation and remodelling

In the months that follow, the new bone is reorganised so that its collagen fibres run in the lines of stress (Fig. 34.3). The bone now returns to its original strength and the fracture is said to be consolidated. In fractures that have been fixed rigidly, the time for consolidation is considerably increased.

For up to 2 years later, the fusiform mass of healing bone is gradually removed and the bone is further remodelled along its whole length in the lines of stress.

CLINICAL FEATURES

History

The history may throw light on the circumstances that led to the injury and the underlying causes. The following are of significance:

- A fall may have been caused by either an accidental loss of balance or by momentary unconsciousness from cardiac or neurological problems which may need to be treated.

- Fracture after trivial injury or stresses and strains which are within the normal range of physical exertion may indicate a pathological fracture.

- The way the injury was sustained should lead to a search for other skeletal injuries from the same cause; a fracture of the os calcis after a fall from a height may be accompanied by vertebral or hip injuries, and a knee injury in a front seat passenger who has been thrown forward in a head-on collision may be associated with a posterior dislocation of the hip.

- Time since injury should be ascertained as accurately as possible because of its association with complications such as infection in an open fracture or with ischaemia distal to a vascular injury.

Unless there is a neurological condition, a limb with a fracture is acutely painful and held as immobile as possible. However, there are circumstances in which a history cannot be obtained, such as unconsciousness or the overriding importance of other injuries; then the history of the injury obtained from others may be of importance.

Clinical findings

Swelling caused by haematoma formation and oedema is usually evident.

Deformity is seen in displaced fractures and is described anatomically as displacement of the distal fragment with respect to the proximal, e.g. anterior or posterior. Varus and valgus are terms also used, but in descriptions of fractures these are best avoided.

Abnormal mobility may be present but should be sought with gentleness.

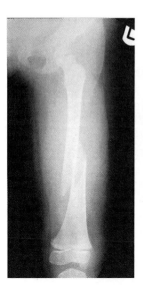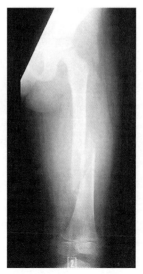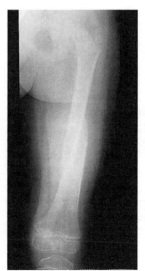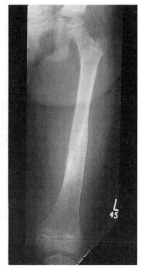

Fig 34.3 **Consolidation/remodelling of fracture site (left to right).**

Crepitus is the grating sensation elicited on palpation as the broken ends of bone grind against each other with movement; it must not be deliberately elicited as it causes intense pain.

Skin integrity must always be assessed: abrasions or mild ischaemia may lead to later breakdown and infection of the fracture.

Vascular perfusion and neurological function distal to the injury must be evaluated in all limb fractures. The presence of arterial pulses must be elicited and recorded. Sensation may be reduced in a glove and stocking manner in vascular insufficiency. Injury to peripheral nerves produces specific neurological deficiencies which must be tested for.

Pelvic fractures may be associated with bladder and urethral injuries and disruption of the muscles of the pelvic floor. Examination for such accompanying injuries is essential.

RADIOLOGICAL INVESTIGATION

If a fracture is suspected, radiographs in two planes at right angles to each other (usually anteroposterior and lateral views) are initially taken and should include the whole length of the fractured bone and the adjacent joints. Only in this way can the full extent of the injury and the associated bone injuries be detected (Fig. 34.4). In some circumstances, additional oblique or tangential views may be required. Computed tomography (CT) and magnetic resonance imaging (MRI) are valuable in the investigation of fractures of the pelvis and spine. Radioisotope bone scanning detects increased vascularity, which begins with the inflammatory phase of healing, and is useful in the early diagnosis of fractures that are not immediately obvious on radiography X-ray because of lack of displacement (e.g. fracture of the scaphoid).

PRINCIPLES OF MANAGEMENT

The management of a patient with a fracture can be summarised by the mnemonic FRIAR (see Box 34.2).

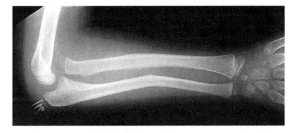

Fig 34.4 **Radiographic examination of a fracture.** The X-ray is of a fracture of the ulna accompanied by anterior dislocation of the radial head at the elbow joint (Monteggia fracture-dislocation). The dislocation would not have been detected without an X-ray that included the elbow joint.

> ### Box 34.2
>
> *Principles of fracture management: (FRIAR)*
>
> **F**irst aid and management of the whole patient – always
>
> **R**eduction – if necessary
>
> **I**mmobilisation – if necessary
>
> **A**ctive
>
> **R**ehabitation – always

First aid and management of the whole patient

Patients who have suffered violence sufficient to fracture part of their skeleton often have injuries to other systems, some which may be life-threatening. In the management of such multiply injured patients, priority should be given to the ABCs – **A**irway maintenance, **B**reathing and **C**irculation. The matter is considered in more detail in Chapter 3. Pain relief is also important and is discussed in Chapter 6.

Reduction

Reduction is manipulation of the fractured bone to restore normal anatomy. Some fractures do not require reduction either because deformity is not present or because its nature is immaterial to the final functional result (e.g. up to 50% displacement of a transverse fracture of the shaft of the tibia is acceptable).

Closed manipulation

This is the preferred initial method. It can be carried out under general anaesthesia, regional anaesthesia or, in some instances, after injection of anaesthetic into the fracture haematoma. Reduction is achieved by:

1. longitudinal traction which dis-impacts any interlocked fragments
2. reversal of the forces that caused deformity.

Reduction must be confirmed by radiography.

Mechanical traction

This method may be used to gradually reduce fractures of the spine or of the femur and also to hold the fracture in position while healing takes place.

Open reduction

Open reduction by operation is necessary when:

- closed reduction fails
- very accurate reduction is required, e.g. a fracture which involves a joint surface

- the fracture has caused a vascular or (sometimes) a nerve injury.

The fracture is manipulated under direct vision and then usually stabilised by internal fixation (see below).

Immobilisation

A fracture is held in reduction to:

- relieve pain
- prevent redisplacement or angulation of the fragments
- avoid shearing movements at the fracture site which damage the delicate capillaries in callus and consequently interfere with the process of union.

Immobilisation is not always necessary, e.g. in fractures of the ribs or metatarsals. In some other injuries, relatively rigid immobilisation is essential if union is to occur, e.g. the scaphoid or the shaft of the ulna.

The methods of immobilisation are summarised in Box 34.3.

External splints

Plaster of Paris (POP) or other casts are, in most circumstances, the standard method. POP is commercially available as bandages coated with hemihydrated calcium sulphate which reacts with water to form a solid cast. Newer synthetic resin materials are available which are stronger, lighter and impervious to water, but they are more expensive and more difficult to apply.

When applying an external cast, a layer of cellulose padding is placed deep to the cast to prevent the plaster from sticking to the hairs and skin and to allow for expansion from swelling at the fracture site. Initial immobilisation should not be by completely encircling the limb because continued swelling can lead to ischaemia distal to the fracture site – compartment syndrome. In consequence, plasters which surround the limb are applied either as a slab on one aspect only held in place by a crepe bandage or as a cylinder which is then immediately split longitudinally. Immobilisation of the adjacent joints above and below is usually necessary to stabilise a fracture managed in a cast but increases the risk of disuse muscle atrophy and joint stiffness.

Any form of immobilisation inevitably causes some muscle atrophy and joint stiffness. The splint must be discarded as soon as union of the fracture is deemed to have occurred. In some long bone fractures, a hinge may be inserted in the splint (functional bracing) as union progresses.

Continuous traction

This method is used when it is difficult to hold the bone reduced with an external splint because the fracture site is surrounded by soft tissue and/or bony points above and below which can be used to gain purchase are absent. Typical examples are fractures of the shaft of the femur and of the lower humerus. Traction of up to 2 kg may be applied with longitudinal adhesive strapping applied to the skin (skin traction) but a careful watch must be kept for damage, especially in the elderly and in patients on steroids. If more force is required, traction may be exerted through a pin inserted into the bone distal to the fracture site (skeletal traction). The pin site must be kept clean to prevent infection tracking down to the bone.

Continuous traction confines the patient to bed and thus increases the risk of pressure sores, chest infection, disuse osteoporosis, hypercalciuria and therefore renal stones. It is best used for the shortest possible period in the young and avoided in the elderly.

Internal fixation

Internal fixation by open operation is used to secure reduction, to ensure it is maintained or to allow earlier mobility of the patient (Fig. 34.5). The advantages of earlier return of function, shorter hospital stay and quicker resumption of work or of pre-injury style of life have to be weighed against the risks of neurovascular damage and of delaying healing by devascularisation of the bone fragments and the introduction of infection. Unless the surgical team is experienced, closed means are preferable for simple fractures. Internal fixation is strongly indicated in patients with:

- multiple injuries
- pathological fractures
- associated neurovascular injury
- fractures where accurate reduction is required (e.g. those involving joints)

Box 34.3

Methods of immobilisation of fractures

External splints
— plaster of Paris, synthetic resins
— specially designed splints

Continuous traction
— applied to the distal fragment usually by some form of skeletal pin but occasionally by adhesive tape applied to the skin

External fixation
— a rigid bridging device held in place by bone pins proximal and distal to the fracture

Internal fixation
— screws, plates and pins inserted at open operation

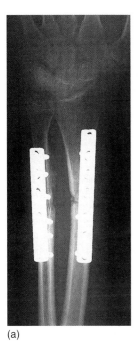
(a)

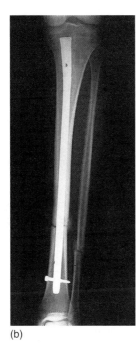
(b)

Fig 34.5 **Open reduction and fixation.** (a) The application of plates to the distal third of both radius and ulna. (b) Intra medullary fixation of a fracture of the distal third of the tibia.

● the need to avoid a long period of immobilisation in bed, e.g. an elderly patient with a fracture of the neck of the femur.

External fixation (Fig. 34.6)
This is mainly used in the management of open or infected fractures (see 'Open fractures,' below). Pins are inserted in the fragments of bone and fixed rigidly to an external device such as a metal bar. The skin overlying the fracture site can be dressed or grafted without disturbing the fracture.

Observation
In the early stages after reduction and immobilisation,

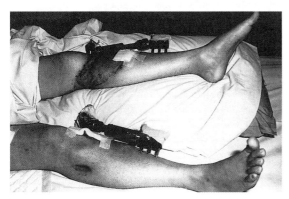

Fig 34.6 **External fixation and management of type III open fracture.**

careful and repeated observation is required to detect insufficient distal blood supply or a neurological injury. A tightly applied circular dressing which becomes soaked with blood and then dries may similarly impair the circulation (see also 'Compartment syndrome'. Suggestive features include:

● persistent or increasing pain
● paraesthesia or tingling in digits
● cyanosis distal to the fracture
● sluggish capillary return
● absent pulses.

Any of these requires removal of all dressings, external splints and casts so that the fracture site can be inspected and necessary remedial action undertaken.

Active rehabilitation
Rehabilitation starts immediately after treatment. The patient is asked to move the injured part as much as the method of fixation allows. The slight movement produced at the fracture site helps to:

● stimulate union
● decrease disuse osteoporosis
● prevent muscle atrophy
● minimise joint stiffness.

All external splints are removed as soon as there is clinical evidence of union and the patient is started on a supervised programme of active exercises to restore function.

Open fractures
The communication with the surface is a pathway along which bacteria can contaminate the fracture site and produce infection. Once bone is infected with pyogenic organisms, the inflammation tends to become chronic, especially if foreign material has been carried into the fracture site at the time of injury. Infection delays and may prevent union and, with some virulent infections such as clostridia (Ch. 9), may cause death. Open fractures are surgical emergencies.

For first aid in all open injuries of bone, the wound is covered with a sterile dressing soaked in normal saline or aqueous iodine. Parenteral broad-spectrum antibiotic therapy is begun at once and attention paid to tetanus prophylaxis.

In types I and II open fractures surgical debridement of the wound with removal of all devitalised tissue and foreign material as soon as possible is essential to prevent sepsis. If treatment on these lines is undertaken within 8 hours of injury, the incidence of sepsis is low. Therefore, internal fixation of type I and II open fractures may be done safely by experienced surgeons operating in ideal conditions. In type III fractures, external trauma causes extensive skin and muscle damage, often with associated injuries to vessels and nerves. The incidence of sepsis is high and internal fixation is usually avoided. After debridement of the wound, external fixation (Fig. 34.6) and repair of neuro-vascular structures is usually followed by many staged procedures to achieve skin cover. Full-thickness skin flaps are best. In the most severe of those injuries (a limb that has been avascular for more than 6 hours or one that has been severely crushed), an amputation both saves life and avoids a long period of invalidity which may have considerable psychological effects.

COMPLICATIONS

In the great majority of fractures, union proceeds according to expectation and function is fully restored. Complications do, however occur, and may be considered in two groups – early or delayed. In both, effects may be local or systemic (Box 34.4).

Infection

This can occur in open fractures or in closed fractures treated by operation.

Haemorrhage

Haemorrhage from the bone marrow, periosteum and surrounding soft tissues may not be immediately clinically obvious but can be considerable and cause reduction in blood volume. As a general rule, blood loss from adult fractures may be estimated as:

- pelvis: 2–3 L
- femur: 1–2 L
- tibia or humerus: 0.5–1 L.

Patients with open or pathological fractures bleed more profusely. Multiple fractures produce cumulative losses which, if unrecognised, are sufficient to cause hypovolaemic shock which is a possible but prevent-able cause of death.

Arterial and venous injury

This can occur in violent injury such as a gunshot wound or from a spike of bone (Fig. 34.7). All types of injury occur. Some bony injuries are commonly associated with vascular damage – supracondylar fractures of the humerus contuse the brachial artery and 50% of knee dislocations give rise to an intimal tear in the popliteal artery.

Distal ischaemia may lead to:

- nerve and muscle necrosis
- total limb death with gangrene, necessitating amputation.

The first line of treatment is to reposition the limb so as to correct gross deformity and remove all occlusive dressings. This may solve the problem but, if the signs of ischaemia do not disappear within 15 minutes, surgical intervention is necessary.

Deep venous thrombosis and pulmonary embolism

These are a common sequelae to many fractures, particularly in the elderly, and are discussed in Chapter 29.

Nerve damage

Nerve damage occurring immediately after fractures is relatively uncommon but, if unrecognised, may lead to

---

Box 34.4

Complications of fracture

Early

Local	*Systemic*
Infection	Hypovolaemic shock
Haemorrhage	Fat embolism
Injury to other structure – arteries, nerves and viscera	Effects of prolonged immobilisation – chest infection, pressure sores, pulmonary embolism
Skin necrosis	
Deep vein thrombosis	
Compartment syndrome	

Late (delayed)

Local	*Systemic*
Malunion	Osteoporosis
Delayed union	Changes in lifestyle and psychological state
Non-union	
Muscle wasting	
Joint stiffness	
Osteoarthritis	
Delayed tendon rupture	
Tardy nerve palsy	
Reflex sympathetic dystrophy	
Myositis ossificans	

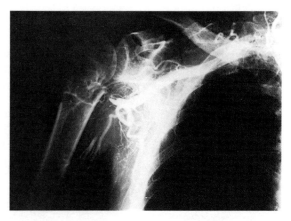

Fig 34.7 **Vascular injury as a consequence of fracture.** A fracture of the surgical neck of the humerus has produced a spike that has injured the distal axillary artery, occlusion of which is shown on the arteriogram.

Table 34.3
Nerve injuries frequently associated with fractures and dislocations

Fracture	Nerve injury
Dislocation of the shoulder	Axillary (5%)
	Other brachial plexus lesions
Shaft of humerus	Radial (10%)
Injuries around the elbow	Median
	Ulnar
Dislocation of the hip	Sciatic (10%)
Injuries around the knee	Common peroneal

permanent loss of function. The common associations are in Table 34.3.

Compartment syndrome

This condition arises because the muscles, vessels and nerves in limbs are held within inelastic osseofascial compartments. Bleeding from a fracture increases the intracompartmental pressure and occludes the venous outflow and hence capillary inflow. The cells first become hypoxic and then swell because of failure of their sodium–potassium pump. There is further rise in intracompartmental pressure and a vicious circle of hypoxia and further swelling ensues. The clinical features are summarised in Box 34.5. An intracompartmental pressure of 30 mmHg is sufficient to impede capillary

---

Box 34.5

Clinical features of compartment syndrome

Early symptoms

Increasing pain

Paraesthesia

Paresis

Early signs

Pain on passive stretching of the muscle groups in the compartment

Palpably tense compartment

Pulses usually normal because arteries traversing the compartment are resistant to a rise in pressure within it

Sluggish capillary filling

Late symptoms

Numbness

Paralysis

Late signs

Muscle contracture

Anaesthesia

Absence of arterial pulses

---

inflow and therefore distal arterial pulses may be present even if compartment syndrome is present.

Irreversible damage to nerves and muscles occurs within a matter of 4–6 hours. The skin overlying the compartment is unaffected but a disabling contracture of the damaged muscles (Volkmann's ischaemic contracture) may result.

Because of the risks of compartment syndrome, pain relief in fractures by the use of local nerve blocks is not recommended because this may mask its early features. Vigilance in detection and prompt treatment are both vital. When a compartment syndrome is suspected, any cast and all dressings are removed. If symptoms do not improve immediately, the compartment is surgically decompressed by division of the overlying skin and fascia (open fasciotomy).

Fat embolism

This is more common in patients with multiple fractures but may follow minor trauma. Its cause is poorly understood: either fat from the marrow of the fractured bone enters the circulation or some as yet unidentified factor causes chylomicrons in the bloodstream to aggregate. In either event, large fat globules are present in the bloodstream and clog capillaries – on the right side of the heart in the pulmonary circulation and, perhaps aided by a subclinical patent foramen ovale, on the arterial side in the brain and skin. Clinically, a few days after injury the patient becomes increasingly confused, develops tachypnoea and mild pyrexia. Skin petechiae may be seen and laboratory investigations usually reveal a reduced P_{O_2} and thrombocytopenia. Fat globules may be detected in the urine. Maintenance of oxygenation is of paramount importance and may require intubation and ventilatory support.

Pressure sores (decubitus ulcers)

Sores occurring as a result of necrosis of skin over the heel, sacrum, ischium and hips are a real risk in patients confined to bed because of skeletal injury (or for other reasons), especially in the debilitated, the elderly and those with spinal cord injury. Prevention is by good nursing care and early mobilisation.

Malunion

This follows imperfect reduction or redisplacement after satisfactory reduction and leads to cosmetic deformity and loss of function (Fig. 34.8). It is prevented by satisfactory primary management but, if established, may require complex corrective procedures.

Delayed union

Union is said to be delayed if the fracture has not united clinically or radiologically at a time when this would have been expected. The fracture may still continue to

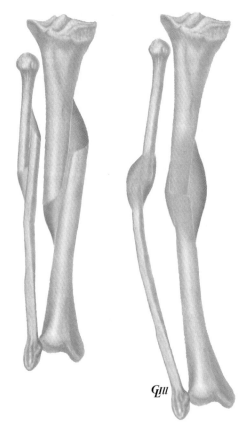

Fig 34.8 **Malunion.**

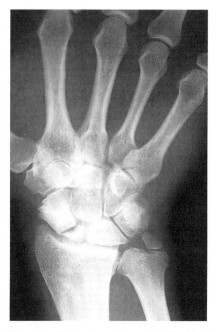

Fig 34.9 **Non-union.** This fracture of the scaphoid has failed to unite. There is a radiological gap between the fragments which can be assumed to be filled with fibrous tissue. There is some, although not much, evidence of sclerosis.

heal slowly until it unites and, provided there are not any adverse factors which require correction, a watching policy is adopted while making sure that optimum conditions for continued healing are present.

Non-union

This is diagnosed when healing has come to a halt before union has occurred (Fig. 34.9). The fracture is now bridged only by fibrous tissue and radiologically the bone ends show signs of reduced vascularity (increased radiodensity – sclerosis) and the medullary cavity may be obliterated. The borderline between delayed union and non-union is difficult to define, although the differentiation may be important for both the patient and the surgeon. Causes of delayed union and non-union are summarised in Box 34.6.

Management is complex: usually a direct operation on the fracture site is indicated with removal of sclerotic bone to increase the blood supply, bone grafting and rigid fixation.

Reflex sympathetic dystrophy (Sudecks's atrophy)

This condition presents after some months as:

- pain
- abnormal sensations (dysaesthesia)

Box 34.6

Causes of delayed union and non-union

- Infection
- Inadequate blood supply to one or both fragments
- Excessive movements at fracture site
- Interposition of soft tissues between the fragments
- Loss of apposition between fragments
- Destruction of bone by another pathological process

- joint stiffness
- thickening of the soft tissues
- abnormal sweating
- loss of hair at the site of injury.

The cause is not known but sympathetic C nerve fibres are said to be overactive. Early active exercises reduce the occurrence of this disorder and are used in its treatment. Guanethidine nerve blocks may speed up recovery by depleting the stores of neurotransmitters.

Myositis ossificans

This is heterotopic bone in the muscles around the fracture. Movement is restricted. The most common site is the elbow and the cause is possibly too early and too vigorous joint movement.

Fractures which involve articular surfaces

If accurate reduction to obtain congruent surfaces is not achieved and maintained, secondary osteoarthritis can develop. Open reduction and internal rigid fixation are thus indicated. Early joint movement should be encouraged to reduce stiffness and (possibly) to promote the healing of articular cartilage.

Fractures in children

The bones of children are more flexible and incomplete fractures of the greenstick type (Fig. 34.1) are common. Turnover of bone is more active in children so that union occurs in approximately half the time taken in adult fractures.

Remodelling in the plane of movement of the joints after a shaft fracture is usually so perfect that eventually the site is indistinguishable in radiographs (Fig. 34.3). Therefore reduction of shaft fractures need not be as accurate as in the adult. However, remodelling is incomplete in mediolateral or lateromedial (varus/valgus) deformities of the elbow and in rotational deformities of the forearm, and accurate reduction should be sought.

Epiphyseal displacement

The growth plate between the epiphysis and metaphysis provides a relatively weak area which is often involved when forces are concentrated near the ends of the bone. Damage to the growth plate may result in arrest of growth and subsequent deformity. Accurate reduction is necessary.

Non-accidental injury (battering)

This condition is part of child abuse and regrettably common. Suspicious features include a delay to take the child to hospital, inadequate or inappropriate explanation of the injury, multiple soft tissue bruises, burns and radiological evidence of previous injuries. A paediatrician should be involved from the outset.

Joint injuries

In *dislocation (luxation)* there is complete loss of contact of the articular joint surfaces (Fig. 34.10), and in *subluxation* there is partial loss of contact. Either may be combined with a fracture.

The clinical features are the same as those of a fracture, i.e.

- pain
- deformity
- loss of function.

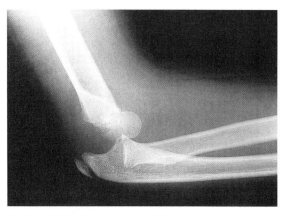

Fig 34.10 **Dislocation of the elbow.** There is complete loss of joint apposition.

The diagnosis is confirmed by radiographs in two planes. The integrity of the surrounding nerves and vessels must be assessed clinically because of the relatively high incidence of associated damage. In addition, time factors are important: the risk of avascular necrosis of the femoral head after a traumatic posterior dislocation of the hip is directly proportional to the time interval between dislocation and reduction. Dislocations are therefore surgical emergencies. Treatment is usually by closed reduction; open reduction is rarely required.

Spinal injuries

Damage to the bony and ligamentous structures of the vertebral column as well as to the enclosed neural elements may occur. It is important to prevent further injury, particularly to the cord, from movement during management. For this purpose, spinal injuries are classified into two types:

- *stable* – the vertebral components will not be displaced by normal movements; an undamaged cord is not in danger
- *unstable* – further displacement and damage may result from movement.

Bony injury to the spine is of the following types:

- Flexion injury produces a crush fracture of the vertebral body which is usually stable.
- If shearing forces are added to flexion, a fracture-dislocation with variable damage to the interarticular facets can occur and may be either stable or unstable. If unstable, injury to the spinal cord and its nerve roots may be primary or take place secondarily because of movement during initial or subsequent management.

- Cord injury without either fracture or dislocation may occur in the more elastic tissues of children or in the spondylitic spine of the elderly.

CLINICAL FEATURES

History

Suspicion of instability of the spine may be aroused from the history of injury and, in a conscious patient, by complaints of pain, decreased muscle power and/or sensation and paraesthesias. An unconscious accident victim should always be assumed to have a spinal injury until proven otherwise.

Physical findings

Injuries to the neurological elements may be complete or incomplete; accurate neurological diagnosis is essential because recovery is more likely if some residual sensation or movement is detectable in the affected area.

Complete neurological injury

Complete neurological injury, such as a transection of the cord, causes complete permanent motor paralysis below the level of injury with corresponding loss of sensation.

Injuries to the lumbar vertebrae which involve only the cauda equina and nerve roots produce:

- flaccid paralysis and eventual wasting of the leg muscles
- loss of sensation in the lower limbs
- variable effects on the bowel and bladder, including loss of reflexes which initiate micturition and defaecation tone.

Complete lesions in the thoracic region result in paraplegia (spastic paralysis of the legs) with:

- reflex spasms
- loss of sensation distal to the lesion
- no voluntary control of bladder, bowel and sexual function, although ultimately automatic function is established.

Injuries to the cervical regions lead to quadriplegia with:

- partial or complete involvement of the arms and hands
- similar effects on organ function to paraplegia.

High cervical lesions lead to:

- phrenic nerve paralysis associated with respiratory failure which may cause immediate or later death
- loss of the potential for an independent life.

Incomplete lesions

These may be the consequence of:

- partial transection
- oedema and bleeding in relation to a spinal fracture or fracture-dislocation.

It is obviously of great importance to recognise that a lesion is incomplete in that efforts to prevent further injury must be rigorous. Although the neurological patterns may be complex, the preservation of any function distal to the established site of injury is an important initial finding; every care must be taken to preserve it. More detailed neurological analysis can follow later.

INVESTIGATION

Accurate imaging is essential. A frequent mistake is not to image the C7/T1 junction clearly – a common site for injury between the mobile cervical and the more fixed thoracic vertebrae and also a difficult area of which to make clear X-rays. The whole spine from the cranio-cervical junction to the lumbosacral articulation should be examined radiologically as other separate fractures occur in 7% of those with one injury. CT scanning demonstrates the extent of injury to the neural arch and the amount of bony neural canal impingement. MRI (Fig. 34.11) outlines the extent of spinal cord compression by bone or intervertebral disc and the type of injury that the cord has sustained such as oedema or haemorrhage.

MANAGEMENT

Management must start at the scene of the accident and may make the difference between recovery or lifelong paralysis. Paramedical staff are trained to apply supportive neck collars and to move patients only in a way that does not threaten further damage. The same must be the case for the surgical team.

Spinal shock

Immediately after a severe spinal injury, a transient depression of all reflex activity is superimposed on either temporary or permanent local neural damage. There is a flacid paralysis of all the distally supplied

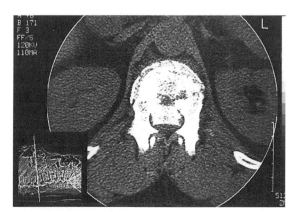

Fig 34.11 **MRI of spinal cord compression.** The image is viewed from below and the posterior aspect of the spine is below. There is a filling defect which is compressing the spinal cord by about a third.

muscles and arterial hypotension caused by vaso-dilatation below the level of injury. Recovery form spinal shock may take a few days to up to 6 weeks and is first evident by return of reflexes, e.g. contraction of the external anal sphincter on stimulation of the perianal skin. Its immediate clinical importance is that the low blood pressure may be confused with hypovolaemia and make evaluation of other injuries and their priority difficult.

Concomitant injuries

Management of other life-threatening conditions, such as head, chest or abdominal trauma, must take precedence over the definitive management of the spinal injury. Reduction of displaced vertebrae is necessary to achieve bony alignment and decrease the distortion of the neural elements and their blood supply and can be achieved either by traction or by operation. Patients with incomplete lesions of the cord and fractures where the bone segments, vertebral disc or a haematoma within the vertebral canal narrow it by more than 50% do better if the canal is surgically decompressed early; the potential for recovery is significant.

General management

Skin

Rigorous attention must be given to the skin that is anaesthetic in an immobile limb. Alteration of position every 2 hours, cleanliness and avoidance of minor trauma are the best ways of avoiding pressure sores.

Bladder

Initially in spinal shock there is acute retention and this should be relieved as soon as possible. Later, bladder 'training' is by intermittent catheterisation which ultimately results in micturition which can be predicted on the basis of time. A few patients may need a permanent indwelling urethral catheter.

Bowel

Attention to diet and the use of aperients are started as early as possible.

Joint contractures

These must be prevented by regular physiotherapy and spasms can be controlled by skeletal muscle relaxants such as baclofen.

Mobilisation and fixation

If the middle and posterior bony and ligamentous supporting complex is intact, the injury is stable and early mobilisation with appropriate supports and braces is undertaken. Those with unstable injuries can be treated either by 6–12 weeks' bed rest or by rigid fixation of the fracture to facilitate nursing and allow earlier rehabilitation.

Rehabilitation

Return of the patient into society is best carried out by a multidisciplinary team working in a spinal injuries unit and it is now feasible for most patients to achieve an independent and fulfilling life.

Peripheral nerve injuries

Transection of a major nerve trunk causes severe disability from paralysis, loss of sensation and sometimes pain. If untreated, atrophy and deformity of the injured part follow.

PATHOLOGICAL FEATURES

The axons of peripheral nerves are cytoplasmic extensions of cell bodies located in the dorsal root ganglia (sensory) or the ventral horn of the spinal cord (motor). They are composed of axoplasm surrounded by a cell membrane. The axons are themselves enclosed in the sheath formed by Schwann cells and may or may not contain myelin.

Types of injury

Neurotmesis

This is division of a nerve trunk and it causes well-defined changes both proximally and distally. Proximally, the axons die back for a distance of about 2 cm and the cell body enlarges with increase in RNA and protein. Sprouting of the divided axon at the division may be evident within a day. Distally, Wallerian degeneration occurs with lysis of axoplasm and fragmentation of myelin sheaths. If the ends of the nerve are apposed, regenerating axons grow into the empty Schwann cell sheath at the rate of 1 mm/day. However, haphazard matching of axonal sprouts with distal sensory receptors and motor units is inevitable. Recovery is therefore always incomplete. If the nerve ends are not in contact, the regenerating axons mingle with proliferating Schwann cells and fibroblasts to form a tangled mass – a neuroma – which may be painful.

When the orderly sequence of regrowth into the distal stump is not achieved, with the passage of time, the activity of the sprouting neurones diminishes, the distal endoneural tubes narrow and the brain forgets how to use the limb. The diagnosis and repair of nerve injuries are, consequently, a matter of urgency.

Axonotmesis

In this type of injury there is damage to axons but the Schwann cell sheath remains intact. It may for example, occur from traction on a nerve. Because the axon is disrupted, Wallerian degeneration occurs, but the potential for recovery is greater than in neurotmesis, as the sprouting neurones do not have to bridge a gap in their sheaths. If the cause is removed, good recovery takes place with time and nerve repair is not required.

Neurapraxia
In this type of injury, there is a physiological block to conduction but the axon is in anatomical continuity. A contusion is one cause – striking the ulna nerve behind the medial epicondyle to cause the well-known funny elbow is a good example. Function is temporarily absent but Wallerian degeneration does not take place and, if the cause is removed, recovery is rapid.

The classification given above into neurotmesis, axonotmesis and neurapraxia (described by Seddon) is useful but it is important to realise that demarcation between different types is not always clear-cut in the individual case.

CLINICAL FEATURES
Early recognition and prompt management of a nerve injury give the patient the best chance of restoring function.

History
After a fracture or dislocation, or any penetrating injury that might conceivably have passed close to a nerve, the history should include specific questions about distal anaesthesia or loss of motor function, because these may not be appreciated by the patient who is more concerned with the bony or soft tissue injury.

Physical findings
A neurological examination for function of the nerves in the vicinity of all fractures, dislocations and lacerations must be done. The commonest reason for failing to detect a nerve injury is failure to suspect one and make a complete assessment. The critical step is to distinguish between non-degenerative and degenerative lesions.

Non-degenerative lesions
These are the result of neurapraxia. Some sensation, e.g. for deep pressure, usually persists. Autonomic function – vasomotor and sudomotor control – is also usually intact. The nerve trunk distal to the injury continues to conduct because the axons beyond the injury are still nourished and this can be established by electrodiagnostic testing.

Degenerative lesions
These follow axonotmesis or neurotmesis and cause a complete loss of all nerve function, including vasomotor and sudomotor control. In consequence, the skin innervated by the damaged nerve is red and dry. The nerve trunk distal to the injury conducts impulses only for the first 3 weeks until Wallerian degeneration has occurred.

The difficulty lies in distinguishing between axonotmesis and neurotmesis. Only time or exposure of the nerve will ultimately be diagnostic. Where a fracture or dislocation has been caused by more than a moderate degree of violence and where there has been wide displacement of the skeletal fragments, then absence of function is assumed to be from rupture of the relevant nerve trunk. Similarly, where a laceration is present over the nerve or a surgeon has been operating in the vicinity, loss of function must be assumed to be from division.

MANAGEMENT
It is better to explore too soon (even if the nerve is found to be intact) than too late. However, life-threatening injuries to the head, chest and abdomen take priority over nerve repair.

Nerve repair
The ideal nerve repair should be performed as a primary procedure in an uncontaminated wound by an experienced surgeon and in an operating room with high quality equipment and lighting. In contaminated wounds, repair is postponed for 3–4 weeks until either the wound is healed or infection has been controlled.

Primary repair is the suture of nerve stumps before a neuroma has had time to form, usually up to 2 weeks after the injury. It gives the best results.

Secondary repair is the later suture of nerve stumps in which a neuroma has formed and requires resection. It is done after any initial wound has healed and oedema and joint stiffness have resolved.

Nerve grafting is required when nerve tissue has been destroyed over a distance that makes direct repair impossible without tension. Nerves commonly used are the sural and the medial cutaneous nerve of the forearm which can be autotransplanted without significant loss of sensation.

Nerve transfer is sometimes indicated. For example, intercostal nerves may be transferred into the stump of an irreparably damaged musculocutaneous nerve and the body learns to use this pathway.

Assessment of recovery
'Tinel's sign' is valuable in the clinical detection of progress. Percussion along the course of a nerve from distal to proximal elicits painful paraesthesia when the area of regeneration is reached. Tinel's sign is initially at the level of injury and advances distally with time. Rehabilitation should be started while recovery is awaited; the range of joint movement should be preserved and the anaesthetic skin protected.

PROGNOSIS
The outcome of nerve repair depends on:

- age
- nerve type

- type of lesion – a clean cut or extensive damage from soft tissue and bony injury
- size of the gap to be bridged
- delay between injury and repair
- surgical skill.

Brachial plexus injuries

AETIOLOGY

Two mechanisms account for nearly all injuries:

- *trauma* – this is of increasing importance because of the contemporary pattern of violence in developed societies
- *obstetric*.

PATHOLOGICAL FEATURES

Adult trauma is usually the outcome of riding motorcycles. The victim is thrown from the machine but holds onto the hand grip while the body rotates. Severe traction/torsion forces are applied to the shoulder girdle and may result in:

- direct tearing of nerve roots from the spinal cord – a preganglionic injury which is usually irreparable
- a wide variety of more distal injuries to the plexus which are more susceptible to repair.

Obstetric injury is usually associated with difficult delivery – shoulder dystocia or a breech presentation – when excessive distraction has been applied to the upper limb.

CLINICAL FEATURES

A brachial plexus injury leads to motor paralysis, loss of sensation and autonomic dysfunction in the area of distribution of the injured part of the plexus.

A preganglionic injury is suggested by:

- a high-speed accident
- an ill-localised sensation of pain in an anaesthetic limb

- sensory loss above the clavicle
- development of deep bruising in the posterior triangle of the neck
- ipsilateral Horner's syndrome
- paralysis of the hemidiaphragm.

Obstetric injuries are difficult to identify but suspicion is aroused if there has been a difficult delivery and the infant displays failure of normal limb movement.

MANAGEMENT

Adult trauma

Brachial plexus reconstruction is a specialised procedure. An injury of the plexus should direct attention to the degree of violence and the possibility of other injuries that threaten life which take higher priority.

When circumstances are right for definitive treatment, nerve exploration and repair are indicated according to the injury that has been sustained. Grafting of the ruptured nerve ends is possible in lesions distal to the trunks of the plexus.

Obstetric injury

In the past, treatment consisted mainly of physiotherapy and delayed tendon transfers. Recent evidence suggests that, in those babies who have not recovered by the age of 3 months, early exploration and grafting gives improved results.

FURTHER READING

Adams JC, Hamblen DL (1999) *Outline of Fractures 11e.* Edinburgh: Churchill Livingstone.

Birch R, Bonney G, Wynn Parry CB, Smith SJM (1998) *Surgical Disorders of the Peripheral Nerves.* Edinburgh: Churchill Livingstone.

McRae R (1994) *Practical Fracture Management.* Edinburgh: Churchill Livingstone.

(2000) *Aids to the Examination of the Peripheral Nervous System 4e.* London: WB Saunders.

35 Principles of paediatric surgery

General principles

Newborns and young infants present with surgical disorders which are uncommon and peculiar to their age group. There are great survival advantages in referring these patients to regional centres where every member of the team is experienced in their special needs. Not only should the surgeon have specific paediatric surgical training, but it is also essential for the anaesthetist to be skilled in the management of the small airway and to be familiar with the physiology and pharmacology of infancy. Successful management is also dependent on nursing skills which can only be learnt, and their standards sustained, in units which accept referrals from a population with at least 20 000 deliveries a year.

Care of the infant during transfer
The priorities in care are:

- temperature control
- nasogastric intubation to keep the stomach empty
- airway protection, e.g. pharyngeal suction for oesophageal atresia (see below) and assisted ventilation via endotracheal tube for respiratory insufficiency
- cardiorespiratory monitoring of pulse rate and oxygen saturation
- intravenous fluids – to provide glucose and sodium; water overload must be avoided; fluid requirements are determined by the infant's age and weight (Table 35.1).

Temperature
Hypothermia is minimised by the use of an incubator and a warming mattress and by an overhead heater in the operating theatre and anaesthetic room. The extremities are wrapped in aluminium foil and the infant nursed in warm cotton wool covered by gauze

Table 35.1
Daily fluid requirement in the first week of life

Day	Fluids (mL/kg per day)
1, 2	60
3, 4	90
5, 6	120
≥ 7	150

Table 35.2
Abnormal losses in infants

Nature of loss	Replacement
Gastric juice	Normal (0.9%) saline
Ileostomy fluid	0.45% saline
Peritoneal exudate	Colloid (4.5% albumin)

(Gamgee), exposing only the operating field. Sick infants may be transferred between hospitals in a transport incubator with other support as detailed below.

Nasogastric intubation

Whenever intestinal obstruction is suspected, a naso-gastric tube large enough to keep the stomach empty (8–10 Fr) is essential to minimise the risk of aspiration of gastric contents into the respiratory tract.

Cardiorespiratory monitoring

Pulse rate and arterial oxygen saturation are sensitive indicators of how the infant is responding to the stresses of illness. Continuous records help to adjust respiratory support and fluid and electrolyte replacement.

Fluid and electrolyte replacement

This is best given as 10% dextrose with 0.18% saline and 10 mmol of potassium added to each 500 mL bag. Additional losses are replaced as outlined in Table 35.2. Babies who require phototherapy for hyperbilirubin-aemia need 20% extra water because of increased insensible loss through the skin.

Intravenous nutrition

If enteral feeding is not possible within 7 days of birth, total parenteral nutrition (TPN) is indicated for mature babies but at a younger age for premature and small-for-dates babies because they are born with very low calorie stores of glycogen and fat.

Intravenous fluids can be delivered via peripheral veins but this necessitates frequent resiting of the cannula. Peripheral administration is not suitable for the hypertonic solutions used in TPN, and central venous catheters, which deliver the fluid directly to the right atrium, are necessary. The risk of thrombophlebitis in peripheral veins has to be balanced against the increased risk of introducing infection through a central line.

Infection in the newborn

Infection is a constant risk for newborns who need to undergo surgical procedures or who require intensive care. Broad-spectrum antibiotics (augmentin or a combination of benzyl penicillin, aminoglycoside and metronidazole) are given intravenously at the start of all operations. Contaminated operations, e.g. when there is a bowel perforation, require 7 days of intravenous antibiotics, and oral nystatin should be given to reduce

colonisation by *Candida* sp. All babies who show clinical evidence of sepsis (raised temperature, tachycardia, failure to feed and leucocytosis) should have blood and surface cultures; many also require cerebrospinal fluid and urine cultures, and intravenous antibiotics should be started immediately and their administration modified in the light of the results of culture.

Prenatal diagnosis

Prenatal ultrasound scanning can alert the obstetrician's attention to many anatomical anomalies, such as anterior abdominal wall defects, diaphragmatic hernia, duodenal atresia and hydronephrosis. This allows planning of postnatal care, with delivery of the baby in a hospital equipped to provide immediate resuscitation and experienced management including nursing care.

Only rarely is it necessary to transfer the mother prenatally to a delivery unit adjacent to a neonatal surgical unit because immediate surgery is not usually indicated (an exception is gastroschisis). It is important to remember that the spectrum of disorders seen in mid-pregnancy (18–20 weeks) may be very different from that seen in newborns, because ultrasound-detected anomalies may be multiple and associated with an abnormal karyotype, which may result in stillbirth. Other apparent fetal anomalies may revert to normality before birth. Fetal chromosomes can be checked, an echocardiogram performed and a scan for detailed mapping of anomalies repeated before a prediction of the findings at birth and their prognosis is reached and postnatal management planned. Fetal medicine is a new and rapidly evolving speciality and fetal surgery, although available in a few centres around the world, has still to establish criteria for intervention; there is little evidence to date that prenatal treatment of structural anomalies is of benefit.

Surgical conditions presenting with respiratory distress

Oesophageal atresia with tracheo-oesophageal fistula

EPIDEMIOLOGY AND NATURE

One in 4000 babies has an oesophageal anomaly, most commonly a mid-oesophageal atresia with a distal tracheo-oesophageal fistula (Fig. 35.1). Three rarer forms are:

- isolated oesophageal atresia, usually with a long gap
- isolated tracheo-oesophageal fistula with an intact oesophagus

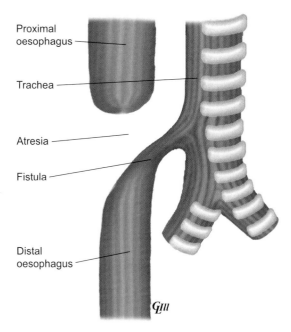

Fig 35.1 **Common variant of oesophageal atresia and tracheo-oesophageal fistula.**

- oesophageal atresia with fistulae to both proximal and distal oesophageal pouches.

Half the infants with oesophageal anomalies have associated abnormalities, mainly of the cardiovascular, renal or skeletal systems. The aetiology is unknown but the embryological abnormality occurs early in pregnancy, about 4 weeks following conception.

CLINICAL FEATURES

In the common form with a blind upper oesophagus, the affected newborn may be able to swallow amniotic fluid via the trachea and the fistula into the stomach, but half of these pregnancies are complicated by polyhydramnios. At birth the infant appears to have excessive pharyngeal mucus because saliva cannot be swallowed. If fed by mouth, a cyanotic episode suggests aspiration into the respiratory tract. Feeding should be avoided when there is suspicion of oesophageal atresia and the diagnosis is confirmed by the passage of a size 10 Fr (3.3 mm) nasogastric tube, which is arrested in the mid-oesophagus. A finer tube curls in the proximal oesophagus and can therefore lead to confusion and misdiagnosis.

INVESTIGATION

A radiograph of the chest shows the tube to be in proximity to the first or second thoracic vertebral body, and gas in the stomach indicates the presence of a distal tracheo-oesophageal fistula.

MANAGEMENT

The initial objective is to keep the upper airway clear with suction and to maintain hydration with intravenous fluids. Transfer to a specialist unit is required. A right thoracotomy is done as soon as the baby is stable; the fistulous opening on the posterior wall of the trachea is repaired and an oesophageal anastomosis fashioned. In 10%, the gap is too wide to permit primary anastomosis and staged surgery is necessary with either a delayed anastomosis, some weeks or months later, or an oesophageal replacement with a gastric or colonic segment.

PROGNOSIS

The outlook for survival is excellent, except in those born very prematurely and those with associated complex cardiac anomalies. However, dysphagia and respiratory complications may continue into adult life and long-term follow-up is necessary.

Diaphragmatic hernia

EPIDEMIOLOGY AND NATURE

Herniation of abdominal viscera through the infant diaphragm occurs in 1 in 2000 live births, most often through a left posterolateral defect, which is a persistence of the embryonic pleuroperitoneal canal. A more severe anomaly is agenesis of the hemidiaphragm, also more common on the left side. Intestine, stomach and spleen may be found in the pleural cavity, and the ipsilateral lung is severely hypoplastic. The mediastinum is displaced away from the hernia, so an apparent dextrocardia is a feature of a left-side diaphragmatic hernia. The cause is unknown.

CLINICAL FEATURES

There is severe respiratory and sometimes circulatory disability at or shortly after birth and breath sounds are absent on the affected side The mediastinum is displaced.

INVESTIGATION

The diagnosis is confirmed by a plain X-ray (Fig. 35.2) which shows a lack of small bowel gas in the abdomen with loops of intestine in the pleural cavity and displacement of the mediastinum. The differential diagnosis includes congenital lung cysts and staphylococcal pneumonia, both being associated with air–fluid spaces in the lung. However, in these conditions, the X-ray shows an intact diaphragm with normal intestinal gas patterns in the abdomen.

MANAGEMENT

Resuscitation requires positive pressure ventilation via an endotracheal tube and a nasogastric tube to decompress the stomach. Assisted respiration via a face mask is contraindicated because this inflates the

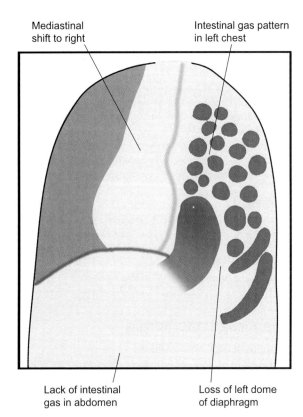

Mediastinal shift to right

Intestinal gas pattern in left chest

Lack of intestinal gas in abdomen

Loss of left dome of diaphragm

Fig 35.2 **Chest and abdominal X-ray in diaphragmatic hernia. Loops of small bowel are present in the left chest and the mediastinum is displaced to the right.**

stomach and small bowel, thereby increasing the size of the space-occupying viscera in the chest. Intravenous analgesia and paralysis increase the efficiency of mechanical ventilation. Infants with more severe pulmonary hypertension require inotropic support with dopamine and pulmonary vasodilatation with nitric oxide and prostacyclin. Extracorporeal membrane oxygenation may be offered to unstable infants with pulmonary hypertension and a right-to-left shunt. Intravenous colloid may be required to expand the circulating blood volume.

Operative repair is delayed until the neonate is stable with good gas exchange and urine output. The defect is exposed through an upper abdominal incision, the contents of the hernia reduced from the thorax and the diaphragmatic defect repaired, if necessary with a prosthetic patch.

PROGNOSIS
The condition still carries a 30% mortality rate, related mainly to severe bilateral pulmonary hypoplasia, but the majority of long-term survivors have no symptoms of pulmonary insufficiency, despite the ipsilateral lung having persistently reduced ventilation and perfusion.

Upper airway obstruction

Cystic hygroma, posterior choanal atresia and a small jaw (micrognathia) are the three main causes.

Cystic hygroma
This condition is of unknown cause. Fluid-filled collections are found in the neck and may extend into the mediastinum or axilla. The presence of respiratory distress requires intubation and surgical removal which may require a long and difficult dissection. Sclerotherapy can also be used to shrink cystic lesions.

Bilateral posterior choanal atresia
This is a bony or membranous obstruction to the nasal passages at the junction of the hard and soft palates. The newborn is an obligatory nasal breather and can suffocate without the assistance of an oropharyngeal tube to maintain a patent airway.

The diagnosis is confirmed by being unable to pass a nasal tube into the pharynx and a CT scan is helpful in defining the extent of the atresia and planning operative repair which is undertaken as soon as possible.

Management. Under a general anaesthetic, the atresia is resected transnasally using a drill. The resulting nasal airway is stented for a minimum of 6 weeks and further resection of tissue may be required.

Micrognathia
A hypoplastic mandible causes obstruction of the pharynx by posterior prolapse of the tongue. Combination of this disorder with a cleft palate is known as the Pierre–Robin syndrome. The respiratory problem is best relieved by a tracheostomy and the defects repaired at a later date.

Neonatal intestinal obstruction

GENERAL CLINICAL FEATURES
The clinical history should include details of maternal illness (diabetes mellitus is common), medication during pregnancy and perinatal events. A history of intestinal obstruction, Hirschsprung's disease (see below) or cystic fibrosis in relatives is noted.

Specific features are:

- bile-stained vomiting
- failure to pass meconium or stools that change to those characteristic of the neonate
- abdominal distension, when the obstruction is distal to the duodenum.

Examination should include a note of any dysmorphic features, such as those found in Down's syndrome where intestinal abnormalities are common (see 'Duodenal atresia' below). In the abdomen, loops of dilated bowel are often visible in distal obstruction and bulky palpable meconium is suggestive of meconium ileus. The site and size of the anus should be recorded and the rectum examined: blood indicates probable ischaemia of the bowel and the explosive passage of meconium and flatus on withdrawal of the finger is suggestive of Hirschsprung's disease.

INVESTIGATION

Plain abdominal X-rays confirm the presence of dilated loops of bowel and indicate if the obstruction is proximal or distal. Free gas, best demonstrated on a right decubitus X-ray (Fig. 35.3), means that intestinal perforation has occurred whereas small bubbles of intramural gas are present in gangrenous necrosis of the bowel wall.

Duodenal atresia

This is the commonest cause of proximal intestinal obstruction – 1 in 10 000 newborns is affected. At least one-third of the infants have Down's syndrome.

The duodenum may be completely closed by a short segment of atresia. Alternatively, partial obstruction may be caused by a stenosis or an incomplete web, usually sited in the second part of the duodenum at the level of the ampulla of Vater.

CLINICAL FEATURES

Vomiting occurs during the first day of life and is usually bile-stained. The abdominal examination in this high obstruction is not usually helpful.

INVESTIGATION AND MANAGEMENT

Abdominal X-ray shows a dilated stomach and proximal duodenum – the 'double-bubble' appearance (Fig. 35.4).

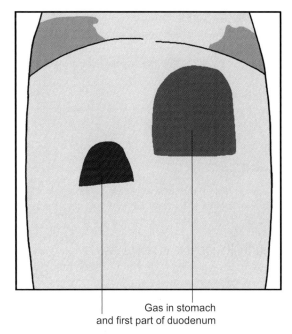

Gas in stomach
and first part of duodenum

Fig 35.4 **'Double bubble' in duodenal atresia.**

These duodenal anomalies can be corrected surgically, care being taken to protect the ampulla.

Volvulus

This condition is the most treacherous small bowel obstruction. The midgut is malrotated and the base of the small bowel mesentery is narrow and unstable. The duodenojejunal junction is found to the right or in the midline; the caecum is mobile on a mesentery and lies close to the midline.

CLINICAL FEATURES

The volvulus most often occurs in the first 4 weeks of life. There is bile-stained vomiting without abdominal distension. Signs of abdominal tenderness and rectal bleeding indicate intestinal ischaemia secondary to occlusion of mesenteric vessels.

MANAGEMENT

Very prompt surgical relief is required or ischaemia of the entire small intestine will be irreversible after 6 hours.

Atresia of the small bowel

Apart from the duodenum, these are more common in the ileum than in the jejunum, but both are relatively rare – fewer than 1 in 10 000 births.

The cause is thought to be a vascular accident in mesenteric vessels late in fetal development.

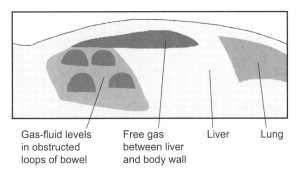

Gas-fluid levels	Free gas	Liver	Lung
in obstructed	between liver		
loops of bowel	and body wall		

Fig 35.3 **Free air in the abdomen on a right decubitus film.**

CLINICAL FEATURES

As in adult small bowel obstruction (Ch. 23), the more distal the obstruction, the greater is the delay in presentation. Otherwise the features are those of obstruction.

MANAGEMENT

Resection of the atresias and anastomosis is usually possible and the outlook is good.

Meconium ileus

In this condition, the tenacious viscid meconium found in 15% of infants with cystic fibrosis obstructs the distal ileum.

CLINICOPATHOLOGICAL FEATURES

The terminal small bowel is full of meconium but the colon is empty and appears undeveloped – a microcolon. However, this is because it has never been filled, rather than there being a developmental defect. Prenatal perforation may take place with sterile peritonitis and local calcification.

There may have been genetic investigations that reveal the likelihood of cystic fibrosis. The infant presents with a distal small bowel obstruction.

INVESTIGATION

A plain X-ray confirms low small bowel obstruction and there may be calcification from sterile perforation. A controlled water-soluble contrast enema (Gastrografin) fills the empty colon and may reflux back through the ileocaecal valve to outline loops of ileum and the inspissated meconium.

The underlying cystic fibrosis is diagnosed by measuring the levels of sodium in several samples of the infant's sweat or by the detection of one of the specific defective genes found on chromosome 7.

MANAGEMENT

When it is possible to fill dilated loops of ileum, the contrast enema may relieve the obstruction because it acts as a lubricating detergent which releases the tenacious meconium. However, in 50% of the infants, meconium ileus is complicated by the presence of an atresia, a volvulus or a perforation, all of which require operative correction. The introduction of feeds postoperatively should include pancreatic enzymes to facilitate the digestion and absorption of fats.

Hirschsprung's disease

EPIDEMIOLOGY AND AETIOLOGY

As already stated, all cases of neonatal intestinal obstruction are rare, but the commonest, which affects 1 in 5000 newborns, is Hirschsprung's disease. The mechanism is failure of development of the myenteric plexus of ganglion cells which implement parasympathetic activity in the wall of the large bowel. The cause is not known but migration from the neural crest has been arrested at varying levels. Most often the aganglionic segment is the distal sigmoid colon and the rectum, but in 10% the entire colon is aganglionic. A number of abnormal genes have been identified in families and patients with Hirschsprung's disease.

CLINICAL FEATURES

Most infants with anything more than a very short segment of aganglionosis present with acute large bowel obstruction at birth or within a few days. The condition is not easy to recognise – there is failure to pass meconium or altered faeces but this may be incomplete. Abdominal distension is uniform but a rectal examination may lead to a deceiving passage of flatus and stool.

INVESTIGATION

Imaging

A contrast enema may demonstrate proximal dilatation of the ganglionic bowel with relative narrowing of the distal aganglionic segment but this may be difficult to interpret.

Biopsy

The diagnosis is confirmed by taking a rectal biopsy of mucosa and submucosa which, suitably stained, demonstrates the lack of ganglion cells in Meissner's submucosal plexus.

MANAGEMENT

The distal obstruction is relieved by a stoma in proximal ganglion-containing bowel (confirmed by biopsy at operation). After a few months, and when the infant is thriving, a definitive operation is performed to excise the aganglionic bowel and anastomose normally innervated colon or ileum to the anorectal junction. Alternatively, the distal obstruction is relieved by daily saline irrigations and a primary definitive operation done without a prior colostomy.

Follow-up through childhood is required to ensure that bowel function is regular. Enterocolitis, often related to *Clostridium difficile* infection, can be fatal in children with Hirschsprung's disease. Any episode of severe diarrhoea requires vigorous resuscitation and treatment.

Anorectal abnormalities

Inspection of the infant's perineum may reveal an abnormality of the anus, which may be:

- Skin-covered anus with a narrow anterior ectopic opening to the skin of the perineum (male) or vulva (female) – either may be corrected by a relatively minor perineal operation.

- Absence of the anal canal and distal rectum with or without a fistula from the mid rectum to the urethra (male) or vagina (female). These higher anorectal anomalies are managed initially with a colostomy; corrective surgery is delayed until the infant is thriving and detailed radiological studies have been performed to establish the extent of the defect and whether or not the urinary tract is involved.

Neonatal necrotising enterocolitis (NEC)

Necrosis of the intestinal wall, affecting the small or large bowel, occurs in about 1 in 1000 infants.

AETIOLOGY

The cause is not fully understood but is related to:

- vascular changes in the splanchnic circulation secondary to exchange transfusions via the umbilical vein
- perinatal stress – hypoxia from the respiratory distress syndrome, cyanotic heart disease or asphyxia.

The disease is commoner in neonates born prematurely and there is often a delay of several days between the initial stress and the onset of the clinical illness which follows the invasion of the damaged bowel wall by bacteria.

CLINICAL FEATURES

Symptoms begin with the infant, who often has the features discussed above, showing evidence of systemic sepsis and failure to absorb gastric feeds. Abdominal distension progresses to tenderness and erythema of the abdominal wall and there is the passage of loose stools which frequently contain blood.

INVESTIGATION

Abdominal X-rays demonstrate dilated loops of bowel but intramural gas (pneumatosis intestinalis) is diagnostic. Free gas in the peritoneum, best seen on a right decubitus X-ray, indicates a perforation, usually in gangrenous intestine.

MANAGEMENT

The management is to stop gastric feeds immediately, investigate for the presence of sepsis and start intravenous broad-spectrum antibiotics against both aerobic and anaerobic intestinal bacteria. A combination of benzylpenicillin, gentamicin and metronidazole is commonly used.

Resuscitation includes intravenous fluids, 10% dextrose in 1/5 normal saline to maintain blood sugar, and colloid or blood to expand the circulating volume.

Ventilation may be required if there is respiratory failure secondary to abdominal distension, sepsis or underlying lung disease. With prompt intensive medical treatment, the majority of infants will improve but require 10 days of TPN before reintroduction of gastric feeds. A laparotomy should be performed if there is:

- suspicion or evidence of a perforation
- failure to respond to medical management including persistent acidosis and thrombocytopenia which are indications of severe necrosis.

At operation, gangrenous bowel is excised and either a primary anastomosis performed or the two viable ends exteriorised as stomas.

OUTCOME

There is an immediate mortality of some 20%, related to very extensive small bowel loss, septicaemia or the complications of extreme prematurity such as intracranial haemorrhage. Longer-term complications in survivors include short bowel syndrome and fibrotic strictures. With an intact ileocaecal valve, 20 cm of small bowel can adapt to achieve adequate absorption but, without an ileocaecal valve or ileum, the jejunum has limited ability to compensate. Late strictures, which present as feeding difficulties or subacute obstruction, are diagnosed by contrast enemas and treated surgically with resection and anastomosis.

Anterior abdominal wall defects and the umbilicus

The most striking examples of anterior abdominal wall defects are all rare and include (Table 35.3):

- exomphalos
- gastroschisis
- exstrophy of the bladder.

Other anomalies are a patent vitellointestinal tract, a patent urachus, true umbilical hernia and the prune belly syndrome (see below).

Exomphalos

This is a central defect with the umbilical cord inserted into a transparent amniotic sac with the vessels spreading out like a tripod (Fig. 35.5). The sac contains loops of bowel and often part of the liver. Associated anomalies include:

- congenital heart disease
- chromosomal abnormalities such as Edward's syndrome (trisomy 18) – dysmorphic features,

Table 35.3
Congenital umbilical anomalies

Descriptive name	Sac	Umbilical cord	Associated abnormalities	Prognosis
Exomphalos	Present	Inserted into sac	Cardiac	Dependent on associated anomalies
			Chromosomal	and size of defect
Gastroschisis	Absent	Inserted into abdominal wall	Intestinal atresias	Excellent, with 90% survival

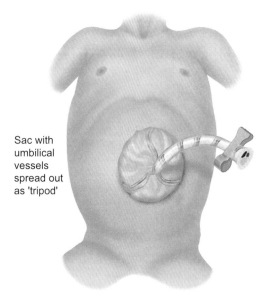

Fig 35.5 'Exomphalos. (a) The umbilical vessels are spread out as a tripod. (b) Exposed loops of matted intestine.

Sac with umbilical vessels spread out as 'tripod'

congential heart disease and severe neurodevelopmental delay
• neonatal hypoglycaemia with the EMG syndrome (exomphalos, macroglossia, gigantism).

Prenatal diagnosis by mid-trimester ultrasound scan is an indication for an echocardiogram and chromosomal analysis of fetal blood or amniotic cells before discussing the prognosis for the fetus with the parents.

MANAGEMENT

Management is by primary closure for smaller defects or the creation of a 'silo' with staged reduction to achieve delayed closure. With major associated anomalies, a non-operative approach, which allows the sac to epithelialise and shrink over a period of months, carries the lowest mortality but requires the longest in-patient stay.

Gastroschisis

This is a defect just to the right of a normally inserted umbilical cord with exposure of herniated loops of intestine, which are foreshortened and covered by a fibrinous exudate (Fig. 35.6). Apart from intestinal atresia, associated anomalies are rare.

MANAGEMENT

Vaginal delivery is preferred and the defect is covered with a sterile transparent bag or clingfilm. A nasogastric tube is indicated to empty the stomach and intravenous antibiotics and fluids, including colloid, are given.

Early operation is recommended to repair the abdominal wall or to create a silo if the abdominal cavity is too small initially to accommodate bowel and other viscera. The prognosis is excellent, although prolonged TPN may be required while waiting for intestinal function to return.

Bladder exstrophy

A rare anomaly, this is more common in boys than in girls. There is an anterior opening of the bladder and urethra with absence of tissue of the subumbilical anterior abdominal wall and separation of the pubic bones. If the bladder epithelium is left exposed into adult life, now a rare event in the West, malignant change may occur. The anomaly requires major reconstruction of the pelvis, bladder and external

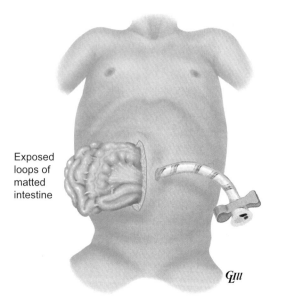

Exposed loops of matted intestine

Fig 35.6 **Gastroschisis.**

genitalia and the infant's problem should be managed in a specialist centre.

Epispadias is a less severe form of the disorder with separation of the pubic bones, a deficient and incontinent bladder neck and a urethral meatus opening on the dorsal aspect of the penis.

Cloacal exstrophy is a more severe anomaly with an open bladder divided in the midline by intestinal stomas. The colon is short and associated with anorectal agenesis. Renal anomalies are common. Again management in a specialist centre is necessary.

Umbilical hernia

This condition is caused by a widening of the natural defect in the linea alba at birth and has a higher incidence in Afro-Caribbean children, and those with Down's syndrome and hypothyroidism.

EMBRYOLOGY AND ANATOMY

The complex folding of the developing embryo results in the formation of the coelomic cavity and the apices of the folds form the umbilical ring through which the midgut communicates with the yolk sac and the connecting stalk (containing the umbilical vein and arteries) passes to the placenta.

The developing gut grows more rapidly than the coelomic capacity and so prolapses into the wide base of the umbilical cord – the extra-embryonic coelom – as a temporary hernia. The abdominal cavity subsequently enlarges, and by the 12th week the herniated intestinal loops return, undergoing rotation as they do so. In normal circumstances, after the return of the gut, the umbilical ring constricts but a defect persists until birth for the passage of the umbilical vessels. After delivery, the umbilical vessels thrombose and fibrous tissue forms and condenses to plug the defect. A congenital umbilical hernia results if the sequence is incomplete.

CLINICAL FEATURES

History
The infant presents with a protrusion that everts the umbilicus and expands when the child cries. Symptoms are absent and invariably the parents are more perturbed by the presence of the lesion than is the owner.

Physical findings
The defect is easily palpable as a sharp-edged hole through which usually little more than omentum protrudes. It is extremely rare for strangulation to take place.

MANAGEMENT
Most of these hernias close spontaneously before the age of 4 years. Very large and persistent umbilical hernias

are closed surgically but this is best delayed until after the first 3 years of life.

Supraumbilical hernia
Defects just above the umbilical cicatrix protrude outwards and downwards into the umbilical skin. These do not close spontaneously and occasionally cause strangulation of bowel. Surgical repair is indicated after the infant's first birthday.

Umbilical granuloma (Table 35.4)

These are moist granulations, pedunculated with a dull irregular surface. They are a superficial persistence of intestinal mucosa or the consequence of sepsis in an infolded umbilical cicatrix. A smooth red moist lesion can be the exposed mucosa of a patent vitellointestinal tract. This rare embryological remnant forms a fistula between the skin and the lumen of the ileum, intermittently leaking small bowel contents. Even more rare is a patent urachus which communicates between the bladder and the umbilicus and leaks urine. The urinary tract should be investigated for other anomalies, particularly bladder outflow obstruction and vesicoureteric reflux.

MANAGEMENT
An umbilical granuloma is cauterised with a silver nitrate stick, best applied to the narrow base, or by ligation of the stalk with a tight ligature (granulomas do not contain pain fibres, so analgesia is not required). A patent vitellointestinal fistula must be surgically excised at a limited laparotomy. A urachal fistula is similarly excised with repair of the bladder dome.

Prune belly syndrome

Absence of the anterior abdominal wall muscles may follow transient but severe prenatal ascites. This is a rare anomaly, seen mostly in boys, and associated with

Table 35.4
Moist lesions at the umbilicus

Condition	Appearance	Management
Granuloma	Dull and irregular surface	Cauterisation or ligation after excluding an underlying, more serious lesion
Patent vitellointestinal tract	Red, smooth and leaking digested milk	Specialised investigation and laparotomy for repair
Patent urachus	Leakage of urine	Urological investigation and repair

bilateral intra-abdominal testes and an abnormal renal tract with gross dilatation and poor function. The skin lies in loose wrinkled folds, with the underlying abdominal wall muscles poorly developed and displaced laterally. The management of the urological problems and renal failure is paramount, but staged orchidopexies and surgical repair of the anterior abdominal wall should be considered.

Abdominal tumours

There are four anatomical groups in infancy and childhood:

- upper abdominal and crossing the midline
- arising in the loin
- arising from the pelvis
- in the right hypochondrium.

Initial investigation of all masses should include a plain abdominal X-ray – calcification is found in many neuroblastomas, hepatoblastomas and teratomas – and an ultrasound scan to differentiate solid from cystic lesions.

Upper abdominal tumours

The usual tumour is a highly malignant *neuroblastoma* in infancy which arises from either the adrenal medulla or the sympathetic ganglia. They have an irregular edge, cross the midline and spread to lymph nodes, bone marrow, liver and skin. Most tumours are advanced at the time of diagnosis with fixation and distant spread from the primary site.

Rarely, a benign *ganglioneuroma* arises from a sympathetic ganglion and this may be cured by total surgical excision.

Retroperitoneal *lymphomas* can also present as central abdominal masses. The diagnosis is confirmed by biopsy and the treatment is by chemotherapy.

Neuroblastoma

Investigation
Catecholamines. Nearly all neuroblastomas produce catecholamines, which are metabolised to vanillyl-mandelic acid (VMA) and homovanyllic acid (HVA), and these substances can be identified in the urine.

Imaging. CT, MRI and bone scans are used to establish the extent of the disease.

Bone marrow biopsy. Identification of neuroblastoma cells in marrow indicates generalised disease.

Other. The *N-myc* gene has been identified on neuroblastoma cells and amplification of this oncogene indicates a poor prognosis for the patient.

Management
Treatment includes chemotherapy, surgery and occasionally radiotherapy, but the majority of patients with advanced tumours are incurable.

Loin tumours

Tumours that arise in the loin and do not cross the midline are usually of renal origin. Cystic lesions include:

- massive hydronephrosis
- hereditary polycystic disease
- sporadic non-functioning multicystic kidney associated with ureteric atresia.

Wilms' tumour
This is the most common cause of a solid renal mass.

Pathological features
It is a malignant nephroblastoma which spreads to adjacent lymph nodes and via the renal vein to the inferior vena cava and so to the lungs. They are occasionally bilateral. Very rarely, a neonate may have a benign mesoblastic nephroma which is cured by excision alone.

Clinical features
The commonest presentation is of a palpable tumour in a child of preschool age. Pain indicates haemorrhage into or rupture of the tumour. Fever and hypertension may be present but haematuria is rare. Left-sided tumours may be associated with varicocele.

Investigation and management
CT establishes the extent of the growth.

Treatment is by radical excision of the tumour with its kidney and the adjacent lymph nodes, chemotherapy and, in some cases, radiotherapy. Over 80% of patients are cured.

Masses arising from the pelvis

A wide variety of swellings fall into this category, including:

- urogenital cyst and neoplasia
- neuroblastoma arising within the pelvic sympathetic ganglia
- presacral teratomas
- ovarian cysts which can be detected by ultrasound prenatally and may resolve before the age of 6 months.

Urogenital cysts and neoplasms
Rhabdomyosarcoma is a mixed solid and cystic malignant tumour that arises from the genitourinary tract. It

may present with haematuria or vaginal bleeding and many can be diagnosed by biopsy through an endoscope.

Treatment includes excision, chemotherapy and radiotherapy, and in the majority leads to cure.

Pelvic neuroblastoma

The characteristics of this growth are similar to neuro-blastoma elsewhere (see above) but have a better prognosis than abdominal neuroblastomas.

Sacrococcygeal teratoma

This is discussed under 'Teratoma' (below).

Ovarian cysts

Cysts that persist into postnatal life may undergo torsion with infarction of the ovary. A massive ovarian cyst with calcification in an older girl is often a mature teratoma and is treated by surgical excision. Malignant ovarian tumours are very rare during childhood but include oestrogen-producing stromal tumours that present with precocious puberty.

Right upper quadrant tumours

Hepatic tumours include:

- benign haemangioma and haemangioendothelioma
- hepatoblastoma.

Benign haemangioma and haemangioendothelioma

Both of these conditions may present with thrombo-cytopenia, which is assumed to be the consequence of turbluent blood flow, or because of the arteriovenous shunt which causes high-output cardiac failure. Their natural history is to regress, but steroids are indicated if complications arise and hepatic artery embolisation or ligation should be considered.

Hepatoblastoma

This is the commonest malignant hepatic tumour and produces alpha-fetoprotein. CT or MRI define the site and extent of the tumours, most of which require chemotherapy before surgical excision is attempted.

Teratoma

Embryonic tumours contain elements of the three germ layers, endoderm, mesoderm and ectoderm. The sacro-coccygeal region is the commonest site in the newborn but they also occur in the gonads of older children. Less common sites are the anterior mediastinum and the neck. Some neonatal sacrococcygeal teratomas are massive – larger than the infant's head. Total excision with the coccyx is recommended within the first few days of life. A less common variant is a teratoma

entirely within the pelvis in the presacral space. When these present later in infancy with bowel or bladder obstruction, they are usually malignant and require chemotherapy in addition to surgical excision. Serial serum alpha-fetoprotein estimations are indicated post-operatively, as rising levels suggest recurrence.

Pyloric stenosis

EPIDEMIOLOGY

Postnatal hypertrophy of the pyloric circular muscle affects 2–3 per 1000 infants in northern Europe but is less common elsewhere in the world. The male:female ratio is 5:1 and the disorder usually develops in the first 6 weeks of life.

AETIOLOGY

The cause is unknown. There is an hereditary effect – the sons of affected mothers have the highest incidence.

CLINICAL FEATURES

Symptoms

There is forceful projectile vomiting between the ages of 2 and 6 weeks. On feeding, the child appears anxious and then vomits but is soon hungry again. As the obstruction is proximal to the point of entry of the bile duct into the duodenum, the vomitus is not bile-stained. When the vomiting is frequent or the diagnosis delayed, there are signs of weight loss and dehydration.

Physical findings

The diagnosis is confirmed by performing a test feed; after emptying the stomach with a nasogastric tube, the infant is offered milk either from the breast or from a bottle. The examiner sits to the child's left and palpates the right hypochondrium with the fingers of the left hand. The hypertrophied and contracted pyloric pseudotumour is felt intermittently as a hard swelling of about 2 × 1cm when the abdominal muscles relax. When the stomach is full, peristalsis may be visible moving from left to right from under the left costal margin.

INVESTIGATION

If the expected mass is not palpated on repeat test feeding and the diagnosis seems likely on the basis of the symptoms, then imaging with ultrasound or a barium meal is performed.

Overfeeding, oesophageal reflux and sepsis such as a urinary tract infection must all be considered as alter-native causes.

MANAGEMENT

The repeated loss of gastric juice may cause metabolic

alkalosis with raised serum bicarbonate and a low serum chloride concentration. This is corrected with intravenous normal saline with added potassium chloride (10–20 mmol of potassium to 500 ml of saline). The renal tubules exchange the potassium for hydrogen ions, which are reabsorbed from the lumen of the tubule. When the infant is well hydrated and has a good urine output, the operation of pyloromyotomy is advised.

Under general anaesthesia, the pyloric muscle is cut longitudinally down to the gastric mucosa; the mucosa pouts and the obstruction is relieved. Postoperatively the infant can be re-established on full feeds within 48 hours.

OUTLOOK

The condition should be managed without mortality and with a wound infection rate below 10%. Other complications are rare. The long-term prognosis for gastric function is excellent.

Intussusception

An intussusception is the invagination of a segment of bowel into an adjacent segment, most often the terminal ileum invaginating into the transverse colon.

EPIDEMIOLOGY

Approximately 2 per 1000 infants are affected and most present between the ages of 3 and 12 months. Boys are affected more frequently than girls, in a ratio of 2:1.

AETIOLOGY

The commonest cause is hyperplasia of a Peyer's patch secondary to a viral infection, usually an adenovirus. The enlarged lymphoid tissue acts as a fixed eccentrically placed bolus in the lumen of the bowel and the gut is invaginated as it tries ineffectively to pass the 'lump' more distally. Invaginated bowel can become strangulated, in which case there are general features of circulatory disturbance. Less commonly in infants, the lead point of the intussusception is a Meckel's diverticulum (Ch. 23), a duplication cyst in the bowel wall or a polyp.

CLINICAL FEATURES

Symptoms

There may be a history of preceding gastroenteritis or an upper respiratory tract infection. Often there has been a change in diet, such as weaning from milk on to some solid food, a few days before the child presents with severe colicky abdominal pain, characterised by flexing the hips and facial pallor. This abdominal colic is accompanied by vomiting and, within 24 hours, the passage of blood from the rectum.

Physical findings

The infant is usually pyrexial and may, if strangulation has occurred, have signs of a poorly perfused peripheral circulation. If the abdomen is relaxed, a sausage-shaped mass may be palpable in the epigastrium or right hypochondrium, but this may be obscured by abdominal tenderness. A rectal examination must be performed to detect rectal bleeding.

Atypical presentation

Although the typical presentation described is easily recognised, a third of instances present atypically, some apparently without pain, and this leads to delay in diagnosis with an increase in morbidity and mortality related to intestinal gangrene, peritonitis and generalised sepsis.

INVESTIGATION

Plain abdominal X-ray may suggest the diagnosis by the presence of a soft tissue shadow in the region of the right transverse colon with an empty distal bowel. Intestinal obstruction with dilated loops of small bowel implies a well established and possibly gangrenous intussusception. Ultrasound scanning will detect the intussusception and is a useful investigation before deciding on transfer to a specialist centre. A contrast enema, with either air or barium, confirms the diagnosis by demonstrating a filling defect.

MANAGEMENT

A contrast enema may also be therapeutic by reducing the intussuscepted bowel so that, if there is free flow into the ileum and several loops are filled, the intussusception has clearly been reduced. The infant must then remain under observation for 48 hours to be certain that the bowel is viable and that the intussusception does not recur.

If the intussusception fails to reduce radiologically or if signs of established small bowel obstruction or peritonitis are present, a laparotomy is required after a period of resuscitation with intravenous fluids, including colloid (approximately 30 mL/kg of 4.5% albumin) and antibiotics against intestinal organisms. The stomach is emptied with a nasogastric tube. The operation is done through a transverse abdominal incision, usually in the right hypochondrium, and the intussusception is delivered and reduced by manual pressure on its distal portion, squeezing the intussuscepted bowel proximally. Traction on the small bowel, in an attempt to pull it out of the colon, tears the bowel and must be avoided. An irreducible intussusception is resected and the same applies if gangrenous bowel is found after reduction has been achieved. Causes other than hypertrophy of Peyer's patches are dealt with. Careful postoperative observation is mandatory in that any deterioration may indicate a late perforation or recurrent intussusception which requires a second procedure.

Although simple reduction does nothing to prevent recurrence, this occurs in fewer than 5% of patients.

The inguinal region and male genitalia

EMBRYOLOGY

The gonad develops from a ridge of tissue on the posterior abdominal wall. The fetal testis descends through the inguinal canal at approximately week 32, sliding down behind a peritoneal pouch, or processus vaginalis, which normally obliterates once descent is complete. Premature male infants may be born with the processus vaginalis patent and the testes undescended.

Undescended testes

EPIDEMIOLOGY

At the age of 1 year, 1.5% of boys have an undescended testis. Most often it is palpable in the groin where it has passed through the external inguinal ring and is lying in a fascial compartment – the superficial inguinal pouch. However, 5% of boys with a testis not present in the scrotum at birth have an impalpable testis, which may be in the:

- inguinal canal
- abdominal cavity
- absent.

Four per cent of term boys have an undescended testis at birth and the incidence rises to 25% in premature births. Most undescended testes at birth will descend during the first few months of life.

CLINICAL FEATURES

The cremasteric reflex can retract the normally positioned testis out of the scrotum when the child is anxious or cold. The reflex is poorly developed at birth and becomes most marked in children of school age. Examination must be carried out in a warm, reassuring atmosphere with the boy lying supine. The index finger of the left hand passes downwards and medially over the inguinal canal, guiding any mobile structure towards the scrotum. With this finger pressing on the pubic tubercle, the cremasteric reflex is controlled and the thumb and index finger of the right hand can then examine the scrotum. Straight leg raising (only possible in the older child) also abolishes the cremasteric reflex. A retractile testis which can be persuaded to reach the bottom of the scrotum is normal, but if on clinical examination it only reaches the neck of the scrotum, it is suspended from a short cord and not fully descended.

MANAGEMENT

The normal retractile testis does not require surgical intervention and reassurance can be reinforced with a repeat examination later in childhood.

An impalpable testis (20% of undescended testes) is proximal to the external inguinal ring. A laparoscopy is indicated to identify the site of the testis either in the inguinal canal or in the abdomen or to verify that it is absent. If the testicular vessels and vas deferens are seen to end short of the internal ring, then the testis is absent, probably as the result of an intrauterine vascular accident or torsion during descent (see below).

Once the anatomical site of the testis has been decided, treatment can be allocated on the basis of the physiological and anatomical state, including possible complications, e.g.:

- reduced fertility
- torsion (see below)
- associated inguinal hernia
- increased risk of malignant change in adult life
- psychological disadvantage of having abnormal genitalia.

Chorionic gonadotrophin

Injections of human chorionic gonadotrophin have a very limited role in the management of an undescended testis but can be useful, particularly in obese boys, to demonstrate that bilateral retractile testes will descend into the scrotum without the need for an operation.

Surgery

Early operation abolishes the risks associated with inguinal hernia and testicular torsion. If done before the age of 4 years, normal fertility is achieved by scrotal placement of the testis from the superficial inguinal pouch, but testes in the inguinal canal or intra-abdominal have reduced spermatogenesis even after corrective surgery. As the increased risk of malignancy is not altered by orchidopexy, orchidectomy should be considered for a school-aged boy with a unilateral intra-abdominal testis when the contralateral testis is of normal size and position.

Orchidopexy is best performed between the ages of 15 months and 4 years. The child is admitted to hospital for day care and the groin explored under general anaesthesia. The testis and spermatic cord are dissected free from any inguinal hernia and a herniotomy done. A gonad lying in the inguinal canal can usually be mobilised to reach the lower scrotum and is placed in a pouch between the scrotal skin and the external spermatic fascia. An impalpable testis, identified at laparoscopy, can be exposed through a higher incision in the iliac fossa but may require staged surgery or even microvascular techniques of reanastomosis of the scrotal vessels to achieve a satisfactory position.

Swellings in the groin

Indirect inguinal hernias

EPIDEMIOLOGY

One in 50 boys is affected but only 1 in 500 girls. Presentation is most commonly in the first year of life, with an increased incidence in infants born prematurely. Irreducibility is common in infants and results in intestinal obstruction and testicular infarction from pressure-occlusion of the testicular vessels as they pass through the inguinal canal. An ovary is the commonest content of an irreducible hernia in a girl and may also infarct.

CLINICAL FEATURES

Symptoms

The mother is usually the first to notice a lump in the groin which disappears when the child is at rest and reappears on activity or straining, e.g. when crying. Mothers are percipient about their children and even if there is nothing obvious on the first examination, the report of an intermittent lump should be taken seriously. Strangulation causes pain and distress and, if bowel is involved, there are features of intestinal obstruction.

Physical findings

The swelling is visible and palpable in the medial part of the inguinal region and extends downwards towards or into the ipsilateral scrotum or labium. In boys it is not possible to get above the swelling to palpate the normal spermatic cord.

DIAGNOSIS

Alternative diagnoses are:

- encysted hydrocele of the cord (see below)
- undescended testis
- femoral or direct inguinal hernia – both are rare.

MANAGEMENT

A *reducible* inguinal hernia is an indication for early elective herniotomy, delayed only by an intercurrent infection or, in premature infants, until a weight of 2 kg has been reached. The operation is usually performed as a day admission and under general anaesthesia. Through a small skin-crease incision, overlying the site of the internal inguinal ring, the hernial sac is isolated and its neck transfixed. Muscle repair is not indicated for indirect inguinal hernia.

An *irreducible* inguinal hernia requires emergency treatment, initially with analgesia and sedation followed by gentle compression of the lump (taxis) which achieves safe reduction of the hernial contents in nine out of 10 infants. Once reduced, the infant remains under observation in hospital until herniotomy is done – best carried out 1 or 2 days later, when oedema of the spermatic cord has subsided. A persistently tender, irreducible hernia requires an emergency operation, which carries an increased risk of both complications and recurrence. Unless there is delay in treatment, it is very rare to encounter gangrenous bowel, but testicular ischaemia and consequent atrophy are complications in up to 10% of boys after a strangulated inguinal hernia.

Hydrocele

AETIOLOGY

The processus vaginalis is usually patent and this has a bearing on treatment. Hydroceles are common in the first year of life and frequently resolve spontaneously as the processus vaginalis obliterates. An encysted hydrocele occurs when the processus vaginalis closes but the cells lining the processus continue to secrete liquid.

There is a painless collection of clear fluid between the two layers of the tunica vaginalis of the testis.

CLINICAL FEATURES

Symptoms

The mother or, in older children, the patient reports an increase in size of one-half of the scrotum; the swelling may vary in size, often enlarging after a warm bath.

Physical findings

The swelling fluctuates. It is possible to palpate the normal spermatic cord above the scrotal swelling. In children, both hydroceles and inguinal hernias transilluminate so that this test is not helpful in differentiating one from the other. In a hydrocele, transillumination demonstrates the position and size of the testis and can identify the very rare testicular tumour or a collection of blood (haematocele) neither of which transmits light.

MANAGEMENT

After the age of 2 years, and if the hydrocele is definitely persistent, an elective operation is recommended to ligate the patent processus vaginalis at the internal inguinal ring. The operation is very similar to that for an indirect inguinal hernia. Scrotal operations, recommended for adult hydroceles (Ch. 32), are not appropriate in children because the processus vaginalis remains open and encysted fluid accumulates in the scrotum.

Torsion of the testis

This condition occurs from prenatal to late adult life with a peak incidence at puberty.

AETIOLOGY

The abnormality is a high position of the tunica vaginalis so that the testicle and distal spermatic cord are suspended free within it. The abnormality has been likened to the clapper of a bell, particularly in that the testis has a horizontal lie. The condition is usually bilateral.

PATHOLOGICAL FEATURES

Prenatal torsion produces an atrophic testicle along the line of descent and the testis is absent. After birth, twisting is usually associated with gangrene which, if untreated, also leads to atrophy.

CLINICAL FEATURES

Perinatal torsion presents with a painless blue swelling in the scrotum, several sizes larger than the contralateral testis.

In childhood or later in life, torsion causes severe pain which is felt in the scrotum and ipsilateral lower abdomen and is usually associated with vomiting. The pain in the iliac fossa may divert attention from the scrotum and so delay the diagnosis. There may have been previous minor episodes.

Physical findings

The cord is shortened and the cremasteric reflex abolished. Palpation of the epididymis and testis is usually impossible because of extreme tenderness. On standing, the contralateral testis has a horizontal lie.

The alternative diagnoses are:

- acute epididymo-orchitis, which is relatively rare and usually associated with urinary tract infection but only likely to cause diagnostic difficulty in the older patient
- torsion of a testicular appendage (hydatid of Morgagni) which is not usually associated with vomiting; the tenderness may be localised to the upper pole of the testis.

MANAGEMENT

In a suspected torsion, urgent exploration is mandatory because within a few hours the ischaemia becomes irreversible and there is no reliable investigation to exclude the diagnosis. The spermatic cord is untwisted and both gonads are fixed by removing the tunica vaginalis and suturing the organs to the inner aspect of the scrotal septum. If a twisted appendage is found, the other side is also explored because the same abnormality is common on the other side. Acute epididymo-orchitis is treated with antibiotics, but exploration on a suspected diagnosis of torsion does no harm and allows for bacteriological sampling of the fluid from the associated inflammatory hydrocele.

Idiopathic scrotal oedema

This is a form of urticarial angio-oedema of uncertain cause.

CLINICAL FEATURES

Symptoms

Bright red oedema of the scrotum or hemiscrotum is observed which often extends posteriorly towards the anus or anteriorly over the inguinal region. The appearance resembles an acute cellulitic infection with some irritation and tenderness. However, fever and pain are not present and antibiotics do not influence the course.

Physical findings

The normal testis is obscured by the intense oedema of the scrotal wall which brilliantly transilluminates.

MANAGEMENT

Reassurance of the often alarmed parents is necessary. There is resolution over 24–48 hours. Antihistamines can speed spontaneous resolution.

The prepuce

Circumcision

For many thousands of years, removal of the prepuce – circumcision – has been part of a religious rite or initiation ceremony, but medical indications for circumcision are uncommon and the role of the operation in reducing the adult incidence of carcinoma of the penis or cervix is not proven. In those with an abnormal urinary tract, such as vesicoureteric reflux, it is possible that circumcision may reduce the risk of urinary tract infections and stone formation.

Forceful and traumatic retraction of the infant's prepuce should be avoided because there are normal preputial adhesions in infancy which separate spontaneously over the first 3 years of life. From this age on, the boy may be encouraged to retract his own prepuce at bath-time. Inability fully to retract the prepuce occurs in over 10% of boys of preschool age but is not an indication for operation because the healthy prepuce will stretch later in childhood. Less than 1% of boys at puberty are unable to retract the prepuce fully and, in these, circumcision should be carefully considered but not necessarily undertaken.

The only absolute medical indications for circumcision are:

- phimosis
- a previous episode of paraphimosis.

The medical contraindications to circumcision are given in Table 35.5.

Phimosis

The opening in the prepuce is narrowed by fibrosis, usually the result of trauma or infection, and the flow

Table 35.5
Contraindications to circumcision

Condition	Reason
Ammoniacal dermatitis	Caused by acid urine not phimosis
	Circumcision may lead to a meatal ulcer
Hypospadias	Prepuce needed for repair
Micropenis or buried penis	Does not help; specialist management required
Ambiguous genitalia	Full investigation necessary to establish gender; skin may be required for reconstruction
Bleeding disorder	Risk of bleeding
Intercurrent infection	Infective complications at suture line

of urine from the external meatus is obstructed. The condition is extremely rare in the first 2 years of life.

CLINICAL FEATURES

Marked ballooning of the prepuce occurs on micturition (some degree of ballooning is normal in the first 2–3 years of life).

The tissue around the preputial meatus is white, fibrotic and thickened. The foreskin cannot be retracted. Inflammation of the skin may be present.

Paraphimosis

In this condition, a prepuce, which is usually fibrotic, retracts and is trapped in the coronal sulcus of the penile shaft, causing oedema of the glans. There is rarely interference with the blood supply.

CLINICAL FEATURES

There may have been previous episodes. There is some pain and swelling of the penile tip which is embarrassing rather than threatening in terms of ischaemia.

The glans is oedematous and sometimes inflamed. The constricting band is usually obvious

MANAGEMENT

The oedema is reduced by firm compression by the hands of the operator over a period of some minutes and manual reduction is then usually possible. Injection of hyaluronidase may assist the dissolution of the swelling. When the oedema and any inflammation have resolved, circumcision is done.

Balanoposthitis

This recurrent subpreputial inflammation with a wide variety of organisms is now relatively uncommon because of improved hygiene. However, where cleanliness is lacking or impossible because the foreskin is fibrotic so that retraction cannot be achieved, it may occur.

CLINICAL FEATURES

Features are of recurrent acute inflammation occasionally with the formation of pus. The episodes make the condition worse by increasing fibrosis.

MANAGEMENT

Once the inflammation has been brought under control, if necessary by slitting the dorsal aspect of the prepuce to release pus (although this is rare), formal circumcision is done.

Redundant prepuce

Occasionally, even though the penis is of normal size, the prepuce is long and redundant and a cause of embarrassment. Circumcision is then indicated.

OPERATION

In children, the operation is done under general anaesthesia with a caudal block for postoperative control of pain. Unipolar diathermy for haemostasis is contraindicated because the passage of the current down the penis to a distant common earth can damage the corpora cavernosa. Bipolar diathermy is allowable. Absorbable sutures are used and the delicate exposed glans protected after the operation by application of soft paraffin or chloramphenicol ointment.

COMPLICATIONS

These include:

- bleeding
- infection
- meatal ulceration progressing to meatal stenosis
- urethral fistula from a suture which has penetrated the penile urethra
- removal of too much penile skin – which leaves the shaft covered by scrotal and abdominal wall skin and causes sexual problems later
- recurrent phimosis which can occur if too little inner preputial skin is excised.

Hypospadias

This condition is a developmental result of failure of closure of the ventral urethra at a varying level in the perineum and along the penile shaft. Minor degrees of hypospadias, with the urethral meatus in the coronal sulcus (see below), are quite common – affecting 1 in 200 boys. The more severe form, with a penoscrotal meatus and severe chordee, is found in 1 in 1000 boys.

PATHOLOGICAL FEATURES

The condition is characterised by:

- a short urethra
- a ventral defect of the prepuce
- ventral curvature of the penis – chordee.

The degrees of hypospadias range from a minor meatal problem through to a perineal meatus.

CLINICAL FEATURES

Identification of the anomaly at birth is important in order to advise the parents that circumcision is contra-indicated (see Table 35.5) and that reconstructive surgery will be required. As the problem is distal to the bladder sphincter, continence is normal but there may be social problems of micturition in the standing position.

MANAGEMENT

This is best done in a specialist centre during infancy, before the child is psychologically aware of his genitalia and before he is expected to stand to micturate. For the more severe anomalies such as ambiguous genitalia and indeterminate gender, investigations are indicated soon after birth.

FURTHER READING

Ashcraft K (2000) *Pediatric Surgery*, 3rd edn. Philadelphia: WB Saunders.

Jones P, Woodward A (1986) *Clinical Paediatric Surgery*, 3rd edn. Oxford: Blackwell Scientific Publications.

MacMahon RA (1991) *An Aid to Paediatric Surgery*, 2nd edn. London: Churchill Livingstone.

Nixon H, O'Donnel B (1992) *Essentials of Paediatric Surgery*, 4th edn. Oxford: Butterworth–Heinemann.

36 Ophthalmology in clinical surgery

The eye is a unique organ because of its specialised function. All ocular structures are transparent to allow the optimal focusing of light; therefore with appropriate instruments the ophthalmologist can examine all structures anterior to and including the retina without resort to special investigations. Moreover, the eye is a window to view the progression of systemic disease.

Evaluation

The non-ophthalmologist can make an effective assessment of the nature and urgency of a presentation from a detailed history and the use of equipment readily available in any A&E department or general practice rooms. Important symptoms and their possible causes are summarised in Table 36.1. Further details are given in the section on common symptoms and signs

Table 36.1
Common symptoms of eye disease

Nature	Type	Causes
Pain	Ocular	Uveitis, acute glaucoma
	Referred	Paranasal sinuses
		Dental
Visual disturbances	Distortion	Disease of the macula
	Photophobia	Uveitis, corneal disease
	Halos	Acute glaucoma
	Flashing lights	Vitreous, retinal disorders, migraines
	Floaters	Vitreous and retinal disorders
	Acute visual loss	Retinal, vascular and neurological disorders
	Chronic visual loss	Media opacities, retinal, vascular and neurological disorders
	Night blindness	Retinal degeneration
Double vision (diplopia)	Monocular	Cataract, refractive errors
	Binocular	Extraocular muscle imbalance
Altered appearance of the eye	Red eye	Conjunctivitis, episcleritis, uveitis, acute glaucoma
	Proptosis	Infection, thyroid eye disease
Lacrimal disturbance	Dry eye	Primary lacrimal failure, Sjögren's syndrome
	Watery eye	Ocular irritation, blocked tear drainage

Table 36.2
Ophthalmic examination

Property examined	Tests and abnormal findings
Visual acuity (normal = 6/6)	At distance
	At near
	Pinhole
Visual field	Confrontation
	Formal perimetry
Ocular motility	Misalignment of visual axis
	Nystagmus
Pupil responses	Unequal size (aniscoria)
	Distortion
	Reaction to light
	Response to accommodation
	Afferent pupil defect
Examination of anterior eye by torch	Redness
	Clarity
	Depth of anterior chamber
Digital tonometry	Subjective hardness of globe
Fundoscopy	Red reflex
	Optic disc
	Macula
	Retinal vessels

Table 36.3
Visual acuity

Snellen acuity	Patient can see	At distance
6/60	60 m line	6 m
6/36	36 m line	6 m
6/24	24 m line	6 m
6/18	18 m line	6 m
6/12	12 m line	6 m
6/9	9 m line	6 m
6/6	6 m line	6 m
6/5	5 m line	6 m
CF	To count fingers	x m
HM	To detect hand movement	x m
PL	To perceive light	

below. Important features of the examination are in Table 36.2.

Physical findings

The items of equipment needed are:

- a Snellen chart of letters that reduce in size so that, to the eye, a letter from the 6 m line seen at 6 m should have the same size as a letter from the 3 m line seen at 3 m
- bright pen torch
- ophthalmoscope.

Visual acuity

Distance. The Snellen chart at 6 m is most commonly used with the subject wearing full refractive correction and bright ambient illumination. Interpretation of results is in Table 36.3.

Pinhole acuity. If a refractive error is uncorrected, confusion may occur as to whether an intrinsic ocular disorder is responsible for poor vision. A pinhole only allows a central ray of light to pass through, undeviated by the eye's focusing system onto the macula area, and therefore the significance of any refractive error is reduced. Pinhole acuity should be measured whenever the acuity, with or without refractive correction, is worse than 6/9.

Movements of the optic globe

The ability to move both globes is tested by asking the eye to follow the examiner's finger while keeping the head steady. The muscles responsible are illustrated in Fig. 36.1.

Visual fields

The *confrontation method* detects significant neurological field defects:

1. Test distance is approximately 1 m.
2. One eye each of both subject and examiner is occluded, which allows comparison between the visual field of the examiner and that of the subject.
3. The subject is asked to steadily fixate the examiner's eye.
4. Finger counting is carried out in all four quadrants: superotemporal, inferotemporal, inferonasal and

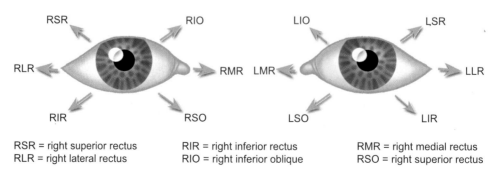

RSR = right superior rectus	RIR = right inferior rectus	RMR = right medial rectus
RLR = right lateral rectus	RIO = right inferior oblique	RSO = right superior rectus

Fig 36.1 **Movements of the optic globe and muscles responsible.**

superonasal; it is best to present, in a static way, one, two or five fingers.

A *hemifield comparison* is also made:

1. Similar distance to the confrontation method.
2. Controlled fixation of the subject on the examiner's eye.
3. The examiner holds up both hands on either side of the vertical meridian and the subject is asked to compare their appearance – is one clearer or darker than the other?

Finally a *kinetic field test* is done using a white hat pin with a 5 mm diameter head. The pin is moved in from the periphery and the point of first detection recorded.

Simple rules of interpretation of the acuity and field tests. The 'rules of the road' are:

- Lesions anterior to the chiasm affect one eye only.
- Lesions at the chiasm most usually damage the crossing nasal fibres from each eye to give rise to defects in the temporal fields on each side (bitemporal field defect).
- Lesions posterior to the chiasm damage the temporal fibres from one eye plus the nasal fibres from the other eye to cause a homonymous defect (i.e. a defect affecting one visual hemifield).

Pupil responses

Abnormal responses are summarised in Table 36.4. Aniscoria is a visible difference between the pupil size of the two eyes, which may be a normal variation in about 20% of the population.

Light reflex (parasympathetic) and pupillary constriction. If all pathways are intact, a light shone on one eye constricts both pupils at an equal rate and to a similar degree (direct and consensual reflexes).

Table 36.4
Abnormal responses of the pupil

Abnormality	Common causes
Dilatation	IIIrd nerve lesion
	Adie pupil (see text)
	Mydriatic drugs
	Iris trauma
Constriction	Horner's sydrome
	Argyll-Robertson pupil
	Drugs – opiates, cholinergic
Failure of accommodation/ convergence	Extrapyramidal disease (Parkinsonism)
	Pineal tumour
Marcus-Gunn pupil	Damage to the anterior visual pathway up to the lateral geniculate nucleus

Pupillary examination

- Observe the sizes of both pupils in bright and dim illumination.
- Shine a bright torch in one eye and observe the direct and consensual light responses.
- A bright light shone into one eye will cause pupillary constriction in both eyes (direct and consensual light response).
- If there is an afferent defect on one side, e.g. a unilateral optic nerve lesion, then the stimulus to constriction when the light is shone on the affected side will be reduced relative to the response when light is shone on the normal side.
- When the torch is swung quickly across from one eye to the other, dwelling for a second on each, the pupils will dilate when light is shone on the affected side – paradoxical dilatation. The side that dilates is described as having a relative afferent pupillary defect (RAPD). This is a very important sign to elicit in the diagnosis of visual loss.
- Ask for fixation first on a distant target, then present a near target at 15 cm and observe the change in pupillary size as fixation is changed.

Ocular motility

The visual acuity must be known to ensure that the subject can fixate on the targets presented.

- Observe for misalignment of the visual axis in the primary position which can easily be determined by shining a torch light from 30 cm away and checking that the reflections on the corneas are central.
- Is nystagmus (involuntary oscillations of the eyes) present?
- Ask the subject to follow a target in the six different directions of gaze.
- Is there a complaint of double vision?

Appearance of external eye

Ocular adnexae (eyelids and periocular area):

- skin lesions
- inflammation
- position of the eyelids – ptosis, retraction, entropion (lid margin turning in) or ectropion (lid margin turning out)
- proptosis
- General facial examination.

Redness of the eye and opacities in the cornea can be easily seen with a torch. Fluorescein staining reveals areas of the cornea denuded of epithelium as bright yellow fluorescence when viewed with a blue light.

Digital tonometry

Intraocular pressure is measured most accurately at the slit lamp using a tonometer. An estimate can be made by digital tonometry. The eyes are palpated through the closed lids over the upper outer angle of the orbit where the tarsal plate is thinnest. A hard eye indicates high pressure and, in the presence of a red, painful eye, may indicate acute angle closure glaucoma.

Fundoscopy

The hand-held direct ophthalmoscope provides a magnified (×15) monocular view of the transparent ocular media (cornea, aqueous, lens and vitreous) and the fundus. The field of view is small, especially through an undilated pupil. The technique should be practised until one can reliably see the optic disc through an undilated pupil, as this forms an important part of any neurological examination.

Technical points are as follows:

- Use a darkened room, ideally with both pupils dilated – common dilators (mydriatics) in adults are an anticholinergic (tropicamide 1%) and a sympathomimetic (phenylephrine 2.5%).
- Use your right eye to examine the subject's right eye and your left for the subject's left, which allows the instrument to be as close as possible to the subject's pupil.
- The green/red free filter in the ophthalmoscope renders the blood vessels black and easier to view.
- An ophthalmoscope contains a sequential arrangement of lenses of different dioptric power which can be rotated clockwise (plus, convergent or black) to compensate for long sight, and anticlockwise (minus, divergent or red) to compensate for short sight in the subject.
- Refractive errors in the observer which normally require glasses can be dealt with by adjusting the diopter strength in the instrument or by keeping on corrective glasses.

The examination starts with the ophthalmoscope 30 cm away from the subject and with observation of the red reflex which fills the pupil. It is formed by the reflection of light from the retina and is impaired by any obstruction to that light, e.g. cataract, vitreous haemorrhage. It proceeds inwards towards the pupil, with one hand on the patient's forehead if necessary to steady the view.

Features to note are the:

- optic disc
- macula
- retinal vessels.

The optic disc. The margin should be sharp and the colour pink. A cup:disc ratio (the cup is the cavity in the centre of the disc) of 0.3 or less is considered normal but a large cup or asymmetry between the two eyes should lead to referral to an ophthalmologist for further investigation.

The macula is the area of central vision which lies approximately 1.5 disc diameters temporal to the optic disc. To examine it, the beam may be directed temporally or the subject asked to look directly at the light. The appearance is of a darker hue than the rest of the retina with a central glistening area which is the reflection from the fovea – the centre of the macula.

Retinal vessels. Note the following:

- size: arteriolar attenuation (hypertension), venous dilatation (venous obstruction)
- crossing over of the retinal vessels for signs of nipping (hypertension)
- microaneurysms (diabetes).

Ophthalmic injuries

Fortunately most injuries to the eye seen in the A&E department are superficial. The question is if and when an ophthalmologist needs to be involved:

- *Any damage to the lacrimal drainage system which involves the lid margin.* An ophthalmologist repairs the lid margin to avoid notching and also determines any damage to lacrimal drainage
- *Blunt injuries.* A history of considerable force e.g. a punch, can cause effects to be transmitted deeper into the eye and should lead to consideration of referral.
- *Blow-out fractures of the orbit.* After a serious blunt injury with or without a fracture to the orbit, a thorough ocular examination is needed. A fracture can cause entrapment of extraocular muscles which can lead to double vision. Sinking of the globe into an enlarged orbital space created by the fracture has the same effect.
- *Suspicion of penetrating injury or possible foreign body.* See below.
- *Chemical injury.* Caustic chemicals, especially alkalis, can penetrate deeply.
- *Contact lenses.* Those with pain, with an acute red eye or with a visible corneal lesion have a high risk of keratitis and must be referred urgently.
- *Recent intraocular procedures.* Trauma may cause breakdown of fragile wounds and infection may have a delayed presentation.
- *Painful orbital swelling (orbital cellulitis).* Particularly in a child, this is an ocular emergency, as the build-up of orbital pressure may compress the optic nerve.

General approach to ocular injuries

CLINICAL FEATURES

Complaints and history

Special attention should be paid to:

- Force applied, including direction and velocity

- what was being done at the time of injury – hammering, other industrial activities
- possible nature of a foreign body.

Physical findings

Be suspicious of an undetected injury, particularly when other and apparently more obvious injuries are present either in the eye or elsewhere; an eyelid laceration can hide a perforated globe which may in turn hide an intracranial injury.

INVESTIGATION

Imaging is most important when a foreign body is suspected: orbital X-ray, CT or (if a non-radio-opaque object is suspected) ultrasound.

GENERAL MANAGEMENT

In a possible penetrating injury, check anti-tetanus status and bring up to date if necessary. (See below for individual injuries.)

Burns

AETIOLOGY

Thermal injury in civilian practice is usually from molten metal. Rapid, reflex eye closure helps to limit the damage. Ultraviolet damage can arise from arc welding, sunlamps or prolonged exposure to high intensities of natural light (skiing or exploring without wearing sunglasses). Chemical burns are usually alkaline and have the devastating effect of saponifying lipid barriers so that they may penetrate into the anterior chamber.

CLINICAL FEATURES

Extensive oedema in the lids and face after a thermal burn may limit examination and give the false impression of blindness until the swelling subsides. Repeated assessment is necessary.

MANAGEMENT

Involvement of the lids in a thermal burn necessitates referral to an ophthalmologist for lid repair. Ultraviolet burns are usually self-limiting and require reassurance that vision will return, as well as pain relief. Chemical burns need copious irrigation with normal saline until the pH is returned to normal and urgent referral to an ophthalmologist to deal with the potentially serious consequences of corneal melt, glaucoma, cataract and phthisis (opacification and atrophy of the cornea).

Orbital injuries

More than 30% of patients who suffer blunt maxillo-facial trauma sustain ocular injuries, of which 3% are blinding. More than 90% of the serious injuries result from midfacial, supraorbital and frontal sinus fractures; 4% of these cause optic nerve damage.

CLINICAL FEATURES

History

The history must include specific questions about:

- diplopia
- decreased vision
- sensory deficits in the skin of the face
- trismus
- rhinorrhoea, which may indicate a compound fracture of the skull.

Physical findings

- Visual acuity
- Pupil and pupil reactions
- Specific features – enophthalmos, subcutaneous emphysema, malar flattening and palpable steps in the orbital rim.

All orbital injuries should be examined by an ophthalmologist and other specialities – maxillofacial and ear, nose and throat should be involved as appropriate. CT is essential to plan surgical repair.

Blunt ocular trauma

Moderate to severe injury may cause immediate or delayed consequences (Table 36.5). All should be seen by an ophthalmologist.

Table 36.5
Effects of blunt trauma

Structure involved	Immediate injury	Delayed injury
Conjunctiva	Subconjunctival haemorrhage	
Cornea	Abrasion Penetrating laceration	
Iris	Rupture, dialysis hyphaema	
Ciliary body and angle	Recession, dialysis	Glaucoma Hyoptony
Vitreous	Haemorrhage	
Retina	Commotio (bruising)	Macula hole
	Macula haemorrhage or hole	Retinal detachment
	Retinal tears/dialysis	Subretinal membranes
Choroid	Rupture	Subretinal membranes
Sclera	Rupture	
Optic nerve	Avulsion	Traumatic neuropathy

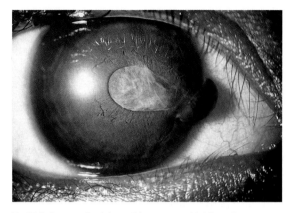

Fig 36.2 **Penetrating injury of the cornea with iris prolapse causing pupillary distortion, and secondary cataract.**

Penetrating or perforating ocular injury

A *penetrating* injury causes cutting or tearing of the walls of the eye. A *perforating* injury is the same but with the addition of entry and exit wounds.

CLINICAL FEATURES
Suspicious appearances are:

- decreased visual acuity
- soft eye
- distorted iris – a teardrop-shaped pupil points towards the site of the perforation (Fig. 36.2).

Ocular foreign bodies

Most foreign bodies in the eye are either trapped underneath the upper lid (subtarsal) or stuck in the cornea.

MANAGEMENT
Removal is by the following steps:

1. Ensure the eye is well anaesthetised with several drops of topical preparation (e.g. amethocaine).
2. Sit the patient at the slit lamp with a warning to keep the forehead firmly against the head rest.
3. Instil a drop of fluorescein to stain any corneal abrasions and enhance the presence of subtarsal foreign bodies and errant contact lenses.
4. Search systematically with a request to look up, down, right and left; evert the upper eyelid for the same purpose and remove foreign bodies with a sterile cotton bud.
5. For a foreign body firmly embedded in the cornea, the ideal instrument is a blunt-tipped burr which can also effectively remove a rust ring which forms around some metallic objects; if this is not available,

a green 18-gauge needle can be used with caution to scrape away the affected tissue.
6. A 1-week course of topical antibiotic (e.g. chloramphenicol) is perscribed.

Intraocular foreign bodies

AETIOLOGY
These may be the consequence of a penetrating injury and can lodge in any part of the eye. Retrieval of foreign bodies from the eye, especially once they have lodged in the posterior segment, requires complicated vitrectomy techniques, often including lens extraction if a traumatic cataract has formed.

Common symptoms of ocular disease

Visual loss may be a reduction of visual acuity (blurring) or loss of visual field, either partial or total. Unilateral symptoms are likely to be from lesions of the eye or the optic nerve; bilateral lesions commonly result from defects proximal to the optic chiasm – in the brain. A summary of visual loss is given in Table 36.6.

Table 36.6
Causes of visual loss

Time course	Painful		Painless
	red eye	white eye	(white eye)
Acute	Trauma	AION – arteriric	CRAO/ BRAO CRVO/BRVO AION – non-arteritic
Subacute	Uveitis Orbital inflammation Acute glaucoma	Optic neuritis	Wet ARMID Uveitis
Gradual	Uveitis	Optic nerve compression	Wet ARMD Dry ARMD Cataract Optic nerve compression Uveitis Chronic glaucoma
Transient	Migraine AION – arteritic		Migraine TIA (amaurosis fugax) Syncope

Acute loss of acuity

Retinal artery occlusion

AETIOLOGY

Central retinal artery occlusion (CRAO) typically occurs in the optic nerve just behind the visible optic nerve head and is usually the result of thrombosis of atheromatous vessels. Rarer causes include vasculitis. Branch retinal artery occlusions (BRAOs) are embolic – 80% are derived from atheromatous disease of the carotid arteries (Ch. 28). Less commonly, calcified material or cholesterol emboli may be released from other sites (valve vegetations and thrombi of cardiac origin). Emboli be visualised on fundoscopy as white or yellow particles lodged at the bifurcations of the retinal arterioles.

CLINICAL FEATURES

History

When the central retinal artery is involved, the visual loss is sudden and painless, and the deficit is profound, with acuity usually reduced to counting fingers (CF) or worse, with even a loss of light perception.

Physical findings

There is a relative afferent pupillary defect (impaired direct light response) and fundoscopy shows a pale retina with attenuated vessels and a cherry red spot at the macula (Fig. 36.3). In around 20%, the macula receives its blood supply from the choroidal circulation via the cilioretinal artery and, in these, a small island of central vision with variable retention of visual acuity may remain but the loss of visual field greatly reduces function.

BRAO affects vision and depends on the location of the vessel affected. A visual field defect (scotoma) results and, when the macula is involved, there is reduced visual acuity.

CRAO typically occurs in the optic nerve just behind the visible nerve head. The usual cause is atheroma

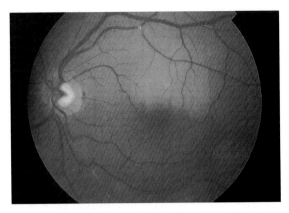

Fig 36.4 **Superior temporal branch retinal artery occlusion (see calcific embolus lodged in bifurcation of retinal arterioles), with cloudy retinal swelling in the distribution of the occluded vessel.**

with embolus of a fibrinoplatelet accumulation (Ch. 28) in the carotid bifurcation from atrial fibrillation or myocardial infarction, but vasculitis (including giant cell arteritis) is another possibility. Cardiovascular assessment is required. Emboli can be seen on fundoscopy as white or yellow particles lodged at bifurcations of the retinal arterioles (Fig. 36.4).

Retinal vein occlusion

AETIOLOGY

Diabetes, hypertension and hyperlipidaemia are the major systemic risk factors.

HISTORY AND FINDINGS

Retinal vein occlusion is experienced as a sudden loss of vision of variable severity. Fundoscopy reveals dilated veins, haemorrhages and cotton wool spots in the affected area of retina. It may be localised, as in branch retinal vein occlusions, or involve all 4 retinal quadrants, often with disc swelling in a case of central retinal vein occlusion.

Anterior ischaemic optic neuropathy (AION)

AETIOLOGY

This is an infarction of the optic nerve head because of closure of the ciliary arteries of supply. Two groups of patients can be identified: 50–60 year-olds and those aged >70 years. Members of the first group are likely to have cardiovascular risk factors such as hypertension and angina caused by thrombosis of atheromatous ciliary vessels. The over-70s may have arteritic AION usually as a result of giant cell arteritis.

CLINICAL FEATURES

A sudden visual loss results which may be total or

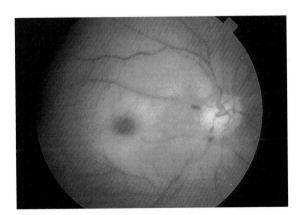

Fig 36.3 **Central retinal artery occlusion with 'cherry red spot'.**

altitudinal (where the inferior or, less commonly, the superior half of the visual field in one eye is lost). Arteritic AION may be accompanied by symptoms of malaise, weight loss, muscle pains and stiffness, temporal headache and scalp tenderness, and jaw or tongue claudication.

There is a relative afferent pupillary defect, and on fundoscopy a pale swollen optic disc is seen.

MANAGEMENT

All patients with acute visual loss thought to be of vascular origin should have an urgent ESR and immediate referral to an ophthalmologist if arteritis is suspected, because high-dose systemic steroids may be required to prevent blindness from involvement of the other eye (see also transient visual loss – 'stuttering amaurosis').

Subacute loss of acuity
Optic neuritis

Visual loss which develops over a few hours to 2–3 days and which is associated with ocular pain exacerbated by ocular movements is characteristic of optic and retrobulbar neuritis. Loss of acuity is variable but may fall to an absence of perception of light. Colour desaturation (i.e. where colours are seen as being washed out) is a prominent early feature. There is a relative afferent pupillary defect and, if the intraocular optic nerve is affected, a swollen optic disc may be noted (Fig. 36.5). More commonly the inflammation is located in the intraorbital optic nerve and fundoscopy is normal (the patient sees nothing and the doctor sees nothing) and the condition is called retrobulbar neuritis.

The most common cause is multiple sclerosis (MS) and patients tend therefore to be in the 20–40 year age group and are more often female. Enquiry and examination for symptoms or signs of previous neurological disease are essential and, if positive, confirm the diagnosis of multiple sclerosis.

Referral to an ophthalmologist or neurologist is indicated for confirmation of eye involvement.

INVESTIGATION AND MANAGEMENT

In isolated optic or retrobulbar neuritis, the extent of investigation is controversial; some recommend a full work-up for signs of subclinical lesions elsewhere in order to make the diagnosis of MS; others feel that, because there is as yet no effective intervention, a 'wait and see' attitude should be adopted. Treatment is also controversial; intravenous corticosteroids shorten the acute episode but have no effect on the extent of final visual recovery or the ultimate prognosis.

PROGNOSIS

After visual loss, some degree of recovery always occurs. In most instances, this takes 4–6 weeks and is full or nearly so although a small residual (subjective) defect is often present. Residual signs include red desaturation, a relative afferent pupillary defect and optic disc pallor, most marked temporally, which develops over a few weeks after an acute episode.

Optic nerve compression

Lesions within the orbit may compress the optic nerve, especially if located posteriorly at the orbital apex where nerves and vessels are crowded together. Many such lesions result in gradual visual loss (see below). Orbital inflammatory disease may, however, be rapidly progressive and is an ophthalmic emergency.

CLINICAL FEATURES

Symptoms include pain; visual loss and diplopia. Signs are of:

- reduced acuity
- loss of colour vision
- a relative afferent pupillary defect
- proptosis
- conjunctival chemosis.

Reduction of ocular motility results either from IIIrd, IVth or VIth cranial nerve damage at the orbital apex or from direct mechanical restriction of ocular movement.

Causes to be considered are:

- acute dysthyroid eye disease (Graves' disease, Ch. 31)
- orbital cellulitis (usually secondary to paranasal sinus disease)
- orbital pseudotumour (idiopathic orbital inflammation which mimics an orbital tumour).

Insidious, unilateral painless visual loss results from compression of the optic nerve by a slowly growing

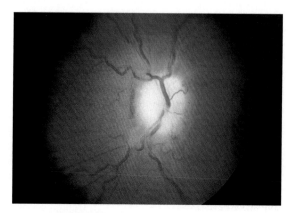

Fig 36.5 **Papilloedema in benign intracranial hypertension**

tumour. In children, this is most commonly an optic nerve glioma, sometimes seen as part of type 1 neuro-fibromatosis. In adults, usually women of 30–50 years, meningioma of the optic nerve sheath or sphenoid wing is most likely.

Fundoscopy shows a pale and sometimes swollen optic disc. Tortuous abnormal vessels on the optic disc (retinochoroidal shunts) are typical of a meningioma.

MANAGEMENT

The patient should be referred to an ophthalmologist who, when the diagnosis is suspected, can confirm it by CT.

Surgical excision often results in damage to the optic nerve. It may be indicated if the sight is already badly damaged and the tumour can be excised whole; otherwise radiotherapy or observation alone may be preferred.

Gradual loss of acuity

Gradual diminution of visual acuity is one of the most common complaints encountered in ophthalmology. By contrast, gradual loss of visual field is rarely noticed by the patient – hence the need for screening programmes for chronic glaucoma). Field loss is usually noticed by the patient only when very extensive, because acuity is retained until late in the disease process.

Cataract

A cataract is an opacity of the lens that interferes with vision. Most are of the idiopathic senile type and the prevalence increases with age (Fig. 36.6). There are many other causes, which include:

- trauma
- uveitis
- metabolic disorders (e.g. diabetes mellitus)
- congenital.

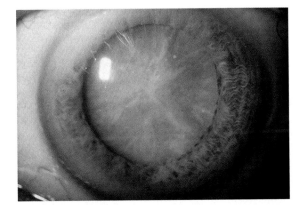

Fig 36.6 **Mature cataract**

In those regions of the world where therapeutic resources are unavailable, cataract is the most common cause of blindness (visual acuity less than 3/60 in the better eye).

CLINICAL FEATURES

Symptoms include:

- gradual blurring of vision
- change in the prescription for glasses – 'second sight' is the myopic shift induced by nuclear sclerotic cataract that may allow a presbyopic patient to resume reading without reading glasses after previously having required them
- glare – most marked in bright sunlight or when confronted by oncoming headlights while driving at night; this is typical of a posterior subcapsular cataract.

A cataract is most easily identified as an obstruction of the red reflex during direct ophthalmoscopy.

MANAGEMENT

Treatment is by extraction and insertion of a prosthetic intraocular lens once the reduction of vision is sufficient to interfere with lifestyle. The threshold for an operation is affected by individual visual needs – driving, occupation and hobbies. Cataract surgery is usually done as a day case under local anaesthesia.

Macular degeneration

Age-related macular degeneration (ARMD) is the most common cause of blindness (visual acuity of less than 3/60 in the better eye) in the developed world. It affects central vision, with reduction of visual acuity and sometimes formation of a central scotoma. There are two types: dry and wet.

Dry ARMD

This is an idiopathic gradual loss of photoreceptors and retinal pigment epithelium in the macular area. Visual loss is gradual, mild to moderate in severity and usually symmetrical. Fundoscopy shows areas of hypo- and hyperpigmentation in the macula. There is no treatment to arrest the process. Management is directed at low vision optical aids to make the most of what residual function exists. Registration as partially sighted or blind is valuable to increase help from community sources.

Wet ARMD

Wet ARMD is again bilateral, although symptoms usually begin on one side. It tends to occur in a younger age group and results from the development of subretinal neovascular complexes 'membranes' that leak serum and may bleed into the retina. Presentation is with

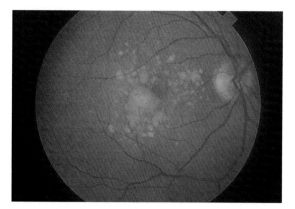

Fig 36.7 **Age related macular degeneration, with large confluent soft drusen.** This eye is at high risk of visual loss from subretinal neovascularisation.

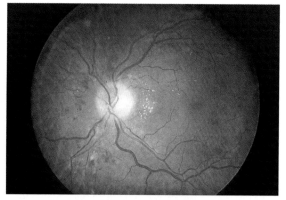

Fig 36.9 **Grade III hypertensive retinopathy.** The concentration of exudates and haemorrhages in the peripapillary area is typical.

more rapid onset of poor vision; central scotomas and visual distortion (see below) are common. Fundoscopy (Fig. 36.7) may reveal dark red blood or grey subretinal elevation (fluid or subretinal membrane) at the macula. Immediate referral to an ophthalmologist is required because sometimes laser photocoagulation can be used to seal off leaking vessels. However, in the majority this is not possible, because such treatment would involve the fovea with a dramatic fall in visual acuity.

Macular oedema

This is a complication of many ophthalmic disorders rather than a separate entity. It is the major cause of visual loss in diabetic retinopathy (Fig. 36.8) and may be the presenting feature of diabetes in non-insulin-dependent disease. Macular oedema may also be seen in ARMD, in uveitis, in hypertensive retinopathy (Fig. 36.9) and as a complication of intraocular surgery.

Another relatively common cause is central serous retinopathy, an idiopathic condition seen most commonly in men of between 20 and 40 years. Choroidal

fluid leaks through the macula to produce a localised serous retinal detachment, which presents with subacute onset of blurring and distortion of the central field characterised by micropsia (objects appear smaller than they actually are). In the great majority, the condition resolves spontaneously, usually within 1–6 months after the onset of symptoms.

Macular hole

This is another degenerative disorder caused by an abnormal vitreoretinal adhesion at the macula which pulls out a circular fragment of retina. The disease is most common in women in the sixth and seventh decades of life and remains unilateral in 90%.

The presenting features are similar to ARMD: visual distortion, reduced acuity and a central scotoma. On fundoscopy a small (approximately one-third of a disc diameter) red round hole over the fovea may be seen. Referral is indicated because surgical intervention may be possible.

Retinal dystrophies

Gradual visual loss in younger patients is uncommon and always warrants ophthalmic referral. There are a large number of hereditary and sporadic retinal and macular dystrophies that may present with reduced acuity and colour or night blindness. Often the gross ophthalmoscopic appearance is normal. Retinitis pigmentosa is the best known of these conditions, in which case the classic mid-peripheral bone spicule pigmentation may indicate the diagnosis (Fig. 36.10).

Uveitis

Acute uveitis (inflammation of the uvea, i.e. the iris [iritis], ciliary body [iridocyclitis] and choroid [posterior

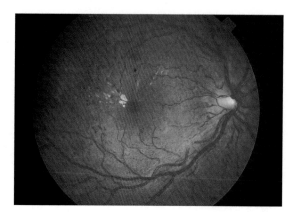

Fig 36.8 **Diabetic maculopathy**

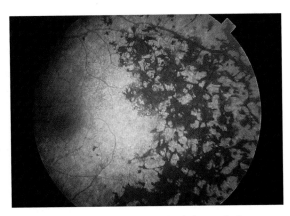

Fig 36.10 **Retinitis pigmentosa with classic bone spicule pigmentation.**

uveitis or choroiditis]) usually presents with a red eye and pain, but chronic uveitis may solely cause visual loss. Chronic anterior uveitis in juvenile rheumatoid arthritis may be asymptomatic until the complications of secondary cataract and (often untreatable) cystoid macular oedema develop. For this reason all children with arthritis must have ophthalmic screening at regular intervals. Intermediate and posterior uveitis may cause gradual or subacute loss of vision, as a result of direct retinal damage, macular oedema or vitritis. The last of these causes a diffuse vitreous haze or floaters (below). All these conditions need specialist assessment. Management is often difficult but may involve periocular or systemic corticosteroids.

Transient loss of vision

This is a common symptom. A careful history often allows benign conditions to be separated from more serious disease.

Syncope

A fall in systemic blood pressure from whatever cause (e.g. Stokes–Adams attack, vasovagal response) can result in, initially, the loss of colour vision (grey-out) and subsequently all vision (blackout), as blood flow to the eyes decreases. Symptoms are bilateral and are usually accompanied by faintness, dizziness and palpitations. Provided blood flow is restored, (e.g. by falling to a horizontal position), both general recovery and visual recovery are likely to be swift.

Migraine

This is a familial vasospastic disorder that may cause neurological symptoms as result of intracranial ischaemia, followed in most instances by headache which is thought to the consequence of compensatory vasodilatation. The most common neurological disturbance is visual, with the appearance of jagged concentric black lines across the visual field (fortification spectra) and a scintillating scotoma. These sensations may last for around 30 minutes and are followed by a severe throbbing ipsilateral hemicranial headache, with debilitation and nausea present for up to several hours, followed by resolution and sleep.

Migraine is, however, protean in its manifestations and should be included in the differential diagnosis of any transient visual disturbance, even without headache, especially in younger patients. If it occurs for the first time after the age of 50, the diagnosis must only be made with caution because an intracranial disorder is possible.

Transient ischaemic attack (TIA)

(See also Ch. 28)

A TIA that involves the central retinal artery circulation has the same cause as a branch retinal arterial occlusion, and those that affect the cerebral hemispheres (embolic disease) usually relate to atheroma of the extra cranial carotid arteries. The patient typically describes a grey curtain moving horizontally upwards or downwards across the vision of one eye; it comes on over seconds to minutes and is likely to resolve within a few minutes (amaurosis fugax – fleeting blindness). Fundoscopy is often normal; alternatively white/yellow refractile emboli may be visible within the retinal arterioles.

The significance of amaurosis fugax is the increased risk of retinal arterial occlusion or stroke. A full assessment is required (Ch. 28). A related symptom is stuttering amaurosis (repeated uniocular episodes of visual loss) which is an occasional precursor of permanent loss of vision in giant cell arteritis.

Loss of visual field

Vascular

All the vascular causes of acute loss of acuity described above can instead present as visual field loss, e.g. with a scotoma in BRAO and BRVO or altitudinal field loss in AION.

Retinal detachment

Retinal detachment may be traumatic; however, in the majority of cases it is spontaneous. The condition is more common in myopes.

PATHOLOGICAL AND PATHOPHYSIOLOGICAL FEATURES

Changes in the vitreous gel (posterior vitreous

detachment) tear a hole in the retina and allow fluid from the vitreous to enter the subretinal space. The neurosensory retina separates from the underlying retinal pigment epithelium so that the detached area of retina ceases to function. The field defect which results mirrors the site of the detachment. Thus a superior detachment (the most common and rapidly progressive) produces an inferior field defect, often referred to as a 'shadow in the vision'.

CLINICAL FEATURES

Symptoms

Visual acuity is retained until the macula is involved in the detachment. This is important, because detachment that is surgically repaired when the macula is still on has a much better visual prognosis than when it has come off. Other symptoms include floaters and photopsia.

Physical findings

The index of suspicion must be high – a myopic spectacle correction is easily detected by looking through the spectacle lens when objects appear smaller. A monocular field defect is usually present. Visual acuity varies depending on the state of the macula. If more than a quarter of the retina has detached, there is a relative afferent pupillary defect. If the detachment is small, fundoscopy may be normal, especially if a direct ophthalmoscope through an undilated pupil is used, because this only affords a small field of view and the detachment starts peripherally. The detachment is seen as an elevated convex area of grey retina which moves with ocular movement and has a wrinkled surface (Fig. 36.11). Therefore, if the history is suggestive but the examination appears to be normal, a referral to an ophthalmologist for more detailed examination is important.

MANAGEMENT

If central vision is retained at the time of diagnosis,

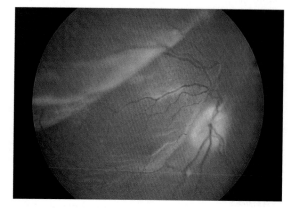

Fig 36.11 **Retinal detachment.**

detachment is an emergency. Treatment is surgical. It involves either an external approach with the application of a compressive buckle to the outside of the eye, or an internal approach with removal of the vitreous gel and usually internal tamponade with gas or liquid. The aim is to oppose the detached retina and underlying retinal pigment epithelium. Adhesion between the two layers is then achieved by the use of laser or cryoprobe to create inflammation and scarring.

Neurological disease

Lesions of the retrochiasmal optic pathway result in bilateral hemianopic visual field defects that obey the vertical meridian. They can usually be easily detected by confrontation testing and need to be specifically sought in all instances of apparently monocular visual loss because a positive finding excludes ocular disease as the cause. In a left homonymous hemianopia, for example, the nasal field defect in the right eye may not be noticed by the patient because it is overlapped by the retained nasal field of the left eye, and it may therefore present as an isolated loss of the left temporal visual field.

Acute-onset hemianopic visual field loss is very likely to be cerebrovascular in origin – 80% of cases are caused by emboli from the extracranial carotid arteries (Ch. 28). Cardiovascular risk factors should therefore be assessed.

Visual distortion

Visual distortion (metamorphopsia) is a symptom restricted to disorders that affect the macula, because it occurs when macular photoreceptors are displaced relative to each other. The result is disruption of macular representation of objects in the central visual field. Altered image size and reduced visual acuity result from the same mechanism.

The formation of a fine membranous scar (epiretinal membrane) may cause metamorphopsia, as may macular oedema from any cause. Detection is easy by asking the patient to examine an Amsler chart, which is a regular grid of black lines on a white background, looked at from a distance of 30 cm. Typically there is distortion and blurring of the grid; the location of worst distortion corresponds to the site of the macular lesion. If an Amsler chart is not available, any straight high-contrast edge will suffice; for example, ask if the edges of a window frame appear straight and regular.

Photopsia

Photopsia refers to the sensation of light arising from non-light stimuli. It may happen when mechanical forces act on the retina: either due to an external force (trauma), which can be transient, or secondary to intraocular disease which is more persistent. The two major intraocular causes are posterior vitreous detachment (see below) and retinal detachment. Mechanical photopsia are unformed visual sensations, as distinct from the structured visual sensations experienced as a result of neurological disease, such as migraine.

Floaters

Floaters are dark spots seen moving in the visual field. They result from opacities with the vitreous gel.

Posterior vitreous detachment

The vitreous gel is increasingly being recognised as a complex structure, rather than simply an amorphous gel, which is reflected in the degenerative changes that are seen in all eyes with increasing age. The gel collapses into itself in places to form denser spots and areas of increased gel mobility, which are of themselves sometimes large enough to be seen as floaters but are not of clinical significance. With further degeneration, a hole may form in the posterior face of the vitreous gel and allow liquefied gel to pass into the retrohyaloid space between the vitreous body and the retina. Movement of the eye will allow the liquid gel to strip the remaining vitreous away from the retina, to create a posterior vitreous detachment (PVD).

Clinical features

There is a sudden onset of floaters, often large and sometimes circular or horseshoe-shaped, which are described as being like a hair or cobweb which obscures vision. Photopsia may precede or accompany the PVD because of traction on the retina from vitreous attachments when the gel collapses. The incidence of PVD increases with age. In the majority, it is annoying but not dangerous. Around 5%, however, sustain damage in the form of a retinal tear as a result of traction. Retinal tears are the major cause of retinal detachments because they allow the liquified vitreous to pass through the hole into the subretinal space and detach it from the retinal pigment epithelium.

Retinal tear

Clinical features of a retinal tear include floaters, persistent photopsia, especially during daylight; and impairment of visual acuity. On fundoscopy the PVD and any vitreous blood may be seen as small, mobile, black spots in the red reflex. However, they are difficult to visualise with the direct ophthalmoscope.

Management of suspected PVD or a retinal tear involves same-day referral to an ophthalmologist for thorough dilated indirect ophthalmoscopy. There is no treatment for the PVD but retinal tears need laser or cryotherapy to seal the tear. Retinal detachments, if present, usually require operation.

Uveitis

Chronic uveitis may lead to organised inflammatory reaction in the vitreous gel which the patient perceives as floaters. The eye is usually painless and the condition may have been present for some time. Visual loss is common, but in intermediate uveitis/pars planitis, where only the region of the ciliary body is inflamed, visual acuity is usually normal, unless and until cystoid macular oedema supervenes.

Ocular pain

While many disorders of the external eye produce ocular discomfort (e.g. conjunctivitis and blepharitis), ocular pain is less common and may indicate serious disease. It is helpful to elicit whether the pain feels superficial (sharp, scratching) or deep (aching, gnawing), as this sometimes distinguishes corneal from intraocular disease. Headache associated with visual symptoms occurs in migraine and giant cell arteritis and should not be confused with ocular pain.

Corneal Abrasion

Defects in the corneal epithelium expose the underlying plexus of naked nerve terminals, cause severe, sharp pain, worse with lid movement, and excessive lacrimation.

CLINICAL FEATURES

History

There is usually a clear history of trauma to the eye, although sometimes an abrasion results from breakdown of healed epithelium at a site of previous injury. This recurrent corneal erosion syndrome has a characteristic pattern of pain on first opening the eyes in the morning, often preceded by short-lived episodes of pain and redness in the few days before the actual abrasion occurs.

Physical findings

Abrasions are identified with guttae fluoroscein 2% stain and cobalt blue light, which shows the abrasion as a fluorescent yellow-green area on the cornea (Fig. 36.12). A blue cover to a penlight torch can be used where a slit lamp is unavailable.

MANAGEMENT

Treatment is with broad-spectrum antibiotic eye drops (usually chloramphenicol 0.5% four times a day for 5 days) with cycloplegia and/or an eye patch if the pain is severe. Simple abrasions do not need referral to an ophthalmologist but should be reviewed after 48 hours to confirm a reduction in size.

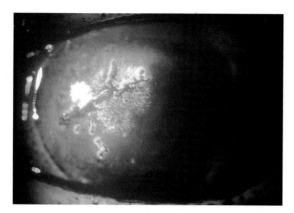

Fig 36.12 **Fluoroscein-stained dendritic ulcer (herpes simplex).**

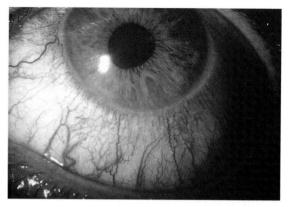

Fig 36.14 **Acute anterior uveitis (iritis) with ciliary flush and a fixed, oval pupil.**

Keratitis

Inflammation of the cornea is usually infective. Herpes virus infections and related immune keratitis are considered below. Most bacteria require a pre-existing epithelial defect to allow them to breach the cornea, but an important exception is *Neisseria gonorrhoeae*; hence the importance of urgent, aggressive treatment in ophthalmia neonatorum. Predisposing conditions include contact lenses (Fig. 36.13), a dry eye and the long-term use of eyedrops that contain corticosteroids. Pain can be severe, partly because of the frequently present secondary uveitis. Suspected keratitis always needs urgent ophthalmic review.

Uveitis

Acute anterior uveitis is inflammation of the iris and/or ciliary body. If only the iris is affected, it may also be called iritis or, if the ciliary body is also involved, iridocyclitis.

AETIOLOGY

There are many possible causes of acute anterior uveitis, including a number of associations with systemic disorders (e.g. HLA B27-positive arthropathies and sarcoidosis). However, in the majority a specific cause is not found.

CLINICAL FEATURES

History

Pain is usually moderate to severe, with photophobia, lacrimation and often reduction of vision.

Physical findings

Redness is most marked around the cornea and typically has a violaceous hue. Miosis is present and the pupil may also be fixed and irregular because of the formation of adhesions between the iris and the lens – posterior synechiae (Fig. 36.14). In most, the condition is unilateral and should be strongly suspected in the presence of any unilateral, persistently painful red eye.

MANAGEMENT

Uveitis always needs specialist attention, even when the diagnosis appears clear, because the efficacy of treatment and the presence of complications such as glaucoma can only be assessed by slit-lamp examination.

Glaucoma

Glaucoma refers to a group of conditions characterised by retinal nerve fibre damage, resulting in typical optic disc changes (cupping) and visual field loss. There are many subgroups, most importantly acute and chronic glaucoma. Raised intraocular pressure is always a feature of acute glaucoma, and most cases of chronic glaucoma also have raised pressure, but to a lesser degree.

Pain is not a feature of chronic open-angle glaucoma (the most common form). However, in acute angle closure glaucoma, the intraocular pressure rises rapidly and dramatically.

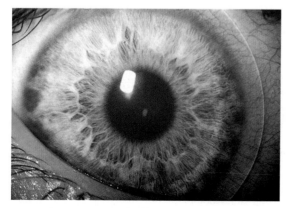

Fig 36.13 **Soft contact lens in-situ.**

CLINICAL FEATURES (ACUTE GLAUCOMA)

The condition is more common with increasing age and is found predominantly in hyperopes (whose glasses magnify images seen through the lens).

The patient is likely to be in distress, with severe pain, blurring of vision and halos around lights. The eye is intensely injected, with clouding of the cornea and a fixed semi-dilated pupil.

MANAGEMENT

Immediate referral is necessary and urgent treatment to lower the pressure is required to alleviate the pain and prevent permanent visual loss due to pressure-induced damage to the retinal nerve fibres as they enter the optic nerve.

Episcleritis and scleritis

Both these conditions present with a red eye and are immune-mediated.

Episcleritis

This is a self-limiting condition characterised by ocular discomfort and diffuse or localised redness. It is rarely associated with underlying disease. If symptoms warrant treatment, a course of oral NSAIDs is usually effective.

Scleritis

This is a much more serious condition that may lead to visual loss. Severe, constant, deep ocular pain is usual. The redness may be localised, diffuse or absent in posterior scleritis. An early ophthalmic opinion should be sought. Scleritis may occur in isolation, but is frequently associated with connective tissue disorders (systemic lupus erythematous, rheumatoid arthritis) or vasculitis.

Orbital pain

It is often very difficult clinically to differentiate between orbital and ocular pain because many describe ocular pain as coming from behind the eye and orbital pain is poorly localised. Orbital inflammatory conditions often lead to secondary scleritis, which adds ocular pain to the clinical picture. Associated features that lead to the suspicion of orbital disease as a cause include proptosis, ophthalmoplegia, ptosis and loss of corneal sensation.

Orbital inflammation

Orbital cellulitis, dysthyroid eye disease and orbital pseudotumour have all been mentioned in the section on visual loss. The severity of pain, inflammatory signs or mass effects vary greatly.

Orbital malignancy

Benign tumours generally present with painless gradual visual loss. Malignant tumours, however, often cause pain as a result of rapid growth or neuronal invasion which is often associated with proptosis and ophthalmoplegia.

Proptosis

The orbit is bounded by bone on all sides except anteriorly. In consequence, any increase in the volume of the intra-orbital contents can only be decompressed by forward displacement of the globe, which causes protrusion of the orbital contents – proptosis. Exophthalmos is a synonymous term but is usually reserved for dysthyroid eye disease (the most common cause of proptosis).

AETIOLOGY

If a lesion is located within the retrobulbar space, bounded by the extraocular muscles (intraconal), the displacement is axial; if extraconal, then non-axial proptosis with mechanical strabismus ensues.

Dysthyroid eye disease and idiopathic orbital inflammation (orbital pseudotumour), orbital cellulitis and other rarer conditions such as tuberculosis and sarcoidosis cause proptosis by increasing the volume of intra-orbital fat and connective tissue and also of the extraocular muscles. Tumours of all kinds may cause proptosis, as may vascular disease such as orbital varices and haemorrhagic cysts. Pulsatile proptosis with enlargement and injection of the conjunctival vessels is the hallmark of a carotid-cavernous fistula, in which the orbital venous system becomes arterialised as a result of an abnormal communication between the ophthalmic artery and the cavernous venous sinus.

Epiphora

Epiphora (excessive production or running of tears) can be difficult to evaluate. Probably the most important question is: Is it constant? Tearing which is only intermittent is unlikely to result from lacrimal duct obstruction. The diagnosis is best approached by considering where the problem may lie:

Lacrimal gland. Primary excessive activity of the gland is very rare but may be seen after injury to the facial nerve with aberrant regeneration (gustatory sweating). Secondary or reflex overactivity is much more common and can result from any painful ocular condition. For

665

Ophthalmology in clinical surgery

chronic epiphora, it is important to examine the lids and ocular surface for irritant lesions such as trichiasis (inturned lashes) and entropion (inturned lid).

Eyelid. Tears are moved across the eye from the superolateral lacrimal gland to the inferomedial drainage system by a combination of gravity and the pumping action of the lids. The mechanism can be upset by ectropion, where the lid margin turns outwards away from the eye; tears spill over the edge and normal apposition of the lacrimal punctum to the pool of tears in the medial canthus is prevented. Even without ectropion, a flaccid orbicularis muscle can impair the pump mechanism and epiphora follows. These changes are commonly involutional in the elderly but may also be seen following VIIth nerve palsy or scarring of the skin of the lower lid.

Lacrimal duct. From the lacrimal punctae, tears drain via the canaliculi to the lacrimal sac and thence to the nasolacrimal duct and the nose. Obstruction at any of these sites causes epiphora. Congenital nasolacrimal duct obstruction affects up to 20% of neonates, but canalisation is completed spontaneously in over 90% by 1 year. When canalisation remains incomplete after this time, probing of the duct usually easily completes the process. In adults, stenosis may be traumatic, infective (e.g. herpes simplex conjunctivitis) or, most commonly, a gradual involutional change. Often a simple explanation of the cause of symptoms is all that is required; however, some require surgery, which can now often be done under local anaesthesia.

Ptosis

This is an abnormally low position of the upper eyelid which may be an isolated problem or the presenting feature of serious neurological disease. It should be differentiated from pseudo-ptosis which is a relative ptosis because of contralateral lid retraction. Ptosis is best considered initially in relation to age.

Congenital ptosis

Infantile ptosis may be the outcome of any of the causes described under subsequent headings but is most commonly dystrophic with abnormal development of the levator muscle. The condition may be unilateral or bilateral. Any significant ptosis in a young child must be urgently referred because of the risk of occlusion amblyopia. This is a failure of development of the cerebral pathways serving the affected eye due to lack of stimulation during the critical period of development. The eye is physically normal, but processing of visual data from the eye is impaired. In infants, a week of occlusion may be significant; once a child is over around 7 years of age, amblyopia can neither develop nor be treated if present.

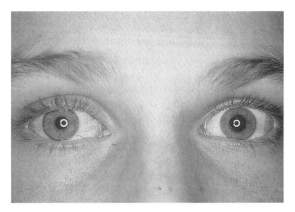

Fig 36.15 **Right Horners syndrome: pupillary miosis and partial ptosis**

Adult

Ptosis in adults of working age may result from a number of causes (Fig. 36.15). Diplopia, rapid muscle fatigue and muscle weakness should be specifically asked for and may indicate myasthenia gravis. The pupil and ocular movements must be examined specifically to look for the down-and-out globe position of a palsy of the IIIrd nerve. In those with diabetes or hypertension, this is commonly a microvascular event; however, the presence of a dilated pupil raises the possibility of an expanding aneurysm of the posterior communicating artery which must be investigated by neuro-imaging. Trauma may also cause ptosis which may not become evident until the initial swelling has died down.

The elderly

The adult causes described above still apply in later life, but the most common cause is degeneration of the attachment of the levator palpebrae superioris aponeurosis to the lid. Five per cent of cataract operations precipitate the condition. There is a drooping upper lid with thin skin and the horizontal upper lid crease lies high up on the lid. In spontaneous instances, the condition is bilateral but not necessarily symmetrical. Operation to reattach the aponeurosis to the lid tissues can be performed under local anaesthetic.

Anisocoria

This is a visible difference in pupil size between the two eyes. It may be a normal variant (seen in 20% of the population at some time, pupillary reactions are normal) or pathological. Pathological causes can be divided into parasympathetic, tonic and sympathetic neurological causes and local (ocular) causes.

Parasympathetic palsy

The innervation of the sphincter pupillae muscle which is responsible for constriction of the pupil (miosis) is by preganglionic parasympathetic axons in the oculomotor nerve with synapses in the ciliary ganglion. The fibres run on the superior border of the nerve within the subarachnoid space where they are vulnerable to compression by intracranial lesions, but their superficial location close to the pial blood vessels spares them from many vascular problems. In consequence, there are two types of lesion: a fixed dilated pupil (surgical), and a pupil-sparing IIIrd (medical)

Tonic (Adie) pupil

This is a dilated pupil with light-near dissociation – the pupil fails to constrict in response to light but does so to accommodation (the near triad of miosis, accommodation and convergence). The lesion is in the ciliary ganglion and is thought to result from viral inflammation. The usual occurrence is in a young woman who presents with blurring of vision because of paresis of accommodation. Regeneration of the nerve results in the return of near vision, but the pupillary responses remain abnormal with a tonic (slow onset and prolonged duration) miosis, initially in response to near vision but which becomes permanent over a few years. The Holmes–Adie syndrome is the association of the tonic pupil with absence of deep tendon reflexes (e.g. knee jerks) which is seen in 60%.

Sympathetic palsy

Horner's syndrome is the triad of partial ptosis, miosis and anhidrosis resulting from a lesion in the sympathetic nervous system. The neuronal pathway originates with preganglionic fibres in the hypothalamus, and then passes through the brain stem and spinal cord to exit in the anterior roots. They ascend in the sympathetic chain and synapse in the superior cervical ganglion. Postganglionic fibres pass from the ganglion into the cervical sympathetic chain and perivascular plexi, and thence to the orbit. Ptosis and miosis are seen in all cases, whereas anhidrosis is absent with lesions affecting postganglionic fibres.

Horner's syndrome may be transient, as in neuralgic migraine/cluster headache where the neuronal plexus around the carotid artery is affected. Otherwise the lesion may be anywhere along the pathway described, and careful examination supplemented by imaging and pharmacological testing may be required to determine the cause. It is particularly important to examine the root of the neck for evidence of apical lung carcinoma (Pancoast's syndrome).

Local causes

Iris damage may result in an unreactive or poorly reactive pupil. Causes include trauma, uveitis and previous acute glaucoma. Pharmacological mydriasis is the commonest cause of an isolated unreactive pupil;

usually the history is apparent, but unprescribed use of eye drops and accidental exposure to mydriatics (e.g. occupational) can also occur. Atropine, the longest-acting mydriatic, has a half-life of around 10 days.

The red eye

Red eye is an initially daunting matter when encountered in primary care or in the A&E department. Provided, however, that the main features of pain and visual symptoms are elicited, the most likely cause can be rapidly narrowed down as shown in Table 36.7 or, where features are suggestive of more serious disease, Table 36.8.

Painless red eye with normal vision

This can only be a subconjunctival haemorrhage (SCH), caused by the rupture of an episcleral vein and producing a bright red area over the sclera. Usually it is localised and the remaining conjunctiva can be seen to be normal; sometimes the bleed is more extensive and swollen conjunctiva can prolapse through the palpebral fissure.

SCHs may be caused by trauma, coughing and straining, clotting disorders or, rarely, hypertension.

Table 36.7
Causes of red eye

	Painless	Uncomfortable	Painful
Normal vision	Subconjunctival haemorrhage	Blepharitis Conjunctivitis Episcleritis	Anterior uveitis Scleritis Keratitis (peri-peripheral)
Reduced vision	None		Anterior uveitis Posterior scleritis Central keratitis

Table 36.8
Features of the dangerous red eye

Symptoms	Physical features
Severe pain	Reduced visual acuity
Photophobia	Unilateral
Loss of vision	Intense injection
Progression of symptoms	Corneal opacity, epithelial defect
	Proptosis
	Loss of red reflex
At risk individual	Neonate
	Immunocompromise
	Contact lenses

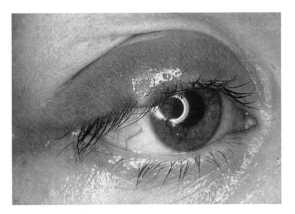

Fig 36.16 **Acute infection of eyelash follicle (stye).**

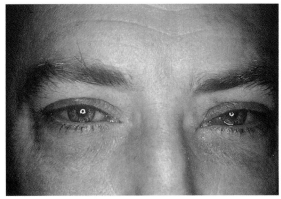

Fig 36.17 **Viral conjunctivitis.** The lids are swollen, the eyes are watering, red and uncomfortable.

However, the great majority are spontaneous. Treatment is not required and the discoloration fades over 1–2 weeks.

Uncomfortable red eye with normal vision

Blepharitis
This is a chronic inflammatory condition that affects the margins of the eyelid. It may be greasy (seborrhoeic) or crusting (staphylococcal), or a combination of both and can be associated with recurrent styes (Fig. 36.16). The complaint is of ocular discomfort, dryness and crusting of the lashes, most noticeable in the mornings. Conjunctival inflammation is mainly inferior from contact with the inflamed lower lid. The cornea may also become involved with a secondary conjunctivitis; more severe cases such as this are often seen in patients with acne rosacea. The main treatment is lid hygiene, with mechanical cleaning of the lid margin using a cotton bud dipped in a dilute solution of baby shampoo or bicarbonate of soda. Artificial tear drops may relieve the symptoms of dryness and topical antibiotics are also often used initially to eliminate or reduce the load of staphylococci.

Conjunctivitis
This is a typical cause of ocular discomfort rather than pain which often begins in one eye but becomes bilateral within a few days. Discharge is an important feature: purulent or mucopurulent is typical in bacterial infection; mucopurulent in chlamydial; mucoid in allergic; and watery in viral (Fig. 36.17). In chlamydial and viral disease, there may be enlarged tender preauricular lymph nodes and conjunctival follicles, visible as small 'rice grains' in the inferior conjunctival fornices.

Bacterial conjunctivitis is commonly caused by Gram-positive cocci, especially *Staphylococcus aureus*. Treatment is with a broad-spectrum topical antibiotic

(e.g. chloramphenicol). Swabs are only required if the infection has not resolved within a week of effective treatment or if the condition is initially severe.

Viral conjunctivitis does not need treatment other than explanation and reassurance because the majority are mild and self-limiting. Adenovirus infection may be more severe and the small proportion that develop keratitis (with visual disturbance and increased pain) require referral for specialist management.

Chlamydial infection is most commonly a sexually transmitted disease in young adults and may be chronic and unilateral. Referral to an ophthalmologist is required for confirmation of the diagnosis. The genitourinary physician is also involved, in order to screen for sexual contacts for *Chlamydia* and other sexually transmitted diseases. Treatment includes topical and systemic tetracyclines.

Episcleritis
See above.

Painful red eyes

Scleritis, keratitis and uveitis are all possible causes of a painful red eye and they are discussed above in the sections on visual loss, floaters and ocular pain.

Diseases with ophthalmic manifestations

Acquired immune deficiency disease (AIDS)

AIDS has a number of ophthalmic manifestations which include primary effects, opportunistic infections and tumours. Only the most important and common are described here. The high incidence of such conditions requires a low threshold for referral for specialist assessment.

Primary effects

The HIV virus has a direct effect on the retinal vasculature, causing cotton wool spots and micro-aneurysms that are very similar to those seen in background diabetic retinopathy. The lesions are asymptomatic and resolve spontaneously and treatment is not required.

Secondary infections

Viral infections

Cytomegalovirus is the major sight-threatening disease in HIV infection and is one of the defining illnesses of AIDS, rarely seen when the CD4 T-cell count is greater than 50 cells/µL. It occurs in approximately 30% of those with AIDS. The virus causes retinitis with white areas of retinal necrosis and often extensive retinal haemorrhages (the pizza-pie appearance). Vision is lost as result of direct retinal destruction, secondary retinal detachment and optic nerve involvement. Treatment initially involves intravenous antiviral agents (ganciclovir is the current first-line agent), with long-term prophylaxis against relapses using intravenous oral or intraocular antivirals.

The recent introduction of protease inhibitors as part of highly active anti-retroviral therapy (HAART) has allowed lymphocyte counts to rise in some patients such that long-term prophylaxis can be safely stopped.

Herpes simplex and varicella zoster viruses may both cause acute fulminating retinitis with a very high incidence of visual loss.

Bacterial infections

Staphylococcal blepharitis. This is common in those with HIV (see also 'Red eye').

Mycobacteria. Tuberculous choroiditis may occur in isolation or with signs of disease elsewhere.

Syphilis has an increased frequency in AIDS because of both the impaired immunity and the common means of transmission. Uveitis is the most common manifestation.

Fungal infections

Candida albicans causes a severe uveitis. It is seen most often in i.v. drug abusers who use unsterilised needles (see Ch. 9).

Cryptococcus neoformans can cause choroiditis in patients with cryptococcal meningitis.

Protozoal infections

Toxoplasmosis. In the immunocompromised, the condition differs from that in the healthy population by being acquired rather than congenital. Creamy white patches on the retina indicate active retinitis and cause visual loss by direct retinal damage. Systemic anti-protozoals are required to control the initial infection and are continued at a lower maintenance dose for life.

Tumours

Kaposi's sarcoma

This is commonly seen on the eyelids or conjunctiva of AIDS patients and is a defining disease. It forms a dark red (or purple) firm mass which may be flat or elevated. In the conjunctiva it may resemble a subconjunctival haemorrhage and must be considered as a possible diagnosis for any such lesion, especially in the young, if persistent for more than 2 weeks.

Rheumatoid Arthritis (RA)

Keratoconjunctivitis sicca

This is an example of secondary Sjögren's syndrome, with autoimmune destruction of the lacrimal gland which leads to dry eye symptoms and corneal damage. The symptoms are distressing and often difficult to control. The mainstay of treatment is ocular lubrication with artificial tears and ointments.

Scleritis and keratitis

Scleritis in rheumatoid arthritis may be acute with a painful red eye and requires urgent referral to an ophthalmologist. More commonly it is chronic, without overt inflammation, eventual scleral thinning and exposure of the underlying uvea (scleromalacia perforans) which renders the eye vulnerable to minor trauma. There is no treatment for scleromalacia.

Keratitis may be painful, with a corneal opacity and conjunctival injection, or a painless non-inflammatory corneal melt which can result in corneal perforation. Again, urgent referral is required.

Iatrogenic disease

Long-term steroid treatment (10 mg/day for more than a year) in rheumatoid arthritis commonly results in cataract.

Systemic lupus erythematosus

Systemic lupus erythematosus (SLE), like RA, may be associated with secondary Sjögren's syndrome. Small vessel vasculitis may present as scleritis, corneal melt, retinal vasculitis or optic nerve infarction. Involvement of the retina or optic nerve implies central nervous system disease, which is a poor prognostic sign. Specialist management, with close liaison between ophthalmologist and rheumatologist, is required.

Iatrogenic disease

Steroids are commonly used in SLE and, as with RA, may cause cataract. Chloroquine and hydroxychloroquine are used, particularly in the control of skin rashes, and can cause a Bull's eye maculopathy which results in irreversible loss of visual acuity. The risk of this complication is much higher with chloroquine than with hydroxychloroquine and is dose-related. Typical dosage regimens of hydroxychloroquine are very unlikely to cause problems within 5 years of beginning the drug. Patients starting on these drugs have a baseline examination by the ophthalmologist and are then warned to stop the drug and seek ophthalmic advice should they subsequently develop visual symptoms or detect a scotoma when viewing an Amsler chart.

Giant cell arteritis (GCA)

This multisystem disorder results in inflammation of medium-sized arteries with an internal elastic lamina. The terms 'temporal' and 'cranial' arteritis refer to the high incidence of involvement of the arteries of the head; systemic disease results in polmyalgia rheumatica. GCA is a disease of the elderly and is very rarely seen in those less than 50 years old.

CLINICAL FEATURES

Symptoms

The patient experiences temporal headache, scalp tenderness (even necrosis) and jaw and tongue claudication. General malaise is usual and muscle stiffness and pain may be present. Visual loss is a late event.

Physical findings

There are often no signs to support the diagnosis. Scalp tenderness on the side of the headache may be present. The ipsilateral superficial temporal artery just in front of the ear may be enlarged, tortuous, tender and non-pulsatile.

INVESTIGATION

The erythrocyte sedimentation rate must be measured urgently. In GCA it is usually elevated; a normal value does not rule out the diagnosis but makes it much less likely. Temporal artery biopsy is usually done to confirm the diagnosis; the histological findings are unaffected by up to a week of steroid treatment, so that treatment of suspected GCA must not be delayed until biopsy can be done.

MANAGEMENT

Hospital admission is usual. Prednisolone 1 mg/kg per day is started orally immediately. If visual loss has occurred or appears imminent ('stuttering amaurosis'), then a loading dose of intravenous hydrocortisone or methyl-prednisolone may be given. The dose is then gradually reduced according to the clinical response. The majority feel subjectively much better after 48 hours of treatment. Steroid therapy is continued at a low dose for around 2 years.

Systemic candidiasis

Candida albicans is a yeast-like organism commonly present as a commensal in the healthy gastrointestinal tract. Candidiasis only becomes an ophthalmic problem in immunocompromised patients (e.g. immunosuppressive drugs, haematological malignancy and AIDS) or if the organism is directly introduced into the bloodstream by non-sterile i.v. drug abuse or the presence of indwelling catheters (especially hyperalimentation following bowel surgery).

CLINICAL FEATURES

Blurring of vision and floaters are the main symptoms of candidal endophthalmitis, i.e. infective inflammation of the internal eye, including the vitreous gel. Pain with a red eye is less common.

Vitreous inflammation may obscure the fundus; when it can be seen, there are usually elevated white chorioretinal lesions. The vitritis is frequently organised into localised masses – the string of pearls. In the minority who have associated anterior uveitis, there is ciliary injection and clouding of the anterior chamber.

INVESTIGATION AND MANAGEMENT

Blood cultures for candidaemia and appropriate investigations to assess immunocompromise are required. Ocular investigation involves anterior chamber and vitreous sampling.

Treatment is with vitrectomy and intravitreal and systemic antifungal agents.

Embolic disease

Emboli which affect the visual system are most commonly thromboemboli and arise from the carotid vessels in the neck. Emboli may result in transient visual loss (transient ischaemic attack), sudden permanent visual loss (retinal artery occlusion) or visual field loss (cerebrovascular disease) (see common symptoms above and Ch. 28).

Graves' disease

This is an autoimmune disorder characterised by the production of thyroid-stimulating immunoglobulins (TSIs) that cause thyrotoxicosis (Ch. 31). Orbital inflammation – dysthyroid eye disease or thyroid ophthalmopathy – is associated. The orbital condition may occasionally be seen in those who are both clinically and biochemically euthyroid.

PATHOLOGICAL FEATURES

Soft tissue inflammation in and around the orbits may produce exophthalmos. If severe, the orbital contents, including the optic nerve, may be compressed and vision is lost. After 1–2 years, the acute inflammation tends to subside, leaving residual chronic fibrotic changes in the orbit and ocular muscles.

CLINICAL FEATURES

Symptoms

In the acute phase, sore red eyes are common. A 'staring eyes' appearance may cause self-embarrassment. When the condition is severe, reduced vision may be noted and, rarely, diplopia.

If the condition reaches a chronic phase, diplopia and the poor appearance of exophthalmos and lid retraction are the main complaints.

Physical findings

In acute disease the conjunctiva are injected, particularly over the insertions of the horizontal recti muscles at 3 and 6 o'clock. There may be chemosis and swelling of the lids. Orbital inflammation increases the volume of the orbit which pushes the globes forwards and can lead to exposure of the cornea; downward movement of the upper eyelids may be restricted so that the sclera above the superior limbus becomes visible. This is most obvious in changing from up-gaze to down-gaze – lid lag. Lid retraction contributes to the staring look and to corneal exposure (Fig. 36.18).

Nerve compression may reduce visual acuity, impair colour vision and cause a relative afferent pupillary defect.

In the later stages, inflammation is replaced by fibrosis which restricts ocular movements. Any direction of squint may occur, but most commonly the limitations are in up-gaze and lateral gaze.

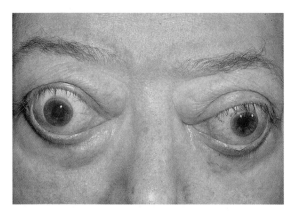

Fig 36.18 **Dysthyroid eye disease, with exophthalmos and strabismus.**

MANAGEMENT

Management of the thyroid state is necessary (Ch. 31). In mild thyroid eye disease, treatment may not be needed. Artificial tears may be necessary to ease the ocular discomfort from corneal exposure.

In more severe disease, immunosuppression with systemic corticosteroids or orbital irradiation may be necessary. Surgical interventions include orbital decompression, strabismus correction and methods of lowering the retracted lids.

Multiple sclerosis

This is a disorder of unknown cause characterised by demyelinating inflammation within the central nervous system, with recurrent attacks in different locations. Ophthalmic presentations are common and include:

- *Optic and retrobulbar neuritis.* This is the most common ophthalmic complication with around 70% having evidence of previous attacks. Optic neuritis may occur in isolation but at least 50% of women and 25% of men with optic neuritis go on to develop MS, the clinical features are described under 'Loss of visual acuity'.
- *Ocular motility disorders.* MS may affect individual nerves to cause paretic strabismus. Brain stem lesions of the medial longitudinal fasciculus cause internuclear ophthalmoplegia (INO – commonly bilateral) which affects horizontal gaze away from the side of the lesion so that the eye ipsilateral to the lesion fails to adduct across the midline while the contralateral eye exhibits nystagmus.
- *Visual field defects.* These are rarely seen but they are the result of a large demyelinating plaque which affects the optic radiations.

Hypertension

Hypertension can cause retinopathy, choroidopathy and optic neuropathy. The changes are most marked in the accelerated hypertension of pre-eclampsia or so-called malignant hypertension. The pathological changes in the eye are usually the consequence of ischaemia with tissue infarction or exudation from a compromised vascular endothelium.

Retinopathy can be graded by the severity and duration of disease. In *chronic disease* (arteriosclerosis):

- Grade 1 – increased arteriolar light reflex
- Grade 2 – deflection of veins at arteriovenous crossings
- Grade 3 – arteriolar narrowing (nipping) at arteriovenous crossings
- Grade 4 – silver wiring of arterioles (increased light reflex and tortuosity of vessels).

In *acute disease*:

- Grade 1 – generalised arteriolar attenuation
- Grade 2 – focal arteriolar attenuation and deflection of veins at arteriovenous crossings
- Grade 3 – hard exudates, flame-shaped haemorrhages and cotton wool spots with arteriolar narrowing (nipping) at arteriovenous crossings
- Grade 4 – grade 3 changes plus silver wiring of arterioles and swelling of the optic disc.

Grade 4 acute retinopathy is usually associated with encephalopathy and requires immediate referral for medical assessment. The fundal changes usually regress after the raised blood pressure has been corrected.

Diabetes

Diabetic retinopathy is a potentially blinding disease and is the leading cause of registration for blindness in the working age population in the UK. It can occur in both Type I and Type II diabetes. Visual loss can occur as a result of macular damage (oedema or ischaemia),vitreous haemorrhage or retinal detachment. The latter two conditions result from proliferative retinopathy (Fig. 36.19) in which retinal ischaemia leads to abnormal neovascularisation. The incidence of retinopathy increases with duration of disease and is reduced by tight control of blood sugar and blood pressure. Argon laser treatment is effective in preventing visual loss from retinopathy, therefore all diabetic patients should be screened for retinopathy. Screening should begin 5 years from diagnosis or at 12 years of age (whichever is the later) in Type I diabetes and at diagnosis in Type II disease.

Sarcoidosis

The eye is (after the lungs and lymph nodes) the most common organ to be affected (20–30%) by this condition. Uveitis is the most common manifestation and granulomatous inflammation can involve the retina and choroid to cause blindness. When this occurs there is a 30% incidence of central nervous system involvement. Granulomas can also affect the eyelid, conjunctiva and the lacrimal gland.

Stevens Johnson syndrome (erythema multiforme major)

This is an acute, generally self-limiting mucocutaneous vesiculobullous disease which tends to affect young healthy individuals. It involves the conjunctiva in 90%, causing mucopurulent conjunctivitis. Lid scarring may follow and lead to misdirection of the eyelashes with corneal damage. In the acute phase, assessment by an ophthalmologist is necessary. Systemic treatment is generally with steroids.

Sickle cell disease

Eye disease in the sickle haemoglobinopathies occurs in the SC and S-Thal forms but rarely in the SS form. The abnormal red blood cells cause vascular obstruction and infarction. The resulting ischaemia may lead to proliferation of abnormal new blood vessels, which may bleed to cause vitreous and retinal haemorrhages and retinal detachment. Once proliferative retinopathy has developed, there is a 3.4% 8-year incidence of visual loss, although the disease may be self-limiting. Most of the retinal changes occur in the retinal periphery, beyond the field of view of a direct ophthalmoscope.

Laser photocoagulation is sometimes required.

Wegener's granulomatosis

This disease is characterised by necrotising granulomas of the upper respiratory tract. The eye can be affected by keratoconjunctivitis sicca, scleritis, corneal melt and orbital involvement. Treatment is by systemic immunosuppression, e.g. cyclophosphamide.

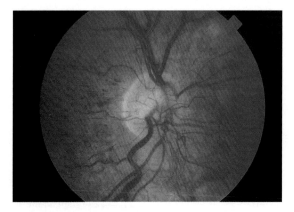

Fig 36.19 **Proliferative diabetic retinopathy, with new vessels growing from the nasal side of the optic disc.**

FURTHER READING

O khravi N (1999) *Manual of Primary Eye Care*. Oxford: Butterworth Heinemann

Kanski J J (1999) *Clinical Ophthalmology*, 4rth edn. Oxford: Butterworth Heinemann

37

Principles of plastic surgery

Unlike other surgical specialties there is no specific territory of the body which is the monopoly of plastic surgery. The plastic surgeon might be regarded as the last of the general surgeons in treating a great variety of problems in many sites (although in general, body cavities are excluded), by means of specialised 'plastic surgery techniques'. Some of these techniques have been in use for many years — there are records of reconstructions of the nose with forehead flaps from India dating back 3000 years. The speciality only developed independently in the last 60 years, triggered specifically by mutilations from trench warfare in the First World War, although the increased mechanisation and high-speed travel of the twentieth century have maintained the need for soft tissue reconstruction.

The demands on the speciality have been even greater as a result of the changing behaviour patterns, and fashions of society. There has been a dramatic increase in sun-induced skin damage, including skin cancer, as a result of the burgeoning package holiday trade and the belief that a suntan is attractive. With greater emphasis on the merits of an improved physical appearance, the demand for aesthetic plastic surgery has also soared. The definition of plastic surgery from the *Union European de Medicins Specialistes* within the EEC has therefore recently been modified as 'surgery intended to restore form and function and to promote well being'.

Defects which require such reconstruction may arise as a result of many different causes in sites all over the body, leading to considerable clinical overlap whereby the plastic surgeon is the member of a team. But while plastic surgery may often be associated with sophisticated reconstructions, the plastic surgeon also manages the commonest tumours of infancy (vascular hamartomata), the commonest form of cancer (skin cancer), the commonest cause of admission to a casualty department (hand and soft tissue injuries) and the commonest cause of prolonged morbidity in the elderly (chronic wounds and decubitus ulcers).

Examples of types of problems involving the plastic surgeon are shown in Table 37.1.

In practical terms, the commonest reconstruction required is the repair of a breach in the skin or a mucosal surface. However, the defect may extend deeper and involve other structures such as muscle, nerve, tendon and bone, and, where possible, these too will need to be corrected to enable full return of function.

Table 37.1
Types of problems involving the plastic surgeon

Aetiology of defect	Example
Congenital abnormality	Cleft lip and palate
Trauma	Lower limb soft tissue loss
Burns	Extensive skin loss
Neoplasia	Intra-oral cancer excision and reconstruction
Degenerative processes	Rheumatoid hand deformities

Plastic surgery techniques

There has been an escalation of surgical technology in the last two decades, supported by advances in anaesthetic and monitoring techniques which have allowed a greater range of reconstructive options. Furthermore, development in instrument technology, including fibreoptics and microsurgery, has increased surgical safety and reliability.

However, regardless of the rich choices available, the surgeon should opt for the simplest and safest surgery in the first instance, turning to more complex and potentially more hazardous procedures only when the simpler methods do not meet the reconstructive and occasionally aesthetic requirements. It is therefore helpful to have a mental picture of a ladder of surgical options, although recent developments have resulted in so many offshoots that the resulting plan resembles more closely a tree (Fig. 37.1).

Spontaneous wound healing

Wound healing is a natural and spontaneous phenomenon which occurs irrespective of (and sometimes despite) the surgeon. Although the basic events of blood clotting, fibrin deposition, organisation and collagen synthesis have been observed for many years, the factors which initiate and control these processes are incompletely understood. The pattern of wound healing may be affected by sophisticated endocrine, pharmacological and physical manipulation, or simply by surgery, but the most important influence on open wounds is the nature in which they are dressed.

Numerous dressings and topical agents are commercially available, some times making extravagant and unproven claims, but there is no evidence that any available dressings accelerate wound healing. They simply provide the optimal environment in which a wound can re-epithelialise. With this in mind, one should select well tried and tested dressings which should also have the properties of being cheap and painless to apply and remove. (See Fig. 37.2).

Some wounds will heal completely without surgical intervention. These not only include small wounds but some large cavernous wounds as might be produced by abscess drainage or excision of a pilonidal sinus. Such wounds may be too heavily contaminated for surgical closure and often contract down surprisingly quickly, particularly if subjected to a negative pressure.

Direct surgical wound closure

The first choice for wound repair is direct closure by suture, a standard and common surgical procedure but one deserving attention to detail to enable the best possible scar. The wound should first be converted to an ellipse whose long axis lies in the same line as the local skin creases (failure to do so is likely to produce unsightly dog ears). The wound is sutured so that the edges are exactly matched and slightly everted while reducing any crushing damage of the tissues with the help of fine toothed forceps or skin hooks. Tension and haematoma must be avoided at all costs by means of meticulous haemostasis and the support of buried intradermal sutures and adhesive tapes. However, the quality of the final scar is determined by the individual's own wound healing properties.

It is unfortunate that a vigorous scar formation is not in the interests of a good cosmetic result. In some patients the normal equilibrium between collagen synthesis and degradation is disturbed. Instead of scar maturation occurring over a twelve month period, collagen may be produced in excess resulting in a red lumpy hypertrophic scar. If there is extension into surrounding tissues a true keloid will result. The management of abnormal scarring following trauma or surgery is not entirely satisfactory but the means available are charted (Table 37.2.).

Skin grafts

If a wound is too wide to be closed directly, grafting is the simplest method of repair. A skin graft is a sheet of skin harvested from elsewhere in the body and comprising either its epidermis and superficial dermis (split thickness graft) or its entire thickness (full thickness graft). The graft is completely detached from the body and, when applied to the wound, depends entirely on the underlying vascular bed for its nutrition by diffusion of metabolites for a few days before its revascularisation by the ingrowth of blood vessels. A skin graft will therefore only 'take' if applied to wounds which can supply the necessary environment. Graft loss will occur if the wound surface dries out, is infected or contains nonvascular necrotic tissue. The spectrum of ability of different tissues to receive a graft is shown in Figure 37.3. Most wounds older than 48 hours will be covered by granulation tissue, whose vascularity will be related to that of the underlying tissue.

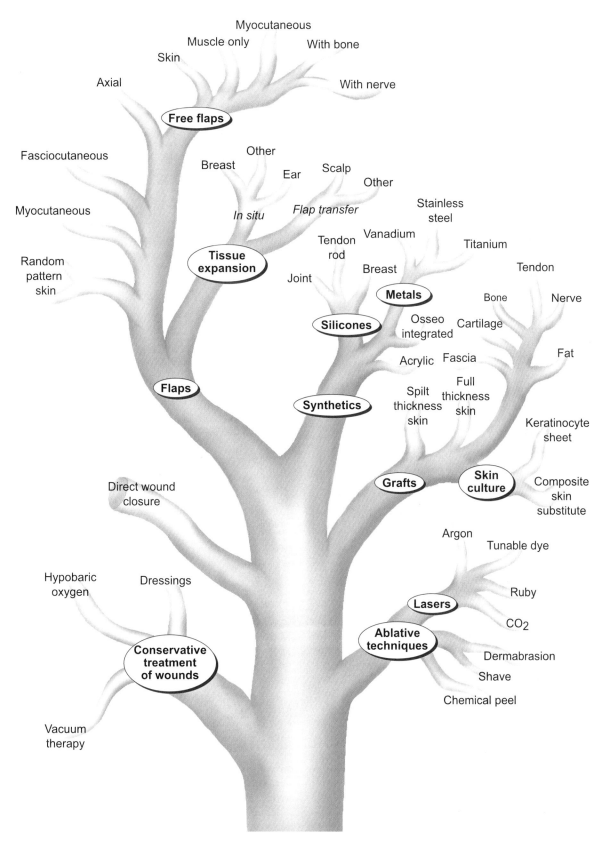

Fig 37.1 'Tree of reconstruction'.

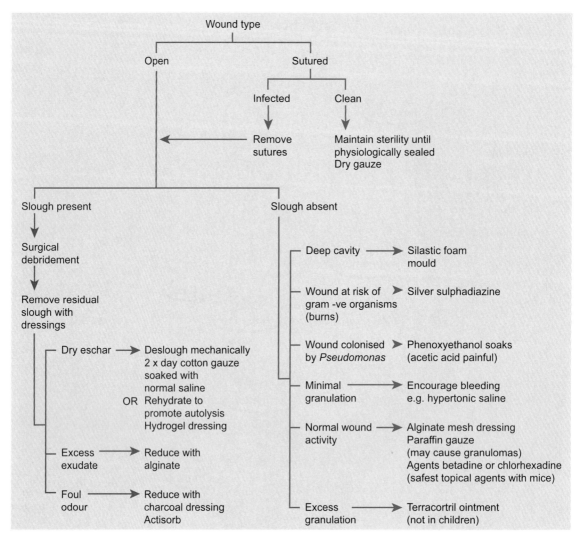

Fig 37.2 Algorithmic flow chart showing choice and examples of dressings in different situations.

Table 37.2
Treatment of unsatisfactory scars

Treatment	Undesirable features of normal scars	Hypertrophic scars	Keloid scars	Pigmented scars	Stretch scars
Surgical Revision	Yes	Yes	Very rarely	Yes	Yes
Topical or intralesional steroid	Rarely	Yes	Yes	No	No
Dermabrasion	Yes	No	No	Yes	No
Injectable bovine collagen	Yes	No	No	No	Yes
External pressure with or without silastic sheet	No	Yes	Yes	No	No
Low-dose radiotherapy	No	No	Yes	No	No
Cosmetic camouflage	Yes	Yes	No	Yes	Yes

Split thickness skin grafts

Split thickness skin grafts are taken with either hand-held graft knives or by powered dermatomes which both cut the superficial layers of the skin 150–300 microns thick. As a large number of epithelial remnants are left behind at the donor site these will, in the same manner as a bad graze, heal within two weeks, provided they are kept free from infection.

'Take' also depends on stability of the graft. Shearing forces which disrupt ingrowing capillary loops must be avoided by immobilising the skin graft with the help of

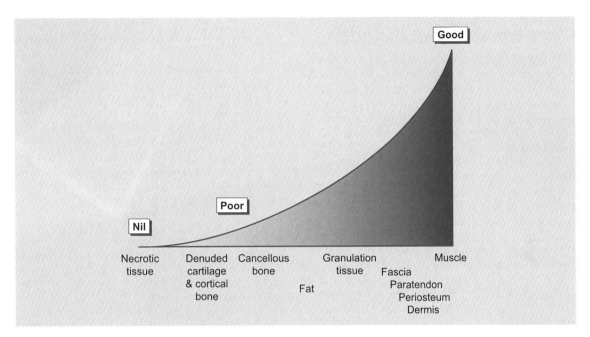

Fig 37.3 Suitability of tissues to receive spilt skin grafts.

a tie-over dressing or by sutures, staples or cyanoacrylate glue.

Large areas of skin can thus be harvested, but as donor sites often heal with some alteration of pigmentation and occasionally with hypertrophic scars, the sites chosen should be inconspicuous, such as the inner thigh or buttock. In the elderly who may have an attenuated dermis, the healing of these donor sites may be considerably delayed. The most acceptable donor site dressing is an alginate mesh which should be left undisturbed for at least 10 days.

The main disadvantage of split skin is that the final appearance is of a patch of unsightly scarring. Also, the wound continues to contract after graft application which may lead to disabling contractures across joints and soft tissue distortion of facial features. Although thin grafts take well, the thinner the graft the more aggressive the contracture.

Given the limited donor sites available for resurfacing extensive defects (like major burns) and the potential morbidity of donor sites, the introduction of the graft mesher proved to be a bonus. The machine cuts slots into the split skin, which enables the graft to be stretched out like a string vest, thereby increasing the area of the original graft. The diamond-shaped slots permit any blood or serum to escape (which might otherwise lift the graft away from its bed) thus reducing the chance of graft failure. Once the graft has taken, each hole heals by secondary intention. However, the disadvantage is that the healed area is like a cobbled surface, implying that it is best suited to inconspicuous recipient beds.

At best, split thickness grafts must be regarded as 'hole fillers' for the repair of large skin defects.

Full thickness skin grafts

For smaller wounds in conspicuous areas a full thickness graft is preferable. Although 'take' of these grafts is less predictable, they retain their original texture with little scarring and contracture, and are particularly suited to the face. However, the colour and texture of the standard postauricular graft is not ideal for all facial areas and one should consider other donor sites such as redundant upper eyelid skin, preauricular and supraclavicular skin to achieve optimum facial skin matching.

Cultured skin

Although not in common usage, there has been considerable clinical experience in the culture of keratinocytes isolated by trypsin from a small split skin graft. These are allowed to proliferate into large sheets of cells on a substrate of fibroblasts. However, such ultrathin layers of cells when applied as a graft were not sufficiently robust to withstand wear and tear and became impractical. The next logical step has been the development of a composite skin substitute which not only has an epithelial surface but a tough adherent dermal layer which raises the possibility of 'off the shelf' banks of skin.

Other types of graft materials

Other tissues available as free grafts for deep tissue defects, contour defects and functional restoration include bone, cartilage, nerve and tendon. Bone is usually harvested from the ilium or rib and cartilage from the ear concha or the rib. For bridging gaps in nerves, a cutaneous nerve such as the sural nerve may be sacrificed, and for tendon reconstruction vestigial tendons such as palmaris longus and plantaris are used (fascia lata is a reasonable substitute in their absence).

Other tissue such as muscle and fat are used only occasionally as their survival is unpredictable. Autografts are preferable (in spite of potential problems at the donor site) on account of their more reliable long-term incorporation. Heterografts and xenografts have the disadvantages of the added expense of denaturing for the sake of reducing antigenicity, while also carrying the higher risk of infection and progressive absorption.

Prostheses

Not only have an enormous range of implantable devices been designed in the last twenty years, but improvements in their composition has rendered them safer with a lower implant failure rate.

Silicone, the most commonly used implant material, is a polymer of silica and oxygen that can take on different physical characteristics from a thin oil to a hard block depending on its degree of polymerisation. It is relatively inert but after implantation, such as in a breast prosthesis or small joint replacement, is characteristically enveloped in a capsule of fibrous tissue of variable thickness lined with smooth mesothelium. An abnormally thick capsule may distort a breast prosthesis and, as yet, this phenomenon is unable to be predicted or prevented.

Other materials used as a bone substitute, either to restore contour such as following loss of the calvarium or for skeletal replacement, include acrylic bone cement and (more commonly) metal such as stainless steel, chrome cobalt and titanium. The recent discovery that bone will produce a very tight bond on a molecular level with titanium even when the latter extends through skin or mucosa has generated 'osseo-integrated' implants as studs on which artificial teeth and, more recently, external facial prostheses can be securely attached.

Flaps

Where a skin graft is impossible or when aesthetics dictate, a defect should be resurfaced with a flap. A flap is a block of tissue which retains an attachment to the body, known as a pedicle, through which it receives its blood supply and innervation as required. An encyclopaedia of flaps have been described according to how they are moved, how they are composed and (of far greater importance) how they are vascularised.

The earliest flaps were simply skin and subcutaneous fat designed without appreciation of the underlying blood supply so that their length and mobility were restricted. More reliable and predictable flaps arose from understanding that the skin obtains its blood supply from three main sources: via direct cutaneous arteries, via perforating vessels of underlying muscles and via tributaries of the vascular plexus within the underlying deep fascia and fascial septa. This has led to the development of three different types of flap (Fig. 37.4).

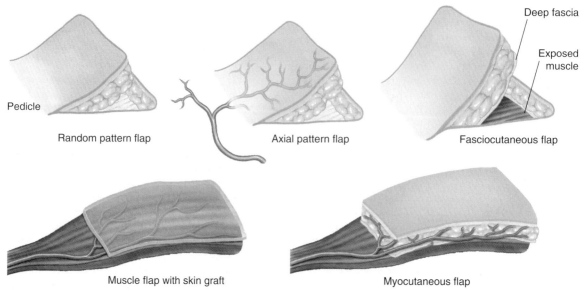

Pedicle

Random pattern flap

Axial pattern flap

Deep fascia

Exposed muscle

Fasciocutaneous flap

Muscle flap with skin graft

Myocutaneous flap

Fig 37.4 The different types of flap.

- Axial pattern flaps have a known cutaneous artery which is included by orientating the flap in the same axis as the vessel, thereby enabling a long and versatile flap. The best known example is the groin flap which has its base over the femoral vessels in the groin and extends laterally following the course of the superficial circumflex iliac artery.
- Fasciocutaneous flaps are similar to skin flaps but also include deep fascia. These are normally used in the limb where there is a very definite layer of well vascularised deep fascia which permit a surviving length two to three times the length of the corresponding skin flap.
- Muscle flaps usually include a polarised blood supply so that the axis of movement can only be at the site of axial arteriovenous penetration. Muscle flaps alone will require epithelial cover in the form of a skin graft, however when the muscle is superficial it is possible to include the overlying skin as a 'composite myocutaneous' flap.

Until a flap is incorporated within the defect it is necessary to be nourished by an intact pedicle even if it bridges across intact skin. After this time the pedicle may be detached and discarded or returned to its original site. It follows that these flaps can only be transferred locally although it is possible to transport them to distant sites by a series of staged and unreliable operations involving their inset into a 'carrier' such as the wrist.

Free tissue transfer

As a result of advances in microsurgery, blood vessels as small as 1 mm can be successfully anastomosed. Thus, a new era of single stage distant flap reconstruction became possible in which the axial vessels of a flap are anastomosed to recipient vessels near the defect. Furthermore, this surgical technology obviates the need for multistaged procedures involving long inpatient stays.

These 'free flaps' permit sophisticated reconstructions in either emergency or elective circumstances. The stages are as follows:

1. Elevation of the flap, islanding it on the vascular pedicle.
2. Preparation of the recipient bed and isolation of healthy recipient vessels (ideally performed by a second team of surgeons).
3. Detachment of the flap followed by anastomosis of donor to recipient vessels.
4. Inset of flap and closure of donor site.

In the hands of an experienced microsurgeon supported by skilled anaesthesia (controlled, high peripheral perfusion is the key), a patency rate of 95% can be expected. Similar techniques are used in the reattachment of any traumatically amputated parts which must be brought swiftly to hospital, preferably cooled in a plastic bag lying within a second plastic bag filled with ice. If the vessels of the part and the recipient site are sufficiently healthy one can safely proceed to replantation and revascularisation using an intervening vein graft, if necessary, to avoid any anastomotic tension.

Tissue expansion

A tissue expander (which consists of an empty silicone ballon connected by a tube to a filler valve) is implanted subcutaneously adjacent to a defect at an initial operation. Over a period of weeks or months the expander is then inflated by serially injecting saline percutaneously into the filler valve thereby distending the overlying skin. When enough skin has been generated the expander is removed and the surplus skin used for reconstruction. The great advantage is that the skin adjacent to the defect is most likely to match that of the area to be reconstructed providing a good aesthetic match. This is particularly important in certain areas where the skin has very specific properties such as the hair bearing scalp.

The method appears to be seductive in its simplicity but in practice there is a 30–40% complication rate including infection, erosion of skin and extrusion. However, tissue expansion still has a place particularly in breast reconstruction and it is the treatment of choice in the reconstruction of the hair-bearing scalp (Fig. 37.5).

Ablative techniques

In the restoration of normal form, surgical reconstruction may be unnecessary if the lesion concerned can be selectively destroyed. Rhinophyma (a condition characterised by massive hypertrophy of cutaneous sebaceous glands of the nose) is effectively treated by shaving alone. Deep epithelial remnants quickly re-epithelialise the surface of the nose. Dermabrasion is a similar technique in which minor irregularities of the skin such as post acne scarring can be improved by abrading the superficial epidermo-dermal layers.

However, the laser is the most sophisticated ablative tool. There are many types of medical laser but those in plastic surgery differ in that they must be very selective in their tissue damage to leave the skin minimally unscarred. The treatment of the intradermal capillary haemangioma (or port wine stain) has been improved initially by an argon laser whose wavelength is similar to that absorbed by haemoglobin so that abnormal vessels could thus be photocoagulated. However, this has been recently superceded by a tuneable dye laser in which a dye is selected which has a wavelength even more specific for haemoglobin. In a similar manner the

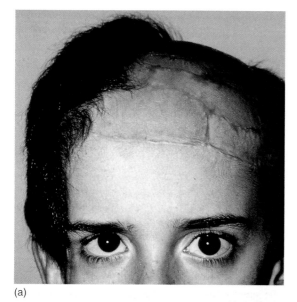

(a)

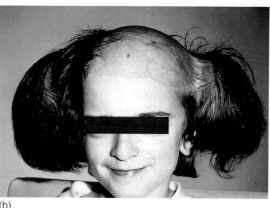

(b)

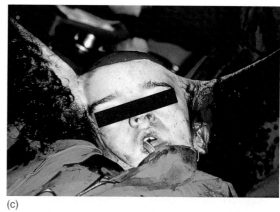

(c)

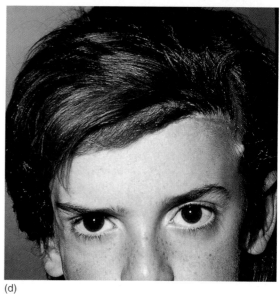

(d)

Fig 37.5 Reconstruction of hair-bearing scalp. **(a)** Following a compound fracture of the right parietal bone with loss of the overlying scalp, a large scalp flap was used to repair this wound. The skin graft used to cover this flap's donor site has left an obvious area of alopecia. **(b)** Following insertion and inflation of two tissue expanders. **(c)** At operation the expanders have been removed and scalp flaps have been raised in the expanded skin prior to excising the skin graft. **(d)** Six weeks after completion of the reconstruction.

indian ink pigment of amateur tattoos may be vapourised by the ruby laser which emits the light of the appropriate wavelength.

Other reconstructive problems

Other problems requiring reconstruction can broadly be divided into those of composite tissue loss and loss of function. In composite loss following the deep resection of a tumour, not only skin cover but loss of mucosal surfaces and intervening tissue including skeletal support must be made good. Here the plastic surgeon is a member of a surgical team either in an excisional role but more commonly in a post-excisional, reconstructive role.

Descriptions of specific reconstruction is beyond the scope of this chapter but the specific aims of reconstruction will be considered for the major branches of the specialty.

Trauma

Trauma has become a multidisciplinary speciality and the plastic surgeon who cares for soft tissues injuries must work as part of a team. Full assessment of the injured patient is essential as other problems may take priority over the soft tissue.

It is important to assess whether tissues are missing or simply displaced. The viability of remaining tissues is then determined and, if avascular such as amputated parts, their suitability for revascularisation. All debris and devitalised tissue must be removed without compromise to allow subsequent reconstruction. However, it is sometimes difficult to judge the viability of tissues especially following injury when they are bruised and swollen. For example, the degloving injury, whereby skin is sheared from the underlying deep fascia, is notoriously difficult to accurately diagnose; the devitalisation of other tissues notably fat occurs some time after an apparently adequate wound toilet. Thus, if there is any doubt about tissue viability, the patient should be returned to theatre for second and third inspections of the wound with necrectomies and surgical toilet as necessary until a clean wound becomes apparent. It can then be closed with the techniques previously discussed.

Congenital abnormalities

Birth defects result from failure of a variety of development processes including formation, fusion, separation and regression of parts. Many abnormalities not only consist of a true shortage of tissues but of an abnormal anatomy of the adjacent tissues.

The treatment of many of these conditions is started at a very young age, varying from the first few days of birth in the case of neonatal cleft repair to repair of hypospadias from nine months. The essential goal is the restoration of as near normal function and appearance by the time the child starts primary school, and as little interference with schooling as possible by any further intervention. Surgery in infancy may interfere with growth of the operated part: thus while the timing of the procedure and meticulous technique are of obvious importance, there must also be careful follow-up in order to monitor any untoward growth changes.

Developments in anaesthesia, diagnostic imaging and neurosurgery have contributed towards safer and more precise correction of major cranio-facial abnormalities. Although these conditions may produce very disfiguring abnormalities, they are not often life threatening and therefore treatment can only be justified if the morbidity is acceptable. Contrary to other sites in the body, much of the facial skeleton can be mobilised, even if this involves devascularisation, and be expected to survive. Once the skeleton has been rigidly fixed in the correct position, possibly with the addition of bone grafts, it is necessary to consider the correction of soft tissue abnormalities. Cranio-facial surgery has developed into a subspecialty in its own right involving a large team headed by plastic and neurosurgeons.

Breast reconstruction

Despite recent trends towards the conservative management of breast cancer there are still indications for mastectomy and there will always be women requesting breast reconstruction. In its simplest terms, breast reconstruction requires the restoration of a skin envelope and the bulk with which to fill it. The former is achieved by a variety of flaps including tissue expansion, and the latter by the bulk of the flap itself or by a silicone prosthetic implant. The restoration of a symmetrical breast with a natural ptosis and projection is sometimes impossible without surgical compromise involving a mastopexy or breast reduction of the other breast.

Some patients will require a nipple areolar reconstruction which can be effected by a variety of local flaps or grafts taken either from the opposite nipple–areolar complex or skin from the upper inner aspect of the thigh.

Hand surgery

Although the priority in hand surgery must always be function, the hand, like the face, is never normally covered and aesthetics must also be born in mind.

The hand is a sophisticated sensate organ composed of highly specialised and compactly organised moving parts with little wasted space. Thus any surgical intervention should be designed to minimise postoperative oedema and scarring to avoid long-term compromise of function in terms of power, range of movement and sensation.

Surgery of the hand is merely the start of treatment. Without dedicated postoperative treatment by physiotherapists, occupational therapists, orthotists and, in particular, the determination of the patient, even the most skillfull surgery may result in an irreversibly stiff hand.

Burns

The initial treatment in patients with major burns is stabilisation by compensating the massive fluid loss which will otherwise produce oligaemic shock. The extent and depth of the burn is assessed to determine which areas are superficially destroyed (i.e. deeper parts of the dermis are viable implying spontaneous healing), or whether the damage is deeper and will require surgical excision. Further assessment is needed to determine whether excision should take place in the first few days to reduce the risk of sepsis while at the same time increasing the risk of oligaemia, or at a later stage when oligaemia is less likely but septicaemia is a greater risk. In both instances the choice of graft is either whole or meshed split skin, or a combination of the two. Once again surgery is only the beginning; not infrequently the subsequent disfigurement and deformity from scarring and contracture and shearing forces involve the patient in multiple surgical procedures over many years.

Decubitus ulcers

These wounds are caused by pressure necrosis of tissues in an immobilised and often debilitated patient. In those patients who are temporarily incapacitated and subsequently become ambulant, the prognosis is good and the defects can be managed conservatively. The majority of ulcers, however, occur in paraplegic patients in tissues over bony prominences subject to chronic pressure when a combination of poor quality and insensate tissues, poor general nutrition and occasionally poor motivation exacerbate the situation.

Treatment is directed to improving the nutritional status with the help of a dietician. Continued pressure must be alleviated by regular turning of the patient with mechanical assistance such as the low air loss bed. These patients are demanding of nursing time and require frequent dressings and repeated necrectomy. Eventually some of these wounds may heal spontaneously though in many the resulting defect is of a size that can only be closed with a local flap. The surgery of decubtus ulcers can be expensive and time consuming and is inadvisable if measures cannot subsequently be taken to prevent any recurrence.

Head and neck surgery

Reconstruction in the head and neck demands the highest possible standards and encapsulates all the principles of restoration of form, appearance and function. In the face the cosmetic result is all important and, with this in mind, the surgeon may well opt for a more complicated method of repair. However, prostheses are indicated when the defect may be beyond the scope of surgical reconstruction or the patient too frail for extensive surgery. The materials of the prosthesis together with the secure fixation with osseointegration or the new biological adhesives has initiated a new era in prosthetic rehabilitation.

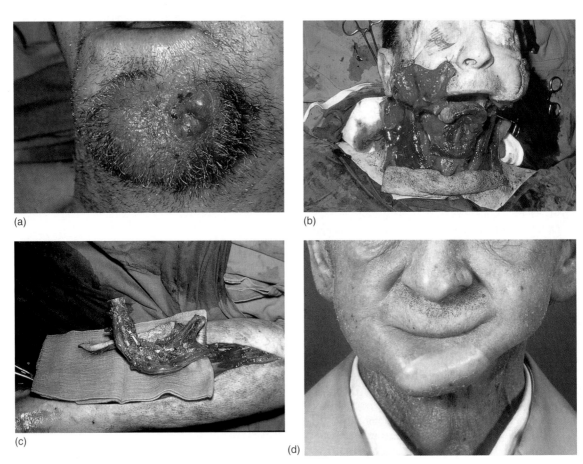

(a)

(b)

(c)

(d)

Fig 37.6 An example of complex intra-oral reconstructive surgery. **(a)** An advanced carcinoma of the floor of mouth invading the chin. **(b)** Defect following bilateral neck dissection and resection of chin skin, mandible from angle to angle, floor of mouth and anterior tongue. **(c)** Free flap raised for reconstruction. A fibular flap will reconstruct the mandible with some overlying skin, vascularised through its deep fascial attachment, which will replace the floor of mouth. Two osteotomies have been made in the bone which has been plated in a design to conform with the resected mandible. **(d)** Four months following surgery there is good bony union. External skin cover was achieved with an axial skin flap from the upper chest (deltopectoral flap).

Conversely intra-oral surgery demands the maintainance and restoration of funtion. Failure to adequately replace lost mucosal surfaces will produce tethering within the mouth which is disastrous when it involves the tongue, resulting in interference with speech and swallowing. Thin and pliable flaps are ideal as they drape the contours of the oral cavity. In many flaps it is possible to include vascularised bone which permits single stage mandibular reconstruction. If part of the lip is resected, dynamic reconstitution of the oral sphincter should be achieved to prevent oral incontinence. An example of complex reconstruction in this region is shown in Figure 37.6.

Aesthetic plastic or cosmetic surgery

In cosmetic surgery there is no obvious surgical pathology. The source of distress may either be variants of normal appearance or the aftermath of normal aging processes, often out of proportion to the degree of physical abnormality as perceived by others. It is therefore essential that the surgeon does not trivialise cosmetic surgery or impart his prejudices on patients,

many of whom enjoy a dramatic improvement in the quality of their lives following appropriate treatment. Meticulous patient selection and detailed discussion of the treatment options are paramount so that the potential benefits and harms can be fully understood. In no other form of surgery is the implementation of fully informed consent more important. In no other form of surgery is there such a thin line between success and failure; between a happy grateful patient and an unhappy, resentful and potentially litigious patient.

FURTHER READING

Aston S, Beasley RW (eds) (1997) *Grabb & Smith's Plastic Surgery*, Boston: Lippincott William & Williams

Burke FD, McGrouther DA, Smith PJ (1990) *Principles of Hand Surgery*. Edinburgh: Churchill Livingstone.

Emmett AJ, O'Rourke MG (1991) *Malignant Skin Tumours*, 2nd edn. Edinburgh: Churchill Livingstone.

McGregor IA (1989) *Fundamental Techniques in Plastic Surgery*, 8th edn. Edinburgh: Churchill Livingstone.

Muir IFK, Barclay TL (1987) *Burns and their Treatment*, 3rd. edn. Oxford Butterworths Heiniman

38 Surgical principles – skin disorders

Introduction

Diagnostic principles

Diagnosis of skin disorders is mainly on the distribution and naked-eye structure of the lesion or rash. The whole skin surface must be examined even if the patient presents with an apparently solitary lesion. It is also important to examine the regional lymph nodes which drain the area involved, particularly in suspected inflammatory or neoplastic conditions.

The majority of those encountered in surgical practice are benign and malignant tumours. However, there is a need to be aware of other conditions which may mimic these and which are also relevant for accurate diagnosis and therapy.

Biopsy

Histological examination is required for final confirmation of a diagnosis or when there is doubt on clinical grounds. Small lesions can be completely excised but larger ones may be initially removed in part before definitive therapy is decided on. It is important, when only partial removal is done, to provide adequate material for interpretation, which usually means a full-thickness (epidermis, dermis and a small amount of subcutaneous tissue) biopsy through the edge of the lesion.

Principles of therapy

Neoplastic lesions must be excised with an adequate margin without primary regard for the cosmetic outcome (e.g. see Melanoma) and their margins checked by histological examination. However, for benign lesions, cosmesis must be given consideration – any incision into collagen (i.e. through the dermis) leaves a scar on healing and this inevitable occurrence must be explained to the patient beforehand. Keloid formation is always a slight possibility and the risk is higher in Afro-Caribbeans.

Lesions in the epidermis can usually be treated by curettage and cautery and so scraped away without damage to collagen and with a consequent good cosmetic result. Superficial lesions can also be dealt with by cryosurgery with a satisfactory cosmetic result.

Caution is required when there is the risk of damage to underlying structures, such as digital nerves and extensor tendons over the dorsal aspect of the fingers. Both can be damaged by injudicious or heavy cryosurgery. Pigmentary change can also follow in Afro-Caribbean and Asian patients. The patient should also be warned of the likelihood of pain and blistering after cryosurgery.

For pedunculated lesions, snip excision across the base is appropriate, although light cautery may be required to control bleeding.

Benign vascular and pigmented lesions are increasingly appropriate for treatment by laser. The emission wavelength of the laser can be matched to the absorption spectrum of the pigment present, e.g. haemoglobin or melanin. Carbon dioxide lasers are more destructive but give immediate haemostasis and vaporise a lesion; they have a role in ablation therapy and increasingly in malignant disease.

Embryology and anatomy

There are three layers to the skin (Fig. 38.1):

- epidermis
- dermis
- hypodermis or subcutaneous tissue.

Epidermis
The epidermis originates from the ectoderm, in contrast to the other two (deeper) layers which are of mesodermal origin. Some epidermal structures – the pilosebaceous unit and nail matrix (see below) – migrate inwards during development and are anatomically

located in the dermis. Similarly, some cells of mesodermal origin, such as melanocytes of neural crest origin, migrate outwards to the epidermis and are located within its basal cell layer.

The interface between the epidermis and dermis is convoluted – the dermal projection of the epidermis is a rete peg and the upward projection of the dermis is a dermal papilla (Fig. 38.2). Between the epidermis and dermis there is a basement membrane zone which is traversed by anchoring fibrils, which are important in the adherence of the two structures.

The epidermis consists of stratified keratinising squamous epithelium. Different layers can be identified histologically and represent stages of the maturation of cell division of the keratinocytes of the basal layer as they migrate towards the surface. Initially, keratin filaments appear in the cytoplasm. As the cells mature further, the cytoplasm becomes progressively replaced by keratin – a structural protein which is surrounded by a phospholipid envelope that is the original cell membrane. As the products of cell division migrate out towards the surface, the cells flatten and by the time they reach the surface they form a laminated structure – the stratum corneum. The epidermal transit time from the basal layer to stratum corneum is about 28 days. Disruption of this smooth transition occurs in inflammatory conditions of the epidermis such a psoriasis and as a result of sun-induced (actinic) damage to the basal cell – a process known as dyskeratosis which makes the affected epidermis unstable.

Other epidermal cells

Melanocytes are of neural crest origin located along the basement membrane, interspersed with the basal keratinocytes. Their shape is dendritic with multiple root-like projections. The number of melanocytes is constant throughout racial groups, but there are differences in their baseline activity of melanin production and the nature of the melanin produced: Celtic races, for example, produce phaeomelanin which gives poorer ultraviolet protection than does melanin. Increased melanin production can be stimulated by ultraviolet light and the cytokines released by inflammatory processes. The melanin is distributed to the surrounding basal cells through the dendrites. Once the melanin granules are taken up by the basal cell, they are dispersed through the cytoplasm and absorb ultraviolet radiation, which protects the nuclei as well as deeper cells from ultraviolet damage. Individuals who are poor at producing melanin and who burn rather than tan are more vulnerable to developing photodamage to the underlying collagen and sun-induced skin tumours.

Immunocompetent cells are of a number of classes. *Langerhans cells* are derived from bone marrow and are closely related to the macrophage. They are located just above the basal layer of keratinocytes in the so-called suprabasal layer. They express HLA receptors on their

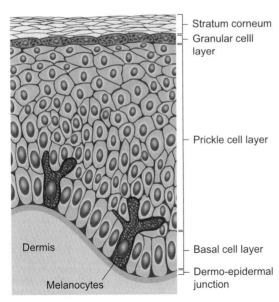

Fig 38.1 **Structure of normal epidermis.**

Stratum corneum
Granular celll layer
Prickle cell layer
Basal cell layer
Dermo-epidermal junction
Dermis
Melanocytes

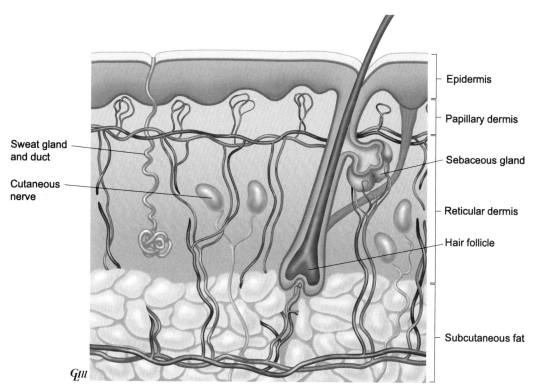

Fig 38.2 **Structure of normal skin.**

Labels: Epidermis, Papillary dermis, Sebaceous gland, Reticular dermis, Hair follicle, Subcutaneous fat, Sweat gland and duct, Cutaneous nerve

surface and are central to the presentation of antigens to other immunologically competent cells. They also, in their own right, release cytokines such as interleukin II. Their prime importance is in immunosurveillance of the skin and mediation of the cutaneous immune response.

Lymphocytes are present in small numbers in normal epidermis – mainly T lymphocytes of both CD4 and CD8 subsets. The T lymphocytes are derived from the thymus, which is of ectodermal origin, and it is believed that they migrate through the epidermis as part of their surveillance of immune function. The interaction between Langerhans cells and lymphocytes makes the epidermis an important component of the body's immune system. This can be disturbed in some inflammatory conditions of the epidermis which are T-cell-mediated, e.g. in psoriasis, which is one of the commonest inflammatory conditions of the epidermis. It appears that T lymphocytes release lymphokines into the epidermis, so increasing keratinocyte proliferation. Antigen-presenting cells and T lymphocytes are important in the cell-mediated (type IV) reaction that mediates contact allergic eczema, such as in an allergic reaction to adhesives used in dressings on wounds.

The epidermal immune system may be suppressed by a number of factors. Ultraviolet light can give rise to suppression of type IV reactions in the skin. Some

cutaneous diseases such as atopic eczema are associated with local immunodeficiency and patients are prone to cutaneous infection with *Staphylococcus aureus*. Also, the epidermal immune system may be suppressed during systemic diseases such as diabetes mellitus, HIV infection and leukaemias.

Merkel cells. These, like the melanocytes, are also of mesodermal origin derived from the neural crest. They function as mechanoreceptors and are found particularly on the digital pads of the fingers.

The dermis

The major component of the dermis is connective tissue composed mainly of collagen fibres within an amorphous ground substance. In addition, there are blood vessels which derive from a deep vascular plexus, sweat glands, nerves, lymphatics and muscle fibres associated with a pilosebaceous unit (see below).

Dermal collagen is produced by fibroblasts which lie between the collagen bundles. It gives the skin elasticity and strength as well as providing support for other structures that lie within it. Changes in collagen occur with ageing and from ultraviolet light, both of which make collagen less flexible and less able to provide support for other structures. Wrinkles result and purpura may also follow from the increased fragility of blood vessels.

Dermal blood vessels arise from a deep arterial plexus which then subdivides into arterioles and finally a capillary loop which supplies the dermal papillae. Blood then drains through a papillary venous network and back into the subcutaneous vessels.

Lymphatic channels can be recognised within the dermis. Their obstruction or failure causes cutaneous lymphoedema.

Dermal nerve fibres are:

- afferent for cutaneous sensation
- efferent vasomotor and also to the sweat glands both of which are important in body temperature control; there is also a supply to the erector pili muscle.

Sweat glands are of two types:

- *Eccrine glands* are present throughout all skin and secrete an aqueous fluid
- *Apocrine glands* occur in the intertriginous areas of the axillae and perineum and in the scalp – their secretion is greasy.

Pilosebaceous units are a combination of a hair shaft, hair follicle and a sebaceous gland. Attached to the hair shaft are muscle fibres of the pili erector muscle. The keratin of the hair shaft is derived from a germinal layer of the hair bulb which lies deep in the dermis. The hair follicle is richly supplied by nerves and blood vessels. The sebaceous glands produce a fatty secretion, sebum, which is discharged into the hair follicle through the pilosebaceous duct (see 'Epidermal cyst').

Nail matrix produces the specialised keratin of the nail plate which grows out beneath the proximal nail fold. The plate is closely adherent to the underlying structures of the nail bed. On either side of the nail plate are the lateral nail folds. Melanocytes can be present in the nail matrix and cause linear pigmented striae within the nails as well as providing the starting place for melanoma. Infection of the nail folds is termed paronychia. The nail plate can grow into the soft nail fold to give rise to an ingrowing nail.

Disorders of the skin

The skin is a large organ – by weight, up to 15% of body mass. It is, along with the mucosal surface of the gastrointestinal tract, with which it is continuous, the interface between the external and internal environment and has a number of important functions in protection and in the maintenance of homeostasis. It is extensively exposed to agents which are actually or potentially noxious, including chemicals, carcinogens and pathogenic organisms. Also, it is at constant risk of physical trauma and subject to a large number of

endogenous diseases such as eczema, lichen planus and psoriasis and may be involved in systemic problems such as vasculitis and granulomatous diseases (sarcoidosis).

Infections

The skin is constantly exposed to infectious agents. Protection is afforded by the physical barrier of the stratum corneum and the very effective immunological barrier of the epidermis.

Host defences may be breached as a result of:

- physical injury, e.g. trauma to the skin or surgical intervention
- endogenous skin disorders – eczema or venous ulceration
- immunosuppression, e.g. HIV infection or leukaemia
- pathogenic organisms that are able to penetrate the normal skin defence mechanisms, e.g. fungal and candidal infection.

Viral infections
Human papillomaviruses

These are a group of RNA viruses. More than 50 subtypes have so far been identified. The skin manifestation is a wart.

EPIDEMIOLOGY AND AETIOLOGY
Warts are common and most people suffer infection at some stage. They are most prevalent in children where they are probably acquired from direct contact or from communal recreation facilities such as swimming pools. Genital and perianal warts are usually found in adults and are most commonly, though not exclusively, acquired as a result of sexual intercourse so that they may coexist with other sexually transmitted diseases.

PATHOLOGICAL FEATURES
The virus infects the basal keratinocyte of the epithelium and the epidermis responds by increased proliferation. In stratified squamous epithelium this gives rise to hyperkeratosis and a hard wart. The characteristic hallmarks of a wart are loss of the normal dermatoglyphics of the skin and thrombosed capillaries that are seen as small black spots which bleed if the overlying hard skin is pared away. On mucosal surfaces, the wart is softer – a soft fleshy papilloma. It is important when assessing patients who present with genital warts to make sure they have not also acquired any other sexually transmitted disease.

CLINICAL FEATURES

History

Cutaneous warts may present suddenly with rapid growth or more gradually creep up on their hosts over weeks, months or even occasionally years. Often tiny excrescences are ignored or scratched away until they are bothersome; itching may be a feature. Larger lesions can become painful, especially if they are on pressure points such as the heel and the ball of the foot. Help is sought for pain or because of the appearance of an exposed area such as the hand or face.

Sexually or non-sexually acquired warts at muco-cutaneous junctions such as the anorectal verge are considered below.

Physical findings

The typical features have been indicated above. Bleeding follows frictional injury or efforts at self-treatment. Multiple warts at the mucocutaneous junction may become infected with inflammation and discomfort.

MANAGEMENT

Prevention

As yet it has not been possible to generate a vaccine that protects patients against warts. Immunotherapy is at present in a trial phase but opens up the possibility for more suitable regimens in the future.

Natural history

Spontaneous resolution is the rule once natural immunity has developed, but this takes longer in adults than in children so that infection may last for many years. The use of local, non-curative and symptom-relieving keratolytic agents for hand and foot warts remains the mainstay of therapy, particularly in children, and keeps the warts comfortable until resolution occurs.

Cryotherapy

The application of liquid nitrogen can destroy the viral-infected tissue which then sloughs. Early resolution in individual lesions follows but there is a high rate of recurrence and the treatment is painful.

Curettage and other destructive measures

More effective physical ablation of the warts can be achieved by curettage, diathermy or laser therapy. All of these are effective but they have to be adapted to the area involved.

Cytotoxic agents

Podophyllin (a compound preparation which contains the agent podophyllotoxin) is particularly helpful in genital warts. However, its application must be closely supervised because it causes soreness and is teratogenic and therefore must not be used during pregnancy.

Intralesional bleomycin has also been successfully used.

Special problems with genital warts

If these proliferate, condylomata acuminatum occurs – a condition which has to be treated with physical destruction such as cautery under general anaesthesia. The main indications for therapy are pain, bleeding and cosmetic appearance.

Molluscum contagiosum

AETIOLOGY AND PATHOLOGICAL FEATURES

This is caused by a pox virus. The individual lesions are smooth and dome-shaped, they have a characteristic central depression or umbilication and, if squeezed, a central white core can be expressed called the molluscum body. Florid molluscum contagiosum may occur in immunosuppressed patients, particularly those with HIV infection. When patients acquire immunity to the virus, the lesions disappear,

MANAGEMENT

Early resolution of individual lesions can be induced by minor trauma such as cryotherapy or superficial diathermy.

Herpesvirus

There are two types of infection:

- herpes simplex (HS), with a number of subtypes
- herpes zoster (HZ).

Herpes simplex

This condition affects any area of skin although the mucous membranes, the lips (HS type 1) and genitalia (HS type 2) are the most common. The patient notices a prodromal tingling of the skin followed by the eruption of clusters of small vesicles. The active lesions are infectious and surgeons must take care to avoid direct contact, which can result in a herpetic whitlow on a finger.

Herpes zoster

This is caused by the varicella virus. The condition is often called shingles by the lay population. The virus lies dormant in the dorsal root ganglia of the CNS and is reactivated along peripheral nerves to produce cutaneous lesions in a dermatomal distribution. Its relevance for surgeons is that the prodromal phase, before the development of vesicles, gives rise to pain in the skin of the affected dermatome which may mimic other cranial nerve lesions or an acute abdomen or sciatic nerve pain.

Bacterial infections

Staphylococcal infections

AETIOLOGY AND PATHOLOGICAL FEATURES

Staphylococcus aureus is a pathogen that may give rise to a primary skin infection – impetigo, furunculosis and acute paronychia – or secondary infection of wounds. Diabetic patients are particularly susceptible and, rarely, a staphylococcal cellulitis may occur.

Impetigo

This condition mainly affects the face and is much more common in children than in adults: presentation is as flaccid blisters underneath the stratum corneum which rupture early on, so giving rise to a raw eroded base. Impetigo is contagious and infected children should be kept away from school. Swabs are taken to determine the antibacterial resistance of the organism in case the condition fails to respond to therapy. If the lesions are localised, topical antistaphylococcal agents such as fusidic acid or mupirocin are effective. If lesions are widespread, they are treated with systemic flucloxacillin.

Furunculosis

This term describes a group of conditions characterised by staphylococcal infection of the hair follicles. Staphylococcal folliculitis is a pyoderma localised to the hair follicle and can be either superficial or deep. A *furuncle* (boil) is a deeply seated inflammatory nodule which develops around a hair follicle from a preceding, more superficial folliculitis. A *carbuncle* is a more extensive and even deeper infiltrating inflammation which occurs in thick and inelastic skin – commonly on the back of the neck.

The acute lesions of furunculosis are characterised by pain and tenderness of the infected area and soft tissue. Localisation of pus gives rise to abscesses. The natural history of the lesions is for the pus to discharge and this to be followed by resolution. Treatment of the early soft tissue phase is with systemic antibiotics. If a deep abscess forms, then surgical drainage is indicated. Carbuncles and ecthyma represent infective gangrene of the deep tissues. The subcutaneous tissues become painful and indurated and drain to the surface through sinuses. Surgical debridement may be necessary, in addition to a course of antibiotics.

Paronychium

This is the term given to inflammation of the nail fold. Infection is usually acquired through loss of the cuticle of the proximal nail fold, sometimes the consequence of a self-inflicted injury at manicure. Paronychia may be acute when caused by *Staphylococcus aureus* infection, or chronic when the result of *Candida* infection whose acquisition is difficult to determine (Fig. 38.3). Treat-

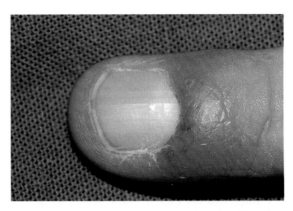

Fig 38.3 **Paronychium showing loss of cuticle and swelling of nail fold.**

ment is by surgical debridement – which may have to include the nail – under local anaesthetic.

Streptococcal infections

Streptococcus pyogenes (beta-haemolytic *Streptococcus* Lancefield group A) causes dermal infections of two types:

- erysipelas – infection in the deep dermis
- cellulitis – full-thickness infection of the skin with involvement of the subcutaneous tissues.

The presentation of both may be that of the systemic features of severe sepsis with rigor and fever but without initial overt evidence of skin involvement. The earliest cutaneous sign is erythema. The leg and face are most commonly affected, although any site may be involved. The infection spreads through the tissue by the release of toxins, giving rise to a brawny erythema spreading across the skin with a sharp well-demarcated edge (Fig. 38.4). If left untreated, the infection will eventually resolve but there is a significant mortality from overwhelming toxaemia and septicaemia.

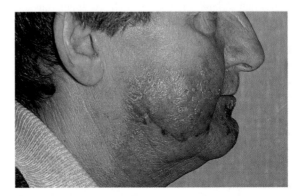

Fig 38.4 **Erysipelas showing indurated red plaque spreading across face.**

The treatment of choice for streptococcal cellulitis is bed rest with intravenous antibiotics. The majority of streptococci are sensitive to penicillin and this is the agent of choice. The fever usually settles within 24–48 hours and the erythema and swelling subside slowly. Streptococcal cellulitis can complicate chronic skin conditions such as venous leg ulceration (Ch. 29) and lymphoedema (Ch. 29). When this occurs, treatment with antibiotics may have to be prolonged to prevent early relapse.

Cutaneous anthrax

AETIOLOGY
This is a rare infection in developed countries caused by the Gram-positive rod *B. anthracis*. It is primarily a disease of animals (especially cattle) but humans may be incidentally involved, usually through their occupation, e.g. those who handle wool or animal hides.

CLINICAL FEATURES
The presentation is with low-grade fever and malaise. A papule develops, often on the back of the hand. The papule evolves into a haemorrhagic blister which gradually turns dark brown to black. There is surrounding non-pitting oedema and, if the condition is untreated, systemic involvement with features of bacterial toxaemia may presage death.

DIAGNOSIS AND MANAGEMENT
The diagnosis is confirmed by aspiration of the pustule and Gram staining, which shows the characteristic large, oblong bacteria.

The organism is usually responsive to the intravenous administration of penicillin, but resistant strains have been identified in Spain, Finland and the USA. Failure to respond to penicillin indicates the likely presence of a resistant strain or the presence of a coexistent staphylococcal cellulitis, although this is rare. The addition of flucloxacillin is effective for penicillin-resistant staphylococcal infection, but expert advice and review of the antibiotic regimen after 48 hours is necessary.

Tumours of the skin

The skin is exposed to chronic irritation and carcinogens. Tumours of the skin, as with any other tissue, can be benign or malignant. The latter may be primary or secondary.

A number of premalignant conditions can be identified and are discussed below. Tumours that derive from the epidermis (ectodermal) have different clinical features from those of the dermis (mesodermal).

Benign tumours of the epidermis
Seborrhoeic warts (basal cell papillomas)
These lesions are common in the elderly.

CLINICAL FEATURES
History
These are rough lesions which may catch on clothing; this or other trauma may cause minor bleeding. The appearance is unattractive and cosmetic distaste is a common reason for presentation.

Physical findings
Raised, well circumscribed lesions may occur anywhere on the body although the trunk is the most common site. They are initially flat with varying amounts of pigmentation. The surface is waxy with superficial clefting and fissuring.

MANAGEMENT
The differential diagnosis of deeply pigmented papillomas from malignant melanoma can be difficult and, if there is doubt, excision biopsy is indicated.

However, if the diagnosis is certain, the growth does not have a dermal component and therefore excision, with subsequent damage to the dermal collagen and scarring, is generally not necessary unless this is the easiest way to get rid of symptoms. Shaving back the lesion or curettage and cautery give a satisfactory cosmetic result with the additional benefit of providing a specimen for histological confirmation of the diagnosis.

Skin tags

These lesions are usually found in sites where skin surfaces rub together and the skin is therefore chronically irritated. There is a loose connective tissue core covered by epidermis which is variably pigmented.

Skin tags are irritated by clothing and bleed as well as causing local symptoms in areas such as the skin surrounding the anus. Patients often present to request removal. The diagnosis is obvious to the naked eye.

Management is by snip excision and cautery, which are carried out under local anaesthetic.

Keratoacanthoma

This lesion arises from squamous epithelium. It is most common on exposed areas of the body and is thought

691

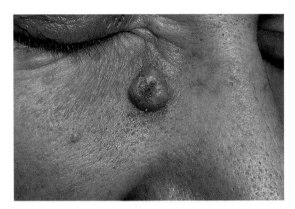

Fig 38.5 **Keratoacanthoma on cheek showing central keratin plug with surrounding acanthotic collar.**

to result from minor trauma. As its name suggests, it has a central keratin plug with a surrounding collar of acanthotic thickened epidermis (Fig. 38.5).

CLINICAL FEATURES

The lesion is characterised by rapid onset and growth. It then enters a static phase, which may last 3–4 months before spontaneous resolution. The appearance of the lesion by itself can be very difficult to distinguish from a squamous cell carcinoma (see below), although the latter usually grows progressively but less rapidly. The same difficulty also occurs on histological examination, but carcinoma always invades the deeper dermis. Treatment is by excision with a margin of surrounding skin and, if there is any remaining doubt about the diagnosis, careful follow-up is indicated.

Solar keratoses

These lesions occur on sun-exposed areas of the skin, often on a background of collagen damage – solar elastosis. Similar changes can occur in the epidermis as a result of exposure to carcinogens such as arsenic. Solar keratoses are areas of damaged basal cells where the normal smooth transition from the basal cell layer is disrupted and the smooth surface is replaced by a scaly keratosis. The surrounding skin can be red and occasionally induration occurs as the lesion becomes more active; progression to a squamous cell carcinoma may take place, although this is rare. At histological examination, there is a variable degree of dysplastic change in the deep epidermis with abnormal mitotic activity which can be very difficult to distinguish from frank carcinoma.

MANAGEMENT

Superficial lesions are dealt with by cryotherapy. If there is any induration of the surrounding area, curettage and cautery are used and the fragments sent

for histological examination. Close follow-up is indicated when the histological diagnosis is uncertain.

Extensive areas of sun damage with multiple solar keratoses can be very difficult to manage by cryotherapy or curettage and cautery. In these circumstances, application of cytotoxic creams such as 5-fluouracil can be helpful in stabilising the epithelium, although this has to be done under close supervision.

Premalignant conditions of the epidermis

Bowen's disease

This is characterised by a well circumscribed scaly plaque (Fig. 38.6), most common on the lower legs although it can occur anywhere on the body including at the anus. The clinical appearance is similar to a solitary patch of psoriasis. Histological examination shows full thickness epidermal dysplasia cells and therefore the condition is potentially malignant although progression is slow.

MANAGEMENT

A variety of methods can be used to treat the condition, including curettage and cautery, the use of topical cytotoxic drugs, excision, cryotherapy, and sometimes superficial radiotherapy. The choice depends on the size of the lesion, its site and the age of the patient.

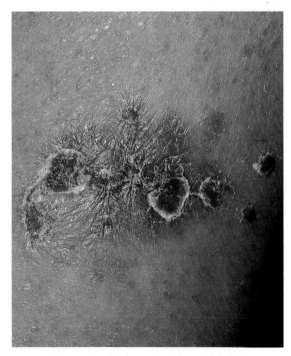

Fig 38.6 **Bowen's disease on leg showing psoriasiform plaque.**

Leucoplakia

In this condition, a fixed white plaque is seen on mucous membranes. The differential diagnosis is from lichen planus – a common inflammatory condition of the skin and mucous membranes – which has a more lace-like appearance, and Candida where the white plaques can be brushed off from the surface mucosa. Oral candidiasis usually occurs in immunocompromised patients, in diabetics or in those on systemic corticosteroid therapy. If there is any doubt, the plaque should be biopsied and, if positive, the area ablated by cryotherapy or laser.

Paget's disease of the nipple

This is discussed in detail in Chapter 27.

Lentigo maligna

This is a rare plaque-like condition which tends to develop in late middle age, most commonly on the cheek, and increases slowly in size with time. Initially the plaque is uniformly pigmented, but as the lesion develops, irregular pigmentation occurs which is the early superficial spreading phase of a malignant melanoma (Fig. 38.7). If left untreated, the melanoma advances and enters a deep invasive phase with the same risk of metastases as melanoma elsewhere.

MANAGEMENT

Smaller lesions should be excised. There is a problem here with lesions that occupy a large area on the cheek and excision is not usually possible without grafting. A graft is unsightly and the condition may be managed expectantly by close and regular follow-up. Action is taken if there is a change in appearance.

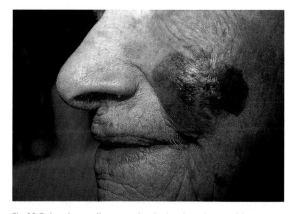

Fig 38.7 **Lentigo maligna on cheek showing plaque with variation in pigmentation.**

Other benign skin tumours

Benign pigmented skin lesions

Freckles

Freckles are areas of the epidermis where melanocytes produce more melanin, usually in response to ultraviolet light. The number of melanocytes is normal and they are quite stable.

Lentigos

Lentigos are an area of the epidermis where the number of melanocytes is increased and melanin production is excessive. They are found in areas of chronic sun exposure and hence are most common on the face, hands and shoulders. If seen in young patients, they are the sites of solar damage and the patient should be advised against unnecessary exposure to the sun.

Pigmented naevus

This term is not necessarily confined to pigmented skin lesions; it may equally refer to blood vessels (vascular naevi). The more correct generic term is a hamartoma. Essentially there is an abnormal collection of a normal skin constituent. Congenital pigmented naevi are rare, often darkly pigmented and may be hairy or papillary. Pigmented naevi may occur anywhere on the skin, including the nail bed where they give rise to linear pigmented stria. According to the clinical and histological features, naevi can be subdivided into five types:

- junctional – at the dermo-epidermal interface
- intradermal – entirely within the dermis
- compound – features of both junctional and intradermal
- blue – deep dermal with considerable pigmentation which gives rise to their colour
- Spitz – juvenile melanoma, reddish brown in colour, usually on the face or limbs of children and young adults; they are benign (but see below).

All of these may develop at any age, although the second decade is the most common. During pregnancy an increase in both size and number of pigmented naevi is common, and pre-existing moles may darken in colour.

A Spitz naevus may undergo rapid growth and for this reason is often removed to exclude malignancy. Histological examination shows large cells which are pleomorphic and can be very difficult to distinguish from those of malignant melanoma. Skilled histological assessment is necessary.

Dermatofibroma

This is a tumour (often multiple) of dermal connective of unknown cause. There have been suggestions that they arise from insect bites. Legs are the most commonly affected sites, and they are more common in women than in men. A small intradermal nodule is present. Pigmentation is usual and the overlying epidermis is tethered to the lesion giving a puckered appearance if the lesion is squeezed. Particularly in the early stages, there may be a considerable vascular component which imparts a reddish brown discoloration. The tissue component is mixed and the lesion may histologically be termed a sclerosing haemangioma. As it matures it becomes pale, although often with a retained surrounding halo of pigmentation. A slow increase in size may occur and excision may be necessary to establish the diagnosis with certainty and, especially with the darker lesions, to exclude melanoma.

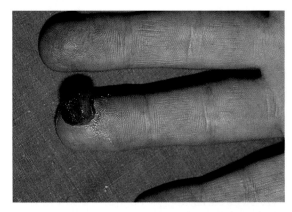

Fig 38.8 **Pyogenic granuloma on finger showing friable vascular tumour.**

Benign abnormalities of the blood vessels

Haemangiomas are distinguished by the size of the blood vessel that is involved.

PATHOLOGICAL FEATURES

Capillary haemangiomas are common and may give rise to salmon pink discoloration on the surface of the skin. The back of the neck is a common site. Other variants include the *port wine stain* on the face, which may be associated with ipsilateral intracranial haemangiomata, giving rise to epilepsy (Sturge–Weber syndrome). *Strawberry naevi* may appear in infancy and grow with age before resolving spontaneously by the early teens. *Campbell de Morgan* spots appear as small cherry papules on the trunk, are very common and of no significance, although they can become increasingly numerous with age and give rise to cosmetic embarrassment. *Pyogenic granulomas* are exuberant granulation tissue, an exaggerated healing response to minor trauma, and are usually found on the finger or the lip (Fig. 38.8). In spite of their name, the lesions are not infective in cause. They are friable and bleed readily. *Glomus tumours* appear as small vascular blebs on the skin. They have a generous nerve supply and are tender, especially if they occur within a confined space such as the nail bed.

Neurofibromas

These are benign tumours of the fibroblasts of the nerve sheath. The usual presentation is a solitary lesion in the area of a peripheral nerve. On clinical examination they are soft and fleshy (Fig. 38.9).

Schwannomas are benign tumours arising from the Schwann cells around the peripheral nerves, are much firmer nodules than neurofibromas and are closely tethered to an identifiable nerve. Pressure on the tumour may cause pain in the area of distribution of

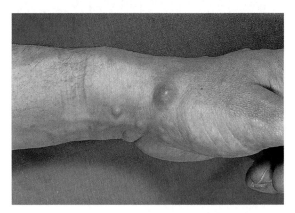

Fig 38.9 **Neurofibroma on wrist showing soft fleshy swelling.**

the nerve and excision has to be performed with great care.

Some patients have multiple neurofibromas, which form part of the syndrome of neurofibromatosis with associated cafe-au-lait spots and axillary freckling. There are sometimes Schwannomas of the larger cranial nerves and phaeochromocytoma.

Benign appendage tumours

Skin appendages, such as sweat glands and hair follicles are a source of benign tumours. Non-specific tumours such as *syringomata* or *trichofolliculomas* are not usually diagnosed clinically but only retrospectively following excision of a non-descript skin nodule. *A cylindroma* is of hair follicle origin and gives rise to a fleshy nodule. They usually occur on the scalp and may become very large, giving rise to what in the past was labelled a turban tumour.

Cysts

A cyst is an epithelial lined cavity usually filled with

thick products of epithelial secretion or of cell breakdown which have undergone degeneration. The most common type originates from the hair follicle.

Pilar or epidermal cyst

This used to be known as a sebaceous cyst. They are found anywhere on the body where hair follicles occur, although the commonest site is the scalp. Many are solitary but multiple lesions occur. The range of size is from a few millimetres to several centimetres. The cyst is located in the deep dermis but is connected to the superficial epithelium through the pilosebaceous duct. A blocked duct may be visible on the surface as a central black punctum. Clinically, they are soft and are mobile over deeper structures.

Epidermal cysts are not usually painful unless they are injured with disruption of the contents into the surrounding dermis where they cause an intense inflammatory reaction. When this occurs, the area swells and becomes tender. Secondary infection also occurs, with *Staphylococcus* being the most common organism.

Uninfected cysts are excised; care must be taken that all abnormal epithelial elements are removed or recurrence is likely. If the lesion has become inflamed, then the contents are best drained and the inflammation allowed to subside, at which point it can be excised.

Dermoid cysts

Congenital

These are rare and arise from abnormalities of development where epithelial remnants occur. They are found in lines of embryological fusion, the midline of the neck, the scalp and the face are common sites. The contents of the cysts include ectodermal structures of hair and sebaceous glands in addition to keratin.

Implantation dermoids

In this condition, a usually insignificant injury drives a fragment of dermis into the subdermal layer from where its secretions cannot escape. The fingertip is the commonest site (rose gardeners), although they may occur at any site of injury.

Lipomas

This is strictly a growth of fat deep to the skin proper. The overlying skin is normal and the lump can be moved in relation to it. Fluctuation can be elicited although the lesion is not cystic. The histological appearance is of a mass of adipose tissue with thin fibroid septa. The size varies and penetration into muscles can occur. Treatment is by excision, parti-

cularly if the lipoma increases in size or becomes tender.

Skin cancer

CLASSIFICATION

There are two clinical types of carcinoma, both of which arise from keratinocytes:

- basal cell carcinoma
- squamous cell carcinoma.

A variety of factors predispose the epidermis towards malignancy:

- exposure to the sun
- immunosuppression either from therapy to prevent rejection of organs or from the effects of HIV
- general carcinogens – arsenic
- topical carcinogens – coal tar
- hereditary disorder – xeroderma pigmentosum, a condition of failure of DNA repair
- chronic inflammation – lupus vulgaris (tuberculosis of the skin) or chronic leg ulcers.

The annual incidence of non-melanoma skin cancer is increasing and basal cell carcinoma is the more common.

Basal cell carcinoma

This generally arises in sites exposed to the sun. Ninety per cent of lesions are on the face.

CLASSIFICATION

There are four clinical types:

- cystic – the most common
- pigmented
- superficial spreading
- morphoeic or sclerotic

PATHOLOGICAL FEATURES

Basal cell carcinomas cause local invasion and destruction of surrounding tissues. They penetrate into subcutaneous tissue and can erode into vital structures such as the orbit and brain. Histologically, the tumour cells have strongly basophilic nuclei and little cytoplasm. Cells at the periphery of the tumour give rise to a palisade pattern reminiscent of normal basal cells. Metastases are extremely rare but may occur as a very late event.

CLINICAL FEATURES

A cystic lesion has fluid-filled spaces and initially presents as a small translucent or pearly nodule which eventually breaks down, usually as the result of minor trauma, to produce an ulcer – a rodent ulcer characterised by a rolled pearly edge with surface telangiectasia (Fig. 38.10).

A pigmented form has characteristic pearly nodules around the edge (Fig. 38.11)

Superficial spreading carcinoma is a scaly plaque, usually on the trunk, with epidermal atrophy; pearly translucent nodules can usually be seen around the periphery of the lesion (Fig. 38.12).

Morphoeic or sclerotic lesions heal by fibrosis and scarring and may be multifocal; they do not look at all like cystic basal cell carcinomas, do not have pearly nodules but appear as a rather depressed plaque of sclerotic skin (Fig. 38.13).

MANAGEMENT

It is important that the tumour is treated adequately on the first occasion to render recurrence unlikely. Treatment depends on the site and size of the lesions at the time of diagnosis. Small lesions can be dealt with by curettage and cautery, although local excision is usually preferred to ensure there is a margin of clearance around the tumour. Larger lesions may require extensive reconstructive surgery or be treated by radiotherapy.

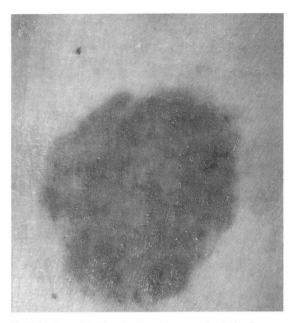

Fig 38.12 **Superficial basal cell carcinoma on back showing spreading flat red plaque.**

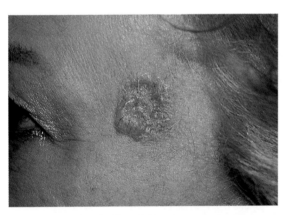

Fig 38.10 **Cystic basal cell carcinoma on temple showing central breakdown and ulceration.**

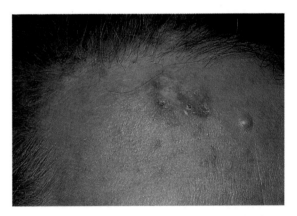

Fig 38.13 **Sclerotic basal cell carcinoma on forehead showing depressed white plaque.**

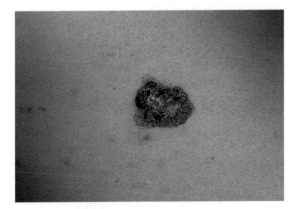

Fig 38.11 **Pigmented basal cell carcinoma showing pigmentation of lesion.**

Cryotherapy can also be employed but runs a significant risk of leaving residual deep in the dermis.

Squamous cell carcinoma

AETIOLOGY AND PATHOLOGICAL FEATURES

Older age groups than those with basal cell carcinoma are usually affected and lesions are also most commonly found on skin repeatedly exposed to ultraviolet light. Industrial carcinogens are also important in their development (ionising radiation, arsenic and chronic exposure to coal tar and mineral oils). Smokers are prone to squamous cell carcinomas of the lip. The origin of the tumour is within the epidermis and the

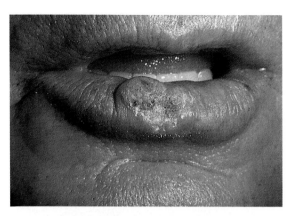

Fig 38.14 **Squamous cell carcinoma on lower lip showing infiltrated keratinised lesion with ulceration.**

cells show some degree of maturation towards keratin formation. Occurrence may be *de novo* or in pre-existing skin lesions such as active solar keratoses, leucoplakia or Bowen's disease. Squamous cell carcinoma invades the dermis and deeper tissues such as bone and cartilage. Metastasis to distant sites via both the lymphatics and the bloodstream takes place, although the second is usually a late and uncommon complication of the disease. Lesions of the lip (Fig. 38.14) and ear are prone to spread early.

CLINICAL FEATURES

The usual presentation is with either an enlarging painless ulcer with a rolled indurated margin or a papillomatous appearance with areas of ulceration, bleeding or serous exudation from secondary infection on the surface. An unexplained area of ulceration or thickening of the lip must be biopsied at once to establish a diagnosis.

MANAGEMENT

Although metastases from squamous cell carcinoma of the skin are rare, there is a need for adequate local treatment to eradicate the tumour once and for all. Most lesions are small and local excision suffices. Problems can occur with larger lesions where reconstruction by grafting or flap procedures (Ch. 37) may be necessary. Where extensive surgery seems likely, radiotherapy can be considered, although long-term sequelae include radiodermatitis, and an unattractive white, avascular scar may make this choice inappropriate for exposed areas such as the face. Tumours on the lip and ear lesions must be treated vigorously from the outset.

Malignant melanoma

This is a highly malignant tumour derived from melanocytes.

EPIDEMIOLOGY AND AETIOLOGY

The majority arise from pigmented naevi but some occur *de novo* in previously normal skin. Melanomas are rare in dark-skinned races and most common in fair-skinned people of Celtic origin. The highest incidence in the world is in northern and western Australia, perhaps because of the exposure of northern hemisphere migrant ethnic groups to ultraviolet light for which their past genetic experience has not prepared them.

The incidence of malignant melanoma has been rising over recent years and it is now, because of the cult of sun exposure for its perceived enhancement of lifestyle, the most rapidly increasing cancer in young adults. Between 1974 and 1987, the number of new cases of malignant melanoma in the UK rose from 1732 to 3599. In 1974, 743 deaths were reported, which increased in 1991 to 1288 – a rise in point prevalence from 21 to 46 per million for men and from 42 to 78 per million for women. In the 15–34 year age group it is the third most common cancer in women (after cervix and breast) and the seventh most common in men (testicular cancer and Hodgkin's disease are first and second).

PATHOLOGICAL FEATURES

All skin areas are vulnerable, although the most commonly affected sites are the lower extremities in women (subungual melanoma in the areas under the nail) and the head and neck in men. Tumours may also arise in the choroid of the eye and in the oral mucosa. The classification of spread is dealt with below under 'Management'. However, the pathways are:

- direct extension into the underlying dermis and thence to the subcutaneous tissues
- satellite nodules – around the lesion and perhaps caused by tumour deposits lodging in the draining lymphatics
- to regional lymph nodes
- blood-borne to distant organs.

CLINICAL CLASSIFICATION

There are five clinical types of malignant melanoma:

- lentigo maligna
- superficial spreading melanoma (Fig. 38.15)
- nodular melanoma (Fig. 38.16)
- acral lentiginous melanoma (Fig. 38.17)
- amelanotic melanoma (Fig. 38.18) – a lesion where the malignant melanocytes are not producing melanin; this is uncommon.

CLINICAL FEATURES

Features that suggest a melanoma

Most patients present with a change in the character of a pre-existing naevus. The features are summarised in Table 38.1.

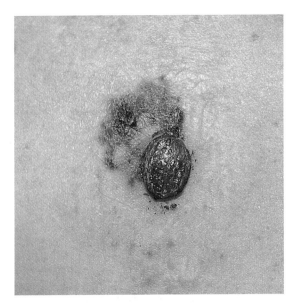

Fig 38.15 **Superficial spreading malignant melanoma showing asymmetry, irregular border and variation in colour with raised nodule developing.**

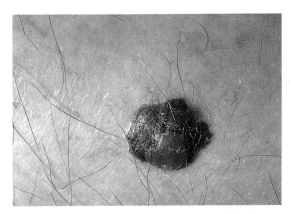

Fig 38.16 **Nodular malignant melanoma showing raised deeply pigmented tumour.**

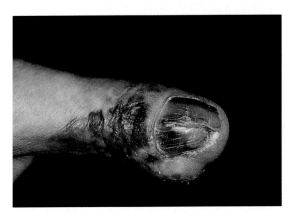

Fig 38.17 **Acral melanoma spreading under nail.**

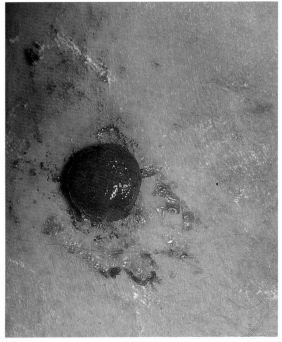

Fig 38.18 **Amelanotic malignant melanoma on neck showing raised non-pigmented tumour.**

Table 38.1
Changes in pigmented lesions indicative of malignant melanoma*

Amercian checklist
A.   Asymmetry of lesion
B.   Irregular Border
C.   Irregular Colour
D.   Diameter > 5 mm

Glasgow Seven point checklist

Major features	**Minor features**
1. Change in size	4. Diameter of lesion > 7 mm
2. Change in shape	5. Inflammation around lesion
3. Change in colour	6. Bleeding of lesion
	7. Mild itching

One major feature indicates removal of lesion

* A feature of both checklists is the presence of a changing lesion which identifies it as being different from other pigmented lesions on the patient.

Other

Malignant melanoma can also present with metastases – localised lymph node enlargement or distant spread such as cerebral deposits.

PROPHYLAXIS

Public awareness campaigns are an important part of the management of the disease. Patients should be persuaded to check their skin regularly for moles that change and should then come early to their doctor if there is concern. Avoidance of unnecessary exposure to the sun by the use of hats, clothing and effective barrier creams is an important message to communicate to the public and should, in the long term, reduce the incidence of both malignant melanoma and other epidermoid cancers.

Patients who are particularly at risk (those with dysplastic naevi or those with a type I skin which burns but never tans in the sun) need to take even greater care with sun protection. Other recognised risk factors include a family history of malignant melanoma, and personal history of previous melanomas. Patients with a large number of pigmented naevi are also thought to be of increased risk.

MANAGEMENT AND PROGNOSIS

Suspicious lesions

Any questionable lesion on either history or physical examination must always be completely excised and sent for histological examination. A more difficult decision is when a patient presents with multiple naevi which are showing variation in the evenness of pigmentation within lesions and between lesions. Patients with this so-called called 'dysplastic naevus syndrome' have a higher than normal risk of developing malignant melanoma. They should be managed by careful photography of the lesions to act as a yardstick for future change and with regular follow-up. Any suspicious lesion should then be excised and examined microscopically.

Established diagnosis

Initial management is by local excision. It is essential to have a clear margin in both periphery and depth (full thickness of the skin but not necessarily subcutaneous tissues). The specimen is then assessed histologically to confirm the diagnosis and to assess depth of invasion.

Histological classification is in one of two ways:

- *Clark's classification* – grades the tumour on the depth within the dermis of malignant invasion (Table 38.2)
- *Breslow thickness* (which has become the widely adopted best criterion for assessment) – penetration of malignant cells by measurement in millimetres from the granular cell layer of the epidermis through to the deepest invading melanocyte

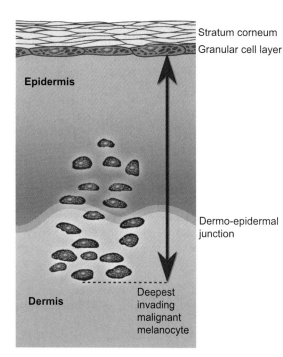

Fig 38.19 **Breslow classification.** The pathologist measures the thickness of the tumour in millimetres as the distance from the granular cell layer of the dermis to the deepest invading melanoma cell.

(Fig. 38.19). Tumours less than 0.76 mm at the time of primary excision carry an excellent prognosis but those that have penetrated greater have a poorer prognosis proportionate to depth. Although the inverse relationship between thickness and survival is generally linear there are occasional melanomas that do not follow the rule. Tumour thickness is the most important prognostic factor but others such as age, sex and size of lesion, metabolic rate, and tumour infiltrating lymphocytes need to be considered.

Further excision can then be planned. Until recently, very wide excision with a skin graft was the normal practice although recent experience suggests that this does not improve the prognosis. Current practice for thin tumours is to excise with a 1 cm margin for each millimetre depth of invasion. Sentinel node biopsy is an important part of staging the tumour and is used in specialised melanoma centres for clinical trial work.

It must be emphasised that malignant melanoma is a curable disease if treated early.

Extensive local tumour

Treatment is by wide excision including subcutaneous tissue down to the deep fascia. Evidence that this enhances survival is not established

Satellite limb lesions

Clinical control can be achieved by either chemo-

Table 38.2
Clark's classification of levels of malignant melanoma

Level I	Lesion confined to epidermis (melanoma in-situ)
Level II	Invasion into upper (papillary) dermis
Level III	Occupation and expansion of papillary dermis by melanoma cells
Level IV	Invasion into deeper (reticular) dermis
Level V	Invasion into subcutaneous fat

Five years survival figures fall steadily with deeper layers.

therapy (see below) or isolated limb perfusion, which uses the technique of oxygenated perfusion to deliver high concentrations of chemotherapeutic agents locally without their potential toxic effects on the body as a whole. There is equivocal evidence on whether survival is increased.

Lymph node involvement

Sentinel node biopsy by which the local draining node is identified by injection of dye or radioisotope at the time of wide excision of the primary tumour and then removed for histological analysis is helpful in assessing local node involvement. If positive, block dissection of the regional nodes is commonly performed. This helps prevent local recurrence but its contribution to survival is unproven and it may cause lymphoedema in the limb with significant morbidity.

Chemotherapy and immunotherapy

Local excision, without lymph node dissection but combined with cytotoxic agents (such as vindesine, dacarbazene), tamoxifen, interferon, interleukin and vaccination have all been used, but controlled trials which attest to the value of various regimens are virtually non-existent.

Targeted monoclonal antibodies against malignant melanocytes which are tagged with a cytotoxic agent are currently in the research phase and offer hope for specific immunotherapy in the future.

Malignant tumours of the dermis

These are rare. The dermis is of mesodermal origin and therefore malignant tumours are classified as sarcomas. They initially present as small nodules which increase in size and may become tender.

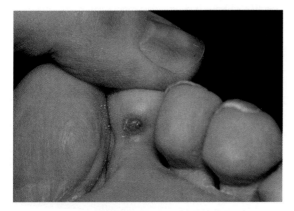

Fig 38.20 **Kaposi's sarcoma showing purple nodule.**

Kaposi's sarcoma

This is a type of haemangiosarcoma which used to be a relatively rare disease and was found most commonly as a small purple nodule usually on a lympho-edematous leg either of an elderly person of central European, Jewish extraction or in sub-Saharan Africa. More recently, however, it has become recognised as an opportunistic tumour in immunosuppressed patients, most commonly those with HIV infections. In this context there are a variety of clinical presentations. The most usual is that of a small purple nodule (Fig. 38.20), but a dusky purple plaque or with mucosal involvement is not uncommon. The treatment is usually surgical excision for small discrete lesions and radiotherapy for larger ones.

Other malignancies of the skin

Lymphoma

These are usually T-cell rather than B-cell lymphomas. Presentation is either with a solitary nodule or, more commonly, with diffuse scaly plaques (mycosis fungoides). The epidermis is atrophic and biopsy confirms the diagnosis of lymphoma with malignant T lymphocytes migrating towards the epidermis – a process known as epidermotropism. In general, only the skin is involved with mycosis fungoides.

As the disease progresses, the lesions become nodular and may eventually ulcerate. Systemic involvement may occur with hepatosplenomegaly and circulating malignant T lymphocytes which may be associated with erythrodermic lymphoma of the skin – the Sézary syndrome.

Treatment of early mycosis fungoides is symptomatic. Photochemotherapy with a combination of the coumarin light-sensitising psoralen and ultraviolet light (PUVA) is very effective. If this fails to control the disease, the use of superficial electron beam therapy or, occasionally, cytotoxic drugs is indicated. If the disease progresses to Sézary syndrome, systemic chemotherapy is undertaken in an attempt to control the disease, although it tends to be poorly responsive.

Secondary carcinoma

The skin may be the site of distant spread of internal carcinoma. Sometimes solitary nodules arise in the skin that are the result of blood-borne metastases or direct involvement through the lymphatics. Biopsy of the lesion usually provides a clue to the site of the primary disorder. Solitary nodules may occur in cancers that are known to spread with single metastases such as thyroid and renal carcinoma.

Cutaneous signs of internal malignancy

The skin is well recognised as a marker for non-metastatic signs of internal malignancy:

- Pruritus may be a presenting feature of myeloproliferative malignancies, particularly in young people – polycythaemia rubra vera, lymphoma
- Deep jaundice from obstruction of the bile duct – carcinoma of the head of the pancreas
- Increased pigmentation – melanocyte-secreting hormone (MSH) in carcinoma of the bronchus
- Finger clubbing
- Unusual annular erythemas such as erythema gyratum repens – carcinoma of the bronchus
- Tylosis (diffuse keratinous thickening) with palmar plantar hyperkeratosis – carcinoma of the oesophagus
- Acanthosis nigricans (a velvety papillomatous appearance in the intertriginous areas of the axillae and groin and around the neck) – upper gastrointestinal tumours
- Acquired ichthyosis – any internal malignancy.

Index

Index

Index

T

Unipolar diathermy, *see* Monopolar diathermy
United Kingdom, United States, breast carcinoma screening, 407
Units of excellence, 10–11
Upper aerodigestive tract, 205–216
Upper limb, arterial disorders, 449–451
Upper oesophageal sphincter, 258
Upper respiratory tract infections, 88
Urachus, anomalies, 556, 641
Urate, *see* Uric acid
Urea
 blood levels, 27, 531
 dehydration, 143
Urease inhibitors, 546
Ureter, 529–530, 546–564
 colic, 529, 552
 perinephric abscess, 540
 tuberculosis, 540
Ureterocele, 549
Urethra
 female, 170
 male, 569–572
 pain, 554
 prostaglandin E1 via, 578
 strictures, 571–572
  micturition, 555
Urethral catheters
 for chronic retention, 566
 placement, 167–170
 postoperative, 94, 96–97
 for spinal cord injury, 562
Urethral valves, 569–570
Urethrography, 555
 trauma, 19
Urge incontinence, 554
 faecal, 377
Uric acid, 585
 normal values, 27
 stones, 545
  geography, 544
Urinalysis, *see* Urine, examination
Urinary calculi, ulcerative colitis, 348
Urinary catheters, *see* Urethral catheters
Urinary tract, 529–579
 infections, 123, 537–541, 556–557
  antibiotics, 123, 124, 537, 538
  postoperative, 96–97
  stones, 544
 rectal carcinoma involvement, 356
Urine
 diversion, 553
 examination, 28, 136, 530–531
  acute abdomen, 319
  arteritis, 430
 5-hydroxy-indolacetic acid, 523
 flow studies, 555, 562
  benign prostatic hyperplasia, 565
 free cortisol, 24-hour, 517
 monitoring, 142–143
 pyelonephritis, 538
 retention
  acute, 565, 566
  chronic, 565, 566
   catheterisation, 169–170
   inguinal hernia surgery, 388
 tuberculosis, 540
 vanillylmandelic acid, 518

Urodynamics, 555–556, 562
Urogenital cysts, 642–643
Urology, 529
Urothelium, *see* Transitional epithelium
Ursodeoxycholic acid, gallstone dissolution therapy, 290
Uterus, fistula to bladder, 561
Uveitis, 660–661, 663
 acute anterior, 664

V

Vaccinations
 health care personnel, 117
 for splenectomy, 115, 298, 299
 tetanus, 21–22, 126
Vacuum erection devices, 578, 579
Vagina
 fistula
  bladder, 561
  diverticular disease, 352
  rectum, 377
 swab for cystitis, 556
Vaginal examination, 555
 acute abdomen, 319
 acute appendicitis, 321
 intestinal obstruction, 330
Vagotomy, 267, 268
Vagus nerve, division, 214
Valgus angulation, 582, 615
Valve of Heister, 276
Valves
 lower limb veins, 463–464
  examination, 467
 urethral, 569–570
Valvulae conniventes, 327–328
Valvular heart disease, 246–252
Valvular lymphoedema, 483
Vancomycin, 121
Vanillylmandelic acid, urinary, 518
Variations, biliary tract, 276
Varicoceles, 575, 578
Varicography, 468
Varicose veins, 463–469
Varus angulation, 582, 615
Vascular catheters, indwelling, complications, 96
Vascular disease, *see* Arterial disease
Vascular ectasias, gastrointestinal haemorrhage, 326
Vasculitis, *see* Arteritis
Vasoconstrictors, 145
Vasodilatation, sepsis, 139
Vasodilators, 145
Vasomotor rhinitis, 229
Vasopressin, 325
 see also Antidiuretic hormone
Vasospastic disorders, *see* Raynaud's phenomenon
Vecuronium, 79, 151
Vegetations, subacute bacterial endocarditis, 247
Veins
 access, 157–164
  asepsis, 156

calcium measurement, 512
 see also Intravenous injections
 disorders, 461–482
  lymphoedema, 483
 draining colon, 344
 grafting with, 437, 448
 interruption for pulmonary embolism, 478
 metastases via, 185
 pressure studies, lower limb, 463, 468
Velocity, blood flow, arterial disease, 435
Venepuncture, 157–159
Venography, ascending, 468, 473–474
Venous claudication, 433
Venous plexuses, anal canal, 365
Venovenous pumping, dialysis, 146
Ventilation, operating departments, 54
Ventilation (respiratory), 144, 145, 166
 airway pressure monitoring, 141
 cardiothoracic surgery, 255
 diaphragmatic hernia, 635–636
 head injury, 488–489
 monitoring, 76
 parenteral nutrition and, 88–89
 see also Breathing
Ventilation scanning, pulmonary embolism, 477
Ventilation tubes (grommets), 223
Ventilation/perfusion mismatch, 81, 88
Ventilators (respiratory), 78
Ventilatory failure, 143
Ventricles (cerebral), drainage, 492–493
Ventricular arrhythmias, cardiac surgery for, 245–246
Ventricular function, assessment, 243–244
Ventriculography (cardiac), technetium-99m red cells, 49
Verner–Morrison syndrome, 521
Vertical banded gastroplasty, 341
Vertical nystagmus, 221
Vertigo, 219
 benign positional, 221
Vesicoureteric reflux, 534, 537, 548–549
 ureteric duplication, 547
Vesicovaginal fistula, 561
Vestibular function, 218, 220–221
 see also Vertigo
Vestibular sedatives, 226
Vestibulo-ocular reflex, 152
Veterans Administration trial, coronary artery disease, 244
Video recording, endoscopy, 46
Video-assisted thoracoscopy, 239–240
Viewing systems, endoscopy, 46
Villous adenoma, rectum, 353
Vinca alkaloids, 190
VIPomas, 521–522
Virchow's node, 311
Virchow's triad, 462
Virilisation, 517–518
Virulence, 113
Viruses
 causing tumours, 192
 conjunctivitis, 668
 parotitis, 211

735